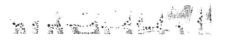

The GALE ENCYCLOPEDIA of MEDICINE

FOURTH EDITION

The GALE ENCYCLOPEDIA of MEDICINE

FOURTH EDITION

VOLUME

2

C–E

LAURIE J. FUNDUKIAN, EDITOR

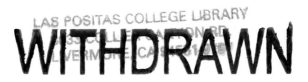

GALE
CENGAGE Learning

Detroit • New York • San Francisco • New Haven, Conn • Waterville, Maine • London

GALE CENGAGE Learning™

Gale Encyclopedia of Medicine, Fourth Edition

Project Editor: Laurie J. Fundukian

Image Editors: Donna Batten and Kristin Key

Editorial: Donna Batten, Kristin Key, Jacqueline Longe, Kristin Mallegg, Brigham Narins, Jeffrey Wilson, Alejandro Valtierra

Product Manager: Kate Hanley

Editorial Support Services: Andrea Lopeman

Indexing Services: Factiva, a Dow Jones Company

Rights Acquisition and Management: Robyn Young

Composition: Evi Abou-El-Seoud

Manufacturing: Wendy Blurton

Imaging: John Watkins

For product information and technology assistance, contact us at
Gale Customer Support, 1-800-877-4253.
For permission to use material from this text or product,
submit all requests online at **www.cengage.com/permissions.**
Further permissions questions can be emailed to
permissionrequest@cengage.com

While every effort has been made to ensure the reliability of the information presented in this publication, Gale, a part of Cengage Learning, does not guarantee the accuracy of the data contained herein. Gale accepts no payment for listing; and inclusion in the publication of any organization, agency, institution, publication, service, or individual does not imply endorsement of the editors or publisher. Errors brought to the attention of the publisher and verified to the satisfaction of the publisher will be corrected in future editions.

Library of Congress Cataloging-in-Publication Data

Gale encyclopedia of medicine—4th ed. Laurie J. Fundukian, editor.
    p. ; cm.
    Other title: Encyclopedia of medicine
    Includes bibliographical references and index.
    ISBN 978-1-4144-8646-8 (set : alk. paper) ISBN 978-1-4144-8647-5 (volume 1 : alk. paper)-- ISBN 978-1-4144-8648-2 (volume 2 : alk. paper)--
ISBN 978-1-4144-8649-9 (volume 3 : alk. paper)-- ISBN 978-1-4144-8650-5 (volume 4 : alk. paper)-- ISBN 978-1-4144-8651-2 (volume 5 : alk. paper)--
ISBN 978-1-4144-8633-8 (volume 6 : alk. paper)--
    1. Internal medicine--Encyclopedias. I. Fundukian, Laurie J. II. Title: Gale Group III. Title: Encyclopedia of medicine.
    [DNLM: 1. Internal Medicine--Encyclopedias--English. 2. Complementary Therapies--Encyclopedias--English. WB 13]

RC41.G35 2011
616.003–dc22   2010053605

Gale
27500 Drake Rd.
Farmington Hills, MI, 48331-3535

ISBN-13: 978-1-4144-8646-8 (set)   ISBN-10: 1-4144-8646-4 (set)
ISBN-13: 978-1-4144-8647-5 (vol. 1)   ISBN-10: 1-4144-8647-2 (vol. 1)
ISBN-13: 978-1-4144-8648-2 (vol. 2)   ISBN-10: 1-4144-8648-0 (vol. 2)
ISBN-13: 978-1-4144-8649-9 (vol. 3)   ISBN-10: 1-4144-8649-9 (vol. 3)
ISBN-13: 978-1-4144-8650-5 (vol. 4)   ISBN-10: 1-4144-8650-2 (vol. 4)
ISBN-13: 978-1-4144-8651-2 (vol. 5)   ISBN-10: 1-4144-8651-0 (vol. 5)
ISBN-13: 978-1-4144-8633-8 (vol. 6)   ISBN-10: 1-4144-8633-2 (vol. 6)

This title is also available as an e-book.
978-1-4144-8691-8
Contact your Gale, a part of Cengage Learning sales representative for ordering information.

Printed in China
1 2 3 4 5 6 7 15 14 13 12 11

CONTENTS

LIST OF ENTRIES

A

Abdominal ultrasound
Abdominal wall defects
Abortion, partial birth
Abortion, selective
Abortion, therapeutic
Abscess
Abscess incision and drainage
Abuse
Acetaminophen
Achalasia
Achondroplasia
Acid phosphatase test
Acne
Acoustic neuroma
Acrocyanosis
Acromegaly and gigantism
Actinomycosis
Acupressure
Acupuncture
Acute kidney failure
Acute lymphangitis
Acute poststreptococcal
  glomerulonephritis
Acute stress disorder
Addiction
Addison's disease
Adenoid hyperplasia
Adenovirus infections
Adhesions
Adjustment disorders
Adrenal gland cancer
Adrenal gland scan

Adrenal virilism
Adrenalectomy
Adrenocorticotropic hormone
  test
Adrenoleukodystrophy
Adult respiratory distress
  syndrome
Aging
Agoraphobia
AIDS
AIDS tests
Alagille syndrome
Alanine aminotransferase test
Albinism
Alcohol-related neurologic
  disease
Alcoholism
Aldolase test
Aldosterone assay
Alemtuzumab
Alexander technique
Alkaline phosphatase test
Allergic bronchopulmonary
  aspergillosis
Allergic purpura
Allergic rhinitis
Allergies
Allergy tests
Alopecia
Alpha-fetoprotein test
Alpha$_1$-adrenergic blockers
Alport syndrome
Altitude sickness
Alzheimer's disease
Amblyopia

Amebiasis
Amenorrhea
Amino acid disorders screening
Aminoglycosides
Amnesia
Amniocentesis
Amputation
Amylase tests
Amyloidosis
Amyotrophic lateral sclerosis
Anabolic steroid use
Anaerobic infections
Anal atresia
Anal cancer
Anal warts
Analgesics
Analgesics, opioid
Anaphylaxis
Anemias
Anesthesia, general
Anesthesia, local
Aneurysmectomy
Angina
Angiography
Angioplasty
Angiotensin-converting enzyme
  inhibitors
Angiotensin-converting enzyme
  test
Animal bite infections
Ankylosing spondylitis
Anorectal disorders
Anorexia nervosa
Anoscopy
Anosmia

B

Behcet's syndrome
Bejel
Bence Jones protein test
Bender-Gestalt test
Benzodiazepines
Bereavement
Beriberi
Berylliosis
Beta$_2$-microglobulin test
Beta blockers
Bile duct cancer
Biliary atresia
Binge eating
Biofeedback
Bipolar disorder
Birth defects
Birthmarks
Bites and stings
Black lung disease
Bladder cancer
Bladder stones
Bladder training
Blastomycosis
Bleeding time
Bleeding varices
Blepharoplasty
Blood-viscosity reducing drugs
Blood clots
Blood culture
Blood donation and registry
Blood gas analysis
Blood sugar tests
Blood typing and crossmatching
Blood urea nitrogen test
Body dysmorphic disorder
Body image
Boils
Bone biopsy
Bone density test
Bone disorder drugs
Bone grafting
Bone growth stimulation
Bone marrow aspiration and
  biopsy
Bone marrow transplantation
Bone scan

Bone x rays
Borderline personality disorder
Botulinum toxin injections
Botulism
Bowel preparation
Bowel resection
Bowel training
Brain abscess
Brain biopsy
Brain tumor
Breast biopsy
Breast cancer
Breast implants
Breast reconstruction
Breast reduction
Breast self-examination
Breast ultrasound
Breastfeeding
Breast-feeding problems
Breech birth
Bronchiectasis
Bronchiolitis
Bronchitis
Bronchodilators
Bronchoscopy
Brucellosis
Bruises
Bruxism
Budd-Chiari syndrome
Buerger's disease
Bulimia nervosa
Bundle branch block
Bunion
Burns
Bursitis
Byssinosis

C

C-reactive protein
Caffeine
Calcium
Calcium channel blockers
Campylobacteriosis
Cancer
Cancer therapy, definitive

Cancer therapy, palliative
Cancer therapy, supportive
Cancer vaccines
Candidiasis
Canker sores
Carbohydrate intolerance
Carbon monoxide poisoning
Carcinoembryonic antigen test
Carcinogens
Cardiac blood pool scan
Cardiac catheterization
Cardiac rehabilitation
Cardiac tamponade
Cardiomyopathy
Cardiopulmonary resuscitation
Cardioversion
Carotid sinus massage
Carpal tunnel syndrome
Cataract surgery
Cat-scratch disease
Cataracts
Catatonia
Catecholamines tests
Catheter ablation
Celiac disease
Cell therapy
Cellulitis
Central nervous system
  depressants
Central nervous system infections
Central nervous system
  stimulants
Cephalosporins
Cerebral amyloid angiopathy
Cerebral aneurysm
Cerebral palsy
Cerebrospinal fluid (CSF)
  analysis
Cerumen impaction
Cervical cancer
Cervical conization
Cervical disk disease
Cervical spondylosis
Cervicitis
Cesarean section
Chagas' disease
Chancroid

D

Dacryocystitis
Death
Debridement
Decompression sickness
Decongestants
Deep vein thrombosis
Defibrillation
Dehydration
Delayed hypersensitivity skin test
Delirium
Delusions
Dementia
Dengue fever
Dental fillings
Dental implants
Dental sealants
Dental trauma
Dental x rays
Depo-Provera/Norplant
Depressive disorders
Dermatitis
Dermatomyositis
DES exposure
Detoxification
Detoxification diets
Deviated septum
Diabetes insipidus
Diabetes mellitus
Diabetic foot infections
Diabetic ketoacidosis
Diabetic neuropathy
Dialysis, kidney
Diaper rash
Diaphragm (birth control)
Diarrhea
Diets
Diffuse esophageal spasm
DiGeorge syndrome
Digital rectal examination
Digoxin
Dilatation and curettage
Diphtheria
Discoid lupus erythematosus
Disk removal

Dislocations and subluxations
Dissociative disorders
Distal pancreatectomy
Diuretics
Diverticulosis and diverticulitis
Dizziness
Doppler ultrasonography
Down syndrome
Drug metabolism/interactions
Drug overdose
Drug therapy monitoring
Drugs used in labor
Dry mouth
Duodenal obstruction
Dysentery
Dysfunctional uterine bleeding
Dyslexia
Dysmenorrhea
Dyspareunia
Dyspepsia
Dysphasia

E

Ear exam with an otoscope
Ear, nose, and throat surgery
Ear surgery
Eating disorders
Echinacea
Echinococcosis
Echocardiography
Ectopic pregnancy
Eczema
Edema
Edwards' syndrome
Ehlers-Danlos syndrome
Ehrlichiosis
Elder abuse
Electric shock injuries
Electrical nerve stimulation
Electrical stimulation of the brain
Electrocardiography
Electroconvulsive therapy
Electroencephalography
Electrolyte disorders
Electrolyte supplements

Electrolyte tests
Electromyography
Electronic fetal monitoring
Electrophysiology study of the heart
Elephantiasis
Embolism
Emergency contraception
Emphysema
Empyema
Encephalitis
Encopresis
Endarterectomy
Endocarditis
Endometrial biopsy
Endometrial cancer
Endometriosis
Endorectal ultrasound
Endoscopic retrograde cholangiopancreatography
Endoscopic sphincterotomy
Endoscopy
Enemas
Enhanced external counterpulsation
Enlarged prostate
Enterobacterial infections
Enterobiasis
Enterostomy
Enterovirus infections
Enzyme therapy
Eosinophilic pneumonia
Epidermolysis bullosa
Epididymitis
Epiglottitis
Epilepsy
Episiotomy
Epstein-Barr virus
Epstein-Barr virus test
Erectile dysfunction
Erectile dysfunction treatment
Erysipelas
Erythema multiforme
Erythema nodosum
Erythroblastosis fetalis
Erythrocyte sedimentation rate

Granuloma inguinale
Group therapy
Growth hormone tests
Guided imagery
Guillain-Barré syndrome
Guinea worm infection
Gulf War syndrome
Gynecomastia (male breast enlargement)

H

H1N1 influenza A
H-2 blockers
Hair transplantation
Hairy cell leukemia
Hallucinations
Hammertoe
Hand-foot-and-mouth disease
Hantavirus infections
Haptoglobin test
Hartnup disease
Hatha yoga
Head and neck cancer
Head injury
Headache
Hearing aids
Hearing loss
Hearing tests with a tuning fork
Heart attack
Heart block
Heart disease
Heart failure
Heart murmurs
Heart surgery for congenital defects
Heart transplantation
Heart valve repair
Heart valve replacement
Heartburn
Heat disorders
Heat treatments
Heavy metal poisoning
Heel spurs
Heimlich maneuver
Helicobacteriosis

Hellerwork
Hematocrit
Hemochromatosis
Hemoglobin electrophoresis
Hemoglobin test
Hemoglobinopathies
Hemolytic-uremic syndrome
Hemolytic anemia
Hemophilia
Hemophilus infections
Hemoptysis
Hemorrhagic fevers
Hemorrhoids
Hepatitis A
Hepatitis, alcoholic
Hepatitis, autoimmune
Hepatitis B
Hepatitis C
Hepatitis D
Hepatitis, drug-induced
Hepatitis E
Hepatitis G
Hepatitis virus tests
Herbalism, traditional Chinese
Herbalism, Western
Hereditary fructose intolerance
Hereditary hemorrhagic telangiectasia
Hernia
Hernia repair
Herniated disk
Hiatal hernia
Hiccups
High-risk pregnancy
Hirschsprung's disease
Hirsutism
Histiocytosis X
Histoplasmosis
Hives
Hodgkin's lymphoma
Holistic medicine
Holter monitoring
Holtzman ink blot test
Homeopathic medicine
Homeopathic medicine, acute prescribing

Homeopathic medicine, constitutional prescribing
Homocysteine
Hookworm disease
Hormone replacement therapy
Hospital-acquired infections
HPV vaccination
Human-potential movement
Human bite infections
Human chorionic gonadotropin pregnancy test
Human leukocyte antigen test
Human papilloma virus
Huntington's disease
Hydatidiform mole
Hydrocelectomy
Hydrocephalus
Hydronephrosis
Hydrotherapy
Hyperaldosteronism
Hyperbaric chamber
Hypercalcemia
Hypercholesterolemia
Hypercoagulation disorders
Hyperemesis gravidarum
Hyperhidrosis
Hyperkalemia
Hyperlipoproteinemia
Hypernatremia
Hyperopia
Hyperparathyroidism
Hyperpigmentation
Hypersensitivity pneumonitis
Hypersplenism
Hypertension
Hyperthyroidism
Hypertrophic cardiomyopathy
Hyphema
Hypnotherapy
Hypoactive sexual desire disorder
Hypocalcemia
Hypochondriasis
Hypoglycemia
Hypogonadism
Hypokalemia
Hypolipoproteinemia

Undernutrition
Undescended testes
Upper GI exam
Ureteral stenting
Urethritis
Uric acid tests
Urinalysis
Urinary anti-infectives
Urinary catheterization
Urinary diversion surgery
Urinary incontinence
Urinary tract infection
Urine culture
Urine flow test
Uterine fibroid embolization
Uterine fibroids
Uveitis

V

Vaccination
Vaginal pain
Vaginismus
Vagotomy
Valsalva maneuver
Valvular heart disease
Varicose veins
Vascular disease
Vascular surgery
Vasculitis
Vasectomy
Vasodilators
Vegetarianism
Vegetative state
Velopharyngeal insufficiency
Vena cava filter
Venography

Venous access
Venous insufficiency
Ventricular aneurysm
Ventricular assist device
Ventricular ectopic beats
Ventricular fibrillation
Ventricular septal defect
Ventricular shunt
Ventricular tachycardia
Vesicoureteral reflux
Vibriosis
Vision training
Visual impairment
Vitamin A deficiency
Vitamin B6 deficiency
Vitamin D deficiency
Vitamin E deficiency
Vitamin K deficiency
Vitamin tests
Vitamin toxicity
Vitamins
Vitiligo
Vitrectomy
Vocal cord nodules and polyps
Vocal cord paralysis
Vomiting
Von Willebrand disease
Vulvar cancer
Vulvodynia
Vulvovaginitis

W

Waldenström's
  macroglobulinemia
Warts
Wechsler intelligence test

Wegener's granulomatosis
Weight loss drugs
West Nile virus
Wheezing
Whiplash
White blood cell count and
  differential
Whooping cough
Wilderness medicine
Wilms' tumor
Wilson disease
Wiskott-Aldrich syndrome
Withdrawal syndromes
Wolff-Parkinson-White
  syndrome
Women's health
Wound culture
Wound flushing
Wounds

X

X-linked agammaglobulinemia
X rays of the orbit

Y

Yaws
Yellow fever
Yersinosis
Yoga

Z

Zellweger syndrome
Zoonosis

PLEASE READ—IMPORTANT INFORMATION

The *Gale Encyclopedia of Medicine, Fourth Edition* is a health reference product designed to inform and educate readers about a wide variety of health topics such as diseases, disorders and conditions, treatments and diagnostic tests, diets, alternative treatments, and prevention. Gale, Cengage Learning believes the product to be comprehensive, but not necessarily definitive. It is intended to supplement, not replace, consultation with a physician or other healthcare practitioners. While Gale, Cengage Learning has made substantial efforts to provide information that is accurate, comprehensive, and up-to-date, Gale, Cengage Learning makes no representations or warranties of any kind, including without limitation, warranties of merchantability or fitness for a particular purpose, nor does it guarantee the accuracy, comprehensiveness, or timeliness of the information contained in this product. Readers should be aware that the universe of medical knowledge is constantly growing and changing, and that differences of opinion exist among authorities. Readers are also advised to seek professional diagnosis and treatment for any medical condition, and to discuss information obtained from this book with their healthcare provider.

INTRODUCTION

The *Gale Encyclopedia of Medicine 4 (GEM4)* is a one-stop source for medical information on common medical disorders, conditions, tests, treatments, drugs, and other health-related topics, including high-profile diseases such as AIDS, Alzheimer's disease, cancer, and heart disease. This encyclopedia avoids medical jargon and uses language that laypersons can understand, while still providing thorough coverage of each topic. The *Gale Encyclopedia of Medicine 4* fills a gap between basic consumer health resources, such as single-volume family medical guides, and highly technical professional materials.

Scope

More than 1,800 full-length articles are included in the *Gale Encyclopedia of Medicine 4*, including disorders/conditions, tests/procedures, and treatments/therapies. Many common drugs are also covered, with generic drug names appearing first and brand names following in parentheses—e.g., acetaminophen (Tylenol). Prominent individuals in medicine are highlighted as sidebar biographies that accompany the main topical essays. Articles follow a standardized format that provides information at a glance. Rubrics include:

Disorders/Conditions	Tests/Treatments
Definition	Definition
Demographics	Purpose
Description	Precautions
Causes and symptoms	Description
Diagnosis	Preparation
Treatment	Aftercare
Prognosis	Risks
Prevention	Normal/abnormal results
Resources	Resources
Key terms	Key terms

In recent years, there has been a resurgence of interest in holistic medicine that emphasizes the connection between mind and body. Aimed at achieving and maintaining good health rather than just eliminating disease, this approach has come to be known as alternative medicine. The *Gale Encyclopedia of Medicine 4* includes a number of essays on alternative therapies, ranging from traditional Chinese medicine to homeopathy and from meditation to aromatherapy. In addition to full essays on alternative therapies, the encyclopedia features specific **Alternative treatment** sections for diseases and conditions that may be helped by complementary therapies. The *Gale Encyclopedia of Medicine 4* also includes entries on diets, nutrition, and general wellness.

Inclusion Criteria

A preliminary list of diseases, disorders, tests, and treatments was compiled from a wide variety of sources, including professional medical guides and textbooks as well as consumer guides and encyclopedias. The general advisory board, made up of public librarians, medical librarians, and consumer health experts, evaluated the topics and made suggestions for inclusion. The list was sorted by category and sent to *GEM4* medical advisors, certified physicians with various medical specialities, for review. Final selection of topics to include was made by the medical advisors in conjunction with the Gale, Cengage Learning editor.

About the Contributors

The essays were compiled by experienced medical writers, including physicians, pharmacists, nurses, and other health care professionals. *GEM4* medical advisors reviewed the completed essays to ensure that they are appropriate, up to date, and medically accurate.

How to Use this Book

The *Gale Encyclopedia of Medicine 4* has been designed with ready reference in mind.

- Straight **alphabetical arrangement** allows users to locate information quickly.

- Bold-faced terms function as **print hyperlinks** that point the reader to related entries in the encyclopedia.

- **Cross-references** placed throughout the encyclopedia direct readers to where information on subjects without entries can be found. Synonyms and acronyms are also cross-referenced.

- Lists of **key terms** are provided where appropriate to define unfamiliar terms or concepts. A **glossary** of key terms is also included at the back of Volume 6.

- Valuable **contact information** for organizations and support groups is included with each entry. The appendix contains an extensive list of organizations arranged in alphabetical order.

- The **resources section** directs users to additional sources of medical information on a topic.

- A comprehensive **general index** allows users to easily target detailed aspects of any topic, including Latin names.

Graphics

The *Gale Encyclopedia of Medicine 4* is enhanced with 765 images, including photos, charts, tables, and detailed illustrations.

ADVISORY BOARD

An advisory board comprised of medical specialists from a variety of backgrounds provided invaluable assistance in the formulation of this encyclopedia. This advisory board performed a myriad of duties, from defining the scope of coverage to reviewing individual entries for accuracy and accessibility. We would therefore like to express our sincere thanks and appreciation for all of their contributions.

CONTRIBUTORS

Margaret Alic, Ph.D.
Science Writer
Eastsound, WA

Janet Byron Anderson
Linguist/Language Consultant
Rocky River, OH

Lisa Andres, M.S., C.G.C.
*Certified Genetic Counselor and
    Medical Writer*
San Jose, CA

Greg Annussek
Medical Writer/Editor
New York, NY

Bill Asenjo, Ph.D.
Science Writer
Iowa City, IA

William Atkins
Medical Writer
Pekin, IL

Sharon A. Aufox, M.S., C.G.C.
Genetic Counselor
Rockford Memorial Hospital
Rockford, IL

Sandra Bain Cushman
*Massage Therapist, Alexander
    Technique Practitioner*
Charlottesville, VA

Howard Baker
Medical Writer
North York, Ontario

Laurie Barclay, M.D.
Neurological Consulting Services
Tampa, FL

Jeanine Barone
Nutritionist, Exercise Physiologist
New York, NY

Julia R. Barrett
Science Writer
Madison, WI

Donald G. Barstow, R.N.
Clincal Nurse Specialist
Oklahoma City, OK

Carin Lea Beltz, M.S.
*Genetic Counselor and Program
    Director*
The Center for Genetic
    Counseling
Indianapolis, IN

Linda K. Bennington, C.N.S.
Science Writer
Virginia Beach, VA

Issac R. Berniker
Medical Writer
Vallejo, CA

Kathleen Berrisford, M.S.V.
Science Writer

Bethanne Black
Medical Writer
Atlanta, GA

Jennifer Bowjanowski, M.S., C.G.C.
Genetic Counselor
Children's Hospital Oakland
Oakland, CA

Michelle Q. Bosworth, M.S., C.G.C.
Genetic Counselor
Eugene, OR

Barbara Boughton
Health and Medical Writer
El Cerrito, CA

Cheryl Branche, M.D.
Retired General Practitioner
Jackson, MS

Michelle Lee Brandt
Medical Writer
San Francisco, CA

Maury M. Breecher, Ph.D.
Health Communicator/Journalist
Northport, AL

Ruthan Brodsky
Medical Writer
Bloomfield Hills, MI

Tom Brody, Ph.D.
Science Writer
Berkeley, CA

Leonard C. Bruno, Ph.D.
Medical Writer
Chevy Chase, MD

Diane Calbrese
*Medical Sciences and Technology
    Writer*
Silver Spring, MD

Richard H. Camer
Editor
International Medical News Group
Silver Spring, MD

Rosalyn Carson-DeWitt, M.D.
Medical Writer
Durham, NC

Laura Jean Cataldo, RN, Ed.D.
Medical Writer
Myersville, MD

Lata Cherath, Ph.D.
Science Writing Intern
Cancer Research Institute
New York, NY

Linda Chrisman
Massage Therapist and Educator
Oakland, CA

Contributors

Lisa Christenson, Ph.D.
Science Writer
Hamden, CT

Geoffrey N. Clark, D.V.M.
Editor
Canine Sports Medicine
  Update
Newmarket, NH

Rhonda Cloos, R.N.
Medical Writer
Austin, TX

Gloria Cooksey, C.N.E
Medical Writer
Sacramento, CA

Amy Cooper, M.A., M.S.I.
Medical Writer
Vermillion, SD

David A. Cramer, M.D.
Medical Writer
Chicago, IL

**Esther Csapo Rastega, R.N.,
  B.S.N.**
Medical Writer
Holbrook, MA

Arnold Cua, M.D.
Physician
Brooklyn, NY

Tish Davidson, A.M.
Medical Writer
Fremont, CA

Dominic De Bellis, Ph.D.
Medical Writer/Editor
Mahopac, NY

Lori De Milto
Medical Writer
Sicklerville, NJ

Robert S. Dinsmoor
Medical Writer
South Hamilton, MA

Stephanie Dionne, B.S.
Medical Writer
Ann Arbor, MI

Martin W. Dodge, Ph.D.
Technical Writer/Editor
Centinela Hospital and Medical
  Center
Inglewood, CA

David Doermann
Medical Writer
Salt Lake City, UT

Stefanie B. N. Dugan, M.S.
Genetic Counselor
Milwaukee, WI

Doug Dupler, M.A.
Science Writer
Boulder, CO

Thomas Scott Eagan
Student Researcher
University of Arizona
Tucson, AZ

Altha Roberts Edgren
Medical Writer
Medical Ink
St. Paul, MN

Karen Ericson, R.N.
Medical Writer
Estes Park, CO

L. Fleming Fallon Jr., M.D., Dr.PH
*Associate Professor of Public
  Health*
Bowling Green State University
Bowling Green, OH

Karl Finley
Medical Writer
West Bloomfield, MI

Faye Fishman, D.O.
Physician
Randolph, NJ

Janis Flores
Medical Writer
Lexikon Communications
Sebastopol, CA

Risa Flynn
Medical Writer
Culver City, CA

Paula Ford-Martin
Medical Writer
Chaplin, MN

Janie F. Franz
Writer
Grand Forks, ND

Sallie Freeman, Ph.D., B.S.N.
Medical Writer
Atlanta, GA

Rebecca J. Frey, Ph.D.
*Research and Administrative
  Associate*
East Rock Institute
New Haven, CT

Cynthia L. Frozena, R.N.
Nurse, Medical Writer
Manitowoc, WI

Jason Fryer
Medical Writer
San Antonio, TX

Ron Gasbarro, Pharm.D.
Medical Writer
New Milford, PA

Julie A. Gelderloos
Biomedical Writer
Playa del Rey, CA

Gary Gilles, M.A.
Medical Writer
Wauconda, IL

Harry W. Golden
Medical Writer
Shoreline Medical Writers
Old Lyme, CT

Debra Gordon
Medical Writer
Nazareth, PA

Megan Gourley
Writer
Germantown, MD

Jill Granger, M.S.
Senior Research Associate
University of Michigan
Ann Arbor, MI

**Melinda Granger Oberleitner, RN,
  DNS**
*Acting Department Head and
  Associate Professor*
Department of Nursing
University of Louisiana at
  Lafayette
Lafayette, LA

Alison Grant
Medical Writer
Averill Park, NY

Elliot Greene, M.A.
*Former president, American
  Massage Therapy Association*

Massage Therapist
Silver Spring, MD

Peter Gregutt
Writer
Asheville, NC

Laith F. Gulli, M.D.
*Consultant Psychotherapist in
    Private Practice*
Lathrup Village, MI

Kapil Gupta, M.D.
Medical Writer
Winston-Salem, NC

Maureen Haggerty
Medical Writer
Ambler, PA

Clare Hanrahan
Medical Writer
Asheville, NC

Ann M. Haren
Science Writer
Madison, CT

Judy C. Hawkins, M.S.
Genetic Counselor
The University of Texas Medical
    Branch
Galveston, TX

Caroline Helwick
Medical Writer
New Orleans, LA

David Helwig
Medical Writer
London, Ontario

Lisette Hilton
Medical Writer
Boca Raton, FL

Katherine S. Hunt, M.S.
Genetic Counselor
University of New Mexico
    Health Sciences Center
Albuquerque, NM

Kevin Hwang, M.D.
Medical Writer
Morristown, NJ

Holly Ann Ishmael, M.S., C.G.C.
Genetic Counselor
The Children's Mercy Hospital
Kansas City, MO

Dawn A. Jacob, M.S.
Genetic Counselor
Obstetrix Medical Group of Texas
Fort Worth, TX

Sally J. Jacobs, Ed.D.
Medical Writer
Los Angeles, CA

Michelle L. Johnson, M.S., J.D.
*Patent Attorney and Medical
    Writer*
Portland, OR

Paul A. Johnson, Ed.M.
Medical Writer
San Diego, CA

Cindy L. A. Jones, Ph.D.
Biomedical Writer
Sagescript Communications
Lakewood, CO

David Kaminstein, M.D.
Medical Writer
West Chester, PA

Beth A. Kapes
Medical Writer
Bay Village, OH

Janet M. Kearney
Freelance Writer
Orlando, FL

Christine Kuehn Kelly
Medical Writer
Havertown, PA

Bob Kirsch
Medical Writer
Ossining, NY

Joseph Knight, P.A.
Medical Writer
Winton, CA

Melissa Knopper
Medical Writer
Chicago, IL

Karen Krajewski, M.S., C.G.C.
Genetic Counselor
Assistant Professor of Neurology
Wayne State University
Detroit, MI

Jeanne Krob, M.D., F.A.C.S.
Physician, Writer
Pittsburgh, PA

Jennifer Lamb
Medical Writer
Spokane, WA

Richard H. Lampert
Senior Medical Editor
W.B. Saunders Co.
Philadelphia, PA

Jeffrey P. Larson, R.P.T.
Physical Therapist
Sabin, MN

Jill Lasker
Medical Writer
Midlothian, VA

Kristy Layman
Music Therapist
East Lansing, MI

Victor Leipzig, Ph.D.
Biological Consultant
Huntington Beach, CA

Brenda Wilmoth Lerner, RN
Medical Editor and Writer
Montrose, AL

Lorraine Lica, Ph.D.
Medical Writer
San Diego, CA

John T. Lohr, Ph.D.
*Assistant Director, Biotechnology
    Center*
Utah State University
Logan, UT

Larry Lutwick, M.D., F.A.C.P.
Director, Infectious Diseases
VA Medical Center
Brooklyn, NY

Suzanne M. Lutwick
Medical Writer
Brooklyn, NY

Nicole Mallory, M.S.
Medical Student
Wayne State University
Detroit, MI

Warren Maltzman, Ph.D.
Consultant, Molecular Pathology
Demarest, NJ

Adrienne Massel, R.N.
Medical Writer
Beloit, WI

Ruth E. Mawyer, R.N.
Medical Writer
Charlottesville, VA

Richard A. McCartney M.D.
Fellow, American College of Surgeons
Diplomat American Board of Surgery
Richland, WA

Bonny McClain, Ph.D.
Medical Writer
Greensboro, NC

Sally C. McFarlane-Parrott
Medical Writer
Ann Arbor, MI

Mercedes McLaughlin
Medical Writer
Phoenixville, CA

Alison McTavish, M. Sc.
Medical Writer and Editor
Montreal, Quebec

Liz Meszaros
Medical Writer
Lakewood, OH

Betty Mishkin
Medical Writer
Skokie, IL

Barbara J. Mitchell
Medical Writer
Hallstead, PA

Mark A. Mitchell, M.D.
Medical Writer
Seattle, WA

Susan J. Montgomery
Medical Writer
Milwaukee, WI

Louann W. Murray, PhD
Medical Writer
Huntington Beach, CA

Bilal Nasser, M. Sc.
Senior Medical Student
Universidad Iberoamericana
Santo Domingo, Domincan Republic

Laura Ninger
Medical Writer
Weehawken, NJ

Nancy J. Nordenson
Medical Writer
Minneapolis, MN

Teresa Odle
Medical Writer
Albuquerque, NM

Lisa Papp, R.N.
Medical Writer
Cherry Hill, NJ

Lee Ann Paradise
Medical Writer
San Antonio, TX

Patience Paradox
Medical Writer
Bainbridge Island, WA

Barbara J. Pettersen
Genetic Counselor
Genetic Counseling of Central Oregon
Bend, OR

Genevieve Pham-Kanter, M.S.
Medical Writer
Chicago, IL

Collette Placek
Medical Writer
Wheaton, IL

J. Ricker Polsdorfer, M.D.
Medical Writer
Phoenix, AZ

Scott Polzin, M.S., C.G.C.
Medical Writer
Buffalo Grove, IL

Elizabeth J. Pulcini, M.S.
Medical Writer
Phoenix, AZ

Nada Quercia, M.S., C.C.G.C.
Genetic Counselor
Division of Clinical and Metabolic Genetics
The Hospital for Sick Children
Toronto, ON, Canada

Ann Quigley
Medical Writer
New York, NY

Robert Ramirez, B.S.
Medical Student

University of Medicine & Dentistry of New Jersey
Stratford, NJ

Kulbir Rangi, D.O.
Medical Doctor and Writer
New York, NY

Esther Csapo Rastegari, Ed.M., R.N./B.S.N.
Registered Nurse, Medical Writer
Holbrook, MA

Toni Rizzo
Medical Writer
Salt Lake City, UT

Martha Robbins
Medical Writer
Evanston, IL

Richard Robinson
Medical Writer
Tucson, AZ

Nancy Ross-Flanigan
Science Writer
Belleville, MI

Anna Rovid Spickler, D.V.M., Ph.D.
Medical Writer
Moorehead, KY

Belinda Rowland, Ph.D.
Medical Writer
Voorheesville, NY

Andrea Ruskin, M.D.
Whittingham Cancer Center
Norwalk, CT

Laura Ruth, Ph.D.
Medical, Science, & Technology Writer
Los Angeles, CA

Karen Sandrick
Medical Writer
Chicago, IL

Kausalya Santhanam, Ph.D.
Technical Writer
Branford, CT

Jason S. Schliesser, D.C.
Chiropractor
Holland Chiropractic, Inc.
Holland, OH

Joan Schonbeck
Medical Writer

Massachusetts Department of
Mental Health
Marlborough, MA

Laurie Heron Seaver, M.D.
Clinical Geneticist
Greenwood Genetic Center
Greenwood, SC

Catherine Seeley
Medical Writer

**Kristen Mahoney Shannon, M.S.,
C.G.C.**
Genetic Counselor
Center for Cancer Risk Analysis
Massachusetts General
Hospital
Boston, MA

Kim A. Sharp, M.Ln.
Writer
Richmond, TX

Judith Sims, M.S.
Medical Writer
Logan, UT

Joyce S. Siok, R.N.
Medical Writer
South Windsor, CT

Jennifer Sisk
Medical Writer
Havertown, PA

Patricia Skinner
Medical Writer
Amman, Jordan

Genevieve Slomski, Ph.D.
Medical Writer
New Britain, CT

Stephanie Slon
Medical Writer
Portland, OR

Linda Wasmer Smith
Medical Writer
Albuquerque, NM

Java O. Solis, M.S.
Medical Writer
Decatur, GA

Elaine Souder, PhD
Medical Writer
Little Rock, AR

Jane E. Spehar
Medical Writer
Canton, OH

Lorraine Steefel, R.N.
Medical Writer
Morganville, NJ

Kurt Sternlof
Science Writer
New Rochelle, NY

Roger E. Stevenson, M.D.
Director
Greenwood Genetic Center
Greenwood, SC

Dorothy Stonely
Medical Writer
Los Gatos, CA

Liz Swain
Medical Writer
San Diego, CA

Deanna M. Swartout-Corbeil, R.N.
Medical Writer
Thompsons Station, TN

Keith Tatarelli, J.D.
Medical Writer

Mary Jane Tenerelli, M.S.
Medical Writer
East Northport, NY

Catherine L. Tesla, M.S., C.G.C.
Senior Associate, Faculty
Dept. of Pediatrics, Division of
Medical Genetics
Emory University School of
Medicine
Atlanta, GA

Bethany Thivierge
Biotechnical Writer/Editor
Technicality Resources
Rockland, ME

Mai Tran, Pharm.D.
Medical Writer
Troy, MI

Carol Turkington
Medical Writer
Lancaster, PA

Judith Turner, B.S.
Medical Writer
Sandy, UT

Amy B. Tuteur, M.D.
Medical Advisor
Sharon, MA

Samuel Uretsky, Pharm.D.
Medical Writer
Wantagh, NY

Amy Vance, M.S., C.G.C.
Genetic Counselor
GeneSage, Inc.
San Francisco, CA

Michael Sherwin Walston
Student Researcher
University of Arizona
Tucson, AZ

Ronald Watson, Ph.D.
Science Writer
Tucson, AZ

James E. Waun, MD, MA, RPh
*Adjunct Assistant Professor of
Clinical Pharmacy*
Ferris State University
East Lansing, MI

Ellen S. Weber, M.S.N.
Medical Writer
Fort Wayne, IN

Ken R. Wells
Freelance Writer
Laguna Hills, CA

Jennifer F. Wilson, M.S.
Science Writer
Haddonfield, NJ

Kathleen D. Wright, R.N.
Medical Writer
Delmar, DE

Jennifer Wurges
Medical Writer
Rochester Hills, MI

Mary Zoll, Ph.D.
Science Writer
Newton Center, MA

Jon Zonderman
Medical Writer
Orange, CA

Michael V. Zuck, Ph.D.
Medical Writer
Boulder, CO

C

C-reactive protein

Definition

C-reactive protein (CRP) is a protein produced by the liver and not normally found in the blood, except for people who smoke, are obese, or have an inflammatory condition somewhere in the body. CRP is measured in samples of blood and reported as ultra-sensitive CRP, US-CRP, or high sensitive CRP, HS-CRP.

Purpose

C-reactive protein appears in response to inflammation, infection, and illnesses such as heart disease, **cancer**, high blood pressure, and connective tissue diseases like **rheumatoid arthritis** and lupus erythematosis.

Individuals vary in the amount of CRP their livers produce. Some people with serious diseases, like rheumatoid arthritis and lupus, may not have elevated blood levels of CRP.

CRP is a sensitive but nonspecific test that signifies inflammation somewhere in the body; it does not help determine where or how serious it is. CRP levels begin rising within a few hours following an injury, surgery, or **heart attack**. Very high CRP levels are found after surgery, acute heart attack, or serious injury. There is a current theory that there is an inflammatory component factor in developing atherosclerotic plaques in the coronary and other major arteries, leading to hardening of the arteries. But, for people at low risk of heart disease, without cardiac symptoms, CRP levels are not useful as screening tests for heart-disease risk.

By taking multiple tests over time, the level of activity of some chronic conditions, like arthritis and other connective tissue diseases, can be followed.

CRP levels are useful in predicting the risk of complications in people with heart or **vascular disease** who have had a **stroke**, heart attack, or coronary treatment procedure like **angioplasty**. But therapy decisions are made on the basis of all clinical findings, not only on CRP levels.

Normal results

Normal CRP test results are zero to one milligram (mg) per liter of blood.

Resources

OTHER

Cleveland Clinic Heart and Vascular Institute. http://my. clevelandclinic.org/health/default.aspx.
MedlinePlus. http://www.nlm.nih.gov/nlmhome.html.

James Waun, MD, RPh

C-section *see* **Cesarean section**
CABG surgery *see* **Coronary artery bypass graft surgery**
CAD *see* **Coronary artery disease**

Caffeine

Definition

Caffeine is a bitter plant alkaloid that acts as a mild central nervous system stimulant and as a diuretic. It is found especially in coffee beans, tea leaves, cacao beans, and kola nuts. Caffeine also is available in capsules and tablets and is added to soft drinks and energy bars and drinks. It is the most widely used psychoactive substance in the world.

Purpose

Caffeine is used to increase mental alertness and temporarily relieve **fatigue**. Throughout the world many people start their days with caffeine. It has been shown to improve short-term memory, enhance concentration, speed-up reaction time, and increase one's capacity for physical labor. These effects are all temporary. Caffeine does not replace the need for rest or sleep; nor does it boost functioning above normal levels. In habitual caffeine users its effects are due, in part, to the prevention of caffeine withdrawal.

In addition to being an ingredient in various foods and beverages such as coffee, tea, soft drinks, and chocolate, caffeine is used medicinally, both alone and as an additive in other drugs. It is added to some **antihistamines** to counteract drowsiness—a common antihistamine side effect. It is added to various over-the-counter (OTC) and prescription painkillers—especially **headache** remedies—to enhance their effectiveness. Some weight-loss medications and supplements also contain caffeine. Prescription citrated caffeine is used to treat breathing problems in premature infants.

Description

About 60 different plants produce caffeine as a natural pesticide against insect predators. The compound was first purified from coffee by the German chemist Friedrich Ferdinand Runge in 1819. In addition to coffee, tea, cacao, and kola nuts, caffeine is derived from yerba mate (*Ilex paraguariensis*) and guarana (*Paullina cupana*) berries.

Humans have consumed caffeine for thousands of years—chewing seeds or leaves of caffeine-producing plants or cooking them to prepare caffeine-containing beverages. Coffee was introduced to Europe from the Middle East in the seventeenth century and soon rivaled alcohol as the social beverage of choice. It is estimated that 90% of North Americans now consume caffeine on a daily basis.

Although caffeine has no nutritional value, the U.S. Food and Drug Administration (FDA) categorizes it as "generally recognized as safe" (GRAS) and recent research suggests that moderate amounts of caffeine may have some health benefits. It is absorbed from the stomach into the bloodstream where it:

- increases heart rate
- temporarily increases blood pressure
- relaxes smooth muscle cells in the airways
- releases fatty acids and glycerol for energy
- easily crosses the blood-brain barrier and affects the levels of neurotransmitters in the brain
- increases urine output

Recommended dosage

Individuals vary greatly in their sensitivity to caffeine and in the length of time that it remains in the body. Caffeine's effects are usually noticeable about 15 minutes after ingestion and typically last several hours. On average, one-half of ingested caffeine is eliminated from the body within three to four hours.

Moderate daily caffeine consumption—300–400 milligrams (mg), about 3–4 cups of coffee—is generally considered to be safe. However it can be difficult to determine an individual's caffeine consumption:

- A large number of products contain caffeine.
- Although caffeine must be listed as an ingredient on U.S. food labels, disclosure of the amount of caffeine per serving is not required.
- The caffeine content of coffees and teas varies greatly depending on the plant source, the location where the plants are grown, and how the beverages are prepared.

Approximate amounts of caffeine is some common products include:

- brewed coffee, 8 ounces (oz) or 240 milliliters (mL): 95–200 mg
- espresso coffee, 1 oz (30 mL): 58–75 mg
- brewed decaffeinated coffee, 8 oz (240 mL): 2–12 mg
- brewed black tea, 8 oz (240 mL): 40–120 mg
- brewed green tea, 8 oz (240 mL): about 15 mg
- decaffeinated tea, 8 oz (240 mL): 1–4 mg
- Mountain Dew, 12 oz (355 mL): 54 mg
- Coca-Cola Classic, 12 oz (355 mL): 35 mg
- Diet Coke, 12 oz (355 mL): 47 mg
- Pepsi, 12 oz (355 mL): 36–38 mg
- Sunkist Orange, regular or diet, 12 oz (355 mL): 41 mg
- Barq's Root Beer, 12 oz (355 mL): 23 mg
- Dr Pepper, 12 oz (355 mL): 42–44 mg
- Sprite, Fanta, 7Up, 12 oz (355 mL): 0 mg
- No Name (formerly Cocaine) energy drink, 8.4 oz (250 mL): 280 mg
- Red Bull energy drink, 8.3 oz (245 mL): 76 mg
- SoBe No Fear energy drink, 8 oz (240 mL): 83 mg
- Hershey's Special Dark Chocolate, 1.45 oz (41 g): 31 mg
- Hershey's Milk Chocolate, 1.55 oz (43 g): 9 mg
- Excedrin extra-strength headache tablet: 65 mg
- NoDoz maximum-strength caffeine tablet: 200 mg

KEY TERMS

Alkaloid—A bitter organic base, such as caffeine or morphine, that contains nitrogen and usually oxygen, often occurs in plant seeds, and usually has physiological activity.

Caffeinism—A group of symptoms caused by excess caffeine.

Diuretic—A medication or other substance that increases urine excretion.

Neurotransmitter—A chemical that transmits impulses between nerve cells.

Stimulant—A drug or other substance that produces a temporary increase in activity or efficiency.

Precautions

Although caffeine is poisonous to dogs, horses, and some birds, in moderate amounts it is not usually harmful to humans and may even have health benefits in adults. However caffeine sensitivity is affected by weight, age, and various medications and there are large individual differences in reactions to caffeine. It is possible to overdose on caffeine and an overdose of caffeine pills is potentially fatal.

The mental and physical benefits of caffeine are temporary and can be followed by a "crash" when the caffeine wears off. Those who use caffeine to stay awake while driving or operating heavy machinery are at risk for accidents from fatigue once the effects dissipate.

Many people quickly develop tolerance to the effects of caffeine, along with mild physical and psychological dependencies. Discontinuing caffeine after regular use can cause withdrawal symptoms, especially headaches, within 12–24 hours. Other withdrawal symptoms can include irritability, **nausea**, inability to concentrate, sleepiness, fatigue, and mild depression. Withdrawal symptoms peak at about 48 hours and can last up to five days. Tapering off on caffeine—such as reducing consumption by one-half cup of coffee (about 50 mg) per day—minimizes or eliminates withdrawal symptoms.

The American Psychiatric Association's *Diagnostic and Statistical Manual of Mental Disorders* recognizes four different syndromes that can result from heavy overuse of caffeine:

- Caffeine intoxication is usually the result of taking caffeine pills (e.g., NoDoz). It is characterized by

mental changes, rambling thoughts and speech, irregular heart beat, and all symptoms associated with caffeine overuse. In severe cases death can result from ventricular fibrillation (unsynchronized contractions of the heart ventricle).

- Caffeine-induced anxiety disorder is severe anxiety that interferes with daily social interactions and occurs after caffeine intoxication or heavy long-term use of caffeine.
- Caffeine-induced sleep disorder is insomnia that requires medical/psychiatric attention and occurs after prolonged caffeine consumption.
- Non-specific caffeine-induced disorder is an otherwise unspecified disorder that is associated with either acute or long-term caffeine consumption.

Pediatric

Children and teens are particularly sensitive to caffeine. Most children obtain their caffeine from soft drinks. Therefore beverages such as water, fruit juice, low-fat milk, or—at the least—caffeine-free sodas should be substituted for caffeine-containing soft drinks. Accidental ingestion of caffeine pills by children is a medical emergency. Coffee drinking often begins during adolescence and many teenagers consume caffeine-containing energy drinks and energy bars as well as coffee, leading to adverse effects.

Geriatric

The elderly also may be particularly sensitive to the adverse effects of caffeine.

Pregnant or breastfeeding

Caffeine has not been shown to cause **birth defects** and moderate amounts are considered safe during **pregnancy**. However caffeine may be eliminated from the body at a much slower rate in pregnant women. It is generally recommended that women limit their caffeine intake to the equivalent of two cups of coffee daily during pregnancy. Women who are having difficulty becoming pregnant should consider eliminating caffeine. Caffeine passes into breast milk and can cause restlessness, irritability, and sleeplessness in infants.

Other conditions and allergies

Patients with high blood pressure may be more susceptible to adverse effects of caffeine. Liver damage slows the elimination of caffeine from the body. Patients with these conditions should carefully monitor their caffeine intake.

Side effects

Caffeinism is a group of symptoms caused by excess consumption of caffeine. Although the amount of caffeine required for these side effects varies with the individual, caffeinism generally develops in people who consume more than about 500 mg daily. Symptoms can be similar to those of caffeine withdrawal and may include:

- restlessness
- irritability
- nervousness
- anxiety
- muscle twitching
- headaches
- insomnia
- racing heart

Interactions

Caffeine may:

- increase the effectiveness of OTC and prescription medicines for migraines and other headaches
- increase urine output in people taking diuretics (water pills)
- take up to six hours to be eliminated from the bodies of women taking oral contraceptives
- be broken down more slowly in patients taking the antibiotics ciprofloxacin (Cipro) and norfloxacin (Noroxin)
- increase the concentration of theophylline in the blood
- increase the risks of ephedra (ma-huang) in herbal teas or banned dietary supplements

Resources

OTHER

Mayo Clinic. http://www.mayoclinic.com.
MedlinePlus. http://www.nlm.nih.gov/medlineplus/ caffeine.html.

ORGANIZATIONS

American Dietetic Association, 120 South Riverside Plaza, Suite 2000, Chicago, IL, 60606-6995, (800) 877-1600, http://www.eatright.org.
American Heart Association, 7272 Greenville Avenue, Dallas, TX, 75231, (800) 242-8721, http://www.american heart.org.
International Food Information Council Foundation, 1100 Connecticut Avenue, NW, Suite 430, Washington, DC, 20036, info@foodinsight.org, www.foodinsight.org.

Tish Davidson, AM
Margaret Alic, PhD

CAH *see* **Congenital adrenal hyperplasia**
Caisson disease *see* **Decompression sickness**
Calcaneal spurs *see* **Heel spurs**
Calcitonin *see* **Bone disorder drugs**

Calcium

Definition

Calcium (Ca) is the most abundant mineral in the body. About 99% of calcium in the body is in bones and teeth. The remaining 1% is in blood and soft tissue. Calcium in body fluids is an electrolyte with a charge of +2. Humans must meet their need for calcium through diet.

Calcium

Age	Recommended dietary allowance (mg)	Tolerable upper intake level (mg)
Children 0–6 mos.	210 (AI)	Not established
Children 7–12 mos.	270 (AI)	Not established
Children 1–3 yrs.	500	2,500
Children 4–8 yrs.	800	2,500
Children 9–13 yrs.	900	2,500
Adolescents 14–18 yrs.	1,300	2,500
Adults 19-50 yrs.	1,000	2,500
Adults 50> yrs.	1,200	2,500
Pregnant women 18≤ yrs.	1,300	2,500
Pregnant women 19≥ yrs.	1,000	2,500
Breastfeeding women 18≤ yrs.	1,300	2,500
Breastfeeding women 19≥ yrs.	1,000	2,500

Food	Calcium (mg)
Yogurt, plain, 1 cup	415
Cheese, mozzarella, 1.5 oz.	372
Sardines with bones, canned in oil, 3 oz.	324
Cheese, cheddar, 1.5 oz.	305
Milk, any type, 1 cup	300
Yogurt with fruit, 1 cup	245–384
Tofu, firm, with calcium sulfate, ½ cup	204
Orange juice, fortified, 6 oz.	200–260
Salmon with bones, canned, 3 oz.	181
Spinach, cooked, ½ cup	120
Beans, white, cooked, ½ cup	113
Instant breakfast drink, powder, prepared with water	105–250
Cereal, fortified, 1 cup	100–1,000
Bok choy, cooked, ½ cup	61
Beans, pinto or red, cooked, ½ cup	43
Bread, whole wheat, 1 slice	20

AI=Adequate intake
mg=milligram

(Table by PreMediaGlobal. Reproduced by permission of Gale, a part of Cengage Learning.)

Purpose

Calcium is essential for

- building and maintaining strong bones and teeth
- muscle contraction
- blood vessel contraction and relaxation
- nerve impulse transmission
- regulating fluid balance in the body

Description

Most calcium in the body is stored in bones and teeth. Here it combines with phosphate to form strong, stable crystals. The remaining 1% is dissolved in body fluids and much of it forms Ca 2+ ions. In the body, these electrically charged particles are called electrolytes. Calcium and other electrolytes are not distributed evenly throughout the body. Dissolved calcium is found mainly in the fluid outside cells (extracellular fluid). Metabolic events cause the movement of calcium across cell membranes result in muscle contraction, nerve impulse transmission, and various chemical reactions. The cell then uses energy to restore the balance of calcium between the inside and outside of the cell membrane, so that the event can be repeated.

To remain healthy, the amount of calcium dissolved in body fluids must be stay within a very narrow range. Bone acts like a calcium bank. Bone is constantly being broken down by cells called osteoclasts and built up again by cells called osteoblasts. This process is called bone remodeling, and it continues throughout an individual's life. When excess calcium is present in the blood, osteoblasts deposit calcium into bones. When too little calcium is in the blood, osteoblasts dissolve calcium from bones and move it into the blood. This process is controlled by parathyroid hormone (PTH) secreted by the parathyroid glands. The parathyroid glands are extremely sensitive to the level of calcium in the blood, and in a healthy individual they are able to maintain the concentration of calcium ions fluctuates very little.

Normal calcium requirements

The United States Institute of Medicine (IOM) of the National Academy of Sciences has developed values called Dietary Reference Intakes (DRIs) for many **vitamins** and **minerals**. The DRIs consist of three sets of numbers. The Recommended Dietary Allowance (RDA) defines the average daily amount of the nutrient needed to meet the health needs of 97–98% of the population. The Adequate Intake (AI) is an estimate set when there is not enough information to

---

---

determine an RDA. The Tolerable Upper Intake Level (UL) is the average maximum amount that can be taken daily without risking negative side effects.

The IOM has not set RDAs for calcium, but instead it has set AI levels for all age groups based on observed and experimental information. However, many studies show that Americans across almost all age groups are not meeting these AI levels. IAs and ULs for calcium are measured in milligrams (mg). The following list gives the recommended AL and UL levels of calcium for each age group.

- adults age 19–50: RDA 1,000 mg; UL 2,500 mg
- adults over age 50: RDA 1,200 mg; UL 2,500 mg

Sources of calcium

In the United States, dairy products—milk, yogurt, and cheese—are the main sources of dietary calcium. Low-fat dairy products, such as skim milk or reduced-fat cheese, contain about the same amount of calcium as whole milk products. Other sources of calcium include canned fish with bones, dark green leafy vegetables, and tofu made with calcium sulfate. Other types of tofu do not contain significant amounts of calcium. Processed foods such as orange juice, breakfast cereal, instant breakfast drinks, and bread are often fortified with calcium. This will be indicated on the label.

The following list gives the approximate calcium content for some common foods:

- milk, any type, 1 cup (8 ounces): 300 mg
- yogurt, plain, 8 ounces: 415 mg
- yogurt with fruit, 8 ounces: 245–384 mg
- cheddar cheese, 1.5 ounces: 305 mg
- mozzarella cheese, 1.5 ounces: 372 mg
- sardines with bones, canned in oil, 3 ounces: 324
- salmon with bones, canned, 3 ounces: 181 mg
- tofu, firm, made with calcium sulfate, 1/2 cup: 204 mg
- pinto or red beans, cooked, 1/2 cup: 43 mg
- white beans, cooked, 1/2 cup: 113 mg
- bok choy, 1/2 cup cooked: 61 mg
- spinach, cooked, 1/2 cup: 120 mg
- bread, whole wheat, 1 slice 20 mg
- orange juice, fortified, 6 ounces: 200–260 mg
- instant breakfast drink, powder prepared with water, 105–250 mg
- breakfast cereal, fortified, 1 cup: 100–1,000 mg

Although experts recommend that people meet as many of their vitamin and mineral needs through diet as possible, it is difficult for many people to get enough calcium from food alone. This is especially true for vegans, who eat no dairy products, adolescent girls who are very calorie conscious and tend to avoid milk and replace it with diet sodas, and people with **lactose intolerance** who cannot easily digest dairy products. Pregnant women and older individuals may also have a hard time eating enough to meet their calcium needs. People who do not get enough calcium through diet can benefit from taking a dietary supplement containing calcium.

Calcium supplements are available over-the-counter. The most common supplements supply calcium in the form of calcium carbonate or calcium citrate. Calcium carbonate is usually the most economical calcium supplement. People who are taking medications to reduce stomach acid may more easily absorb calcium citrate. Some supplements combine calcium and vitamin D because vitamin D helps the body absorb calcium. No calcium supplement contains enough calcium meet the entire daily adequate intake, because the pill would be too large to swallow. In addition, the body absorbs calcium best in doses of 500 mg or less. People who need more than 500 mg of supplemental calcium should divide the dose in half to be taken morning and evening.

Calcium deficiency

Calcium deficiency, called **hypocalcemia**, can occur because of inadequate calcium intake, excess calcium excretion by the kidney (usually caused by kidney damage), the inability to adequately absorb calcium, or because of interactions between calcium and some prescription drugs. People at highest risk of calcium deficiency are teenagers, women past the age of **menopause**, individuals who are lactose intolerant, vegans, and people with kidney (renal) damage.

Calcium deficiency rarely shows up in blood tests because calcium is withdrawn from the bones to maintain blood levels of calcium. The bones then become less dense, weaker, and more likely to break. This condition is called **osteoporosis** and it is most noticeable in the elderly who have a high rate of broken bones resulting from falls. Osteoporosis is a part of **aging**, but eating a healthy diet high in calcium, getting adequate vitamin D, and doing weight-bearing exercises regularly can delay its onset. Severe calcium deficiency, is usually caused by a medical condition rather than inadequate calcium intake. It causes symptoms such as **muscle cramps**, **tingling** in the fingers, lethargy, convulsions, heart rhythm abnormalities, and **death**. These symptoms can also be caused by many other diseases.

Calcium excess

Calcium excess is called **hypercalcemia**. It usually results from poor kidney function (renal failure) or from a malignant **cancer** tumor. It can also be caused by very large supplemental doses of vitamin D. Very rarely is hypercalcemia caused by too much calcium from food or dietary supplements. High levels of calcium interfere with the absorption of other minerals such as iron, zinc, magnesium, and phosphorous. People with hypercalcemia usually have multiple medical problems and are under the supervision of a physician.

Precautions

People of all ages, races, and gender need to be alert to getting enough calcium in their diet. Building strong, dense bones begins in childhood and adolescence, even though the results cannot be seen until old age. People mentioned previously as being at especially high risk of low dietary calcium intake should investigate taking a calcium supplement.

Interactions

Absorption of calcium is affected by several conditions.

- Age. Infants absorb as much as 60% of the calcium in their digestive system. This decreases to 15–20% in adulthood, and even less in old age.
- Amount of calcium consumed. The more calcium consumed at one time, the less efficient absorption

becomes. Calcium from supplements should be spaced out during the day for maximum absorption.

- Vitamin D. The presence of vitamin D improves calcium absorption. Vitamin D deficiency can worsen calcium deficiency.
- Plant products. Phytic found in beans and oxalic acid found in spinach and leafy greens decrease the amount of calcium absorbed from those foods, but does not affect the absorption of calcium from other foods present at the same time in the intestine. Fiber such as wheat bran also reduced calcium absorption.

Prescription medications can also affect or be affected by the absorption of calcium. These include:

- digoxin
- fluroquinolones
- levothyroxine
- tetracycline antibiotics
- anticonvulsants
- thiazide-type diuretics
- glucacorticoids
- mineral oil
- stimulant laxatives
- antacids

People taking these drugs should check with their healthcare provider or pharmacist about potential adjustments in their medications or calcium intake.

Complications

No complications are expected when healthy people take calcium in amounts equal to the AI level and less than the UL level. Some people experience gas, **nausea**, and abdominal discomfort from calcium supplements. Taking the supplement with meals, taking smaller doses spread out over the day, or changing the type of supplement usually solves this problem. Complications of excess calcium and calcium deficiency were discussed previously.

Resources

BOOKS

Fragakis, Allison. *The Health Professional's Guide to Popular Dietary Supplements.* Chicago: American Dietetic Association, 2003.

Gaby, Alan R., ed. *A-Z Guide to Drug-Herb-Vitamin Interactions Revised and Expanded 2nd Edition: Improve Your Health and Avoid Side Effects When Using Common Medications and Natural Supplements Together.* New York: Three Rivers Press, 2006.

Lieberman, Shari and Nancy Bruning. *The Real Vitamin and Mineral Book: The Definitive Guide to Designing Your Personal Supplement Program,* 4th ed. New York: Avery, 2007.

Pressman, Alan H. and Sheila Buff. *The Complete Idiot's Guide to Vitamins and Minerals,* 3rd ed. Indianapolis, IN: Alpha Books, 2007.

Rockwell, Sally. *Calcium Rich & Dairy Free: How to Get Calcium Without the Cow.* Pomeroy, WA: Health Research Books, 2005.

Rucker, Robert B., ed. *Handbook of Vitamins.* Boca Raton, FL: Taylor & Francis, 2007.

PERIODICALS

Familydoctor.org. "Vitamins and Minerals: What You Should Know." *American Family Physician.* December 2006. familydoctor.org/863.xml

OTHER

Harvard School of Public Health. "Calcium & Milk." Harvard University, December 13, 2004. http://www.hsph.harvard.edu/nutritionsource/calcium.html

Mayo Clinic Staff. "Calcium supplements: Do Men Need Them Too?" MayoClinic.com, January 4, 2007. http://www.mayoclinic.com/health/calcium-supplements/AN00420

Medline Plus. "Calcium." U. S. National Library of Medicine, March 14, 2007. http://www.nlm.nih.gov/medlineplus/calcium.html

Office of Dietary Supplements. "Dietary Supplement Fact Sheet: Calcium." National Institutes of Health. http://ods.od.nih.gov/factsheets/Calcium-Consumer

National Institute of Arthritis and Musculoskeletal and Skin Diseases (NIAMS). "Calcium Supplements: What to Look For." NIAMS, April 2005. http://www.niams.nih.gov/bone/hi/calcium_supp.htm

ORGANIZATIONS

American Dietetic Association, 120 South Riverside Plaza, Suite 2000, Chicago, IL, 60606-6995, (800) 877-1600, http://www.eatright.org.

International Food Information Council, 1100 Connecticut Avenue, NW Suite 430, Washington, DC, 20036, (202) 296-6540, (202) 296-6547, http://www.ific.org.

Linus Pauling Institute, Oregon State University, 571 Weniger Hall, Corvallis, OR, 97331-6512, (541) 717-5075, (541) 737-5077, http://lpi.oregonstate.edu.

National Institutes of Health Osteoporosis and Related Bone Diseases National Resource Center, 2 AMS Circle, Bethesda, MD, 20892-3676, (202) 223-0344, 202, 466-4325, (800) 624-BONE, http://www.niams.nih.gov/bone.

Office of Dietary Supplements, National Institutes of Health, 6100 Executive Blvd., Room 3B01, MSC 7517, Bethesda, MD, 20892-7517, (301) 435-2920, (301) 480-1845, http://ods.od.nih.gov.

Tish Davidson, A.M.

Calcium carbonate *see* **Antacids**

Calcium channel blockers

Definition

Calcium channel blockers are medicines that slow the movement of calcium into the cells of the heart and blood vessels. This, in turn, relaxes blood vessels, increases the supply of oxygen-rich blood to the heart, and reduces the heart's workload.

Purpose

Calcium channel blockers are used to treat high blood pressure, to correct abnormal heart rhythms, and to relieve the type of chest **pain** called **angina** pectoris. Physicians also prescribe calcium channel blockers to treat panic attacks and **bipolar disorder** (manic depressive illness) and to prevent **migraine headache**.

Precautions

Seeing a physician regularly while taking calcium channel blockers is important. The physician will check to make certain the medicine is working as it should and will watch for unwanted side effects. People who have high blood pressure often feel perfectly fine. However, they should continue to see their prescribing physician even when they feel well so that he can keep a close watch on their condition. They should also continue to take their medicine even when they feel fine.

Calcium channel blockers will not cure high blood pressure, but will help to control the condition. To avoid the serious health problems associated with high blood pressure, patients may have to take this type of medication for the rest of their lives. Furthermore, the blockers alone may not be enough. People with high blood pressure may also need to avoid certain foods and keep their weight under control. The health care professional who is treating the condition can offer advice as to what measures may be necessary. Patients being treated for high blood pressure should not change their **diets** without consulting their physicians.

Anyone taking calcium channel blockers for high blood pressure should not take any other prescription or over-the-counter medication without first checking with the prescribing physician, as some of these drugs may increase blood pressure.

Some people feel drowsy or less alert than usual when taking calcium channel blockers. Anyone who takes these drugs should not drive, use machines, or do anything else that might be dangerous until they have found out how the drugs affect them.

People who normally have chest pain when they **exercise** or exert themselves may not have the pain when they are taking calcium channel blockers. This could lead them to be more active than they should be. Anyone taking calcium channel blockers should therefore consult with the prescribing physician concerning how much exercise and activity may be considered safe.

Some people get headaches that last for a short time after taking a dose of this medication. This problem usually goes away during the course of treatment. If it does not, or if the headaches are severe, the prescribing physician should be informed.

Patients taking certain calcium channel blockers may need to check their pulse regularly, as the drugs may slow the pulse too much. If the pulse is too slow, circulation problems may result. The prescribing physician can show patients the correct way to check their pulse.

This type of medication may cause the gums to swell, bleed, or become tender. If this problem occurs, a medical physician or dentist should be consulted. To help prevent the problem, care should be taken when brushing and flossing the teeth. Regular dental check-ups and cleanings are also recommended.

Older people may be unusually sensitive to the effects of calcium channel blockers. This may increase the chance of side effects.

Special conditions

People with certain medical conditions or who are taking certain other medicines may develop problems if they also take calcium channel blockers. Before taking these drugs, the prescribing physician should be informed about any of these conditions:

ALLERGIES. Anyone who has had a previous unusual reaction to any calcium channel blocker should let his or her physician know before taking the drugs again. The physician should also be notified about any **allergies** to foods, dyes, preservatives, or other substances.

PREGNANCY. The effects of taking calcium channel blockers during **pregnancy** have not been studied in humans. However, in studies of laboratory animals, large doses of these drugs have been reported to cause **birth defects**, **stillbirth**, poor bone growth, and other problems when taken during pregnancy. Women who are pregnant or who may become pregnant should check with their physicians before using these drugs.

BREASTFEEDING. Some calcium channel blockers pass into breast milk, but there have been no reports of problems in nursing babies whose mothers were taking this type of medication. However, women who need to take this medicine and want to breastfeed their babies should check with their physicians.

OTHER MEDICAL CONDITIONS. Calcium channel blockers may worsen heart or blood vessel disorders.

The effects of calcium channel blockers may be greater in people with kidney or **liver disease**, as their bodies are slower to clear the drug from their systems.

Certain calcium channel blockers may also cause problems in people with a history of heart rhythm problems or with depression, Parkinson's disease, or other types of parkinsonism.

USE OF CERTAIN MEDICINES. Taking calcium channel blockers with certain other drugs may affect the way the drugs work or may increase the chance of side effects.

As with most medications, certain side effects are possible and some interactions with other substances may occur.

Side effects

Side effects are not common with this medicine, but some may occur. Minor discomforts, such as **dizziness**, lightheadedness, flushing, **headache**, and **nausea**, usually go away as the body adjusts to the drug and do not require medical treatment unless they persist or they are bothersome.

If any of the following side effects occur, the prescribing physician should be notified as soon as possible:

- breathing problems, coughing or wheezing
- irregular, fast, or pounding heartbeat
- slow heartbeat (less than 50 beats per minute)
- skin rash
- swollen ankles, feet, or lower legs

Other side effects may occur. Anyone who has unusual symptoms after taking calcium blockers should contact the prescribing physician.

Interactions

Calcium channel blockers may interact with a number of other medications. When this happens, the effects of one or both of the drugs may change or the risk of side effects may increase. Anyone who takes calcium channel blockers should not take any other prescription or non-prescription (over-the-counter) medicines without first checking with the prescribing physician. Substances that may interact with calcium channel blockers include:

- Diuretics (water pills). This type of medicine may cause low levels of potassium in the body, which may increase the chance of unwanted effects from some calcium channel blockers.
- Beta-blockers, such as atenolol (Tenormin), propranolol (Inderal), and metoprolol (Lopressor), used to treat high blood pressure, angina, and other conditions.

Also, eye drop forms of beta blockers, such as timolol (Timoptic), used to treat glaucoma. Taking any of these drugs with calcium channel blockers may increase the effects of both types of medicine and may cause problems if either drug is stopped suddenly.

- Digitalis heart medicines. Taking these medicines with calcium channel blockers may increase the action of the heart medication.
- Medicines used to correct irregular heart rhythms, such as quinidine (Quinidex), disopyramide (Norpace), and procainamide (Procan, Pronestyl). The effects of these drugs may increase if used with calcium channel blockers.
- Anti-seizure medications such as carbamazepine (Tegretol). Calcium channel drugs may increase the effects of these medicines.
- Cyclosporine (Sandimmune), a medicine that suppresses the immune system. Effects may increase if this drug is taken with calcium channel blockers.
- Grapefruit juice may increase the effects of some calcium channel blockers.

This list does not include every drug that may interact with calcium channel blockers. The prescribing physician or pharmacist will advise as to whether combining calcium channel blockers with any other prescription or nonprescription (over-the-counter) medication is appropriate or not.

Description

Calcium channel blockers are available only with a physician's prescription and are sold in tablet, capsule, and injectable forms. Some commonly used calcium channel blockers include amlopidine (Norvasc), diltiazem (Cardizem), isradipine (DynaCirc), nifedipine (Adalat, Procardia), nicardipine (Cardene), and verapamil (Calan, Isoptin, Verelan).

The recommended dosage depends on the type, strength, and form of calcium channel blocker and the condition for which it is prescribed. Correct dosage is determined by the prescribing physician and further information can be obtained from the pharmacist.

Calcium channel blockers should be taken as directed. Larger or more frequent doses should not be taken, nor should doses be missed. This medicine may take several weeks to noticeably lower blood pressure. The patient taking calcium channel blockers should keep taking the medicine, to give it time to work. Once it begins to work and symptoms improve, it should continue to be taken as prescribed.

This medicine should not be discontinued without checking with the prescribing physician. Some conditions may worsen when patients stop taking calcium channel blockers abruptly. The prescribing physician will advise as to how to gradually taper down before stopping the medication completely.

Risks

A report from the European Cardiology Society in 2000 found that patients taking certain calcium channel blockers had a 27% greater risk of **heart attack**, and a 26% greater risk of **heart failure** than patients taking other high blood pressure medicines. However, there are many patients affected by conditions that still make calcium channel blockers the best choice for them. The patient should discuss this issue with the prescribing physician.

Normal results

The expected result of taking a calcium channel blocker is to either correct abnormal heart rhythms, return blood pressure to normal, or relieve chest pain.

Resources

BOOKS

Beers, Mark H., Robert S. Porter, and Thomas V. Jones, eds. *The Merck Manual of Diagnosis and Therapy*. 18th ed. Whitehouse Station, NJ: Merck Research Laboratories, 2006.

Deanna M. Swartout-Corbeil, R.N.

Calcium imbalance *see* **Hypercalcemia; Hypocalcemia**

Calcium polycarbophil *see* **Laxatives**

California flower essences *see* **Flower remedies**

Calluses *see* **Corns and calluses**

Calorie-modified diet *see* **Diets**

Calymmatobacteriosis *see* **Granuloma inguinale**

Campylobacter jejuni infection *see* **Campylobacteriosis**

Campylobacteriosis

Definition

Campylobacteriosis refers to infection by the group of bacteria known as *Campylobacter*. The term comes from the Greek word meaning "curved rod" referring to the bacteria's curved shape. The most common disease caused by these organisms is **diarrhea**, which most often affects children and younger adults. *Campylobacter* infections account for a substantial percent of food-borne illness encountered each year.

Description

There are over 15 different subtypes, all of which are curved Gram-negative rods. *C. jeuni* is the subtype that most often causes gastrointestinal disease. However, some species such as *C. fetus* produce disease outside the intestine, particularly in those with altered immune systems, such as people with **AIDS**, **cancer**, and **liver disease**.

Campylobacter are often found in the intestine of animals raised for food products and pets. Infected animals often have no symptoms. Chickens are the most common source of human infection. It is estimated that 1% of the general population is infected each year.

Causes and symptoms

Improper or incomplete food preparation is the most common way the disease is spread, with poultry accounting for over half the cases. Untreated water and raw milk are also potential sources.

The incubation period after exposure is from one to 10 days. A day or two of mild **fever**, muscle aches, and **headache** occur before intestinal symptoms begin. Diarrhea with or without blood and severe abdominal cramps are the major intestinal symptoms. The severity of symptoms is variable, ranging from only mild fever to **dehydration** and rarely **death** (mainly in the very young or old). The disease usually lasts about one week, but persists longer in about 20% of cases. At

KEY TERMS

Antibiotic—A medication that is designed to kill or weaken bacteria.

Anti-motility medications—Medications such as loperamide (Imodium), dephenoxylate (Lomotil), or medications containing codeine or narcotics which decrease the ability of the intestine to contract. This can worsen the condition of a patient with dysentery or colitis.

Fluoroquinolones—A relatively new group of antibiotics that have had good success in treating infections with many Gram-negative bacteria. One drawback is that they should not be used in children under 17 years of age, because of possible effect on bone growth.

Food-borne illness—A disease that is transmitted by eating or handling contaminated food.

Gram-negative—Refers to the property of many bacteria that causes them to not take up color with Gram's stain, a method which is used to identify bacteria. Gram-positive bacteria which take up the stain turn purple, while Gram-negative bacteria which do not take up the stain turn red.

Guillain-Barré syndrome—Progressive and usually reversible paralysis or weakness of multiple muscles usually starting in the lower extremities and often ascending to the muscles involved in respiration. The syndrome is due to inflammation and loss of the myelin covering of the nerve fibers, often associated with an acute infection.

Meninges—Outer covering of the spinal cord and brain. Infection is called meningitis, which can lead to damage to the brain or spinal cord and even death.

Oral Rehydration Solution (ORS)—A liquid preparation developed by the World Health Organization that can decrease fluid loss in persons with diarrhea. Originally developed to be prepared with materials available in the home, commercial preparations have recently come into use.

Stool—Passage of fecal material; a bowel movement.

least 10% will have a relapse, and some patients will continue to pass the bacteria for several weeks.

Complications

Dehydration is the most common complication. Especially at the extremes of age, this should be watched for and treated with either Oral Rehydration Solution or intravenous fluid replacement.

Infection may also involve areas outside the intestine. This is unusual, except for infections with *C. fetus*. *C. fetus* infections tend to occur in those who have diseases of decreased immunity such as AIDS, cancer, etc. This subtype is particularly adapted to protect itself from the body's defenses.

Areas outside the intestine that may be involved are:

- Nervous system involvement either by direct infection of the meninges (outer covering of the spinal cord and brain) or more commonly by producing the Guillain-Barré syndrome (progressive and reversible paralysis or weakness of many muscles). In fact, *Campylobacter* may be responsible for 40% of the reported cases of this syndrome.
- Joint inflammation can occur weeks later (leading to an unusual form of arthritis).
- Infection of vessels and heart valves is a special characteristic of *C. fetus*. Immunocompromised patients

may develop repeated episodes of passage of bacteria into the bloodstream from these sites of infection.
- The gallbladder, pancreas, and bone may be affected.

Diagnosis

Campylobacter is only one of many causes of acute diarrhea. Culture (growing the bacteria in the laboratory) of freshly obtained diarrhea fluid is the only way to be certain of the diagnosis.

Treatment

The first aim of treatment is to keep up **nutrition** and avoid dehydration. Medications used to treat diarrhea by decreasing intestinal motility, such as Loperamide or Diphenoxylate are also useful, but should only be used with the advice of a physician. **Antibiotics** are of value, if started within three days of onset of symptoms. They are indicated for those with severe or persistent symptoms. Either an erythromycin type drug or one of the **fluoroquinolones** (such as ciprofloxacin) for five to seven days are the accepted therapies.

Prognosis

Most patients with *Campylobacter* infection rapidly recover without treatment. For certain groups of patients, infection becomes chronic and requires repeated courses of antibiotics.

Prevention

Good hand washing technique as well as proper preparation and cooking of food is the best way to prevent infection.

Resources

OTHER

Centers for Disease Control. http://www.cdc.gov.

ORGANIZATIONS

Centers for Disease Control and Prevention (CDC), 1600 Clifton Road, Atlanta, GA, 30333, (800) 232-4636, cdcinfo@cdc.gov, http://www.cdc.gov.

David Kaminstein, MD

Cancer

Definition

Cancer is not just one disease, but a large group of over 100 diseases. Its two main characteristics are uncontrolled growth of the cells in the human body and the ability of these cells to migrate from the original site and spread to distant sites. If the spread is not controlled, cancer can result in **death**.

Demographics

About 1.5 million Americans are diagnosed with cancer annually. One out of every four deaths in the United States is from cancer. More than 562,000 people in the United States are anticipated to die of cancer in 2009. This equates to more than 1,500 deaths from

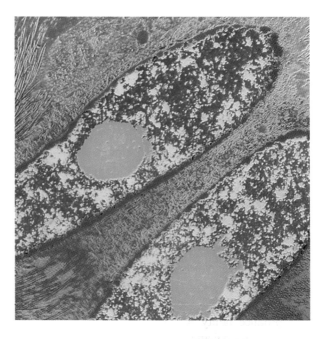

A transmission electron micrograph (TEM) of two spindle cell nuclei from a human sarcoma. Sarcomas are cancers of the connective tissue (bone, nerves, smooth muscle). *(Dr. Brian Eyden/SPL/Photo Researchers, Inc.)*

cancer per day. Overall, cancer death rates for both men and women have decreased since 2004. However, cancer ranks as the number one cause of death in persons under the age of 85 and ranks second only to heart disease as a cause of death overall in the United States.

Since the occurrence of cancer increases as individuals age, most of the cases are seen in adults, middle-aged or older. Seventy-seven percent of all cancers are diagnosed in people who are older than 55 years of age. The probability of an American male developing an invasive cancer or dying from cancer in his lifetime is 1 in 2; for American females the probability is 1 in 3. The most common cancers are skin cancer, lung cancer, **colon cancer**, **breast cancer** (in women), and **prostate cancer** (in men). In addition, cancer of the kidneys, ovaries, uterus, pancreas, bladder, rectum, and blood and lymph node cancer (leukemias and lymphomas) are also included among the 12 major cancers that affect most Americans.

Although most cancer occurs in adults, in the United States cancer is still responsible for more deaths in children under age 20 than any other disease. Each year, about 12,500 new cases of cancer are diagnosed in children compared to 1.5 million new cases annually in adults. About 2,300 children die of cancer in the U.S. each year. In general, children respond better to cancer treatment than adults do. Advances in treatment have resulted in better outcomes and increased long-term survival rates for children. Eighty

Common pathogens and associated cancers	
Causative agent	**Type(s) of cancer**
Viruses	
Epstein-Barr virus	Burkitt's lymphoma
Hepatitis B	Liver cancer
Hepatitis C	Liver cancer
Human immunodeficiency virus (HIV)	Kaposi's sarcoma, lymphoma
Papillomaviruses	Cervical cancer
Bacteria	
Helicobacter pylori	Stomach cancer, lymphomas

(Table by PreMediaGlobal. Reproduced by permission of Gale, a part of Cengage Learning.)

percent of children newly diagnosed with cancer now live at least 5 years compared to about 60% in the mid-1970s. However, the incidence of cancer in children, especially acute lymphocytic leukemia and brain cancer, has increased steadily for the past 30 years.

Description

Cancer, by definition, is a disease of the genes. A gene is a small part of DNA, which is the master molecule of the cell. Genes make proteins, which are the ultimate workhorses of the cells. These proteins allow the body to carry out all the many processes that permit an individual to function—to breathe, think, and move.

Throughout people's lives, the cells in their bodies are growing, dividing, and replacing themselves. Many genes produce proteins that are involved in controlling the processes of cell growth and division. An alteration (mutation) to the DNA molecule can disrupt the genes and produce faulty proteins. This causes the cell to become abnormal and lose its restraints on growth. The abnormal cell begins to divide uncontrollably and eventually forms a new growth known as a tumor or neoplasm (medical term for cancer meaning "new growth").

In a healthy individual, the immune system can recognize the neoplastic cells and destroy them before they get a chance to divide. However, some mutant cells may escape immune detection and survive to become tumors or cancers.

Tumors are of two types, benign or malignant. A benign tumor is not considered cancer. It is typically slow-growing, does not spread or invade surrounding tissue, and once it is removed, does not usually recur. A malignant tumor, by contrast, is cancer. It invades surrounding tissue and spreads to other parts of the body. If the cancer cells have spread to the surrounding tissues, even after the malignant tumor is removed, it generally recurs.

A majority of cancers are caused by changes in the cell's DNA because of damage to the environment. Environmental factors that are responsible for causing the initial mutation in the DNA are called **carcinogens**, of which there are many types.

Some cancers have a genetic or inherited basis. In other words, individuals can inherit faulty DNA from a parent, which could predispose the person to getting cancer. While there is scientific evidence that both factors (environmental and genetic) play a role, less than 10% of all cancers are strictly linked to hereditary factors. Cancers that are known to have a hereditary link are breast cancer, colon cancer, **ovarian cancer**, and uterine cancer. Besides genes, certain physiological traits could be inherited and could contribute to

cancers. For example, inheriting fair skin makes a person more likely to develop skin cancer, but only if that person also has prolonged exposure to intensive sunlight.

There are several different types of cancers:

- Carcinomas are cancers that arise in the epithelium (the layer of cells covering the body's surface and lining the internal organs and various glands). Ninety percent of human cancers fall into this category. Carcinomas can be subdivided into two types: adenocarcinomas (those that develop in an organ or a gland) and squamous cell carcinomas (those that originate in the skin).
- Melanomas also originate in the skin, usually in the pigment cells (melanocytes).
- Sarcomas are cancers of the supporting tissues of the body, such as bone, muscle, and blood vessels.
- Cancers of the blood and lymph glands are called leukemias and lymphomas, respectively.
- Gliomas are cancers of the nerve tissue.

Risk factors

The major risk factors for cancer are related to: tobacco and alcohol use, dietary factors, sexual and reproductive behavior, exposure to infectious agents, family history, occupation, and environmental factors including pollution.

Causes and symptoms

According to estimates of the American Cancer Society (ACS), approximately 40% of cancer deaths in 2009 were anticipated to be due to tobacco and excessive alcohol use. An additional one-third of the deaths were expected to be related to being overweight, being obese, lacking physical activity, and having poor **nutrition**. Many of the one million skin cancers diagnosed in 2009 were believed to be a direct result of over-exposure to ultraviolet light from the sun's rays.

Tobacco

Eighty to 90% of lung cancer cases occur in smokers. **Smoking** has also been shown to be a contributory factor in cancers of the upper respiratory tract, esophagus, larynx, bladder, pancreas, and probably liver, stomach, breast, and kidney as well. In the 2000s, scientists also confirmed that secondhand smoke (or passive smoking) can increase one's risk of developing cancer.

Alcohol

Excessive consumption of alcohol is a risk factor in certain cancers, such as **liver cancer**. Alcohol, in combination with tobacco, significantly increases the chances that an individual will develop mouth, pharynx, larynx, and esophageal cancers.

Diet

Thirty-five percent of all cancers are due to dietary causes. Excessive intake of fat leading to **obesity** has been associated with cancers of the breast, colon, rectum, pancreas, prostate, gall bladder, ovaries, and uterus.

Sexual and reproductive behavior

The human papillomavirus (HPV), which is sexually transmitted, has been shown to cause cancer of the cervix. Having multiple sexual partners and becoming sexually active at an early age have been shown to increase one's chances of contracting HPV. In addition, it has also been shown that women who do not have children or have children later in life have an increased risk for both ovarian and breast cancer.

Infectious agents

Between 1985 and 2005, scientists obtained evidence to show that approximately 15% of the world's cancer deaths can be traced to viruses, bacteria, or parasites. The most common cancer-causing pathogens and the cancers associated with them were shown previously in table form.

Family history

Certain cancers such as breast, colon, ovarian, and uterine cancer recur generation after generation in some families. A few cancers, such as the **eye cancer retinoblastoma**, a type of colon cancer, and a type of breast cancer known as early-onset breast cancer, have been shown to be linked to certain genes that can be tracked within a family. It is, therefore, possible that inheriting particular genes makes a person susceptible to certain cancers.

Occupational hazards

There is evidence to show that certain occupational hazards account for 4% of all cancer deaths. For example, asbestos workers have an increased incidence of lung cancer. Similarly, a higher likelihood of getting **bladder cancer** is associated with dye, rubber, and gas workers; skin and lung cancer with smelters, gold miners, and arsenic workers; leukemia with glue and varnish workers; liver cancer with PVC manufacturers; and lung, bone, and bone marrow cancer with radiologists and uranium miners.

Environment

Radiation is believed to cause 1 to 2% of all cancer deaths. Ultra-violet radiation from the sun accounts for a majority of melanoma deaths. Other sources of radiation are x rays, radon gas, and ionizing radiation from nuclear material.

Pollution

Several studies have shown a link between asbestos and cancer. Chlorination of water may account for a small rise in cancer risk. However, the main danger from pollution occurs when dangerous chemicals from industries escape into the surrounding environment. It has been estimated that 1% of cancer deaths are due to air, land, and water pollution.

Symptoms

Cancer is a progressive disease and goes through several stages. Each stage may produce a number of symptoms. Some symptoms are produced early and may occur due to a tumor that is growing within an organ or a gland. As the tumor grows, it may press on the nearby nerves, organs, and blood vessels. This causes **pain** and some pressure, which may be the earliest warning signs of cancer.

Despite the fact that there are over 100 different types of cancers, producing very different symptoms, the American Cancer Society (ACS) has established the following seven symptoms as possible warning signals of cancer:

- changes in the size, color, or shape of a wart or a mole
- a sore that does not heal
- persistent cough, hoarseness, or sore throat
- a lump or thickening in the breast or elsewhere
- unusual bleeding or discharge
- chronic indigestion or difficulty in swallowing
- any change in bowel or bladder habits

Many other diseases besides cancer can produce the same symptoms. However, it is important to have these symptoms checked, as soon as possible, especially if they linger. The earlier a cancer is diagnosed and treated, the better the chance of cure. Many cancers such as breast cancer may not have any early symptoms. Therefore, it is important to undergo routine screening tests such as breast self-exams and mammograms.

Diagnosis

Examination

Diagnosis of many cancers begins with a thorough **physical examination** and a complete medical history.

Cancer incidence and mortality, 2010[1]		
Type of cancer	Number of new diagnoses	Number of deaths
Breast cancer	207,090	39,840
Cervical cancer[2]	12,200	4,210
Colorectal cancer	142,570	51,370
Lung cancer	222,520	157,300
Non-Hodgkin lymphoma	65,540	20,210
Ovarian cancer	21,880	1,385
Prostate cancer	217,730	32,050
Skin cancer, melanoma	68,130	8,700
Skin cancer, non-melanoma	2,000,000	2,000
Testicular cancer	8,480	350

[1]Numbers are estimates
[2]Invasive

SOURCE: American Cancer Society.

(Table by PreMediaGlobal. Reproduced by permission of Gale, a part of Cengage Learning.)

The doctor will observe, feel, and palpate (apply pressure by touch) different parts of the body in order to identify any variations from the normal size, feel, and texture of the organ or tissue.

As part of the physical exam, the doctor will inspect the patient's mouth. By focusing a light into the mouth, the physician will look for abnormalities in color, moisture, surface texture, or presence of any thickening or sore in the lips, tongue, gums, the hard palate on the roof of the mouth, and the throat. To detect **thyroid cancer**, the doctor will observe the front of the neck for swelling. He may gently manipulate the neck and palpate the front and side surfaces of the thyroid gland (located at the base of the neck) to detect any nodules or tenderness. As part of the physical examination, the doctor will also palpate the lymph nodes in the neck, under the arms, and in the groin. Many illnesses and cancers cause a swelling of the lymph nodes.

The doctor may conduct a thorough examination of the skin to look for sores that have been present for more than three weeks and that bleed, ooze, or crust; irritated patches that may itch or hurt; and any change in the size of a wart or a mole.

Examination of the female pelvis is used to detect cancers of the ovaries, uterus, cervix, and vagina. In the visual examination, the doctor looks for abnormal discharges or the presence of sores. Then, using gloved hands the physician palpates the internal pelvic organs such as the uterus and ovaries to detect any abnormal mass. Breast examination includes visual observation where the doctor looks for any discharge, unevenness, discoloration, or scaling. The doctor palpates both breasts to feel for masses or lumps.

For males, inspection of the testicles, rectum and the prostate is also included in the physical examination. The doctor inserts a gloved finger into the rectum and rotates it slowly to feel for any growths, tumors, or other abnormalities. The doctor also conducts an examination of the testes, in which the doctor observes the genital area and looks for swelling or other abnormalities. The testicles are palpated to identify any lumps, thickening, or differences in the size, weight, and firmness.

Tests

The doctor may order diagnostic tests if an abnormality has been detected on physical examination, or if the patient has some symptom that could be indicative of cancer.

Laboratory studies of sputum (sputum cytology), blood, urine, and stool can detect abnormalities that may indicate cancer. Sputum cytology is a test in which the phlegm that is coughed up from the lungs is microscopically examined. It is often used to detect lung cancer. Many blood tests used for cancer detection are typically easy to perform. The blood sample is obtained by a lab technician or a doctor by inserting a needle into a vein and is relatively painless. Blood tests can be either specific or non-specific. Often, in certain cancers, the cancer cells release particular proteins (called **tumor markers**) and blood tests can be used to detect the presence of these tumor markers. However, with a few exceptions, tumor markers are not used for routine screening of cancers, because several noncancerous conditions also produce positive results. Blood tests are generally more useful in monitoring the effectiveness of the treatment, or in following the course of the disease and detecting recurrent disease.

Imaging tests such as **computed tomography scans** (CT scans), **magnetic resonance imaging** (MRI), ultrasound, and fiberoptic scope examinations help the doctors determine the location of the tumor even if it is deep within the body. Conventional x rays are often used for initial evaluation because they are relatively cheap, painless, and easily accessible. In order to increase the information obtained from a conventional x ray, air or a dye (such as barium or iodine) may be used as a contrast medium to outline or highlight parts of the body.

The most definitive diagnostic test is the biopsy, wherein a piece of tissue is surgically removed for microscope examination. Besides confirming a cancer, the biopsy also provides information about the type of cancer, the stage it has reached, the aggressiveness of the cancer, and the extent of its spread. Since a biopsy

Benign—Mild, nonmalignant. Recovery is favorable with treatment.

Biopsy—The surgical removal and microscopic examination of living tissue for diagnostic purposes.

Bone marrow—Spongy material that fills the inner cavities of the bones. The progenitors of all the blood cells are produced in this bone marrow.

Carcinogen—Any substance capable of causing cancer by mutating the cell's DNA.

Chemotherapy—Treatment with certain anticancer drugs.

Epithelium—The layer of cells covering the body's surface and lining the internal organs and various glands.

Hormone therapy—Treatment of cancer by inhibiting the production of hormones such as testosterone and estrogen.

Immunotherapy—Treatment of cancer by stimulating the body's immune defense system.

Malignant—A general term for cells and the tumors they form that can invade and destroy other tissues and organs.

Metastasis—The spread of cancer from one part of the body to another.

Radiation therapy—Treatment using high-energy radiation from x-ray machines, cobalt, radium, or other sources.

Sore—An open wound, bruise, or lesion on the skin.

Tumor—An abnormal growth resulting from a cell that lost its normal growth control restraints and started multiplying uncontrollably.

X rays—High-energy radiation used in high doses, either to diagnose or treat disease.

provides the most accurate analysis, it is considered the gold standard of diagnostic tests.

Screening examinations conducted regularly by healthcare professionals can result in the detection of cancers of the breast, colon, rectum, cervix, prostate, testis, tongue, mouth, and skin at early stages, when treatment is more likely to be successful. Some of the routine screening tests recommended by the ACS are **sigmoidoscopy** (for colorectal cancer), **mammography** (for breast cancer), pap smear (for **cervical cancer**), and the PSA test (for prostate cancer). Self-examinations for cancers of the breast, testis, mouth, and skin can also help in detecting the tumors before the symptoms become serious.

A revolution in molecular biology and cancer genetics has contributed a great deal to the development of several tests designed to assess the risk of getting cancers. These new techniques include **genetic testing**, in which molecular probes are used to identify mutations in certain genes that have been linked to particular cancers. As of 2009, however, there remain some limitations to genetic testing and its utility appeared ambiguous, emphasizing the need to develop better strategies for early detection.

Treatment

Treatment and prevention of cancers continues to be the focus of a great deal of research as of 2010.

Research into new cancer therapies includes cancer-targeting **gene therapy**, **cancer vaccines**, and other targeted therapies such as monoclonal antibodies. Most new therapies take years of clinical testing and research.

The aim of cancer treatment is to remove all or as much of the tumor as possible and to prevent the recurrence or spread of the primary tumor. While devising a treatment plan for cancer, the likelihood of curing the cancer has to be weighed against the side effects of the treatment. If the cancer is very aggressive and a cure is not possible, then the treatment should be aimed at relieving the symptoms and controlling the cancer for as long as possible.

Cancer treatment can take many different forms, and is typically tailored to the individual patient. The decision as to which type of treatment is the most appropriate depends on the type and location of cancer, the extent to which it has already spread, the patient's age, sex, general health status, and personal treatment preferences. The major types of treatment are: surgery, radiation, **chemotherapy**, biological therapy, targeted therapy, hormone therapy, and bone-marrow and **stem cell transplantation**.

Surgery

Surgery is the removal of a visible tumor and is the most frequently used cancer treatment. It is most effective when a cancer is small and/or confined to one area of the body.

Surgery can be used for many purposes:

- Treatment. Treatment of cancer by surgery involves removal of the tumor to cure the disease. This is typically done when the cancer is localized to a discrete area. Along with the cancer, some part of the normal surrounding tissue is also removed to ensure that no cancer cells remain in the area. Since cancer usually spreads via the lymphatic system, adjoining lymph nodes may be examined and sometimes are removed as well.

- Preventive surgery. Preventive or prophylactic surgery involves removal of an abnormal looking area that is likely to become malignant over time. For example, 40% of people with a colon disease known as ulcerative colitis ultimately die of colon cancer. Rather than live with the fear of developing colon cancer, these people may choose to have the colon removed which reduces the risk of developing colon cancer significantly.

- Diagnostic purposes. The most definitive tool for diagnosing cancer is a biopsy. Sometimes, a biopsy can be performed by inserting a needle through the skin. However, at other times, the only way to obtain a tissue sample for biopsy is by performing a surgical operation.

- Cytoreductive surgery is a procedure in which the doctor removes as much of the cancer as possible and then treats the remaining area with radiation therapy or chemotherapy or both.

- Palliative surgery is aimed at minimizing symptoms associated with cancer. Usually, in such cases, the tumor is so large or has spread so much that removing the entire tumor is not an option. For example, a tumor in the abdomen may be so large that it may press on and block a portion of the intestine, interfering with digestion and causing pain and vomiting.

- Debulking surgery can be used to remove a part of the blockage and to relieve associated symptoms. In tumors that are dependent on hormones, removal of the organs that secrete the hormones is an option. For example, in prostate cancer, the release of testosterone by the testicles stimulates the growth of cancerous cells. Hence, a man may undergo an orchiectomy (removal of testicles) to slow the progress of the disease. Similarly, in a type of aggressive breast cancer, removal of the ovaries (oophorectomy) stops the synthesis of hormones from the ovaries and may slow the progression of the cancer.

Radiation therapy

Radiation kills tumor cells. Radiation is used alone in cases in which a tumor is unsuitable for surgery. More often, it is used in conjunction with surgery and chemotherapy. Radiation can be either external or internal. In the external form, the radiation is aimed at the tumor from outside the body. In internal radiation (also known as brachytherapy), a radioactive substance in the form of pellets or liquid is placed at the cancerous site by means of a pill, injection, or insertion in a sealed container.

Chemotherapy

Chemotherapy is the use of drugs to kill cancer cells. It destroys the hard-to-detect cancer cells that have spread and are circulating in the body. Chemotherapeutic drugs can be given in many forms. The most common administration methods include oral (by mouth) or intravenous administration. Chemotherapy may be given alone or in conjunction with surgery, radiation, or both.

When chemotherapy is used before surgery or radiation, it is known as primary chemotherapy or neoadjuvant chemotherapy. An advantage of neoadjuvant chemotherapy is that since the cancer cells have not been exposed to anti-cancer drugs, they are especially vulnerable. It can, therefore, be used effectively to reduce the size of the tumor for surgery or target it for radiation. The more common use of chemotherapy is adjuvant therapy, which is given to enhance the effectiveness of other treatments. For example, after surgery, adjuvant chemotherapy is given to destroy any cancerous cells that still remain in the body.

Biological and targeted therapies

Biological and targeted therapies use the body's own immune system to destroy cancer cells. As of 2009, this form of treatment was being intensively studied in clinical trials. Many newer agents are used to treat a variety of cancers. The various agents being tested in clinical trials and used as treatment modalities include substances produced by the body (such as the interferons, interleukins, and growth factors), monoclonal antibodies, and vaccines. Unlike traditional vaccines, cancer vaccines do not prevent cancer. Instead, they are designed to treat people who already have the disease. Cancer vaccines work by boosting the body's immune system and training the immune cells to specifically destroy cancer cells.

Hormone therapy

Hormone therapy is standard treatment for some types of cancers that are hormone-dependent and grow faster in the presence of particular hormones. These include cancer of the prostate, breast, and uterus. Hormone therapy involves blocking the production or action of these hormones. As a result, the growth of the tumor slows, and survival may be extended.

Bone marrow, stem cell, and cord blood transplantation

The bone marrow is the tissue within the bone cavities that contains blood-forming cells. Healthy bone marrow tissue constantly replenishes the blood supply and is essential to life.

A bone marrow transplant is the removal of marrow from one person and the transplant of the blood-forming cells either to the same person or to someone else. Bone-marrow transplantation, while not a therapy in itself, is often used to "rescue" patients, by allowing those with cancer to undergo aggressive therapy. Stem cell transplants have been performed to replace bone marrow that has been destroyed by cancer, chemotherapy, or **radiation therapy**. Stem cells are specialized cells in the bone marrow from which the body receives a constant source of blood cells. Stem cells may also be harvested from umbilical cords, a process that is referred to as a cord blood transplant. Some cancers in which stem cell transplants may be used include leukemia, lymphoma, and **multiple myeloma**.

Alternative treatment

There are a multitude of alternative treatments available to help the person with cancer. They can be used in conjunction with, or separate from, surgery, chemotherapy, and radiation therapy. Alternative treatment of cancer is a complicated arena and a trained health practitioner should be consulted.

Although the effectiveness of complementary therapies such as **acupuncture** in alleviating cancer pain has not been clinically proven, many cancer patients find it safe and beneficial. Bodywork therapies such as massage and **reflexology** ease muscle tension and may alleviate side effects such as **nausea and vomiting**. Homeopathy and herbal remedies used in Chinese traditional herbal medicine also have been shown to alleviate some of the side effects of radiation and chemotherapy and are recommended by many doctors.

Certain foods, including many vegetables, fruits, and grains, are believed to offer protection against various cancers. However, isolation of the individual constituent of vegetables and fruits that are anti-cancer agents has proven difficult. In laboratory studies, **vitamins** such as A, C, and E, as well as compounds such as isothiocyanates and dithiolthiones found in broccoli, cauliflower, and cabbage, and beta-carotene found in carrots have been shown to protect against cancer. Studies have shown that eating a diet rich in fiber as found in fruits and vegetables reduces the risk of colon cancer. **Exercise** and a low fat diet help control weight and reduce the risk of endometrial, breast, and colon cancer.

Cancer treatment team

Many different specialists generally work together as a team to treat cancer patients. An oncologist is a physician who specializes in cancer care. The oncologist provides chemotherapy, hormone therapy, and any other non-surgical treatment that does not involve radiation. The oncologist often serves as the primary physician and coordinates the patient's treatment plan.

The radiation oncologist specializes in using radiation to treat cancer, whereas the surgical oncologist performs the operations needed to diagnose or treat cancer. Gynecologist-oncologists and pediatric-oncologists, as their titles suggest, are physicians involved with treating women's and children's cancers, respectively. Many other specialists also may be involved in the care of a cancer patient. For example, radiologists specialize in the use of x rays, ultrasounds, CT scans, MRI imaging and other techniques that are used to diagnose cancer. Hematologists specialize in disorders of the blood and are consulted in case of blood cancers and bone marrow cancers. The samples that are removed for biopsy are sent to a laboratory, where a pathologist examines them to determine the type of cancer and extent of the disease. There are many other specialties, and virtually any type of medical or surgical specialist may become involved with care of the cancer patient should it become necessary.

Prognosis

Lifetime risk is the phrase that cancer researchers use to refer to the probability that an individual over the course of a lifetime will develop cancer or die from it. In the United States, men have a one in two lifetime risk of developing cancer, and for women the risk is one in three. Overall, African Americans are more likely to develop cancer than whites. African Americans are also 30% more likely to die of cancer than whites.

Many cancers are curable if detected and treated in their early stages. A cancer patient's prognosis is affected by many factors, particularly the type of

JANET D. ROWLEY (1925–)

Janet Davison Rowley was born in New York City on April 5, 1925, to Ethel Mary (Ballantyne) and Hurford Henry Davison. Rowley attended the University of Chicago, earning her B.S. degree in 1946 and her M.D. degree in 1948. She also married Donald A. Rowley in 1948, and the couple ultimately had four sons. Rowley completed both her internship and residency at Chicago hospitals before returning to the University of Chicago Medical School where she conducted research from 1962-1969. She became an associate professor, and finally, in 1977, earned her position as a full professor.

Rowley's research has focused on understanding cancer, with special emphasis on its cytogenetic causes. Her development and use of Giemsa and quinacrine stains enabled Rowley to discover oncogenes and to ultimately show a consistent shifting or translocation of genetic material in chronic myeloid leukemia cells. Rowley's discoveries and continued research have shown that malignant cells in humans undergo this translocation and deletion of genes that cause tumors to grow. Her research has given oncologists new pathways to explore concerning gene therapies for the treatment of cancer.

Co-editor and co-founder of the journal, *Genes, Chromosomes and Cancer*, Rowley has published an abundance of materials including *Chromosome Changes in Leukemia* (1978), *Genes and Cancer* (1984), and *Advances in Understanding Genetic Changes in Cancer* (1992). Rowley has also received many awards and honors for her work and research.

In 1984, Dr. Rowley was made the Blum-Riese Distinguished Service Professor at the University of Chicago, a position she still holds, as well as serving as the interim deputy dean for science since 2001. In 1998, she was one of three scientists awarded the prestigious Lasker Award for their work on translocation. She has published more than 400 articles and continues her research at the University of Chicago.

cancer the patient has, the stage of the cancer, the extent to which it has metastasized, and the aggressiveness of the cancer. In addition, the patient's age, general health status, and the effectiveness of the treatment being pursued are important factors.

To help predict the future course and outcome of the disease and the likelihood of recovery from the disease, doctors often use statistics. The five-year survival rates are the most common measures used. The number refers to the proportion of people with cancer who are expected to be alive five years after initial diagnosis compared with a similar population that is free of cancer. It is important to note that while statistics can give some information about the average survival experience of cancer patients in a given population, they cannot be used to indicate individual prognosis because no two patients are exactly alike.

Prevention

According to nutritionists and epidemiologists from leading universities in the United States, a person can reduce the chances of getting cancer by following some simple guidelines:

- eating plenty of vegetables and fruits
- exercising vigorously for at least 30 minutes on 5 or more days every week. Forty-five to sixty minutes of moderate to vigorous physical activity is preferable.
- avoiding excessive weight gain
- avoiding tobacco (even secondhand smoke)
- decreasing or avoiding consumption of animal fats and red meats
- avoiding excessive amounts of alcohol
- avoiding the midday sun (between 11 a.m. and 3 p.m.) when the sun's rays are the strongest
- avoiding risky sexual practices
- avoiding known carcinogens in the environment or work place

Resources

BOOKS

Bradbury, Robert H, ed. *Cancer*. New York: Springer, 2007.

Geffen, Jeremy R. *The Journey through Cancer: Healing and Transforming the Whole Person*. New York: Three Rivers Press, 2006.

Visel, Dave. *Living with Cancer: A Practical Guide*. New Brunswick, NJ: Rutgers University Press, 2006.

Weinberg, Robert A. *The Biology of Cancer*. New York: Garland Science, 2007.

PERIODICALS

Jemal, A., Siegel, R., Ward, E., et al. "Cancer Statistics 2009." *CA: A Cancer Journal for Clinicians* 59(2009): 225–249.

OTHER

"Cancer Facts and Figures 2009." http://www.cancer.org/downloads/STT/500809web.pdf. [cited September 20, 2009].

ORGANIZATIONS

American Cancer Society, 250 Williams Street, Atlanta, GA, 30303-1002, (800) ACS-2345, https://www.cancer.org/.

National Cancer Institute, 6116 Executive Blvd., Room 3036A, Bethesda, MD, 20892-8322, (800) 422-6237, http://www.cancer.gov.

National Coalition for Cancer Survivorship, 1010 Wayne Avenue, 5th Floor, Suite 300, Silver Spring, MD, 20910, (888) 650-9127, http://www.canceradvocacy.org/.

Rosalyn Carson-DeWitt, MD
Teresa G. Odle
Melinda Oberleitner, R.N., D.N.S.

Cancer chemotherapy drugs *see* **Anticancer drugs**

Cancer therapy, definitive

Definition

Definitive **cancer** therapy is a treatment plan designed to control and potentially cure cancer using one or a combination of interventions including surgery, radiation, **chemotherapy**, biological or targeted therapies.

Purpose

The primary purpose of definitive care is to establish a cure and to destroy and remove all cancer cells from the person diagnosed with cancer.

Surgery

Surgery is not only a diagnostic tool, but is also used for **tumor removal**. The surgeon usually identifies potential candidates for tumor removal which typically occurs during a surgical procedure. Surgery can be curative for some stomach, genital/urinary, thyroid, breast, skin, and central nervous system cancers. The best chance for a surgical cure is usually with the first operation. It is essential that the cancer surgeon (oncologic surgeon) be experienced in the specific procedure.

Radiation therapy

Radiation therapy is administered to many cancer patients during the course of treatment of cancer. This type of treatment can be used as the sole method of cure for tumors in the mouth and neighboring structures in the oral cavity, vagina, prostate, cervix, esophagus, Hodgkin's disease, and certain types of cancer in the spinal cord and brain. Research and clinical trials have demonstrated that combination treatment is typically more effective than radiation therapy alone.

Chemotherapy

Chemotherapy is curative treatment strategy for some cancers. It is most effective against **choriocarcinoma**, cancer of the testis, some types of lymphomas, and cancer of skeletal muscles.

Biological and targeted therapies

Biological therapies and targeted therapies offer a newer and promising direction for cancer control and cure. Targeted therapies interfere with the actions of specific molecules involved in the growth and progression of cancerous tumors. One type of targeted therapy is directed toward stopping angiogenesis, which is the development of a blood supply to the tumor. Usually when cancer cells grow they manage to derive a blood supply that allows passage of nutrients promoting continuation of abnormal cancer growth. Treatment that focuses on destroying these blood vessels is called antiangiogenesis therapy. Cutting off the blood supply has been shown to destroy tumors, since this stops the flow of essential nutrients required for cancer growth.

Other examples of targeted therapies include use of certain growth factors which can stimulate self-destructive pathways in cancer cells (apoptosis) and **gene therapy**, which is directed toward inhibiting specific cellular signals that promote cancer cell multiplication.

Description

Surgery

Surgical removal of the tumor must be performed with care and accuracy. The surgeon must avoid over-manipulation of the surgical field. Too much movement within the area can cause cancer cell displacement into surrounding tissue. If this occurs and no further treatment is administered, the tumor may grow again. The surgeon also should perform an assessment concerning tissue removal around the cancer site. Tissue around the site may not seem cancerous by visual inspection, but adjacent structures may have cancer cells which can only be detected microscopically. Surrounding tissue removal is usually part of the operative procedure. Pieces of tumor and the surrounding area are analyzed microscopically during the operation for cell type. An adequate resection (removal of tissue) will reveal normal cells in the specimens analyzed from areas bordering the cancerous growth.

Surgery can also help to decrease the tumor bulk (size) and, along with other treatment measures, may provide a cure for certain cancers. Surgery generally works best on slow-growing cancers.

Not only can surgery be curative for some cancers, but it is an essential diagnostic tool. Examples of diagnostic procedures which can be done in the surgical environment include an aspiration biopsy, in which a needle is inserted to extract (aspirate) fluid contained inside a cancerous growth; a needle biopsy in which the surgeon uses a specialized needle to obtain a core tissue specimen; an incision biopsy which removes a section from a large tumor; and an excision biopsy, a procedure which removes the entire tumor. The surgeon also can take samples of neighboring lymph nodes. Cancer in surrounding lymph nodes is an important mechanism for distant spread of cancer to other areas. If microscopic analysis determines the presence of cancer cells in lymph nodes, the surgeon may decide to perform a more aggressive surgical approach.

Radiation therapy

Similar to surgical intervention, radiation therapy is a localized treatment. It involves the administration of ionizing radiation to a solid tumor location. This generates reactive oxygen molecules, causing the destruction of DNA in local cells. There are three commonly used radiation therapy beams: gamma rays from a linear accelerator machine produce a focused beam; orthovoltage rays are of less energy, thus penetrate less and typically deliver higher doses to superficial tissues (efficient for treating skin cancers); and megavoltage rays are high energy producing beams that can penetrate deeply situated internal organs, while sparing extensive skin damage.

Brachytherapy delivers radiation internally by placing radioactive materials such as radioactive seeds and pellets within close proximity or directly into the cancerous tumor. Teletherapy delivers radiation to a specific area of the body using a machine which delivers a beam of radiation from a source which is external to the body.

Chemotherapy

Chemotherapy drugs work by disrupting cancer cell division which leads to cell **death**. Combining several different chemotherapy agents with different mechanisms of action and different toxicity profiles often results in more effective therapy and is known as combination chemotherapy. Chemotherapy is considered to be systemic therapy because it is typically administered via the blood and circulates through the entire body. The choice of chemotherapeutic agents depends on the specific type of cancer and the effectiveness of that drug(s) on the specific cancer being treated.

Curative chemotherapy usually requires multiple administrations of the chemotherapy drug over several months. This is referred to as a treatment cycle.

Biologic or targeted therapy

Targeted therapies, as the name implies, are designed to target specific molecular flaws of cancer cells. Some drugs in this classification target specific proteins produced by cancer cells, some target cancer cell communication pathways in an attempt to disrupt the pathways, some work to inhibit new blood vessel growth required to sustain a tumor, while other drugs target the pathways in cancer cells which facilitate the ability of cancer cells to metastasize.

Biologic therapies primarily function to alter the patient's response to cancer. These treatments tend to stimulate specific immune cells or immune chemicals to destroy cancer cells.

Precautions

Surgical resection requires an experienced surgeon and surgical team, preoperative assessment, imaging studies, and delicate operative technique. Care should be taken during the procedure to avoid unnecessary tumor manipulation, which can cause cancer cells to infiltrate adjacent structures. If manipulation is excessive, cells can enter nearby areas for future re-growth. Accurate isolation of the tumor also can help avoid contamination of the surgical area. Early ligation of the blood supply to the tumor is an essential component of a surgical cure.

Radiation therapy requires extensive treatment planning and imaging. Care must be taken to localize the cancer treatment field while attempting to spare normal tissue from the effects of radiation. This requires image monitoring and exact positioning during radiation treatment sessions.

Chemotherapy usually causes destruction of normal cells, and some cancer cells can develop immunity or become refractory to the effects of chemotherapy. These agents must be administered only by clinicians who are experienced and who have been educated specifically in the administration of these very potent drugs. Side effects and patient tolerance issues typically are anticipated and dosages may have to be specifically altered.

Biological or targeted therapies may cause patient toxicity resulting in extensive side effects. The side effect profile of biologic or targeted agents is usually different from the side effect profile of chemotherapy agents. Side effects of biologic or targeted agents are usually specific to the classification of the drug while some drugs have their own unique side effects.

KEY TERMS

Bone marrow suppression—A decrease in cells responsible for providing immunity, carrying oxygen, and those responsible for normal blood clotting.

DNA—The molecule responsible for cell multiplication.

Titrate—To analyze the best end point (for dose) for a medication.

Preparation

For all treatment modalities imaging studies, biopsy, and constant blood analysis is essential before, during, and after treatments. Surgical candidates should undergo extensive pre-operative evaluation with imaging studies, blood chemistry analysis, stabilized health status, and readiness of staff for any potential complications and cell biopsy analysis. Patients with other pre-existing chronic disease may require intensive post-operative monitoring.

Prior to radiotherapy, the patient undergoes extensive imaging studies. Additional planning strategies include beam localization to spare normal tissues, calibration of fractionated doses, and specific positioning during treatment sessions.

Patients who receive curative chemotherapy should be informed of possible side effects associated with the chemotherapeutic agent. Patients should also be informed of temporary lifestyle changes and medications that may offer some symptomatic relief.

Patients undergoing biologic or targeted therapies should be advised of potential side effects, treatment cycles, and specific tests for monitoring progress.

Aftercare

Patients will typically be evaluated by imaging studies, blood analysis, **physical examination**, and will be observed for response to treatment. These follow-up visits usually occur at specific time intervals during the course of treatment. Surgical patients may require closer observation during the initial post-operative period to avoid potential complications. **Reconstructive surgery** can be considered to improve appearance and restore function. Certain surgical procedures (such as flaps and microsurgery of blood vessels) can restore new tissues to a previous surgery site.

Risks

Surgical risks

Surgical therapy can be both disfiguring and disabling. Any surgical procedure contains a risk for complications during and after the procedure in the post-operative period. Patients are monitored very closely during and after surgery to minimize the risk of complications.

Radiation risks

Many normal tissues can be adversely affected by radiation therapy. Side effects from radiation therapy are dependent on the area being treated. Some of the more common side effects which can occur shortly after a treatment cycle include **nausea**, **vomiting**, **fatigue**, loss of appetite, and bone marrow suppression (a decrease in the cells that provide defense against infections and those that carry oxygen to cells). Radiation therapy also can cause skin changes in the skin in the treatment field, difficulty swallowing, oral gum disease, and **dry mouth**. Additionally, radiation therapy can cause damage to local structures within the irradiated field.

Chemotherapy risks

Many commonly utilized chemotherapy agents cause bone marrow suppression as a side effect of treatment. Additionally, cells called platelets—important for normal blood clotting—may be significantly lowered, causing patients to bleed. This may be problematic enough to limit the treatment course. Bone marrow suppression can increase susceptibility to infection. Some chemotherapy agents may also cause **infertility**. Patients commonly have bouts of **nausea and vomiting** shortly after a treatment session. Rapidly multiplying normal cells also are affected such as skin cells (causing blistering and ulceration) and hair cells causing loss of hair, a condition called **alopecia**.

Biologic therapy risks

Biologic therapies can cause patients to develop suppression of cells that help the body fight against infection. As with all other treatment methods for cancer, patients will be screened very carefully to determine if the benefits of the treatment outweigh the potential risks to the patient.

Resources

BOOKS

Halperin, E. C., C. A. Perez, and L. W. Brady, eds. *Principles and Practice of Radiation Oncology, 5th Edition*. Philadelphia: Lippincott, Williams & Wilkins, 2008.

Wilkes, G. M., and M. Barton-Burke. *2009 Oncology Nursing Drug Handbook*. Boston, MA: Jones and Bartlett Publishers, 2009.

PERIODICALS

Printz, C. "Shorter Radiation Treatments Might Equal or Surpass Traditional Radiation." *Cancer* (May 15, 2010); 116(10):2289.

Ricevuto, E., G. Bruera, and P. Marchetti. "General Principles of Chemotherapy." *European Review of Med Pharmacol Sci.* (April 2010);14(4):269–71.

OTHER

"Chemotherapy Principles." American Cancer Society. June 17, 2009 [cited June 26, 2010]. http://www.cancer.org. docroot/ETO/eto_1_3_Chemotherapy_Principles.asp

"Targeted Cancer Therapies." National Cancer Institute. June 21, 2010 [cited June 26, 2010]. http://www.cancer. gov/cancertopics/factsheet/Therapy/targeted

Laith Farid Gulli, M.D.
Nicole Mallory, M.S.
Melinda Granger Oberleitner, RN,
DNS, APRN, CNS

Cancer therapy, palliative

Definition

Palliative **cancer** therapy is treatment specifically designed to help improve symptoms at the end of life associated with advanced and/or terminal cancer. **Palliative care** has evolved to become an integral component of cancer care and is typically provided by a team of multidisciplinary health care professionals.

Demographics

Currently, it is estimated that approximately 40% of patients diagnosed with cancer—about 550,000 people per year in the United States—will die from their cancer. The end-of-life care of many of these patients will be delivered by professionals skilled in hospice or palliative cancer care.

Description

Palliative care is directed at improving symptoms associated with advanced and incurable cancer. The five major precepts of palliative care, which were delineated as part of the Robert Wood Johnson Foundation-funded Last Acts campaign to improve quality of care at the end of life, include:

- respect for patient wishes and goals related to end-of-life decisions

- provision of comprehensive end-of-life care

- integration of care delivery from a multidisciplinary perspective

- incorporating the caregiver in to the plan of care at the end of life

- developing adequate support systems for the patient, caregiver, and family

Palliative care can include surgery, **radiation therapy**, **chemotherapy**, hormone therapy, and other specialized therapies, as well as treatment of symptoms resulting from cancer, and providing relief from side effects of treatment. The primary objective of palliative care is to improve the quality of the remainder of a patient's life. Treatment usually involves a combination of modalities (multimodality approach) and numerous specialists typically are involved in the treatment planning process. Therapeutic planning usually involves careful coordination with the treatment team. The approach to palliative care also involves easing psychosocial problems and typically incorporates an emphasis on the patient's family.

Causes and symptoms

Some signs of advanced cancer include extreme **fatigue** and weakness that is progressive, unexplained weight loss, **pain**, and **shortness of breath**, especially if the cancer has spread to the lungs.

There is the potential for a wide range of symptoms as the cancer progresses to the advanced or terminal phase. These symptoms include pain, myoclonus, dyspnea, **anxiety**, **delirium**, and noisy breathing or "rattle" among a variety of other symptoms.

Pain is one of the common symptoms associated with cancer. Approximately 75% of terminal cancer patients have pain. Pain is a subjective symptom and thus it cannot be measured using technological approaches. Pain can be assessed using numeric scales (from 1 to 10, 1 is rated as no pain while 10 is severe) or by rating specific facial expressions associated with various levels of pain. The majority of cancer patients experience pain as a result of tumor mass that compresses neighboring nerves, bone, or soft tissues, or from direct nerve injury (neuropathic pain). Pain can occur from affected nerves in the ribs, muscles, and internal structures such as the abdomen (cramping type pain associated with obstruction). Many patients also experience various types of pain as a direct result of follow-up tests, treatments (surgery, radiation, and chemotherapy) and diagnostic procedures (i.e., biopsy).

Diagnosis

Patients typically are informed that their diagnosis is terminal and treatments are directed to improve quality of life and ease suffering at the end of life.

Examination

The physician may perform a **physical examination** to help confirm advanced cancer based on the signs and symptoms the patient is experiencing. Results of this physical exam may include evidence of fluid in the lungs or abdominal area. An enlarged liver may be palpated by the physician, or external lumps that are comprised of tumor may be able to be seen and palpated on various areas of the body.

Tests

Blood test results that may confirm advanced cancer include elevated levels of **tumor markers** in the blood, elevated **liver function tests** and liver enzymes, and elevated or decreased white blood cells, red blood cells, and/or platelets, among other findings.

Imaging tests such as x rays and CT, MRI, **PET**, bone, and ultrasound scans may be conducted to determine the location and spread of the cancer.

A comprehensive palliative care assessment should be conducted to evaluate the following:

- benefits and risks associated with continuing treatments and therapies directed at controlling the cancer
- physical symptoms and problems such as pain, anorexia, dyspnea, nausea/vomiting, constipation, fatigue, weakness, alterations with sleep, and delirium, as well as other problems
- psychosocial symptoms and problems including spiritual needs
- the patient's and family's goals and wishes related to end-of-life care
- educational level to determine information needs and requirements
- the impact of cultural beliefs on preferences related to end-of-life care

Treatment

Surgery can be utilized for palliation after careful evaluation and planning. The use of surgery in these cases may reduce the tumor bulk and help improve the quality of life by relieving pain, alleviating obstruction, or controlling bleeding. Radiation therapy for terminal cancer patients can also alleviate pain, bleeding, and obstruction of neighboring areas. A combination of radiation therapy and bisphosphanates offers palliative relief to patients with metastatic bone disease (metastatic disease is cancer that has spread beyond the original site or organ to other areas of the body). Chemotherapy may be helpful to reduce tumor size and provide some reduction to metastatic disease. Long-term chemotherapy patients develop drug resistance, a situation that renders chemotherapeutic treatments ineffective. If this occurs, patients usually are given a second-line medication or, if admission criteria are met, they may participate in an experimental research protocol. Palliative treatments and terminal cancer in combination can cause many symptoms that can become problematic. These symptoms commonly include pain, **nausea, vomiting**, difficulty breathing, **constipation, dehydration**, agitation, and delirium. The palliative treatment-planning goal focuses on reducing these symptoms.

Surgery for **tumor removal**, biopsy, or size reduction is associated with postoperative pain and local nerve damage, which may be both severe and difficult to alleviate. Chemotherapy and radiation therapy also can produce nerve damage and severe pain. Additionally, patients with malignant cancer are susceptible to infections such as herpes, **pneumonia**, urinary tract infections, and wound **abscess**, all of which can cause severe pain. Pain associated with cancer and/or treatments can significantly impair the patient's abilities to perform daily tasks and hence impair quality of life. These complications may negatively impact the patient's psychological well-being.

Drugs

Drugs that may be used in palliative care include:

- opioids, benzodiazepines, glycopyrrolate, and scopolamine—used to treat dyspnea in advanced cancer
- appetite stimulants such as megestrol acetate, medroprogesterone acetate, and steroids—used to ameliorate the effects of anorexia/cachexia
- antiemetics such as prochlorperazine, haloperidol, metoclorpramide, 5-HT3 receptor antagonists, and others—used to treat nausea and vomiting
- biscodyl, glycerine suppositories, polyethylene glycol, lactulose, magnesium hydroxide, magnesium cirate, and/or methylnaltrexone—used to treat constipation in advanced cancer
- haloperidol, risperidone, olanzapine, or quetiapine fumarate—used in the treatment of delirium at the end of life

Prognosis

Palliative cancer care is typically offered to patients with six months to one year of life expectancy.

Prevention

Currently, the only way to prevent a cancer from spreading and developing into an advanced or incurable cancer is to detect the cancer prior to metastatic spread and to initiate treatment for the cancer as soon as possible after diagnosis.

Resources

BOOKS

Esper, P. "Principles and Issues in Palliative Care." In *Cancer Nursing Principles and Practice,* 6th ed. Yarbro, C.H., Frogge, M.H., & Goodman, M. eds. Boston, MA: Jones and Bartlett Publishers, 2005.

Paice, J. "Delivery of Comfort Care." In *Cancer Nursing Principles and Practice,* 6th ed. Yarbro, C.H., Frogge, M.H., & Goodman, M. eds. Boston, MA: Jones and Bartlett Publishers, 2005.

PERIODICALS

"Bisphosphanates, Radiation Therapy Can Be Used for Metastatic Bone Disease." *Cancer Weekly* October 28, 2003: 112.

Cimino, James E. "The Role of Nutrition in Hospice and Palliative Care of the Cancer Patient." *Topics in Clinical Nutrition* July-September 2003: 154–158.

Chochinov, H.M."Dying, Dignity, and New Horizons in Palliative End-of-Life Care."*CA: A Cancer Journal for Clinicians* 56(2006):84–103.

Holland, J.C., Andersen, B., & Breitbark, W.S., et al. "Distress Management."*Journal of the National Comprehensive Cancer Network* 5(2007): 66–98.

OTHER

"Overview: Advanced Cancer." *American Cancer Society Cancer Reference Information* . February 26, 2009. http://www.cancer.org/docroot/CRI/content/ CRI_2_2_3X_ Advanced_Cancer_Overview [cited September 7, 2009].

"Palliative Care."*National Comprehensive Cancer Network Practice Guidelines in Oncology – v.1.2009.* http://www. nccn.org./professionals/physician_gls/PDF/palliative. pdf [cited September 7, 2009].

ORGANIZATIONS

American Cancer Society, 250 Williams Street, Atlanta, GA, 30303-1002, (800) ACS-2345, https://www.cancer.org/.

American Pain Society, 4700 W. Lake Ave., Glenview, IL, 60025, (847) 375-4715, (866) 574-2654, info@ampainsoc. org, http://www.ampainsoc.org/.

National Cancer Institute, 6116 Executive Blvd., Room 3036A, Bethesda, MD, 20892-8322, (800) 422-6237, http://www.cancer.gov.

Laith Farid Gulli, M.D.
Nicole Mallory, M.S.
Melinda Granger Oberleitner, R.N., D.N.S., A.P.R.N., C.N.S.

Cancer therapy, supportive

Definition

Supportive **cancer** therapy is the use of medicines to counteract unwanted effects of cancer treatment.

Purpose

Along with their beneficial effects, many cancer treatments produce uncomfortable and sometimes harmful side effects. For example, cancer drugs may cause **nausea** or **vomiting**. They also may destroy red or white blood cells, resulting in a low blood count. Fortunately, many of these side effects can be relieved with other medicines.

Description

Different kinds of drugs are used for different purposes in supportive cancer therapy. To relieve **nausea and vomiting**, a physician may prescribe dolasetron (Anzemet), granisetron (Kytril) or ondansetron (Zofran). Drugs called colony stimulating factors are used to help the bone marrow make new white blood cells to replace those destroyed by cancer treatment. Examples of colony stimulating factors are filgrastim (Neupogen) and sargramostim (Leukine). Another type of drug, epoetin (Epogen, Procrit), stimulates the bone marrow to make new red blood cells and help patients overcome anemia. It is a synthetically made version of human erythropoietin that is made naturally in the body and has the same effect on bone marrow.

Some physicians who treat cancer recommend that their patients use **marijuana** to relieve nausea and **vomiting**. This practice is controversial for several reasons. Using marijuana, even for medicinal purposes, is illegal in most states. Also, most of the evidence that marijuana effectively relieves nausea and vomiting comes from reports of people who have used it, not from carefully designed scientific studies called clinical trials. An oral medication that contains one of the active ingredients of marijuana is available with a physician's prescription and sometimes is used to treat nausea and vomiting in patients undergoing cancer treatment. However, the drug, dronabinol (Marinol), takes longer to work than smoked marijuana and may be difficult for patients with nausea and vomiting to swallow and keep down.

In 1997, the National Institutes of Health issued a report calling for more research into medical uses of marijuana. The panel of experts who wrote the report also recommended that researchers investigate other ways of getting the active ingredients of marijuana into the body, such as nasal sprays, skin patches and inhalers. In 2000, the American Cancer Society funded research into a skin patch. A 2003 report said that a University of Kentucky researcher had applied for a patent for the patch which used synthetic cannabinoids.

Patients who want to use marijuana to relieve side effects of cancer treatment should talk to their physicians and should carefully consider the benefits and risks, both medical and legal.

Recommended dosage

The recommended dosage depends on the type of supportive cancer therapy. The physician who prescribed the drug or the pharmacist who filled the prescription can recommend the correct dosage.

Precautions

Dolasetron, granisetron, and ondansetron

If severe nausea and vomiting occur after taking these medications, patients should check with a physician.

The use of ondansetron after abdominal surgery may cover up symptoms of stomach problems.

People with **liver disease** may be more likely to have side effects from ondansetron.

Colony stimulating factors

Certain cancer drugs reduce the body's ability to fight infections. Although colony stimulating factors help restore the body's natural defenses, the process takes time. Getting prompt treatment for infections is important, even while taking this medicine. A patient should call the physician at the first sign of illness or infection, such as a **sore throat**, **fever**, or chills.

Seeing a physician regularly while taking this medicine is important. This will give the physician a chance to make sure the medicine is working and to check for unwanted side effects.

People with certain medical conditions may have problems if they take colony stimulating factors. In people who have **kidney disease**, liver disease, or conditions caused by inflammation or immune system problems, colony stimulating factors may make these problems worse. People with heart disease may be more likely to have side effects such as water retention and heart rhythm problems when they take these drugs. And people with lung disease may be more likely to

have **shortness of breath**. Anyone who has any of these medical conditions should check with his or her physician before using colony stimulating factors.

Epoetin

This medicine may cause seizures (convulsions), especially in people with a history of seizures. Anyone who takes these drugs should not drive, use machines or do anything else that might be dangerous if they have had a seizure.

Epoetin helps the body make new red blood cells, but it cannot do its job unless there is plenty of iron in the body. The physician may recommend taking iron supplements or certain **vitamins** that help get iron into the body. Following the physician's orders to make sure the body has enough iron for this medicine makes it work. Iron supplements should not be taken unless they are prescribed by a physician.

In studies of laboratory animals, epoetin taken during **pregnancy** caused **birth defects**, including damage to the bones and spine. However, the drug has not been reported to cause problems in human babies whose mothers take it. Women who are pregnant or who may become pregnant should check with their physicians for the most up-to-date information on the safety of taking this medicine during pregnancy.

People with certain medical conditions may have problems if they take this medicine. For example, the chance of side effects may be greater in people with high blood pressure, heart or blood vessel disease, or a history of **blood clots**. Epoetin may not work properly in people who have bone problems or sickle cell anemia.

Research continues on the benefits of epoetin as a supportive cancer therapy. One 2003 report said new research showed doubt as to its effectiveness in treating anemia, while other reports confirmed it worked well. In mid-2003, a new large clinical trial (CREATE) was beginning in England to help determine epoetin's effectiveness.

Dronabinol

This medicine contains sesame oil and one of the active ingredients of marijuana. Anyone who has had allergic or unusual reactions to sesame oil or marijuana products should let his or her physician know before taking dronabinol.

Because dronabinol works on the central nervous system, it may add to the effects of alcohol and other drugs that slow down the central nervous system. Examples of these drugs are **antihistamines**, cold medicine, allergy medicine, sleep aids, medicine for seizures, tranquilizers, some **pain** relievers, and **muscle relaxants**. Dronabinol also may add to the effects of anesthetics, including those used for dental procedures. Anyone taking dronabinol should not drink alcohol and should check with his or her physician before taking any of the drugs listed previously.

This drug makes some people feel drowsy, dizzy, lightheaded or "high," with a sense of well-being. Because of these possible reactions, anyone who takes dronabinol should not drive, use machines or do anything else that might be dangerous until they have found out how the drug affects them. The **dizziness** and lightheadedness are especially likely when getting up after sitting or lying down. Getting up gradually and holding onto something for support should lessen the problem.

In laboratory studies, giving high doses of dronabinol to pregnant animals increased the risk of the unborn baby's **death**. The medicine's effects on pregnant women have not been studied. Women who are pregnant or who may become pregnant should check with their physicians before taking this medicine.

Dronabinol passes into breast milk and may affect nursing babies whose mothers take the medicine. Women who are **breastfeeding** their babies should check with their physicians before using dronabinol.

Because of its possible mind-altering effects, dronabinol should be used with care in children and older people. Both children and older people should be watched carefully when they are taking this medicine.

Using dronabinol may worsen some medical conditions, including high blood pressure, heart disease, **bipolar disorder**, and **schizophrenia**.

General precautions for all types of supportive cancer therapy

Anyone who previously has had unusual reactions to drugs used in supportive cancer therapy should let his or her physician know before taking the drugs again. The physician should also be told about any **allergies** to foods, dyes, preservatives, or other substances.

Side effects

Dolasetron, granisetron, and ondansetron

The most common minor side effects are **headache**, dizziness or lightheadedness, drowsiness, **dry mouth**, **diarrhea**, **constipation**, abdominal pain or stomach cramps, and unusual tiredness or weakness. These problems usually do not require medical treatment.

A physician should be notified as soon as possible if fever occurs after taking granisetron.

If any of these symptoms occur after taking ondansetron, the patient should check with a physician immediately:

- breathing problems or wheezing
- chest pain or tightness in chest
- skin rash, hives or itching

Colony stimulating factors

As this medicine starts to work, it may cause mild pain in the lower back or hips. This is nothing to worry about, and it will usually go away within a few days. If the pain is too uncomfortable, the physician may prescribe a painkiller. A physician needs to know if the painkiller does not help.

Other possible side effects include headache, joint or muscle pain, and skin rash or **itching**. These side effects usually go away as the body adjusts to the medicine and do not need medical treatment. If they continue or interfere with normal activities, a physician should be notified.

Epoetin

This medicine may cause flu-like symptoms, such as muscle aches, bone pain, fever, chills, shivering, and sweating, within a few hours after it is taken. These symptoms usually go away within 12 hours. If they do not, or if they are troubling, a physician should be told. Other possible side effects that do not need medical attention are diarrhea, nausea or vomiting, and tiredness or weakness.

Certain side effects should be brought to a physician's attention as soon as possible. These include headache, vision problems, increased blood pressure, fast heartbeat, weight gain, and swelling of the face, fingers, lower legs, ankles, or feet.

Anyone who has chest pain or seizures after taking epoetin should check with a physician immediately.

Dronabinol

Side effects such as dizziness, drowsiness, confusion and clumsiness or unsteadiness usually do not need medical attention unless they are long-lasting or they interfere with normal activities.

Other side effects or signs of overdose should have immediate medical attention. These include:

- fast or pounding heartbeat
- constipation

KEY TERMS

Bipolar disorder—A severe mental illness in which a person has extreme mood swings, ranging from a highly excited state — sometimes with a false sense of well-being — to depression

Bone marrow—Soft tissue that fills the hollow centers of bones. Blood cells and platelets (disk-shaped bodies in the blood that are important in clotting) are produced in the bone marrow.

Hallucination—A false or distorted perception of objects, sounds, or events that seems real. Hallucinations usually result from drugs or mental disorders.

Immune system—The body's natural defenses against disease and infection.

Inflammation—Pain, redness, swelling, and heat that usually develop in response to injury or illness.

Schizophrenia—A severe mental disorder in which people lose touch with reality and may have illogical thoughts, delusions, hallucinations, behavioral problems, and other disturbances.

Sickle cell anemia—An inherited disorder in which red blood cells contain an abnormal form of hemoglobin, a protein that carries oxygen. The abnormal form of hemoglobin causes the red cells to become sickle- or crescent-shaped. The misshapen cells may clog blood vessels, preventing oxygen from reaching tissues and leading to pain, blood clots and other problems. Sickle cell anemia is most common in people of African descent and in people from Italy, Greece, India, and the Middle East.

- trouble urinating
- red eyes
- slurred speech
- mood changes, including depression, nervousness, or anxiety
- confusion
- forgetfulness
- changes in sight, smell, taste, touch, or hearing
- a sense that time is speeding up or slowing down
- hallucinations

General advice on side effects for all types of supportive cancer therapy

Other side effects are possible with any type of supportive cancer therapy. Anyone who has unusual symptoms during or after treatment with these drugs should get in touch with his or her physician.

Interactions

Anyone who has supportive cancer therapy should let the physician know all other medicines he or she is taking. Some combinations of drugs may interact, which may increase or decrease the effects of one or both drugs or may increase the risk of side effects. Patients should ask their physician if the possible interactions can interfere with drug therapy or cause harmful effects.

Resources

PERIODICALS

"CREATE Trial Providing Valuable Information on Epoetin Treatment for Anemia." *Hematology Week* August 25, 2003: 10.
"Doubts Over Epoetin in Cancer." *SCRIP World Pharmaceutical News* October 24, 2003: 24.
"Researcher Working on Medical Patch to Deliver Marijuana–like Drug." *Cancer Weekly* September 9, 2003: 126.

Nancy Ross-Flanigan
Teresa G. Odle

Cancer vaccines

Definition

Cancer vaccines are biological response modifiers that stimulate the immune system. Cancer preventative vaccines are substances that prevent healthy people from developing cancer by targeting infectious organisms that contribute to cancer development. They work in the same way as traditional vaccines (e.g., **mumps, measles, rubella, polio**). Cancer treatment vaccines are a method of treating cancer involving administration of one or more substances characteristic of the cancer, called antigens, often in combination with factors that boost immune function. This induces the patient's immune system to attack and eliminate the cancerous cells.

Purpose

In 2006, the U.S. Food and Drug Administration (FDA) approved the cancer preventative vaccine, Gardasil, that protects against certain human papilloma viruses associated with the development of **cervical cancer**. A second preventative cancer vaccine called Cervarix, which also protects against certain human papilloma viruses, has been approved in Europe, but is not, as of 2010, available in the United States. The only other cancer preventative vaccine approved in the United States is the **hepatitis B** vaccine (HBV or HepB). It is an injection that protects individuals from contracting hepatitis B, a serious disease that contributes to the development of **liver cancer**.

Cancer treatment vaccines are in clinical trials in the United States, but as of 2010, none have been approved by the FDA. Most cancer vaccines are a method of treating cancer that has already occurred and are given to patients already diagnosed with cancer. As a cancer treatment method, the ultimate goal of most cancer vaccines is the elimination of tumor or cancerous cells from the body. Other cancer vaccines are given after the use of more traditional treatments, such as **chemotherapy**, radiation, or surgery, with the aim of suppressing the recurrence of the cancer.

Description

There are four general types of cancer vaccines, those that use whole tumor cells, those that use only one substance derived from the tumors, those using more than one substance derived from tumors, and those that administer primed cells from the patient's immune system.

Whole cell vaccines

Whole cell vaccines are autologous when they contain only inactivated tumor cells from the patient's own tumors. The cells have been isolated from the tumor and made to grow in the laboratory, a process known as creating a cell line. Allogeneic whole cell vaccines are made from inactivated tumor cells isolated from one or more other people. The main advantage to autologous vaccines is the direct relation between the vaccine and the tumor target. However, because of the screening of self antigens away from a body's own immune system, immune response to tumor antigens in autologous whole cells vaccines can be low.

Allogeneic vaccines avoid some of the problems of autologous vaccines. First, cell lines do not have to be created for each patient, a labor-intensive process that can have highly variable results. Second, the same vaccine can be given to all patients, making the response to the vaccine more predictable. Third, using a pool of tumor cells can increase the possibility of having the full repertoire of the tumor antigens in the vaccine. This helps to overcome the ability of tumor cells to escape notice by the immune system. Finally, by using well-characterized cell lines, it is much easier for the researcher to add genetic

modifications that increase the immune system's response to the cells.

Isolated antigen vaccines

There are many kinds of vaccines that deliver only a portion of the tumor cell that will elicit an immune response, called an antigen. Some antigens are unique to a cancer type, some are unique to an individual tumor, while a very few are found in more than one cancer type. For example, vaccines against telomerase and human chorionic gonadotripin (hCG), two proteins produced by many cancers, have been developed, raising hopes for the development of a universal cancer vaccine.

The most common kind of antigen used in cancer vaccines is a protein or a part of a protein. The protein can actually be isolated from the tumor cells, or more commonly, produced in large quantity using genetic engineering techniques. When a part of a protein is used, experimental efforts generally preceded the vaccine production to determine what parts of the protein most often are the target of immune responses. Parts of proteins that elicit immune responses are called epitopes.

Antigens do not necessarily have to be proteins. Immune responses are also mounted against the carbohydrate (sugar) molecules present on the surface of the proteins. Tumor proteins can have unusual carbohydrate structures that set them apart from cells of normal tissue. Carbohydrates are also found in abundant numbers on the surface of the tumor cells. Accordingly, researchers have developed cancer vaccines that combine the tumor-characteristic carbohydrates anchored on protein bases. These vaccines are being tested for their ability to reduce the recurrence of **prostate cancer**.

Vaccines can also contain the naked genetic material encoding the protein (either deoxyribose nucleic acid, DNA, or ribose nucleic acid, RNA). After the genetic material gains entry to the cell, the cellular machinery uses it to produce the antigen and an immune response is mounted against it. Animal studies have found that these types of vaccines are very dependent on the particular antigen and the mode of administration of the vaccine. A unique method of delivery used with DNA or RNA vaccines is the coating of tiny gold beads with the genetic material and shooting the beads into the skin.

Genetically engineered viruses can also be used to bring the DNA or RNA into the cell. When used in this way the viruses are called viral vectors. One example of a viral vector being used as a cancer vaccine is based on the adenovirus. When viruses are used as vectors they have been altered to no longer cause disease, but they do retain the ability to infect human cells. Instead of making new viruses, the infected cells make the desired antigen, and the body responds against it. Viral vectors can also carry the genetic instructions for factors, called cytokines, which boost the immune system's response to the antigen. This process of using a virus that no longer causes a disease but promotes the creation of antigens is used to develop vaccines to prevent cancer from developing. As of 2010, there are two types of preventative vaccines for cancer; hepatitis B virus for the prevention of liver cancer and human papillomavirus vaccine, which reduces one of the main causes of cervical cancer.

Antigen-presenting cell (APC) vaccines

Vaccines can also be made that contain cells from the patient's own immune system called antigen-presenting cells (APCs). These cells play a central role in the development of an immune response against a particular antigen. Specifically, APCs ingest the antigen and present them to the T cells, a type of immune cells responsible for targeting and killing cells seen as foreign to the body. If T cells are exposed to the antigen by an APC, as opposed to seeing the antigen on the cell itself, they are more strongly activated. That is, more T cells that specifically attack that antigen are produced and the immune response against the foreign cell is stronger.

Dendritic cells are a type of APC that is most effective in activating T cells. For this reason, they are often the kind of cells used in APC vaccines. Unfortunately, the number of dendritic cells circulating in the blood at any one time is relatively low. New techniques have been developed that allow that small number of dendritic cells to be isolated and then stimulated outside the body to result in a usable number. During stimulation, the dendritic cells are exposed to the tumor antigen, a process known as priming. When injected into the body, the dendritic cells are primed to recruit large numbers of T cells specific against the tumor antigen.

Cytokines and adjuvants

Since tumor cells are able to escape detection by the immune system, an important component of many cancer vaccines is the addition of biological factors or chemical adjuvants to help boost immune response. One type of adjuvant is a cytokine, a factor normally produced by cells of the immune system to help recruit cells to the site of the foreign cells or help T cells function. Examples of cytokines used in vaccines are granulocyte/macrophage colony stimulating factor (GM-CSF, or sargramostim), the interleukins (especially IL-2), the interferons (INFs), and tumor necrosis factor alpha (TNF-α).

Adjuvants are chemical additions to vaccines that help boost the response to the contained cells or antigens. Adjuvants are derived from a variety of sources and can be isolated from animals, plants, or are synthetic chemical compounds. Several adjuvants in use with cancer vaccines are keyhole lympocianin (KLH, derived from shell-dwelling sea animals), incomplete Freud's adjuvant (IFA, mineral oil and an emulsifying agent), and QS-21 (a chemical derived from the soapbark tree).

Administration

The particular administration method and schedule varies for each clinical trial. Administration methods include intradural (injection within the skin), subcutaneous (injection below the skin), injection into the lymph nodes, or intravenous (injection into the veins). Typically, vaccines are administered as a series of several doses (initial challenge and boosters). Many clinical trials utilize various administration methods and timing strategies in order to determine the best means of inducing an anti-tumor immune response. Preventative vaccines are usually given in a series of three injections.

Risks

The greatest risk with cancer vaccines is that there will be no immune response and the treatment will be ineffective. Serious adverse reactions to the antigens, such as the attack of healthy cells, are theoretically possible, but these fears have not materialized. Other than some mild adverse reactions, such as **fever** and redness of the skin at the injection site, vaccine treatment appears relatively low-risk in the traditional sense.

Precautions

No vaccine has yet been approved by the FDA for the treatment of cancer. Accordingly, vaccines are not standard treatments and other more traditional treatments should be investigated first. Vaccines are available only through participation in clinical trials. Each trial has its own criteria that limits who can participate. Many cancers have a current trial for one or more types of vaccines.

Most vaccine trials test the response of the disease with and without the vaccine or the effect of substances added to the vaccine, called adjuvants. Such trials usually only accept patients who have already tried the standard treatment methods. Others test a standard treatment method with and without the addition of the

KEY TERMS

Adjuvant—A substance added to a vaccine to increase the immune system's response to the vaccine contents.

Allogeneic—A type of vaccine made up of tumor cells derived from persons other than the patient.

Antigen—A substance characteristic of a tumor that evokes an immune response.

Antigen presenting cell—A cell of the immune system that ingests antigens and exposes them to cells of the immune system in a way that activates the cells to seek out and destroy any other cells displaying that antigen.

Autologous—A type of vaccine made up of tumor cells from the patient's own tumor.

Cytokine—A substance made by cells of the immune system that increases the response to a foreign substance.

Dendritic cell—A special type of antigen-presenting cell that is effective in stimulating T cells.

Epitope—A portion of a protein or other molecule that is the specific target of an immune response.

Hepatitis B—A virus that is spread through blood and sexual contact and causes hepatitis. Hepatitis causes the liver to inflame and can cause liver cancer.

Human papillomavirus (HPV)—A virus that causes abnormal tissue growth. Certain types of HPV can cause cervical and other types of cancer such as anal and vaginal cancer.

vaccine. A very few compare the standard treatment to the vaccine.

Looking at cancer vaccines overall, this treatment method has been more successful eliminating very small tumors rather than getting rid of a large tumor load. If the size of the tumor is significant, a more realistic goal is to shrink the tumor and reduce its effect on the patient's body, rather than total elimination of the cancer.

The complexity of the human immune system has made it very difficult to develop an effective vaccine. Tumors have strategies to evade detection by the immune system. Most notably, they mimic the outward appearance and antigens of the body's own cells. The immune system's built-in lack of response against "self" allows the tumor to escape notice by the body. Now fully aware of this phenomenon, researchers are

working to develop methods of circumventing this problem to develop a highly effective vaccine system.

There has been a huge success with preventative cancer vaccines. A vaccine introduced in 2006 protects against four HPV viruses that cause 70% of cervical cancers and 90% of **genital warts**. The vaccine is most effective when given before a female becomes sexually active. It is recommended for all women ages 11–18 and may be given as young as age 9. Women ages 19–26 also may be vaccinated at the discretion of their physician. The vaccine is given in three doses over a six-month period and is covered by most health insurance programs.

Universal childhood **vaccination** against hepatitis B has been practiced in the United States since 1991. Hepatitis B vaccine usually is the first vaccine a child receives, most often while still in the hospital within 24 hours after birth. The second and third HBV immunizations are administered by the age of 18 months in conjunction with other routine childhood vaccinations.

The Centers for Disease Control and Prevention (CDC) estimates that before the launch of the infant HBV immunization program, about 33,000 American children of non-infected mothers acquired hepatitis B by the age of ten. This number has substantially decreased. In 2007, 4,519 cases of acute Hepatitis B in the United States were reported, the lowest ever recorded. However, this number is thought to be about a ten-fold underestimate because many new cases do not cause symptoms and are not reported.

Preparation

Before enrolling in a clinical trial, patients should discuss the potential benefits and risks with their doctor. Clinical trials can be located by contacting the research institutes directly or by searching the Internet. The National Cancer Institute is a good resource for information about clinical trials for cancer treatment. Patients should talk to their doctor about receiving preventative cancer vaccines.

Aftercare

One of the most striking advantages of vaccines compared to other cancer treatments is the relatively low incidence of side effects. If IFN is used as an immunoadjuvant, patients sometimes experience flu-like symptoms. However, other than some soreness at the site of injection, vaccine patients generally have no adverse reactions to this kind of treatment.

It is possible to have an allergic reaction to the HPV or hepatitis B vaccine or to experience some swelling or soreness around the injection site. Patients should contact their doctor if they have any unusual reactions to the vaccines.

Results

For each trial, a very small percentage of patients have complete, partial, or mixed response to experimental cancer treatment vaccines. A few others show a stabilization of the disease where deterioration of the condition would be expected. As traditional treatments were often unsuccessful with these patients, these results are significant. However, the very low rate of success underscores the complexity of the human immune system, the number of variables in the vaccine method, and the amount of research necessary to develop an effective vaccine treatment for this disease.

Resources

BOOKS

Arthur, Allen. *Vaccine: The Controversial Story of Medicine's Greatest Lifesaver*. New York: W.W. Norton, 2007.

Dizon, Don S., and Michael L. Krychman. *Questions & Answers About Human Papilloma Virus (HPV)*. Sudbury, MA: Jones and Bartlett Publishers, 2011.

Miller, Neil Z. *Vaccine Safety Manual for Concerned Families and Health Practitioners*. 2nd ed. Santa Fe, NM: New Atlantean Press, 2010.

Offit, Paul A. *Vaccinated: One Man's Quest to Defeat the World's Deadliest Diseases*. New York: Collins, 2007.

Orentas, Rimas, et al., eds. *Cancer Vaccines and Tumor Immunity*. Hoboken, NJ: Wiley-Interscience, 2008.

OTHER

"Cervical Cancer." U.S Department of Health and Human Services. May 18, 2010. http://www.women shealth.gov/FAQ/cervical-cancer.cfm (accessed June 6, 2010).

"National Cancer Institute Fact Sheet: Cancer Vaccines." National Cancer Institute. April 17, 2009. http://www. cancer.gov/cancertopics/factsheet/Therapy/cancer-vaccines (accessed June 6, 2010).

"Treating and Preventing Cancer with Vaccines." National Cancer Institute. March 12, 2006. http://www.cancer. gov/clinicaltrials/learning/cancervaccines (accessed June 6, 2010).

"Vaccines." Centers for Disease Control and Prevention (CDC). March 30, 2010. http://www.cdc.gov/vaccines (accessed June 6, 2010).

"Vaccines, Blood and Biologics: Vaccines." U.S. Food and Drug Administration. March 29, 2010. http://www. fda.gov/BiologicsBloodVaccines/Vaccines/defaul. htm (accessed June 6, 2010).

ORGANIZATIONS

American Cancer Society, 1599 Clifton Rd., NE, Atlanta, GA, 30329, (404) 320-3333, (800) ACS-2345, http://www.cancer.org.

Cancer Research and Prevention Foundation, 1600 Duke Street, Suite 500, Alexandria, VA, 22314, (703) 836-4412, (800) 227-2732, info@preventcancer.org, http://www.preventcancer.org.

Centers for Disease Control and Prevention (CDC), 1600 Clifton Road, Atlanta, GA, 30333, (404) 639-3534, (800) CDC-INFO (800-232-4636). TTY: (888) 232-6348, inquiry@cdc.gov, http://www.cdc.gov.

National Cancer Institute Public Inquires Office, 6116 Executive Boulevard, Room 3036A, Bethesda, MD, 20892-8322, (800) 4-CANCER (800-422-6237). TTY: (800) 332-8615, http://www.cancer.gov.

National Vaccine Information Center, 407-H Church Street, Vienna, VA, 22180, (703) 938-0342, (703) 938-5768, contactNVIC@gmail.com, http://www.nvic.org.

National Vaccine Program Office, 200 Independence Avenue, SW Room 715-H, Washington, DC, 20201, (202) 619-0257, (877) 696-6775, (409) 772-5208, http://www. hhs.gov/nvpo/.

World Health Organization, Avenue Appia 20, 1211 Geneva 27, Switzerland, + 22 41 791 21 11, + 22 41 791 31 11, info@who.int, http://www.who.int.

Michelle Johnson, MS, JD
Tish Davidson, AM
Paul Checchia, MD

Candida albicans infection *see* **Candidiasis**

Candidiasis

Definition

Candidiasis is an infection caused by a species of the yeast *Candida*, usually *Candida albicans*. This is a common cause of vaginal infections in women. Also, *Candida* may cause mouth infections in people with reduced immune function, or in patients taking certain **antibiotics**. *Candida* can be found in virtually all normal people but causes problems in only a fraction. In recent years, however, several serious categories of candidiasis have become more common, due to overuse of antibiotics, the rise of **AIDS**, the increase in organ transplantations, and the use of invasive devices (catheters, artificial joints, and valves)—all of which increase a patient's susceptibility to infection.

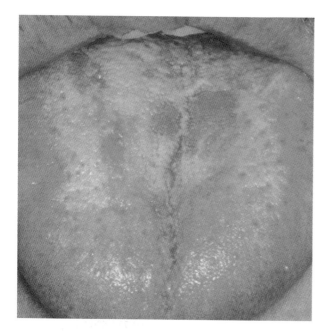

This patient's tongue is infected with candidiasis. *(Custom Medical Stock Photo, Inc. Reproduced by permission.)*

Demographics

The candida organism is present in the oropharyngeal areas in 30 to 55% of healthy young adults. About 75% of women are infected with vaginal candidiasis at least one time in their lifetime. The candida species is now the fourth most commonly isolated organism from blood cultures and is the most common cause of fungal infection in patients whose immune systems are compromised.

Risk factors

Patients at high risk for the development of candidiasis include patients who are often extremely ill.

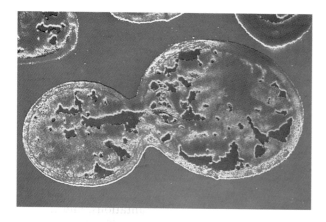

A transmission electron microscopy (TEM) of *Candida albicans.* *(Custom Medical Stock Photo, Inc. Reproduced by permission.)*

Patients in neonatal, pediatric, and adult intensive care units are considered to be at high risk. Other high risk patients are patients who are immunosuppressed due to **chemotherapy**, **radiation therapy**, severe trauma, and organ transplantation. Patients undergoing procedures such as recent surgery, hemodialysis, **urinary catheterization**, central **venous access** device placement, and those on mechanical ventilation for longer than 3 days are at high risk for the development of invasive or systemic candidiasis.

Neonates and older adults over the age of 65 years are at highest risk for infection with the candida organism.

Description

Vaginal candidiasis

Over one million women in the United States develop vaginal yeast infections each year. It is not life-threatening, but it can be uncomfortable and frustrating.

Oral candidiasis

This disorder, also known as thrush, causes white, curd-like patches in the mouth or throat.

Deep organ candidiasis

Also known as invasive candidiasis, deep organ candidiasis is a serious systemic infection that can affect the esophagus, heart, blood, liver, spleen, kidneys, eyes, and skin. Like vaginal and oral candidiasis, it is an opportunistic disease that strikes when a person's resistance is lowered, often due to another illness. There are many diagnostic categories of deep organ candidiasis, depending on the tissues involved.

Causes and symptoms

Vaginal candidiasis

Most women with vaginal candidiasis experience severe vaginal **itching**. They also have a discharge that often looks like cottage cheese and has a sweet or bread-like odor. The vulva and vagina can be red, swollen, and painful. Sexual intercourse can also be painful.

Oral candidiasis

Whitish patches can appear on the tongue, inside of the cheeks, or the palate. Oral candidiasis typically occurs in people with abnormal immune systems. These can include people undergoing chemotherapy for **cancer**, people taking immunosuppressive drugs to protect transplanted organs, or people with HIV infection.

Deep organ candidiasis

Anything that weakens the body's natural barrier against colonizing organisms—including stomach surgery, **burns**, nasogastric tubes, and catheters—can predispose a person for deep organ candidiasis. Rising numbers of AIDS patients, organ transplant recipients, and other individuals whose immune systems are compromised help account for the dramatic increase in deep organ candidiasis in recent years. Patients with granulocytopenia (deficiency of white blood cells) are particularly at risk for deep organ candidiasis.

Diagnosis

Often clinical appearance gives a strong suggestion about the diagnosis. Generally, a clinician will take a sample of the vaginal discharge or swab an area of oral plaque, and then inspect this material under a microscope. Under the microscope, it is possible to see characteristic forms of yeasts at various stages in the lifecycle.

Fungal blood cultures should be taken for patients suspected of having deep organ candidiasis. However, blood cultures may not detect up to 50% of cases of disseminated candidiasis. A more specific test to detect Beta-glucan, a fungal cell wall component, is the serum Beta-D-glucan detection assay. This test has shown to be highly specific in detecting fungal infections.

A tissue biopsy of suspected infected areas may also be helpful in confirming a diagnosis of systemic or disseminated candidiasis.

Treatment

Vaginal candidiasis

In most cases, vaginal candidiasis can be treated successfully with a variety of over-the-counter antifungal creams or suppositories. These include Monistat, Gyne-Lotrimin, and Mycelex. However, infections often recur. However, a single 150 mg dose of oral fluconazole (Diflucan) has been shown to as effective or better than topical antifungal agents when treating acute cases of vaginal candidiasis.

Oral candidiasis

This is usually treated with prescription lozenges or mouthwashes. Some of the most-used prescriptions are nystatin mouthwashes (Nilstat or Nitrostat) and clotrimazole lozenges. Other treatment options include amphotericin B oral suspension or treatment with systemic azole medications such as fluconazole (Diflucan), itraconazole (Sporonox), or posaconazole (Noxafil) for more severe oral infections.

Deep organ candidiasis

Guidelines for the treatment of invasive candidiasis were revised in 2009 by the Infectious Diseases Society of America (ISDA). The guidelines include the recommended use of drugs such as caspofungin (Cancidas), micafungin (Mycamine), and anidulafungin (Eraxis), which are classified as echinocandins, and the drugs voriconazole (Vfend) and posaconazole (Noxafil), which are classified as triazoles. Lipid formulations of amphotericin B are also recommended in the treatment of systemic fungal infections caused by candida organisms. Treatment with fluconazole (Diflucan) continues to be recommended as first line treatment for invasive candidiasis in non-neutropenic patients.

Alternative treatment

Home remedies for vaginal candidiasis include vinegar douches or insertion of a paste made from *Lactobacillus acidophilus* powder into the vagina. In theory, these remedies will make the vagina more acidic and therefore less hospitable to the growth of *Candida*. Fresh garlic (*Allium sativum*) is believed to have antifungal action, so incorporating it into the diet or inserting a gauze-wrapped, peeled garlic clove into the vagina may be helpful. The insert should be changed twice daily. Some women report success with these remedies; they should try a conventional treatment if an alternative remedy isn't effective.

Prognosis

Vaginal candidiasis

Although most cases of vaginal candidiasis are cured reliably, these infections can recur. To limit recurrences, women may need to take a prescription anti-fungal drug or take other anti-fungal drugs on a preventive basis.

Oral candidiasis

These infections can also recur, sometimes because the infecting *Candida* develops resistance to one drug. Therefore, a physician may need to prescribe a different drug.

Deep organ candidiasis

The prognosis depends on the category of disease as well as on the condition of the patient when the infection strikes. Patients who are already suffering from a serious underlying disease are more susceptible to deep organ candidiasis that spreads throughout the body.

Mortality rates for disseminated candidiasis have not improved significantly over the years. It is estimated that as many as 30 to 40% of patients diagnosed with severe cases of systemic candidiasis will die from infection with this pathogen.

Prevention

Because *Candida* is part of the normal group of microorganisms that co-exist with all people, it is impossible to avoid contact with it. Good vaginal hygiene and good **oral hygiene** might reduce problems, but they are not guarantees against candidiasis.

Because hospital-acquired (nosocomial) deep organ candidiasis is on the rise, people need to be made aware of it. Patients should be sure that catheters and other medical devices are properly maintained and used for the shortest possible time lengths.

Resources

PERIODICALS

Guery, B. P., M. C. Arendrup, G. Auzinger, et al. "Management of Invasive Candidiasis and Candidemia in Adult Non-Neutropenic Intensive Care Unit Patients: Part I. Epidemiology and Diagnosis." *Intensive Care Med.* (Jan 2009);35(1): 55–62.

Pappas, P. G. "Invasive Candidiasis." *Infect Dis Clin North Am.* (Sept 2006);20(3):485–506.

Pappas, P. G., Kauffman, C.A., Andes, D., Benjamin, D.K. Jr., Calandra, T.F., Edwards, J.E.Jr., et al. "Clinical Practice Guidelines for the Management of Candidiasis: 2009 Update by the Infectious Diseases Society of America." *Clin Infect Dis.* (Mar 1, 2009); 48(5): 503–35.

OTHER

Hildalgo, J. A. and J. A. Vazquez, J.A. "Candidiasis." eMedicine Infectious Diseases. January 11, 2010 [cited June 26, 2010]. http://www.emedicine.medscape.com

Richard H. Lampert
Melinda Granger Oberleitner, RN, DNS, APRN, CNS

Candidosis *see* **Candidiasis**

Canker sores

Definition

Canker sores are small white or yellowish sores or ulcers that develop inside the mouth. They are painful, self-healing, and can recur.

Description

Canker sores occur on the inside of the mouth, usually on the inside of the lips, cheeks, and/or soft palate. They also can occur on the tongue and in the throat. Often, several canker sores will appear at the same time and may be grouped in clusters. Canker sores appear as a whitish, round area with a red border. The sores are painful and sensitive to touch. The average canker sore is about .25 inch (60 mm) in diameter, although they can occasionally be larger. Canker sores are not infectious.

Approximately 20% of Americans experience recurring canker sores. They are more common in women than in men. Women are more likely to have canker sores at certain times during their menstrual period, suggesting that they may be influenced by female hormones.

Canker sores are sometimes confused with **cold sores**. Cold sores are caused by herpes simplex virus. This disease, also known as oral herpes or **fever** blisters, can occur anywhere on the body. Most commonly, herpes infection occurs on the outside of the lips and the gums, and much less frequently on the inside the mouth. Unlike canker sores, cold sores are infectious.

Causes and symptoms

The exact cause of canker sores is uncertain; however, they seem to be related to a localized immune reaction. Other proposed causes for this disease are trauma to the affected areas from toothbrush scrapes or dental cleanings, **stress**, hormones, and **food allergies**. They may also be related to nutritional deficiencies.

Canker sores commonly tend to appear in response to stress. The initial symptom is a **tingling** or mildly painful, **itching** sensation in the area where the sore will appear. After one to three days, a small red swelling appears. The sore is round and whitish in color with a grayish colored center. Usually, there is a red ring of inflammation surrounding the sore. The main symptom is **pain**. Canker sores can be very painful, especially if the tongue touches them repeatedly. They last for one to two weeks and heal on their own.

Diagnosis

Canker sores are diagnosed by observation of the blister. A distinction between canker sores and cold sores must be made because cold sores are infectious, and herpes infection can be transmitted to other people. The two sores can usually be distinguished

---

KEY TERMS

Inflammation—A local reaction to tissue injury or damage, usually characterized by pain, swelling, and redness.

Ulcer—A site of damage to the skin or mucous membrane that is characterized by the formation of pus, death of tissue, and is frequently accompanied by an inflammatory reaction.

---

visually, and there are specific diagnostic tests for herpes infection.

Treatment

Since canker sores heal by themselves, treatment is not usually necessary. Pain relief remedies, such as over-the-counter topical anesthetics, may be used to reduce the pain of the sores. The use of corticosteroid ointments sometimes speeds healing. Avoidance of spicy or acidic foods can help reduce the pain associated with canker sores.

Alternative treatment

Alternative therapies for canker sores are aimed at healing existing sores and preventing their recurrence. Several herbal remedies, including calendula (*Calendula officinalis*), myrrh (*Commiphora molmol*), and goldenseal (*Hydrastis canadensis*), may be helpful in the treatment of existing sores. Compresses soaked in teas made from these herbs are applied directly to the sores. The tannic acid in a tea bag can also help dry up the sores when the wet tea bag is used as a compress. Taking dandelion (*Taraxacum officinale*) tea or capsules may help heal sores and prevent future outbreaks. Since canker sores are often brought on by stress, such stress-relieving techniques as **meditation**, **guided imagery**, and certain **acupressure** exercises may help prevent canker sores or lessen their severity.

Prognosis

There is no cure for canker sores. They do not get larger or occur more frequently with age.

Resources

OTHER

"Canker Sores." *Medline Plus Encyclopedia, National Institutes of Health* December 18, 2006 [cited December 17, 2008]. http://www.nlm.nih.gov/medlineplus/ency/article/000998.htm

"Fever Blisters and Canker Sores." *National Institute of Dental and Cranioascial Research.* July 1992 [cited December 17, 2008]. http://www.pueblo.gsa.gov/cic_text/health/fever-blister/fever-canker.html

John T. Lohr, Ph.D.
Tish Davidson, A.M.

Captopril *see* **Angiotensin-converting enzyme inhibitors**

Carbamazepine *see* **Anticonvulsant drugs**

Carbidopa *see* **Antiparkinson drugs**

Carbohydrate intolerance

Definition

Carbohydrate intolerance is the inability of the body to completely process carbohydrates (a classification that includes sugars and starches) into a source of energy for the body, usually because of the deficiency of an enzyme needed for digestion.

Demographics

The rate of **lactose intolerance**, the inability to digest the sugar found in milk, is widespread and varies with ethnicity. About one-quarter of white Americans are thought to be lactose intolerant, of which half are thought to lack the enzyme lactase needed to digest lactose. The rate is lowest in people of Northern European ancestry (about 5%, increasing to 30% of Central Europeans and 70% of Southern Europeans. About 90% of Asians and Africans are lactose intolerant. Often intolerance increases as the individual moves from infancy through childhood and into adulthood. In addition, according to a poll done for the pharmaceutical company GlaxoSmithKline, about 30% of Americans show symptoms of complex carbohydrate intolerance.

Description

Carbohydrates are the primary source of energy for the body and, along with fats and proteins, one of the three major nutrients in the human diet. Carbohydrates are classified according to their structure based on the number of basic sugar (saccharide) units they contain.

A monosaccharide is the simplest carbohydrate and is called a simple sugar. Simple sugars include glucose (the form in which sugar circulates in the blood), fructose (found in fruit and honey), and galactose (produced by the digestion of milk). These simple sugars are important because they can be absorbed by the small intestine.

Two simple sugars linked together make a disaccharide. The disaccharide sugars present in the diet are maltose (a product of the digestion of starch), sucrose (table sugar), and lactose (the sugar in milk). These disaccharides must be broken down by enzymes into two simple sugars in order for them to be absorbed by the intestine. Polysaccharides are much more complex carbohydrates made up of many simple sugars, the most important of which are glycogen, which is stored in the liver, and starch.

Digestion of sugars

Digestion of food begins in the mouth, moves on to the stomach, and then into the small intestine. Along the way, specific enzymes are needed to process different types of sugars. An enzyme is a substance that acts as a catalyst to produce chemical changes without being changed itself. The enzymes lactase, maltase, and isomaltase (or sucrase) are needed to break down the disaccharides; when one or more enzymes is produced in inadequate amounts, the result is carbohydrate intolerance. Adult lactose intolerance is the most common of all enzyme deficiencies. Deficiencies in enzymes other than lactase are extremely rare.

Types of intolerance

Carbohydrate intolerance can be primary or secondary. Primary deficiency is caused by an enzyme defect present at birth or developed over time. The most common carbohydrate intolerance is lactose intolerance. Secondary deficiencies are caused by a disease or disorder of the intestinal tract; they disappear when the disease is treated. These include protein deficiency, **celiac disease**, and some intestinal infections.

Causes and symptoms

Enzymes play an important role in breaking down carbohydrates into forms that can pass through the intestine and be used by the body. Cooked starch is broken down in the mouth to a disaccharide by amylase, an enzyme in the saliva. The disaccharides maltose, sucrose, and lactose cannot be absorbed until they have been separated into simple sugar molecules by their corresponding enzymes present in the cells lining the intestinal tract. If this process is not completed, digestion is interrupted.

KEY TERMS

Celiac disease—A disease, occurring in both children and adults, which is caused by a sensitivity to gluten, a protein found in grains. It results in chronic inflammation and shrinkage of the lining of the small intestine.

Digestion—The mechanical, chemical, and enzymatic process in which food is converted into the materials suitable for use by the body.

Enzyme—A substance produced by the body to assist in a chemical reaction. In carbohydrate intolerance, lack of an enzyme makes it impossible for one type of sugar to be broken down into a simpler form so that it can be absorbed by the intestines and used by the body.

Lactase—The enzyme needed to break down lactose, the sugar found in milk.

Metabolism—All the physical and chemical changes that take place within an organism.

Nutrient—Food or another substance that supplies the body with the elements needed for metabolism.

Sugars—Carbohydrates having the general composition of one part carbon, two parts hydrogen, and one part oxygen.

Although not common, a deficiency in the enzymes needed to digest lactose, maltose, and sucrose is sometimes present at birth. Intestinal lactase enzymes usually decrease naturally with age, but this happens to varying degrees. Because of the uneven distribution of enzyme deficiency based on race and ethnic heritage, especially in lactose intolerance, genetics are believed to play a role in the cause of primary carbohydrate intolerance.

Digestive diseases such as celiac disease and tropical sprue (which affect absorption in the intestine), as well as intestinal infections and injuries, can reduce the amount of enzymes produced. In **cancer** patients, for example, treatment with **radiation therapy** or **chemotherapy** may affect the cells in the intestine that normally secrete lactase, leading to secondary carbohydrate intolerance.

The severity of the symptoms depends on the extent of the enzyme deficiency, and range from a feeling of mild bloating to severe **diarrhea**. In the case of a lactase deficiency, undigested milk sugar remains in the intestine, where bacteria normally present in the intestine then ferment it. These bacteria produce gas, cramping, bloating, or a "gurgly" feeling in the abdomen. In a

growing child, the main symptoms are diarrhea and a failure to gain weight. In an individual with lactase deficiency, gastrointestinal distress begins about 30 minutes to two hours after eating or drinking foods containing lactose. Food intolerances should not be confused with **food allergies**, which cause a biochemical allergic response in the body, but the symptoms of **nausea**, cramps, bloating, and diarrhea can be similar.

Sugars that are not broken down into one of the simplest forms cause the body to push fluid into the intestines, which results in watery diarrhea (osmotic diarrhea). Diarrhea may sweep other nutrients out of the intestine before they can be absorbed, causing **malnutrition**.

Diagnosis

Tests

Carbohydrate intolerance can be diagnosed using oral tolerance tests. The carbohydrate being investigated is given by mouth in liquid form and several blood levels are measured and compared to normal values. This helps evaluate the individual's ability to digest the sugar.

To identify lactose intolerance in children and adults, the hydrogen breath test is used to measure the amount of hydrogen in the breath. The patient drinks a beverage containing lactose and the breath is analyzed at regular intervals. If undigested lactose in the large intestine (colon) is fermented by bacteria, various gases are produced. Hydrogen is absorbed from the intestines and carried by the bloodstream into the lungs where it is exhaled. Normally there is very little hydrogen detectable in the breath, so its presence indicates faulty digestion of lactose.

When lactose intolerance is suspected in infants and young children, many pediatricians recommend simply changing from cow's milk to soy formula and watching for improvement. If needed, a stool sample can be tested for acidity. The inadequate digestion of lactose will result in an increase of acid in the waste matter excreted by the bowels and the presence of glucose.

Treatment

Traditional

Carbohydrate intolerance caused by temporary intestinal diseases disappears when the condition is successfully treated. In primary conditions, no treatment exists to improve the body's ability to produce the enzymes, but symptoms can be controlled by diet.

For those individuals who are sensitive to even very small amounts of lactose, the lactase enzyme is available without a prescription. It comes in liquid form for use with milk. The addition of a few drops to a quart of milk will reduce the lactose content by 70% after 24 hours in the refrigerator. Heating the milk speeds up the process, and doubling the amount of lactase liquid will result in milk that is 90% lactose free. Chewable lactase enzyme tablets are also available. Three to six tablets taken before a meal or snack will aid in the digestion of solid foods. Lactose-reduced milk and other products are also available in stores. The milk contains the same nutrients as regular milk.

Because the degree of lactose intolerance varies so much, treatment should be tailored for the individual. Young children showing signs of intolerance should avoid milk products; infants should switch to soy-based formula. Older children and adults can adjust their intake of lactose depending on how much and what they can tolerate. For some, a small glass of milk will not cause problems, while others may be able to handle ice cream or aged cheeses such as cheddar or Swiss, but not other dairy products. Generally, small amounts of lactose-containing foods taken throughout the day are better tolerated than a large amount consumed all at once.

Because dairy products are an important source of **calcium**, people who reduce or severely limit their intake of dairy products may need to consider other ways to consume an adequate amount of calcium in their **diets**.

Prognosis

With good dietary management, individuals with carbohydrate intolerance can lead normal lives with minimal discomfort.

Prevention

Since the cause of the enzyme deficiency leading to carbohydrate intolerance is unknown, there is no way to prevent this condition.

Resources

OTHER

Complex Carbohydrate Intolerance Center Information Center. GalaxoSmithKline. 2010. http://www.preventcci.com/default.aspx

Guandalini, Stefano, et al. Lactose Intolerance. eMedicine.com March 30, 2010. http://emedicine.medscape.com/article/930971-overview

Lactose Intolerance. MedlinePlus. June 8, 2010. http://www.nlm.nih.gov/medlineplus/lactoseintolerance.html

ORGANIZATIONS

American Gastroenterological Association (AGA), 4930 Del Ray Avenue, Bethesda, MD, 20814, (310) 654-2055, (301) 654-5920, www.gastro.org.

National Institute of Diabetes and Digestive and Kidney Diseases (NIDDK), National Institutes of Health, 2 Information Way, Bethesda, MD, 20892, (800) 891-5389. TTY: (866) 569-1162, nddic@niddk.nih.gov, http://digestive.niddk.nih.gov.

Karen Ericson, RN
Tish Davidson, AM

Carbon monoxide poisoning

Definition

Carbon monoxide (CO) poisoning occurs when carbon monoxide gas is inhaled. CO is a colorless, odorless, highly poisonous gas that is produced by incomplete combustion. It is found in automobile exhaust fumes, faulty stoves and heating systems, fires, and cigarette smoke. Other sources include woodburning stoves, kerosene heaters, improperly ventilated water heaters and gas stoves, and blocked or poorly maintained chimney flues. CO interferes with the ability of the blood to carry oxygen. The result is **headache**, **nausea**, convulsions, and finally **death** by asphyxiation.

Description

Carbon monoxide, sometimes called coal gas, has been known as a toxic substance since the third century B.C. It was used for executions and suicides in early Rome. Today it is the leading cause of accidental poisoning in the United States. According to the *Journal of the American Medical Association*, 2,000 Americans die each year from accidental exposure to CO, and another 2,300 from intentional exposure (**suicide**). An additional 10,000 people seek medical attention after exposure to CO. The Consumer Products Safety Commission eported in 2004 that about 64% of unintentional CO poisoning deaths occur in the home.

Anyone who is exposed to CO will become sick, and the entire body is involved in CO poisoning. A developing fetus can also be poisoned if a pregnant woman breathes CO gas. Infants, people with heart or lung disease, or those with anemia may be more seriously affected. People such as underground parking garage attendants who are exposed to car exhausts in a confined area are more likely to be poisoned by CO. Firemen also run a higher risk of inhaling CO.

Causes and symptoms

Normally when a person breathes fresh air into the lungs, the oxygen in the air binds with a molecule called hemoglobin (Hb) that is found in red blood cells. This allows oxygen to be moved from the lungs to every part of the body. When the oxygen/hemoglobin complex reaches a muscle where it is needed, the oxygen is released. Because the oxygen binding process is reversible, hemoglobin can be used over and over again to pick up oxygen and move it throughout the body.

Inhaling carbon monoxide gas interferes with this oxygen transport system. In the lungs, CO competes with oxygen to bind with the hemoglobin molecule. Hemoglobin prefers CO to oxygen and accepts it more than 200 times more readily than it accepts oxygen. Not only does the hemoglobin prefer CO, it holds on to the CO much more tightly, forming a complex called carboxyhemoglobin (COHb). As a person breathes CO contaminated air, more and more oxygen transportation sites on the hemoglobin molecules become blocked by CO. Gradually, there are fewer and fewer sites available for oxygen. All cells need oxygen to live. When they don't get enough oxygen, cellular metabolism is disrupted and eventually cells begin to die.

The symptoms of CO poisoning and the speed with which they appear depend on the concentration of CO in the air and the rate and efficiency with which a person breathes. Heavy smokers can start off with up to 9% of their hemoglobin already bound to CO, which they regularly inhale in cigarette smoke. This makes them much more susceptible to environmental CO. The Occupational Safety and Health Administration (OSHA) has established a maximum permissible exposure level of 50 parts per million (ppm) over eight hours.

With exposure to 200 ppm for two to three hours, a person begins to experience headache, **fatigue**, nausea, and **dizziness**. These symptoms correspond to 15–25% COHb in the blood. When the concentration of COHb reaches 50% or more, death results in a very short time. Emergency room physicians have the most experience diagnosing and treating CO poisoning.

The symptoms of CO poisoning in order of increasing severity include:

- headache
- shortness of breath
- dizziness
- fatigue

- mental confusion and difficulty thinking
- loss of fine hand-eye coordination
- nausea and vomiting
- rapid heart rate
- hallucinations
- inability to execute voluntary movements accurately
- collapse
- lowered body temperature (hypothermia)
- coma
- convulsions
- seriously low blood pressure
- cardiac and respiratory failure
- death

In some cases, the skin, mucous membranes, and nails of a person with CO poisoning are cherry red or bright pink. Because the color change doesn't always occur, it is an unreliable symptom to rely on for diagnosis.

Although most CO poisoning is acute, or sudden, it is possible to suffer from chronic CO poisoning. This condition exists when a person is exposed to low levels of the gas over a period of days to months. Symptoms are often vague and include (in order of frequency) fatigue, headache, dizziness, sleep disturbances, cardiac symptoms, apathy, nausea, and memory disturbances. Little is known about chronic CO poisoning, and it is often misdiagnosed.

Diagnosis

The main reason to suspect CO poisoning is evidence that fuel is being burned in a confined area, for example a car running inside a closed garage, a charcoal grill burning indoors, or an unvented kerosene heater in a workshop. Under these circumstances, one or more persons suffering from the symptoms listed previously strongly suggests CO poisoning. In the absence of some concrete reason to suspect CO poisoning, the disorder is often misdiagnosed as **migraine headache**, **stroke**, psychiatric illness, **food poisoning**, alcohol poisoning, or heart disease.

Concrete confirmation of CO poisoning comes from a carboxyhemoglobin test. This blood test measures the amount of CO that is bound to hemoglobin in the body. Blood is drawn as soon after suspected exposure to CO as possible.

Other tests that are useful in determining the extent of CO poisoning include measurement of other arterial blood gases and pH; a **complete blood count**; measurement of other blood components such as **sodium**, potassium, bicarbonate, urea nitrogen, and lactic acid; an electrocardiogram (ECG); and a **chest x ray**.

Treatment

Immediate treatment for CO poisoning is to remove the victim from the source of carbon monoxide gas and get him or her into fresh air. If the victim is not breathing and has no pulse, **cardiopulmonary resuscitation** (CPR) should be started. Depending on the severity of the poisoning, 100% oxygen may be given with a tight fitting mask as soon as it is available.

Taken with other symptoms of CO poisoning, COHb levels of over 25% in healthy individuals, over 15% in patients with a history of heart or lung disease, and over 10% in pregnant women usually indicate the need for hospitalization. In the hospital, fluids and electrolytes are given to correct any imbalances that have arisen from the breakdown of cellular metabolism.

In severe cases of CO poisoning, patients are given hyperbaric **oxygen therapy**. This treatment involves placing the patient in a chamber breathing 100% oxygen at a pressure of more than one atmosphere (the normal pressure the atmosphere exerts at sea level). The increased pressure forces more oxygen into the blood. Hyperbaric facilities are specialized, and are usually available only at larger hospitals.

Prognosis

The speed and degree of recovery from CO poisoning depends on the length and duration of exposure to the gas. The half-life of CO in normal room air is four to five hours. This means that, in four to five hours, half of the CO bound to hemoglobin will be replaced with oxygen. At normal atmospheric pressures, but breathing 100% oxygen, the half-life for the elimination of CO from the body is 50–70 minutes. In hyperbaric therapy at three atmospheres of pressure, the half-life is reduced to 20–25 minutes.

Although the symptoms of CO poisoning may subside in a few hours, some patients show memory problems, fatigue, confusion, and mood changes for two to four weeks after their exposure to the gas.

Prevention

Carbon monoxide poisoning is preventable. Particular care should be paid to situations where fuel is burned in a confined area. Portable and permanently installed carbon monoxide detectors that sound a warning similar to smoke detectors are available for less than $50. Specific actions that will prevent CO poisoning include:

KEY TERMS

Carboxyhemoglobin (COHb)—Hemoglobin that is bound to carbon monoxide instead of oxygen.

Hemoglobin (Hb)—A molecule that normally binds to oxygen in order to carry it to our cells, where it is required for life.

Hypothermia—Development of a subnormal body temperature.

pH—A measurement of the acidity or alkalinity of a fluid. A neutral fluid, neither acid nor alkali, has a pH of 7.

- stopping smoking. Smokers have less tolerance to environmental CO

- having heating systems and appliances installed by a qualified contractor to assure that they are properly vented and meet local building codes

- inspecting and properly maintaining heating systems, chimneys, and appliances

- not using a gas oven or stove to heat the home

- not burning charcoal indoors

- making sure there is good ventilation if using a kerosene heater indoors

- not leaving cars or trucks running inside the garage

- keeping car windows rolled up when stuck in heavy traffic, especially if inside a tunnel

Resources

PERIODICALS

"Silencing the Silent Killer." *USA Today Magazine* March 2004: 77.

OTHER

"Carbon Monoxide Headquarters." Wayne State University School of Medicine. http://www.coheadquarters.com/CO1.htm.

ORGANIZATIONS

American Lung Association, 1301 Pennsylvania Ave. NW, Suite 800, Washington, DC, 20001, (202) 758-3355, (202) 452-1805, (800) 548-8252, info@lungusa.org, http://www.lungusa.org/.

Tish Davidson, A.M.
Teresa G. Odle

Carbunculosis *see* **Boils**

Carcinoembryonic antigen test

Definition

The carcinoembryonic antigen (CEA) test is a laboratory blood study. CEA is a substance that is normally found only during fetal development, but may reappear in adults who develop certain types of **cancer**. CEA is produced when there is rapid multiplication of epithelial cells such as those of the digestive track. CEA is also found in the blood of individuals who are chronic smokers.

Purpose

The CEA test is ordered for patients with known cancers. It is most commonly ordered when a patient has a cancer of the gastrointestinal system. These include cancer of the colon, rectum, stomach (gastric cancer), esophagus, liver, or pancreas. It is also used with cancers of the breast, lung, or prostate.

The CEA level in the blood is one of the factors that doctors consider when determining the prognosis, or most likely outcome of a cancer. In general, a higher CEA level predicts a more severe disease, one that is less likely to be curable. But it does not give clear-cut information. The results of a CEA test are considered along with other laboratory and/or imaging studies to follow the course of the disease.

Once treatment for the cancer has begun, CEA tests have a valuable role in monitoring the patient's progress. A decreasing CEA level means therapy is effective in fighting the cancer. A stable or increasing CEA level may mean the treatment is not working, and/or that the tumor is growing. It is important to understand that serial CEA measurements, several done over a period of time, are the most useful. A single test result is difficult to evaluate, but a number of tests, done weeks apart, shows trends in disease progression or regression.

Certain types of cancer treatments, such as hormone therapy for **breast cancer**, may cause the CEA level to go up. This elevation does not accurately reflect the state of the disease. It is sometimes referred to as a "flare response." Recognition that a rise in CEA may be temporary and due to therapy is significant. If this possibility is not taken into account, the patient may be unnecessarily discouraged. Further, treatment that is actually effective may be stopped or changed prematurely.

CEA tests are also used to help detect recurrence of a cancer after surgery and/or other treatment has been completed. A rising CEA level may be the first sign of cancer return, and may show up months before other studies or patient symptoms would raise concern. Unfortunately, this does not always mean the recurrent cancer can be cured. For example, only a small percentage of patients with colorectal cancers and rising CEA levels benefit from another surgical exploration. Those with recurrence in the same area as the original cancer, or with a single metastatic tumor in the liver or lung, have a chance that surgery will eliminate the disease. Patients with more widespread return of the cancer are generally not treatable with surgery. The CEA test will not separate the two groups.

Patients who are most likely to benefit from non–standard treatments, such as bone marrow transplants, may be determined on the basis of CEA values, combined with other test results. CEA levels may be one of the criteria for determining whether the patient will benefit from more expensive studies, such as CT scan or MRI.

Description

Determination of the CEA level is a laboratory blood test. Obtaining a specimen of blood for the study takes only a few minutes. CEA testing should be covered by most insurance plans.

The CEA test is not a screening test for cancer. It is not useful for detecting the presence of cancer since many cancers do not produce an increased CEA level. Some noncancerous diseases, such as hepatitis, inflammatory bowel disease, **pancreatitis**, and obstructive pulmonary disease, may cause an elevated CEA level.

Preparation

No preparation is required.

Aftercare

No specific aftercare measures are required. Results will be sent to the healthcare provider who ordered the test originally. The health care provider will then discuss results with the patient.

Risks

There are no complications or side effects of this test. However, the results of a CEA study should be interpreted with caution. A single test result may not yield clinically useful information. Several studies over a period of months may be needed.

Another concern is the potential for false positive or false negative results. A false positive result means the test shows an abnormal value when cancer is not present. A false negative means the test reveals a normal value when cancer actually is present.

Results

The absolute numbers that are considered normal vary from one laboratory to another. Any results reported should come with information regarding the testing facility's normal range.

Abnormal results

A single abnormal CEA value may be significant, but must be regarded cautiously. In general, very high CEA levels indicate more serious cancer, with a poorer chance for cure. But some benign diseases and certain cancer treatments may produce an elevated CEA test. Cigarette **smoking** will also cause the CEA level to be abnormally high.

Resources

BOOKS

Van Leeuwen, A.M., and D.J. Poelhuis-Leth. *Davis's Comprehensive Handbook of Laboratory and Diagnostic Tests with Nursing Implications*. 3rd ed. Philadelphia: F.A. Davis Co., 2009.

PERIODICALS

Iwanicki-Caron, I., et al. "Usefulness of Serum Carcinoembryonic Antigen Kinetic for Chemotherapy Monitoring in Patients with Unresectable Metastasis of Colorectal Cancer." *Journal of Clinical Oncology* 26, no. 22 (August 1, 2008): 3681–3886.

Ellen S. Weber, MSN
Melinda Granger Oberleitner
RN, DNS, APRN, CNS

Carcinogens

Definition

Carcinogens are substances capable of causing **cancer**. The United States Environmental Protection Agency (EPA) classifies many substances on the basis of their potential for causing cancer. Classifications are based on results of studies on animals or experience with humans. Classification categories refer to epidemiological studies, which are studies to identify the factors controlling the presence or absence of a disease.

Description

Group A, or Human Carcinogens, are substances for which there is a relationship between the substance and cancer that has been conclusively demonstrated through epidemiological studies of humans. Group B, or Probable Human Carcinogens are composed of two types of carcinogens. There is sufficient evidence from animal studies and limited epidemiological studies that B1 carcinogens cause cancer. B2 carcinogens are classified on the basis of sufficient evidence from animal studies only; epidemiological data are inadequate or nonexistent. Group C or Possible Human Carcinogens are substances where there is limited evidence from animal studies and no human epidemiological data. Group D or Not Classifiable as to Human Carcinogenicity are substances for which information is inadequate or completely lacking, so no assessment of the substance's cancer–causing potential is possible. Group E or Evidence of Noncarcinogenicity for Humans are substances that have tested negative in at least two adequate animal cancer tests in different species and in adequate epidemiological and animal studies.

As of 2010, the International Agency for Research on Cancer (IARC) has determined that the following list of agents and mixtures are carcinogenic to humans.

- Acetaldehyde associated with consumption of alcoholic beverages
- Acid mists, strong inorganic
- Aflatoxins (naturally occurring)
- 4–Aminobiphenyl
- Alcoholic beverages
- Aluminium production
- Areca nut
- Aristolochic acid
- Aristolochic acid–containing plants
- Arsenic and arsenic compounds
- Asbestos, all forms

- Auramine production
- Azathioprine
- Benzene (used in nail polish remover, varnishes, airplane dopes, lacquers, and as a solvent)
- Benzidine and benzidine dyes
- Benzopyrene
- Betel quid with and without tobacco
- Beryllium and beryllium compounds
- N,N–Bis (2–Chloreothyl)–2–Naphthylamine (Chlomophaozine)
- Bis(chloromethyl) ether and technical grade chloromethyl methyl ether
- Busulphan (Myleran)
- 1, 3–Butadiene
- Cadmium and cadmium compounds
- Chlorambucil
- Chlornaphazine)
- Chromium and certain chromium compounds
- Clonorchis sinensis, infection with
- Coal, indoor emissions and gasification
- Coal–tar distillation
- Coke production
- Cyclophosphamide
- Cyclosporin (ciclosporin)
- Diethystilbestrol (DES)
- Epstein–Barr virus
- Erionite
- Estrogen therapy, postmenopausal
- Estrogen–progesterone combined menopausal therapy
- Estrogen–progesterone combined oral contraceptives
- Ethanol in alcoholic beverages
- Ethylene oxide
- Etoposide
- Etoposide in combination with cisplatin and bleomycin
- Fission products, including strontium–90
- Formaldehyde
- Haematite underground mining
- Helicobacter pylori, infection with
- *Helicobacter pylori* (infection)
- Hepatitis B and C virus (chronic infection)
- HIV virus type 1
- Human papillomavirus (HPV) types 16, 18, 31, 33, 35, 39, 45, 51, 52, 56, 58, 59
- Human T–cell lypmhotropic virus type 1
- Ionizing radiation of all types
- Iron and steel founding occupational exposure
- Isopropyl alcohol manufacture using strong acids
- Kaposi sarcoma herpes virus
- Leather dust
- Magenta production
- Melphalan
- Methoxsalen with ultraviolet A radiation
- Mineral oils which are untreated or mildly treated
- MOPP and other combined chemotherapy especially alkylating agents
- 2–Naphthylamine
- Neutron radiation
- Nickel compounds
- N–Nitrosonornicotine (NNN) and 4–1–1–butanone (NNK)
- *Opisthorchis viverrini* (infection)
- Painter, occupational exposure
- 3,4,5,3,4–Pentachlorobiphenyl (PCB–126)
- 2,3,4,7,8–Pentachlorodibenzofuran
- Phenacetin and phenacetin–containing analgesic mixtures
- Phosphorus–32
- Plutonium
- Radioiodines, such as I–131
- Radionuclides, alpha– and beta–particle emission when internally deposited
- Radium–224, 226, and 228
- Radon–222
- Rubber industry (certain occupations)
- Salted fish, Chinese style
- Schistosoma haematobium, infection with
- Semsustine–3–1–nitrosurea, Methyl–CCNU
- Shale oils
- Silica
- Solar radiation
- Soot
- Sulfur mustard
- Tamoxifen (There is also evidence that this agent protects against contralateral breast cancer.)
- 2,3,7,8–Tetrachlorodibenzo–para–dioxin
- Thiotepa
- Thorium–232
- Tobacco, smoking, smokeless, and second–hand smoke
- Ortho–Toluidine
- Treosulfan
- Ultraviolet radiation encompassing UVA, UVB, and UVC
- Ultraviolet–emitting tanning devices
- Vinyl chloride

- Wood dust
- X- and Gamma radiation

Resources

BOOKS

Meister, Kathleen. *America's War on "Carcinogens": Reassessing the Use of Animal Tests Predict Human Cancer Risk.* Washington, DC: American Council on Science, 2005.

PERIODICALS

Gallo, V., et al. "Validation of Biomarkers for the Study of Environmental Carcinogens: A Review." *Biomarkers.* 13(5) (Aug. 2008): 505–34.

OTHER

American Cancer Society. "Known and Probable Carcinogens." October 8, 2008. http://www.cancer.org/docroot/PED/content/PED_1_3x_Known_and_Probable_Carcinogens.asp?sitearea = PED (accessed September 9, 2010).
International Agency for Research on Cancer. "IARC Monographs on the Evaluation of Carcinogenic Risks to Humans, Agents Classified by the IARC Monographs, Volumes 1–100." May 27, 2010 http:www.monographs.iarc.fr/ENG/Classification/index.php (accessed September 9, 2010).

ORGANIZATIONS

American Cancer Society, (800) ACS–2345, TTY (866) 228–4327, http://www.cancer.org.
United States Environmental Protection Agency (EPA), 1200 Pennsylvania Ave., NW, Washington, DC, 20460, (202) 272–0167, http://www.epa.gov.

Melinda Granger Oberleitner, RN, DNS, APRN,CNS

Carcinoid tumors *see* **Neuroendocrine tumors**

Cardiac arrest *see* **Sudden cardiac death**

Cardiac arrhythmias *see* **Arrhythmias**

Cardiac blood pool scan

Definition

A cardiac blood pool scan is a non-invasive test that uses a mildly radioactive marker to observe the functioning of the left ventricle of the heart.

Purpose

The left ventricle is the main pump for distributing blood through the body. A cardiac blood pool scan is used to determine how efficiently the left ventricle is working. The scan can detect aneurysms of the left ventricle, motion abnormalities caused by damage to the heart wall, cardiac shunts between the left and right ventricle, and coronary occlusive artery disease.

Precautions

Pregnant women are the only patients who should not participate in a cardiac blood pool scan. However, the accuracy of the results may be affected if the patient moves during imaging, has had other recent nuclear scans, or has an irregular heartbeat.

Description

A cardiac blood pool scan is sometimes called equilibrium radionuclide angiocardiography or gated (synchronized) cardiac blood pool imaging. A **multiple-gated acquisition (MUGA) scan** is a variation of this test.

To perform a cardiac blood pool scan, the patient lies under a special gamma scintillation camera that detects radiation. A protein tagged with a radioactive marker (usually technetium-99m) is injected into the patient's forearm.

The camera is synchronized with an electrocardiogram (ECG) to take a picture at specific times in the cycle of heart contraction and relaxation. When data from many sequential pictures is processed by a computer, a doctor can analyze whether the left ventricle is functioning normally.

The patient needs to remain silent and motionless during the test. Sometimes the patient is asked to **exercise**, then another set of pictures is taken for comparison. This test normally takes about 30 minutes.

Preparation

No changes in diet or medication are necessary. An ECG will probably be done before the test.

Aftercare

The patient may resume normal activities immediately.

Risks

Cardiac blood pool scans are a safe and effective way of measuring left ventricle function. The only risk is to the fetus of a pregnant woman.

Normal results

A computer is used to process the information from the test, then the results are analyzed by a doctor. A normally functioning left ventricle will contract symmetrically, show even distribution of the radioactively tagged protein, and eject about 55–65% of volume of blood it holds on each contraction.

Abnormal results

Patients with damage to the ventricle or heart wall will show an uneven distribution of the radiopharmaceutical. The volume of blood ejected in each contraction will be less than 55%.

Resources

BOOKS

Pagana, Kathleen Deska, and Timothy J. Pagana.*Mosby's Manual of Diagnostic and Laboratory Tests*. 4th ed. St. Louis: Mosby, 2009.

Tish Davidson, A.M.

Cardiac catheterization

Definition

Cardiac catheterization (also called heart catheterization) is a diagnostic procedure which does a comprehensive examination of how the heart and its blood vessels function. One or more catheters is inserted through a peripheral blood vessel in the arm (antecubital artery or vein) or leg (femoral artery or vein) with x-ray guidance. This procedure gathers information such as adequacy of blood supply through the coronary arteries, blood pressures, blood flow throughout chambers of the heart, collection of blood samples, and x rays of the heart's ventricles or arteries.

A test that can be performed on either side of the heart, cardiac catheterization checks for different functions in both the left and right sides. When testing the heart's right side, tricuspid and pulmonary valve function are evaluated, in addition to measuring pressures of and collecting blood samples from the right atrium, ventricle, and pulmonary artery. Left-sided heart catheterization is performed by way of a catheter through an artery which tests the blood flow of the coronary arteries, function of the mitral and aortic valves, and left ventricle.

Purpose

The primary reason for conducting a cardiac catheterization is to diagnose and manage persons known or suspected to have heart disease, a frequently fatal condition that leads to 1.5 million heart attacks annually in the United States.

Symptoms and diagnoses that may lead to performing this procedure include:

- chest pain, characterized by prolonged heavy pressure or a squeezing pain
- abnormal treadmill stress test
- myocardial infarction, also known as a heart attack
- congenital heart defects, or heart problems that originated from birth
- a diagnosis of valvular-heart disease
- a need to measure the heart muscle's ability to pump blood

Typically performed along with **angiography**, a technique of injecting a dye into the vascular system to outline the heart and blood vessels, a catheterization can aid in the visualization of any blockages, narrowing, or abnormalities in the coronary arteries. If these signs are visible, the cardiologist may assess the patient's need and readiness for coronary bypass surgery, or perhaps a less invasive approach, such as dilation of a narrowed blood vessel either surgically or with the use of a balloon (**angioplasty**).

When looking at the left side of the heart, fluoroscopic guidance also allows the following diagnoses to be assessed:

- enlargement of the left ventricle

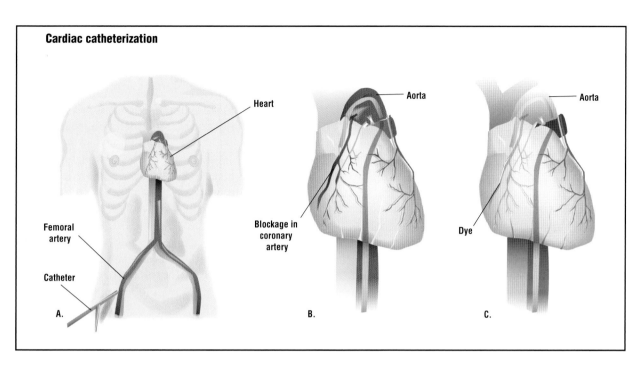

Cardiac catheterization

During cardiac catheterization, a catheter is fed into the femoral artery of the upper leg (A). The catheter is fed up to coronary arteries to an area of blockage (B). A dye is released, allowing visualization of the blockage (C). *(Illustration by PreMediaGlobal. Reproduced by permission of Gale, a part of Cengage Learning.)*

- ventricular aneurysms (abnormal dilation of a blood vessel)
- narrowing of the aortic valve
- insufficiency of the aortic or mitral valve
- the detour of blood from one side of the heart to the other due to septal defects (also known as shunting)

Precautions

Cardiac catheterization is categorized as an "invasive" procedure which involves the heart, its valves, and coronary arteries, in addition to a large artery in the arm or leg. Due to the nature of the test, it is important to evaluate for the following conditions before considering this procedure:

- A diagnosis of a bleeding disorder, poor kidney function, or debilitation. Any of these pre-existing conditions typically raises the risk of the catheterization procedure and may be reason to cancel the procedure.
- A diagnosis of heart valve disease. If this is detected, antibiotics may be given before the test to prevent inflammation of the membrane which lines the heart (endocarditis).

Description

To understand how a cardiac catheterization is able to diagnose and manage heart disease, the basic workings of the heart muscle must also be understood. Just as the body relies on a constant supply of blood to aid in its everyday functions, so does the heart. The heart is made up of an intricate web of blood vessels (coronary arteries) that ensure an adequate supply of blood rich in oxygen and nutrients. It is easy to see how an abnormality in any of these arteries can be detrimental to the heart's function. These abnormalities cause the heart's blood flow to decrease and result in the condition known as **coronary artery disease** or coronary insufficiency.

Catheterization is a valuable tool in detecting and treating abnormalities of the heart. Through the use of fluoroscopic (x-ray) guidance, a catheter, which may resemble a balloon-tipped tube, is strung through the veins or arteries into the heart, so the cardiologist can monitor a body's various functions at each moment.

Generally a test that lasts two to three hours, a patient should expect the following prior to and during the catheterization procedure:

- A mild sedative may be given that will allow the patient to relax but remain conscious during the test.
- An intravenous needle will be inserted in the arm to administer medication. Electrodes will be attached to the chest to enable the painless procedure known as an electrocardiograph.

- Prior to inserting a catheter into an artery or vein in the arm or leg, the incision site will be made numb by injecting a local anesthetic. When the anesthetic is injected it may feel like a pin-prick followed by a quick stinging sensation. Pressure may also be experienced as the catheter travels through the blood vessel.
- After the catheter is guided into the coronary-artery system, a dye (also called a radiocontrast material) is injected to aid in the identification of any abnormalities of the heart. During this time, the patient may experience a hot, flushed feeling or a quickly passing nausea. Coughing or breathing deeply aids in any discomfort.
- Medication may be given during the procedure if chest pain is experienced, and nitroglycerin may also be administered to allow expansion of the heart's blood vessels.
- When the test is complete, the physician will remove the catheter and close the skin with several sutures or tape.

Preparation

Prior to the cardiac catheterization procedure, it is important to relay information to the physician or nurse regarding **allergies** to shellfish (such as shrimp or scallops) which contain iodine, iodine itself, or the dyes that are commonly used in other diagnostic tests.

Because this procedure is categorized as a surgery, the patient will be instructed not to eat or drink anything for at least six hours prior to the test. Just before the test begins, the patient will urinate and change into a hospital gown, then lie flat on a padded table that may also be tilted in order for the heart to be examined from a variety of angles.

Aftercare

While cardiac catheterization may be performed on an out-patient basis, a patient may require close monitoring following the procedure while remaining in the hospital for at least 24 hours. The patient will be instructed to rest in bed for at least eight hours immediately after the test. If the catheter was inserted into a vein or artery in the leg or groin area, the leg will be kept extended for four to six hours. If a vein or artery in the arm was used to insert the catheter, the arm will need to remain extended for a minimum of three hours.

The patient should expect a hard ridge to form over the incision site that diminishes as the site heals. Bluish discoloration under the skin at the point of insertion should also be expected but fades in two weeks. It is also not uncommon for the incision site to bleed during the first 24 hours following surgery. If this should happen, the patient should apply pressure to the site with a clean tissue or cloth for 10–15 minutes.

Risks

Similar to all surgical procedures, the cardiac catheterization test does involve some risks. Complications that may occur during the procedure include

- cardiac arrhythmias (an irregular heart beat)
- pericardial tamponade (a condition that causes excess pressure in the pericardium which affects the heart due to accumulation of excess fluid)
- the rare occurrence of myocardial infarction (heart attack) or stroke may also develop due to clotting or plaque rupture of one or more of the coronary or brain arteries.

Before left-side catheterization is performed, the anticoagulant medication heparin may be administered. This drug helps decrease the risk of the development of a blood clot in an artery (thrombosis) and **blood clots** traveling throughout the body (embolization).

The risks of the catheterization procedure increase in patients over the age of 60, those who have severe **heart failure**, or persons with serious **valvular heart disease**.

Normal results

Normal findings from a cardiac catheterization will indicate no abnormalities of heart chamber size or configuration, wall motion or thickness, the direction of blood flow, or motion of the valves. Smooth and regular outlines on the x ray indicate normal coronary arteries.

An essential part of the catheterization is measuring intracardiac pressures, or the pressure in the heart's chambers and vessels. Pressure readings that are higher than normal are significant for a patient's overall diagnosis. The pressure readings that are lower, other than those which are produced as a result of **shock**, typically are not significant.

An ejection fraction, or a comparison of how much blood is ejected from the heart's left ventricle during its contraction phase with a measurement of blood remaining at the end of the left ventricle's relaxation phase, is also determined by performing a catheterization. The cardiologist will look for a normal ejection fraction reading of 60–70%.

Abnormal results

Cardiac catheterization provides valuable still and motion x-ray pictures of the coronary arteries that help in diagnosing coronary artery disease, poor heart function, disease of the heart valves, and septal defects (a defect in the septum, the wall that separates two heart chambers).

The most prominent sign of coronary artery disease is the narrowing or blockage in the coronary

KEY TERMS

Aneurysm—An abnormal dilatation of a blood vessel, usually an artery. It can be caused by a congenital defect or weakness in the vessel's wall.

Angiography—In cardiac catheterization, a picture of the heart and coronary arteries is seen after injecting a radiopaque substance (often referred to as a dye) throughout the veins and arteries.

Angioplasty—An alternative to vascular surgery, a balloon catheter is used to mechanically dilate the affected area of the artery and enlarge the constricted or narrowed segment.

Aortic valve—The valve between the heart's left ventricle and ascending aorta that prevents regurgitation of blood back into the left ventricle.

Catheter—A tube made of elastic, elastic web, rubber, glass, metal, or plastic used to evacuate or inject fluids into the body. In cardiac catheterization, a long, fine catheter is used for passage through a blood vessel into the chambers of the heart.

Coronary bypass surgery—A surgical procedure which places a shunt to allow blood to travel from the aorta to a branch of the coronary artery at a point past an obstruction.

Left anterior descending coronary artery (LAD)—One of the heart's coronary artery branches from the left main coronary artery which supplies blood to the left ventricle.

Mitral valve—The bicuspid valve which is between the left atrium and left ventricle of the heart.

Pulmonary valve—The heart valve which is positioned between the right ventricle and the opening into the pulmonary artery.

Shunt—A passageway (or an artificially created passageway) that diverts blood flow from one main route to another.

Tricuspid valve—The right atrioventricular valve of the heart.

arteries, with narrowing that is greater than 70% considered significant. A clear indication for intervention (by angioplasty or surgery) is a finding of significant narrowing of the left main coronary artery and/or blockage or severe narrowing in the high, left anterior descending coronary artery.

A finding of impaired wall motion is an additional indicator of coronary artery disease, aneurysm, an enlarged heart, or a congenital heart problem. Using the findings from an ejection fraction test which measures wall motion, cardiologists look at an ejection fraction reading under 35% as increasing the risk of complications while also decreasing a successful long term or short term outcome with surgery.

Detecting the difference in pressure above and below the heart valve can verify heart valve disease. The greater narrowing correlates with the higher pressure difference.

To confirm septal defects, a catheterization measures oxygen content on both the left and right sides of the heart. The right heart pumps unoxygenated blood to the lungs, and the left heart pumps blood that contains oxygen from the lungs to the rest of the body. Right side elevated oxygen levels indicate left-to-right atrial or **ventricular shunt**. A left side that experiences decreased oxygen indicates a right-to-left shunt.

ORGANIZATIONS

American Heart Association National Center, 7272 Greenville Avenue, Dallas, TX, 75231, (800) 242-8721, Review.personal.info@heart.org.
National Heart Lung and Blood Institute Health Information Center, P.O. Box 30105, Bethesda, MD, 20824-0105, (301) 592-8573, (240) 629-3246, http://www.nhlbinih.gov.

Beth A. Kapes

Cardiac compression *see* **Cardiac tamponade**

Cardiac conduction disorder *see* **Heart block**

Cardiac mapping *see* **Electrophysiology study of the heart**

Cardiac rehabilitation

Definition

Cardiac **rehabilitation** is a comprehensive **exercise**, education, and behavioral modification program designed to improve the physical and emotional condition of patients with heart disease.

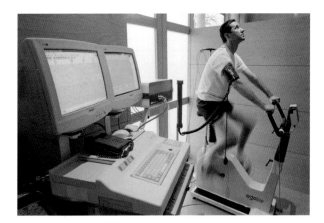

Man undergoing cardiac rehabilitation after receiving a heart transplant. *(RAJAU/PHANIE/Photo Researchers, Inc.)*

Purpose

Heart attack survivors, bypass and **angioplasty** patients, and individuals with **angina**, congestive **heart failure**, and heart transplants are all candidates for a cardiac rehabilitation program. Cardiac rehabilitation is prescribed to control symptoms, improve exercise tolerance, and improve the overall quality of life in these patients.

Precautions

A cardiac rehabilitation program should be implemented and closely monitored by a trained team of healthcare professionals.

Description

Cardiac rehabilitation is overseen by a specialized team of doctors, nurses, and other healthcare professionals. Members of the cardiac rehabilitation team may include a dietician or nutritionist, physical therapist, exercise physiologist, psychologist, vocational counselor, occupational therapist, and social worker. The program frequently begins in a hospital setting and continues on an outpatient basis after the patient is discharged over a period of six to 12 months.

Components of a cardiac rehabilitation program vary by individual clinical need, and each program will be carefully constructed for the patient by his or her rehabilitation team.

- Exercise. Exercise programs typically start out slowly, with simple range-of-motion arm and leg exercises. Walking and stair climbing soon follow. Blood pressure is carefully monitored before and after exercise sessions, and patients are taught how to measure their heart rate and evaluate any possible cardiac

symptoms during each session. Patients with advanced coronary disease may require continuous ECG monitoring throughout their exercise sessions. Once discharged from the hospital, the patient works with his cardiac team to create an individual exercise plan.

- Diet. Cardiac patients will work with a nutritionist or dietician to develop a low-fat, low-cholesterol diet plan. Patients with high blood pressure may be put on a salt-restricted diet and instructed to limit alcohol intake. Weight loss may also be a goal with obese cardiac patients.

- Counseling. A psychologist or social worker can help cardiac patients with issues that may be contributing to their heart condition, such as stress and anxiety. Relaxation techniques may be taught to patients to help them deal with these feelings. Cardiac patients frequently experience a period of depression, and group or individual counseling can be beneficial in overcoming these feelings. Vocational counselors can assist cardiac patients in returning to the workforce.

- Education. The patient and family should be fully educated on the physical limitations of the patient, his recommended diet and exercise plan, his emotional status, and the lifestyle changes required to improve the patient's overall health.

- Smoking cessation. Cardiac patients who smoke are twice as likely to have a heart attack in the following five years than non-smoking patients. These patients are strongly encouraged to enroll in a smoking cessation program, which typically includes patient education and behavioral counseling. Nicotine replacement therapy, which uses nicotine patches, nose spray, or gum to wean patients off of cigarettes, may also be part of the program. Antidepressants and anti-anxiety medication may be helpful in some cases.

Aftercare

Long-term maintenance is a critical feature of cardiac rehabilitation. Patients require support from their healthcare team, family, and friends to continue the lifestyle changes they implemented during the rehabilitation period.

Risks

The risks of another heart attack during cardiac rehabilitation are slight, and greatly reduced by careful, continuous monitoring of the physical status of the patient.

Normal results

The outcome of the cardiac rehabilitation program depends on a number of variables, including patient follow-through, type and degree of heart disease, and the availability of an adequate support network for the patient. Patients who successfully complete the program will ideally reach an age-appropriate level of physical activity and be able to return to the workforce and/or other daily activities.

ORGANIZATIONS

American Heart Association National Center, 7272 Greenville Avenue, Dallas, TX, 75231, (800) 242-8721, Review. personal.info@heart.org.

Paula Anne Ford-Martin

Cardiac tamponade

Definition

Cardiac tamponade occurs when the heart is squeezed by fluid that collects inside the sac that surrounds it.

Description

The heart is surrounded by a sac called the pericardium. When this sac becomes filled with fluid, the liquid presses on the heart, preventing the lower chambers of the heart from properly filling with blood.

Because the lower chambers (the ventricles) cannot fill with the correct amount of blood, less than normal amounts of blood reach the lungs and the rest of the body. This condition is very serious and can be fatal if not treated.

Causes and symptoms

Fluid can collect inside the pericardium and compress the heart when the kidneys do not properly remove waste from the blood, when the pericardium swells from unknown causes, from infection, or when the pericardium is damaged by **cancer**. Blunt or penetrating injury from trauma to the chest or heart can also result in cardiac tamponade when large amounts

> ## KEY TERMS
>
> **Pericardiocentesis**—A procedure used to drain fluid out of the sac surrounding the heart. This is done by inserting a needle through the chest and into the sac.

of blood fill the pericardium. Tamponade can also occur during heart surgery.

When the heart is compressed by the surrounding fluid, three conditions occur: a reduced amount of blood is pumped to the body by the heart, the lower chambers of the ventricles are filled with a less than normal amount of blood, and higher than normal blood pressures occur inside the heart, caused by the pressure of the fluid pushing in on the heart from the outside.

When tamponade occurs because of trauma, the sound of the heart beats can become faint, and the blood pressure in the arteries decreases, while the blood pressure in the veins increases.

In cases of tamponade caused by more slowly developing diseases, **shortness of breath**, a feeling of tightness in the chest, increased blood pressure in the large veins in the neck (the jugular veins), weight gain, and fluid retention by the body can occur.

Diagnosis

When cardiac tamponade is suspected, accurate diagnosis can be life-saving. The most accurate way to identify this condition is by using a test called an echocardiogram. This test uses sound waves to create an image of the heart and its surrounding sac, making it easy to visualize any fluid that has collected inside the sac.

Treatment

If the abnormal fluid buildup in the pericardial sac is caused by cancer or **kidney disease**, drugs used to treat these conditions can help lessen the amount of fluid collecting inside the sac. Drugs that help maintain normal blood pressure throughout the body can also help this condition; however, these drugs are only a temporary treatment. The fluid within the pericardium must be drained out to reduce the pressure on the heart and restore proper heart pumping.

The fluid inside the pericardium is drained by inserting a needle through the chest and into the sac itself. This allows the fluid to flow out of the sac, relieving the abnormal pressure on the heart. This procedure is called **pericardiocentesis**. In severe cases, a tube (catheter) can be inserted into the sac or a section of the sac can be surgically cut away to allow for more drainage.

Prognosis

This condition is life-threatening. However, drug treatments can be helpful, and surgical treatments can successfully drain the trapped fluid, though it may reaccumulate. Some risk of **death** exists with surgical drainage of the accumulated fluid.

ORGANIZATIONS

American Heart Association National Center, 7272 Greenville Avenue, Dallas, TX, 75231, (800) 242-8721, Review. personal.info@heart.org.

Dominic De Bellis, PhD

Cardiac tumors *see* **Myxoma**
Cardiogenic shock *see* **Shock**

Cardiomyopathy

Definition

Cardiomyopathy is a chronic disease of the heart muscle (myocardium), in which the muscle is abnormally enlarged, thickened, and/or stiffened. The weakened heart muscle loses the ability to pump blood effectively, resulting in irregular heartbeats (**arrhythmias**) and possibly even **heart failure**.

Description

Cardiomyopathy, a disease of the heart muscle, primarily affects the left ventricle, which is the main pumping chamber of the heart. The disease is often associated with inadequate heart pumping and other heart function abnormalities. Cardiomyopathy is not common (affecting about 50,000 persons in the United States) but it can be severely disabling or fatal. Severe cases may result in heart failure and will require a heart transplant for patient survival. Cardiomyopathy is a heart condition that not only affects middle-aged and elderly persons, but can also affect infants, children, and adolescents.

There are four major types of cardiomyopathy:

- Dilated (congestive cardiomyopathy). This is the most common form of the disease. The heart cavity is enlarged and stretched (cardiac dilation), which results in weak and slow pumping of the blood, which in turn can result in the formation of blood clots. Abnormal heart rhythms (arrhythmias) and disturbances in the electrical conduction processes in the heart may also occur. Most patients with this type of cardiomyopathy develop congestive heart failure. There is also a genetically-linked cardiac disease, Barth syndrome, that can cause dilated cardiomyopathy. This syndrome affects male children, and is usually diagnosed at birth or within the first few months of life. Pregnant women during the last trimester of pregnancy or after childbirth may develop a type of dilated cardiomyopathy referred to as peripartum cardiomyopathy.

- Hypertrophic cardiomyopathy. With this type of cardiomyopathy, the muscle mass of the left ventricle enlarges, or hypertrophies. In hypertrophic obstructive cardiomyopathy (HOCM), the septum (wall) between the two heart ventricles (the pumping chambers) becomes enlarged and obstructs blood flow from the left ventricle. The thickened wall can also distort one leaflet of the mitral valve, which results in leakage. HOCM is most common in young adults. HOCM is often hereditary, caused by genetic mutations in the affected person's DNA. The disease is either inherited through one parent who is a carrier or through both parents who each contribute a defective gene. HOCM is also referred to as asymmetrical septal hypertrophy (ASH) or idiopathic hypertrophic subaortic stenosis (IHSS). In another form of hypertrophic cardiomyopathy, non-obstructive cardiomyopathy, the enlarged heart muscle does not obstruct the blood flow through the heart.

- Restrictive cardiomyopathy. This is a less common type of cardiomyopathy, in which the heart muscle of the ventricles becomes rigid. Restrictive cardiomyopathy affects the diastolic function of the heart, that is, it affects the period when the heart is relaxing between contractions. Since the heart cannot relax adequately between contractions, it is harder for the ventricles to fill with blood between heartbeats. This type of cardiomyopathy is usually the result of another disease.

- Arrhythmogenic right ventricular cardiomyopathy (ARVC). ARVC is very rare and is believed to be an inherited condition. With ARVC, heart muscle cells become disorganized and damaged and are replaced by fatty tissues. The damage appears to be a result of the body's inability to remove damaged cells. The damaged cells are replaced with fat, leading to abnormal electrical activity (arrhythmias) and abnormal heart contractions. ARVC is the most common cause of sudden death in athletes.

Causes and symptoms

Cardiomyopathy may be caused by many different factors, including viral infections (e.g., **myocarditis**), heart attacks, **alcoholism**, long-term, severe high blood pressure, genetic neuromuscular diseases (e.g., muscular dystrophies and ataxias), genetic metabolic disorders, complications from **AIDS**, and other reasons that have not yet been identified (idiopathic cardiomyopathy). Cardiomyopathy caused by heart attacks (referred to as ischemic cardiomyopathy) results from scarring in the heart muscle. Larger **scars** or more numerous heart attacks increases the risk that ischemic cardiomyopathy will develop. Alcoholic cardiomyopathy usually develops about 10 years after sustained, heavy alcohol consumption. Other toxins that may cause cardiomyopathy include drugs and radiation exposure.

The major symptoms of cardiomyopathy include:

- shortness of breath
- temporary and brief loss of consciousness, especially after engaging in activity
- lightheadedness, especially after engaging in activity
- decreased ability to tolerate physical exertion
- fatigue
- dizziness
- palpitations, that is, the sensation of feeling the heart beat
- chest pain (angina), whereby there is a feeling of sharp and unrelenting pressure in the middle of the chest (especially experienced by persons whose cardiomyopathy is a result of a previous heart attack)
- high blood pressure

Other symptoms that may be associated with cardiomyopathy include:

- abdominal swelling or enlargement
- swelling of legs or ankles
- low amount of urine during the daytime, but a need to urinate at night
- decreased alertness and difficulty concentrating
- cough
- loss of appetite

Diagnosis

A complete **physical examination** and health history review by a health care provider is recommended if a person is suspected to have cardiomyopathy. The examination may reveal the presence of an irregular heartbeat, heart murmur, or other abnormal heart and breath sounds.

Various invasive and non-invasive tests are performed as diagnostic tools for cardiomyopathy. An echocardiogram is the most informative noninvasive test for diagnosing the type of cardiomyopathy and the degree of dysfunction in the heart muscle. High frequency sound waves produce moving images of the beating heart on a video screen, which allows the measurement of muscle thickness, size, pumping ability, degree of obstruction, chamber size, and heart valve movement.

The use of non-invasive radiation-based imaging procedures, such as chest radiography, computed tomography (CT), or **magnetic resonance imaging** (MRI) procedures show the size, shape, and structure of the heart. If dilated cardiomyopathy is suspected, one of these techniques is performed first to see if the heart is enlarged and whether there is any fluid accumulation in the lungs.

An electrocardiogram (EKG) is a non-invasive procedure where electrodes are placed on the person's limbs and chest wall to provide a graphic record of the electrical activity of the heart. This test can show the amount of heart enlargement and reveal abnormal heart rhythms. Children with a normal echocardiogram may have an abnormal EKG, indicating that they may be a carrier of the cardiomyopathy gene and may develop the disease later in life. A person may also wear a Holter monitor, which is an external device that continuously records heart rhythms. The monitor can identify irregular heart rhythms associated with dilated, hypertrophic, or **restrictive cardiomyopathy**.

Genetic studies may help in understanding the cause of cardiomyopathy, since the disease may be a symptom of another genetic disorder. If a child under the age of 4 has cardiomyopathy, metabolic screening should be performed, for certain metabolic disorders with cardiomyopathy as a symptom can be controlled with a change in diet, drug therapy, or by a bone marrow transplant, which may reduce or reverse the progression of the cardiomyopathy. Since cardiomyopathy can be inherited and present initially without signs or symptoms, relatives of a patient with the disease should be screened periodically for evidences of the disease.

Invasive procedures, which involve the use of anesthesia, are used to determine the severity of the disease. In the radionuclide ventriculogram procedure, a low-dose radioactive material is injected into a vein and flows to the heart. The heart is photographed with a special camera to assess the contraction and filling of the ventricles at rest and with activity. **Cardiac**

catheterization involves insertion of thin, flexible plastic tubes (catheters) into the heart from a blood vessel in the groin area. A dye is then injected that can indicate blood pressures, blood flow within the heart, and blockages in the arteries. Although rarely used, a heart muscle biopsy, where the doctor removes a few, tiny pieces of the heart for laboratory studies, can aid in diagnosing possible infections in the heart or metabolic abnormalities. An electrophysiology study is similar to heart catheterization. Catheters with fine wires are inserted through veins in the groin area into the heart. Electrical stimuli applied through the wires can indicate abnormal conduction pathways, arrhythmias, effectiveness of drugs, and the need for an implanted defibrillator.

Treatment

Although there is a long list of possible causes for cardiomyopathy, few are directly treatable or curable. Therefore, most therapy is directed toward treating the effects of the disease on the heart. If cardiomyopathy is diagnosed at an advanced stage, a critically ill patient will require immediate life-saving measures such as placement of a breathing tube and administration of medicines to improve heart function and blood pressure. Once the patient is stabilized, long-term therapy needs, such as oral medication, **pacemakers**, surgery, or **heart transplantation**, will be identified.

Initial treatments for cardiomyopathy for patients diagnosed in the earlier stages of cardiomyopathy include drug therapy to relieve heart failure, to decrease oxygen requirements and workload of the heart (by relaxing the arteries in the body), and to regulate abnormal heartbeats. Drugs that help the heart contract include **digoxin** for at-home use and dopamine, dobutamine, and milrinone for in-hospital use. **Diuretics** help relieve fluid overloads in heart failure. **Vasodilators**, ACE-inhibitors, and **beta blockers** dilate blood vessels in the body and lower blood pressure, thus reducing the workload for the heart. For patients at risk of developing **blood clots**, anticoagulation medication or blood thinners such as heparin or coumadin are prescribed along with diuretics such as Lasix and aldactone to relieve venous congestion. These drugs may result in side effects, so the patient must be carefully monitored to prevent complications.

When drugs are not effective or when arrhythmias require regulation, a pacemaker or a defibrillator may be implanted surgically into the patient. The procedures for implanting both devices involves placing a small mechanical device under the skin of the chest or abdomen with wire leads threaded through veins to the heart. A pacemaker is used to monitor and stabilize slow heartbeats, while a defibrillator ("an emergency room in the heart") detects and treats fast and potentially lethal heart rhythms. Since sudden **death** may occur in patients with cardiomyopathy, defibrillators are often recommended for persons who show evidence of arrhythmias.

For heart failure symptoms associated with restricted blood flow from the ventricles, septal **myomectomy**, which is considered major heart surgery, is sometimes recommended. This procedure involves surgical removal of the part of the thickened septal muscle that blocks the blood flow. In some cases, the mitral valve is replaced with an artificial valve. However, the procedure does not prevent sudden death due to hear arrhythmias nor does it stop the disease from progressing.

Since cardiomyopathy often becomes progressively worse, the heart can reach a state where it no longer responds to medication or to surgery. The treatment of "last resort" is a heart transplant, when the patient exhibits severe heart failure symptoms. A transplant can cure the symptoms of heart failure, but the surgery carries significant risks, such as infection, organ rejection, and side effects of required medications.

There are surgical procedures that can be implemented to sustain life until a transplant donor becomes available. Left **Ventricular Assist Device** (LVAD) provides mechanical circulatory support, while Dynamic Cardiomyoplasty is a procedure whereby a skeletal-muscular flap, created from a patient's chest muscle, is first taught to contract and then is wrapped around the heart to aid in contraction.

Alternative treatment

Alternative treatments are directed toward control of the effects of heart disease. **Exercise**, diet, **nutrition**, herbal therapies, **stress reduction**, and other life style changes (e.g., cessation of **smoking**) can all be used to complement conventional treatments. Certain herbs such as fox glove (*Digitalis purpurea*) and lily of the valley (*Convallaria majalis*) contain cardiac glycosides that make them particularly potent and may cause dangerous side effects. Their use should be supervised only be a qualified medical herbalist, with the concurrence of the primary conventional health care provider. Even the use of less potent herbs that improve cardiac function, such as hawthorn (*Crataegus laevigata*), should be approved by the conventional health care provider and administered under the supervision of a medical herbalist.

KEY TERMS

Arrhythmia—An abnormal rhythm or irregularity of the heartbeat. The heartbeat may either be too fast (tachycardia) or too slow (bradicardia). Arrhythmias may cause symptoms such as palpitation or light-headedness, but many have more serious consequences, including sudden death.

Congestive heart failure—Potentially lethal condition in which congestion develops in the lungs that is produced by a heart attack, poorly controlled or uncontrolled hypertension, or disease processes that weaken the heart.

Hypertrophy—Literally means an increase in the muscle mass (or weight) of the heart.

Mitral valve leaflets—The mitral valve is made up of two valve leaflets (the anteromedial leaflet and the posterolateral leaflet) and a ring around the valve, known as the mitral valve annulus. The orientation of the two leaflets resembles a bishop's miter, which is where the valve receives its name.

Myocardium—The muscular wall of the heart located between the inner endocardial layer and the outer epicardial layer.

Noninvasive—Refers to tests that generally do not invade the integrity of the body, such as echocardiography or electrocardiography. (Cardiac catheterization, on the other hand, in which catheters are introduced through blood vessels into the heart, is an example of an invasive test).

Septum (ventricular septum)—That portion of the heart wall that divides the right and left ventricles.

Ventricles—The two main (lower) pumping chambers of the heart; the right and left ventricles pump blood to the lungs and aorta, respectively.

maintaining a healthy weight, exercising regularly, eating a well-balanced nutritious diet, and avoiding or minimizing smoking.

Resources

BOOKS

Dilated Cardiomyopathy: A Medical Dictionary, Bibliography, and Annotated Research Guide to Internet Resources. San Diego, CA: Icon Health Publications, 2004.

Maron, Barry J., and Salberg, Lisa. *Hypertrophic Cardiomyopathy: For Patients, Their Families, and Interested Physicians.* 2nd ed. New York: Wiley/Blackwell, 2006.

Maron, Barry J., ed. *Diagnosis and Management of Hypertrophic Cardiomyopathy.* New York: Wiley/Blackwell, 2004.

PERIODICALS

Ommen, Steve R., and Nishimura, Rick A. *"A Physician's Guide to the Treatment of Hypertrophic Cardiomyopathy."HeartViews* 1(10): 393–401.

OTHER

Cleveland Clinic Heart Center. http://www.clevelandclinic.org/heartcenter/pub/guide/disease/hcm.asp.

National Heart, Blood, and Lung Institute, National Institutes of Health, NHLBI Health Information Center, P.O. Box 30105, Bethesda, MD 20824-0105. Telephone: (301) 592 8573; http://www.nhlbi.nih.gov.

ORGANIZATIONS

American Heart Association National Center, 7272 Greenville Avenue, Dallas, TX, 75231, (800) 242-8721, Review. personal.info@heart.org.

Children's Cardiomyopathy Foundation, P.O. Box 547, Tenafly, NJ, 07670, 201, 227-7016, (866) 808-2873, info@childrenscardiomyopathy.org, http://www.childrenscardiomyopathy.org.

Hypertrophic Cardiomyopathy Association, 328 Green Pond Rd. ; P.O. Box 306, Hibernia, NJ, 07842, (973) 983-7429, (973) 983-7870, support@4hcma.org, http://www. 4hcm.org/.

Judith Sims

Prognosis

Long-term prognosis can be unpredictable, as there can be a wide range of severities and outcomes associated with the disease. There is no cure, but some symptoms and complications can be managed and controlled with medication and implantable devices or with a heart transplant.

Prevention

Prevention of cardiomyopathy is focused on controlling risk factors for heart disease, which includes

Cardiopulmonary resuscitation

Definition

Cardiopulmonary resuscitation, commonly called CPR, is a lifesaving procedure performed when a person has stopped breathing or a person's heart has stopped beating.

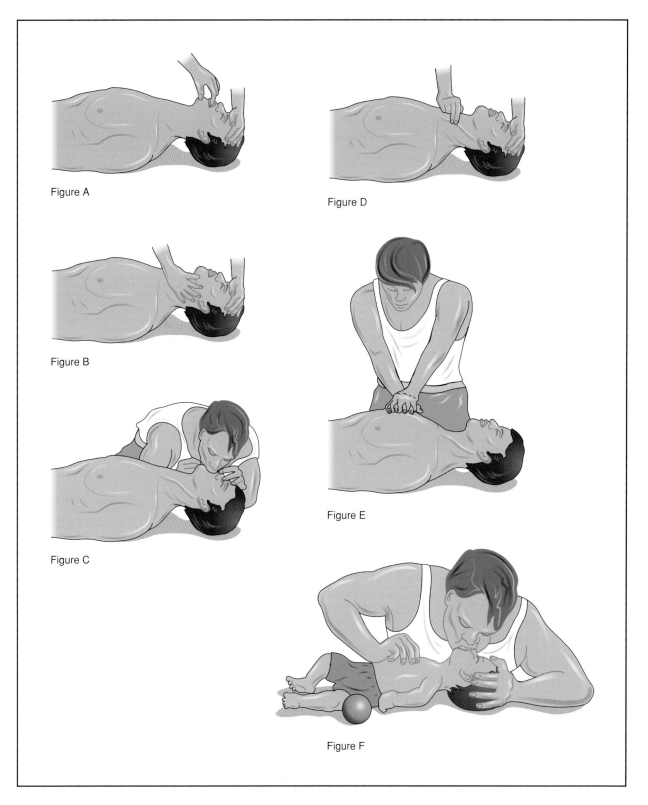

Figure A

Figure B

Figure C

Figure D

Figure E

Figure F

Call 911 and immediately start CPR with compressions. Push hard on the center of the chest 30 times (E) at a rate of 100 compressions/minute. If you're trained in CPR, continue by opening the airway with a head tilt (B). Pinch the victim's nose shut, inhale normally, and create an airtight seal between your mouth and the victim's (C). Give two short breaths and watch for chest rise. Continue compressions and breaths until trained help arrives. *(Illustration by Electronic Illustrators Group. Reproduced by permission of Gale, a part of Cengage Learning.)*

Purpose

The purpose of CPR is to bring oxygen to the individual's lungs and to keep blood circulating so oxygen gets to every part of the body. When a person is deprived of oxygen, permanent brain damage can begin in as little as four minutes and **death** can follow only minutes later. When performed quickly enough, CPR can save lives in such emergencies as **heart attack** or sudden cardiac arrest, electric shock, **near-drowning**, **drug overdose**, and other conditions in which the heart has stopped and there is no breathing.

Description

In 2010, over 300,000 Americans were expected to die of sudden cardiac arrest. Some of these people could be saved by the immediate application of CPR. In October of 2010, the instructions for performing CPR by people who have not received formal CPR training or who are not healthcare professionals was changed.

There are three physical symptoms that indicate a potential need for CPR to be performed immediately and for emergency medical support to be called: unconsciousness, absence of breathing, and no pulse detected (absence of heartbeat).

Unconsciousness

Unconsciousness is the loss of all awareness and failure to respond to questions, touch, or gentle shaking. When unconscious, a person cannot cough or clear the throat, which may allow the windpipe to become blocked, causing suffocation and death. People with a major illness or injury or who have had recent surgery are at risk for losing consciousness. Alcohol or drug overdose also can cause unconsciousness.

Individuals who are unconscious and *not breathing* need immediate CPR. Individuals who are unconscious and breathing (e.g., a traumatic **head injury**) need emergency medical care, and should be watched to assure that their breathing continues. If the person is conscious, he or she may be **choking** and need other medical help but *does not* need CPR. Fainting is a brief period of unconsciousness, which may occur from **dehydration** (lack of body fluids), low blood pressure, low blood sugar, excessive bleeding, or emotional distress. This is a temporary condition. Again, the individual may need medical help but does not normally need CPR because people who faint normally continue to breathe without assistance.

Failure to breathe

Apnea is the lack of spontaneous breathing. The individual may become limp and lifeless, have a seizure, or turn bluish (a sign of inadequate oxygen). Prolonged apnea is called respiratory arrest. In children, this can quickly lead to cardiac arrest in which the heart stops beating. In adults, cardiac arrest usually happens first, followed by respiratory arrest. In adults, common causes of apnea and respiratory arrest include choking, drug overdose, near-drowning, head injury, and cardiac arrest. In children, the causes may be different, such as **prematurity**, swelling of the airways (e.g., an **asthma** attack, an allergic reaction), choking on a foreign object, seizures, regurgitating food or near-drowning.

No pulse detected

If the rescuer is unable to detect a pulse or has difficulty feeling a pulse, it may be due to cardiac arrest (i.e., the heart has stopped beating). Not all rescuers are adept at finding a pulse either in the wrist or the carotid artery of the neck. Rescuers who are uncertain about whether there is a pulse should err on the side of caution and begin CPR.

Medical help and possibly CPR are needed immediately if any of these three symptoms are found. Time is critical. A local emergency number should be called immediately. If more than one person is available to help, one person can call the local emergency medical service (911 in the United States), while the other person begins CPR. If needed, the emergency dispatcher (the person who picks up emergency calls) can give step-by-step CPR instructions over the telephone.

Performing CPR

The explanation below is not a substitute for CPR training and is intended as a descriptive guideline only.

In 2010 the American Heart Association recommended that the three traditional steps for performing CPR be re-ordered for lay people who have had little or no training in CPR. This change applies to performing CPR on adults, children, and infants, but not on newborns. Formerly the steps were (in order): clear the airways, check for breathing, and begin chest compressions. This was known as the A-B-C method of CPR.

The 2010 recommendations have changed the order. Chest compressions should begin *first*, followed by clearing the airways and checking for breathing if the rescuer is adequately trained. There are two reasons for this change. First, most people have residual oxygen in their lungs from their last breath. It is most important that the blood be kept circulating continuously through chest compressions so that this oxygen reaches the brain without delay. Second, many lay people are reluctant to do mouth-to-mouth breathing on a stranger. After reviewing multiple studies that examined the outcome of CPR done by lay people, the American Heart Association has determined that chest compressions alone (hands-only CPR) are almost as effective as chest compressions with breathing, and that breathing need not be done by people untrained in CPR. The American Heart Association hopes that this change will encourage more bystanders to come to the aid of a cardiac arrest victim and potentially save more lives.

The steps to be followed in CPR by a layperson are as follows:

- If the victim appears to be unconscious, he or she should be shaken or tapped gently to check for any sign of consciousness. If there is no response, the rescuer should call emergency medical services immediately, or (preferably) send someone else to call for help. If the rescuer is alone, he or she should call for emergency services before beginning CPR.

- The victim should be placed on his or her back on a level surface such as the ground or the floor unless there is some sign of neck or back injuries, in which case the individual should not be moved. It is better to err on the side of caution and not move the individual if there is any question about whether moving will cause additional damage.

- The rescuer then places the heel of one hand in the middle of the chest, putting the other hand on top of the first, interlacing the fingers, and pressing down so that the chest is compressed by at two inches. Hard and fast compressions are essential if CPR is to be effective. The rescuer should not worry about damaging the breastbone or ribs. (These will heal; death is permanent.) When performing compressions, the rescuer should keep the elbows straight, center his or her shoulders over the individual, develop an up-and-down rhythm, and keep the hands firmly on the individual's chest. Compressions should be done on the center of the chest midway between the nipples. Compressions should be hard and fast at a rate of *at least* 100 times per minute. That is about the same rhythm as the beat of the Bee Gee's song "Stayin' Alive." Compressions should continue at this rate until the victim begins to breathe spontaneously or until trained medical help arrives.

If the rescuer has been trained in CPR, he or she may jut the victim's jaw forward, tilt the head back,

KEY TERMS

Apnea—A period of no breathing, sometimes sudden, sometimes prolonged.

Arrest—A sudden stopping of the function of a body organ, such as no breathing (respiratory arrest) or no beating of the heart (cardiac arrest).

Cardiopulmonary—Involving both heart and lungs.

Circulation—The passage of blood and delivery of oxygen through the veins and arteries of the body.

Respiratory—Referring to breathing in and breathing out, and the function of the lungs.

Resuscitation—Reviving an unconscious person or restoring breathing.

and open the mouth. Using the finger, the rescuer should clear any debris from inside the mouth. The rescuer then should put his or her ear to the victim's open mouth, look for chest movement, listen for air flowing through the mouth or nose, and feel for air on his or her cheek. If there is no breathing, the rescuer pinches the individual's nose shut, makes a seal over the individual's mouth with his or her own mouth, and gives the individual two puffs of breath big enough to make the chest rise. If the chest does not rise, the individual's head should be repositioned to help ensure the tongue is kept away from the windpipe, then the rescuer should try again to give a breath. Chest compressions should continue with two puffs of breath given for every 50 compressions (two puffs per minute) until help arrives or the victim begins breathing spontaneously.

Benefits

Successful CPR is a life-saving procedure. It can restore breathing and circulation in the individual. Medical attention is required immediately even if successful CPR has been performed and the individual is breathing freely.

Precautions

Rescuers should observe the following:

- Do not leave the individual alone.
- Do not give the individual anything to eat or drink.
- Avoid moving the individual's head or neck if spinal injury is a possibility. To check for breathing when

spinal injury is suspected, the rescuer should only listen for breath by the individual's mouth and watch the chest for movement.

- Do not place a pillow under the individual's head.

Preparation

As CPR is performed in emergency situations, there is no time to prepare the recipient for the procedure. It is necessary to place lay the recipient on a flat surface facing up before administering compressions.

Training in CPR is the best preparation the rescuer. Training is not difficult or expensive. The American Heart Association provides CPR instruction for the community, schools, and workplace, along with health care settings. Courses vary from short programs to teach laypersons the basics of CPR to advanced cardiac life support certification for healthcare professionals. CPR is taught as part of many first aid courses.

In addition, the American Heart Association has a 22-minute long self-directed program called CPR Anytime in an effort to prepare the public and people who would not otherwise attend a CPR course to be able to respond to an emergency with core CPR skills. CPR Anytime does not lead to certification, but research has shown that the program is effective in quickly training the lay public and could prove to be a valuable tool in increasing the overall number of CPR-prepared individuals.

Aftercare

When CPR is initiated, emergency responders have ideally already been notified and are on the way to the scene. It is important to stay with the affected person and continue CPR until breathing and circulation are restored and/or emergency medical personnel arrive. When emergency personnel assume care of the individual, the person who initially provided CPR can often be helpful by providing information to emergency responders.

Risks

Minor injuries such as bruising can occur with chest compressions. Sometimes chest compressions can result in one or more breaks in the ribs and accompanying damage to internal organs, especially in young children, the elderly, or debilitated persons. The American Heart Association states, however, that in the event of a suspected cardiac arrest, even CPR performed by an untrained bystander who receives instructions from an emergency dispatcher is more beneficial than the risk of injury in a person who is actually not in cardiac arrest.

Training and certification

Local medical personnel, staff at hospitals and fire departments, and members of the American Heart Association teach CPR courses for the community, schools, and workplaces, along with more extensive courses for allied health professionals. Courses vary from short programs to teach laypersons the basics of CPR to advanced cardiac life support certification for healthcare professionals. Certification must be renewed on a regular basis by taking a refresher course.

Prevention

People with serious health conditions can follow these general guidelines:

- Risk factors that contribute to heart disease should be reduced or eliminated. People can reduce risks if they stop smoking, lower blood pressure and cholesterol, lose excess weight, and reduce stress.
- Illegal recreational drugs should be avoided.
- Seeing a doctor regularly and being aware of any disease conditions or risk factors can help prevent or complicate illness, as can seeking and following the doctor's advice about diet and exercise.

Resources

PERIODICALS

American Heart Association. "2010 American Heart Association Guidelines for Cardiopulmonary Resuscitation and Emergency Cardiovascular Care Science." *Circulation* 122: (2010) S640–S656.S http://circ.ahajournals.org/content/vol122/18_suppl_3/#____AMERICAN_HEART_ASSOCIATION_GUIDELINES_FOR_CARDIOPULMONARY_RESUSCITATION__AND_EMERGENCY_CARDIOVASCULAR_CARE_SCIENCE

OTHER

"A New Order for CPR, spelled C-A-B." American Heart Association. http://www.newsroom.heart.org/index.php?s = 43&item = 1139 (accessed December 22, 2010).

American Heart Association. *Emergency Cardiovascular Care.* http://www.americanheart.org/presenter.jhtml?identifier = 3011764 (accessed February 5, 2010).

"CPR." MedlinePlus. December 1, 2010 [accessed December 1, 2010]. http://www.nlm.nih.gov/medlineplus/cpr.html

ORGANIZATIONS

American Heart Association, 7272 Greenville Avenue, Dallas, TX, 75231, (800) 242-8721, http://www.americanheart.org.

L Lee Culvert, Ph.D.
Tish Davidson AM

Cardioversion

Definition

Cardioversion refers to the process of restoring the heart's normal rhythm by applying a controlled electric shock to the exterior of the chest.

Purpose

When the heart beats too fast, blood no longer circulates effectively in the body. Cardioversion is used to stop this abnormal beating so that the heart can begin normal rhythm and pump more efficiently.

Precautions

Not all unusual heart rhythms (called **arrhythmias**) are dangerous or fatal. **Atrial fibrillation** and **atrial flutter** often revert to normal rhythms without the need for cardioversion. Healthcare providers may also try to correct the heart rhythm with medication or recommend a lifestyle change before trying cardioversion. However, **ventricular tachycardia** lasting more than 30 seconds and **ventricular fibrillation** require immediate cardioversion.

Description

Elective cardioversion is usually scheduled ahead of time. After arriving at the hospital, an intravenous (IV) catheter will be placed in the arm and oxygen will be given through a face mask. A short-acting general anesthetic will be administered through the vein. During the two or three minutes of anesthesia, the doctor will apply two paddles to the exterior of the chest and administer the electric shock. It may be necessary to give the shock two or three times to obtain normal rhythm.

Preparation

Medication to thin the blood is usually given for at least three weeks before elective cardioversion. Food intake should be stopped eight hours before the procedure.

Aftercare

Medical personnel will monitor the heart rhythm for a few hours, after which the patient is usually sent home. It is advisable to arrange for transportation home, because drowsiness may last several hours. The doctor may prescribe anti-arrhythmic medication to prevent the abnormal rhythm from returning.

KEY TERMS

Atrial fibrillation—A condition in which the upper chamber of the heart quivers instead of pumping in an organized way.

Atrial flutter—A rapid pulsation of the upper chamber of the heart that interferes with normal function.

Ventricular fibrillation—A condition in which the lower chamber of the heart quivers instead of pumping in an organized way.

Ventricular tachycardia—A rapid heart beat, usually over 100 beats per minute.

Risks

Cardioverters have been in use for many years and the risks are few. Those unlikely risks that remain include those instances when the device delivers greater or lesser power than expected or when power setting and control knobs are not set correctly. Unfortunately, in a number of cases, the heart prefers its abnormal rhythm and reverts to it despite cardioversion.

Normal results

Most cardioversions are successful and, at least for a time, restore the normal heart rhythm.

ORGANIZATIONS

American Heart Association National Center, 7272 Greenville Avenue, Dallas, TX, 75231, (800) 242-8721, Review. personal.info@heart.org.

Dorothy Elinor Stonely

Carisoprodol *see* **Muscle relaxants**

Carotid artery surgery *see* **Endarterectomy**

Carotid Doppler ultrasound *see* **Doppler ultrasonography**

Carotid endarterectomy *see* **Endarterectomy**

Carotid sinus massage

Definition

Carotid sinus massage involves rubbing the large part of the arterial wall at the point where the common carotid artery, located in the neck, divides into its two main branches.

KEY TERMS

Angina pectoris—Chest pain usually caused by a lack of oxygen in the heart muscle.

Arrhythmia—Any deviation from a normal heart beat.

Atrial fibrillation—A condition in which the upper chamber of the heart quivers instead of pumping in an organized way.

Atrial flutter—Rapid, inefficient contraction of the upper chamber of the heart.

Carotid artery—One of the major arteries supplying blood to the head and neck.

Tachycardia—A rapid heart beat, usually over 100 beats per minute.

Purpose

Sinus, in this case, means an area in a blood vessel that is bigger than the rest of the vessel. This is a normal dilation of the vessel. Located in the neck just below the angle of the jaw, the carotid sinus sits above the point where the carotid artery divides into its two main branches. Rubbing the carotid sinus stimulates an area in the artery wall that contains nerve endings. These nerves respond to changes in blood pressure and are capable of slowing the heart rate. The response to this simple procedure often slows a rapid heart rate (for example, **atrial flutter** or atrial tachycardia) and can provide important diagnostic information to the physician.

Description

The patient will be asked to lie down, with the neck fully extended and the head turned away from the side being massaged. While watching an electrocardiogram monitor, the doctor will gently touch the carotid sinus. If there is no change in the heart rate on the monitor, the pressure is applied more firmly with a gentle rotating motion. After massaging one side of the neck, the massage will be repeated on the other side. Both sides of the neck are never massaged at the same time.

Preparation

No special preparation is needed for carotid sinus massage.

Aftercare

No aftercare is required.

Risks

The physician must be sure there is no evidence of blockage in the carotid artery before performing the procedure. Massage in a blocked area might cause a clot to break loose and cause a **stroke**.

Normal results

Carotid sinus massage will slow the heart rate during episodes of atrial flutter, fibrillation, and some tachycardias. It has been known to stop the arrhythmia completely. If the procedure is being done to help diagnose **angina** pectoris, massaging the carotid sinus may make the discomfort go away.

Resources

BOOKS

Fuster, Valentin, et al. *Hurst's the Heart*. 12th ed. New York: McGraw Hill Professional, 2007.

Dorothy Elinor Stonely

Carpal tunnel syndrome

Definition

Carpal tunnel syndrome is a disorder caused by compression at the wrist of the median nerve supplying the hand, causing **numbness and tingling**.

Description

The carpal tunnel is an area in the wrist where the bones and ligaments create a small passageway for the median nerve. The median nerve is responsible for both sensation and movement in the hand, in particular the thumb and first three fingers. When the median nerve is compressed, an individual's hand will feel as if it has "gone to sleep."

Women between the ages of 30 and 60 have the highest rates of carpal tunnel syndrome. Research has demonstrated that carpal tunnel syndrome is a very significant cause of missed work days due to **pain**. In 1995, about $270 million was spent on sick days taken for pain from repetitive motion injuries.

Causes and symptoms

Compression of the median nerve in the wrist can occur during a number of different conditions, particularly those conditions which lead to changes in fluid accumulation throughout the body. Because

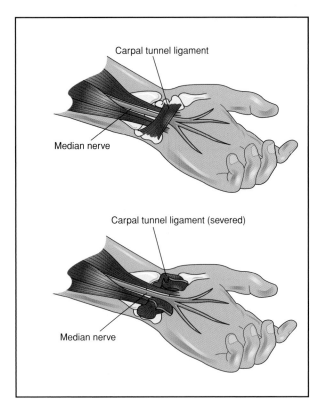

Carpal tunnel ligament

Median nerve

Carpal tunnel ligament (severed)

Median nerve

The most severe cases of carpal tunnel syndrome may require surgery to decrease the compression of the median nerve and restore its normal function. This procedure involves severing the ligament that crosses the wrist, thus allowing the median nerve more room and decreasing compression. *(Illustration by Electronic Illustrators Group. Reproduced by permission of Gale, a part of Cengage Learning.)*

the area of the wrist through which the median nerve passes is very narrow, any swelling in the area will lead to pressure on the median nerve. This pressure will ultimately interfere with the nerve's ability to function normally. **Pregnancy**, **obesity**, arthritis, certain thyroid conditions, diabetes, and certain pituitary abnormalities all predispose to carpal tunnel syndrome. Other conditions which increase the risk for carpal tunnel syndrome include some forms of arthritis and various injuries to the arm and wrist (including **fractures**, sprains, and **dislocations**). Furthermore, activities which cause an individual to repeatedly bend the wrist inward toward the forearm can predispose to carpal tunnel syndrome. Certain jobs which require repeated strong wrist motions carry a relatively high risk of carpal tunnel syndrome. Injuries of this type are referred to as "repetitive motion" injuries, and are more frequent among secretaries doing a lot of typing, people working at computer keyboards or cash registers, factory workers, and some musicians.

Symptoms of carpal tunnel syndrome include **numbness**, burning, **tingling**, and a prickly pin-like sensation over the palm surface of the hand, and into the thumb, forefinger, middle finger, and half of the ring finger. Some individuals notice a shooting pain which goes from the wrist up the arm, or down into the hand and fingers. With continued median nerve compression, an individual may begin to experience muscle weakness, making it difficult to open jars and hold objects with the affected hand. Eventually, the muscles of the hand served by the median nerve may begin to grow noticeably smaller (atrophy), especially the fleshy part of the thumb. Untreated, carpal tunnel syndrome may eventually result in permanent weakness, loss of sensation, or even **paralysis** of the thumb and fingers of the affected hand.

Diagnosis

The diagnosis of carpal tunnel syndrome is made in part by checking to see whether the patient's symptoms can be brought on by holding his or her hand in position with wrist bent for about a minute. Wrist x rays are often taken to rule out the possibility of a tumor causing pressure on the median nerve. A physician examining a patient suspected of having carpal tunnel syndrome will perform a variety of simple tests to measure muscle strength and sensation in the affected hand and arm. Further testing might include electromyographic or nerve conduction velocity testing to determine the exact severity of nerve damage. These tests involve stimulating the median nerve with electricity and measuring the resulting speed and strength of the muscle response, as well as recording speed of nerve transmission across the carpal tunnel.

Treatment

Carpal tunnel syndrome is initially treated with splints, which support the wrist and prevent it from flexing inward into the position which exacerbates median nerve compression. Some people get significant relief by wearing such splints to sleep at night, while others will need to wear the splints all day, especially if they are performing jobs which **stress** the wrist. Ibuprofen or other **nonsteroidal anti-inflammatory drugs** may be prescribed to decrease pain and swelling. When carpal tunnel syndrome is more advanced, injection of **steroids** into the wrist to decrease inflammation may be necessary.

The most severe cases of carpal tunnel syndrome may require surgery to decrease the compression of the median nerve and restore its normal function. Such a

KEY TERMS

Carpal tunnel—A passageway in the wrist, created by the bones and ligaments of the wrist, through which the median nerve passes.

Electromyography—A type of test in which a nerve's function is tested by stimulating a nerve with electricity, and then measuring the speed and strength of the corresponding muscle's response.

Median nerve—A nerve which runs through the wrist and into the hand. It provides sensation and some movement to the hand, the thumb, the index finger, the middle finger, and half of the ring finger.

repair involves cutting that ligament which crosses the wrist, thus allowing the median nerve more room and decreasing compression. This surgery is done almost exclusively on an outpatient basis and is often performed without the patient having to be made unconscious. Careful injection of numbing medicines (**local anesthesia**) or nerve blocks (the injection of anesthetics directly into the nerve) create sufficient numbness to allow the surgery to be performed painlessly, without the risks associated with **general anesthesia**. Recovery from this type of surgery is usually quick and without complications.

Prognosis

Without treatment, continued pressure on the median nerve puts an individual at risk for permanent disability in the affected hand. Most people are able to control the symptoms of carpal tunnel syndrome with splinting and anti-inflammatory agents. For those who go on to require surgery, about 95% will have complete cessation of symptoms.

Prevention

Prevention is generally aimed at becoming aware of the repetitive motions which one must make which could put the wrist into a bent position. People who must work long hours at a computer keyboard, for example, may need to take advantage of recent advances in "ergonomics," which try to position the keyboard and computer components in a way that increases efficiency and decreases stress. Early use of a splint may also be helpful for people whose jobs increase the risk of carpal tunnel syndrome.

Resources

PERIODICALS

Seiler, John Gray. "Carpal Tunnel Syndrome: Update on Diagnostic Testing and Treatment Options." *Consultant* 37, no. 5 (May 1997): 1233.

Rosalyn Carson-DeWitt, MD

Casts *see* **Immobilization**

Cataract surgery

Definition

Cataract surgery is a procedure performed to remove a cloudy (natural) lens from the eye; usually an intraocular (artificial) lens is implanted at the same time. The removed lens, sometimes also called a crystalline lens, is called a cataract because the originally clear lens has turned cloudy. An ophthalmologist (commonly called an eye surgeon) usually performs such surgeries on an outpatient basis within a surgical center, hospital, or other professional medical facility. The commonly performed procedure, which takes less than an hour, is generally safe and nearly risk free.

Demographics

Nearly all cataract surgeries are performed on older people. As the eyes age, **cataracts** form on the lens of the eyes, which cause blurry vision, difficulties looking at bright lights, and other such vision problems. According to the National Institutes of Health, over 50% of people in the United States over the age of 80 years have a cataract or have had cataract surgery. Normally, people will have cataract surgery when the eyes degrade enough so that it is increasingly difficult to carry out daily activities of life. Often times, people, especially elderly adults, have other eye problems, such as **macular degeneration**, which are difficult to treat when cataracts are present. In such cases, it is often advisable to have the cataracts removed.

Purpose

The purpose of cataract surgery is to restore clear vision. It is indicated when cloudy vision due to cataracts has progressed to such an extent that it interferes with normal daily activities. Other symptoms of cataracts include colors that fade, excessive glare, inability to see well at night, double vision, and numerous changes in vision prescriptions (for **eye glasses** or contacts). It is one of the most commonly performed surgical procedures in the world.

Precautions

Cataract surgery is not performed on both eyes at once. To avoid risking blindness in both eyes in the event of infection or other catastrophe, the first eye is allowed to heal before the cataract is removed from the second eye.

The presence of cataracts can mask additional eye problems, such as retinal damage, that neither doctors nor patients are aware of prior to surgery. Since such conditions will continue to impair sight after cataract removal if they are not identified and treated, the eventual outcome of cataract surgery will depend on the outcome of other problems.

In 1997 and 1998, evidence that cataract surgery can contribute to the progression of age-related macular degeneration (ARMD) was published. ARMD is the degeneration of the central part of the retina. However, as of 2010, studies have not shown such a conclusive relationship. Whether cataract surgery contributes to the progression of ARMD is still up to debate in the medical community. Accordingly, ARMD patients with cataracts must weigh the possible risks of the loss of central vision, within four or five years, against short-term improvement. When an ARMD patient chooses cataract surgery, the surgeon should shield the retina against bright light to protect it from possible light-induced damage during surgery and install an intraocular lens capable of absorbing ultraviolet and blue light, which seem to do the most damage.

Description

Just before the start of the surgery, eye drops are placed in the eye to dilate the pupil. Local anesthetics are provided to de-sensitive (numb) the area around the eye. A sedative may be provided for anxious patients so they can relax. The patient will remain awake during the surgery but may feel sleepy.

There are two types of cataract surgery: intracapsular and extracapsular. Intracapsular surgery is the removal of both the lens and the thin capsule that surround the lens. This type of surgery was common before 1980, but it has since been displaced by extracapsular surgery. Removal of the capsule requires a large incision and does not allow comfortable intraocular lens implantation. Thus, people who undergo intracapsular cataract surgery have long recovery periods and have to wear very thick glasses.

Extracapsular cataract surgery is the removal of the lens where the capsule is left in place. Each year in the United States, over a million cataracts are removed this way. Physicians and researchers continue to improve cataract surgery methods. Research from France in 2003 said that cataract removal and non-penetrating glaucoma surgery can be combined in glaucoma patients.

There are two methods for extracapsular cataract surgery. The usual technique is phacoemulsification. A tiny incision (about 0.12-inch, or 3-millimeter, long) is made next to the cornea (the eye's outer covering) in the front of the eye, and an ultrasonic probe is used to break up (emulsify) the cataract into minute pieces, which are then removed by suction. Stitches may or may not be used to close the small incision point.

When the lens is too hard to be emulsified ultrasonically, the surgeon will use a slightly different technique called extracapsular extraction, which requires a larger incision. The extracapsular extraction is performed during phacoemulsification. During the process, an incision—one with a length of about 0.37 inch (9 millimeters) long—is made, and the whole lens (without its capsule) is removed through the incision. In this method, stitches are usually necessary. Both kinds of extracapsular cataract surgery leave the back of the capsule intact, so a silicone or plastic intraocular lens can be stably implanted in about the same location as the original lens.

The surgery takes about 30 to 60 minutes for one eye. Once completed the patient will have a clear, artificial lens implanted into the empty capsule. The implant, called an intraocular lens (IOL), is made of acrylic, plastic, or silicone. There are a variety of different IOLs that can be implanted. Some are flexible, while others rigid. Some are made so they block ultraviolet (UV) radiation, while others function like bifocal or trifocal eye glasses.

Preparation

Patients must have a pre-operation **eye examination**, which will include ultrasound analysis to make sure the retina (the innermost layer of the eye, containing the light receptors) is intact and also to measure eye curvature so that a lens with the proper correction can be implanted. The patient also will have a pre-operative **physical examination**. In addition, patients start a course of antibiotic eye drops or ointment the day before surgery. Medications taken by the patient may be stopped under the advice of the surgeon. Such medications include any that may cause increased bleeding during surgery.

About 12 hours before the surgery, the physician may ask you to stop eating or drinking. The medical staff will also ask the patient to arrange for someone to remain at the surgical site to drive the patient home afterwards.

KEY TERMS

Age-related macular degeneration (ARMD)— Degeneration of the macula (the central part of the retina where the rods and cones are most dense) that leads to loss of central vision in people over 60 years of age.

Cataract—Progressive opacity or clouding of an eye lens, which obstructs the passage of light to the retina.

Cornea—Clear outer covering of the front of the eye.

Intraocular lens—Lens made of silicone or plastic placed within the eye; can be corrective.

Retina—Innermost layer at the back of the eye, which contains light receptors, the rods and cones.

Aftercare

Proper post-operative care is especially important after cataract surgery. Patients will need someone to drive them home after the surgery and should not bend over or lift anything up for a few days after the surgery, or do anything strenuous for about two weeks. The sight through the repaired eye will be blurry over the first few days after surgery as the eye adjusts to the new lens. Patients should refrain from rubbing or pressing the eye, should wear glasses to protect their eye, and should wear a shield while sleeping so the eye will not be rubbed or bumped accidentally.

The patient will usually continue their antibiotic for two to three weeks and will also take anti-inflammatory medication for about the same length of time. If the patient experiences inflammation, redness, or **pain**, they should seek immediate medical treatment to avoid serious complications. If complications do not occur, the patient will normally visit the doctor a few days after the surgery and, then again, after a week and finally after a month.

Any type of after care is not necessary for the intraocular lens itself. It becomes a permanent part of the eye. The eye should be completely healed within eight weeks of the surgery.

Risks

Cataract surgery itself is quite safe and is almost always treated successfully; over 90% of the time, complications do not occur. However, complications can occur and should be noted by anyone thinking about cataract surgery. Possible complications include intraocular infection (endophthalmitis), central retinal inflammation (macular **edema**), post-operative glaucoma, **retinal detachment**, bleeding under the retina (choroidal hemorrhage), and tiny lens fragments in the back (vitreous) cavity of the eye, all of which can lead to loss of sight.

If the following symptoms occur, contact your doctor immediately:

• Nausea, vomiting, or disproportionate amount of coughing

• Loss of vision in the eye

• Redness in the eye

• Excessive, persistent pain (especially if pain medications are being used)

• Flashes of light or floaters (spots) on the front of the eye.

An added risk of complications can also occur when other diseases are present. Such diseases may prevent an otherwise successful surgery from being completed satisfactorily. In such cases, vision may not be improved due to diseases present within the body, and especially those diseases of the eyes, such as glaucoma. Consequently, it may be wise to treat such diseases before having cataract surgery.

Since increased use of the phacoemulsification method of cataract surgery, researchers have noted a decline in cases of infection (endophthalmitis). This probably is because injectable intraocular lenses do not make contact with the ocular surface. In 2004, the FDA approved a new capsular tension ring for use in cataract surgery that helps prevent lens dislocation and other possible complications of surgery.

After cataract surgery, some patients develop posterior capsule opacification (PCO). This complication occurs when the back of the lens capsule becomes cloudy and sight is again degraded. However, if this happens, then a procedure called yttrium-aluminum-garnet (YAG) laser capsulotomy can be performed. The procedure allows light to pass through the clouded capsule, which solves the problem.

Normal results

Ordinarily, according to the National Institutes of Health, about 95% of patients experience improved visual acuity and improved perception of the vividness of colors, leading to increased abilities in many activities, including reading, needlework, driving, golf, and tennis, for example. This improvement in sight should be apparent within a few days after the surgery. In addition, sometimes implanted corrective lenses eliminate the need for eyeglasses or **contact lenses**. Researchers and manufacturers also continue to work to improve the lenses available in cataract surgeries, so that eventual vision and outcome are improved.

Resources

PERIODICALS

"Cataract Removal, Nonpenetrating Glaucoma Surgery Can Be Combined." *Biotech Week* September 13, 2003: 133.

"FDA Approves Stabil Eyes Capsular Tension Rig for Cataract Surgery." *Biotech Week* May 26, 2004: 23.

Groves, Nancy. "Advances in Cataract Surgery Driven by Technology; Surgeons Able to Achieve Better Outcomes with New IOL, Viscoadaptive Devices." *Ophthalmology Times* April 1, 2004: 39.

Mayer, E., et al. "A 10-year Retrospective Survey of Cataract Surgery and Endophthalmitis in a Single Yey Unit: Injectable Lenses Lower the Incidence of Endophthalmitis." *British Journal of Ophthalmology* July 2003: 867–873.

OTHER

"Cataract in Adults: A Patient's Guide." *National Library of Medicine Page.* http://text.nlm.nih.gov.

"Patient Information." *Digital Journal of Ophthalmology.* http://www.djo.harvard.edu/site.php?url = /patients/pi.

ORGANIZATIONS

American Academy of Ophthalmology (AAO), P. O. Box 7424, San Francisco, CA, 94120-7424, (415) 561-8500, (415) 561-8500, http://www.aao.org.

American Society of Cataract and Refractive Surgery, 4000 Legato Road, Suite 700, Fairfax, VA, 22033, (703) 591-2220, (703) 591-0614, http://www.ascrs.org.

Lorraine Lica, PhD
Teresa G. Odle

Cat-bite infection *see* **Animal bite infections**

Cat-scratch disease

Definition

Cat-scratch disease is an uncommon infection that typically results from a cat's scratch or bite. Most sufferers experience only moderate discomfort and find that their symptoms clear up without any lasting harm after a few weeks or months. Professional medical treatment is rarely needed.

Description

Cat-scratch disease (also called cat-scratch **fever**) is caused by the *Bartonella henselae* bacterium, which is found in cats around the world and is transmitted from cat to cat by fleas. Researchers have discovered that large numbers of North American cats carry antibodies for the disease (meaning that the cats have been infected at some point in their lives). Some parts of North America have much higher rates of cat infection than others, however. *Bartonella henselae* is uncommon or absent in cold climates, which fleas have difficulty tolerating, but prevalent in warm, humid places such as Memphis, Tennessee, where antibodies were found in 71% of the cats tested. The bacterium, which remains in a cat's bloodstream for several months after infection, seems to be harmless to most cats, and normally an infected cat will not display any symptoms. Kittens (cats less than one year old) are more likely than adult cats to be carrying the infection.

Bartonella henselae can infect people who are scratched or (more rarely) bitten or licked by a cat. It cannot be passed from person to person. Although cats are popular pets found in about 30% of American households, human infection appears to be rare. One study estimated that for every 100,000 Americans there are only 2.5 cases of cat-scratch disease each year (2.5/100,000). It is also unusual for more than one family member to become ill; a Florida investigation discovered multiple cases in only 3.5% of the families studied. Children and teenagers appear to be the most likely victims of cat-scratch disease, although the possibility exists that the disease may be more common among adults than previously thought.

Causes and symptoms

The first sign of cat-scratch disease may be a small blister at the site of a scratch or bite three to 10 days after injury. The blister (which sometimes contains pus) often looks like an insect bite and is usually found on the hands, arms, or head. Within two weeks of the blister's appearance, lymph nodes near the site of injury become swollen. Often the infected person develops a fever or experiences **fatigue** or headaches. The symptoms usually disappear within a month, although the lymph nodes may remain swollen for several months. Hepatitis, **pneumonia**, and other dangerous complications can arise, but the likelihood of cat-scratch disease posing a serious threat to health is very small. **AIDS** patients

KEY TERMS

Acetaminophen—A drug for relieving pain and fever.

AIDS—Acquired immunodeficiency syndrome. A disease that attacks the immune system.

Antibiotics—A category of manufactured substances used to combat infection.

Antibodies—Special substances created by the body to combat infection.

Bacterium—A tiny organism. Some bacteria cause disease.

Hepatitis—A disease that inflames the liver.

Immune system—A body system that combats disease.

Immunocompromised—Having a damaged immune system.

Lymph nodes—Small, kidney-shaped organs that filter a fluid called lymph.

Pneumonia—A disease that inflames the lungs.

Pus—A thick yellowish or greenish fluid.

and other immunocompromised people face the greatest risk of dangerous complications.

Occasionally, the symptoms of cat-scratch disease take the form of what is called Parinaud's oculoglandular syndrome. In such cases, a small sore develops on the palpebral conjunctiva (the membrane lining the inner eyelid), and is often accompanied by **conjunctivitis** (inflammation of the membrane) and swollen lymph nodes in front of the ear. Researchers suspect that the first step in the development of Parinaud's oculoglandular syndrome occurs when *Bartonella henselae* bacteria pass from a cat's saliva to its fur during grooming. Rubbing one's eyes after handling the cat then transmits the bacteria to the conjunctiva.

Diagnosis

A family doctor should be called whenever a cat scratch or bite fails to heal normally or is followed by a persistent fever or other unusual symptoms such as long-lasting bone or joint **pain**. The appearance of painful and swollen lymph nodes is another reason for consulting a doctor. When cat-scratch disease is suspected, the doctor will ask about a history of exposure to cats and look for evidence of a cat scratch or bite and swollen lymph nodes. A blood test for *Bartonella henselae* may be ordered to confirm the doctor's diagnosis.

Treatment

For otherwise healthy people, rest and over-the-counter medications for reducing fever and discomfort (such as **acetaminophen**) while waiting for the disease to run its course are usually all that is necessary. **Antibiotics** are prescribed in some cases, particularly when complications occur or the lymph nodes remain swollen and painful for more than two or three months, but

there is no agreement among doctors about when and how they should be used. If a lymph node becomes very swollen and painful, the family doctor may decide to drain it.

Prognosis

Most people recover completely from a bout of cat-scratch disease. Further attacks are rare.

Prevention

Certain common–sense precautions can be taken to guard against the disease. Scratches and **bites** should be washed immediately with soap and water, and it is never a good idea to rub one's eyes after handling a cat without first washing one's hands. Children should be told not to play with stray cats or make cats angry. Immunocompromised people should avoid owning kittens, which are more likely than adult cats to be infectious. Because cat-scratch disease is usually not a life-threatening illness and people tend to form strong emotional bonds with their cats, doctors do not recommend getting rid of a cat suspected of carrying the disease.

Resources

PERIODICALS

Smith, David L. "Cat-Scratch Disease and Related Clinical Syndromes." *American Family Physician* April 1997: 1783.

Howard Baker

Cat-scratch fever *see* **Cat-scratch disease**

CAT scan *see* **Computed tomography scans**

Cataracts

Definition

A cataract is a cloudiness or opacity in the normally transparent crystalline lens of the eye. This cloudiness can cause a decrease in vision and may lead to eventual blindness.

Description

The human eye has several parts. The outer layer of the eyeball consists of a transparent dome-shaped cornea and an opaque, white sclera. The cornea and sclera help protect the eye. The next layer includes the iris, pupil, and ciliary body. The iris is the colored part of the eye and the pupil is the small dark round hole in the middle of the iris. The pupil and iris allow light into the eye. The ciliary body contains muscles that help in the eye's focusing ability. The lens lies behind the pupil and iris. It is covered by a cellophane-like capsule. The lens is normally transparent, elliptical in shape, and somewhat elastic. This elasticity allows the lens to focus on both near and far objects. The lens is attached to the ciliary body by fibers (zonules of Zinn). Muscles in the ciliary body act on the zonules, which then change the shape of the lens. This process is called accommodation—the lens focuses images to help make vision clear. As people age, the lens hardens and changes shape less easily. As a result, the accommodation process becomes more difficult, making it harder to see things up close. This generally occurs around the age of 40 and continues until about age 65. The condition is called **presbyopia**. It is a normal condition of **aging**, generally resulting in the need for reading glasses.

The lens is made up of approximately 35% protein and 65% water. As people age, degenerative changes

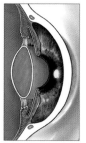
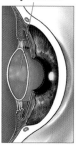

Normal lens (transparent)   Lens clouded by cataract

Cut section of the eye

Normal eye compared to an eye with a cataract. (© *Nucleus Medical Art, Inc/Alamy.*)

in the lens's proteins occur. Changes in the proteins, water content, enzymes, and other chemicals are some of the reasons for the formation of a cataract.

The major areas of the lens are the nucleus, the cortex, and the capsule. The nucleus is in the center of the lens, the cortex surrounds the nucleus, and the capsule is the outer layer. Opacities can occur in any area of the lens. Cataracts, then, can be classified according to location (nuclear, cortical, or posterior subcapular cataracts). The density and location of the cataract determine the amount of vision affected. If the cataract forms in the area of the lens directly behind the pupil, vision may be significantly impaired. A cataract that occurs on the outer edges or side of the lens will create less of a visual problem.

Cataracts in the elderly are so common that they are thought to be a normal part of the aging process. Between the ages of 52 and 64, there is a 50% chance of having a cataract, while at least 70% of those 70 and older are affected. In 2004, it was revealed that blacks are twice as likely to develop cataracts as whites. Cataracts associated with aging (senile or age-related cataracts) most often occur in both eyes, with each cataract progressing at a different rate. Initially, cataracts may not affect vision. If the cataract remains small or at the periphery of the lens, the visual changes may be minor.

Cataracts that occur in people other than the elderly are much less common. Congenital cataracts occur very rarely in newborns. Genetic defects or an infection or disease in the mother during **pregnancy** are among the causes of congenital cataracts. Traumatic cataracts may develop after a foreign body or trauma injures the lens or eye. Systemic illnesses, such as diabetes, may result in cataracts. Cataracts can also occur secondary to other eye diseases—for example, an inflammation of the inner layer of the eye (**uveitis**)

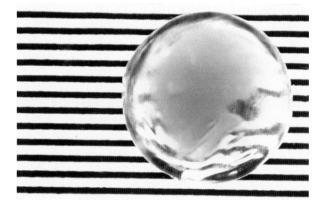

A dense cataract on lens of eye. (© *Margaret Cubberly/ Phototake. — All rights reserved.*)

or glaucoma. Such cataracts are called complicated cataracts. Toxic cataracts result from chemical toxicity, such as steroid use. Cataracts can also result from exposure to the sun's ultraviolet (UV) rays.

Causes and symptoms

Recent studies have been conducted to try to determine whether diet or the use of **vitamins** might have an effect on the formation of cataracts in older people. The results have been mixed, with some studies finding a connection and other studies finding none. Much interest has been focused on the use of antioxidant supplements as a protection against cataracts. Antioxidant vitamins such as vitamins A, C, E, and beta-carotene help the body clean-up oxygen-free radicals. Some vitamins are marketed specifically for the eyes. Patients should speak to their doctors about the use of such vitamins.

Smoking and alcohol intake have been implicated in cataract formation. Some studies have determined that a diet high in fat will increase the likelihood of cataract formation, while an increase in foods rich in **antioxidants** will reduce the incidence. More research is needed to determine if diet, smoking, alcohol consumption, or vitamins have any connection to the formation of cataracts.

There are several common symptoms of cataracts:

- gradual, painless onset of blurry, filmy, or fuzzy vision
- poor central vision
- frequent changes in eyeglass prescription
- changes in color vision
- increased glare from lights, especially oncoming headlights when driving at night
- "second sight" improvement in near vision (no longer needing reading glasses), but a decrease in distance vision
- poor vision in sunlight
- presence of a milky whiteness in the pupil as the cataract progresses.

Diagnosis

Both ophthalmologists and optometrists may detect and monitor cataract growth and prescribe prescription lenses for visual deficits. However, only an ophthalmologist can perform cataract extraction.

Cataracts are easily diagnosed from the reporting of symptoms, a visual acuity exam using an eye chart, and by examination of the eye itself. Shining a penlight into the pupil may reveal opacities or a color change of the lens even before visual symptoms have developed.

An instrument called a slit lamp is basically a large microscope. This lets the doctor examine the front of the eye and the lens. The slit lamp helps the doctor determine the location of the cataract.

Some other diagnostic tests may be used to determine if cataracts are present or how well the patient may potentially see after surgery. These include a glare test, potential vision test, and contrast sensitivity test.

Treatment

For cataracts that cause no symptoms or only minor visual changes, no treatment may be necessary. Continued monitoring and assessment of the cataract is needed by an ophthalmologist or optometrist at scheduled office visits. Increased strength in prescription eyeglasses or **contact lenses** may be helpful. This may be all that is required if the cataract does not reduce the patient's quality of life.

Cataract surgery—the only option for patients whose cataracts interfere with vision to the extent of affecting their daily lives—is the most frequently performed surgery in the United States. It generally improves vision in over 90% of patients. Some people have heard that a cataract should be "ripe" before being removed. A cataract is considered ripe or mature when the lens is completely opaque. Most cataracts are removed before they reach this stage. Sometimes cataracts need to be removed so that the doctor can examine the back of the eye more carefully. This is important in patients with diseases that may affect the eye. If cataracts are present in both eyes, only one eye at a time should be operated on. Healing occurs in the first eye before the second cataract is removed, sometimes as early as the following week. A final eyeglass prescription is usually given about four to six weeks after surgery. Patients will still need reading glasses. The overall health of the patient needs to be considered in making the decision to operate. However, age alone need not preclude effective surgical treatment of cataracts. People in their nineties can have successful return of vision after **cataract surgery**.

Surgery to remove cataracts is generally an outpatient procedure. A local anesthetic is used and the procedure lasts about one hour. Removal of the cloudy lens can be done by several different procedures. The three types of cataract surgery available are:

- Extracapsular cataract extraction. This type of cataract extraction is the most common. The lens and the front portion of the capsule are removed. The back part of the capsule remains, providing strength to the eye.
- Intracapsular cataract extraction. The lens and the entire capsule are removed. This method carries an

KEY TERMS

Aphakia—Absence of the lens of the eye.

Ciliary body—A structure in the eye that contains muscles that will affect the focusing of the lens.

Glaucoma—Disease of the eye characterized by increased pressure of the fluid inside the eye. Untreated, glaucoma can lead to blindness.

Phacoemulsification—Surgical procedure to remove a cataract using sound waves to disintegrate the lens which is then removed by suction.

Retina—The innermost layer of the eyeball. Images focused onto the retina are then sent to the brain.

Ultraviolet radiation (UV)—Invisible light rays that may be responsible for sunburns, skin cancers, and cataract formation.

Uveitis—Inflammation of the uvea. The uvea is a continuous layer of tissue that consists of the iris, the ciliary body, and the choroid. The uvea lies between the retina and sclera.

increased risk for detachment of the retina and swelling after surgery. It is rarely used.

• Phacoemulsification. This type of extracapsular extraction needs a very small incision, resulting in faster healing. Ultrasonic vibration is applied to the lens to break it up into very small pieces which are then aspirated out of the eye with suction by the ophthalmologist. A new liquid technique that its inventor says may one day replace ultrasound has been invented, but has not yet been proven in clinical trials.

A replacement lens is usually inserted at the time of the surgery. A plastic artificial lens called an intraocular lens (IOL) is placed in the remaining posterior lens capsule of the eye. When the intracapsular extraction method is used, an IOL may be clipped onto the iris. Contact lenses and cataract glasses (aphakic lenses) are prescribed if an IOL was not inserted. A folding IOL is used when phacoemulsification is performed to accommodate the small incision.

Antibiotic drops to prevent infection and **steroids** to reduce inflammation are prescribed after surgery. An eye shield or glasses during the day will protect the eye from injury while it heals. During the night, an eye shield is worn. The patient returns to the doctor the day after surgery for assessment, with several follow-up visits over the next two months to monitor the healing process.

Prognosis

The success rate of cataract extraction is very high, with a good prognosis. A visual acuity of 20/40 or better may be achieved. If an extracapsular cataract extraction was performed, a secondary cataract may develop in the remaining back portion of the capsule. This can occur one to two years after surgery. YAG capsulotomy is most often used for this type of cataract. YAG stands for yttrium aluminum garnet, the name of the laser used for this procedure. This is a painless

outpatient procedure and requires no incision. The laser beam makes a small opening in the remaining back part of the capsule, allowing light through.

In a very small percentage (3–5%) of surgical cataract extractions, complications occur. Infections, swelling of the cornea (**edema**), bleeding, **retinal detachment**, and the onset of glaucoma have been reported. Some problems may occur one to two days, or even several weeks, after surgery. Any haziness, redness, decrease in vision, **nausea**, or **pain** should be reported to the surgeon immediately.

Prevention

Preventive measures emphasize protecting the eyes from UV radiation by wearing glasses with a special coating to protect against UV rays. Dark lenses alone are not sufficient. The lenses must protect against UV light (specifically, UV-A and UV-B). Antioxidants may also provide some protection by reducing free radicals that can damage lens proteins. A healthy diet rich in sources of antioxidants, including citrus fruits, sweet potatoes, carrots, green leafy vegetables, and/or vitamin supplements may be helpful. In 2004, research in England revealed that **nonsteroidal anti-inflammatory drugs** (over-the counter pain killers such as **aspirin**) may help decrease risk of cataracts by as much as 43%. When taking certain medications, such as steroids, more frequent eye exams may be necessary. Patients should speak to their doctors to see if medications may affect their eyes.

Resources

PERIODICALS

"Blacks May Have Higher Incidence of Cataract." *Review of Optometry* April 15, 2004: 12.
"Research Suggests Aspirin Helps Combat Cataracts." *Health & Medicine Week* June 21, 2004: 724.
Talsma, Julia. "Liquefication Device Provides Safe Removal of All Cataracts: Lens Emulsified with BSS Micropulses

Using Reusable Titanium Handpiece with Smooth Polymer Tip." *Ophthlamology Times* June 1, 2004: 50.

ORGANIZATIONS

American Academy of Ophthalmology (AAO), P. O. Box 7424, San Francisco, CA, 94120-7424, (415) 561-8500, (415) 561-8500, http://www.aao.org.

American Optometric Association, 243 North Lindbergh Blvd., St. Louis, MO, 63141, (314) 991-4100, (314) 991-4101, (800) 365-2219, http://www.aoa.org/.

Lighthouse International, 111 East 59th Street, New York, NY, 10022-120, (212) 821-9200, (212) 821-9707, (800) 829-0500, info@lighthouse.org, http://www.lighthouse.org.

Prevent Blindness America, 211 West Wacker Drive, Suite 1700, Chicago, IL, 60606, (800) 331-2020, http://www.preventblindness.org.

Cynthia L. Frozena, RN
Teresa G. Odle

Catatonia

Definition

Catatonia is a condition marked by changes in muscle tone or activity associated with a large number of serious mental and physical illnesses. There are two distinct sets of symptoms that are characteristic of this condition. In catatonic stupor the individual experiences a deficit of motor (movement) activity that can render him/her motionless. Catatonic excitement, or excessive movement, is associated with violent behavior directed toward oneself or others.

Features of catatonia may also be seen in Neuroleptic Malignant Syndrome (NMS) which is an uncommon (but potentially lethal) reaction to some medications used to treat major mental illnesses. NMS is considered a medical emergency since 25% of untreated cases result in **death**. Catatonia can also be present in individuals suffering from a number of other physical and emotional conditions such as drug intoxication, depression, and **schizophrenia**. It is most commonly associated with **mood disorders**.

Description

In catatonic stupor, motor activity may be reduced to zero. Individuals avoid bathing and grooming, make little or no eye contact with others, may be mute and rigid, and initiate no social behaviors. In catatonic excitement the individual is extremely hyperactive although the activity seems to have no purpose. Violence toward him/herself or others may also be seen.

NMS is observed as a dangerous side effect associated with certain neuroleptic (antipsychotic) drugs such as haloperidol (Haldol). It comes on suddenly and is characterized by stiffening of the muscles, **fever**, confusion, and heavy sweating.

Catatonia can also be categorized as intrinsic or extrinsic. If the condition has an identifiable cause, it is designated as extrinsic. If no cause can be determined following **physical examination**, laboratory testing, and history taking, the illness is considered to be intrinsic.

Causes and symptoms

The causes of catatonia are largely unknown although research indicates that brain structure and function are altered in this condition. While this and other information point to a physical cause, none has yet been proven. A variety of medical conditions also may lead to catatonia including head trauma, cerebrovascular disease, **encephalitis**, and certain metabolic disorders. NMS is an adverse side effect of certain **antipsychotic drugs**.

A variety of symptoms are associated with catatonia. Among the more common are echopraxia (imitation of the gestures of others) and echolalia (parrot-like repetition of words spoken by others). Other signs and symptoms include violence directed toward him/herself, the assumption of inappropriate posture, selective **mutism**, negativism, facial grimaces, and animal-like noises.

Catatonic stupor is marked by immobility and a behavior known as *cerea flexibilitas* (waxy flexibility) in which the individual can be made to assume bizarre (and sometimes painful) postures that they will maintain for extended periods of time. The individual may become dehydrated and malnourished because food and liquids are refused. In extreme situations such individuals must be fed through a tube. Catatonic excitement is characterized by hyperactivity and violence; the individual may harm him/herself or others. On rare occasions, **isolation** or restraint may be needed to ensure the individual's safety and the safety of others.

Diagnosis

Recognition of catatonia is made on the basis of specific movement symptoms. These include odd ways of walking such as walking on tiptoes or ritualistic pacing, and rarely, hopping and skipping. Repetitive odd movements of the fingers or hands, as well as

KEY TERMS

Barbiturates—A group of medicines that slow breathing and lower the body temperature and blood pressure. They can be habit forming and are now used chiefly for anesthesia.

Benzodiazipines—This group of medicines is used to help reduce anxiety (especially before surgery) and to help people sleep.

Electroconvulsive therapy—This type of therapy is used to treat major depression and severe mental illness that does not respond to medications. A

measured dose of electricity is introduced into the brain in order to produce a convulsion. Electroconvulsive therapy is safe and effective.

Mutism—The inability or refusal to speak.

Negativism—Behavior characterized by resistance, opposition, and refusal to cooperate with requests, even the most reasonable ones.

Neuroleptic drugs—Antipsychotic drugs, including major tranquilizers, used in the treatment of psychoses like schizophrenia.

imitating the speech or movements of others also may indicate that catatonia is present. There are no laboratory or other tests that can be used to positively diagnose this condition, but medical and neurological tests are necessary to rule out underlying lesions or disorders that may be causing the symptoms observed.

Treatment

Treatment of catatonia includes medications such as benzodiazipines (which are the preferred treatment) and rarely **barbiturates**. Antipsychotic drugs may be appropriate in some cases, but often cause catatonia to worsen. **Electroconvulsive therapy** may prove beneficial for clients who do not respond to medication. If these approaches are unsuccessful, treatment will be redirected to attempts to control the signs and symptoms of the illness.

Prognosis

Catatonia usually responds quickly to medication interventions.

Prevention

There is currently no known way to prevent catatonia because the cause has not yet been identified. Research efforts continue to explore possible origins. Avoiding excessive use of neuroleptic drugs can help minimize the risk of developing catatonic-like symptoms.

Resources

BOOKS

Frisch, Noreen Cavan, and Lawrence E. Frisch.*Psychiatric Mental Health Nursing*. 4th ed. Clifton Park, NY: Delmar Publishers, 2011.

Donald G. Barstow, RN

Catecholamines tests

Definition

Catecholamines is a collective term for the hormones epinephrine, norepinephrine, and dopamine. Manufactured chiefly by the chromaffin cells of the adrenal glands, these hormones are involved in readying the body for the "fight-or-flight" response (also known as the alarm reaction). When these hormones are released, the heart beats stronger and faster, blood pressure rises, more blood flows to the brain and muscles, the liver releases stores of energy as a sugar the body can readily use (glucose), the rate of breathing increases and airways widen, and digestive activity slows. These reactions direct more oxygen and fuel to the organs most active in responding to stress–mainly the brain, heart, and skeletal muscles.

Purpose

Pheochromocytoma (a tumor of the chromaffin cells of the adrenal gland) and tumors of the nervous system (neuroblastomas, ganglioneuroblastomas, and ganglioneuromas) that affect hormone production can cause excessive levels of different catecholamines to be secreted. This results in constant or intermittent high blood pressure (**hypertension**). Episodes of high blood pressure may be accompanied by symptoms such as **headache**, sweating, **palpitations**, and **anxiety**. The catecholamines test can be ordered, then, to determine if high blood pressure and other symptoms are related to improper hormone secretion and to identify the type of tumor causing elevated catecholamine levels.

KEY TERMS

Dopamine—Dopamine is a precursor of epinephrine and norepinephrine.

Epinephrine—Epinephrine, also called adrenaline, is a naturally occurring hormone released by the adrenal glands in response to signals from the sympathetic nervous system. These signals are triggered by stress, exercise, or by emotions such as fear.

Ganglioneuroma—A ganglioneuroma is a tumor composed of mature nerve cells.

Neuroblastoma—Neuroblastoma is a tumor of the adrenal glands or sympathetic nervous system. Neuroblastomas can range from being relatively harmless to highly malignant.

Norepinephrine—Norepinephrine is a hormone secreted by certain nerve endings of the sympathetic nervous system, and by the medulla (center) of the adrenal glands. Its primary function is to help maintain a constant blood pressure by stimulating certain blood vessels to constrict when the blood pressure falls below normal.

Pheochromocytoma—A pheochromocytoma is a tumor that originates from the adrenal gland's chromaffin cells, causing overproduction of catecholamines, powerful hormones that induce high blood pressure and other symptoms.

Description

The catecholamines test can be performed on either blood or urine. If performed on blood, the test may require one or two samples, depending on the physician's request. The first blood sample will be drawn after the patient has been lying down in a warm, comfortable environment for at least 30 minutes. If a second sample is needed, the patient will be asked to stand for 10 minutes before the blood is drawn. Instead of a venipuncture, which can be stressful for the patient, possibly increasing catecholamine levels in the blood, a plastic or rubber tube-like device called a catheter may be used to collect the blood samples. The catheter would be inserted in a vein 24 hours in advance, eliminating the need for needle punctures at the time of the test.

It may take up to a week for a lab to complete testing of the samples. Because blood levels of catecholamines commonly go up and down in response to such factors as temperature, **stress**, postural change, diet, **smoking**, **obesity**, and many drugs, abnormally high blood test results should be confirmed with a 24-hour urine test. In addition, catecholamine secretion from a tumor may not be steady, but may occur periodically during the day, and potentially could be missed when blood testing is used. The urine test provides the laboratory with a specimen that reflects catecholamine production over an entire 24-hour period. If urine is tested, the patient or a healthcare worker must collect all the urine passed over the 24-hour period.

Preparation

It is important that the patient refrain from using certain medications, especially cold or allergy remedies, for two weeks before the test. Certain foods—including bananas, avocados, cheese, coffee, tea, cocoa, beer, licorice, citrus fruit, vanilla, and Chianti—must be avoided for 48 hours prior to testing. However, people should be sure to get adequate amounts of vitamin C before the test, because this vitamin is necessary for catecholamine formation. The patient should be **fasting** (nothing to eat or drink) for 10 to 24 hours before the blood test and should not smoke for 24 hours beforehand. Some laboratories may call for additional restrictions. As much as possible, the patient should try to avoid excessive physical **exercise** and emotional stress before the test, because either may alter test results by causing increased secretion of epinephrine and norepinephrine.

Patients collecting their own 24-hour urine samples will be given a container with special instructions. The urine samples must be refrigerated.

Risks

Risks for the blood test are minimal, but may include slight bleeding from the venipuncture site, **fainting** or feeling lightheaded after blood is drawn, or blood accumulating under the puncture site (hematoma). There are no risks for the urine test.

Normal results

Reference ranges are laboratory-specific, vary according to methodology of testing, and differ between blood and urine samples. If testing is done by the method called High Performance Liquid Chromatography (HPLC), typical values for blood and urine follow.

Reference ranges for blood catecholamines

Supine (lying down): Epinephrine less than 50 pg/mL, norepinephrine less than 410 pg/mL, and dopamine less than 90 pg/mL. Standing: Values for blood specimens taken when the subject is standing are higher than the ranges for supine posture for norepinephrine and epinephrine, but not for dopamine.

Reference ranges for urine catecholamines

Epinephrine 0–20 micrograms per 24 hours; norepinephrine 15–80 micrograms per 24 hours; dopamine 65–400 micrograms per 24 hours.

Abnormal results

Depending on the results, high catecholamine levels can indicate different conditions and/or causes:

- High catecholamine levels can help to verify pheochromocytoma, neuroblastoma, or ganglioneuroma. An aid to diagnosis is the fact that an adrenal medullary tumor (pheochromocytoma) secretes epinephrine, whereas ganglioneuroma and neuroblastoma secrete norepinephrine.
- Elevations are possible with, but do not directly confirm, thyroid disorders, low blood sugar (hypoglycemia), or heart disease.
- Electroshock therapy, or shock resulting from hemorrhage or exposure to toxins, can raise catecholamine levels.
- In the patient with normal or low baseline catecholamine levels, failure to show an increase in the sample taken after standing suggests an autonomic nervous system dysfunction (the division of the nervous system responsible for the automatic or unconscious regulation of internal body functioning).

Resources

BOOKS

Pagana, Kathleen Deska, and Timothy J. Pagana. *Mosby's Manual of Diagnostic and Laboratory Tests*. 4th ed. St. Louis: Mosby, 2009.

Janis O. Flores

▌Catheter ablation

Definition

Catheter ablation of an irregular heartbeat involves having a tube (a catheter) inserted into the heart through which electrical energy is sent to either reset the heartbeat or stop the heart from beating so a mechanical pacemaker can be put in place.

Purpose

Irregular heartbeats can occur in healthy people without causing any dangerous symptoms or requiring medical attention. Slight changes in the normal patterns of heartbeats often reset themselves without notice.

But when the heartbeat is greatly disrupted–either because of traumatic injury, disease, **hypertension**, surgery, or reduced blood flow to the heart caused by blockages in the blood vessels that nourish the heart– the condition must be recognized and treated immediately. Otherwise, it can be fatal.

Various drugs can be used to control and help reset these abnormal heart rhythms (**arrhythmias**). The technique of catheter ablation (meaning tube-guided removal) is used to interrupt the abnormal contractions in the heart, allowing normal heart beating to resume. **Atrial fibrillation and flutter** and **Wolff-Parkinson-White syndrome** are two of the most common disorders treated with catheter ablation.

Precautions

The improper correction of abnormal heartbeats can cause additional arrhythmias and can be fatal. Abnormalities in different areas of the heart cause different types of irregular heartbeats; the type of arrhythmia must be clearly defined before this procedure can be properly done.

Description

Catheter ablation involves delivering highly focused heat (or radio frequency energy) to specific areas of the heart. Radio frequency energy is very rapidly alternating electrical current that is produced at the tip of the catheter that is placed inside the heart. At the same time as the catheter is inserted, a second electrode is placed on the patient's skin. When the catheter is energized, the body conducts the energy from the catheter's tip, through the heart and to the electrode on the skin's surface, completing the circuit.

Although very little electricity is given off by the catheter, the instrument does generate a large amount of heat. This heat is absorbed by the heart tissue, causing a small localized burn and destroying the tissue in contact with the catheter tip; in this way, small regions of heart tissue are burned in a controlled manner. This controlled destruction of small sections

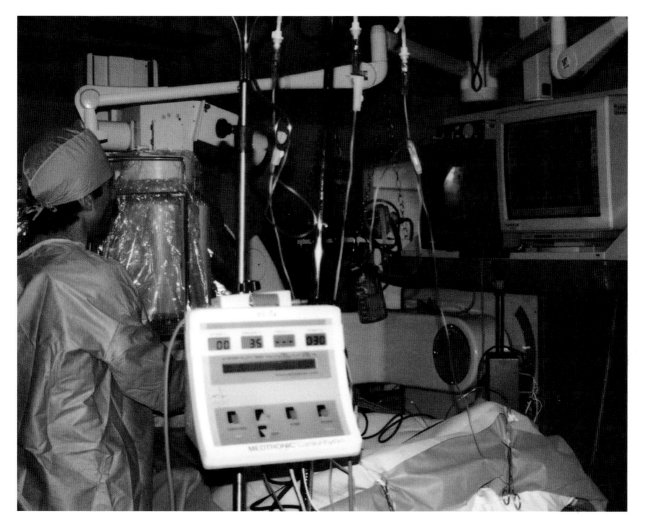

During catheter ablation, a long flexible tube called a catheter is inserted into a vein in the patient's groin and guided toward the heart. A special x-ray machine called a fluoroscope helps the electrophysiologist visualize correct placement. *(Collette Placek. Reproduced by permission.)*

of heart muscle actually kills the nerve cells causing the irregular heartbeat, stopping the nerve signals that are passing through this section of the heart. This usually causes the irregular heartbeat to be reset into a normal heartbeat.

Preparation

People can undergo this procedure by having **general anesthesia** or by taking medicines to make them relaxed and sleepy (sedatives) along with painkillers. Once the type of irregular heartbeat is identified and these medicines are given, the catheter is inserted through a blood vessel and into the heart. Importantly, correct placement of the catheter is visualized by using a specialized type of x-ray machine called a fluoroscope.

Aftercare

Being sure the patient is comfortable during and after this procedure is very important. However, because each person may have a different arrhythmia and possibly other medical problems as well, each patient's needs must be evaluated individually.

Risks

Overall, fewer than 5% of people having this procedure experience complications. The most common complications are usually related to blood vessel injury when the catheter is inserted and to different heart-related problems due to the moving of the catheter within the heart. However, in general, this technique is safe and can control many different heart arrhythmias.

Normal results

Depending upon the type of irregular heartbeat being treated, either the normal heartbeat resumes after treatment or the ability of the heart to beat on its own is lost, requiring the insertion of a pacemaker to stimulate the heart to beat regularly.

Abnormal results

Additional irregular heartbeats can occur as a result of this procedure, as can damage to the blood vessels that feed the heart. Because this procedure requires the use of the x-ray machine called a fluoroscope, there is exposure to x-ray radiation, but it is doubtful that this is harmful in adult patients. The risk versus benefit is considered with pediatric patients.

ORGANIZATIONS

American Heart Association National Center, 7272 Greenville Avenue, Dallas, TX, 75231, (800) 242-8721, Review.personal.info@heart.org.

Dominic De Bellis, PhD

Cat's cry syndrome *see* **Cri du chat syndrome**

CBC *see* **Blood count**

CEA test *see* **Carcinoembryonic antigen test**

CEB *see* **Chronic fatigue syndrome**

Cefaclor *see* **Cephalosporins**

Cefadroxil *see* **Cephalosporins**

Cefixime *see* **Cephalosporins**

Cefprozil *see* **Cephalosporins**

Cefurox *see* **Cephalosporins**

Celiac disease

Definition

Celiac disease is a disease of the digestive system that damages the small intestine and interferes with the absorption of nutrients from food.

Demographics

Celiac disease may be discovered at any age, from infancy through adulthood. The disorder is more commonly found among white Europeans or in people of European descent. It is very unusual to find celiac disease in African or Asian people. The exact incidence of the disease is uncertain. Estimates vary from one in 5,000, to as many as one in every 300 individuals with this background. The prevalence of celiac disease seems to be different from one European country to another, and between Europe and the United States. This may be due to differences in diet and/or unrecognized disease. A recent study of random blood samples tested for celiac disease in the United States showed one in 250 testing positive. It is clearly underdiagnosed, probably due to the symptoms being attributed to another problem, or lack of knowledge about celiac disease by physicians and laboratories.

Because celiac disease has a hereditary influence, close relatives (especially first degree relatives, such as children, siblings, and parents) have a higher risk of being affected with the condition. The chance that a first degree relative of someone with celiac disease will have the disease is about 10%.

As more is learned about celiac disease, it becomes evident that there are many variations which may not produce typical symptoms. It may even be clinically "silent," where no obvious problems related to the disease are apparent.

Description

Celiac disease occurs when the body reacts abnormally to gluten, a protein found in wheat, rye, barley, and possibly oats. When someone with celiac disease eats foods containing gluten, that person's immune system causes an inflammatory response in the small intestine, which damages the tissues and results in an impaired ability to absorb nutrients from foods. The inflammation and malabsorption create wide–ranging problems in many systems of the body. Since the body's own immune system causes the damage, celiac disease is classified as an autoimmune disorder. Celiac

Celiac disease

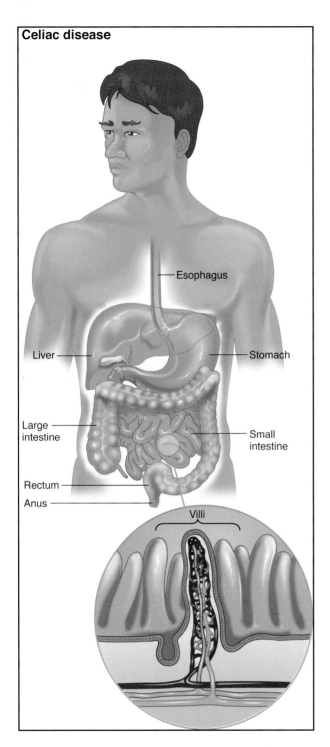

Esophagus

Liver

Stomach

Large
intestine

Small
intestine

Rectum

Anus

Villi

When people with celiac disease eat foods or use products containing gluten, their immune system responds by damaging or destroying villi in the intestine. Villi allows nutrients from food to be absorbed into the bloodstream; without healthy villi, a person becomes malnourished, regardless of the quantity of food eaten. *(Illustration by Electronic Illustrators Group. Reproduced by permission of Gale, a part of Cengage Learning.)*

disease may also be called sprue, nontropical sprue, gluten sensitive enteropathy, celiac sprue, and adult celiac disease.

Each person with celiac disease is affected differently. When food containing gluten reaches the small intestine, the immune system begins to attack a substance called gliadin, which is found in the gluten. The resulting inflammation causes damage to the delicate finger–like structures in the intestine, called villi, where food absorption actually takes place. This damage is referred to as villus atrophy. The patient may experience a number of symptoms related to the inflammation and the chemicals it releases, and/or the lack of ability to absorb nutrients from food, which can cause **malnutrition**.

Risk factors

People with **autoimmune disorders** are more at risk for celiac disease. Since it can run in families, risk is also increased if there is a family history of the condition.

Many disorders are associated with celiac disease, though the nature of the connection is unclear. One type of **epilepsy** is linked to celiac disease. Once their celiac disease is successfully treated, a significant number of these patients have fewer or no seizures. Patients with **alopecia** areata, a condition where hair loss occurs in sharply defined areas, have been shown to have a higher risk of celiac disease than the general population. There appears to be a higher percentage of celiac disease among people with **Down syndrome**, but the link between the conditions is unknown.

Several conditions attributed to a disorder of the immune system have been associated with celiac disease. People with insulin dependent diabetes (type I) have a much higher incidence of celiac disease. One source estimates that as many as one in 20 insulin–dependent diabetics may have celiac disease. Patients with juvenile chronic arthritis, some thyroid diseases, and IgA deficiency are also more likely to develop celiac disease.

There is an increased risk of intestinal lymphoma, a type of **cancer**, in individuals with celiac disease. Successful treatment of the celiac disease seems to decrease the chance of developing lymphoma.

Causes and symptoms

The exact cause of celiac disease is unknown. It can run in families and has a genetic basis, but the pattern of inheritance is complicated. The type of inheritance pattern that celiac disease follows is called multifactorial (caused by many factors, both genetic and environmental). Researchers think that several factors must exist in order for the disease to occur. First, the patient must have a genetic predisposition to develop the disorder. Then, something in their environment acts as a stimulus to trigger their immune system, causing the disease to become active for the first time. For conditions with multifactorial inheritance, people without the genetic predisposition are less likely to develop the condition with exposure to the same triggers. Or, they may require more exposure to the stimulus before developing the disease than someone with a genetic predisposition. Several factors may provoke a reaction including surgery, especially gastrointestinal surgery; a change to a low fat diet, which has an increased number of wheat–based foods; **pregnancy**; **childbirth**; severe emotional **stress**; or a viral infection. This combination of genetic susceptibility and an outside agent leads to celiac disease.

Each person with celiac disease is affected differently. When food containing gluten reaches the small intestine, the immune system begins to attack a substance called gliadin, which is found in the gluten. The resulting inflammation causes damage to the delicate finger–like structures in the intestine, called villi, where food absorption actually takes place. The patient may experience a number of symptoms related to the inflammation and the chemicals it releases, and or the lack of ability to absorb nutrients from food, which can cause malnutrition.

The most commonly recognized symptoms of celiac disease relate to the improper absorption of food in the gastrointestinal system. Many patients with gastrointestinal symptoms will have **diarrhea** and fatty, greasy, unusually foul–smelling stools. The patient may complain of excessive gas (flatulence), distended abdomen, weight loss, and generalized weakness. Not all people have digestive system complications; some people only have irritability or depression. Irritability is one of the most common symptoms in children with celiac disease.

Not all patients have these problems. Unrecognized and untreated celiac disease may cause or contribute to a variety of other conditions. The decreased ability to digest, absorb, and utilize food properly (malabsorption) may cause anemia (low red blood count) from iron deficiency or easy bruising from a lack of vitamin K. Poor mineral absorption may result in **osteoporosis**, or "brittle bones," which may lead to bone **fractures**. Vitamin D levels may be insufficient and bring about a "softening" of

bones (osteomalacia), which produces **pain** and bony deformities, such as flattening or bending. Defects in the tooth enamel, characteristic of celiac disease, may be recognized by dentists. Celiac disease may be discovered during medical tests performed to investigate **failure to thrive** in infants, or lack of proper growth in children and adolescents. People with celiac disease may also experience **lactose intolerance** because they do not produce enough of the enzyme lactase, which breaks down the sugar in milk into a form the body can absorb. Other symptoms can include, **muscle cramps**, **fatigue**, delayed growth, **tingling** or **numbness** in the legs (from nerve damage), pale sores in the mouth (called aphthus ulcers), tooth discoloration, or missed menstrual periods (due to severe weight loss).

A distinctive, painful skin rash, called **dermatitis** herpetiformis, may be the first sign of celiac disease. Approximately 10% of patients with celiac disease have this rash, but it is estimated that 85% or more of patients with the rash have the disease.

Diagnosis

Examination

Because of the variety of ways celiac disease can manifest itself, it is often not diagnosed promptly. Its symptoms are similar to many other conditions including **irritable bowel syndrome**, **Crohn's disease**, ulcerative **colitis**, **diverticulosis**, intestinal infections, **chronic fatigue syndrome**, and depression. The condition may persist without diagnosis for so long that the patient accepts a general feeling of illness as normal. This leads to further delay in identifying and treating the disorder. It is not unusual for the disease to be identified in the course of medical examinations for seemingly unrelated problems.

Tests

If celiac disease is suspected, a blood test can be ordered. This test looks for the antibodies to gluten (called antigliadin, anti–endomysium, and antireticulin) that the immune system produces in celiac disease. Antibodies are chemicals produced by the immune system in response to substances that the body perceives to be threatening. Some experts advocate not just evaluating patients with symptoms, but using these blood studies as a screening test for high–risk individuals, such as those with relatives (especially first degree relatives) known to have the disorder. An abnormal result points toward celiac disease, but further tests are needed to confirm the diagnosis. Because celiac disease affects the ability of the body to absorb nutrients from food, several tests may be ordered to look for nutritional deficiencies. For example, doctors may order a test of iron levels in the blood because low levels of iron (anemia) may accompany celiac disease. Doctors may also order a test for fat in the stool, since celiac disease prevents the body from absorbing fat from food.

Procedures

If celiac disease is suspected, a biopsy (removal of a tiny piece of tissue surgically) of the small intestine can be performed. This is usually done by a gastroenterologist, a physician who specializes in diagnosing and treating bowel disorders. It is generally performed in the office, or in a hospital's outpatient department. The patient remains awake, but is sedated. A narrow tube, called an endoscope, is passed through the mouth, down through the stomach, and into the small intestine. A small sample of tissue is taken and sent to the laboratory for analysis. If it shows a pattern of tissue damage characteristic of celiac disease, the diagnosis is established.

The patient is then placed on a gluten–free diet (GFD). The physician will periodically recheck the level of antibodies in the patient's blood. After several months, the small intestine is biopsied again. If the diagnosis of celiac disease was correct (and the patient followed the rigorous diet), healing of the intestine will be apparent. Most experts agree that it is necessary to follow these steps in order to be sure of an accurate diagnosis.

Treatment

Traditional

The only treatment for celiac disease is a gluten–free diet. This may be easy for the doctor to prescribe, but difficult for the patient to follow. For most people, adhering to this diet will stop symptoms and prevent damage to the intestines. Damaged villi can be functional again in three to six months. This diet must be followed for life. For people whose symptoms are cured by the gluten–free diet, this is further evidence that their diagnosis is correct.

Gluten is present in any product that contains wheat, rye, barley, or oats. It helps make bread rise, and gives many foods a smooth, pleasing texture. In addition to the many obvious places gluten can be found in a normal diet, such as breads, cereals, and pasta, there are many hidden sources of gluten. These include ingredients added to foods to improve texture or enhance flavor and products used in food packaging. Gluten may even be present on surfaces used for food preparation or cooking.

Fresh foods that have not been artificially processed, such as fruits, vegetables, and meats, are permitted as part of a GFD. Gluten–free foods can be found in health food stores and in some supermarkets. Mail–order food companies often have a selection of gluten–free products. Help in dietary planning is available from dieticians (health care professionals specializing in food and **nutrition**) or from support groups for individuals with celiac disease. There are many cookbooks on the market specifically for those on a GFD.

Treating celiac disease with a GFD is almost always completely effective. Gastrointestinal complaints and other symptoms are alleviated. Secondary complications, such as anemia and osteoporosis, resolve in almost all patients. People who have experienced lactose intolerance related to their celiac disease usually see those symptoms subside as well. Although there is no risk and much potential benefit to this treatment, it is clear that avoiding all foods containing gluten can be difficult.

Experts emphasize the need for lifelong adherence to the GFD to avoid the long–term complications of this disorder. They point out that although the disease may have symptom–free periods if the diet is not followed, silent damage continues to occur. Celiac disease cannot be "outgrown" or cured, according to medical authorities.

Prognosis

Treating celiac disease with a strict GFD is almost always completely effective. Gastrointestinal complaints and other symptoms are alleviated. Secondary complications, such as anemia and osteoporosis, resolve in almost all patients. People who have experienced lactose intolerance related to their celiac disease usually see those symptoms subside as well.

Patients with celiac disease must adhere to a strict GFD throughout their lifetime. Once the diet has been followed for several years, individuals with celiac disease have similar mortality rates as the general population. However, about 10% of people with celiac disease develop a cancer involving the gastrointestinal tract (both carcinoma and lymphoma).

There are a small number of patients who develop a refractory type of celiac disease, where the GFD no longer seems effective. Once the diet has been thoroughly assessed to ensure no hidden sources of gluten are causing the problem, medications may be prescribed. **Steroids** or **immunosuppressant drugs** are often used to try to control the disease. It is unclear whether these efforts meet with much success.

Prevention

There is no way to prevent celiac disease. However, the key to decreasing its impact on overall health is early diagnosis and strict adherence to the prescribed gluten–free diet.

Resources

BOOKS

Dowler Shepard, Jules E. *The First Year: Celiac Disease and Living Gluten–Free: An Essential Guide for the Newly Diagnosed.* Philadelphia, PA: Da Capo Lifelong Books, 2008.

Green, Peter, and Rory Jones. *Celiac Disease: A Hidden Epidemic.* New York, NY: William Morrow, 2010.

Hasselbeck, Elisabeth. *The G–Free Diet: A Gluten–Free Survival Guide.* New York, NY: Center Street, 2009.

Libonati, Cleo J. *Recognizing Celiac Disease: Signs, Symptoms, Associated Disorders & Complications.* Ambler, PA: Gluten Free Works Publishing, 2007.

Llewelyn Bower, Sylvia. *Celiac Disease: A Guide to Living with Gluten Intolerance.* New York, NY: Demos Medical Publishing, 2006.

Tessmer, Kimberly A. *Tell Me What to Eat If I Have Celiac Disease: Nutrition You Can Live With.* Franklin Lakes, NJ: Career Press, 2009.

PERIODICALS

Chang, H. J., et al. "JAMA patient page, Celiac disease." *JAMA* 302, no. 11 (September 2009): 1248.

Cottingham, K. "Toward a better understanding of celiac disease." *Journal of Proteome Research* 8, no. 4 (April 2009): 1620.

Green, P. H. "Mortality in celiac disease, intestinal inflammation, and gluten sensitivity." *JAMA* 302, no. 11 (September 2009): 1225–1226

Malterre, T. "Digestive and nutritional considerations in celiac disease: could supplementation help?" *Alternative Medicine Review* 14, no. 3 (September 2009): 247–257

Plot, L., et al. "Infections may have a protective role in the etiopathogenesis of celiac disease." *Annals of the New York Academy of Sciences* 1173 (September 2009): 670–6748.

Roma, E., et al. "Changing pattern in the clinical presentation of pediatric celiac disease: a 30–year study." *Digestion* 80, no. 3 (2009): 185–191.

OTHER

"Celiac Disease." *National Digestive Diseases Information Clearinghouse.* Information Page. http://digestive.niddk.nih.gov/ddiseases/pubs/celiac (accessed October 24, 2009)

"Celiac Disease." *Medline Plus.* Health Topic. http://www.nlm.nih.gov/medlineplus/celiacdisease.html (accessed October 24, 2009)

"Celiac Disease." *FamilyDoctor.* Information Page. http://familydoctor.org/online/famdocen/home/common/digestive/disorders/236.printerview.html (accessed October 24, 2009)

"What I Need to Know About Celiac Disease." *National Digestive Diseases Information Clearinghouse.* Information Page. http://digestive.niddk.nih.gov/ddiseases/pubs/celiac_ez (accessed October 24, 2009)

"What Is Celiac Disease?" *Celiac Sprue Association.* Information Page. http://www.csaceliacs.org/celiac_defined.php (accessed October 24, 2009)

ORGANIZATIONS

American Celiac Disease Alliance, 2504 Duxbury Place, Alexandria, VA, 22308, (703) 622-3331, info@americanceliac.org, http://www.americanceliac.org.

Celiac Disease Foundation, 13251 Ventura Boulevard, #1, Studio City, CA, 91604, (818) 990–2354, (818) 990–2379, cdf@celiac.org, http://www.celiac.org.

Celiac Sprue Association/USA Inc., P.O. Box 31700, Omaha, NE, 68131–0700, (877) 272–4272, (402) 558–1347, celiacs@csaceliacs.org, http://www.csaceliacs.org.

Children's Digestive Health and Nutrition Foundation, P.O. Box 6, Flourtown, PA, 19031, (215) 233-0808, (215) 233-3918, mstallings@naspghan.org, http://www.cdhnf.org.

Gluten Intolerance Group of North America, 31214 124th Avenue SE, Auburn, WA, 98092-3667, (253) 833-6655, (253) 833-6675, info@gluten.net, http://www.gluten.net.

National Foundation for Celiac Awareness, 224 South Maple Street, Ambler, PA, 19002-0544, (215) 325-1306, info@celiaccentral.org, http://www. celiaccentral.org.

Judith Sims, MS
Amy Vance, MS, CGC

Cell therapy

Definition

Cell therapy is the transplantation of human or animal cells to replace or repair damaged tissue.

Purpose

The purpose of cell therapy is to introduce cells into the body that will grow and replace damaged tissue. Cell therapy differs from conventional stem cell therapy in that the cells injected into the body in cell therapy are already differentiated (e.g., muscle cells, gland cells), whereas conventional stem cell therapy utilizes undifferentiated, usually embryonic cells. Cell therapy has long been used by alternative medicine practitioners who have claimed great benefits; these have not been replicated by conventional medical practitioners.

Description

The theory behind cell therapy has been in existence for several hundred years. The first recorded discussion of the concept of cell therapy can be traced to Phillippus Aureolus Paracelsus (1493-1541), a German-Swiss physician and alchemist who wrote in his *Der grossen Wundartzney* (Great Surgery Book) in 1536 that "the heart heals the heart, lung heals the lung, spleen heals the spleen; like cures like." Paracelsus and many of his contemporaries agreed that the best way to treat an illness was to use living tissue to restore the ailing. In 1667, at a laboratory in the palace of Louis XIV, Jean-Baptiste Denis (1640–1704) attempted to transfuse blood from a calf into a mentally ill patient. Since blood **transfusion** is, in effect, a form of cell therapy, this could be the first documented case of this procedure. However, the first recorded attempt at non-blood cellular therapy occurred in 1912 when German physicians attempted to treat children with **hypothyroidism** (underactive thyroid gland), with thyroid cells.

In 1931, Dr. Paul Niehans (1882–1971), a Swiss physician, became known as "the father of cell therapy" quite by chance. After a surgical accident by a colleague, Niehans attempted to replace a patient's severely damaged parathyroid glands with those of a steer. When the patient began to rapidly deteriorate before the transplant could take place, Niehans decided to dice the steer's parathyroid gland into fine pieces, mix the pieces in a saline solution, and inject them into the dying patient. He reported that immediately the patient began to improve and, in fact, lived for another 30 years.

Cell therapy as alternative medicine

Cell therapy as performed by alternative medicine practitioners is very different from the controlled research done by conventional stem cell medical researchers. Alternative practitioners refer to their form of cell therapy by several other different names including xenotransplant therapy, glandular therapy, and fresh cell therapy. The procedure involves the injection of either whole fetal xenogenic (animal) cells (e.g., from sheep, cows, pigs, and sharks) or cell extracts from human tissue. Several different types of cells may be administered simultaneously.

Just as Paracelsus's theory of "like cures like," the types of cells that are administered correspond in some way with the organ or tissue in the patient that is failing. In other words, the cells are not species specific, but only organ specific. Alternative practitioners cannot explain how this type of cell therapy works, but proponents claim that the injected cells travel to the similar organ from which they were taken to revitalize and stimulate that organ's function and regenerate its cellular structure. Supporters of cellular treatment believe that embryonic and fetal animal tissue contain active therapeutic agents distinct from **vitamins**, **minerals**, hormones, or enzymes. This theory and these claims are rejected by practitioners of conventional medicine.

Proponents of cell therapy claim that it has been used successfully to rebuild damaged cartilage in joints, repair spinal cord injuries, strengthen a weakened immune system, treat autoimmune diseases such as **AIDS**, and help patients with neurological disorders such as **Alzheimer's disease**, Parkinson's disease, and **epilepsy**. Further claims of positive results have been made in the treatment of a wide range of chronic conditions such as arteriosclerosis, congenital defects, and **sexual dysfunction**. The therapy has also been used to treat **cancer** patients at a number of clinics in Tijuana, Mexico. Most of these claims are anecdotal. None of these application is supported by well-designed, controlled clinical studies.

Cell therapy as conventional medicine

Cell therapy in conventional medicine is still in the research and early clinical trial stage. This research is an outgrowth of stem cell research, and is performed in government-regulated laboratories by traditionally trained scientists. Embryonic stem cells are cells taken from an embryo before they have differentiated (specialized) into such specific cell types as muscle cells, nerve cells, or skin cells. In laboratory test tube and animal experiments, stem cells often can be manipulated into differentiating into specific types cells that have the

KEY TERMS

Anaphylactic shock—A severe allergic reaction that causes blood pressure drop, racing heart, swelling of the airway, rash, and possibly convulsions.

Culturing—To grow cells in a special substance, or media, in the laboratory.

Encephalitis—Inflammation of the brain that is often fatal.

Xenotransplant—Transplantation of animal cells or tissues into a human.

potential to replace differentiated cells in damaged organs. For example, in early 2008, researchers at the Diabetic Research Institute at the University of Miami in Florida were able to convert embryonic stem cells into insulin-producing cells and use them to treat insulin-dependent diabetes in mice.

Stem cells also have been found in bone marrow, and work is underway to see if other cells can be manipulated into transforming into differentiated cells. In January 2009, researchers at Northwestern University's Feinberg School of Medicine in Chicago announced that they had used a patient's own bone marrow stem cells to improve early symptoms of **multiple sclerosis**. Researchers noted improvement only in patients with early symptoms; in earlier research those with advanced symptoms had not improved. Other researchers are working on treating symptoms of **muscular dystrophy** with fully differentiated myoblasts (a kind of muscle cell) with mixed results. Still other are working with using cartilage cells (chondrocyte cells) to repair cartilage in joints such as the knee.

Stem cell therapy has potential to treat a wide range of diseases and disorders, but it is, for the most part, still in the test tube and animal research stage of development. Because of the ethical questions raised when the harvesting of stem cells destroys embryos, the United States has placed restrictions on some human stem cell research. These restrictions, however, do not apply to research that does not destroy embryos. However, much stem cell research is being carried out in other countries, especially Thailand, South Korea, and China, where fewer restrictions are placed on obtaining human stem cells for experimentation. A list of FDA-approved clinical trials involving stem cell therapy can be found at http://www.clinicaltrials.gov.

Preparations

Alternative practitioners use several processes to prepare cells for use. One procedure involves extracting cells from the patient and then culturing them in a laboratory until they multiply to the level needed for transplantation back into the same patient. Another procedure uses freshly removed fetal animal tissue that has been processed and suspended in a saline (salt water) solution. The preparation of fresh cells then may be either injected immediately into the patient or preserved by being freeze-dried or deep-frozen in liquid nitrogen before being injected. Injected cells may or may not be tested for pathogens, such as bacteria, viruses, or parasites, before use. Conventional cell therapy researchers work in laboratories where the growing environment of the cells is highly controlled and monitored to prevent contamination.

Precautions

Many forms of cell therapy in the United States are highly experimental procedures. Patients should approach any cell therapy treatments with extreme caution, inquire about their proven efficacy and legal use in the United States or their home country, and should only accept treatment only from a licensed physician who should educate the patient completely on the risks and possible side effects involved with cell therapy. These same cautions apply for patients interested in participating in FDA-approved clinical trials of cell therapy treatments.

Side effects

Because cell therapy encompasses a wide range of treatments and applications and many of these treatments are unproven and highly experimental, the full range of possible side effects of the treatments is not yet known. Anaphylactic shock, immune system reactions, and **encephalitis** are just a few of the known reported side effects in some patients to date.

Patients undergoing cell therapy treatments which use cells transplanted from animals or other humans run the risk of cell rejection, in which the body recognizes the cells as a foreign substance and uses immune system cells to attack and destroy them. Some forms of cell therapy use special coatings on the cells in an attempt to trick the immune system into recognizing the new cells as native to the body. There is also the chance of the cell solution transmitting a bacterial, viral, fungal, or parasitic infection to the patient. Careful screening and testing of cells for pathogens can reduce this risk.

PAUL NIEHANS (1882–1971)

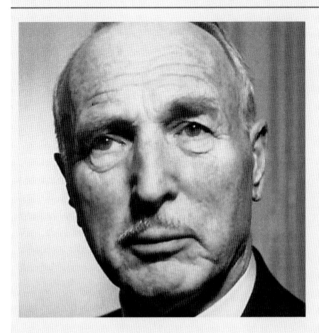

(© Bettmann/Corbis.)

Paul Niehans was born and raised in Switzerland. His father, a doctor, was dismayed when he entered the seminary, but Niehans quickly grew dissatisfied with religious life and took up medicine after all. He first studied at Bern, then completed an internship in Zurich.

Niehans enlisted in the Swiss Army in 1912. When war erupted in the Balkans, Niehans set up a hospital in Belgrade, Yugoslavia. The war provided him the opportunity to treat numerous patients, gaining a firsthand knowledge of the body and its workings.

Since 1913, Niehans had been intrigued with Alexis Carrel's experiments concerning the adaptive abilities of cells, though Niehans himself specialized in glandular transplants and by 1925 was one of the leading glandular surgeons in Europe.

Niehans referred to 1931 as the birth year of cellular therapy. That year, he treated a patient suffering from tetany whose parathyroid had been erroneously removed by another physician. Too weak for a glandular transplant, the patient was given injections of the parathyroid glands of steer, and she soon recovered. Niehans made more injections, even experimenting on himself, and reported he could cure illnesses through injections of live cells extracted from healthy animal organs. He believed adding new tissue stimulated rejuvenation and recovery.

Niehans treated Pope Pious XII with his injections and was nominated to the Vatican Academy of Science following the pope's recovery.

Niehans remained a controversial figure throughout his life. As of 2010, the Clinique Paul Niehans in Switzerland, founded by his daughter, continued his work. http://www.paulniehans.ch/clinic.htm

Research and general acceptance

Cell therapy as alternative healers practice it is generally rejected as effective by the traditionally-trained scientific community. Most of the claims made for these therapies are based on anecdotal evidence and are not backed by controlled clinical trials. While some mainstream cell therapy procedures have shown some success in clinical studies, others are still largely unproven, including cell therapy for cancer treatment. Until large, controlled human clinical studies are performed on cell therapy procedures, they will remain fringe treatments.

Resources

BOOKS

Steenblock, David, and Anthony G. Payne. *Umbilical Cord Stem Cell Therapy: The Gift of Healing from Healthy Newborns.* Laguna Beach, CA: Basic Health Publications, 2006.

PERIODICALS

Pollack, Andrew. "Stem Cell Therapy Controls Diabetes in Mice." *New York Times.* February 21, 2007.

OTHER

"Cellular Therapy." *Quackwatch.* 2003 [cited February 2, 2009]. http://www.quackwatch.com/01QuackeryRelated Topics/Cancer/cellular.html

"Multiple Sclerosis 'Reversed' with Stem Cell Therapy." *New Scientist Health.* January 30, 2009 [cited February 2, 2009]. http://www.newscientist.com/article/dn16509-multiple-sclerosis-reversed-with-stem-cell-therapy.html

ORGANIZATIONS

Alternative Medicine Foundation, P. O. Box 60016, Potomac, MD, 20859, (301) 340-1960, http://www.amfoundation.org.

Center for Cell and Gene Therapy. Baylor College of Medicine, One Baylor Plaza, Houston, TX, 77030, (713) 798-4028, (888) 550-9288, gradappboss@bcm.edu, http://www.bcm.edu/genetherapy/.

Paula Anne Ford-Martin
Tish Davidson, A. M.

Cellulitis

Definition

Cellulitis is a spreading bacterial infection just below the skin surface. It is most commonly caused by *Streptococcus pyogenes* or *Staphylococcus aureus*.

Description

The word "cellulitis" actually means "inflammation of the cells." Specifically, cellulitis refers to an infection of the tissue just below the skin surface. In humans, the skin and the tissues under the skin are the most common locations for microbial infection. Skin is the first defense against invading bacteria and other microbes. An infection can occur when this normally strong barrier is damaged due to surgery, injury, or a burn. Even something as small as a scratch or an insect bite allows bacteria to enter the skin, which may lead to an infection. Usually, the immune system kills any invading bacteria, but sometimes the bacteria are able to grow and cause an infection.

Once past the skin surface, the warmth, moisture, and nutrients allow bacteria to grow rapidly. Disease-causing bacteria release proteins called enzymes which cause tissue damage. The body's reaction to damage is inflammation which is characterized by **pain**, redness, heat, and swelling. This red, painful region grows bigger as the infection and resulting tissue damage spread. An untreated infection may spread to the lymphatic system (**acute lymphangitis**), the lymph nodes (**lymphadenitis**), the bloodstream (**bacteremia**), or into deeper

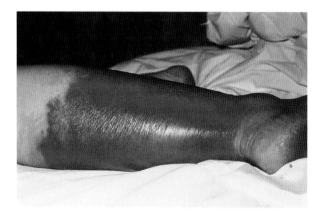

This person's lower leg is swollen and inflamed due to cellulitis. Cellulitis is a *Streptococcus* bacterial infection of the skin and the tissues beneath it. The face, neck, or legs are common sites of cellulitis. *(Custom Medical Stock Photo, Inc. Reproduced by permission.)*

tissues. Cellulitis most often occurs on the face, neck, and legs.

Orbital cellulitis

A very serious infection, called **orbital cellulitis**, occurs when bacteria enter and infect the tissues surrounding the eye. In 50–70% of all cases of orbital cellulitis, the infection spreads to the eye(s) from the sinuses or the upper respiratory tract (nose and throat). Twenty-five percent of orbital infections occur after surgery on the face. Other sources of orbital infection include a direct infection from an eye injury, from a dental or throat infection, and through the bloodstream.

Infection of the tissues surrounding the eye causes redness, swollen eyelids, severe pain, and causes the eye to bulge out. This serious infection can lead to a temporary loss of vision, blindness, brain abscesses, inflammation of the brain and spinal tissues (**meningitis**), and other complications. Before the discovery of **antibiotics**, orbital cellulitis caused blindness in 20% of patients and **death** in 17% of patients. Antibiotic treatment has significantly reduced the incidence of blindness and death.

Causes and symptoms

Although other kinds of bacteria can cause cellulitis, it is most often caused by *Streptococcus pyogenes* (the bacteria that causes **strep throat**) and *Staphylococcus aureus*. *Streptococcus pyogenes* is the so-called "flesh-eating bacteria" and, in rare cases, can cause a dangerous, deep skin infection called necrotizing fasciitis. Orbital cellulitis may be caused by bacteria which cannot grow in the presence of oxygen (anaerobic bacteria). In children, *Haemophilus influenzae* type B frequently causes orbital cellulitis following a sinus infection.

Streptococcus pyogenes can be picked up from a person who has strep throat or an infected sore. Other cellulitis-causing bacteria can be acquired from direct contact with infected sores. Persons who are at a higher risk for cellulitis are those who have a severe underlying disease (such as **cancer**, diabetes, and **kidney disease**), are taking steroid medications, have a reduced immune system (because of **AIDS**, organ transplant, etc.), have been burned, have insect **bites**, have reduced blood circulation to limbs, or have had a leg vein removed for coronary bypass surgery. In addition, chicken pox, human or animal bite **wounds**, skin wounds, and recent surgery can put a person at a higher risk for cellulitis.

The characteristic symptoms of cellulitis are redness, warmth, pain, and swelling. The infected area appears as a red patch that gets larger rapidly within the first 24 hours. A thick red line which progresses toward the heart may appear indicating an infection of the lymph vessels (lymphangitis). Other symptoms which may occur include **fever**, chills, tiredness, muscle aches, and a general ill feeling. Some people also experience **nausea**, **vomiting**, stiff joints, and hair loss at the infection site.

The characteristic symptoms of orbital cellulitis are eye pain, redness, swelling, warmth, and tenderness. The eye may bulge out and it may be difficult or impossible to move. Temporary loss of vision, pus drainage from the eye, chills, fever, headaches, **vomiting**, and a general ill feeling may occur.

Diagnosis

Cellulitis may be diagnosed and treated by a family doctor, an **infectious disease** specialist, a doctor who specializes in skin diseases (dermatologist), or in the case of orbital cellulitis, an eye doctor (ophthalmologist). The diagnosis of cellulitis is based mainly on the patient's symptoms. The patient's recent medical history is also used in the diagnosis.

Laboratory tests may be done to determine which kind of bacteria is causing the infection but these tests are not always successful. If the skin injury is visible, a sterile cotton swab is used to pick up a sample from the wound. If there is no obvious skin injury, a needle may be used to inject a small amount of sterile salt solution into the infected skin, and then the solution is withdrawn. The salt solution should pick up some of the bacteria causing the infection. A blood sample may be taken from the patient's arm to see if bacteria have entered the bloodstream. Also, a blood test may be done to count the number of white blood cells in the blood. High numbers of white blood cells suggest that the body is trying to fight a bacterial infection.

For orbital cellulitis, the doctor may often perform a special x-ray scan called computed tomography scan (CT). This scan enables the doctor to see the patient's head in cross-section to determine exactly where the infection is and see if any damage has occurred. A CT scan takes about 20 minutes.

Treatment

Antibiotic treatment is the only way to battle this potentially life-threatening infection. Mild to moderate cellulitis can be treated with the following antibiotics taken every four to eight hours by mouth:

- penicillins (Bicillin, Wycillin, Pen Vee, V-Cillin)

KEY TERMS

Inflammation—A local, protective response to tissue injury. It is characterized by redness, warmth, swelling, and pain.

Necrotizing fasciitis—A destructive infection which follows severe cellulitis and involves the deep skin and underlying tissues.

Sinuses—Air cavities found in the bones of the head. The sinuses which are connected to the nose are prone to infection.

- erythromycin (E-Mycin, Ery-Tab)
- cephalexin (Biocef, Keflex)
- cloxacillin (Tegopen)

Other medications may be recommended, such as **acetaminophen** (Tylenol) or ibuprofen (Motrin, Advil) to relieve pain, and **aspirin** to decrease fever.

A normally healthy person is usually not hospitalized for mild or moderate cellulitis. General treatment measures include elevation of the infected area, rest, and application of warm, moist compresses to the infected area. The doctor will want to see the patient again to make sure that the antibiotic treatment is effective in stopping the infection.

Persons at high risk for severe cellulitis will probably be hospitalized for treatment and monitoring. Antibiotics may be given intravenously to patients with severe cellulitis. Complications such as deep infection, or bone or joint infections, might require surgical drainage and a longer course of antibiotic treatment. Extensive tissue destruction may require **plastic surgery** to repair. In cases of orbital cellulitis caused by a sinus infection, surgery may be required to drain the sinuses.

Prognosis

Over 90% of all cellulitis cases are cured after seven to ten days of antibiotic treatment. Persons with serious disease and/or those who are taking immunosuppressive drugs may experience a more severe form of cellulitis which can be life threatening. Serious complications include blood poisoning (bacteria growing in the blood stream), meningitis (brain and spinal cord infection), tissue death (necrosis), and/or lymphangitis (infection of the lymph vessels). Severe cellulitis caused by *Streptococcus pyogenes* can lead to destructive and life-threatening necrotizing fasciitis.

Prevention

Cellulitis may be prevented by wearing appropriate protective equipment during work and sports to avoid skin injury, cleaning cuts and skin injuries with antiseptic soap, keeping wounds clean and protected, watching wounds for signs of infection, taking the entire prescribed dose of antibiotic, and maintaining good general health. Persons with diabetes should try to maintain good blood sugar control.

Resources

PERIODICALS

Lewis, Ronald T. "Soft Tissue Infections." *World Journal of Surgery* 22, no. 2 (February 1998): 146-51.

Belinda Rowland, PhD

Central Mississippi Valley disease *see* **Histoplasmosis**

Central nervous system depressants

Definition

Central nervous system (CNS) depressants are drugs that reduce brain activity.

Purpose

These drugs are used to treat **anxiety**, muscle tension, **pain**, **insomnia**, acute **stress** reactions, panic attacks, and seizure disorders. In higher doses, some of them produce **coma** and anesthesia.

Description

Throughout history, humans have sought relief from anxiety and insomnia by using substances that induce a drowsy or calming effect. CNS depressants include a wide range of drugs such as alcohol, the most widely used depressant, **narcotics**, **barbiturates** (Amytal, Nembutal, Seconal), **benzodiazepines** (Ativan, Halcion, Librium, Valium, Xanax), chloral hydrate, Buspirone (Buspar) and Zolpidem (Ambien). Street names for illegal CNS depressants include Reds, Yellows, Blues, Barbs, and Downers.

Precautions

- Most CNS depressants have the potential to be physically and psychologically addictive.
- The body tends to develop tolerance for CNS depressants, and larger doses are needed to achieve the same effects.
- Sudden withdrawal from some CNS depressants can produce rebound insomnia or anxiety, occasionally resulting in life-threatening seizures.
- When depressant medications is discontinued, it should be done gradually to give the body time to adjust.
- The difference is small between effective doses and overdoses for some CNS depressants, such as barbiturates.
- Elderly people are subject to more profound and prolonged effects from CNS depressants.

Side effects

Adverse effects include confusion, **dizziness**, slurred speech, loss of muscle coordination, and impaired thinking and judgment.

Interactions

Interactions with benzodiazepines (Xanax, Ativan, Valium) include:

- These drugs can increase the effects of narcotics and other pain management medications.
- Antifungal drugs, Diflucan, Nizoral, Sporanox, greatly increase and prolong the effects of benzodiazepines.
- Anti-seizure medications, like Tegretol, can decrease the effectiveness of benzodiazepines.
- Cimetidine (Tagamet) can increase the effectiveness of benzodiazepines.
- Calcium channel blockers, like Cardizem, can increase and prolong the effects of benzodiazepines.
- Grapefruit juice can increase the effects of benzodiazepines.
- Macrolide antibiotics (erythromycin, Biaxin) can increase and prolong the effects of benzodiazepines.
- Modifinil (Provigil) may reduce the effects of benzodiazepines.
- AIDS and antiretroviral drugs may increase and prolong the effects of benzodiazepines.

Resources

BOOKS

Bezchlibnyk–Butler, et al.*Clinical Handbook of Psychotropic Drugs.* Ashland, OH: Hogrefe & Huber, 2009.

ORGANIZATIONS

American Society of Addiction Medicine, 4601 N. Park Avenue, Upper Arcade #101, Chevy Chase, MD, 20815, (301) 656-3920, (301) 656-3815, email@asam.org, http://www.asam.org.

National Institute on Drug Abuse, 6001 Executive Blvd., Room 5213, Bethesda, MD, (301) 443-1124, information @nida.nih.gov, http://drugabuse.gov.

Ann Quigley
James Waun, MD, RPh

Central nervous system infections

Definition

The central nervous system, or CNS, comprises the brain, the spinal cord, and associated membranes. Under some circumstances, bacteria may enter areas of the CNS. If this occurs, abscesses or empyemas may be established.

Description

In general, the CNS is well defended against infection. The spine and brain are sheathed in tough, protective membranes. The outermost membrane, the dura mater, and the next layer, the arachnoid, entirely encase the brain and spinal cord. However, these defenses are not absolute. In rare cases, bacteria gain access to areas within the CNS.

Bacterial infection of the CNS can result in abscesses and empyemas (accumulations of pus). Abscesses have fixed boundaries, but empyemas lack definable shape and size. CNS infections are classified according to the location where they occur. For example, a spinal epidural **abscess** is located above the dura mater, and a cranial subdural **empyema** occurs between the dura mater and the arachnoid.

As pus and other material from an infection accumulate, pressure is exerted on the brain or spinal cord. This pressure can damage the nervous system tissue, possibly permanently. Without treatment, a CNS infection is fatal.

Causes and symptoms

Typically, bacterial invasion results from the spread of a nearby infection; for example, a chronic sinus or middle ear infection can extend beyond its initial site. Bacteria may also be conveyed to the CNS from distant sites of infection by the bloodstream. In rare cases, head trauma or surgical procedures introduce bacteria directly into the CNS. The source of infection cannot always be identified.

Specific symptoms of a CNS infection hinge on its exact location, but may include severe **headache** or back **pain**, weakness, sensory loss, and **fever**. An individual may report a stiff neck, **nausea** or **vomiting**, and tiredness or disorientation. There is a potential for seizures, **paralysis**, or **coma**.

Diagnosis

Examination

Physical symptoms, such as a fever and intense backache or a fever, severe headache, and stiff neck, raise the suspicion of a CNS infection.

Tests

Blood tests may indicate the presence of an infection but do not pinpoint its location. CT scans or MRI scans of the brain and spine can provide definitive diagnosis, with an MRI scan being the most sensitive.

Procedures

A **lumbar puncture** and analysis of the cerebrospinal fluid can help diagnose an epidural abscess; however, the procedure can be dangerous in cases of subdural empyema.

Treatment

A two-pronged approach is taken to treat CNS infections. First, antibiotic therapy against an array of potential infectious bacteria is begun. The second stage involves surgery to drain the infected site.

Although some CNS infections have been resolved with **antibiotics** alone, the more aggressive approach is often preferred. Surgery allows immediate relief of pressure on the brain or spinal cord, as well as an opportunity to collect infectious material for bacterial identification. Once the bacterial species is identified, drug therapy can be altered to a more specific antibiotic. Surgery may not be an option in some cases, such as when there are numerous sites of infection or when infection is located in an inaccessible area of the brain.

Prognosis

The fatality rate associated with CNS infections ranges from 10% to as high as 40%. Some survivors experience permanent CNS damage, resulting in partial paralysis, speech problems, or seizures. Rapid diagnosis and treatment are essential for a good prognosis. With prompt medical attention, an individual may recover completely.

KEY TERMS

Abscess—A pus-filled area with definite borders.

Arachnoid—One of the membranes that sheathes the spinal cord and brain; the arachnoid is the second-layer membrane.

Cerebrospinal fluid—Fluid that is normally found in the spinal cord and brain. Abnormal levels of certain molecules in this fluid can indicate the presence of infection or damage to the central nervous system.

Computed tomography scan (CT)—Cross-sectional x rays of the body are compiled to create a three-dimensional image of the body's internal structures.

Dura mater—One of the membranes that sheathes the spinal cord and brain; the outermost layer.

Empyema—A pus-filled area with indefinite borders.

Lumbar puncture—A procedure in which a needle is inserted into the lower spine to collect a sample of cerebrospinal fluid.

Magnetic resonance imaging (MRI)—An imaging technique that uses a large circular magnet and radio waves to generate signals from atoms in the body. These signals are used to construct images of internal structures.

Prevention

Treatment for pre-existing infections, such as sinus or middle ear infections, may prevent some cases of CNS infection. Since some CNS infections are of unknown origin, not all are preventable.

Resources

BOOKS

Donaghy, Michael., ed. *Brain's Diseases of the Nervous System*. New York: Oxford University Press, 2009.

Murdoch, Bruce E. *Acquired Speech and Language Disorders*. 2nd ed. Hoboken, NJ: Wiley, 2010.

ORGANIZATIONS

Center for Disability Information and Referral, Indiana Institute on Disability and Community, 2853 East Tenth Street, Bloomington, IA, 47408-2696, (812) 855-9396, http://www.iidc.indiana.edu/cedir.

Centers for Disease Control and Prevention (CDC), 1600 Clifton Road, Atlanta, GA, 30333, (404) 498-1515, (800) 311-3435, http://www.cdc.gov.

National Institute of Neurological Disorders and Stroke (NINDS), P.O. Box 5801, Bethesda, MD, 20824, (301) 496-5751, (800) 352-9424, http://www.ninds.nih.gov.

Julia Barrett
Laura Jean Cataldo, RN, EdD

Central nervous system stimulants

Definition

Central nervous system (CNS) stimulants are medicines that stimulate the release of excitatory chemicals (primarily norepinephrine) from nerve cells, increasing brain and nerve activity.

Purpose

By increasing brain and nerve activity, these drugs increase wakefulness and speed thinking and physical processes.

The most commonly used central nervous system stimulant is **caffeine**.

Central nervous system stimulant drugs are used to treat daytime lethargy and sleepiness and, paradoxically, attention deficit and hyperactivity disorders, presumably by improving the ability to organize, focus and concentrate mental activities.

Examples of central nervous system stimulants include modafinil (Provigil), sibutramine (Meridia), mistures of dextroamphetamines (Adderal), and methylphenidate (Ritalin, Concerta).

Description

With the exception of caffeine, which is available in a host of consumer products, these drugs are highly regulated, Class II **narcotics**.

These drugs are available in tablets, capsules, liquids, and patches.

Pregnancy and nursing

Studies on pregnant animals showed fetal teratogenic effects. They are not used in pregnant women unless the benefits outweigh potential risks. Nursing mothers pass small amounts of these drugs through their milk to babies,

Precautions

Children with structural abnormalities or diseases of the heart are at risk for sudden **death** from taking these drugs. Before starting on them, they should have a careful cardiac evaluation.

Adults with heart abnormalities or diseases are at risk for sudden death, **stroke**, **heart attack**, or sudden death from taking these drugs. Before starting on them, they should have a careful cardiac evaluation.

These drugs can increase blood pressure and should be taken with caution by anyone who has **hyperthyroidism** or high blood pressure.

These drugs may increase manic episodes in people with bipolar manic-depressive disorder, and aggressive behavior, **psychosis** or thought disorders. They may increase the likelihood of seizures in people with **seizure disorder**.

These drugs should be used with caution by people who have a history of alcohol or drug **abuse**.

These drugs may produce drug-dependency and should not be withdrawn abruptly after prolonged use.

The brain adjusts and becomes tolerant to these drugs, so increasing doses are often needed to maintain the desired effects.

These drugs are not approved for use in children under the age of six; their use has been associated with growth retardation.

Side effects

- Angina, heart attack, and increased heart rate and arrhythmias
- High blood pressure
- Agitation and restlessness
- Confusion
- Headache
- Sleeplessness
- Anger and aggression
- Abdominal pain
- Decreased appetite
- Nausea, vomiting, and diarrhea
- Anemia

Drug interactions

When taken with **monoamine oxidase inhibitors** (MAOI) (Marplan, Nardil, Parnate), these drugs can produce dangerously high blood pressure.

Withdrawal syndrome

Abruptly stopping these drugs after prolonged use may result in extreme **fatigue**, depression, and **sleep disorders**.

James Waun, MD, RPh

Central retinal artery occlusion *see*
  Retinopathies
Central retinal vein occlusion *see*
  Retinopathies

Cephalosporins

Definition

Cephalosporins are antibiotic medications, in the beta-lactam (penicillin) family, that kill bacteria or prevent their growth.

Purpose

These drugs are used to treat bacterial infections in the middle ear, nose, throat, lungs, sinuses, urinary system, and skin.

They are sometimes used as alternatives to penicillin to prevent infections in people who have a history of heart damage and are susceptible to infections while undergoing dental and other procedures.

These drugs will *not* cure or prevent colds, flu, and other viral infections.

Description

Cephalosporin examples include cefaclor (Ceclor), cefadroxil (Duricef), cefazolin (Ancef, Kefzol, Zolicef), cefixime, (Suprax), cefoxitin (Mefoxin), cefprozil (Cefzil), ceftazidime (Ceptaz, Fortaz, Tazicef, Tazideme), cefuroxime (Ceftin), and cephalexin (Keflex).

Available only by prescription, these medicines come in tablet, capsule, liquid, eye and ear drop, and injectable forms.

Recommended dosage

The dosage depends on the form of drug used and the reason for its use.

All **antibiotics** should be taken exactly as directed for as long as directed. They should not be stopped if or when symptoms improve.

Some cephalosporins work best when taken on an empty stomach; others should be taken after meals. Read the advice tags on prescription labels or ask your pharmacists if there are special instructions regarding food.

PREGNANCY. Cephalosporins pass through the placenta. While there are no well controlled studies on their possible risks to developing fetuses, caution is advised.

BREASTFEEDING. Cephalosporins passes into breast milk in small amounts and may affect the bowels of nursing babies.

OTHER MEDICAL CONDITIONS. Before using cephalosporins, people with any of these medical problems should make sure their physicians are aware of their conditions:

- Penicillin allergy. Cephalosporins are related to penicillins; people with a history of severe reactions to penicillin may also have allergic reactions to cephalosporins.
- Chronic kidney disease. The dose of cephalosporins may need to be reduced in people who have chronic kidney disease.
- Bleeding problems. Cephalosporins may increase the chance of bleeding in people with a history of bleeding problems.
- Liver disease and chronic malnutrition. Long term use of cephalosporins may lead to bleeding problems.

Side effects

- Headache, confusion, agitation, dizziness, and fatigue
- Skin rash or itching
- Joint aches or pains
- Fever
- Abdominal cramps, upset stomach, nausea, diarrhea
- Vaginal itching or discharge
- Unusual bruising or bleeding

Drug interactions

Cephalosporins may increase the blood levels of metformin used to treat type 2 diabetes.

Probenecid, used to treat chronic **gout**, may increase the blood levels of cephalosporins, increasing the possibility of diarrhea as an adverse effect.

Cephalosporins may increase the blood thinning effects of warfarin (Coumadin).

James Waun, MD. RPh

Cerebral abscess *see* **Brain abscess**

Cerebral amyloid angiopathy

Definition

Cerebral amyloid angiopathy (CAA) is also known as congophilic angiopathy or cerebrovascular **amyloidosis**. It is a disease of small blood vessels in the brain in which deposits of amyloid protein in the vessel walls may lead to **stroke**, brain hemorrhage, or **dementia**. Amyloid protein resembles a starch and is deposited in tissues during the course of certain chronic diseases.

Description

CAA may affect patients over age 45, but is most common in patients over age 65, and becomes more common with increasing age. Men and women are equally affected. In some cases, CAA is sporadic but it may also be inherited as an autosomal dominant condition (a form of inheritance in which only one copy of a gene coding for a disease need be present for that disease to be expressed; if either parent has the disease, a child has a 50% chance of inheriting the disease). CAA is responsible for 5–20% of brain hemorrhage, and up to 30% of lobar hemorrhages localized to one lobe of the brain. CAA may be found during an **autopsy** in over one-third of persons over age 60, even though they may not have had brain hemorrhage, stroke, or other manifestations of the disease during life. In **Alzheimer's disease**, CAA is more common than in the general population, and may occur in more than 80% of patients over age 60.

Causes and symptoms

The cause of amyloid deposits in blood vessels in the brain in sporadic CAA is not known. In hereditary CAA, genetic defects, typically on chromosome 21, allow accumulation of amyloid, a protein made up of units called beta-pleated sheet fibrils. The fibrils tend to clump together, so that the amyloid cannot be dissolved and builds up in the brain blood vessel walls. One form of amyloid fibril subunit proteins is the amyloid beta protein.

Different theories have been suggested for the source of amyloid beta protein in the brain. The systemic theory suggests that amyloid beta protein in the blood stream is deposited in blood vessels in the brain, causing weakness in the blood vessel wall and breakdown in the blood-brain barrier. Normally, the blood-brain barrier keeps proteins and other large molecules from escaping from the blood vessel to the brain tissue. When there is breakdown of the blood-brain barrier, amyloid beta protein leaks through the blood vessel wall, and is deposited in the brain substance, where it forms an abnormal structure called a neuritic plaque.

A second, more likely theory is that amyloid fibrils that form amyloid beta protein are produced by perivascular microglia, or support cells in contact with the brain blood vessel wall. The third theory is that the brain tissue gives rise to amyloid beta protein. Both the nerve cells and the glia are known to produce amyloid precursor protein, which increases with **aging** and with cell **stress**.

Bleeding into the brain may occur as tiny blood vessels carrying amyloid deposits become heavier and more brittle, and are therefore more likely to burst with minor trauma or with fluctuating blood pressure. Aneurysms, or ballooning of the blood vessel wall, may develop, and may also rupture as the stretched wall becomes thinner and is under more pressure. Amyloid deposits may destroy smooth muscle cells or cause inflammation in the blood vessel wall. This may also cause the blood vessel to break more easily.

The most common form of CAA is the sporadic form associated with aging. This type of CAA usually causes lobar hemorrhage, which may recur in different lobes of the brain. The frontal lobe (behind the forehead) and parietal lobe (behind the frontal lobe) are most often affected; the temporal lobe (near the temple) and occipital lobe (at the back of the brain) are affected less often; and the cerebellum (under the occipital lobe) is rarely affected. Approximately 10–50% of hemorrhages in sporadic CAA involve more than one lobe.

Symptoms of lobar hemorrhage in CAA include sudden onset of **headache**, neurologic symptoms such as weakness, sensory loss, visual changes, or speech problems, depending on which lobe is involved; and decreased level of consciousness (a patient who is difficult to arouse), **nausea**, and **vomiting**. Sporadic CAA may be associated with symptoms unrelated to lobar hemorrhage. Petechial hemorrhages (tiny hemorrhages involving many small vessels) may produce recurrent, brief neurologic symptoms secondary to seizures or decreased blood flow, or may produce rapidly progressive dementia (loss of memory and other brain functions) that worsens in distinct steps rather than gradually. Over 40% of patients with hemorrhage secondary to CAA also have dementia.

Genetic factors play a role in certain types of CAA and in diseases associated with CAA:

- Dutch type of hereditary cerebral hemorrhage with amyloidosis (build up of amyloid protein in blood vessels): autosomal dominant, with a genetic mutation involving the amyloid precursor protein. Onset is at age 40–60 with headaches, brain hemorrhage often in the parietal lobe, strokes, and dementia. More than half of patients die from their first hemorrhage. Patients with the Dutch type of CAA may produce an abnormal anticoagulant, or blood thinner, which makes hemorrhage more likely.

- Flemish type of hereditary cerebral hemorrhage with amyloidosis: autosomal dominant, with a mutation involving the amyloid precursor protein. Symptoms include brain hemorrhage or dementia.

- Familial Alzheimer's disease: autosomal dominant, comprising 5–10% of all Alzheimer's disease cases (a brain disease in which death of nerve cells leads to progressive dementia).

- Down Syndrome: caused by trisomy 21 (three rather than two copies of chromosome 21), causing excess amyloid precursor protein gene. Children with Down syndrome are mentally handicapped and may have heart problems.

- Icelandic type of hereditary cerebral hemorrhage with amyloidosis: autosomal dominant, with mutation in the gene coding for cystatin C. Symptoms often begin at age 30–40 with multiple brain hemorrhages, dementia, paralysis (weakness), and death in 10–20 years. Headache occurs in more than half of patients, and seizures occur in one-quarter. Unlike most other forms of CAA, most hemorrhages involve the basal ganglia deep within the brain. (Basal ganglia are islands of tissues in the cerebellum part of the brain.)

- Familial oculo-leptomeningeal amyloidosis: autosomal dominant with unknown gene defect(s), described in Japanese, Italian, and North American families. Symptoms can include dementia, ataxia (problems with coordination), spasticity (limb stiffness), strokes, seizures, peripheral neuropathy (disease affecting the nerves supplying the limbs), migraine, spinal cord problems, blindness, and deafness. Brain hemorrhage is rare as the amyloid protein is deposited in blood vessels in the eye and meninges (brain coverings), but not in the brain itself. In Italian families with the disease, patients may be affected as early as 20–30 years of age.

- British type of familial amyloidosis: autosomal dominant with unknown gene defect(s), associated with progressive dementia, spasticity, and ataxia. Brain stem, spinal cord, and cerebellum all exhibit amyloid deposits, but hemorrhage typically does not occur.

Diagnosis

As in most neurologic diseases, diagnosis is made most often from the patient's history, with careful inquiry into family history and the patient's onset

KEY TERMS

Amyloid—Amyloid protein resembles a starch and is deposited in tissues during the course of certain chronic diseases.

Ataxia—Problems with coordination and walking.

Autosomal dominant—A form of inheritance in which only one copy of a gene coding for a disease need be present for that disease to be expressed. If either parent has the disease, a child has a 50% chance of inheriting the disease.

Chromosome—A cellular structure containing genetic information in the form of DNA.

Dementia—Loss of memory and other higher functions, such as thinking or speech, lasting six months or more.

Hemorrhage—Bleeding, or escape of blood through ruptured or unruptured blood vessel walls.

Lobar hemorrhage—Bleeding into one of the lobes of the brain.

Seizure—Epileptic convulsion, fit, or attack.

Spasticity—Limb stiffness related to disease of the brain or spinal cord.

Sporadic—A form of disease found in persons without a family history of the disease.

Stroke—Sudden neurological deficit related to impaired blood supply to the brain.

and pattern of symptoms, as well as neurologic examination. Brain computed tomography scan (CT) or **magnetic resonance imaging** (MRI) may identify lobar hemorrhage, stroke, or petechial hemorrhages, and are important in excluding arteriovenous malformation, **brain tumor**, or other causes of hemorrhage. **Angiography** (x-ray study of the interior of blood vessels and the heart) is not helpful in diagnosis of CAA, but may be needed to exclude aneurysm. **Brain biopsy** (surgical removal of a small piece of brain tissue) may show characteristic amyloid deposits, but is rarely performed, as the risk may not be justifiable in the absence of effective treatment for CAA. If diagnosis is uncertain, biopsy may be needed to rule out conditions which are potentially treatable. Definite diagnosis requires microscopic examination of brain tissue, either at biopsy, at autopsy, or at surgery when brain hemorrhage is drained. **Lumbar puncture** to examine cerebrospinal fluid proteins may show characteristic abnormalities, but is not part of the routine exam. In familial forms, genetic analysis may be helpful.

CAA with hemorrhage must be distinguished from other types of brain hemorrhage. In CAA, hemorrhage typically occurs in the lobar region, often ruptures into the subarachnoid space between the brain and its coverings, and occurs at night. In hemorrhage related to high blood pressure, hemorrhage is usually deeper within the brain, ruptures into the ventricles or cavities deep inside the brain, and occurs during daytime activities. Other causes of brain hemorrhage are **arteriovenous malformations**, trauma, aneurysms, bleeding into a brain tumor, **vasculitis** (inflammation of blood vessels), or bleeding disorders.

Treatment

Although there is no effective treatment for the underlying disease process of CAA, measures can be taken to prevent brain hemorrhage in patients diagnosed with CAA. High blood pressure should be treated aggressively, and even normal blood pressure can be lowered as much as tolerated without side effects from medications. Blood thinners such as Coumadin, antiplatelet agents such as **aspirin**, or medications designed to dissolve **blood clots** may cause hemorrhage in patients with CAA, and should be avoided if possible. If these medications are required for other conditions, such as heart disease, the potential benefits must be carefully weighed against the increased risks.

Seizures, or recurrent neurologic symptoms thought to be seizures, should be treated with anti-epileptic drugs, although Depakote (**sodium** valproate) should be avoided because of its antiplatelet effect. Anti-epileptic drugs are sometimes given to patients with large lobar hemorrhage in an attempt to prevent seizures, although the benefit of this is unclear.

Once brain hemorrhage has occurred, the patient should be admitted to a hospital (ICU) for neurologic monitoring and control of increased pressure within the brain, blood pressure control, and supportive medical care. Antiplatelet agents and blood thinners should be discontinued and their effects reversed, if possible. Surgery may be needed to remove brain hemorrhage, although bleeding during surgery may be difficult to control.

CAA may be rarely associated with cerebral vasculitis, or inflammation of the blood vessel walls. In these cases treatment with **steroids** or immune system suppressants may be helpful. Without tissue examination, vasculitis cannot be diagnosed reliably, and probably coexists with CAA too rarely to justify steroid treatment in most cases.

Prognosis

Since CAA is associated with progressive blood vessel degeneration, and since there is no effective treatment, most patients have a poor prognosis. Aggressive neurosurgical management allows increased survival following lobar hemorrhage, but 20–90% of patients die from the first hemorrhage or its complications, which include progression of hemorrhage, brain **edema** (swelling) with herniation (downward pressure on vital brain structures), seizures, and infections such as **pneumonia**. Many survivors have persistent neurologic deficits related to the brain lobe affected by hemorrhage, and are at risk for additional hemorrhages, seizures, and dementia. Prognosis is worse in patients who are older, or who have larger hemorrhages or recurrent hemorrhages within a short time.

Resources

PERIODICALS

Neau, J. P., et.al. "Recurrent Intracerebral Hemorrhage." *Neurology* 49, no. 1 (1997): 106–113.

Laurie Barclay, MD

Cerebral aneurysm

Definition

A cerebral aneurysm occurs at a weak point in the wall of a blood vessel (artery) that supplies blood to the brain. Because of the flaw, the artery wall bulges outward and fills with blood. This bulge is called an aneurysm. An aneurysm can rupture, spilling blood into the surrounding body tissue. A ruptured cerebral aneurysm can cause permanent brain damage, disability, or **death**.

Description

A cerebral aneurysm can occur anywhere in the brain. Aneurysms can have several shapes. The saccular aneurysm, once called a berry aneurysm, resembles a piece of fruit dangling from a branch. Saccular aneurysms are usually found at a branch in the blood vessel where they balloon out by a thin neck. Saccular cerebral aneurysms most often occur at the branch points of large arteries at the base of the brain. Aneurysms may also take the form of a bulge in one wall of the artery–a lateral aneurysm–or a widening of the entire artery–a fusiform aneurysm.

The greatest danger of aneurysms is rupture. Approximately 50–75% of stricken people survive an aneurysmal rupture. A ruptured aneurysm spills blood into the brain or into the fluid-filled area that surrounds the brain tissue. Bleeding into this area, called the subarachnoid space, is referred to as **subarachnoid hemorrhage** (SAH). About 25,000 people suffer a SAH each year. It is estimated that people with unruptured aneurysm have an annual 1–2% risk of hemorrhage. Under age 40, more men experience SAH. After age 40, more women than men are affected.

Most people who have suffered a SAH from a ruptured aneurysm did not know that the aneurysm even existed. Based on **autopsy** studies, medical researchers estimate that 1–5% of the population has some type of cerebral aneurysm. Aneurysms rarely occur in the very young or the very old; about 60% of aneurysms are diagnosed in people between ages 40 and 65.

Some aneurysms may have a genetic link and run in families. The genetic link has not been completely proven and a pattern of inheritance has not been determined. Some studies seem to show that first-degree relatives of people who suffered aneurysmal SAH are more likely to have aneurysms themselves. These studies reported that such immediate family members were four times more likely to have aneurysms than the general population. Other studies do not confirm these findings. Better evidence links aneurysms to certain rare diseases of the connective tissue. These diseases include **Marfan syndrome, pseudoxanthoma elasticum, Ehlers-Danlos syndrome**, and fibromuscular dysplasia. **Polycystic kidney disease** is also associated with cerebral aneurysms.

These diseases are also associated with an increased risk of aneurysmal rupture. Certain other conditions raise the risk of rupture, too. Most aneurysms that rupture are a half-inch or larger in diameter. Size is not the only factor, however, because smaller aneurysms also rupture. Cigarette **smoking**, excessive alcohol consumption, and recreational drug use (for example, use of **cocaine**) have been linked with an increased risk. The role, if any, of high blood pressure has not been determined. Some studies have implicated high blood

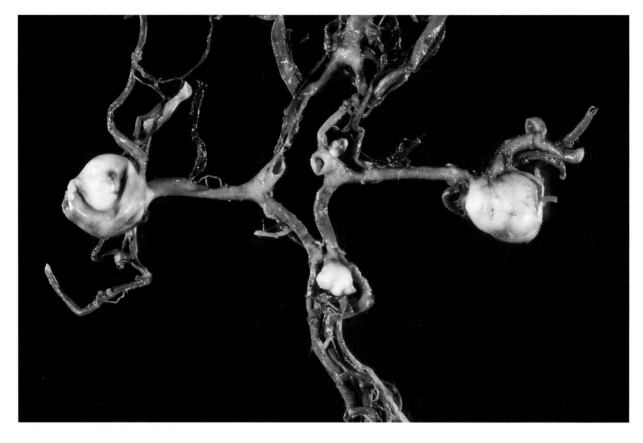

Three aneurysms can be seen in this section of a cerebral artery removed from a human brain. *(© Martin Rotker/Phototake. — All rights reserved.)*

pressure in aneurysm formation and rupture, but people with normal blood pressure also experience aneurysms and SAHs. High blood pressure may be a risk factor but not the most important one. **Pregnancy**, labor, and delivery also seem to increase the possibility that an aneurysm might rupture, but not all doctors agree. Physical exertion and use of **oral contraceptives** are not suspected causes for aneurysmal rupture.

Causes and symptoms

Cerebral aneurysms can be caused by brain trauma, infection, hardening of the arteries (**atherosclerosis**), or abnormal rapid cell growth (neoplastic disease), but most seem to arise from a congenital, or developmental, defect. These congenital aneurysms occur more frequently in women. Whatever the cause may be, the inner wall of the blood vessel is abnormally thin and the pressure of the blood flow causes an aneurysm to form.

Most aneurysms go unnoticed until they rupture. However, 10–15% of unruptured cerebral aneurysms are found because of their size or their location. Common warning signs include symptoms

that affect only one eye, such as an enlarged pupil, a drooping eyelid, or **pain** above or behind the eye. Other symptoms are a localized **headache**, unsteady gait, a temporary problem with sight, double vision, or **numbness** in the face.

Some aneurysms bleed occasionally without rupturing. Symptoms of such an aneurysm develop gradually. The symptoms include headache, **nausea**, **vomiting**, neck pain, black-outs, ringing in the ears, **dizziness**, or seeing spots.

Eighty to ninety percent of aneurysms are not diagnosed until after they have ruptured. Rupture is not always a sudden event. Nearly 50% of patients who have aneurysmal SAHs also experience "the warning leak phenomenon." Persons with warning leak symptoms have sudden, atypical headaches that occur days or weeks before the actual rupture. These headaches are referred to as sentinel headaches. Nausea, **vomiting**, and dizziness may accompany sentinel headaches. Unfortunately, these symptoms can be confused with tension headaches or migraines, and treatment can be delayed until rupture occurs.

When an aneurysm ruptures, most victims experience a sudden, extremely severe headache. This headache is typically described as the worst headache of the victim's life. **Nausea and vomiting** commonly accompany the headache. The person may experience a short loss of consciousness or prolonged **coma**. Other common signs of a SAH include a stiff neck, **fever**, and a sensitivity to light. About 25% of victims experience neurological problems linked to specific areas of the brain, swelling of the brain due to fluid accumulation (**hydrocephalus**), or seizure.

Diagnosis

Based on the clinical symptoms, a doctor will run several tests to confirm an aneurysm or an SAH. A computed tomography scan (CT) of the head is the initial procedure. A **magnetic resonance imaging** test (MRI) may be done instead of a CT scan. MRI, however, is not as sensitive as CT for detecting subarachnoid blood. A CT scan can determine whether there has been a hemorrhage and can assist in pinpointing the location of the aneurysm. The scan is most useful when it is done within 72 hours of the rupture. Later scans may miss the signs of hemorrhage.

If the CT scan is negative for a hemorrhage or provides an unclear diagnosis, the doctor will order a **cerebrospinal fluid (CSF) analysis**, also called a **lumbar puncture**. In this procedure, a small amount of cerebrospinal fluid is removed from the lower back and examined for traces of blood and blood-breakdown products. If this test is positive, cerebral **angiography** is used to map the brain's blood vessels and the damaged area. The angiography is done to pinpoint the aneurysm's location. About 15% of people who experience SAH have more than one aneurysm. For this reason, angiography should include both the common carotid artery that feeds the front of the brain and the vertebral artery that feeds the base of the brain. Occasionally, the angiography fails to find the aneurysm and must be repeated. If seizures occur, **electroencephalography** (EEG) may be used to measure the electrical activity of the brain.

Treatment

Unruptured aneurysm

If an aneurysm has not ruptured and is not causing any symptoms, it may be left untreated. Because there is a 1–2% chance of rupture per year, the cumulative risk over a number of years may justify surgical treatment. However, if the aneurysm is small or in a place that would be difficult to reach, or if the person who has the aneurysm is in poor health, the surgical

treatment may be a greater risk than the aneurysm. Risk of rupture is higher for people who have more than one aneurysm. Unruptured aneurysm would probably be treated with a surgical procedure called the clip ligation, as described in the following text.

Ruptured aneurysm

The primary treatment for a ruptured aneurysm involves stabilizing the victim's condition, treating the immediate symptoms, and promptly assessing further treatment options, especially surgical procedures. The patient may require mechanical ventilation, oxygen, and fluids. Medications may be given to prevent major secondary complications such as seizures, rebleeding, and vasospasm (narrowing of the affected blood vessel). Vasospasm decreases blood flow to the brain and causes the death of nerve cells. A drug such as nimodipine (Nimotop) may help prevent vasospasm by relaxing the smooth muscle tissue of the arteries. Even with treatment, however, vasospasm may cause **stroke** or death.

To prevent further hemorrhage from the aneurysm, it must be removed from circulation. In general, surgical procedures should be performed as soon as possible to prevent rebleeding. The chances that aneurysm will rebleed are greatest in the first 24 hours, and vasospasm usually does not occur until 72 hours or more after rupture. If the patient is in poor condition or if there is vasospasm or other complication, surgical procedures may be delayed. The preferred surgical method is a clip ligation in which a clip is placed around the base of the aneurysm to block it off from circulation. Surgical coating, wrapping, or trapping of the aneurysm may also be performed. These procedures do not completely remove the aneurysm from circulation, however, and there is some risk that it may rebleed in the future. Newer techniques that look promising include balloon embolization, a procedure that blocks the aneurysm with an inflatable membrane introduced by means of a catheter inserted through the artery.

Prognosis

An unruptured aneurysm may not cause any symptoms over an entire lifetime. Surgical clip ligation will ensure that it won't rupture, but it may be better to leave the aneurysm alone in some cases. Familial cerebral aneurysms may rupture earlier than those without a genetic link.

The outlook is not as good for a person who suffers a ruptured aneurysm. Fifteen to twenty-five percent of people who experience a ruptured aneurysm do not survive. An additional 25–50% die as a

KEY TERMS

Congenital—Existing at birth.

Ehlers-Danlos syndrome—A rare inheritable disease of the connective tissue marked by very elastic skin, very loose joints, and very fragile body tissue.

Embolization—A technique to stop or prevent hemorrhage by introducing a foreign mass, such as an air-filled membrane (balloon), into a blood vessel to block the flow of blood.

Fibromuscular dysplasia—A disorder that causes unexplained narrowing of arteries and high blood pressure.

Magnetic resonance angiography—A noninvasive diagnostic technique that uses radio waves to map the internal anatomy of the blood vessels.

Marfan syndrome—An inheritable disorder that affects the skeleton, joints, and blood vessels. Major indicators are excessively long arms and legs, lax joints, and vascular defects.

Nimodipine (Nimotop)—A calcium-channel blocker, that is, a drug that relaxes arterial smooth muscle by slowing the movement of calcium across cell walls.

Polycystic kidney disease—An abnormal condition in which the kidneys are enlarged and contain many cysts.

Pseudoxanthoma elasticum—A hereditary disorder of the connective, or elastic, tissue marked by premature aging and breakdown of the skin and degeneration of the arteries that leads to hemorrhages.

Subarachnoid hemorrhage (SAH)—Loss of blood into the subarachnoid space, the fluid-filled area that surrounds the brain tissue.

Vasospasm—Narrowing of a blood vessel caused by a spasm of the smooth muscle of the vessel wall.

---

result of complications associated with the hemorrhage. Of the survivors, 15–50% suffer permanent brain damage and disability. These conditions are caused by the death of nerve cells. Nerve cells can be destroyed by the hemorrhage itself or by complications from the hemorrhage, such as vasospasm or hydrocephalus. Hydrocephalus, a dilatation (expansion) of the fluid-filled cavity surrounding the brain, occurs in about 15% of cases. Immediate medical treatment is vital to prevent further complications and brain damage in those who survive the initial rupture. Patients who survive SAH and aneurysm clipping are unlikely to die from events related to SAH.

Prevention

There are no known methods to prevent an aneurysm from forming. If an aneurysm is discovered before it ruptures, it may be surgically removed. CT or MRI angiography may be recommended for relatives of patients with familial cerebral aneurysms.

Resources

OTHER

Bernadini, Gary L. "Intracerebral Aneurysms." *Columbia University Health Sciences Page.* http://cpmcnet.columbia.edu.

"The Brain Aneurysm Report." *Neurosurgical Service Page.* Harvard Medical School. http://neurosurgery.mgh.harvard.edu/abta/primer.htm.

ORGANIZATIONS

Brain Aneurysm Foundation, 66 Canal St, Boston, MA, 02114, (999) 272-4602, office@bafound.org, http://www.bafound.org.

Julia Barrett

Cerebral angiography *see* **Angiography**

Cerebral palsy

Definition

Cerebral palsy (CP) is the term used for a group of nonprogressive disorders of movement and posture caused by abnormal development of, or damage to, motor control centers of the brain. CP is caused by events before, during, or after birth. The abnormalities of muscle control that define CP are often accompanied by other neurological and physical abnormalities.

Demographics

As of 2009, United Cerebral Palsy (UCP) estimates that some 764,000 children and adults in the United States display one or more of the symptoms of cerebral palsy. Approximately 8,000 babies and infants are diagnosed with the condition each year. In addition, some

1,500 preschool age children are recognized each year to have cerebral palsy.

Description

Voluntary movement (walking, grasping, chewing, etc.) is primarily accomplished using muscles that are attached to bones, known as the skeletal muscles. Control of the skeletal muscles originates in the cerebral cortex, the largest portion of the brain. Palsy means **paralysis**, but may also be used to describe uncontrolled muscle movement or tension (hypertonia). Therefore, cerebral palsy encompasses any disorder of abnormal movement and paralysis caused by abnormal function of the cerebral cortex. In truth, however, CP does not include conditions due to progressive disease or degeneration of the brain. For this reason, CP is also referred to as static (nonprogressive) encephalopathy (disease of the brain). Also excluded from CP are any disorders of muscle control that arise in the muscles themselves and/or in the peripheral nervous system (nerves outside the brain and spinal cord).

CP is not a specific condition, but is more accurately considered a description of a broad but defined group of neurological and physical problems.

The severity of CP is quite variable. Some people with CP may have only minor difficulty with fine motor skills, such as grasping and manipulating items with their hands. A severe form of CP could involve significant muscle problems in all four limbs, **mental retardation**, seizures, and difficulties with vision, speech, and hearing.

Muscles that receive abnormal messages from the brain may be constantly contracted and tight (spastic), exhibit involuntary writhing movements (athetosis), or have difficulty with voluntary movement (dyskinesia). There can also be a lack of balance and coordination with unsteady movements (ataxia). A combination of any of these problems may also occur. Spastic CP and mixed CP constitute the majority of cases. Effects on the muscles can range from mild weakness or partial paralysis (*paresis*), to complete loss of voluntary control of a muscle or group of muscles (*plegia*). CP is also designated by the number of limbs affected. For instance, affected muscles in one limb is monoplegia, both arms or both legs is diplegia, both limbs on one side of the body is hemiplegia, and in all four limbs is quadriplegia. Muscles of the trunk, neck, and head may be affected as well.

Risk factors

Babies born prematurely or at low birth weights are at higher risk for cerebral palsy.

Two factors are involved in the risk for CP associated with **prematurity**. First, premature babies are at higher risk for various CP–associated medical complications, such as intracerebral hemorrhage, infection, and difficulty in breathing, to name a few. Second, the onset of **premature labor** may be induced, in part, by complications that have already caused neurologic damage in the fetus. A combination of both factors almost certainly plays a role in some cases of CP. The tendency toward premature delivery tends to run in families, but the genetic mechanisms are far from clear.

An increase in multiple birth pregnancies in recent years, especially in the United States, is blamed on the increased use of fertility drugs. As the number of fetuses in a **pregnancy** increases, the risks for abnormal development and premature delivery also increase. Children from twin pregnancies have four times the risk of developing CP as children from singleton pregnancies, owing to the fact that more twin pregnancies are delivered prematurely. The risk for CP in a child of triplets is up to 18 times greater. Furthermore, recent evidence suggests that a baby from a pregnancy in which its twin died before birth is at increased risk for CP.

Causes and symptoms

CP can be caused by a number of different mechanisms at various times—from several weeks after conception, through birth, to early childhood. For many years, it was accepted that most cases of CP were due to brain injuries received during a traumatic birth, known as birth asphyxia. However, research has shown that only 5–10% of CP can be attributed to birth trauma. Causes can be grouped into those that occur during pregnancy (prenatal), those that happen around the time of birth (perinatal), and those that occur after birth (postnatal).

Prenatal causes

Although much has been learned about human embryology in the last couple of decades, a great deal remains unknown. Studying prenatal human development is difficult because the embryo and fetus develop in a closed environment—the mother's womb. However, the relatively recent development of a number of prenatal tests has opened a window on the process. Add to that more accurate and complete evaluations of newborns, especially those with problems, and a clearer picture of what can go wrong before birth is possible.

The complicated process of brain development before birth is susceptible to many chance errors that can result in abnormalities of varying degrees. Some of these errors will result in structural anomalies of the brain, while others may cause undetectable, but significant, abnormalities in how the cerebral cortex is "wired." An abnormality in structure or wiring is sometimes hereditary, but is most often due to chance, or a cause unknown at this time. Whether and how much genetics played a role in a particular brain abnormality depends to some degree on the type of anomaly and the form of CP it causes.

Several maternal–fetal infections are known to increase the risk for CP, including **rubella** (German **measles**, now rare in the United States), cytomegalovirus (CMV), and **toxoplasmosis**. Each of these infections is considered a risk to the fetus only if the mother contracts it for the first time during that pregnancy. Even in those cases, though, most babies will be born normal. Most women are immune to all three infections by the time they reach childbearing age, but a woman's immune status can be determined using the TORCH (Toxoplasmosis, Rubella, Cytomegalovirus, and Herpes) test before or during pregnancy.

Just as a **stroke** can cause neurologic damage in an adult, so too can this type of event occur in the fetus. A burst blood vessel in the brain followed by uncontrolled bleeding (coagulopathy), known as intracerebral hemorrhage, could cause a fetal stroke, or a cerebral blood vessel could be obstructed by a clot (**embolism**). Infants who later develop CP, along with their mothers, are more likely than other mother–infant pairs to test positive for factors that put them at increased risk for bleeding episodes or **blood clots**. Some **coagulation disorders** are strictly hereditary, but most have a more complicated basis.

A teratogen is any substance to which a woman is exposed that has the potential to harm the embryo or fetus. Links between a drug or other chemical exposure during pregnancy and a risk for CP are difficult to prove. However, any substance that might affect fetal brain development, directly or indirectly, could increase the risk for CP. Furthermore, any substance that increases the risk for premature delivery and low birth weight, such as alcohol, tobacco, or **cocaine**, among others, might indirectly increase the risk for CP.

The fetus receives all nutrients and oxygen from blood that circulates through the placenta. Therefore, anything that interferes with normal placental function might adversely affect development of the fetus, including the brain, or might increase the risk for premature delivery. Structural abnormalities of the placenta, premature detachment of the placenta from the uterine

wall (abruption), and placental infections (chorioamnionitis) are thought to pose some risk for CP.

Certain conditions in the mother during pregnancy might pose a risk to fetal development leading to CP. Women with autoimmune anti–thyroid or anti–phospholipid (APA) antibodies are at slightly increased risk for CP in their children. A potentially important clue uncovered recently points toward high levels of cytokines in the maternal and fetal circulation as a possible risk for CP. Cytokines are proteins associated with inflammation, such as from infection or **autoimmune disorders**, and they may be toxic to neurons in the fetal brain. More research is needed to determine the exact relationship, if any, between high levels of cytokines in pregnancy and CP. A woman has some risk of developing the same complications in more than one pregnancy, slightly increasing the risk for more than one child with CP.

Serious physical trauma to the mother during pregnancy could result in direct trauma to the fetus as well, or injuries to the mother could compromise the availability of nutrients and oxygen to the developing fetal brain.

Perinatal causes

Birth asphyxia significant enough to result in CP is now uncommon in developed countries. Tight nuchal cord (umbilical cord around the baby's neck) and prolapsed cord (cord delivered before the baby) are possible causes of birth asphyxia, as are bleeding and other complications associated with **placental abruption** and **placenta previa** (placenta lying over the cervix).

Infection in the mother is sometimes not passed to the fetus through the placenta, but is transmitted to the baby during delivery. Any such infection that results in serious illness in the newborn has the potential to produce some neurological damage.

Postnatal causes

The remaining 15% of CP is due to neurological injury sustained after birth. CP that has a postnatal cause is sometimes referred to as acquired CP, but this is only accurate for those cases caused by infection or trauma.

Incompatibility between the Rh blood types of mother and child (mother Rh negative, baby Rh positive) can result in severe anemia in the baby (**erythroblastosis fetalis**). This may lead to other complications, including severe **jaundice**, which can cause CP. Rh disease in the newborn is now rare in developed countries due to routine screening of maternal blood type and treatment of pregnancies at risk. The routine, effective treatment of jaundice due to other causes has also made it an infrequent cause of CP in developed countries. Rh blood type poses a risk for recurrence of Rh disease if treatment is not provided.

Serious infections that affect the brain directly, such as **meningitis** and **encephalitis**, may cause irreversible damage to the brain, leading to CP. A **seizure disorder** early in life may cause CP, or may be the product of a hidden problem that causes CP in addition to seizures. Unexplained (idiopathic) seizures are hereditary in only a small percentage of cases. Although rare in infants born healthy at or near term, intracerebral hemorrhage and brain embolism, like fetal stroke, are sometimes genetic.

Physical trauma to an infant or child resulting in brain injury, such as from **abuse**, accidents, or near drowning/suffocation, might cause CP. Likewise, ingestion of a toxic substance such as lead, mercury, poisons, or certain chemicals could cause neurological damage. Accidental overdose of certain medications might also cause similar damage to the central nervous system.

Prematurity and multiple birth pregnancy

Advances in the medical care of premature infants in the last 20 years have dramatically increased the rate of survival of these fragile newborns. However, as gestational age at delivery and birth weight of a baby decrease, the risk for CP dramatically increases. A term pregnancy is delivered at 37–41 weeks gestation. The risk for CP in a preterm infant (32–37 weeks) is increased about five–fold over the risk for an infant born at term. Survivors of extremely preterm births (less than 28 weeks) face as much as a fifty–fold increase in risk. About 50% of all cases of CP now being diagnosed are in children who were born prematurely.

Symptoms

By definition, the defect in cerebral function causing CP is nonprogressive. However, the symptoms of CP often change over time. Most of the symptoms of CP relate in some way to the aberrant control of muscles. To review, CP is categorized first by the type of movement/postural disturbance(s) present, then by a description of which limbs are affected, and finally by the severity of motor impairment. For example, spastic diplegia refers to continuously tight muscles that have no voluntary control in both legs, while athetoid quadraparesis describes uncontrolled writhing movements and muscle weakness in all four limbs. These three-part descriptions are helpful in providing a general picture, but cannot give a complete description of any one person with CP. In addition, the various "forms" of CP do not occur with equal frequency-spastic diplegia is seen in more individuals than is athetoid quadraparesis. CP can also be loosely categorized as mild, moderate, or severe, but these are very subjective terms with no firm boundaries between them.

A muscle that is tensed and contracted is hypertonic, while excessively loose muscles are hypotonic. Spastic, hypertonic muscles can cause serious orthopedic problems, including **scoliosis** (spine curvature), hip dislocation, or **contractures**. A contracture is shortening of a muscle, aided sometimes by a weak-opposing force from a neighboring muscle. Contractures may become permanent, or "fixed," without some sort of intervention. Fixed contractures may cause postural abnormalities in the affected limbs. Clenched fists and contracted feet (equinus or equinovarus) are common in people with CP. Spasticity in the thighs causes them to turn in and cross at the knees, resulting in an unusual method of walking known as a "scissors gait." Any of the joints in the limbs may be stiff (immobilized) due to spasticity of the attached muscles.

Athetosis and dyskinesia often occur with spasticity, but do not often occur alone. The same is true of ataxia. It is important to remember that "mild CP" or "severe CP" refers not only to the number of symptoms present, but also to the level of involvement of any particular class of symptoms.

Mechanisms that can cause CP are not always restricted to motor–control areas of the brain. Other neurologically based symptoms may include:

- mental retardation/learning disabilities
- behavioral disorders
- seizure disorders
- visual impairment
- hearing loss
- speech impairment (dysarthria)
- abnormal sensation and perception

These problems may have a greater impact on a child's life than the physical impairments of CP, although not all children with CP are affected by other problems. Many infants and children with CP have growth impairment. About one–third of individuals with CP have moderate–to–severe mental retardation, one–third have mild mental retardation, and one–third have normal intelligence.

KEY TERMS

Asphyxia—Lack of oxygen. In the case of cerebral palsy, lack of oxygen to the brain.

Ataxia—A deficiency of muscular coordination, especially when voluntary movements are attempted, such as grasping or walking.

Athetosis—A condition marked by slow, writhing, involuntary muscle movements.

Cerebral palsy—Movement disability resulting from nonprogressive brain damage.

Coagulopathy—A disorder in which blood is either too slow or too quick to coagulate (clot).

Contracture—A tightening of muscles that prevents normal movement of the associated limb or other body part.

Cytokine—A protein associated with inflammation that, at high levels, may be toxic to nerve cells in the developing brain.

Diplegia—Paralysis affecting like parts on both sides the body, such as both arms or both legs.

Dorsal rhizotomy—A surgical procedure that cuts nerve roots to reduce spasticity in affected muscles.

Dyskinesia—Impaired ability to make voluntary movements.

Hemiplegia—Paralysis of one side of the body.

Hypotonia—Reduced or diminished muscle tone.

Quadriplegia—Paralysis of all four limbs.

Serial casting—A series of casts designed to gradually move a limb into a more functional position.

Spastic—A condition in which the muscles are rigid, posture may be abnormal, and fine motor control is impaired.

Spasticity—Increased muscle tone, or stiffness, which leads to uncontrolled, awkward movements.

Static encephalopathy—A disease of the brain that does not get better or worse.

Tenotomy—A surgical procedure that cuts the tendon of a contracted muscle to allow lengthening.

Diagnosis

Examination

Diagnosing CP in an infant is often a difficult and slow process that takes time to establish with certainty, as there are other health problems that can mimic the condition. The physician may suspect that the infant has CP because of a history of difficulties at birth, seizures, feeding problems, or low muscle tone. Detailed medical and developmental history, including the history of the pregnancy and delivery, medications taken by the mother during fetal development, infections, and fetal movement are all considered. A detailed family history, including the mother's history of **miscarriage**, relatives with similar conditions, ethnic background, and consanguinity (marriage between close blood relatives) can also prove helpful.

The signs of CP are not usually noticeable at birth. Children normally progress through a predictable set of developmental milestones through the first 18 months of life. Children with CP, however, tend to develop these skills more slowly because of their motor impairments, and delays in reaching milestones are usually the first symptoms of CP. Babies with more severe cases of CP are normally diagnosed earlier than others.

Selected developmental milestones, and the ages for normally acquiring them, are given in the following list. If a child does not acquire the skill by the age shown in parentheses, there is some cause for concern.

- Sits well unsupported—6 months (8–10 months)
- Babbles—6 months (8 months)
- Crawls—9 months (12 months)
- Finger feeds, holds bottle—9 months (12 months)
- Walks alone—12 months (15–18 months)
- Uses one or two words other than dada/mama—12 months (15 months)
- Walks up and down steps—24 months (24–36 months)
- Turns pages in books; removes shoes and socks—24 months (30 months)

Children do not consistently favor one hand over the other before 12–18 months, and doing so may be a sign that the child has difficulty using the other hand. This same preference for one side of the body may show up as asymmetric crawling or, later on, favoring one leg while climbing stairs.

It must be remembered that children normally progress at somewhat different rates, and slow beginning accomplishment is often followed by normal development. Other causes for developmental delay—some benign, some serious—should be excluded before considering CP as the answer. CP is nonprogressive, so continued loss of previously acquired milestones indicates that CP is not the cause of the problem.

Tests

No one test is diagnostic for CP, but certain factors increase suspicion. The Apgar score measures a baby's condition immediately after birth. Babies that have low Apgar scores are at increased risk for CP. Presence of abnormal muscle tone or movements may indicate CP, as may the persistence of infantile reflexes. Imaging of the brain using ultrasound, x rays, MRI, and/or CT scans may reveal a structural anomaly. Some brain lesions associated with CP include scarring, cysts, expansion of the cerebral ventricles (**hydrocephalus**), periventricular leukomalacia (an abnormality of the area surrounding the ventricles), areas of dead tissue (necrosis), and evidence of an intracerebral hemorrhage or blood clot. Ultrasound in the neonate (newborn) is also used as it provides information about the structures of the brain as well as diagnostic information on possible hemorrhage or hypoxic–ischemic (lack of oxygen) injury. Blood and urine biochemical tests, as well as genetic tests, may be used to rule out other possible causes, including muscle and peripheral nerve diseases, mitochondrial and metabolic diseases, and other inherited disorders. Evaluations by a pediatric developmental specialist and a geneticist may be of benefit.

Treatment

Cerebral palsy cannot be cured, but many of the disabilities it causes can be managed through planning and timely care. Treatment for a child with CP depends on the severity, nature, and location of the primary muscular symptoms, as well as any associated problems that might be present. Optimal care of a child with mild CP may involve regular interaction with only a physical therapist and occupational therapist, whereas care for a more severely affected child may include visits to multiple medical specialists throughout life. With proper treatment and an effective plan, most people with CP can lead productive, happy lives.

Parents of a child newly diagnosed with CP are not likely to have the necessary expertise to coordinate the full range of care their child will need. Although knowledgeable and caring medical professionals are indispensable for developing a care plan, a potentially more important source of information and advice is other parents who have dealt with the same set of difficulties. Support groups for parents of children with CP can be significant sources of both practical advice and emotional support. Many cities have support groups that can be located through the United Cerebral Palsy Association, and most large medical centers have special multidisciplinary clinics for children with developmental disorders.

Traditional

Spasticity, muscle weakness, coordination, ataxia, and scoliosis are all significant impairments that affect the posture and mobility of a person with CP. Physical and occupational therapists work with the patient and the family to maximize the ability to move affected limbs, develop normal motor patterns, and maintain posture. Assistive technology such as wheelchairs, walkers, shoe inserts, crutches, and braces are often required. A speech therapist and high–tech aids, such as computer–controlled communication devices, can make a tremendous difference in the life of those who have speech impairments.

Daily range of motion (ROM) exercises are important to prevent or delay contractures (fixed, rigid muscles) secondary to spasticity, and to maintain mobility of joints and soft tissues. Stretching exercises are performed to increase motion. Progressive resistance exercises also increase strength. Age–appropriate play and adaptive toys and games using the desired exercises are important to elicit the child's full cooperation. Strengthening knee extensor muscles helps to improve crouching and stride length. Postural and motor control training is important following the normal developmental sequence of children (i.e., achieve head and neck control if possible before advancing to trunk control).

Occupational therapists keep the child's developmental age in mind and use adaptive equipment as needed to help attain these milestones. For example, if a child is developmentally ready to stand and explore the environment, but is limited by lack of motor control, a stander or modified walker is used. Performance based upon previous success is encouraged to maintain the child's interest and cooperation. Assistive devices and durable medical equipment help attain function that may not be possible otherwise. Orthotic devices frequently are required to maintain functional joint position especially in persons who are non–ambulatory. Frequent reevaluation of orthotic devices is important as children quickly outgrow them and can develop skin irritation from improper use of orthotic devices.

Recreational therapy, especially hippotherapy (horseback riding therapy) is frequently a well–liked activity of parents and patients alike to help with muscle tone, range of motion, strength, coordination, and balance. Hippotherapy also offers many potential cognitive, physical, and emotional benefits. Incorporation of play into all of a child's therapies is important. The child should view physical and **occupational therapy** as fun, not work. Caregivers should seek fun and creative ways to stimulate children, especially those who have decreased ability to explore their own environments.

Drugs

Before fixed contractures develop, muscle–relaxant drugs such as diazepam (Valium), dantrolene (Dantrium), and baclofen (Lioresal) may be prescribed. Botulinum toxin (Botox), a newer and highly effective treatment, is injected directly into the affected muscles. Alcohol or phenol injections into the nerve controlling the muscle are another option. Multiple medications are available to control seizures, and athetosis can be treated using medications such as trihexyphenidyl HCl (Artane) and benztropine (Cogentin).

Alternative

Fixed contractures are usually treated with either serial casting or surgery. The most commonly used surgical procedures are tenotomy, tendon transfer, and dorsal rhizotomy. In tenotomy, tendons of the affected muscle are cut and the limb is cast in a more normal position while the tendon regrows. Alternatively, tendon transfer involves cutting and reattaching a tendon at a different point on the bone to enhance the length and function of the muscle. A neurosurgeon performing dorsal rhizotomy carefully cuts selected nerve roots in the spinal cord to prevent them from stimulating the spastic muscles. Neurosurgical techniques in the brain such as implanting tiny electrodes directly into the cerebellum, or cutting a portion of the hypothalamus, have very specific uses and have had mixed results.

Clinical trials

Many clinical trials for the treatment of cerebral palsy are currently sponsored by the National Institutes of Health (NIH) and other agencies. In 2009, NIH reported 53 on–going or recently completed studies.

A few examples include:

- The evaluation of the effectiveness of hyperbaric oxygen treatments and the potential longer term effects in children between the ages of 3 and 8 yrs with spastic CP. (NCT00290186)

- The classification of types of hypertonia in patients with cerebral palsy. (NCT00123708)
- A study of the radiographic and clinical outcomes of scoliosis surgical treatment in patients with CP. (NCT00680264)
- A study on how the muscle architecture of the quadriceps muscles in CP adapts to two separate training programs. (NCT00629070)
- The effectiveness of acupuncture as complementary therapy for CP. (NCT00221247)
- The effects of botulinum toxin injections on walking and on the changes it causes in the muscle, brain and spinal cord of CP patients. (NCT00503620)
- The assessment of the predictive value of generalized movements in preterm and term infants who are at risk for development of cerebral palsy. (NCT00749008)

Clinical trial information is constantly updated by NIH and the most recent information on CP trials can be found at: http://clinicaltrials.gov.

Prognosis

The prognosis of persons with CP varies according to the severity of the disorder. Some children have only mild problems in muscle tone and no problems with daily activities, while others are unable to purposefully move any part of the body. Regression, or worsening of long–term symptoms, is not characteristic of CP. If regression occurs, it is necessary to look for a different cause of the child's problems. In order for a child to be able to walk, a major cascade of events in motor control have to occur. A child must be able to hold up his head before he can sit up on his own, and he must be able to sit independently before he can walk on his own. It is generally assumed that if a child is not sitting up by himself by age four or walking by age eight, he will never be an independent walker. But a child who starts to walk at age three will certainly continue to walk unless he has a disorder other than CP.

In people with severe CP, motor problems often lead to medical complications, including more frequent and serious infections, severe breathing problems, feeding intolerance, and skin breakdown. These medical complications can lead to frequent hospitalizations and a shortened life expectancy. **Epilepsy** also occurs in about a third of children with CP and is more frequent in patients with spastic quadriplegia or mental retardation. Cognitive impairment occurs more frequently in CP than in the general population, and mental delays or some form of learning disability has been estimated to occur in over two thirds of CP cases.

Prevention

Research in the early 2000s is focused on the possible benefits of recognizing and treating coagulopathies and inflammatory disorders in the prenatal and perinatal periods in order to reduce the incidence of CP and other congenital diseases. The use of magnesium sulfate in pregnant women with **preeclampsia** or threatened preterm delivery may reduce the risk of CP in very preterm infants. Finally, the risk of CP can be decreased through good maternal **nutrition**, avoidance of drugs and alcohol during pregnancy, and prevention or prompt treatment of infections.

Resources

BOOKS

Bower, Eva. *Finnie's Handling the Young Child with Cerebral Palsy at Home,* 4th ed., Woburn, MA: Butterworth–Heinemann, 2008.

Enck, Becky. *Walking Hand in Hand with Cameron, Together We Can!: One Family's Journey with Cerebral Palsy.* Bloomington, IN: iUniverse, 2008.

Gage, James R., et al, editors. *The Identification and Treatment of Gait Problems in Cerebral Palsy.* London, UK: Mac Keith Press, 2009.

Grimm, James. *The Heart's Alphabet: Daring to Live with Cerebral Palsy.* Minneapolis, MN: BookMobile, 2007.

Hinchcliffe, Archie. *Children with Cerebral Palsy: A Manual for Therapists, Parents and Community Workers.* Thousand Oaks, CA: Sage Publications, 2007.

Martin, Sieglinde. *Teaching Motor Skills to Children with Cerebral Palsy and Similar Movement Disorders: A Guide for Parents and Professionals.* Bethesda, MD: Woodbine House, 2006.

Miller, Freeman, and Steven J. Bachrach. *Cerebral Palsy: A Complete Guide for Caregiving,* 2nd edition, Baltimore, MD: The Johns Hopkins University Press, 2006.

Miller, Freeman, editor. *Physical Therapy of Cerebral Palsy.* New York, NY: Springer, 2007.

PERIODICALS

Berker, A. N., and M. S. Yalcin. "Cerebral palsy: orthopedic aspects and rehabilitation." *Pediatric Clinics of North America* 55, no. 5 (October 2008): 1209–1225.

Fasoli, S. E., et al. "Upper limb robotic therapy for children with hemiplegia." *American Journal of Physical Medicine & Rehabilitation* 87, no. 11 (November 2008): 929–936.

Koop, S. E. "Scoliosis in cerebral palsy." *Developmental Medicine and Child Neurology* 51, suppl. 4 (October 2009): 92–98.

Kuperminc, M. N., and R. D. Stevenson. "Growth and nutrition disorders in children with cerebral palsy." *Developmental Disabilities Research Reviews* 14, no. 2 (2008): 137–146.

Moore, A. P., et al. "Two-year placebo-controlled trial of botulinum toxin A for leg spasticity in cerebral palsy." *Neurology* 71, no. 2 (July 2008): 122–128.

Newey, C. "Improving care for children with cerebral palsy." *Pediatric Nursing* 20, no. 7 (2008): 20–23.

Oppenheim, W. L. "Complementary and alternative methods in cerebral palsy." *Developmental Medicine and Child Neurology* 51, suppl. 4 (October 2009): 122–129.

Surman, G., et al. "Children with cerebral palsy: severity and trends over time." *Paediatric and Perinatal Epidemiology* 23, no. 6 (November 2009): 513–521.

Wiart, L., et al. "Stretching with children with cerebral palsy: what do we know and where are we going?" *Pediatric Physical Therapy* 20, no. 2 (2008): 173–178.

Willoughby, K. L., et al. "Two hands are better than one: bimanual skill development in children with hemiplegic cerebral palsy." *Developmental Medicine and Child Neurology* 31, no. 24 (October 2009): 1971–1979.

OTHER

"Cerebral Palsy." *Medline Plus.* Health Topic. http://www.nlm.nih.gov/medlineplus/cerebralpalsy.html (accessed October 31, 2009).

"Cerebral Palsy." *MOD.* Fact Sheet. http://www.marchofdimes.com/professionals/14332_1208.aspx (accessed October 31, 2009).

"Cerebral Palsy." *Mayo Clinic.* Information Page. http://www.mayoclinic.com/print/cerebral-palsy/DS00302/METHOD=print&DSECTION=all (accessed October 31, 2009).

"Cerebral Palsy Information Page." *NINDS.* Information Page. http://www.ninds.nih.gov/disorders/cerebral_palsy/cerebral_palsy.htm (accessed October 31, 2009).

"CP in the News." *Cerebral Palsy International Foundation.* News Archive. http://cpirf.org/stories/category/cp-news (accessed October 31, 2009).

ORGANIZATIONS

Cerebral Palsy International Research Foundation, 1025 Connecticut Avenue, Suite 701, Washington, DC, 20036, (202) 496-5060, nmaher@cpirf.org, http://www.cpirf.org.

Children's Hemiplegia and Stroke Assocn. (CHASA), 4101 West Green Oaks Blvd., Suite 305, Arlington, TX, 76016, (817) 492-4325, info437@chasa.org, http://www.hemi-kids.org.

Children's Neurobiological Solutions (CNS) Foundation, 1726 Franceschi Road, Santa Barbara, CA, 93101, (805) 898-4442, (866) CNS-5580, info@cnsfoundation.org, http://www.cnsfoundation.org.

March of Dimes Foundation, 1275 Mamaroneck Avenue, White Plains, NY, 10605, (914) 428-7100, (888) MODIMES, (914) 428-8203, askus@marchofdimes.com, http://www.marchofdimes.com.

National Institute of Neurological Disorders and Stroke (NINDS), PO Box 5801, Bethesda, MD, 20824, (301) 496-5751, (800) 352-9424, http://www.ninds.nih.gov.

Pedal with Pete, PO Box 274, Kent, OH, 44240, (800) 304-PETE, (330) 673-1240, petezeid@aol.com, http://www.pedalwithpete.com.

United Cerebral Palsy (UCP), 1660 L Street, NW, Suite 700, Washington, DC, 20036, (202) 776-0406, (800) USA-5UCP, (202) 776-0414, national@ucp.org, http://www. ucp.org.

Scott J. Polzin, MS, CGC
Francisco de Paula Careta
Luri Drummond Louro, MS, CGC
Monique Laberge, PhD

Cerebrospinal fluid (CSF) analysis

Definition

Cerebrospinal fluid (CSF) analysis is a laboratory test to examine a sample of the fluid surrounding the brain and spinal cord. This fluid is a clear, watery liquid that protects the central nervous system from injury and cushions it from the surrounding bone structure. It contains a variety of substances, particularly glucose (sugar), protein, and white blood cells from the immune system. The fluid is withdrawn through a needle in a procedure called a **lumbar puncture**.

Purpose

The purpose of a CSF analysis is to diagnose medical disorders that affect the central nervous system. Some of these conditions include:

- viral and bacterial infections, such as meningitis, West Nile virus, herpes virus, and encephalitis
- tumors or cancers of the nervous system
- syphilis, a sexually transmitted disease
- bleeding (hemorrhaging) around the brain and spinal cord
- multiple sclerosis, a disease that affects the myelin coating of the nerve fibers of the brain and spinal cord
- Guillain-Barré syndrome, an inflammation of the nerves
- early-onset Alzheimer's disease; the levels of two substances known as amyloid beta (1–42) and phosphorylated tau in CSF appear to be useful diagnostic markers for early-onset Alzheimer's

CSF analysis is also used in forensic investigations to identify the presence of illicit drugs (e. g., heroin) or poisons in the bodies of murder, accidental overdose, or **suicide** victims.

Precautions

In some circumstances, a lumbar puncture to withdraw a small amount of CSF for analysis may lead to serious complications. Lumbar puncture should be performed only with extreme caution, and only if the benefits are thought to outweigh the risks, in certain conditions. For example, in people who have blood clotting (coagulation) or bleeding disorders, lumbar puncture can cause bleeding that can compress the spinal cord. If there is a large **brain tumor** or other mass, removal of CSF can cause the brain to droop down within the skull cavity (herniate), compressing the brain stem and other vital structures, and leading to irreversible brain damage or **death**. These problems are easily avoided by checking blood coagulation through a blood test and by doing a computed tomography scan (CT) or **magnetic resonance imaging** (MRI) scan before attempting the lumbar puncture. In addition, a lumbar puncture procedure should never be performed at the site of a localized skin infection on the lower back because the infection may be introduced into the CSF and may spread to the brain or spinal cord.

Description

The procedure to remove cerebrospinal fluid is called a lumbar puncture, or spinal tap, because the area of the spinal column used to obtain the sample is in the lumbar spine, or lower section of the back. In rare instances, such as a spinal fluid blockage in the middle of the back, a doctor may perform a spinal tap in the neck. The lower lumbar spine (usually between the vertebrae known as L4–5) is preferable because the spinal cord stops near L2, and a needle introduced below this level will miss the spinal cord and encounter only nerve roots, which are easily pushed aside.

A lumbar puncture takes about 30 minutes. Patients can undergo the test in a doctor's office, laboratory, or outpatient hospital setting. Sometimes it requires an inpatient hospital stay. If the patient has spinal arthritis, is extremely uncooperative, or obese, it may be necessary to introduce the spinal needle using x-ray guidance.

In order to get an accurate sample of cerebrospinal fluid, it is critical that a patient is in the proper position. The spine must be curved to allow as much space as possible between the lower vertebrae, or bones of the back, for the doctor to insert a lumbar puncture needle between the vertebrae and withdraw a small amount of fluid. The most common position is for the patient to lie on his or her side with the back at the edge of the exam table, head and chin bent down, knees drawn up to the chest, and arms clasped around the knees. (Small infants and people who are obese may need to curve their spines

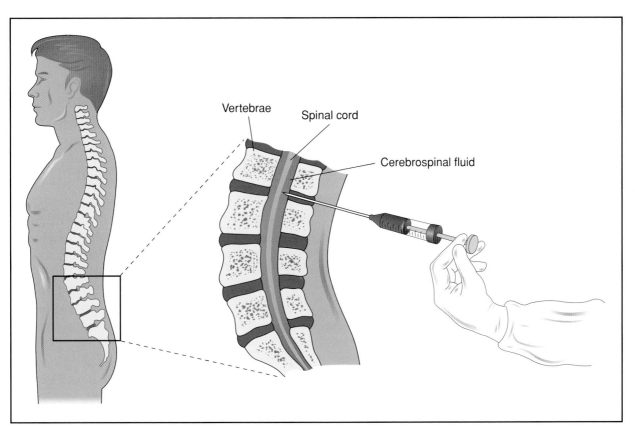

Vertebrae   Spinal cord

Cerebrospinal fluid

During a lumbar puncture, or spinal tap, a procedure in which cerebrospinal fluid is aspirated, the physician inserts a hollow, thin needle in the space between two vertebrae of the lower back and slowly advances it toward the spine. The cerebrospinal fluid pressure is then measured and the fluid is withdrawn for laboratory analysis. *(Illustration by Electronic Illustrators Group. Reproduced by permission of Gale, a part of Cengage Learning.)*

in a sitting position.) People should talk to their doctor if they have any questions about their position because it is important to be comfortable and to remain still during the entire procedure. In fact, the doctor will explain the procedure to the patient (or guardian) so that the patient can agree in writing to have it done (informed consent). If the patient is anxious or uncooperative, a short-acting sedative may be given.

During a lumbar puncture, the doctor drapes the back with a sterile covering that has an opening over the puncture site and cleans the skin surface with an antiseptic solution. Patients receive a local anesthetic to minimize any **pain** in the lower back.

The doctor inserts a hollow, thin needle in the space between two vertebrae of the lower back and slowly advances it toward the spine. A steady flow of clear cerebrospinal fluid, normally the color of water, will begin to fill the needle as soon as it enters the spinal canal. The doctor measures the cerebrospinal fluid pressure with a special instrument called a manometer and withdraws several vials of fluid for laboratory analysis. The amount of fluid collected depends

on the type and number of tests needed to diagnose a particular medical disorder.

In some cases, the doctor must remove and reposition the needle. This occurs when there is not an even flow of fluid, the needle hits bone or a blood vessel, or the patient reports sharp, unusual pain.

Preparation

Patients can go about their normal activities before a lumbar puncture. Experts recommend that patients relax before the procedure to release any muscle tension, since the lumbar puncture needle must pass through muscle tissue before it reaches the spinal canal. A patient's level of relaxation before and during the procedure plays a critical role in the test's success.

Aftercare

After the procedure, the doctor covers the site of the puncture with a sterile bandage. Patients must avoid sitting or standing and remain lying down for as long as six hours after the lumbar puncture. They

KEY TERMS

Encephalitis—An inflammation or infection of the brain and spinal cord caused by a virus or as a complication of another infection.

Guillain-Barré syndrome—An inflammation involving nerves that affect the extremities. The inflammation may spread to the face, arms, and chest.

Forensic—Referring to legal procedures or courts of law. Forensic medicine is the branch of medicine that obtains, analyzes, and presents medical evidence in criminal cases.

Immune system—Protects the body against infection.

Manometer—A device used to measure fluid pressure.

Meningitis—An infection or inflammation of the membranes or tissues that cover the brain and spinal cord, caused by bacteria or a virus.

Multiple sclerosis—A disease that destroys the covering (myelin sheath) of nerve fibers of the brain and spinal cord.

Spinal canal—The cavity or hollow space within the spine that contains cerebrospinal fluid.

Vertebrae—The bones of the spinal column. There are 33 along the spine, with five (called L1–L5) making up the lower lumbar region.

---

should also drink plenty of fluid to help prevent lumbar puncture **headache**, which is discussed in the next section.

Risks

For most people, the most common side effect after the removal of CSF is a headache. This occurs in 10–30% of adult patients and in up to 40% of children. It is caused by a decreased CSF pressure related to a small leak of CSF through the puncture site. These headaches usually are a dull pain, although some people report a throbbing sensation. A stiff neck and **nausea** may accompany the headache. Lumbar puncture headaches typically begin within two days after the procedure and persist from a few days to several weeks or months.

Since an upright position worsens the pain, patients with a lumbar puncture headache can control the pain by lying in a flat position and taking a prescription or non-prescription pain relief medication, preferably one containing **caffeine**. In rare cases, the puncture site leak is "patched" using the patient's own blood.

People should talk to their doctor about complications from a lumbar puncture. In most cases, this test to analyze CSF is a safe and effective procedure. Some patients experience pain, difficulty urinating, infection, or leakage of cerebrospinal fluid from the puncture site after the procedure.

Normal results

Normal CSF is clear and colorless. It may be cloudy in infections; straw- or yellow-colored if there is excess protein, as may occur with **cancer** or inflammation; blood-tinged if there was recent bleeding; or yellow to brown (xanthochromic) if caused by an older instance of bleeding.

A series of laboratory tests analyze the CSF for a variety of substances to rule out possible medical disorders of the central nervous system. The following are normal values for commonly tested substances:

- CSF pressure: 50–180 mm H_2O
- glucose: 40%–85 mg/dL
- protein: 15–50 mg/dL
- leukocytes (white blood cells) total less than 5 per mL
- lymphocytes: 60–70%
- monocytes: 30–50%
- neutrophils: none

Normally, there are no red blood cells in the CSF unless the needle passes though a blood vessel on route to the CSF. If this is the case, there should be more red blood cells in the first tube collected than in the last.

Abnormal results

Abnormal test result values in the pressure or any of the substances found in the cerebrospinal fluid may suggest a number of medical problems including a tumor or spinal cord obstruction; hemorrhaging or bleeding in the central nervous system; infection from bacterial, viral, or fungal microorganisms; or an inflammation of the nerves. It is important for patients to review the results of a cerebrospinal fluid analysis with their doctor and to discuss any treatment plans.

Resources

BOOKS

Beers, Mark H., Robert S. Porter, and Thomas V. Jones, eds. *The Merck Manual of Diagnosis and Therapy*. 18th ed. Whitehouse Station, NJ: Merck Research Laboratories, 2006.

PERIODICALS

Boivin, G. "Diagnosis of Herpesvirus Infections of the Central Nervous System." *Herpes* 11, Supplement 2 (June 2004): 48A–56A.

Roos, K. L. "West Nile Encephalitis and Myelitis." *Current Opinion in Neurology* 17 (June 2004): 343–346.

Schoonenboom, N. S., Y. A. Pijnenburg, C. Mulder, et al. "Amyloid Beta(1-42) and Phosphorylated Tau in CSF as Markers for Early-Onset Alzheimer Disease." *Neurology* 62 (May 11, 2004): 1580–1584.

Sharma, A. N., L. S. Nelson, and R. S. Hoffman. "Cerebrospinal Fluid Analysis in Fatal Thallium Poisoning: Evidence for Delayed Distribution into the Central Nervous System." *American Journal of Forensic Medicine and Pathology* 25 (June 2004): 156–158.

Wyman, J., and S. Bultman. "Postmortem Distribution of Heroin Metabolites in Femoral Blood, Liver, Cerebrospinal Fluid, and Vitreous Humor." *Journal of Analytical Toxicology* 28 (May–June 2004): 260–263.

ORGANIZATIONS

American Academy of Neurology, 1080 Montreal Ave., St. Paul, MN, 5516, (651) 695-2717, (651) 695-2791, (800) 879-1960, memberservices@aan.com, http://www.aan.com/.

American College of Forensic Examiners International (ACFEI), 2750 East Sunshine, Springfield, MO, 65804, (417) 881-3818, (417) 881-4702, (800) 423-9737, http://www.acfei.com.

Martha Floberg Robbins
Rebecca J. Frey, PhD

Cerebrovascular accident *see* **Stroke**

Cerebrovascular amyloidosis *see* **Cerebral amyloid angiopathy**

Cerumen impaction

Definition

Cerumen impaction is a condition in which earwax has become tightly packed in the external ear canal to the point that the canal is blocked.

Description

Cerumen impaction develops when earwax accumulates in the inner part of the ear canal and blocks the eardrum. It affects between 2% and 6% of the general population in the United States. Impaction does not happen under normal circumstances because cerumen is produced by glands in the outer part of the ear canal; it is not produced in the inner part. The cerumen traps sand or dust particles before they reach the ear drum. It also protects the outer part of the ear canal because it repels water. The slow movement of the outer layer of skin of the ear canal carries cerumen toward the outer opening of the ear. As the older cerumen reaches the opening of the ear, it dries out and falls away.

Causes and symptoms

Cerumen is most likely to become impacted when it is pushed against the eardrum by cotton-tipped applicators, hair pins, or other objects that people put in their ears; and when it is trapped against the eardrum by a hearing aid. Less common causes of cerumen impaction include overproduction of earwax by the glands in the ear canal, or an abnormally shaped ear canal.

The most important symptom of cerumen impaction is partial loss of hearing. Other symptoms are **itching**, **tinnitus** (noise or ringing in the ears), a sensation of fullness in the ear, and **pain**.

Diagnosis

The diagnosis of impacted cerumen is usually made by examining the ear canal and eardrum with an otoscope, an instrument with a light attached that allows the doctor to look into the canal.

Treatment

Irrigation is the most common method of removing impacted cerumen. It involves washing out the ear canal with water from a commercial irrigator or a syringe with a catheter attached. Although some doctors use Water Piks to remove cerumen, most do not recommend them because the stream of water is too forceful and may damage the eardrum. The doctor may add a small amount of alcohol, hydrogen peroxide, or other antiseptic. The water must be close to body temperature; if it is too cold or too warm, the patient may feel dizzy or nauseated. After the ear has been irrigated, the doctor will apply antibiotic ear drops to protect the ear from infection.

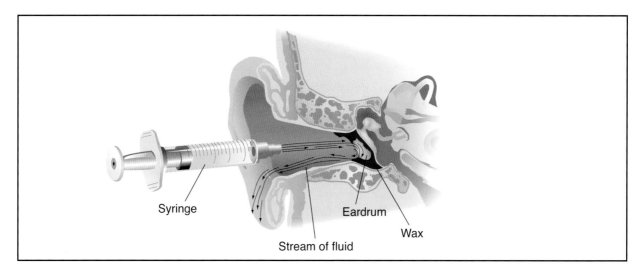

Ear wax is removed by flushing the ear canal with warm fluid. *(Illustration by Argosy, Inc. Reproduced by permission of Gale, a part of Cengage Learning.)*

Irrigation should not be used to remove cerumen if the patient's eardrum is ruptured or missing; if the patient has a history of chronic **otitis media** (inflammation of the middle ear) or a **myringotomy** (cutting the eardrum to allow fluid to escape from the middle ear); or if the patient has hearing in only one ear.

If irrigation cannot be used or fails to remove the cerumen, the patient is referred to an ear, nose, and throat (ENT) specialist. The specialist can remove the wax with a vacuum device or a curette, which is a small scoop-shaped surgical instrument.

Some doctors prescribe special ear drops, such as Cerumenex, to soften the wax. The most common side effect of Cerumenex is an allergic skin reaction. Over-the-counter wax removal products include Debrox or Murine Ear Drops. A 3% solution of hydrogen peroxide may also be used. These products are less likely to irritate the skin of the ear.

Alternative treatment

One alternative method that is sometimes touted as a way to remove impacted cerumen is ear candling. Ear candling involves the insertion of a burning candle or a cone of wax-soaked linen or cotton into the affected ear. The person lies on his or her side with the affected ear uppermost. A collecting plate is placed on the ear to catch melted wax. The cone or candle is threaded through a hole in the plate into the ear canal and lit. A variation on this technique involves blowing herbal smoke into the ear through homemade pottery cones. Practitioners of ear candling claim that the heat from the burning candle or smoke creates a vacuum that draws out the impacted cerumen. Some also claim that ear candling improves hearing, relieves sinus infections, cures earache or swimmer's ear, stops tinnitus, or purifies the mind. None of these claims are true. Ear candling is not recognized as an acceptable alternative practice by naturopaths, homeopaths, practitioners of Native American medicine, or any other authority on complementary and alternative medicine.

Ear candling is not only an ineffective way to remove impacted cerumen, it can actually damage the ear. According to a 1996 survey of 122 otolaryngologists (doctors who specialize in treating ear, nose, and throat disorders) in the Spokane area, the doctors reported 21 severe ear injuries resulting from ear candling, including 13 cases of external **burns**, 7 cases of ear canal obstruction from melted candle wax, and 1 case of eardrum perforation. Ear candles cannot legally be sold as health devices in the United States because they do not have Food and Drug Administration (FDA) approval. A similar ban is in effect in Canada. Ear candles are, however, available over the Internet and in some health food stores with the labeling "for entertainment only."

Prognosis

In most cases, impacted cerumen is successfully removed by irrigation with no lasting side effects.

Cerumen—The medical term for earwax.

Curette—A small scoop-shaped surgical instrument that can be used to remove cerumen if irrigation does not work or cannot be used.

Ear candling—An alternative method for removing impacted cerumen with a lighted hollow cone of paraffin or beeswax. It does not work, and is not considered an acceptable treatment for any ear problem or disorder.

Impaction—A condition in which earwax has become tightly packed in the outer ear to the point that the external ear canal is blocked.

Irrigation—The technique of removing cerumen from the ear canal by flushing it with water.

Myringotomy—Surgical cutting of the ear drum to allow fluid to escape from the middle ear.

Otitis media—Inflammation of the middle ear. Patients who have had recurrent otitis media should not have cerumen removed by irrigation.

Tinnitus—A sensation of noise or ringing in the ears. Tinnitus may be a symptom of cerumen impaction.

Irrigation can, however, lead to infection of the outer or the middle ear if the patient has a damaged or absent ear drum. Patients who try to remove earwax themselves with hair pins or similar objects run the risk of perforating the ear drum or damaging the fragile skin covering the ear canal, causing bleeding and the risk of infection.

Prevention

The best method of cleaning the external ear is to wipe the outer opening with a damp washcloth folded over the index finger, without going into the ear canal itself. Two techniques have been recommended to prevent cerumen from reaccumulating in the ear. The patient may place two or three drops of mineral oil into each ear once a week, allow it to remain for two or three minutes, and rinse it out with warm water; or place two drops of Domeboro otic solution in each ear once a week after showering.

Patients who wear **hearing aids** should have their ears examined periodically for signs of cerumen accumulation.

Resources

BOOKS

Beers, Mark H., MD, and Robert Berkow, MD, editors. "External Ear: Obstructions." Section 7, Chapter 83 In *The Merck Manual of Diagnosis and Therapy.* Whitehouse Station, NJ: Merck Research Laboratories, 2002.

Jackler, Robert K., MD, and Michael J. Kaplan, MD. "Cerumen Impaction." In "Ear, Nose, & Throat." *Current Medical Diagnosis & Treatment 2001*, edited by L. M. Tierney, Jr., MD, et al., 40th ed. New York: Lange Medical Books/McGraw-Hill, 2001.

PERIODICALS

Crummer, R. W., and G. A. Hassan. "Diagnostic Approach to Tinnitus." *American Family Physician* 69 (January 1, 2004): 120–126.

Ernst, E. "Ear Candles—A Triumph of Ignorance Over Science." *Journal of Laryngology and Otology* 118 (January 2004): 1–2.

Whatley, V. N., C. L. Dodds, and R. I. Paul. "Randomized Clinical Trial of Docusate, Triethanolamine Polypeptide, and Irrigation in Cerumen Removal in Children." *Archives of Pediatrics and Adolescent Medicine* 157 (December 2003): 1177–1180.

OTHER

Health Canada/Santé Canada. *It's Your Health: Ear Candling.* Ottawa: Health Canada/Santé Canada, 2002.

ORGANIZATIONS

American Academy of Family Physicians (AAFP), 11400 Tomahawk Creek Parkway, Leawood, KS, 66211-2672, (913) 906-6000, (800) 274-2237, http://www.aafp.org.

American Academy of Otolaryngology, Head and Neck Surgery, One Prince St., Alexandria, VA, 22314-3357, (703) 836-4444, http://www.entnet.org.

Rebecca J. Frey, PhD
Tish Davidson, AM

Cervical biopsy *see* **Cervical conization**

Cervical cancer

Definition

Cervical **cancer** is a disease of the female reproductive system in which the cells lining the cervix (the area between the uterus body and vagina) become abnormal, start to grow uncontrollably, and form invasive tumors. Caught in its early stages, cervical cancer is highly curable; left untreated it can be fatal.

Demographics

In 2009, the American Cancer Society projected that about 11,270 new cases of invasive cervical cancer would be diagnosed in the United States, and about 4,700 American women would die from the disease. Although the median age for diagnosis of cervical cancer in the United States between 2000 and 2004 was 48, almost half of new cases of serious cervical cancer and deaths from cervical cancer are in women aged 65 and older. Rarely is cervical cancer diagnosed in women under age 20. In the United States poor and minority women have the highest rates of cervical cancer and cervical cancer deaths, most likely because they have less access to screening tests and healthcare.

Internationally, about half a million new cases of cervical cancer are diagnosed each year, at least three–quarters of which are in developing countries. In the developing world, cervical cancer is the second most common cancer in women and the third most common cause of cancer **death**, with nearly 300,000 women dying annually.

Description

There are two types of cervical cancers. They are named after type of cell that becomes cancerous. Between 80% and 90% of cervical cancers are squamous cell carcinomas. Squamous cells are thin, flat cells of the surfaces of the skin, the cervix, and linings of various organs. Squamous cell carcinoma originates in the squamous cells on the surface of the ectocervix, the part of the cervix that is next to the vagina. Most of the remaining 10–20% of cervical cancers are adenocarcinomas. This cancer originates in the mucus–producing cells of the inner cervix, or endocervix, the part of the cervix nearest the body of the uterus. Occasionally, cervical cancer may have characteristics of both types of carcinomas. This condition is called adenosquamous carcinoma or mixed carcinoma. In the United States adenocarcinomas have become increasingly common since the 1980s.

Cervical cancer usually is slow to develop. The initial abnormalities that occur in some cervical cells are not cancerous, and not every woman who has abnormal cervical cells develops cancer. The precancerous cells form a lesion called dysplasia. Dysplasia is a common condition, and the abnormal cells often disappear without treatment. Moderate to severe dysplasia may be called carcinoma in situ or non–invasive cervical cancer.

In some women, precancerous cells continue to change and become cancerous. This process often takes years, although it occasionally can happen within one year. When the abnormal cells become malignant (cancerous), they start to grow uncontrollably and invade the deeper layers of the cervix, becoming an invasive cervical cancer. Non–invasive cervical cancer is about four times more common than invasive cervical cancer.

Screening for cervical cancer is done with a **Pap test** or smear, in which cells are scraped from the cervix and examined for abnormalities under a microscope. In the United States and other developed countries, the rate of cervical cancer has declined steadily since the mid–1950s with widespread use of routine Pap tests. Because cervical cancer develops slowly, early detection makes cervical cancer highly treatable.

Risk factors

Risk factors for cervical cancer include:
- sexual intercourse before age 16
- numerous sexual partners
- sexual partners who have had many sexual partners
- giving birth to seven or more children
- smoking cigarettes
- a weakened immune system.

Diethylstilbestrol (DES), which was given to pregnant women in the United States between 1940 and 1971, may increase the risk of a rare type of cervical cancer in women who were exposed to the drug before birth.

Causes and symptoms

Infection with the human papilloma viruses (HPVs) is associated with about 90% of all cervical cancers. However, HPV infection is very common and only a small number of women with untreated HPV develop cervical cancer There are more than 80 types of HPV. About 30 of these types can be

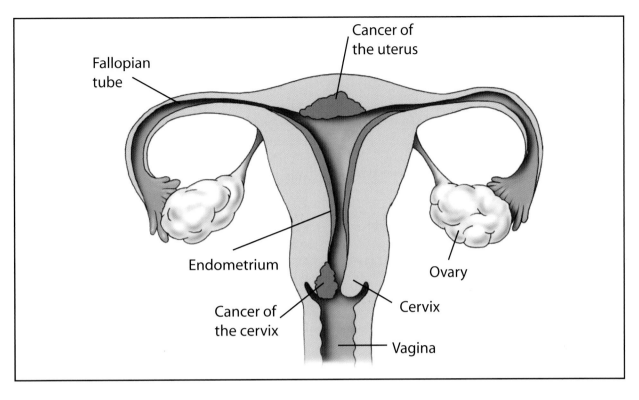

Illustrated anatomy of the female reproductive system showing cervical and uterine cancers. *(Illustration by Frank Forney. Reproduced by permission of Gale, a part of Cengage Learning.)*

transmitted sexually, including those that cause **genital warts** (papillomas). About half of sexually transmitted HPVs are associated with cervical cancer. These high–risk HPVs produce a protein that may cause cervical epithelial cells to grow uncontrollably. The virus also makes a second protein that interferes with tumor (cell growth) suppressors that are produced by the human immune system. HPV–16 or HPV–18 are associated with about 90% of invasive cervical cancers.

Although cervical cancer often has no signs or symptoms, possible signs and symptoms include:

- menstrual bleeding that is unusually prolonged or heavy
- vaginal bleeding between periods or after sexual intercourse, douching, or a pelvic exam
- bleeding after menopause
- painful sexual intercourse
- pelvic pain.

Diagnosis

Pap test

Most often, cervical cancer is first detected with a Pap test that is performed as part of a regular pelvic examination. The vagina is spread with a metal or plastic instrument called a speculum. A swab is used to remove mucus and cells from the cervix. This sample is sent to a laboratory for microscopic examination.

The Pap test is a screening tool rather than a diagnostic tool. It is very efficient at detecting cervical abnormalities. The Bethesda System commonly is used to report Pap test results. A negative test means that no abnormalities are present in the cervical tissue. A positive Pap test describes abnormal cervical cells as low–grade or high–grade squamous intraepithelial lesions (SILs), depending on the extent of dysplasia. About 5–10% of Pap tests show at least mild abnormalities. However, a number of factors other than cervical cancer can cause abnormalities, including inflammation from bacteria or yeast infections. A few months after the infection is treated, the Pap test is repeated.

Biopsy

Following an abnormal Pap test, a **colposcopy** is usually performed. The physician uses a magnifying scope to view the surface of the cervix. The cervix may be coated with an iodine solution that causes normal cells to turn brown and abnormal cells to turn white or yellow. This procedure is called a Schiller test. If any

Adenocarcinoma—Cervical cancer that originates in the mucus–producing cells of the inner or endocervix.

Biopsy—Removal of a small sample of tissue for examination under a microscope; used for the diagnosis and treatment of cervical cancer and precancerous conditions.

Carcinoma in situ—Cancer that is confined to the cells in which it originated and has not spread to other tissues.

Cervix—The narrow, lower end of the uterus forming the opening to the vagina.

Colposcopy—Diagnostic procedure using a hollow, lighted tube (colposcope) to look inside the cervix and uterus.

Conization—Cone biopsy; removal of a cone–shaped section of tissue from the cervix for diagnosis or treatment.

Dysplasia—Abnormal cellular changes that may become cancerous.

Endocervical curettage—Biopsy performed with a curette to scrape the mucous membrane of the cervical canal.

Human papilloma virus (HPV)—A group of viruses that cause abnormal cell growth (warts or papillomas); some types can cause cervical cancer.

Hysterectomy—Removal of the uterus.

Interferon—Potent immune–defense protein produced by viral–infected cells. Manufactured interferon is used as an anticancer and antiviral drug.

Laparoscopy—Insertion of a tube through a very small surgical incision to remove tissue.

Loop electrosurgical excision procedure (LEEP)—Cone biopsy performed with a wire that is heated by electrical current.

Lymph nodes—Small, bean–shaped masses of tissue scattered along the lymphatic system that act as filters and immune monitors, removing fluids, bacteria, or cancer cells that travel through the lymph system. Cancer cells in the lymph nodes are a sign that the cancer has spread, and that it might recur.

Pelvic exenteration—Extensive surgery to remove the uterus, ovaries, pelvic lymph nodes, part or all of the vagina, and the bladder, rectum, and/or part of the colon.

Squamous cells—Thin, flat cells of the surfaces of the skin and cervix and linings of various organs.

Squamous intraepithelial lesion (SIL)—Abnormal growth of squamous cells on the surface of the cervix.

Vaginal stenosis—Narrowing of the vagina due to a build–up of scar tissue.

---

abnormal areas are observed, a colposcopic biopsy may be performed. A biopsy is the removal of a small piece of tissue for microscopic examination by a pathologist.

Other types of cervical biopsies may be performed. An endocervical curettage is a biopsy in which a narrow instrument called a curette is used to scrape tissue from inside the opening of the cervix. A cone biopsy, or conization, is used to remove a cone–shaped piece of tissue from the cervix. In a cold knife cone biopsy, a surgical scalpel or laser is used to remove the tissue. A loop electrosurgical excision procedure (LEEP) is a cone biopsy using a wire that is heated by an electrical current. Cone biopsies can be used to determine whether abnormal cells have invaded below the surface of the cervix. They also can be used to treat many precancers and very early cancers. Biopsies may be performed using a local or **general anesthesia**. They may cause cramping and bleeding.

Diagnosing the cancer stage

Following a diagnosis of cervical cancer, various procedures may be used to stage the disease (determine how far the cancer has spread). For example, additional pelvic exams may be performed under anesthesia.

Several procedures help to determine if cervical cancer has invaded the urinary tract. With **cystoscopy**, a lighted tube with a lens is inserted through the urethra (the urine tube from the bladder to outside the body) and into the bladder to examine these organs for cancerous cells. Tissue samples may be removed for microscopic examination by a pathologist. **Intravenous urography** (intravenous pyelogram or IVP) is an x ray of the urinary system, following the injection of special dye. The kidneys remove the dye from the bloodstream and the dye passes into the ureters (the tubes from the kidneys to the bladder) and bladder. IVP can detect a blocked ureter caused by the spread of cancer to the pelvic lymph nodes.

A procedure called proctoscopy or **sigmoido-scopy** is similar to cystoscopy. It is used to determine whether the cancer has spread to the rectum or lower part of the large intestine.

Computed tomography (CT or CAT) scans, ultrasound, or other imaging techniques may be used to determine the spread of cancer to various parts of the body. With a CT scan, an x–ray beam rotates around the body, taking images from various angles. It is used to determine if the cancer has spread to the lymph nodes. **Magnetic resonance imaging** (MRI), which uses a magnetic field to image the body, sometimes is used for evaluating the spread of cervical cancer. Chest x rays may be used to detect cervical cancer that has spread to the lungs.

Cancer staging

The FIGO system of staging

Staging the cancer is important, as treatment depends in large part on how far the cancer has developed and spread. The International Federation of Gynecologists and Obstetricians (FIGO) system usually is used to stage cervical cancer:

- Stage 0: Carcinoma in situ; non–invasive cancer that is confined to the layer of cells lining the cervix.
- Stage I: Cancer that has spread into the connective tissue of the cervix but is confined to the uterus.
- Stage IA: Very small cancerous area that is visible only with a microscope.
- Stage IA1: Invasion area is less than 0.1 in (0.3 mm) deep and 0.3 in (7 mm) wide.
- Stage IA2: Invasion area is 0.1–0.2 in (3–5 mm) deep and less than 0.3 in (7 mm) wide.
- Stage IB: Cancer can be seen without a microscope or is deeper than 0.2 in (5 mm) or wider than 0.3 in (7 mm).
- Stage IB1: Cancer is no larger than 2 in (4 cm).
- Stage IB2: Stage IB cancer is larger than 2 in (4 cm).
- Stage II: Cancer has spread from the cervix but is confined to the pelvic region.
- Stage IIA: Cancer has spread to the upper region of the vagina, but not to the lower one–third of the vagina.
- Stage IIB: Cancer has spread to the parametrial tissue adjacent to the cervix.
- Stage III: Cancer has spread to the lower one–third of the vagina or to the wall of the pelvis and may be blocking the ureters.
- Stage IIIA: Cancer has spread to the lower vagina but not to the pelvic wall.

- Stage IIIB: Cancer has spread to the pelvic wall and/ or is blocking the flow of urine through the ureters to the bladder.
- Stage IV: Cancer has spread to other parts of the body.
- Stage IVA: Cancer has spread to the bladder or rectum.
- Stage IVB: Cancer has spread to distant organs such as the lungs.
- Recurrent: Following treatment, cancer has returned to the cervix or some other part of the body.

Treatment

Sometimes cervical cancer must be treated immediately, but more often there is time to get a second opinion. In addition to the stage of the cancer, factors such as a woman's age, general health, and preferences may influence the choice of treatment. The exact location of the cancer within the cervix and the type of cervical cancer also are important considerations.

The standard treatments for cervical cancer are surgery, **radiation therapy**, and **chemotherapy**. Studies have shown that a combination of radiation therapy and chemotherapy reduces the death rate by 30–50%.

Treatment of precancer and carcinoma in situ

Most low–grade SILs that are detected with Pap tests revert to normal without treatment. Most high–grade SILs require treatment. Treatments to remove precancerous cells include:

- cold knife cone biopsy
- LEEP
- cryosurgery (freezing the cells with a metal probe)
- cauterization or diathermy (burning off the cells)
- laser surgery (burning off the cells with a laser beam)

These methods also may be used to treat cancer that is confined to the surface of the cervix (stage 0) and other early–stage cervical cancers in women who may want to become pregnant. They may be used in conjunction with other treatments. These procedures may cause bleeding or cramping. All of these treatments require close follow–up to detect any recurrence of the cancer.

Surgery

Surgical treatments include:

- conization
- LEEP
- laser surgery for a surface lesion or tumor
- cryosurgery

- total vaginal hysterectomy (removal of the uterus and cervix through the vagina)
- total abdominal hysterectomy (removal of the uterus and cervix through a large abdominal incision)
- total laparoscopic hysterectomy (removal of the uterus and cervix with a laparoscope through a small abdominal incision)
- bilateral salpingo–oophorectomy (removal of the ovaries and fallopian tubes)
- radical hysterectomy (removal of the uterus, cervix, a portion of the vagina, and possibly the ovaries, fallopian tubes, and nearby lymph nodes)
- pelvic exenteration (removal of the uterus, cervix, ovaries, nearby lymph nodes, lower colon, rectum, and bladder, with construction of artificial openings for collecting feces and urine and possible plastic surgery to construct an artificial vagina).

Radiation

External radiation therapy uses high–energy x rays applied to the outside of the body to kill cancer cells. With internal radiation therapy thin tubes or implants containing a radioactive substance are placed in the vagina for a few hours or up to three days, two or more times over a period of several weeks.

Radiation therapy to the pelvic region can have many side effects:

- skin reaction in the area of treatment
- fatigue
- upset stomach and loose bowels
- vaginal stenosis (narrowing of the vagina due to build–up of scar tissue) leading to painful sexual intercourse
- premature menopause in young women
- problems with urination

Chemotherapy

Chemotherapy uses one or more drugs to kill cancer cells. It is used to treat disease that has spread beyond the cervix. The common drugs used for cervical cancer are cisplatin (Platinol), 5–fluorouracil (Efudex, Adrucil, Fluoroplex), ifosfamide (Ifex), paclitaxel (Taxol), and topotecan (Hycamtin). These drugs may be injected or taken by mouth.

The side effects of chemotherapy depend on a number of factors, including the type of drug, the dosage, and the length of the treatment. Side effects may include:

- nausea and vomiting
- fatigue
- changes in appetite
- hair loss (alopecia)
- mouth or vaginal sores
- infections
- menstrual cycle changes
- premature menopause
- infertility
- bleeding or anemia (low red blood cell count) With the exception of **menopause** and **infertility**, most of the side effects are temporary.

Treatment by stage

Common treatment options by stage are:

- O—conization; LEEP; laser surgery; cryosurgery; total hysterectomy for women who cannot or do not want to have children; internal radiation therapy for women who cannot have surgery
- IA—conization; total hysterectomy with or without bilateral salpingo–oophorectomy; radical hysterectomy with removal of lymph nodes; internal radiation therapy
- IB, IIA—combination internal and external radiation therapy; radical hysterectomy with removal of lymph nodes, possibly followed by radiation therapy and chemotherapy; radiation therapy plus chemotherapy
- IIB, III, IVA—internal and external radiation therapy and chemotherapy
- IVB—radiation therapy to relieve symptoms and improve quality of life; chemotherapy
- recurrent—pelvic exenteration followed by radiation therapy and chemotherapy; chemotherapy to relieve symptoms and improve quality of life.

Complementary and alternative treatment

Many complementary and alternative medicine (CAM) treatments claim to help prevent or cure various cancers. Complementary therapies are those used in addition to traditional Western medicine, while alternative therapies are used in place of conventional Western medicine. CAM treatments include **acupuncture**, bodywork therapies such as massage and **reflexology**, homeopathy, and herbal remedies used in **traditional Chinese medicine** or **Ayurvedic medicine** (traditional Indian medicine). Complementary and alternative treatment of cancer is a complicated arena. In some cases CAM is effective in relieving or reducing the symptoms associated with cancer and cancer treatment. Nevertheless, CAM treatments may interact with each other and with conventional treatments in ways that are not always well understood but that may alter the expected treatment results. In the United States, the National Center for Complementary and Alternative Medicine (NCCAM) within the National Institutes of Health supervises clinical trials of many CAM cancer therapies. Individuals should discuss all CAM therapies with their physician before beginning a treatment.

Certain foods, mainly vegetables, fruits, and grains, are believed by many people to offer protection against various cancers. As of 2007, the American Cancer Society (ACS) recommended a diet high in fruits, vegetables, and whole grains and low in calories and fats as the best way to maintain health. The ACS does not recommend taking mega–doses of any dietary supplements to cure or reduce the risk any cancer.

Prognosis

For cervical cancers that are diagnosed in the pre–invasive stage, the five–year–survival rate is almost 100%. When cervical cancer is detected in the early invasive stages, approximately 91% of women survive five years or more. Stage IVB cervical cancer is not considered curable. The five–year–survival rate for all cervical cancers combined is about 70%. The death rate from cervical cancer in the United States continues to decline by about 2% each year. Women over age 65 account for 40–50% of all deaths from cervical cancer.

Prevention

A vaccine introduced in 2006, Gardasil®, protects against four HPV viruses that cause 70% of cervical cancers and 90% of genital **warts**. The vaccine is most effective when given before a female becomes sexually active. It is recommended for all women ages 11–18 and may be given as young as age nine. Women ages 19–26 also may be vaccinated at the discretion of their physician. The vaccine is given in three doses over a six–month period and is covered by most health insurance programs. A second vaccine, Cervarix, was released in 2009 and protects against two types of HPV.

Since **vaccination** does not provide complete protection against all HPV viruses, sexual behaviors can put women at risk for HPV infection and cervical cancer. These behaviors include:

- sexual intercourse at age 16 or younger
- partners who began having intercourse at a young age
- multiple sexual partners

- sexual partners who have had multiple partners ("high–risk males")
- a partner who has had a previous sexual partner with cervical cancer

HPV infection may not produce any symptoms, so sexual partners may not know that they are infected. However, Pap tests can detect the infection. A DNA screening test for HPV can be done at the same time as the Pap test. **Condoms** do not necessarily prevent HPV infection.

Infection with the human **immunodeficiency** virus (HIV) that causes acquired immunodeficiency syndrome (**AIDS**) is a risk factor for cervical cancer. Women who test positive for HIV may have impaired immune systems that cannot correct precancerous conditions. Furthermore, sexual behavior that puts women at risk for HIV infection, also puts them at risk for HPV infection. There is some evidence suggesting that another sexually transmitted virus, the **genital herpes** virus, also may be involved in cervical cancer.

Smoking may double the risk of cervical cancer. Chemicals produced by tobacco smoke can damage the DNA of cervical cells. The risk increases with the number of years a woman smokes and the amount she smokes. A 2003 study also linked smoking to poorer outcomes and survivals in cervical cancer patients.

Most cases of cervical cancers are preventable, since they start with easily detectable precancerous changes. Therefore, the best prevention for cervical cancer is to have regular Pap tests. The American Cancer Society recommends that women begin having Pap tests about three years after first having sexual intercourse, but no later than 21 years of age. Women should continue screening every year with regular Pap tests until age 30. Once a woman has had three normal results in a row, she may get screened every two to three years. A doctor may suggest more frequent screening if a woman has certain risk factors for cervical cancer. Women who have had total hysterectomies including the removal of the cervix and those over age 70 who have had three normal results generally do not need to continue having Pap tests under these guidelines.

The National Breast and Cervical Cancer Early Detection Program provides free or low–cost Pap tests and treatment for women without health insurance, for older women, and for members of racial and ethnic minorities. The program is administered through individual states, under the direction of the Centers for Disease Control and Prevention.

Resources

BOOKS

Dizon, Don S. *100 Questions & Answers About Cervical Cancer.* Sudbury, MA: Jones and Bartlett, 2009.

Markovic, Nenad and Olivera Markovic. *What Every Woman Should Know About Cervical Cancer.* New York: Springer, 2008.

Spencer, Juliet V. *Cervical Cancer.* New York: Chelsea House, 2007.

OTHER

MedlinePlus. "Cervical Cancer." United States National Library of Medicine. June 2, 2009. http://www.nlm.nih.gov/medlineplus/cervicalcancer.html (accessed August 31, 2010).

ORGANIZATIONS

American Cancer Society, 1599 Clifton Rd., NE, Atlanta, GA, 30329, (404) 320–3333, (800) ACS–2345, http://www.cancer.org.

American Social Health Association, National HPV and Cervical Cancer Prevention Resource Center, PO Box 13827, Research Triangle Park, NC, 27709, (919) 361–8400, (800) 227–8922, (919) 361–8425, http://www.ashastd.org/hpvccrc.

Cancer Research and Prevention Foundation, 1600 Duke Street, Suite 500, Alexandria, VA, 22314, (703) 836–4412, (800) 227–2732, info@preventcancer.org, http://www.preventcancer.org.

Gynecologic Cancer Foundation, 230 W. Monroe, Suite 2528, Chicago, IL, 60606, (312) 578–1439, (800) 444–4441, (312) 578–9769, info@thegcf.org, http://www.wcn.org/gcf.

National Cancer Institute, NCI Public Inquiries Office, 6116 Executive Blvd., Room 3036A, Bethesda, MD, 20892–8322, (800) 4–CANCER, http://www.cancer.gov.

Margaret Alic, Ph.D.
Tish Davidson, A.M.

Cervical conization

Definition

Cervical conization is both a diagnostic and treatment tool used to detect and treat abnormalities of the cervix. It is also known as a cone biopsy or cold knife cone biopsy.

Purpose

Cervical conization is performed if the results of a cervical biopsy have found a precancerous condition in the cervix. The cervix is the small cylindrical organ at the lower part of the uterus, which separates the uterus from the vagina. Cervical conization also may be performed if there is an abnormal cervical smear test (**Pap test**). A biopsy is a diagnostic test in which tissue or cells are removed from the body and examined under a microscope, primarily to look for **cancer** or other abnormalities.

Precautions

As with any operation that is performed under **general anesthesia**, the patient must not eat or drink anything for six to eight hours before surgery.

Description

The patient lies on the table with her legs raised in stirrups, similar to the position when having a Pap test. The patient is given general anesthesia, and the vagina is held open with an instrument called a speculum. Using a scalpel or laser the doctor removes a cone-shaped piece of the cervix containing the area with abnormal cells. The resulting crater is repaired by stitching flaps of tissue over the wound. Alternatively, the wound may be left open, and heat or freezing is used to stop bleeding.

Once the tissue has been removed, it is examined under a microscope for signs of cancer. If cancer is present, other tests will be needed. Surgery will be performed to remove the cervix and uterus (**hysterectomy**) and other treatments may be used as well. If the abnormal cells are precancerous, a laser can be used to destroy them.

Cold knife cone biopsy used to be the preferred treatment for removing abnormal cells in the cervix. Now, most cone biopsies are performed using **laser surgery**. Cold knife cone biopsy is generally used only for special situations. For example, if a biopsy did not remove all the abnormal cells, the cold knife cone procedure allows the physician to remove what's left.

Aftercare

An overnight stay in the hospital may be required. After the test, the patient may feel some cramps or discomfort for about a week. Women should not have sex, use tampons, or douche until after seeing their physician for a follow up appointment (a week or more after the procedure).

Risks

Because cone biopsies carry risks such as bleeding and problems with subsequent pregnancies, they have been replaced with newer technologies except in a few circumstances.

About one in 10 women experience bleeding from the vagina about two weeks after the biopsy. There is also a slight risk of infection or perforation of the uterus. In a few women, the cervical canal becomes narrowed or completely blocked, which can later interfere with the movement of sperm. This can impair a woman's fertility.

If too much muscle tissue has been removed, the procedure can lead to an **incompetent cervix**, which can be a problem with subsequent pregnancies. An incompetent cervix cannot seal properly to maintain a **pregnancy**. If untreated, the condition increases the odds of **miscarriage** or **premature labor**.

Cervical conization also may temporarily alter cervical cells, which can make a Pap smear test hard to interpret accurately for three or four months.

Normal results

This procedure is only performed if an abnormality is known or suspected.

Abnormal results

The presence of precancerous or cancerous cells in the cervix.

ORGANIZATIONS

NCI Office of Communications and Education, 6116 Executive Blvd., Suite 300, Bethesda, MD, 20892-8322, (800) 4-CANCER (422-6237), cancergovstaff@mail.nih.gov, http://www.cancer.gov/aboutnci/cis.

Carol A. Turkington

Cervical disk disease

Definition

Cervical disk disease refers to a gradual deterioration of the spongy disks in the top part of the spine.

Description

The spine is made up of 33 bones called vertebrae separated by spongy rings of elastic material. These rings, known as disks, are often compared to shock absorbers because they help to cushion the vertebrae. Just as importantly, they also make it possible to turn the head and neck. Over time, these disks slowly become flattened and less elastic due to everyday wear and tear. When this process occurs in the disks of the neck, it is referred to as cervical disk disease. Other general terms for this process include degenerative disk disease and intervertebral disk disease.

Cervical disk disease affects everyone to some degree, often without causing any bothersome symptoms. However, this condition can also lead to specific problems related to nerve functioning. For example, the outer edge of a disk may tear, allowing the gelatinous material inside to bulge outward (**herniated disk**). This can put pressure on nerves that exit the spine. Two adjacent vertebrae may rub together (sometimes resulting in bone spurs) that can also pinch these nerves. In other cases, the inner part of the ring may push on the spinal cord itself, which passes through the disk. Any of these situations can cause **pain** and limit movement. While symptoms primarily affect the neck, they can also occur in other parts of the body.

Causes and symptoms

Cervical disk disease is a gradual process that occurs with **aging**, though poor posture, repeated lifting, and tobacco use can hasten its course. Symptoms include pain when moving the neck and limited neck movement. The condition can also affect the hand, shoulder, and arm resulting in pain, numbness/tingling, and weakness. If the spinal cord itself is affected, these symptoms may occur in the legs. Loss of bowel or bladder control may also occur.

Diagnosis

Cervical disk disease is typically diagnosed by an orthopedist or a neurologist. After taking a medical history and conducting a **physical examination**, the doctor will recommend an imaging procedure to

KEY TERMS

Bone spur—An overgrowth of bone.

Cervical—Relating to the top part of the spine that is composed of the seven vertebrae of the neck and the disks that separate them.

Computed tomography (CT) scan—An imaging procedure that produces a three-dimensional picture of organs or structures inside the body.

Magnetic resonance imaging—A type of imaging that uses magnetic fields to generate a picture of internal structures.

Myelography—An imaging procedure involving the injection of a radioactive dye into the fluid surrounding the spine. A myelography can be used to detect herniated disks, nerve root damage, and other problems affecting the cervical spine.

Neurologist—A doctor who specializes in disorders of the brain and central nervous system.

Orthopedist—A doctor who specializes in disorders of the musculoskeletal system.

gather more information about the nature of the problem. This may include a CT scan, an MRI, or **myelography**. In addition, an electromyogram (EMG) may be used to evaluate the functioning of nerves in the arms, hands, or legs. Cervical disk disease is typically covered by medical insurance.

Treatment

Treatment usually involves **physical therapy**, several weeks of drug therapy with **nonsteroidal anti-inflammatory drugs** (NSAIDs), and limited use of a cervical collar (to reduce neck movement). Neck **traction** and **heat treatments** may also be recommended. In some cases, **steroids** or anesthetic drugs may be injected into the spinal canal to help alleviate symptoms. Aside from these measures, maintaining good posture and placing a pillow under the neck and head during sleep can be helpful. Treatment may last anywhere from several weeks to three months or more. Neck surgery is not usually advised unless other therapies have failed.

Alternative treatment

Acupuncture, therapeutic massage, and **yoga** are believed by some practitioners of alternative medicine to have generalized pain-relieving effects. However, any therapy that involves manipulating the neck is not recommended and be approved by primary doctor beforehand.

Prognosis

In most people symptoms go away within three months if not sooner. A smaller number may require surgery to correct the problem.

Prevention

While some degree of disk degeneration is inevitable, people can reduce their risk by practicing good posture (during sitting, standing, and lifting), performing neck-stretching exercises, maintaining an ideal weight, and quitting **smoking**.

ORGANIZATIONS

American Academy of Orthopaedic Surgeons, 6300 North River Road, Rosemont, IL, 60018-4262, (847) 823-7186, (847) 823-8125, pemr@aaos.org, http://www.aaos.org.

Greg Annussek

Cervical osteoarthritis *see* **Cervical spondylosis**

Cervical spondylosis

Definition

Cervical spondylosis refers to common age-related changes in the area of the spine at the back of the neck. With age, the vertebrae (the component bones of the spine) gradually form bone spurs, and their shock-absorbing disks slowly shrink. These changes can alter the alignment and stability of the spine. They may go unnoticed, or they may produce problems related to pressure on the spine and associated nerves and blood vessels. This pressure can cause weakness, **numbness**, and **pain** in various areas of the body. In severe cases, walking and other activities may be compromised.

Description

As it runs from the brain down the back, the spinal cord is protected by ringlike bones, called vertebrae, stacked one upon the other. The vertebrae are not in direct contact with one another, however. The intervening spaces are filled with structures called disks. The disks are made up of a tough, fibrous outer tissue with an inner core of elastic or gel-like tissue.

One of the most important functions of disks is protecting the vertebrae and the nerves and blood vessels between the vertebrae. The disks also lend flexibility to the spinal cord, facilitating movements such as turning the head or bending the neck. As people age, disks gradually become tougher and more unyielding. Disks also shrink with age, which reduces the amount of padding between the vertebrae.

As the amount of padding shrinks, the spine loses stability. The vertebrae react by constructing osteophytes, commonly known as bone spurs. There are seven vertebrae in the neck; development of osteophytes on these bones is sometimes called cervical **osteoarthritis**. Osteophytes may help to stabilize the degenerating backbone and help protect the spinal cord.

By age 50, 25–50% of people develop cervical spondylosis; by 75 years of age, it is seen in at least 70% of people. Although shrunken vertebral disks, osteophyte growth, and other changes in their cervical spine may exist, many of these people never develop significant problems.

However, about 50% of people over age 50 experience neck pain and stiffness due to cervical spondylosis. Of these people, 25–40% have at least one episode of cervical radiculopathy, a condition that arises when osteophytes compress nerves between the vertebrae. Another potential problem occurs if osteophytes, degenerating disks, or shifting vertebrae narrow the spinal canal. This pressure compresses the spinal cord and its blood vessels, causing cervical spondylitic myelopathy, a disorder in which large segments of the spinal cord are damaged. This disorder affects fewer than 5% of people with cervical spondylosis. Symptoms of both cervical spondylitic myelopathy and cervical radiculopathy may be present in some people.

Causes and symptoms

As people age, shrinkage of the vertebral disks prompts the vertebrae to form osteophytes to stabilize the back bone. However, the position and alignment of the disks and vertebrae may shift despite the osteophytes. Symptoms may arise from problems with one or more disks or vertebrae.

Osteophyte formation and other changes do not necessarily lead to symptoms, but after age 50, half of the population experiences occasional neck pain and stiffness. As disks degenerate, the cervical spine becomes less stable, and the neck is more vulnerable to injuries, including muscle and ligament strains. Contact between the edges of the vertebrae can also cause pain. In some people, this pain may be referred–that is, perceived as occurring in the head, shoulders, or chest, rather than the neck. Other symptoms may include vertigo (a type of **dizziness**) or ringing in the ears.

The neck pain and stiffness can be intermittent, as can symptoms of radiculopathy. Radiculopathy refers to compression on the base, or root, of nerves that lead away from the spinal cord. Normally, these nerves fit comfortably through spaces between the vertebrae. These spaces are called intervertebral foramina. As the osteophytes form, they can impinge on this area and gradually make the fit between the vertebrae too snug.

The poor fit increases the chances that a minor incident, such as overdoing normal activities, may place excess pressure on the nerve root, sometimes referred to as a pinched nerve. Pressure may also accumulate as a direct consequence of osteophyte formation. The pressure on the nerve root causes severe shooting pain in the neck, arms, shoulder, and/or upper back, depending on which nerve roots of the cervical spine are affected. The pain is often aggravated by movement, but in most cases, symptoms resolve within four to six weeks.

Cervical spondylosis can cause cervical spondylitic myelopathy through stenosis- or osteophyte-related pressure on the spinal cord. **Spinal stenosis** is a narrowing of the spinal canal—the area through the center of the vertebral column occupied by the spinal cord. Stenosis occurs because of misaligned vertebrae and out-of-place or degenerating disks. The problems created by spondylosis can be exacerbated if a person has a naturally narrow spinal canal. Pressure against the spinal cord can also be created by osteophytes forming on the inner surface of vertebrae and pushing against the spinal cord. Stenosis or osteophytes can compress the spinal cord and its blood vessels, impeding or choking off needed nutrients to the spinal cord cells; in effect, the cells starve to **death**.

With the death of these cells, the functions that they once performed are impaired. These functions may include conveying sensory information to the brain or transmitting the brain's commands to voluntary muscles. Pain is usually absent, but a person may experience leg numbness and an inability to make the legs move properly. Other symptoms can include clumsiness and weakness in the hands, stiffness and weakness in the legs, and spontaneous twitches in the legs. A person's ability to walk is affected, and a wide-legged, shuffling gait is sometimes adopted to compensate for the lack of sensation in the legs and the accompanying, realistic fear of falling. In very few cases, bladder control becomes a problem.

Diagnosis

Cervical spondylosis is often suspected based on the symptoms and their history. Careful neurological examination can help determine which nerve roots are involved, based on the location of the pain and numbness, and the pattern of weakness and changes in reflex responses. To confirm the suspected diagnosis, and to rule out other possibilities, imaging tests are ordered. The first test is an x ray. X rays reveal the presence of osteophytes, stenosis, constricted space between the vertebrae, and misalignment in the cervical spine–in short, an x ray confirms that a person has cervical spondylosis. To demonstrate that the condition is causing the symptoms, more details are needed. Other imaging tests, such as **magnetic resonance imaging** (MRI) and computed tomography **myelography**, help assess effects of cervical spondylosis on associated nerve tissue and blood vessels.

An MRI may be preferred, because it is a noninvasive procedure and does not require injecting a contrast medium as does computed tomography myelography. MRIs also have greater sensitivity for detecting disk problems and spinal cord involvement, and the test allows the physician to create images of a larger area from various angles. However, these images may not show enough detail about the vertebrae themselves. Computed tomography myelography yields a superior image of the bones involved in cervical spondylosis. Added benefits include that it takes less time to perform and tends to be less expensive than an MRI. A good diagnosis may be reached with either a computed tomography myelography or an MRI, but sometimes complementary information from both tests is necessary. Nerve conduction velocity, electromyogram (EMG), and/or somatosensory evoked potential testing may help to confirm which nerve roots are involved.

Treatment

When possible, conservative treatment of symptoms is preferred. Conservative treatment begins with rest–either restricting normal activities to a less strenuous level or bed rest for three to five days. If rest is not adequate to relieve symptoms, a cervical orthosis may be prescribed, such as a soft cervical collar or stiffer neck brace to restrict neck movement and shift some of the head's weight from the neck to the shoulders. Cervical **traction** may also be suggested, either at home with the advice of a physical therapist or in a health-care setting.

Pain is treated with **nonsteroidal anti-inflammatory drugs**, such as **aspirin** or ibuprofen. If these drugs are ineffective, a short-term prescription for **corticosteroids** or **muscle relaxants** may be given. For chronic pain, **tricyclic antidepressants** can be prescribed. Although these drugs were developed to treat depression, they are also effective in treating pain. Once any pain is resolved, exercises to strengthen neck muscle and preserve flexibility are prescribed.

If the pain is severe, a short treatment of epidural corticosteroids may be prescribed with discretion. A corticosteroid such as prednisone can be combined with an anaesthetic and injected with a long needle into the space between the damaged disk and the covering of the nerve and spinal cord. Injection into the cervical epidural space relieves severe pain that is not managed with conventional treatment. Frequent use of this treatment is not medically recommended and is used only if the more conservative therapy is not effective.

If pain is continuous and does not respond to conservative treatment, surgery may be suggested. Surgery is usually not recommended for neck pain, but it may be necessary to address radiculopathy and myelopathy. Surgery is particularly recommended for people who have already developed moderate to severe symptoms of myelopathy, although age or poor health may prohibit that recommendation. The specific details of the surgery depend on the structures involved, but the overall goal is to relieve pressure on the nerve root, spinal cord, or blood vessels and to stabilize the spine.

Alternative treatment

Alternative therapy is not meant to replace conventional medical treatment, but it can be a useful adjunct. Its main roles are to relieve tension, manage pain, and strengthen neck and back muscles. Massage is one way to relieve tension, and **yoga** provides the additional benefit of strengthening muscles. **Chiropractic** and **acupuncture** have been reported to relieve the pain associated with disk problems, although great care needs to be taken to avoid exacerbating them. Practitioners of the **Alexander technique** or the **Feldenkrais method** can provide

KEY TERMS

Alexander technique—A technique developed by Frederick Alexander that focuses on the variations in body posture, muscles, and breathing. Defects in these functions can lead to stress, nervous tension or possible loss of function.

Bone spur—Also called an osteophyte, it is an outgrowth or ridge that forms on a bone.

Cervical—Referring to structures within the neck.

Computed tomography myelography—This medical procedure combines aspects of computed tomography scanning and plain-film myelography. A CT scan is an imaging technique in which cross-sectional x rays of the body are compiled to create a three-dimensional image of the body's internal structures. Myelography involves injecting a water-soluble substance into the area around the spine to make it visible on x rays. In computed tomography myelography or CT myelography, the water-soluble substance is injected, but the imaging is done with a CT scan.

Disk—A ringlike structure that fits between the vertebrae in the spine to protect the bones, nerves, and blood vessels. The outer layer is a tough, fibrous tissue, and the inner core is composed of more elastic tissue.

Feldenkrais method—A therapy based on creating a good self image by correction and improvements of body movements.

Magnetic resonance imaging (MRI)—An imaging technique that uses a large circular magnet and radio waves to generate signals from atoms in the body. These signals are used to construct images of internal structures.

Myelopathy—A disorder in which the tissue of the spinal cord is diseased or damaged.

Orthosis—An external device, such as a splint or a brace, that prevents or assists movement.

Osteophyte—Also referred to as bone spur, it is an outgrowth or ridge that forms on a bone.

Radiculopathy—Sometimes referred to as a pinched nerve, it refers to compression of the nerve root–the part of a nerve between vertebrae. This compression causes pain to be perceived in areas to which the nerve leads.

Spine—A term for the backbone that includes the vertebrae, disks, and spinal cord as a whole.

Stenosis—A condition in which a canal or other passageway in the body is constricted.

Traction—A medical treatment that exerts a pulling or extending force. Used for cervical problems, it relieves pressure on structures between the vertebrae and muscular tension.

Vertebrae—The ringlike component bones of the spine.

---

instruction on correct posture and **exercise** that may help prevent further symptoms. Vitamin and mineral supplementation along with herbal therapies and homeopathy can help build and rebalance the weakened structure.

Prognosis

The gradual progression of cervical spondylosis cannot be stopped; however, it doesn't always cause symptoms. For the individuals who do experience problems, conservative treatment is very effective in managing the symptoms. Nearly all people with neck pain, approximately 75% of persons with radiculopathy, and up to 50% of people with myelopathy find relief through therapy alone. For the remaining people with radiculopathy or myelopathy, surgery may be recommended. Surgery is deemed successful in 70–80% of cases.

Prevention

Since cervical spondylosis is part of the normal **aging** process, not much can be done to prevent it. It may be possible to ward off some or all of the symptoms by engaging in regular physical exercise and limiting occupational or recreational activities that place pressure on the head, neck, and shoulders. The best exercises for the health of the cervical spine are non-contact activities, such as swimming, walking, or yoga. Once symptoms have already developed, the emphasis is on symptom management rather than prevention.

Resources

PERIODICALS

McCormack, Bruce M., and Phillip R. Weinstein. "Cervical Spondylosis: An Update." *Western Journal of Medicine* 165 (July-August 1996): 43.

Julia Barrett

Cervicitis

Definition

Cervicitis is an inflammation of the cervix.

Description

Cervicitis is a inflammation of the cervix (the opening into the uterus). This inflammation can be chronic and may or may not have an identified cause.

Causes and symptoms

The most common cause of cervicitis is infection, either local or as a result of various **sexually transmitted diseases**, such as chlamydia or **gonorrhea**. Cervicitis can also be caused by birth control devices such as a cervical cap or diaphragm, or chemical exposure. Other risk factors include multiple sexual partners or cervical trauma following birth. In post-menopausal women, cervicitis is sometimes related to a lack of estrogen.

Although a woman may not notice any signs of infection, symptoms of cervicitis include the following:

- persistent unusual vaginal discharge
- abnormal bleeding, either between periods or following sexual intercourse
- painful sexual intercourse
- vaginal pain
- frequent need to urinate
- burning or itching in the vaginal area

Diagnosis

The standard method of diagnosing cervicitis is through a pelvic examination or a Pap smear. During the **pelvic exam**, the physician usually swabs the affected area, and then sends the tissue sample to a laboratory. The laboratory tries to identify the specific organism responsible for causing the cervicitis. A biopsy to take a sample of tissue from the affected area is sometimes required in order to rule out **cancer**. **Colposcopy**, a procedure used to look at the cervix under a microscope, may also be used to rule out cancer.

Treatment

The first course of treatment for cervicitis is usually **antibiotics**. If these medicines do not cure the cervicitis, other treatment options include:

- Loop Electrosurgical Excision Procedure (LEEP)
- cryotherapy

- electrocoagulation
- laser treatment

Prognosis

Cervicitis will usually be cured when the course of therapy is complete. Severe cases, however, may last for a few months, even after the therapy is complete. If the cervicitis was caused by a sexually transmitted disease, both partners should be treated with medication.

Prevention

Practicing safe sexual behavior, such as monogamy, is one way of lowering the prevalence of cervicitis. In addition, women who began sexual activity at a later age have been shown to have a lower incidence of cervicitis. Another recommendation is to use a latex condom consistently during intercourse. If the cervicitis is caused by any sexually transmitted disease, the patient is advised to notify all sexual partners.

Resources

BOOKS

Domino, Frank J., et al., eds. *The 5–Minute Clinical Consult.* 18th ed. Philadelphia: Lippincott Williams & Wilkins, 2009.

Mandell, Gerald L., et al. *Mandell, Douglas, and Bennett's Principles and Practice of Infectious Diseases.*

McPhee, Stephen, and Maxine Papadakis. *Current Medical Diagnosis and Treatment, 2010,* 49th ed. New York: McGraw–Hill Medical, 2009.

PERIODICALS

Malik, S. N., et. al. "Benign Cellular Changes in Pap Smears. Causes and Significance." *Acta Cytologica* January–February 2001: 5–8.

ORGANIZATIONS

American College of Obstetricians and Gynecologists (ACOG), PO Box 96920, Washington, DC, 20090-6920, (202) 638-5577, http://www.acog.org.

Kim A. Sharp, M.Ln.

Cesarean section

Definition

A cesarean section is a surgical procedure in which incisions are made through a woman's abdomen and uterus to deliver her baby.

Purpose

Cesarean sections, also called c-sections or cesarean deliveries, are performed whenever abnormal conditions complicate labor and vaginal delivery, threatening the life or health of the mother or the baby. Dystocia, or difficult labor, is the other common cause of c-sections. According the National Center for Health Statistics, about 32%, or more than 1.4 million babies were delivered by cesarean section in the United States in 2007. The procedure is often used in cases where the mother has had a previous c-section.

The most common reason for performing cesarean section is that the woman has had a previous c-section. The "once a cesarean, always a cesarean" rule originated when the uterine incision was made vertically (termed a classical incision); the resulting scar was weak and had a risk of rupturing in subsequent deliveries. Today, the incision is usually made horizontally across the lower end of the uterus (called a low transverse incision), resulting in reduced blood loss and a decreased chance of rupture. This kind of incision allows many women to have a vaginal birth after a cesarean (VBAC).

The second most common reason that a c-section is performed is difficult **childbirth** due to non-progressive labor (dystocia). Difficult labor is commonly caused by one of the three following conditions: abnormalities in the mother's birth canal; abnormalities in the position of the fetus; or abnormalities in the labor, including weak or infrequent contractions. The mother's pelvic structure may not allow adequate passage for birth. When the baby's head is too large to fit through the pelvis, the condition is called cephalopelvic disproportion (CPD).

About 12% of c-sections are performed to deliver a baby in a breech presentation (buttocks or feet first). Breech presentation is found in about 3% of all births.

In about 9% of cases, c-sections are performed in response to fetal distress, which refers to any situation that threatens the baby such as the umbilical cord wrapped around the baby's neck. This may appear on the fetal heart monitor as an abnormal heart rate or rhythm. Fetal brain damage can result from oxygen deprivation. Fetal distress is often related to abnormalities in the position of the fetus or abnormalities in the birth canal, causing reduced blood flow through the placenta.

Other serious conditions may indicate the need for a cesarean section. One is prolapse of the umbilical cord; the cord is pushed into the vagina ahead of the baby and becomes compressed, cutting off blood flow to the baby. Another is **placental abruption**, whereby the placenta separates from the uterine wall before the baby is born, cutting off blood flow to the baby. The risk of this is especially high in multiple births (twins, triplets, etc.). A third factor is **placenta previa**, in which the placenta covers the cervix partially or completely, making vaginal delivery impossible. In some cases requiring c-section, the baby is in a transverse position, lying horizontally across the pelvis, perhaps with a shoulder in the birth canal.

The mother's age or health may make delivery by c-section the safer choice, especially in cases of maternal diabetes, **hypertension**, **genital herpes**, malignancies of the genital tract, and **preeclampsia** (high blood pressure related to **pregnancy**).

Choosing cesarean section

The incidence of cesarean section has increased greatly in the United States, rising from 21% in the 1990s to 32% in the 2000s. The greatest percentage increase is in cesarean sections that arise less from medical need and more from changes in obstetrical practice. This has occurred despite studies showing that babies born by cesarean section are at higher risk for neonatal complications.

There are a number of reasons why a woman and her obstetrician might choose a c-section in the absence of the usual indications. These include:

- Convenience. A scheduled c-section would allow a woman to choose the time and date of delivery to avoid conflicting with work or family obligations.

- Fear of childbirth. A woman might fear the pain of labor and delivery and feel that a scheduled c-section would allow her to circumvent it.

- Avoiding risks of vaginal delivery. Certain risks inherent to vaginal delivery (urinary or rectal incontinence, sexual dysfunction, dystocia) are

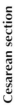

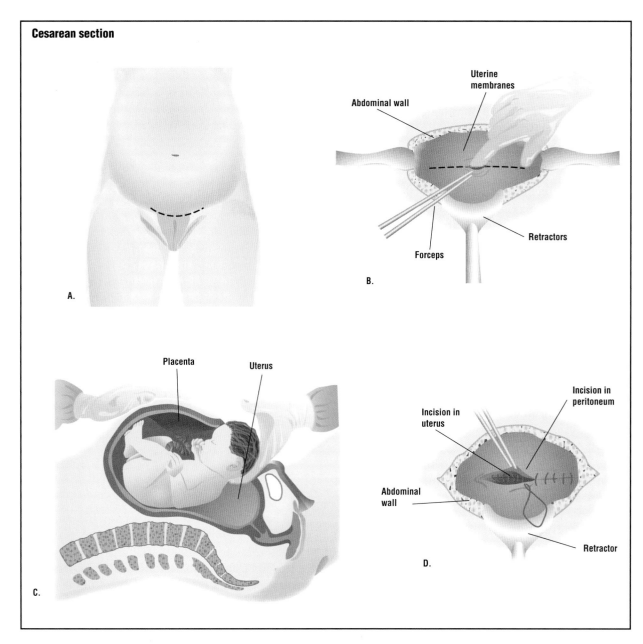

Cesarean section

To remove a baby by cesarean section, an incision is made into the abdomen, usually just above the pubic hairline (A). The uterus is located and divided (B), allowing for delivery of the baby (C). After all the contents of the uterus are removed, the uterus is repaired and the rest of the layers of the abdominal wall are closed (D). *(Illustration by PreMediaGlobal. Reproduced by permission of Gale, a part of Cengage Learning.)*

avoided in a c-section. On the other hand, risks also exist with a cesarean section.

Demographics

Women of higher socioeconomic status are more likely to have a c-section than women who live in low-income families. C-section rates are highest among non-Hispanic white women, followed in decreasing order by Asian American women, African American women, and Hispanic women.

Internationally there is a large variation in the incidence of cesarean section. In most of the well-developed world, the rate is about 21% of births. In less-developed countries, the rate is around 14% and in still developing countries where medical care is limited, the rate drops to about 2%. Internationally, the type of health care provided also affects the rate of

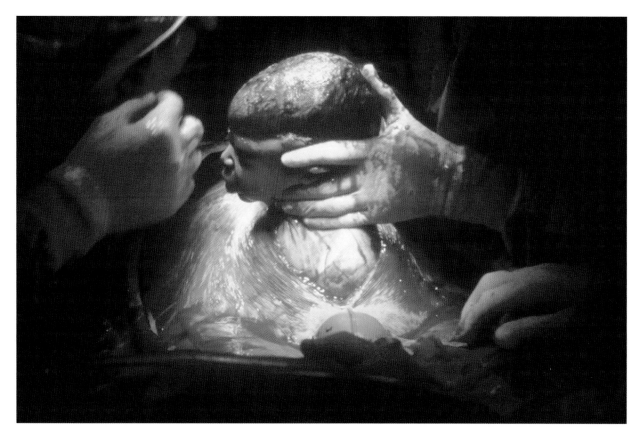

This baby is being delivered by cesarean section. *(Custom Medical Stock Photo, Inc. Reproduced by permission.)*

this procedure. For example, in South America, the rate of cesarean sections among women who receive public health care is about 28% compared to a rate of 75% for those who have private health care.

Description

Regional anesthesia, either a spinal or epidural, is the preferred method of **pain** relief during a c-section. The benefits of regional anesthesia include allowing the mother to be awake during the surgery, avoiding the risks of **general anesthesia**, and allowing early contact between mother and child. Spinal anesthesia involves inserting a needle into a region between the vertebrae of the lower back and injecting numbing medications. An epidural is similar to a spinal except that a catheter is inserted so that numbing medications may be administered continuously. Some women experience a drop in blood pressure when a regional anesthetic is administered; this can be countered with fluids and/or medications.

In some instances, use of general anesthesia may be indicated. General anesthesia can be administered more rapidly in the case of an emergency (e.g., severe fetal distress). If the mother has a coagulation (blood clotting) disorder that would be complicated by a drop in blood pressure (a risk with regional anesthesia), general anesthesia is an alternative. A major drawback of general anesthesia is that the procedure carries with it certain risks such as pulmonary aspiration and failed intubation. The baby may also be affected by anesthetics since they cross the placenta; this effect is generally mild if delivery occurs within 10 minutes after anesthesia is administered.

Once the patient has received anesthesia, the abdomen is washed with an antibacterial solution, and a portion of the pubic hair may be shaved. The first incision opens the abdomen. Infrequently, it will be vertical from just below the navel to the top of the pubic bone or, more commonly, it will be a horizontal incision across and above the pubic bone (informally called a "bikini cut").

The second incision opens the uterus. In most cases, a transverse incision is made. This is the favored type because it heals well and makes it possible for a woman to attempt a vaginal delivery in the future. The classical incision is vertical. Because it provides a larger

KEY TERMS

Breech presentation—The condition in which the baby enters the birth canal with its buttocks or feet first.

Cephalopelvic disproportion (CPD)—The condition in which the baby's head is too large to fit through the mother's pelvis.

Classic incision—In a cesarean section, an incision made vertically along the uterus.

Dystocia—Failure to progress in labor, either because the cervix will not dilate (expand) further or (after full dilation) the head does not descend through the mother's pelvis.

Hematoma—A collection of blood localized to an organ, tissue, or space of the body.

Low transverse incision—Incision made horizontally across the lower end of the uterus.

Placenta previa—The placenta totally or partially covers the cervix, preventing vaginal delivery.

Placental abruption—Separation of the placenta from the uterine wall before the baby is born, cutting off blood flow to the baby.

Preeclampsia—A pregnancy-related condition that causes high blood pressure and swelling.

Prolapsed cord—The umbilical cord is pushed into the vagina ahead of the baby and becomes compressed, cutting off blood flow to the baby.

Respiratory distress syndrome (RDS)—Difficulty breathing; found in infants with immature lungs.

Transverse presentation—The baby is laying sideways across the cervix instead of head first.

VBAC—Vaginal birth after cesarean.

opening than a low transverse incision, it is used in the most critical situations such as placenta previa. However, the classic incision causes more bleeding, a greater risk of abdominal infection, and a weaker scar.

Once the uterus is opened, the amniotic sac is ruptured, and the baby is delivered. The time from the initial incision to birth is typically five minutes. The umbilical cord is clamped and cut, and the newborn is evaluated. The placenta is removed from the mother, and her uterus and abdomen are stitched closed (surgical staples may be used instead in closing the outermost layer of the abdominal incision). From birth through suturing may take 30–40 minutes; the entire surgical procedure may be performed in less than one hour.

Diagnosis/Preparation

There are several ways that obstetricians and other doctors diagnose conditions that may make a c-section necessary. Ultrasound testing reveals the positions of the baby and the placenta and may be used to estimate the baby's size and gestational age. Fetal heart monitors, in use since the 1970s, transmit any signals of fetal distress. Oxygen deprivation may be determined by checking the amniotic fluid for meconium (feces); a lack of oxygen may cause an unborn baby to defecate. Oxygen deprivation may also be determined by testing the pH of a blood sample taken from the baby's scalp; a pH of 7.25 or higher is normal, between 7.2 and 7.25 is suspicious, and below 7.2 is a sign of trouble.

When a c-section becomes necessary, the mother is prepped for surgery. A catheter is inserted into her bladder and an intravenous (IV) line is inserted into her arm. Leads for monitoring the mother's heart rate, rhythm, and blood pressure are attached. In the operating room, the mother is given anesthesia, usually a regional anesthetic (epidural or spinal), making her numb from below her breasts to her toes. In some cases, a general anesthetic will be administered. Surgical drapes are placed over the body, except the head; these drapes block the direct view of the procedure.

Aftercare

A woman who undergoes a c-section requires both the care given to any new mother and the care given to any patient recovering from major surgery. She should be offered pain medication that does not interfere with **breastfeeding**. She should be encouraged to get out of bed and walk around eight to 24 hours after surgery to stimulate circulation (thus avoiding the formation of **blood clots**) and bowel movement. She should limit climbing stairs to once a day, and avoid lifting anything heavier than the baby. She should nap as often as the baby sleeps, and arrange for help with the housework, meals, and care of other children. She may resume driving after two weeks, although some doctors recommend waiting for six weeks, the typical recovery period from major surgery.

The aftereffects of a c-section vary, depending on the woman's age, physical fitness, and overall health. Following this procedure, a woman commonly experiences gas pains, incision pain, and uterine contractions (also common in vaginal delivery). Her hospital stay may be two to four days. Breastfeeding the baby is encouraged, taking care that it is in a position that keeps the baby from resting on the mother's incision.

As the woman heals, she may gradually increase appropriate exercises to regain abdominal tone. Full recovery may be achieved in four to six weeks.

Risks

Because a c-section is a surgical procedure, it carries more risk to both the mother and the baby. The maternal **death** rate is less than 0.02%, but that is four times the maternal death rate associated with vaginal delivery. Complications occur in less than 10% of cases.

The mother is at risk for increased bleeding (a c-section may result in twice the blood loss of a vaginal delivery) from the two incisions, the placental attachment site, and possible damage to a uterine artery. The mother may develop infection of the incision, the urinary tract, or the tissue lining the uterus (endometritis); infections occur in approximately 7% of women after having a c-section. Less commonly, she may receive injury to the surrounding organs such as the bladder and bowel. When a general anesthesia is used, she may experience complications from the anesthesia. Very rarely, she may develop a wound hematoma at the site of either incision or other blood clots leading to pelvic **thrombophlebitis** (inflammation of the major vein running from the pelvis into the leg) or a pulmonary embolus (a blood clot lodging in the lung).

Undergoing a c-section may also inflict psychological distress on the mother, beyond hormonal mood swings and **postpartum depression** ("baby blues"). The woman may feel disappointment and a sense of failure for not experiencing a vaginal delivery. She may feel isolated if the father or birthing coach is not with her in the operating room, or if an unfamiliar doctor treats her rather than her own doctor or midwife. She may feel helpless from a loss of control over labor and delivery with no opportunity to actively participate. To overcome these feelings, the woman must understand why the c-section was necessary. She must accept that she could not control the unforeseen events that made the c-section the optimum means of delivery, and recognize that preserving the health and safety of both her and her child was more important than her delivering vaginally. Women who undergo a c-section should be encouraged to share their feelings with others. Hospitals can often recommend support groups for such mothers. Women should also be encouraged to seek professional help if negative emotions persist.

Babies born by cesarean section have an increased risk of breathing problems, especially if they are delivered before 39 weeks of pregnancy.

The prognosis for a successful vaginal birth after a cesarean (VBAC) may be at least 75%, especially when the c-section involved a low transverse incision in the uterus and there were no complications during or after delivery. However, very few American women attempt to give birth vaginally after a cesarean delivery.

Morbidity and mortality rates

Surgical injuries to the ureter or bowel occur in approximately 0.1% of c-sections. The risk of infection to the incision ranges from 2.5% to 15%. Urinary tract infections occur in 2–16% of patients post-c-section. The risk for developing a deep-vein thrombosis is three to five times higher in patients undergoing c-section than vaginal delivery.

Of the hundreds of thousands of women in the United States who undergo a c-section each year, about 500 die from serious infections, hemorrhaging, or other complications. The overall maternal mortality rate is estimated to be between 6 and 22 deaths per 100,000 births; approximately one-third of maternal deaths that occur after c-section can be attributed to the procedure. These deaths may be related to the health conditions that made the operation necessary, and not simply to the operation itself.

Special considerations

When a c-section is being considered because labor is not progressing, the mother should first be encouraged to walk around to stimulate labor. Labor may also be stimulated with the drug oxytocin. A woman should receive regular prenatal care and be able to alert her doctor to the first signs of trouble. Once labor begins, she should be encouraged to move around and to urinate. The doctor should be conservative in diagnosing dystocia and fetal distress, taking a position of "watchful waiting" before deciding to operate.

Approximately 3% of babies present at term in the breech position. Before opting to perform an elective c-section, the doctor may first attempt to reposition the baby; this is called external cephalic version. The doctor may also try a vaginal breech delivery, depending on the size of the mother's pelvis, the size of the baby, and the type of breech position the baby is in. However, a c-section is safer than a vaginal delivery when the baby is 8 lb (3.6 kg) or larger, in a breech position with the feet crossed, or in a breech position with the head hyperextended.

A vaginal birth after cesarean (VBAC) is an option for women who have had previous c-sections and are interested in a trial of labor (TOL). TOL is a purposeful attempt to deliver vaginally. The success rate for VBAC in patients who have had a prior low transverse uterine incision is approximately 70%. The most severe risk associated with TOL is uterine rupture: 0.2–1.5% of attempted VBACs among women with a low transverse uterine scar will end in uterine rupture, compared to 12% of women with a classic uterine incision. To minimize this risk, the American College of Obstetricians and Gynecologists (ACOG) recommends that VBAC be limited to women with full-term pregnancies (37–40 weeks) who have only had one previous low transverse c-section.

Resources

BOOKS

Jukelevics, Nicette. *Understanding the Dangers of Cesarean Birth: Making Informed Decisions.* Westport, CT: Praeger, 2008.

Knight, Mary Beth. *Strategies for the C-Section Mom.* Avon, MA: Adams Media, 2010.

PERIODICALS

Wilmink, F. A., et al. "Neonatal Outcome Following Elective Cesarean Section Beyond 37 Weeks of Gestation: A 7-Year Retrospective Analysis of a National Registry." *American Journal of Obstetrics and Gynecology* 202 no. 3 (March 2010): 250.

OTHER

Cesarean Section. MedlinePlus. May 4, 2010. http://www.nlm.nih.gov/medlineplus/cesareansection.html

C-Section. Mayo Foundation for Education and Research. January 20, 2009. http://www.mayoclinic.com/health/c-section/my00214

ORGANIZATIONS

American College of Obstetricians and Gynecologists, P.O. Box 96920, Washington, DC, 20090-6920, (202) 638-5577, http://www.acog.org.

Association of Women's Health, Obstetric, and Neonatal Nurses, 2000 L St., NW, Suite. 740, Washington, DC, 20036, (202) 261-2400, (800) 673-8499. Toll free in Canada (800) 245-0231, (202) 728-0575, customer service@ awhonn.org, http://www.awhonn.org.

Bethany Thivierge
Stephanie Dionne Sherk
Tish Davidson, A.M.

Cestodiasis *see* **Tapeworm diseases**

CFS *see* **Chronic fatigue syndrome**

CGD *see* **Chronic granulomatous disease**

Chagas' disease

Definition

Chagas' disease is named after Dr. Carlos Chagas who first found the organism in the early 1900s. It involves damage to the nerves that control the heart, digestive and other organs, and eventually leads to damage to these organs. Worldwide, Chagas' disease affects over 15 million persons, and kills 50,000 each year. Researchers believe that the parasite that causes the disease is only found in the Americas.

Description

When a person is infected with Chagas' disease, the parasite known as *Trypanosoma cruzi* first causes a mild, short-lived period of "acute" illness; then after a long period without symptoms, the effects of the infection begin to appear. The heart, esophagus, and colon are most frequently involved. These organs become unable to contract properly, and begin to stretch or dilate.

Causes and symptoms

T. cruzi is carried by insects or bugs known as reduviid or "kissing bugs." These insects are very common in Central and South America where they inhabit poorly constructed houses and huts. The insects deposit their waste material, exposing inhabitants to the parasites. The parasites then enter the body by way of a cut or via the eyes or mouth. *T. cruzi* can also be transmitted by blood **transfusion**. Eating uncooked, contaminated food or **breastfeeding** can also transmit the disease. The reduviids, in turn, become infected with the parasite by biting infected animals and humans.

There are three phases related to infection:

- Acute phase lasts about two months, with non-specific symptoms of low grade fever, headache, fatigue, and enlarged liver or spleen.
- Indeterminate phase lasts 10–20 years, during which time no symptoms occur, but the parasites are reproducing in various organs.
- Chronic phase is the stage when symptoms related to damage of major organs (heart, esophagus, colon) begin.

In the chronic phase, irregularities of heart rhythm, **heart failure**, and **blood clots** cause weakness, **fainting**, and even sudden **death**.

Esophageal symptoms are related to difficulty with swallowing and chest **pain**. Because the esophagus does not empty properly, food regurgitates into the lungs causing **cough**, **bronchitis**, and repeated bouts of **pneumonia**. Inability to eat, weight loss, and **malnutrition** become a significant factor in affecting survival.

Involvement of the large intestine (colon) causes **constipation**, distention, and abdominal pain.

Diagnosis

The best way to diagnose acute infection is to identify the parasites in tissue or blood. Occasionally it is possible to culture the organism from infected tissue, but this process usually requires too much time to be of value. In the chronic phase, antibody levels can be measured. Efforts to develop new, more accurate tests are ongoing.

Treatment

In most cases treatment of symptoms is all that is possible. Present medications can reduce the duration and severity of an acute infection, but are only 50% effective, at best, in eliminating the organisms.

Cardiac effects are managed with **pacemakers** and medications. Esophageal complications require either endoscopic or surgical methods to improve esophageal emptying, similar to those used to treat the disorder known as **achalasia**. Constipation is treated by increasing fiber and bulk **laxatives**, or removal of diseased portions of the colon.

Prognosis

Those patients with gastrointestinal complications often respond to some form of treatment. Cardiac problems are more difficult to treat, particularly since transplant would rekindle infection.

Prevention

Visitors traveling to areas of known infection should avoid staying in mud, adobe, or similar huts. Mosquito nets and insect repellents are useful in helping to avoid contact with the bugs. Blood screening is not always effective in many regions where infection is common. It is necessary to carefully screen people who have emigrated from Central and South America before they make blood donations.

Resources

OTHER

Centers for Disease Control. http://www.cdc.gov.

David Kaminstein, MD

Chalazion *see* **Eyelid disorders**

Chancroid

Definition

Chancroid is a sexually transmitted disease caused by a bacterial infection that is characterized by painful sores on the genitals.

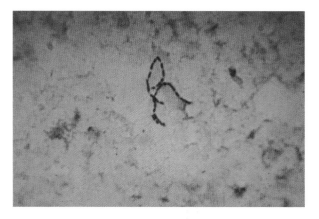

A close-up view of a chancroid specimen. *(Custom Medical Stock Photo, Inc. Reproduced by permission.)*

Description

Chancroid is an infection of the genitals that is caused by the bacterium *Haemophilus ducreyi*. Chancroid is a sexually transmitted disease, which means that it is spread from person to person almost always by sexual contact. However, there have been a few cases in which healthcare providers have become infected through contact with infected patients.

Common locations for chancroid sores (ulcers) in men are the shaft or head of the penis, foreskin, the groove behind the head of the penis, the opening of the penis, and the scrotum. In women, common locations are the labia majora (outer lips), labia minora (inner lips), perianal area (area around the anal opening), and inner thighs. It is rare for the ulcer(s) to be on the vaginal walls or cervix. In about 50% of the patients with chancroid, the infection spreads to either or both of the lymph nodes in the groin.

Chancroid is most commonly found in developing and third world countries. In the United States, the most common cause of genital ulcers is **genital herpes**, followed by **syphilis**, and then chancroid. There are about 1,500 cases of chancroid in the United States per year and it occurred primarily in African Americans, Hispanic Americans, and Native Americans. There are occasional localized outbreaks of chancroid in the United States. In addition, the practice of exchanging sex for drugs has lead to a link between crack **cocaine** use and chancroid.

Even though the incidence of chancroid in the United States decreased in the 1990s, there is an alarming connection between chancroid and human **immunodeficiency** virus (HIV) infection. HIV causes **AIDS** (acquired immunodeficiency syndrome) and is easily spread from person to person through chancroid ulcers. Uncircumcised men with chancroid ulcers have a 48% risk of acquiring HIV from sexual contact. Women with chancroid ulcers are also at a greater risk of being infected with HIV during sexual contact. Genital ulcers seem to act as doorways for HIV to enter and exit.

Causes and symptoms

Haemophilus ducreyi is spread from person to person by vaginal, anal, and oral sexual contact. Uncircumcised men are about three times more likely than circumcised men to become infected following exposure to *Haemophilus ducreyi*. Having unprotected sex, exchanging sex for drugs, and having unprotected sex with a prostitute are other risk factors. Many cases of chancroid in the United States occur in persons who had traveled to countries where the disease is more common.

Chancroid occurs when *Haemophilus ducreyi* penetrates the skin through an injury, like a scratch or cut. Once past the skin surface, the warmth, moisture, and nutrients allow bacteria to grow rapidly. The first sign of chancroid is a small, red papule that occurs within three to seven days following exposure to the bacteria, but may take up to one month. Usually within one day, the papule becomes an ulcer. The chancroid ulcer is painful, bleeds easily, drains a grey or yellowish pus, and has sharply defined, ragged edges. They can vary in size from an eighth of an inch to two inches in diameter. Men usually have only one ulcer, but women often have four or more. Sometimes "kissing" ulcers occur when one ulcer spreads the bacterial infection to an opposite skin surface. For example, kissing ulcers can form on the lips of the labia majora. Alternatively, women may not have any external sores but may experience painful urination, intercourse, and/or bowel movements and may have a vaginal discharge or rectal bleeding.

Signs that the infection has spread to the lymph node appear about one week after the formation of the genital ulcer. Lymph nodes are small organs in the lymphatic system that filter waste materials from nearly every organ in the body. This lymph node infection is called "lymphadenitis" and the swollen, painful lymph node is called a "bubo." The bubo, which appears as a red, spherical lump, may burst through the skin, releasing a thick pus and forming another ulcer.

Diagnosis

Chancroid may be diagnosed and treated by urologists (urinary tract doctors for men), gynecologists (for women), and **infectious disease** specialists. Part of the diagnosis of chancroid involves ruling out genital herpes and syphilis because genital ulcers are also symptoms of these diseases. The appearance of these three diseases can be close enough to be confusing. However, the presence of a pus-filled lump in the groin of a patient with a genital ulcer is highly specific for chancroid.

For a clear-cut diagnosis of chancroid, *Haemophilus ducreyi* must be isolated from the ulcer. To do this, a sterile cotton swab is wiped over the ulcer to obtain a pus sample. In the laboratory, the sample is put into special media and placed in an incubator. *Haemophilus ducreyi* takes from two to five days to grow in the laboratory. In addition, the pus may be examined under the microscope to see which bacteria are in the ulcer. A sample of the pus may also be tested to see if the herpes virus is present. A blood sample will probably be taken from the patient's arm to test for the presence of antibodies to the bacteria that causes syphilis.

Treatment

The only treatment for chancroid is **antibiotics** given either once or for several days. Antibiotics taken by mouth for one to two weeks include erythromycin (E-Mycin, Ery-Tab), amoxicillin plus clavulanic acid (Augmentin), co-trimoxazole (Bactrim, Septra), or ciprofloxacin (Cipro). Antibiotics given in one dose include ceftriaxone (Rocephin), spectinomycin (Trobicin), co-trimoxazole, or ofloxacin (Floxin).

The ulcer(s) may be cleaned and soaked to reduce the swelling. Salt solution **dressings** may be applied to the ulcer(s) to reduce the spread of the bacteria and prevent additional ulcers. A serious infection of the foreskin may require **circumcision**. Pus would be removed from infected lymph nodes by using a needle and syringe. Very large buboes may require surgical drainage.

Prognosis

Without treatment, chancroid may either go away quickly or patients may experience the painful ulcers for many months. A complete cure is obtained with antibiotic treatment. Severe ulcers may cause permanent **scars**. Severe scarring of the foreskin may require circumcision. Urethral fistulas (abnormal passageways from the urine tube to the skin) may occur and requires corrective surgery.

Prevention

The best prevention for chancroid is to use a condom during sexual intercourse. Chancroid can also be prevented by abstinence (avoidance of any sexual contact) and by being in a monogamous relationship with a disease-free partner. To prevent the spread of chancroid, it is important that all sexual contacts of the patient are identified and treated.

ORGANIZATIONS

Planned Parenthood Federation of America, 434 West 33rd St., New York, NY, 10001, (212) 541-7800, (212) 245-1845, (800) 230-7526, http://www.plannedparenthood.org.

Belinda Rowland, PhD

Change of life *see* **Menopause**

Character disorders *see* **Personality disorders**

Charcoal, activated

Definition

Activated charcoal is a fine black odorless and tasteless powder made from wood or other materials that have been exposed to high temperatures in an airless environment. The powder is treated (activated) with oxidizing gas or other chemicals to increase its ability to adsorb various substances. Activated charcoal is pure carbon that absorbs particles and gases in the body's digestive system.

Activated charcoal has been used since ancient times to cure various ailments and poisonings, and its healing effects have been documented since 1550 B.C. by the Egyptians. In the 1980s, it was rediscovered as an oral treatment for **poisoning** and drug overdoses.

Description

Activated charcoal is not absorbed from the stomach or intestines and binds or adsorbs most drugs and poisons. Its most important use in humans is in treating **drug overdose** and poisoning. It is also sometimes used to treat **diarrhea** or excessive gas. It can be used to treat poisoned pets and animals. Other possible uses, in treating viruses, bacteria, bacterial toxic byproducts, snake venoms, and other substances, have not been supported by clinical studies. By adding water to the powder to make a paste, activated charcoal can be used as an external application to reduce **pain** and **itching** from **bites and stings**.

Poisons and drug overdoses

It is estimated that one million children accidentally overdose every year on medications, thinking they are candies, or eat, drink, or inhale poisonous household products. Infants and toddlers are at the greatest risk for accidental poisoning. Activated charcoal can absorb large quantities of poisons quickly in the intestines, is non-toxic, may be stored indefinitely, and can be conveniently administered at home. Charcoal binds irritating or toxic substances in the stomach and intestines, preventing their absorption, so they can be excreted in the stool. When poisoning is suspected, the local poison control center should always be contacted for instructions. They may recommend using activated charcoal, which should be available at home so that it can be immediately given to the poisoned child or pet. For severe poisoning, several doses of activated charcoal may be needed.

Activated charcoal is used in adults who have accidentally taken too much medication, or attempted **suicide** by intentionally taking a drug overdose.

Intestinal disorders

In the past, activated charcoal was a popular remedy for flatus (intestinal gas). But more recent studies have not shown its value. Other measures, like dietary changes or **biofeedback** training, are more effective in relieving patients' symptoms.

Charcoal has been used to treat other intestinal disorders like diarrhea, **constipation**, and cramps. There is little evidence to support these uses. Frequent use may decrease absorption of essential nutrients and cause constipation. So a laxative should be taken if several doses of charcoal are taken.

Other uses

Activated charcoal has been used to clean skin **wounds** and adsorb waste materials from the gastrointestinal tract. When used with other remedies such as aloe vera, acidophilus, and psyllium, charcoal helps keep symptoms of ulcerative **colitis** under control. While charcoal shows some anti-aging activity in rats, it is doubtful if it has the same effect in humans.

Apart from its medicinal applications, activated charcoal is used by biologists to cool cell suspensions; by public health physicians to filter disease organisms from drinking water; and by environmental scientists to remove organic pollutants from ocean sediments.

Recommended dosage

For poisoning

Activated charcoal is available without prescription. In cases of accidental poisoning or drug overdose, always call a poison control center for advice. If both syrup of **ipecac** and charcoal are recommended, ipecac should be given first to induce **vomiting**, and charcoal given only after **vomiting** stops. Activated charcoal may be mixed with a liquid and drunk, or put into a stomach tube. Activated charcoal is available as 1.1 oz (33 mL) and 0.5 oz (15 mL) containers as pre-mixed slurries, or as containers to which water or soda pop can be added. It is a good idea to keep activated charcoal at home for the immediate treatment of poisonings.

For acute poisoning, the dosage is as follows:

- Infants (under 1 year of age): 1 g/kg
- Children (1–12 years of age): 15–30 g or 1–2 g/kg with at least 8 oz of water
- Adults: 30–100 g or 1–2 g/kg with at least 8 oz of water

For diarrhea

Charcoal can be taken as tablets or capsules with water, or sprinkled onto foods. The dosage for treatment of diarrhea in adults is 520–975 mg after each meal and up to 5 g per day.

Precautions

Parents should keep activated charcoal on hand for emergencies.

Charcoal should not be given together with syrup of ipecac as it will adsorb the ipecac. It should not be taken until after the vomiting from ipecac stops.

Some activated charcoal products contain sorbitol, a sweetener and laxative that can cause **nausea**, vomiting, and diarrhea. These products should not be used in infants.

Charcoal may interfere with the absorption of medications and nutrients such as **vitamins** or **minerals**. It should not be taken for at least two hours after other medications.

Charcoal should not be used to treat poisonings caused by lye or other corrosives, strong acids, or petroleum products like gasoline or cleaning fluids. In those cases, charcoal may cause treatment for the condition to be delayed. It is also not effective in lithium, cyanide, iron, ethanol, or methanol overdoses or poisonings.

Chocolate syrup, sherbet, or ice cream may improve the taste of charcoal, but they may prevent it from working properly.

Activated charcoal may produce abdominal pain or swelling, and can complicate intestinal bleeding or obstruction.

Charcoal may be less effective in people with slow digestion.

KEY TERMS

Adsorption—The binding of a chemical (e.g., drug or poison) to a solid material such as activated charcoal or clay.

Antidote—A remedy to counteract unwanted effects from medications or poisons.

Flatus—Gas or air in the digestive tract.

Charcoal should not be given for more than three or four days for treatment of diarrhea, as it may interfere with normal **nutrition**.

Charcoal should not be used in children under three years of age to treat diarrhea or gas.

Activated charcoal should be kept out of reach of children.

Side effects

Charcoal may cause constipation when taken for a drug overdose or accidental poisoning. A laxative should be taken after the crisis is over.

Activated charcoal normally causes stools to turn black.

Patients should consult a doctor if they have pain or swelling of the stomach.

Interactions

Chocolate syrup, ice cream, or sherbet mixed may prevent charcoal from working properly.

Resources

BOOKS

Beers, Mark H., Robert S. Porter, and Thomas V. Jones, eds. *The Merck Manual of Diagnosis and Therapy*. 18th ed. Whitehouse Station, NJ: Merck Research Laboratories, 2006.

Mack, Daniel. *EMT Field Guide*. Sudbury, MA: Jones & Bartlett, 2011.

Wilson, Billie A., et al. *Nurses Drug Guide 2008*. Upper Saddle River, NJ: Prentice Hall, 2008.

PERIODICALS

Azpiroz, F., and J. Serra. "Treatment of Excessive Intestinal Gas." *Current Treatment Options in Gastroenterology* 7 (August 2004): 299–305.

Ho, K. T., R. M. Burgess, M. C. Pelletier, et al. "Use of Powdered Coconut Charcoal as a Toxicity Identification and Evaluation Manipulation for Organic Toxicants in Marine Sediments." *Environmental Toxicology and Chemistry* 23 (September 2004): 2124–2131.

Littlejohn, C. "Management of Intentional Overdose in A&E Departments." *Nursing Times* 100 (August 17, 2004): 38–43.

Matsui, T., J. Kajima, and T. Fujino. "Removal Effect of the Water Purifier for Home Use Against *Cryptosporidium parvum* Oocysts." *Journal of Veterinary Medical Science* 66 (August 2004): 941–943.

Morris, G. J., and H. E. Richens. "Improved Methods for Controlled Rapid Cooling of Cell Suspensions." *Cryo Letters* 25 (July-August 2004): 265–272.

Osterhoudt, K. C., E. R. Alpern, D. Durbin, et al. "Activated Charcoal Administration in a Pediatric Emergency Department." *Pediatric Emergency Care* 20 (August 2004): 493–498.

ORGANIZATIONS

American Society of Health-System Pharmacists (ASHP), 7272 Wisconsin Avenue, Bethesda, MD, 20814, (301) 657-3000, (866) 279-0681, http://www.ashp.org.

United States Food and Drug Administration (FDA), 10903 New Hampshire Ave, Silver Spring, MD, 02993-0002, (888) 463-6332, http://www.fda.gov.

Rebecca J. Frey, PhD
James E. Waun, MD. RPh

Charcot Marie Tooth disease

Definition

Charcot Marie Tooth disease (CMT) is the name of a group of inherited disorders of the nerves in the peripheral nervous system (nerves throughout the body that communicate motor and sensory information to and from the spinal cord) causing weakness and loss of sensation in the limbs.

Description

CMT is named for the three neurologists who first described the condition in the late 1800s. It is also known as hereditary motor and sensory neuropathy, and is sometimes called peroneal muscular atrophy, referring to the muscles in the leg that are often affected. The age of onset of CMT can vary anywhere from young childhood to the 50s or 60s. Symptoms typically begin by the age of 20. For reasons yet unknown, the severity in symptoms can also vary greatly, even among members of the same family.

Although CMT has been described for many years, it is only since the early 1990s that the genetic cause of many of the types of CMT have become known.

Therefore, knowledge about CMT has increased dramatically within a short time.

The peripheral nerves

CMT affects the peripheral nerves, those groups of nerve cells carrying information to and from the spinal cord. CMT decreases the ability of these nerves to carry motor commands to muscles, especially those furthest from the spinal cord located in the feet and hands. As a result, the muscles connected to these nerves eventually weaken. CMT also affects the sensory nerves that carry information from the limbs to the brain. Therefore people with CMT also have sensory loss. This causes symptoms such as not being able to tell if something is hot or cold or difficulties with balance.

There are two parts of the nerve that can be affected in CMT. A nerve can be likened to an electrical wire, in which the wire part is the axon of the nerve and the insulation surrounding it is the myelin sheath. The job of the myelin is to help messages travel very fast through the nerves. CMT is usually classified depending on which part of the nerve is affected. People who have problems with the myelin have CMT type 1 and people who have abnormalities of the axon have CMT type 2.

Specialized testing of the nerves, called nerve conduction testing (NCV), can be performed to determine if a person has CMT1 or CMT2. These tests measure the speed at which messages travel through the nerves. In CMT1, the messages move too slowly, but in CMT2 the messages travel at the normal speed.

Demographics

CMT has been diagnosed in people from all over the world. It occurs in approximately one in 2,500 people, which is about the same incidence as **multiple sclerosis**. It is the most common type of inherited neurologic condition.

Causes and symptoms

CMT is caused by changes (mutations) in any one of a number of genes that carry the instructions to make the peripheral nerves. Genes contain the instructions for how the body grows and develops before and after a person is born. There are probably at least 15 different genes that can cause CMT. However, many have not yet been identified.

CMT types 1 and 2 can be broken down into subtypes based upon the gene that is causing CMT. The subtypes are labeled by letters, so there is

CMT1A, CMT1B, etc. Therefore, the gene with a mutation that causes CMT1A is different from the gene that causes CMT1B.

Types of CMT

CMT1A. The most common type of CMT is called CMT1A. It is caused by a mutation in a gene called peripheral myelin protein 22 (PMP22) located on chromosome 17. The job of this gene is to make a protein (PMP22) that makes up part of the myelin. In most people who have CMT, the mutation that causes the condition is a duplication (doubling) of the PMP22 gene. Instead of having two copies of the PMP22 gene (one on each chromosome) there are three copies. It is not known how this extra copy of the PMP22 gene causes the observed symptoms. A small percentage of people with CMT1A do not have a duplication of the PMP22 gene, but rather have a point mutation in the gene. A point mutation is like a typo in the gene that causes it to work incorrectly.

HEREDITARY NEUROPATHY WITH LIABILITY TO PRESSURE PALSIES (HNPP). HNPP is a condition that is also caused by a mutation in the PMP22 gene. The mutation is a deletion. Therefore, there is only one copy of the PMP22 gene instead of two. People who have HNPP may have some of the signs of CMT. However, they also have episodes where they develop weakness and problems with sensation after compression of certain pressure points such as the elbows or knee. Often these symptoms will resolve after a few days or weeks, but sometimes they are permanent.

CMT1B. Another type of CMT, called CMT1B, is caused by a mutation in a gene called myelin protein zero (MPZ) located on chromosome 1. The job of this gene is to make the layers of myelin stick together as they are wrapped around the axon. The mutations in this gene are point mutations because they involve a change (either deletion, substitution, or insertion) at one specific component of a gene.

CMTX. Another type of CMT, called CMTX, is usually considered a subtype of CMT1 because it affects the myelin, but it has a different type of inheritance than type 1 or type 2. In CMTX, the CMT–causing gene is located on the X chromosome and is called connexin 32 (Cx32). The job of this gene is to code for a class of protein called connexins that form tunnels between the layers of myelin.

CMT2. There are at least five different genes that can cause CMT type 2. Therefore, CMT2 has subtypes A, B, C, D, and E. As of early 2001, scientists have narrowed in on the location of most of the CMT2 causing genes. However, the specific genes and the mutations have not yet been found for most types. Very recently, the gene for CMT2E has been found. The gene is called neurofilament-light (NF-L). Because it has just been discovered, not much is known about how mutations in this gene cause CMT.

CMT3. In the past a condition called Dejerine-Sottas disease was referred to as CMT3. This is a severe type of CMT in which symptoms begin in infancy or early childhood. It is now known that this is not a separate type of CMT and in fact people who have onset in infancy or early childhood often have mutations in the PMP22 or MPZ genes.

CMT4. CMT4 is a rare type of CMT in which the nerve conduction tests have slow response results. However, it is classified differently from CMT1 because it is passed through families by a different pattern of inheritance. There are five different subtypes and each has only been described in a few families. The symptoms in CMT4 are often severe and other symptoms such as deafness may be present. There are three different genes that have been associated with CMT4 as of early 2001. They are called MTMR2, EGR2, and NDRG1. More research is required to understand how mutations in these genes cause CMT.

Inheritance

CMT1A and 1B, HNPP, and all of the subtypes of CMT2 have autosomal dominant inheritance. Autosomal refers to the first 22 pairs of chromosomes that are the same in males and females. Therefore, males and females are affected equally in these types. In a dominant condition, only one gene of a pair needs to have a mutation in order for a person to have symptoms of the condition. Therefore, anyone who has these types has a 50%, or one in two, chance of passing CMT on to each of their children. This chance is the same for each **pregnancy** and does not change based on previous children.

CMTX has X-linked inheritance. Since males only have one X chromosome, they only have one copy of the Cx32 gene. Thus, when a male has a mutation in his Cx32 gene, he will have CMT. However, females have two X chromosomes and therefore have two copies of the Cx32 gene. If they have a mutation in one copy of their Cx32 genes, they will only have mild to moderate symptoms of CMT that may go unnoticed. This is because their normal copy of the Cx32 gene does make normal myelin.

Females pass on one or the other of their X chromosomes to their children—sons or daughters. If a woman with a Cx32 mutation passes her normal X chromosome, she will have an unaffected son or daughter who will not pass CMT on to his or her children. If the woman passes the chromosome with Cx32 mutation on she will have an affected son or daughter, although the daughter will be mildly affected or have no symptoms. Therefore, a woman with a Cx32 mutation has a 50%, or a one in two, chance of passing the mutation to her children: a son will be affected, and a daughter may only have mild symptoms.

When males pass on an X chromosome, they have a daughter. When they pass on a Y chromosome, they have a son. Since the Cx32 mutation is on the X chromosome, a man with CMTX will always pass the Cx32 mutation on to his daughters. However, when he has a son, he passes on the Y chromosome, and therefore the son will not be affected. Therefore, an affected male passes the Cx32 gene mutation on to all of his daughters, but to none of his sons.

CMT4 has autosomal recessive inheritance. Males and females are equally affected. In order for a person to have CMT4, they must have a mutation in both of their CMT-causing genes—one inherited from each parent. The parents of an affected person are called carriers. They have one normal copy of the gene and one copy with a mutation. Carriers do not have symptoms of CMT. Two carrier parents have a 25%, or one in four, chance of passing CMT on to *each* of their children.

The onset of symptoms is highly variable, even among members of the same family. Symptoms usually progress very slowly over a person's lifetime. The main problems caused by CMT are weakness and loss of sensation mainly in the feet and hands. The first symptoms are usually problems with the feet such as high arches and problems with walking and running. Tripping while walking and sprained ankles are common. Muscle loss in the feet and calves leads to "foot drop" where the foot does not lift high enough off the ground when walking. Complaints of cold legs are common, as are cramps in the legs, especially after **exercise**.

In many people, the fingers and hands eventually become affected. Muscle loss in the hands can make fine movements such as working buttons and zippers difficult. Some patients develop tremor in the upper limbs. Loss of sensation can cause problems such as **numbness** and the inability to feel if something is hot or cold. Most people with CMT remain able to walk throughout their lives.

Diagnosis

Diagnosis of CMT begins with a careful **neurological exam** to determine the extent and distribution of weakness. A thorough family history should be taken at this time to determine if other people in the family are affected. Testing may also be performed to rule out other causes of neuropathy.

A nerve conduction velocity test should be performed to measure how fast impulses travel through the nerves. This test may show characteristic features of CMT, but it is not diagnostic of CMT. Nerve conduction testing may be combined with **electromyography** (EMG), an electrical test of the muscles.

A nerve biopsy (removal of a small piece of the nerve) may be performed to look for changes characteristic of CMT. However, this testing is not diagnostic of CMT and is usually not necessary for making a diagnosis.

Definitive diagnosis of CMT is made only by **genetic testing**, usually performed by drawing a small amount of blood. As of early 2001, testing is available to detect mutations in PMP22, MPZ, Cx32, and EGR2. However, research is progressing rapidly and new testing is often made available every few months. All affected members of a family have the same type of CMT. Therefore once a mutation is found in one affected member, it is possible to test other members who may have symptoms or are at risk of developing CMT.

Prenatal diagnosis

Testing during pregnancy to determine whether an unborn child is affected is possible if genetic testing in a family has identified a specific CMT-causing mutation. This can be done after 10–12 weeks of pregnancy using a procedure called **chorionic villus sampling** (CVS). CVS involves removing a tiny piece of the placenta and examining the cells. Testing can also be done by **amniocentesis** after 16 weeks gestation by removing a small amount of the amniotic fluid surrounding the baby and analyzing the cells in the fluid. Each of these procedures has a small risk of **miscarriage** associated with it, and those who are interested in learning more should check with their doctor or genetic counselor. Couples interested in these options should obtain **genetic counseling** to carefully explore all of the benefits and limitations of these procedures.

Treatment

There is no cure for CMT. However, physical and **occupational therapy** are an important part of CMT treatment. **Physical therapy** is used to preserve range of motion and minimize deformity caused by muscle shortening, or contracture. Braces are sometimes used to improve control of the lower extremities that can

KEY TERMS

Axon—Skinny, wire-like extension of nerve cells.

Myelin—A fatty sheath surrounding nerves in the peripheral nervous system, which helps them conduct impulses more quickly.

Nerve conduction testing—Procedure that measures the speed at which impulses move through the nerves.

Neuropathy—A condition caused by nerve damage. Major symptoms include weakness, numbness, paralysis, or pain in the affected area.

Peripheral nerves—Nerves throughout the body that carry information to and from the spinal cord.

help tremendously with balance. After wearing braces, people often find that they have more energy because they are using less energy to focus on their walking. Occupational therapy is used to provide devices and techniques that can assist tasks such as dressing, feeding, writing, and other routine activities of daily life. Voice-activated software can also help people who have problems with fine motor control.

It is very important that people with CMT avoid injury that causes them to be immobile for long periods of time. It is often difficult for people with CMT to return to their original strength after injury.

There is a long list of medications that should be avoided if possible by people diagnosed with CMT such as hydralazine (Apresoline); megadoses of vitamin A, B_6, and D; Taxol; and large intravenous doses of penicillin. Complete lists are available from the CMT support groups. People considering taking any of these medications should weigh the risks and benefits with their physician.

Prognosis

The symptoms of CMT usually progress slowly over many years, but do not usually shorten life expectancy. The majority of people with CMT do not need to use a wheelchair during their lifetime. Most people with CMT are able to lead full and productive lives despite their physical challenges.

Resources

BOOKS

Hannigan, Steve. *Inherited Metabolic Diseases: A Guide to 100 Conditions.* Oxford, UK; New York: Radcliffe, 2007 .

OTHER

GeneClinics. University of Washington, Seattle. www.
geneclinics.org.
*HNPP—Hereditary Neuropathy with Liability to Pressure
Palsies*. http://www.hnpp.org.
OMIM—Online Mendelian Inheritance in Man. www.ncbi.
nlm.nih.gov/Omim.

ORGANIZATIONS

Charcot Marie Tooth Association (CMTA), 2700 Chestnut
Parkway, Chester, PA, 19013-4867, (610) 499-9264,
(610) 499-9267, (800) 606-2682, info@charcot-mariet-
tooth.org, http://www.charcot-marie-tooth.org.
Muscular Dystrophy Association, 3300 East Sunrise
Drive, Tucson, AZ, 85718, (800) 572-1717, http://
www.mdausa.org.
The Neuropathy Association, Inc, 60 East 42nd Street, Suite
942, New York, NY, 10165, (212) 692-0662, (212) 692-
0668, info@neuropathy.org, http://www.neuropathy.
org.

Karen M. Krajewski, MS, CGC

Charcot's joints

Definition

Charcot's joints is a progressive degenerative disease of the joints caused by nerve damage resulting in
the loss of ability to feel **pain** in the joint and instability
of the joint.

Description

Charcot's joints, also called neuropathic joint disease, is the result of two conditions present in the joint.
The first factor is the inability to feel pain in the joint
due to nerve damage. The second factor is that injuries
to the joint go unnoticed leading to instability and
making the joint more susceptible to further injury.
Repeated small injuries, strains, and even **fractures**
can go unnoticed until finally the joint is permanently
destroyed. Loss of the protective sensation of pain is
what leads to the disintegration of the joint and often
leads to deformity in the joint.

Although this condition can affect any joint, the
knee is the joint most commonly involved. In individuals with **diabetes mellitus**, the foot is most commonly
affected. The disease can involve only one joint or it
may affect two or three joints. More than three affected
joints is very rare. In all cases, the specific joint(s)
affected depends on the location of the nerve damage.

Causes and symptoms

Many diseases and injuries can interfere with the
ability to feel pain. Conditions such as diabetes mellitus, spinal injuries and diseases, **alcoholism**, and even
syphilis can all lead to a loss of the ability to feel pain
in some areas. Lack of pain sensation may also be
congenital.

The symptoms of Charcot's joints can go unnoticed for some time and may be confused with **osteoarthritis** in the beginning. Swelling and stiffness in a
joint without the expected pain, or with less pain than
would be expected, are the primary symptoms of this
condition. As the condition progresses, however, the
joint can become very painful due to fluid build-up
and bony growths.

Diagnosis

Charcot's joints is suspected when a person with a
disease that impairs pain sensation exhibits painless
swelling and/or stiffness in a joint. Standard x rays will
show damage to the joint, and may also show abnormal bone growth and **calcium** deposits. Floating bone
fragments from previous injuries may also be visible.

Treatment

In the early stages of Charcot's joints, braces to
stabilize the joints can help stop or minimize the damage. When the disease has progressed beyond braces,
surgery can sometimes repair the joint. If the damage
is extensive, an artificial joint may be necessary.

Prognosis

Treatment of the disease causing loss of pain perception may help to slow the damage to the joints.

Prevention

Preventing or effectively managing the underlying
disease can slow or in some cases reverse joint damage,
but the condition cannot be prevented.

Resources

BOOKS

Burgener, Francis A., Martti Kormano, and Tomi Pudas.
*Bone and Joint Disorders: Differential Diagnosis in
Conventional Radiology*. Stuttgart; New York: Thieme,
2006.

Dorothy Elinor Stonely

Charley horse *see* **Muscle spasms and
cramps**

Chelation therapy

Definition

Chelation therapy is an intravenous treatment designed to bind heavy metals in the body in order to treat heavy metal toxicity. Proponents claim it also treats **coronary artery disease** and other illnesses that may be linked to damage from free radicals (reactive molecules).

Purpose

The benefits of EDTA chelation for the treatment of **lead poisoning** and excessively high **calcium** levels are undisputed. The claims of benefits for those suffering from **atherosclerosis**, coronary artery disease, and other degenerative diseases are more difficult to prove. Reported uses for chelation therapy include treatment of **angina**, **gangrene**, arthritis, **multiple sclerosis**, Parkinson's disease, **psoriasis**, and **Alzheimer's disease**. Improvement is also claimed for people experiencing diminished sight, hearing, smell, coordination, and sexual potency.

Description

Origins

The term chelation is from the Greek root word "chele," meaning "claw." Chelating agents, most commonly diamine tetraacetic acid (EDTA), were originally designed for industrial applications in the early 1900s. It was not until the World War II era that the potential for medical therapy was realized. The initial intent was to develop antidotes to poison gas and radioactive contaminants. The need for widespread therapy of this nature did not materialize, but more practical uses were found for chelation. During the following decade, EDTA chelation therapy became standard treatment for people suffering from lead poisoning. Patients who had received this treatment claimed to have other health improvements that could not be attributed to the lead removal only. Especially notable were comments from those who had previously suffered from **intermittent claudication** and angina. They reported suffering less **pain** and **fatigue**, with improved endurance, after chelation therapy. These reports stimulated further interest in the potential benefits of chelation therapy for people suffering from atherosclerosis and coronary artery disease.

If the preparatory examination suggests that there is a condition that could be improved by chelation therapy, and there is no health reason why it shouldn't be used, then the treatment can begin. The patient is generally taken to a comfortable treatment area, sometimes in a group location, and an intravenous line is started. A solution of EDTA together with **vitamins** and **minerals** tailored for the individual patient is given. Most treatments take three to four hours, as the infusion must be given slowly in order to be safe. The number of recommended treatments is usually between 20 and 40. They are given one to three times a week. Maintenance treatments can then be given at the rate of once or twice a month. Maximum benefits are reportedly attained after approximately three months after a treatment series. The cost of therapy is considerable, but it is a fraction of the cost of an expensive medical procedure like cardiac bypass surgery. Intravenous vitamin C and mercury chelation therapies are also offered.

Preparations

A candidate for chelation therapy should initially have a thorough history and physical to define the type and extent of clinical problems. Laboratory tests will be done to determine whether there are any conditions present that would prevent the use of chelation. Patients who have preexisting **hypocalcemia**, poor liver or kidney function, congestive **heart failure**, **hypoglycemia**, **tuberculosis**, clotting problems, or potentially allergic conditions are at higher risk for complications from chelation therapy. A Doppler ultrasound may be performed to determine the adequacy of blood flow in different regions of the body.

Precautions

It is important for people who receive chelation therapy to work with medical personnel who are experienced in the use of this treatment. Treatment should not be undertaken before a good physical, lifestyle evaluation, history, and any laboratory tests necessary are performed. The staff must be forthcoming about test results and should answer any questions the patient may have. Evaluation and treatment should be individualized and involve assessment of kidney function before each treatment with chelation, since the metals bound by the EDTA are excreted through the kidneys.

Although EDTA binds harmful, toxic metals like mercury, lead, and cadmium, it also binds some essential nutrients of the body, such as copper, iron, calcium, zinc, and magnesium. Large amounts of zinc are lost during chelation. Zinc deficiency can cause impaired immune function and other harmful effects. Supplements of zinc are generally given to patients undergoing chelation, but it is not known whether this is adequate to prevent deficiency. Also, chelation therapy does not replace proper **nutrition**, **exercise**, and appropriate medications or surgery for specific diseases or conditions.

Side effects

Side effects of chelation therapy are reportedly unusual, but are occasionally serious. Mild reactions may include, but are not limited to, local irritation at the infusion site, skin reactions, **nausea**, **headache**, **dizziness**, hypoglycemia, **fever**, leg cramps, or loose bowel movements. Some of the more serious complications reported have included hypocalcemia, kidney damage, decreased clotting ability, anemia, bone marrow damage, insulin **shock**, **thrombophlebitis** with **embolism**, and even rare deaths. However, some doctors feel that the latter groups of complications occurred before the safer method currently used for chelation therapy was developed.

Research and general acceptance

EDTA chelation is a highly controversial therapy. The treatment is approved by the United States Food and Drug Administration (FDA) for lead poisoning and seriously high calcium levels. However, for the treatment of atherosclerotic heart disease, EDTA chelation therapy is not endorsed by the American Heart Association (AHA), the FDA, the National Institutes of Health (NIH), or the American College of Cardiology. The AHA reports that there are no adequate, controlled, published scientific studies using currently approved scientific methods to support this therapy

for the treatment of coronary artery disease. However, a pooled analysis from the results of over 70 studies showed positive results in all but one.

Resources

OTHER

Cranton, Elmer. *EDTA Chelation therapy*. April 12, 2008. http://www.drcranton.com/chelation.htm.
Green, Saul. *Quackwatch: Chelation therapy*. 2000. http://www.quackwatch.com/01QuackeryRelatedTopics/chelation.html.

ORGANIZATIONS

American Heart Association National Center, 7272 Greenville Avenue, Dallas, TX, 75231, (800) 242-8721, Review.personal.info@heart.org.
The American College for Advancement in Medicine, 8001 Irvine Center Drive, Ste 825, Irvine, CA, 92619, (949) 309-3538, (600) 532-3688, http://www.acamnet.org.

Judith Turner

Chemical debridement *see* **Debridement**
Chemical peel *see* **Skin resurfacing**
Chemobrasion *see* **Skin resurfacing**

Chemonucleolysis

Definition

Chemonucleolysis is a medical procedure that involves the dissolving of the gelatinous cushioning material in an intervertebral disk by the injection of an enzyme such as chymopapain.

Purpose

Between each vertebra lies a disk of cushioning material that keeps the spinal bones from rubbing together and absorbs some of the shock to the spine from body movements. In the center of the disk is soft, gelatinous material called the nucleus pulposus (NP). The NP is surrounded by a tough fibrous coating. Sometimes when the back is injured, this coating can weaken and bulge or tear to allow the NP to ooze out. When this happens, it is called a herniated nucleus pulposus (HNP), or—in common language—a **herniated disk**.

When the disk bulges or herniates, it can put pressure on nerves which originate in the spinal column, and go to other parts of the body. This causes lower back **pain**, and/or pain to the hips, legs, arms, shoulders, and neck, depending on the location of the herniated disk. Chemonucleolysis uses chymopapain, an enzyme derived from papyrus, to dissolve the disk material that has been displaced because of injury. Herniated disks are the cause of only a small proportion of cases of lower back pain, and chemonucleolysis is appropriate for only some cases of HNP.

Chemonucleolysis is a conservative alternative to disk surgery. There are three types of disk injuries. A protruded disk is one that is intact but bulging. In an extruded disk, the fibrous wrapper has torn and the NP has oozed out, but is still connected to the disk. In a sequestered disk, a fragment of the NP has broken loose from the disk and is free in the spinal canal. Chemonucleolysis is effective on protruded and extruded disks, but not on sequestered disk injuries. In the United States, chymopapain chemonucleolysis is approved only for use in the lumbar (lower) spine. In other countries, it has also been used successfully to treat cervical (upper spine) hernias.

Other indications that a patient is a good candidate for chemonucleolysis instead of surgery include:

- the patient is 18–50 years of age
- leg pain is worse than lower back pain
- other conservative treatments have failed
- The spot where the herniated disk presses on the nerve has been pinpointed by myelography, computed tomography scan (CT scan), or magnetic resonance imaging (MRI)
- the patient wishes to avoid surgery

Precautions

There are some situations in which chemonucleolysis should not be performed. Chymopapain is derived from the papaya. About 0.3% of patients are allergic to chymopapain and go into life-threatening shock when exposed to the enzyme. Chemonucleolysis should not be performed on patients allergic to chymopapain or papaya. It also should not be done:

- when the patient is pregnant
- if the disk is sequestered
- if the patient has had several failed back operations
- if a spinal cord tumor is present
- if the patient has a neurological disease such as multiple sclerosis

Other conditions may affect the appropriateness of chemonucleolysis, including **hypertension**, **obesity**, diabetes, and a family history of **stroke**.

KEY TERMS

Chymopapain—An enzyme from the milky white fluid of the papaya, used for medical purposes in chemonucleolysis.

Myelography—An x-ray test that evaluates the subarachnoid space of the spine.

Nucleus pulposus (NP)—An elastic, pulpy mass in the center of each vertebral disk.

Description

A small gauge needle is placed in the center of the affected disk. Chymopapain is introduced into the disk. The patient needs to remain still.

Preparation

Patients will need tests such as a myelogram or CT scan to pinpoint the herniated disk. Some doctors medicate the patient 24 hours prior to the operation in order to decrease the chances of post-operative lower back stiffness.

Aftercare

Patients may feel lower back stiffness, which goes away in few weeks. Heavy lifting and sports activities should be avoided for at least three months.

Risks

The greatest risk is that the patient may be allergic to chymopapain. The **death** rate for chemonucleolysis is only 0.02%. Complications overall are five to 10 times less than with conventional surgery, and the failure rate is roughly comparable to the failure rate in conventional disk surgery.

Normal results

Many patients feel immediate relief from pain, but, in about 30% of patients, maximal relief takes six weeks. The long term (seven to 20 years) success rate averages about 75%, which is comparable to the success rate for conventional surgery.

Resources

PERIODICALS

Erstad, Shannon, MBA, MPH. "Chemonucleolysis for Herniated Disc." WebMD, July 21, 2008. http://www.webmd.com/back-pain/chemonucleolysis-for-herniated-disc (accessed November 23, 2010).

Tish Davidson, A.M.

Chemotherapy

Definition

Chemotherapy is treatment of **cancer** with **anti-cancer drugs**.

Purpose

The main purpose of chemotherapy is to kill cancer cells. It usually is used to treat patients with cancer that has spread from the place in the body where it started (metastasized). Chemotherapy destroys cancer cells anywhere in the body. It even kills cells that have broken off from the main tumor and traveled through the blood or lymph systems to other parts of the body.

Chemotherapy can cure some types of cancer. In some cases, it is used to slow the growth of cancer cells or to keep the cancer from spreading to other parts of the body. When a cancer has been removed by surgery, chemotherapy may be used to keep the cancer from coming back (adjuvant therapy). Chemotherapy also can ease the symptoms of cancer, helping some patients have a better quality of life.

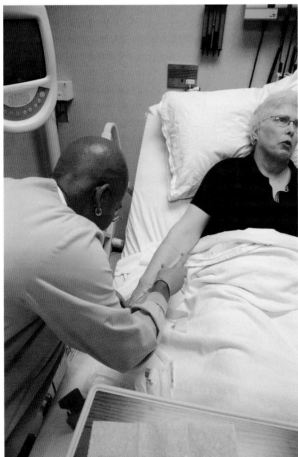

Woman undergoing a clinical trial to test a new chemotherapy treatment. (© Jim West/Alamy.)

Description

Numerous chemotherapy drugs are currently available to treat cancer and many more are being tested for their ability to destroy cancer cells. Most chemotherapy drugs interfere with a cell's ability to grow or multiply. Although these drugs affect all cells in the body, many useful treatments are most effective against rapidly growing cells. Cancer cells of some tumor types grow more quickly than most other body cells. Other cells that grow fast are cells of the bone marrow that produce blood cells, cells in the stomach and intestines, and cells of the hair follicles. Therefore, the most common side effects of chemotherapy are linked to the treatment's effects on other fast growing cells.

Types of chemotherapy drugs

Chemotherapy drugs are classified based on how they work. Drugs that kill cancer cells in a specific part of the cell cycle are called cell cycle specific agents:

- Antimetabolites interfere with the production of DNA and keep cells from growing and multiplying. An example of an antimetabolite is 5-fluorouracil (5-FU).
- Vinca alkaloids prevent cells from dividing normally. Vinblastine and vincristine are plant alkaloids obtained from the periwinkle plant.
- Epipodophyllotoxins work by damaging the cell prior to cell division. Drugs such as etoposide and teniposide are categorized as epipodophyllotoxins.
- Taxanes cause cell death by interfering with actions critical to cell function and by arresting cell division. Paclitaxel (Taxol) and docetaxel (Taxotere) are members of this drug group.
- Epothilones work similarly to the taxanes in causing cell death. Ixabepilone (Ixempra) is classified as an epothilone.
- Camptothecins such as toptecan (Hycamtin) and irinotecan (Camptosar) work in the synthesis phase of the cell cycle to cause cell death.
- Miscellanous agents include L-asparinginase (ELSPAR), which exerts its activity in the first growth phase of cell division, and bleomycin (Blenoxane), which works in the second growth phase to arrest cancer cell division.

Chemotherapy drug categories classified as having cell cycle nonspecific mechanisms of action include:

- alkylating drugs that kill cancer cells by directly attacking DNA, the genetic material of the genes. Cyclophosphamide is an alkylating drug.
- antitumor antibiotics that are made from natural substances such as fungi in the soil. They interfere with important cell functions, including production of DNA and cell proteins. Doxorubicin (Adriamycin) and thiotepa belong to this group of chemotherapy drugs.

Combination chemotherapy

Chemotherapy usually is given in addition to other cancer treatments, such as surgery and **radiation therapy**. When given with other treatments, it is called adjuvant chemotherapy. An oncologist decides which chemotherapy drug or combination of drugs will work best for each patient. The use of two or more chemotherapy drugs together often works better than a single drug for treating cancer. This is called combination chemotherapy. Scientific studies of different drug combinations (clinical trials) help doctors learn which combinations work best for each type of cancer.

How chemotherapy is given

Chemotherapy is administered in different ways, depending on the drugs to be given and the type of cancer. Doctors decide the dose of chemotherapy drugs considering many factors, among them being the patient's height and weight.

Oral chemotherapy is given by mouth in the form a pill, capsule, or liquid. This is the easiest method and can usually be done at home.

Intravenous (IV) chemotherapy is injected into a vein. A small needle is inserted into a vein on the hand or lower arm. The needle usually is attached to a small tube called a catheter, which delivers the drug from an IV bag or bottle.

Intramuscular (IM) chemotherapy is injected into a muscle. Chemotherapy given by intramuscular injection is absorbed into the blood more slowly than IV chemotherapy. Because of this, the effects of IM chemotherapy may last longer than chemotherapy given intravenously. Chemotherapy also may be injected subcutaneously (SQ or SC), which means under the skin. Because of the toxic effects of many chemotherapy drugs on tissue, intramuscular and subcutaneous administration of these drugs is not common. Injection of chemotherapy directly into the cancer is called intralesional (IL) injection.

Chemotherapy may be given by a catheter or port temporarily inserted into a central, large vein or body cavity. A port is a small reservoir or container that is placed in a vein or under the skin in the area where the drug will be given. These methods eliminate the need for repeated injections and may allow patients to spend less time in the hospital while receiving chemotherapy. Intraperitoneal (IP) chemotherapy is administered into the abdominal cavity through a catheter or port. Chemotherapy given by catheter or port into the spinal fluid is called intrathecal (IT) administration. Catheters and ports may be placed in the chest cavity, bladder, or pelvis, depending on the location of the cancer to be treated.

Topical chemotherapy is given as a cream or ointment applied directly to the cancer. This method is more common in treatment of certain types of skin cancer.

Treatment location and schedule

Patients may receive chemotherapy in the doctor's office, or as an inpatient or outpatient at the hospital.

How often and how long chemotherapy is given depends on the type of cancer, how patients respond to the drugs, patients' health and ability to tolerate the drugs, and the types of drugs given. Chemotherapy administration may take only a few minutes or may last as long as several hours. Chemotherapy may be given daily, weekly, or monthly. A rest period may follow a course of treatment before the next course begins. In combination chemotherapy, more than one drug may be given at a time, or they may be given alternately, one following the other.

Precautions

There are many different types of chemotherapy drugs. Oncologists, doctors who specialize in treating cancer, determine which drugs are best suited for each patient. This decision is based on the type of cancer, the patient's age and health, and other drugs the patient is taking. Some patients should not be treated with certain chemotherapy drugs. Age and other conditions may affect the drugs with which a person may be treated. Heart disease, **kidney disease**, and diabetes are conditions that may limit the choice of treatment drugs.

Preparation

A number of medical tests are done before chemotherapy is started. The oncologist will determine how much the cancer has spread from the results of x rays

KEY TERMS

Adjuvant therapy—Treatment given after surgery or radiation therapy to prevent the cancer from coming back.

Alkaloid—A type of chemical commonly found in plants and often having medicinal properties.

Alkylating drug—A drug that kills cells by directly damaging DNA.

Antiemetic—A medicine that helps control nausea; also called an anti-nausea drug.

Antimetabolite—A drug that interferes with a cell's growth or ability to multiply.

Platelets—Blood cells that function in blood clotting.

and other imaging tests and from samples of the tumor taken during surgery or biopsy.

Blood tests give the doctor important information about the function of the blood cells and levels of chemicals in the blood. A **complete blood count** (CBC) is commonly done before and regularly during treatment. The CBC shows the numbers of white blood cells, red blood cells, and platelets in the blood. Because chemotherapy affects the bone marrow, where blood cells are made, levels of these cells often drop during chemotherapy. The white blood cells and platelets are most likely to be affected by chemotherapy. A drop in the **white blood cell count** means the immune system cannot function properly. Low levels of platelets can cause a patient to bleed easily from a cut or other wound. A low red blood cell count can lead to anemia (deficiency of red blood cells) and **fatigue**.

When a chemotherapy treatment takes a long time, the patient may prepare for it by wearing comfortable clothes. Bringing a book to read or a tape to listen to may help pass the time and ease the **stress** of receiving chemotherapy. Some patients bring a friend or family member to provide company and support during treatment.

Sometimes, patients taking chemotherapy drugs known to cause **nausea** are given medications called anti-emetics before chemotherapy is administered. Anti-emetic drugs help to lessen feelings of nausea. Two anti-nausea medications that may be used are Kytril and Zofran.

Other ways to prepare for chemotherapy and help lessen nausea are:

- regularly eating nutritious foods and drinking lots of fluids
- eating and drinking normally until about two hours before chemotherapy
- eating high carbohydrate, low-fat foods and avoiding spicy foods

Aftercare

Tips for helping to control side effects after chemotherapy include:

- following any instructions given by the doctor or nurse
- taking all prescribed antinausea medications
- eating small amounts of bland foods
- drinking lots of fluids
- getting plenty of rest

Some patients find it helps to breathe fresh air or get mild **exercise**, such as taking a walk.

Risks

Chemotherapy drugs are toxic to normal cells as well as cancer cells. A dose that will destroy cancer cells will probably cause damage to some normal cells. Doctors adjust doses to do the least amount of harm possible to normal cells. Some patients feel few or no side effects, and others may have more serious side effects. In some cases, a dose adjustment may be required to reduce or stop a side effect.

Some chemotherapy drugs have more side effects than others. The most common side effects are:

- nausea and vomiting
- loss of appetite
- hair loss
- anemia and fatigue
- infection
- easy bleeding or bruising
- sores in the mouth and throat
- neuropathy and other damage to the nervous system
- kidney damage

Nausea and vomiting are common, but can usually be controlled by **antinausea drugs**, drinking fluids, and avoiding spicy foods. Loss of appetite may be due to nausea or the stress of undergoing cancer treatment.

Some chemotherapy drugs cause hair loss, but it is almost always temporary.

Low blood cell counts caused by the effect of chemotherapy on the bone marrow can lead to anemia, infections, and easy bleeding and bruising.

Patients with anemia have too few red blood cells to deliver oxygen and nutrients to the body's tissues. Anemic patients feel tired and weak. If red blood cell levels fall too low, a blood **transfusion** may be given.

Patients receiving chemotherapy are more likely to get infections. This happens because their infection-fighting white blood cells are reduced. It is important to take measures to avoid getting infections. When the white blood cell count drops too low, the doctor may prescribe medications called colony stimulating factors that help white blood cells grow.

Platelets are blood cells that make the blood clot. When patients do not have enough platelets, they may bleed or bruise easily, even from small injuries. Patients with low blood platelets should take precautions to avoid injuries. Medicines such as **aspirin** and other **pain** relievers can affect platelets and slow down the clotting process.

Chemotherapy can cause irritation and dryness in the mouth and throat. Painful sores may form that can bleed and become infected. Precautions to avoid this side effect include getting dental care before chemotherapy begins, brushing the teeth and gums regularly with a soft brush, and avoiding mouth washes that contain salt or alcohol.

Normal results

The main goal of chemotherapy is to cure cancer. Many cancers are cured by chemotherapy. It may be used in combination with surgery and/or radiation therapy to keep a cancer from spreading to other parts of the body. Some widespread, fast-growing cancers are more difficult to treat. In these cases, chemotherapy may slow the growth of the cancer cells.

Doctors can tell if the chemotherapy is working by the results of medical tests. **Physical examination**, blood tests, and x rays are all used to check the effects of treatment on the cancer.

The possible outcomes of chemotherapy are:

- Complete remission or response. The cancer completely disappears. The course of chemotherapy is completed and the patient is tested regularly for a recurrence.
- Partial remission or response. The cancer shrinks in size but does not disappear. The same chemotherapy may be continued or a different combination of drugs may be tried.
- Stabilization. The cancer does not grow or shrink. Other therapy options may be explored. A tumor may remain stabilized for many years.
- Progression. The cancer continues to grow. Other therapy options may be explored.

- A secondary malignancy may develop as a result of being treated with some chemotherapy agents, and that second cancer may need additional chemotherapy or other treatment.

Resources

OTHER

"Chemotherapy Principles: An In-Depth Discussion." American Cancer Society. June 17, 2009. http://www.cancer.org/docroot/ETO/content/ETO_1_4X_What_Is_Chemotherapy.asp?sitearea=ETO (accessed October 3, 2010).

"Understanding Chemotherapy." National Cancer Institute. November 24, 2008 [cited June 26, 2010]. http://www.cancer.gov/cancertopics/chemo-side-effects/understandingchemo (accessed October 3, 2010).

ORGANIZATIONS

American Cancer Society, (800) 227-2345, http://www.cancer.org.

National Cancer Institute, Building 31, Room 10A31, 31 Center Drive, MSC 2580, Bethesda, MD, 20892-2580, (800) 422-6237, http://www.cancer.gov.

Toni Rizzo
Teresa G. Odle
Melinda Granger Oberleitner, RN,
DNS, APRN, CNS

Chest drainage therapy

Definition

Chest drainage therapy involves the removal of air, blood, pus, or other secretions from the chest cavity.

Purpose

Chest drainage therapy is done to relieve pressure on the lungs, and remove fluid that could promote infection. Installing a chest drainage tube can be either an emergency or a planned procedure.

Removing air or fluids from the chest involves the insertion of a tube through the skin and the muscles between the ribs, and into the chest cavity. This cavity is also called the pleural space. Insertion of this tube is called thoracostomy, and chest drainage therapy is sometimes called thoracostomy tube drainage.

Conditions that may need to be treated by chest drainage therapy include **emphysema** (air in the tissues of the lungs), **tuberculosis**, and spontaneous **pneumothorax** (air in the chest cavity) that causes more than a

25% collapse of the lung. Other conditions include **cancer** that causes excessive secretions, **empyema** (pus in the thoracic cavity), or hemothorax (blood in the thoracic cavity). Almost all chest drainage therapy is done to drain blood from the chest cavity after lung or heart surgery. In cases where the lung is collapsed, removing fluids by chest drainage therapy allows the lung to reinflate.

Oftentimes an x ray is performed prior to treatment to determine whether the problem is either fluid or air in the pleural space. Sometimes a procedure called **thoracentesis** is performed in an effort to avoid inserting a chest drainage tube. In this procedure a needle with a catheter is inserted into the pleural space and fluid is removed. When fluid continues to accumulate, chest drainage therapy is usually the next step. This is especially true when there is a lung infection underlying the fluid build-up.

Precautions

Chest drainage therapy is not done if a collapsed lung is not life-threatening. It also should be avoided for patients who have blood clotting problems.

Description

Most patients are awake when the chest drainage tube is inserted. They are given a sedative and a local anesthetic. Chest drainage tubes are usually inserted between the ribs. The exact location depends on the type of material to be drained and its location in the lungs.

An incision is made in the skin and through the muscles between the ribs. A chest tube is inserted and secured in place. The doctor connects one end of the tube to the chest drainage system.

The chest drainage system must remain sealed to prevent air from entering the chest cavity through the tube. One commonly used system is a water-seal drainage system, comprised of three compartments that collect and drain the fluid or air without allowing air to backflow into the tube. An alternative to this system is to connect the tube to a negative suction pump.

Once the tube and drainage system are in place, a **chest x ray** is done to confirm that the tube is in the right location, and that it is working. In some cases it may be necessary to insert more than one tube to drain localized pockets of fluid that have accumulated.

KEY TERMS

Empyema—Pus in the pleural cavity.

Hemothorax—Blood in the pleural cavity.

Pleural cavity—The area of the chest that includes the lining of the chest cavity, the space the lungs are located in, and the membrane covering of the lungs.

Spontaneous pneumothorax—Air in the chest cavity that occurs because of disease or other naturally occurring cause. Air and blood together in this space is called a pneumohemothorax.

Preparation

A chest x ray is usually done before the chest drainage tube is inserted. Sometimes fluid becomes trapped in isolated spaces in the lung, and it is necessary to do an ultrasound to determine where to locate the drainage tube. **Computed tomography scans** (CT) are useful in locating small pockets of fluids caused by cancer or tuberculosis.

Aftercare

Normally after the material has been removed from the chest cavity and the situation is resolved, the chest drainage tube is removed. In cases where the reason for the tube was air in the pleural cavity, the tube is clamped and left in place several hours before it is removed to make sure no more air is leaking into the space. If the patient is on mechanical ventilation, the tube is often left in place until a respirator is no longer necessary. Chest drainage therapy is usually done in conjunction with treating the underlying cause of the fluid build-up.

The fluid that has been drained is examined for bacterial growth, cancer cells, pus, and blood to determine the underlying cause of the condition and appropriate treatment.

Risks

Problems can arise in the insertion of the tube if the membrane lining the chest cavity is thick or if it has many **adhesions**. The tube will not drain correctly if the chest cavity contains **blood clots** or thick secretions that are often associated with infections. Excessive bleeding may occur during the insertion and positioning of the tube. Infection may result from the procedure. **Pain** is also a common complication.

Normal results

The gas, pus, or blood is drained from the chest cavity, and the lungs reinflate or begin to function more efficiently. The site at which the tube was inserted heals normally.

Resources

BOOKS

McPhee, Stephen, and Maxine Papadakis.*Current Medical Diagnosis and Treatment, 2010*, 49th ed. New York: McGraw–Hill Medical, 2009.

Tish Davidson, A.M.

Chest pain *see* **Angina**

Chest physical therapy

Definition

Chest **physical therapy** is the term for a group of treatments designed to improve respiratory efficiency, promote expansion of the lungs, strengthen respiratory muscles, and eliminate secretions from the respiratory system.

Purpose

The purpose of chest physical therapy, also called chest physiotherapy, is to help patients breathe more freely and to get more oxygen into the body. Chest physical therapy includes postural drainage, chest percussion, chest vibration, turning, deep breathing exercises, and coughing. It is usually done in conjunction with other treatments to rid the airways of secretions. These other treatments include suctioning, nebulizer treatments, and the administration of expectorant drugs.

Chest physical therapy can be used with newborns, infants, children, and adults. People who benefit from chest physical therapy exhibit a wide range of problems that make it difficult to clear secretions from their lungs. Some people who may receive chest physical therapy include people with **cystic fibrosis** or neuromuscular diseases like **Guillain-Barré syndrome**, progressive muscle weakness (**myasthenia gravis**), or **tetanus**. People with lung diseases such as **bronchitis**, **pneumonia**, or **chronic obstructive pulmonary disease** (COPD) also benefit from chest physical therapy. People who are likely to aspirate their mucous secretions because of diseases such as **cerebral palsy** or **muscular dystrophy** also receive chest physical therapy, as do some people

who are bedridden, confined to a wheelchair, or who cannot breathe deeply because of postoperative **pain**.

Precautions

Chest physical therapy should not be performed on people with

- bleeding from the lungs
- neck or head injuries
- fractured ribs
- collapsed lungs
- damaged chest walls
- tuberculosis
- acute asthma
- recent heart attack
- pulmonary embolism
- lung abscess
- active hemorrhage
- some spine injuries
- recent surgery, open wounds, or burns

Description

Chest physical therapy can be performed in a variety of settings including critical care units, hospitals, nursing homes, outpatient clinics, and at the patient's home. Depending on the circumstances, chest physical therapy may be performed by anyone from a respiratory care therapist to a trained member of the patient's family. Different patient conditions warrant different levels of training.

Chest physical therapy consists of a variety of procedures that are applied depending on the patient's health and condition. Hospitalized patients are reevaluated frequently to establish which procedures are most effective and best tolerated. Patients receiving long term chest physical therapy are reevaluated about every three months.

Turning

Turning from side to side permits lung expansion. Patients may turn themselves or be turned by a caregiver. The head of the bed is also elevated to promote drainage if the patient can tolerate this position. Critically ill patients and those dependent on mechanical respiration are turned once every one to two hours around the clock.

Coughing

Coughing helps break up secretions in the lungs so that the mucus can be suctioned out or expectorated.

Patients sit upright and inhale deeply through the nose. They then exhale in short puffs or coughs. Coughing is repeated several times a day.

Deep breathing

Deep breathing helps expand the lungs and forces better distribution of the air into all sections of the lung. The patient either sits in a chair or sits upright in bed and inhales, pushing the abdomen out to force maximum amounts of air into the lung. The abdomen is then contracted, and the patient exhales. Deep breathing exercises are done several times each day for short periods.

Postural drainage

Postural drainage uses the force of gravity to assist in effectively draining secretions from the lungs and into the central airway where they can either be coughed up or suctioned out. The patient is placed in a head or chest down position and is kept in this position for up to 15 minutes. Critical care patients and those depending on mechanical ventilation receive postural drainage therapy four to six times daily. Percussion and vibration may be performed in conjunction with postural drainage.

Percussion

Percussion is rhythmically striking the chest wall with cupped hands. It is also called cupping, clapping, or tapotement. The purpose of percussion is to break up thick secretions in the lungs so that they can be more easily removed. Percussion is performed on each lung segment for one to two minutes at a time.

Vibration

As with percussion, the purpose of vibration is to help break up lung secretions. Vibration can be either mechanical or manual. It is performed as the patient breathes deeply. When done manually, the person performing the vibration places his or her hands against the patient's chest and creates vibrations by quickly contracting and relaxing arm and shoulder muscles while the patient exhales. The procedure is repeated several times each day for about five exhalations.

Preparation

The only preparation needed for chest physical therapy is an evaluation of the patient's condition and determination of which chest physical therapy techniques would be most beneficial.

KEY TERMS

Coughing—Coughing helps break up secretions in the lungs so that the mucus can be suctioned out or expectorated. Patients sit upright and inhale deeply through the nose. They then exhale in short puffs or coughs. Coughing is repeated several times per day.

Deep breathing—Deep breathing helps expand the lungs and forces better distribution of the air into all sections of the lung. The patient either sits in a chair or sits upright in bed and inhales, pushing the abdomen out to force maximum amounts of air into the lung. The abdomen is then contracted, and the patient exhales. Deep breathing exercises are done several times each day for short periods.

Percussion—This consists of rhythmically striking the chest wall with cupped hands. It is also called cupping, clapping, or tapotement. The purpose of percussion is to break up thick secretions in the lungs so that they can be more easily removed. Percussion is performed on each lung segment for one to two minutes at a time.

Postural drainage—This technique uses the force of gravity to assist in effectively draining secretions from the lungs and into the central airway where they can either be coughed up or suctioned out. The patient is placed in a head or chest down position and is kept in this position for up to 15 minutes. Critical care patients and those depending on mechanical ventilation receive postural drainage therapy four to six times daily. Percussion and vibration may be performed in conjunction with postural drainage.

Turning—Turning from side to side permits lung expansion. Patients may turn themselves or be turned by a caregiver. The head of the bed is also elevated to promote drainage if the patient can tolerate this position. Critically ill patients and those dependent on mechanical respiration are turned once every one to two hours around the clock.

Vibration—The purpose of vibration is to help break up lung secretions. Vibration can be either mechanical or manual. It is performed as the patient breathes deeply. When done manually, the person performing the vibration places his or her hands against the patient's chest and creates vibrations by quickly contracting and relaxing arm and shoulder muscles while the patient exhales. The procedure is repeated several times each day for about five exhalations.

Aftercare

Patients practice **oral hygiene** procedures to lessen the bad taste or odor of the secretions they spit out.

Risks

Risks and complications associated with chest physical therapy depend on the health of the patient. Although chest physical therapy usually poses few problems, in some patients it may cause

- oxygen deficiency if the head is kept lowered for drainage
- increased intracranial pressure
- temporary low blood pressure
- bleeding in the lungs
- pain or injury to the ribs, muscles, or spine
- vomiting
- inhaling secretions into the lungs
- heart irregularities

Normal results

The patient is considered to be responding positively to chest physical therapy if some, but not necessarily all, of these changes occur:

- increased volume of sputum secretions
- changes in breath sounds
- improved vital signs
- improved chest x ray
- increased oxygen in the blood as measured by arterial blood gas values
- patient reports of eased breathing

ORGANIZATIONS

Cystic Fibrosis Foundation, 6931 Arlington Road, 2nd floor, Bethesda, MD, 20814, (301) 951-4422, (301) 951-6378, (800) 344-4823, info@cff.org, http://www.cff.org.

Tish Davidson, A.M.

Chest radiography *see* **Chest x ray**

Chest x ray

Definition

A chest x ray is a procedure used to evaluate organs and structures within the chest for symptoms of disease. Chest x rays include views of the lungs, heart, small portions of the gastrointestinal tract,

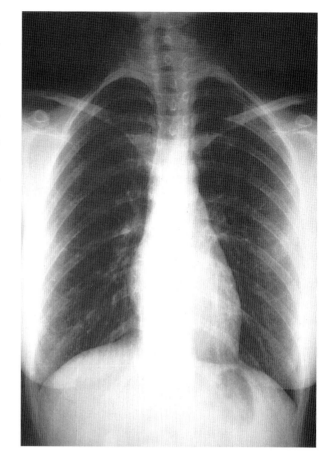

Normal adult chest x ray. *(Custom Medical Stock Photo, Inc. Reproduced by permission.)*

thyroid gland, and the bones of the chest area. X rays are a form of radiation that can penetrate the body and produce an image on an x-ray film. Another name for the film produced by x rays is radiograph.

Purpose

Chest x rays are ordered for a wide variety of diagnostic purposes. In fact, this is probably the most frequently performed type of x ray. In some cases, chest x rays are ordered for a single check of an organ's condition, and at other times, serial x rays are ordered to compare to previous studies. Some common reasons for chest x rays include the following.

Pulmonary disorders

Chest films are frequently ordered to diagnose or rule out **pneumonia**. One type, **tuberculosis**, can be observed on chest x rays, as can cardiac disease and damage to the ribs or lungs. Other pulmonary disorders such as **pneumothorax** (presence of air or gas in

KEY TERMS

Bronchi—Plural of bronchus. The air passages in the lungs through which inhaled air passes on its way through the lungs.

Diaphragm—The large muscle that is located between the abdomen and the chest area. The diaphragm aids in breathing.

Gastrointestinal—The digestive organs and structures, including the stomach and intestines.

Interstitial lung disease—About 180 diseases fall into this category of breathing disorders. Injury or foreign substances in the lungs (such as asbestos fibers) as well as infections, cancers, or inherited disorders may cause the diseases. They can lead to breathing or heart failure.

Lymphoid—Tissues relating to the lymphatic system. A thin, yellowish fluid called lymph fluid, travels throughout the body. The lymphatic system helps control fluids in the body.

Portable chest x ray—An x ray procedure taken by equipment that can be brought to the patient. The resulting radiographs may not be as high in quality as stationary x-ray radiographs, but allow a technologist to come to the patient.

Pulmonary—Refers to the lungs and the breathing system and function.

Serial x rays—A number of x rays performed at set times in the disease progression or treatment intervals. The radiographs will be compared to one another to track changes.

Sternum—Also referred to as the breast bone, this is the long flat bone in the middle of the chest.

Thorax—The chest area, which runs between the abdomen and neck and is encased in the ribs.

X ray—A form of electromagnetic radiation with shorter wavelengths than normal light. X rays can penetrate most structures.

the chest cavity outside the lungs) or **emphysema** may be detected or evaluated through the use of chest x ray.

Cancer

A chest x ray may be ordered by a physician to check for possible tumors of the lungs, lymphoid tissue, or bones of the thorax. These may be primary tumors, or the areas in which **cancer** originates in the body. X rays also check for secondary spread of cancer from another organ to the chest.

Cardiac disorders

While less sensitive than **echocardiography**, chest x ray can be used to check for disorders such as congestive **heart failure** or **pulmonary edema**.

Other

Chest x rays are used to see foreign bodies that may have been swallowed or inhaled, and to evaluate response to treatment for various diseases. Often the chest x ray is also used to verify correct placement of chest tubes or catheters. Chest x rays can be used to check for fluid surrounding the lungs (**pleural effusion**).

Description

Routine chest x rays consist of two views, the frontal view (referred to as posterioranterior or PA) and the lateral (side) view. It is preferred that the patient stand for this exam, particularly when studying collection of fluid in the lungs.

During the actual time of exposure, the technologist will ask the patient to hold his or her breath. It is very important in taking a chest x ray to ensure there is no motion that could detract from the quality and sharpness of the film image. The procedure will only take a few minutes and the time patients must hold their breath is a matter of a few seconds.

The chest x ray may be performed in a physician's office or referred to an outpatient radiology facility or hospital radiology department. In some cases, particularly for patients who cannot get out of bed, a portable chest x ray may be taken. Portable films are sometimes of poorer quality than those taken with permanent equipment, but are the best choice for some patients or situations when the patient cannot be moved or properly positioned for the chest x ray. Patients confined to bed may be placed in as upright a position as possible to get a clear picture, particularly of chest fluid.

Preparation

There is no advance preparation necessary for chest x rays. Once the patient arrives in the exam area, a hospital gown will replace all clothing on the upper body and all jewelry must be removed.

Aftercare

No aftercare is required by patients who have chest x rays.

Risks

The only risk associated with chest x ray is minimal exposure to radiation, particularly for pregnant women and children. Those patients should use protective lead aprons during the procedure. Technologists are cautioned to check carefully for possible dislodging of any tubes or monitors in the chest area from the patient's placement during the exam.

Normal results

A radiologist, or physician specially trained in the technique and interpretation of x rays, will evaluate the results. A normal chest x ray will show normal structures for the age and medical history of the patient. Findings, whether normal or abnormal, will be provided to the referring physician in the form of a written report.

Abnormal findings on chest x rays are used in conjunction with a physician's physical exam findings, patient medical history, and other diagnostic tests, including laboratory tests, to reach a final diagnosis. For many diseases, chest x rays are more effective when compared to previous chest x-ray studies. The patient is asked to help the radiology facility in locating previous chest radiographs from other facilities.

Pulmonary disorders

Pneumonia shows up on radiographs as patches and irregular areas of density (from fluid in the lungs). If the bronchi (air passages in the lungs which are usually not visible) can be seen, a diagnosis of bronchial pneumonia may be made. Shifts or shadows in the hila (lung roots) may indicate enlarged lymph nodes of a malignancy. Widening of the spaces between ribs and increased lucency of the lung fields suggests emphysema. Other pulmonary diseases may also be detected or suspected through chest x ray.

Cancer

In nearly all patients with lung cancer, some sort of abnormality can be seen on a chest radiograph. Hilar masses (enlargements at that part of the lungs where vessels and nerves enter) are one of the more common symptoms as are abnormal masses and fluid buildup on the outside surface of the lungs or surrounding areas. Interstitial lung disease, which is a large category of disorders, many of which are related to exposure of substances (such as asbestos fibers), may be detected on a chest x ray as increased prominence of the interstitial pattern, often in the lower portions of the lungs.

Other

Congestive heart failure and other cardiac diseases may be indicated on the view of a heart and lung in a chest radiograph. **Fractures** of the sternum and ribs are sometimes detected as breaks on the chest x ray, though often dedicated bone films are needed. In some instances, the radiologist's view of the diaphragm may indicate an abdominal problem. Foreign bodies that may have been swallowed or inhaled can usually be located by the radiologist, as they will look different from any other tissue or structure in the chest. Serial chest x rays may be ordered to track changes over a period of time, usually to evaluate response to therapy of a malignancy.

ORGANIZATIONS

American Lung Association, 1740 Broadway, New York, NY, 10019, (800) 586-4872, http://www.lungusa.org.

National Heart, Lung and Blood Institute, P.O. Box 30105, Bethesda, MD, 20824-0105, (301) 251-1222, http://www.nhlbi.nih.gov.

Teresa Odle
Lee Shratter, MD
Brenda W. Lerner

Chickenpox

Definition

Chickenpox is a common and highly contagious childhood disease that also occasionally affects adults. It is caused by the varicella–zoster virus. Chickenpox produces an itchy, blistery rash that typically lasts about a week and is sometimes accompanied by **fever** or other symptoms.

Demographics

Chickenpox is a common **infectious disease** with an estimated 60 million cases occurring annually worldwide. In temperate regions, the disease usually affects children under age 10; in tropical regions, adult cases are more common. The rate of infection is independent of race or gender, but is much lower in countries where **vaccination** against the disease is practiced. For example, before a vaccine against chickenpox was introduced in the United States in 1995, about 99% of the population got chickenpox by age 30. A decade after the vaccine was introduced, only about 10% of Americans who had not already had chickenpox got the disease.

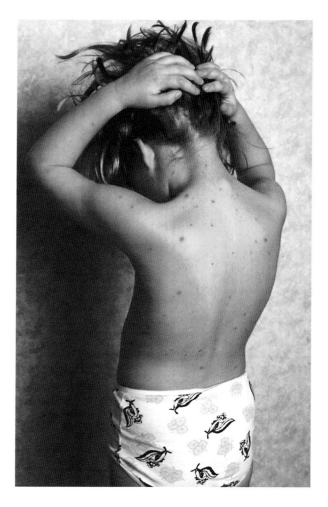

A five-year-old girl with chickenpox. The first symptom of the disease is the rash that is evident on the girl's back and neck. The rash and the mild fever that accompanies it should disappear in a week or two. *(Jim Selby/Photo Researchers, Inc.)*

Description

Chickenpox is very contagious. The virus is transmitted through either direct contact or coughing and sneezing. A person with chickenpox is contagious from one to two days before the outbreak of the chickenpox rash to about six days after the rash erupts. After being exposed, a person will show symptoms of chickenpox within 10–21 days. Individuals normally get chickenpox only once in a lifetime.

Most cases of chickenpox contracted by healthy children are mild, with the child experiencing seven to 10 days of discomfort. However, in children who are immunocompromised, such as those with leukemia, **AIDS**, or who are undergoing immunosuppression therapy in connection with an organ transplant, chickenpox can have serious complications including **death**. For

example, the number of children with leukemia who die of complications from chickenpox is estimated at 7% to 28%. This compares to a death rate of about seven in every 100,000 healthy children. Abnormalities may occur in the fetuses of women who develop chickenpox during the first 22 weeks of **pregnancy**.

Risk factors

The greatest risk factor for acquiring chickenpox is the failure to vaccinate; almost every unvaccinated person exposed to the virus develops chickenpox. It may not be safe to vaccinate some children with compromised immune systems, leaving them highly vulnerable to both the disease and severe complications including death. Pregnant women who develop chickenpox during the first half of their pregnancy put the fetus at risk for **birth defects**.

Causes and symptoms

Chickenpox is caused by the varicella–zoster virus, a member of the herpes virus family. It easily spreads through the air or by direct contact with an infected person.

A case of chickenpox usually starts without warning or with only a mild fever and a slight feeling of illness. Within a few hours or days, small red spots begin to appear on the scalp, neck, or upper half of the trunk. After a further 12–24 hours, the spots typically become itchy, fluid–filled bumps called vesicles, which continue to appear for the next two to five days. In any area of skin, lesions in a variety of stages can be seen. These blisters can spread to cover much of the skin, and in some cases may be found inside the mouth, nose, ears, vagina, or rectum. Some people develop only a few blisters, but in most cases the number reaches 250–500.

The blisters soon begin to form scabs and fall off. Scarring usually does not occur unless the blisters have been scratched and become infected. Occasionally a minor and temporary darkening of the skin (called **hyperpigmentation**) develops around some of the blisters. The degree of itchiness can range from barely noticeable to extreme. Some people who contract chickenpox also have headaches, abdominal **pain**, or a fever. Full recovery usually takes five to 10 days after the first symptoms appear. The most severe cases of the disease tend to be found among adolescents and adults.

Although for most people chickenpox is no more than a matter of a few days of discomfort, some groups are at risk for developing complications, the most

Acetaminophen—A drug for relieving pain and fever. Tylenol is the most common example.

Acyclovir—An antiviral drug used for combating chickenpox and other herpes viruses.

Dehydration—Excessive water loss by the body.

Encephalitis—A rare viral infection that causes inflammation in the membranes lining the brain.

Hepatitis—A disease that causes inflammation of the liver and serious liver damage.

Immune system—A mechanism that protects the body from foreign substances, foreign cells, and pathogens (viruses, bacteria). The thymus, spleen, lymph nodes, white blood cells, including the B cells and T cells, and antibodies are involved in the immune response, which aims to destroy these foreign bodies.

Immunocompromised—Having a damaged immune system.

Passive immunity—Immunity produced by providing a person with antibodies from another source than self. Infants are born with passive immunity acquired from their mothers.

Pneumonia—A disease that causes inflammation of the lungs. It can be caused by a bacterium or a virus.

Pus—A thick yellowish or greenish fluid containing inflammatory cells. Usually caused by bacterial infection.

Reye's syndrome—A rare but often fatal disease that involves the brain, liver, and kidneys. It may be brought on by giving salicylates to children (but not adults) who have a viral infection.

Salicylates—A group of drugs that includes aspirin and related compounds. Salicylates are used to relieve pain, reduce inflammation, and lower fever.

Shingles—A disease also called herpes zoster that causes a rash and a very painful nerve inflammation. An attack of chickenpox eventually gives rise to shingles in about 20% of the population.

Vaccination—Injection of a killed or weakened microbe in order to stimulate the immune system against the microbe, thereby preventing disease. Vaccinations, or immunizations, work by stimulating the immune system, the natural disease–fighting system of the body. The healthy immune system is able to recognize invading bacteria and viruses and produce substances (antibodies) to destroy or disable them. Vaccinations prepare the immune system to ward off a disease. To immunize against viral diseases, the virus used in the vaccine has been weakened or killed.

Varicella–zoster immune globulin (VZIG)—A substance that can reduce the severity of chickenpox symptoms.

Virus—A tiny particle that can cause infections by duplicating itself inside a cell using the cell's own reproductive mechanisms. Antibiotics are generally ineffective against viruses, though antiviral drugs exist for some viruses, including chickenpox.

common of which are bacterial infections of the blisters, **pneumonia**, **dehydration**, **encephalitis**, and hepatitis:

- Infants. Complications occur much more often among children less than one year old than among older children. The threat is greatest to newborns, who are more at risk of death from chickenpox than any other group. Under certain circumstances, children born to mothers who contract chickenpox just before delivery develop the disease and face an increased possibility of dangerous complications, including brain damage and death. If the infection occurs during the first half of pregnancy, there is a small risk of the baby being born with congenital abnormalities.

- Immunocompromised children. Children whose immune systems have been weakened by a genetic disorder, disease, or medical treatment usually experience the most severe symptoms of any group. They have the second–highest rate of death from chickenpox.

- Adults and children age 15 and older. Among this group, typical symptoms of chickenpox tend to be more severe, and the risk of complications is much higher than among young children. Adults are ten times more likely than children to require hospitalization from chickenpox.

Diagnosis

For otherwise healthy children, especially those with recent exposure to the disease, diagnosis usually can be made at home, by a school nurse, or by a doctor if the child's parent or caregiver is unsure that the disease is chickenpox. A doctor should be called immediately if:

- The child has a chronic disease or is undergoing a treatment that weakens the immune system.
- The child's fever goes above 102°F (38.9°C) or takes more than four days to disappear.
- The child's blisters appear infected. Signs of infection include pus drainage or excessive redness, warmth, tenderness, or swelling.
- The child seems nervous, confused, unresponsive, or unusually sleepy; complains of a stiff neck or severe headache; shows signs of poor balance or has trouble walking; finds bright lights hard to look at; is having breathing problems or is coughing a lot; is complaining of chest pain; is vomiting repeatedly; or is having convulsions. These may be signs of Reye's syndrome or encephalitis, two rare but potentially very dangerous conditions.

Treatment

Home remedies

Treatment usually takes place at home and focuses on reducing discomfort and fever. The individual should drink plenty of fluids and eat simple, nutritious foods. Soups, herbal teas, and fruit juices are good choices. If mouth blisters make eating or drinking an unpleasant experience, cold drinks and soft, bland foods can ease the discomfort.

Applying wet compresses or bathing in cool or lukewarm water once a day can help the itch. Adding four to eight ounces of baking soda or one to two cups of oatmeal to the bath may help ease **itching**. Oatmeal bath packets are sold by pharmacies. Only mild soap should be used in the bath. Patting, not rubbing, is recommended for drying off to prevent irritating the blisters. Calamine lotion also helps to reduce itchiness. Because scratching can cause blisters to become infected and lead to scarring, a child's nails should be cut short. Older children need to be warned not to scratch. For babies, light mittens or socks on the hands can help guard against scratching.

Drugs

Fever and discomfort can be reduced by **acetaminophen** (Tylenol, Tempera). **Aspirin** and any medications that contain aspirin or other salicylates must not be used for children with chickenpox because they appear to increase the chances of developing **Reye's syndrome**. The best idea is to consult a doctor or pharmacist if unsure about which medications are safe.

Because chickenpox is a viral disease, **antibiotics** are ineffective against it, although antibiotics may be prescribed if blisters become infected.

Children who are immunocompromised or healthy children who develop serious complications are often treated with the antiviral drug acyclovir (Zovirax), which is given intravenously. This drug may also be used under certain circumstances in adolescents and adults with chickenpox.

A substance called varicella–zoster immune globulin (VZIG), which reduces the severity of chickenpox symptoms, may be used to treat immunocompromised children and others at high risk of developing complications. VZIG is produced from a **gamma globulin** from blood of recently infected individuals. It provides some degree of passive immunity when administered by injection within 96 hours of known or suspected exposure to the disease. It is not useful if given more than 96 hours after exposure.

Alternative

Alternative practitioners recommend a variety of treatments with the aim of reducing discomfort, strengthening the immune system, and speeding healing. An alternative practitioner should be consulted about the best choice for each individual.

SUPPLEMENTS. Vitamin A may help to heal damaged skin. Vitamin C and bioflavonoids may help to reduce fever and stimulate the immune system. Zinc stimulates the immune system and is thought to promote healing; however zinc can cause **nausea and vomiting**. **Calcium** and magnesium may help to relieve restlessness and sleeping difficulties, but magnesium has a laxative effect at high doses.

HERBALS AND CHINESE MEDICINE. The following herbals may used internally (ingested) to treat chickenpox:

- Echinacea and goldenseal (*Hydrastis canadensis*) support the immune system and soothe skin and mucous membranes. Echinacea is also thought to have antiviral properties.
- Chamomile tea is a sleep aid.
- Chinese cucumber (*Trichosanthes kirilowii*) root tea is used to relieve symptoms of chickenpox.
- Elder flower, peppermint, and yarrow may reduce fever.
- Garlic has antiviral activity.
- Mullein (*Verbascum thapsus*).
- Yin Qiao Jie Du Wan (Honeysuckle and Forsythia Pill).

- Ban Lan Gen Chong Ji (Isatis Infusion).

The following herbals are used externally (applied to skin) to treat chickenpox:

- Aloe leaf, calendula, and plantain relieve the itching of the chickenpox rash.
- Turmeric powder mixed with lime juice treats chickenpox rash.
- Garlic helps clear skin infection.

OTHER ALTERNATIVE REMEDIES. Homeopathic remedies are selected on a case–by–case basis. Some common remedy choices are apis, aconitum, belladonna, calendula, antimonium tartaricum, pulsatilla, *Rhus toxicodendron*, and sulphur.

The **acupressure** points Four Gates, Large Intestine 11, Spleen 10, and Stomach 36 help alleviate symptoms associated with chickenpox.

Alternative treatments should be used with care, as the benefits of many such treatments have not been confirmed by scientific research.

Prognosis

Most cases of chickenpox run their course within a week. Although complications from chickenpox generally are rare, the most common one is bacterial infection of the skin, initiated at the site of a chickenpox blister that has broken or was scratched open. Other complications include viral or bacterial pneumonia and rarely encephalitis (swelling of the brain). Anyone with a weakened immune system, lung diseases, **eczema** or other skin conditions, infants under one year of age, premature infants whose mothers have not had chickenpox, and newborns whose mothers had chickenpox around the time of delivery are at highest risk for developing complications are.

After symptoms subside, the varicella–zoster virus lies dormant in nerve cells where it may be reactivated years later by disease or age–related weakening of the immune system. The result is **shingles** (herpes zoster), a very painful rash and nerve inflammation, that develops in between 10% and 20% of all people who have ever had chickenpox. Shingles is particularly common in people over age 50. Shingles cause **numbness**, itching, or severe pain in skin areas where the affected nerve root is located. Within about three days cause clusters of blisters to form along the affected nerve. The blisters last two to three weeks. A vaccine against shingles is recommended for individuals age 60 and older.

Prevention

Vaccination against the varicella–zoster virus is the best way of preventing chickenpox. Vaccination has been proven to be about 85% effective for preventing all cases of chickenpox and about 95% effective in preventing severe cases. Side effects of the vaccine normally are limited to occasional soreness or redness at the injection site. The United States Centers for Disease Control and Prevention (CDC) guidelines state that the vaccine should be given to all children (with the exception of certain high–risk groups) at 12–18 months of age, preferably when they receive their measles–mumps–rubella (MMR) vaccine. For older children, up to age 12, the CDC recommends vaccination when a reliable determination that the child in question has already had chickenpox cannot be made. Vaccination also is recommended for any older child or adult considered susceptible to the disease, particularly those, such as health care workers and women of childbearing age.

A single dose of the vaccine was once thought sufficient for children up to age 12; older children and adults received a second dose four to eight weeks later. However, an outbreak at a daycare center in 2000 brought concern in the medical community about the permanence of immunity and the necessity of a second vaccination for younger children, since many of the affected children had already received a single dose of the vaccine. Since 2006, a second dose of the vaccine has become standard.

The chickenpox vaccine is not recommended for pregnant women, and women should delay pregnancy for three months following a complete vaccination. The vaccine is useful when given early after exposure to chickenpox and, if given in the midst of the incubation period, it may be preventative.

While there was initial concern regarding the vaccine's safety and effectiveness when first released, the vaccination has gained acceptance, and many states require it for admittance into daycare or public school. In 2004, 87.5% of toddlers ages 19–35 months in the United States were immunized; up nearly 20% from 2000.

The vaccine was approved for use in Australia in 2000 and is recommended for children starting at age 18 months. Between 2000 and 2006, 1.3 million doses of the vaccine have been given in Australia, with 342 reports of adverse effects and 115 reports of the vaccine' giving only partial protection, according to the Australian Adverse Drug Reaction Committee.

Resources

BOOKS

Corlett, William Thomas. *A Treatise on the Acute, Infectious Exanthemata, Including Variola, Rubeola, Scarlatina, Rubella, Varicella, and Vaccina.* Whitefish, MT: Kessinger Publishing LLC, 2007.

Sears, Robert. *The Vaccine Book: Making The Right Decision for Your Child.* New York: Little, Brown, 2007.

PERIODICALS

Bond, Deborah. and Mooney, Janice. "A Literature Review Regarding the Management of Varicella-Zoster Virus." *Musculoskeletal Care.* 8(2) (March 19, 2010): 118–22.

Muscarella, Maria. "Chickenpox Remedies: Maria Muscarella Offers Soothing Herbal Solutions." *New Life Journal.* (April 2007): 35.

OTHER

Mayo Clinic. "Chickenpox." Mayo Foundation for Medical Education and Research. (September 5, 2008). http://mayoclinic.com/health/chickenpox/DS00053 (accessed September 17, 2010).

MedlinePlus. "Chickenpox." U.S. National Library of Medicine. (January 27, 2010). http://www.nlm.nih.gov/medlineplus/chickenpox.html (accessed September 17, 2010).

ORGANIZATIONS

American Academy of Family Physicians (AAFP), PO Box 11210, Shawnee Mission, KS, 66207, (913) 906–6000, (800) 274–2237, (913) 906–6075, http://familydoctor.org.

American Academy of Pediatrics (AAP), 141 Northwest Point Blvd., Elk Grove Village, IL, 60007–1098, (847) 434–4000, (847) 434–8000, http://www.aap.org.

Centers for Disease Control and Prevention (CDC), 1600 Clifton Rd., Atlanta, GA, 30333, (404) 639–3534, (800) CDC–INFO ((800) 232–4636). TTY: (888) 232–6348, inquiry@cdc.gov, http://www.cdc.gov.

Ken Wells
Tish Davidson, A.M.

Child abuse

Definition

Child abuse, sometimes called child maltreatment, describes four types of actions toward children: physical abuse, **sexual abuse**, psychological abuse, and neglect. In many cases, the same child experiences more than one type of abuse. The abusers can be parents or other family members, caregivers such as teachers or babysitters, acquaintances (including other children), and (in very rare instances) strangers.

Demographics

Child abuse was once viewed as a minor social problem affecting only a handful of American children. However, in the late twentieth century, issues of child welfare came under scrutiny by the media, law enforcement, and the helping professions. This increase in public and professional awareness led to a sharp rise in the number of reported cases of child abuse. Today child abuse is recognized as a problem that occurs among households of all racial, ethnic, and income levels, although the incidence of reported cases is higher in low-income households where adult caregivers experience greater financial **stress** and social difficulties, have less education and less understanding of child development, and may have less access to social services. In addition, children of parents who are substance abusers are more likely to experience abuse than children living in households where there is no **substance abuse**. Many child abusers were themselves abused as children.

Statistically, it is difficult to find reliable national figures for cases of child abuse because each state keeps its own records and has its own definitions of what constitutes abuse. Child abuse almost always occurs in private, and because abuse often is hidden from view and its victims may be too young or too frightened to speak out, experts suggest that its true prevalence is probably greater than the official data indicate. However, based on information states reported to the United States Department of Health and Human Services Administration for Children and Families, in 2007 Child Protective Services (CPS) investigated almost reports of child maltreatment of 3.5 million children. Of these, approximately 794,000 children were documented victims. Fifty-nine percent were victims of neglect, 10.8% of physical abuse, 7.6% of sexual abuse, 4.2% of psychological maltreatment, less than 1% of medical neglect, and 13.1 percent were victims of multiple maltreatments. Victims were split almost evenly between girls and boys.

Nearly 70% of abused children were maltreated by a parent, and almost three-quarters of these children were victims of repeated maltreatment. In addition, the National Child Abuse and Neglect Data System (NCANDS) reported that an estimated 1,760 children (2.35 children per 100,000) died from an injury where abuse or neglect was the cause or a contributing factor. Of these, more than 75% were under age 4, with the largest number of deaths occurring in infants under one year old.

Child abuse signs and symptoms

Although these signs do not necessarily indicate that a child has been abused, they may help adults recognize that something is wrong. The possibility of abuse should be investigated if a child shows a number of these symptoms, or any of them to a marked degree:

Sexual abuse

Being overly affectionate or knowledgeable in a sexual way inappropriate to the child's age
Medical problems such as chronic itching, pain in the genitals, or venereal diseases
Other extreme reactions, such as depression, self-mutilation, suicide attempts, running away, overdoses, or anorexia
Personality changes, such as becoming insecure or clingy
Regressing to younger behavior patterns such as thumb sucking or bringing out discarded cuddly toys
Sudden loss of appetite or engaging in compulsive eating
Being isolated or becoming withdrawn
Inability to concentrate
Lack of trust or fear toward someone they know well, such as not wanting to be alone with a babysitter or specific family member
Starting to wet the bed again or having nightmares
Anxiety about clothing being removed
Suddenly starting to draw sexually explicit pictures
Trying to be "ultra-good" or perfect; overreacting to criticism

Physical abuse

Unexplained recurrent injuries or burns
Improbable excuses or refusal to explain injuries
Wearing clothes to cover injuries, even in hot weather
Refusal to undress for gym
Bald patches
Chronic running away
Fear of medical help or examination
Self-destructive tendencies
Aggression toward others
Fear of physical contact; shrinking back if touched
Admitting that they are punished, but the punishment is excessive (such as a child being beaten every night to make him/her study)
Fear of suspected abuser being contacted

Psychological abuse

Physical, mental, and psychological developmental lags
Sudden speech disorders
Continual self-depreciation (e.g., "I'm stupid, ugly, worthless," etc.)
Overreaction to mistakes
Extreme fear of any new situation
Inappropriate response to pain (e.g., "I deserve this")
Neurotic behavior (e.g., rocking, hair twisting, self-mutilation)
Extremes of passivity or aggression

Neglect

Constant hunger
Poor personal hygiene
No social relationships
Constant tiredness
Poor state of clothing
Compulsive scavenging
Emaciation
Untreated medical problems
Destructive tendencies

A child may be subjected to a combination of different kinds of abuse. It is also possible that a child may show no outward signs and hide what is happening from everyone.

(Table by PreMediaGlobal. Reproduced by permission of Gale, a part of Cengage Learning.)

Description

Physical abuse

Physical abuse is nonaccidental infliction of physical injury to a child. Legal definitions of physical child abuse vary from state to state, but injuries requiring medical attention typically are regarded as abusive. Physical abuse takes many forms, including cuts, **bruises**, **burns**, broken bones, **poisoning**, and internal injuries. Nonetheless, difficulties associated with defining the line between discipline and abuse are well known. Many states explicitly note that spanking "when administered in a reasonable manner" does not constitute abuse. Thus, how severely parents can inflict physical punishment upon their children without it being considered abusive remains subject to interpretation.

The physical abuser is usually a family member or other caregiver, and is likely to be male. The injuries can be inflicted by punching, kicking, biting, burning, beating, or use of a weapon such as a baseball bat or knife. A rare form of physical abuse is **Munchausen syndrome** by proxy, in which a caregiver (most often the mother) seeks attention by intentionally making the child sick or appear to be sick.

Sexual abuse

Children are sexually abused when they experience contact that is for the sexual gratification of an adult or a significantly older or dominant child when they are younger than the legal age of consent or at a stage of development at which they do not possess sufficient maturity to understand the nature of the acts and therefore to provide informed consent. Abusers may use coercion or deceptive manipulation, but often physical force is not necessary since the perpetrator is likely to be someone with whom the child has a trusting relationship and who is in a position of authority over the child. In many states, sexual activity is automatically assumed to be abuse when a defined age difference exists between the older abuser and the younger (minor) victim independent of any consent the victim may have given.

Sexual behaviors can include touching breasts, genitals, and buttocks while the victim is either dressed or undressed. Sexual abuse behavior also includes cunnilingus, fellatio, or penetration of the vagina or anus with sexual organs or objects. Sexual abuse does not have to involve any actual touching. Children can be coerced into disrobing and exposing themselves or watching adults disrobe or engage in sexual activity. Pornographic photography or videography also are forms of sexual abuse of children.

The U.S. Department of Justice estimates that one in six victims of a **sexual assault** is under age 12. Sexual abuse victims can be either boys or girls. Most, but not all, perpetrators are male. Despite publicity surrounding cases where a child is sexually assaulted by a stranger, almost all sexual abuse against children is perpetrated by a family member (e.g. father, stepfather, aunt, uncle, sibling, cousin) or family intimate (e.g., live-in lover or friend of the parent). Perpetrators go to great lengths to conceal sexual abuse. Children who have been sexually abused may not report the behavior due to threats, shame, or to a lack of understanding of what has happened.

Rape is the most violent form of sexual abuse. Rape is the perpetration of an act of sexual intercourse when:

- will is overcome by force or fear (from threats, use of weapons, or use of drugs).
- mental impairment renders the victim incapable of rational judgment.
- if the victim is below the legal age established for consent. According the U.S. Department of Justice, 54% of all rapes are of women under age 18.

Psychological abuse

Abuse of children is not limited to the physical body. Psychological abuse encompasses rejecting, ignoring, criticizing, belittling, humiliating, threatening the child with violence, or otherwise terrorizing the child, all of which have the effect of eroding the child's self-esteem and sense of security. It also can include isolating the child from friends or other family members or destroying the child's property.

Psychological abuse may be the result of actions not directed specifically at the child. The prevalence of domestic violence exposes children to intimidating and frightening scenes every day. Many children live in homes where domestic violence is an ongoing problem that they witness regularly often as a result of being "caught in the middle" of a parental altercation. Children who observe violence react with many of the same psychological symptoms as children who have experienced it directly. Psychological abuse often accompanies other types of abuse. It is difficult to prove and rarely is reported.

Neglect

Neglect is the failure to satisfy a child's basic needs. About 60% of cases of maltreatment documented by CPS involve neglect. Neglect can assume many forms. Physical neglect is the failure (beyond the constraints imposed by poverty) to provide adequate food, clothing, shelter, or supervision. Children may live in filthy conditions or situations where food is not provided, or where they develop infections or other medical conditions that go untreated. Failure to send children to school or otherwise provide for their education may also be considered neglect. Psychological neglect is the failure to satisfy a child's normal psychological needs and/or behavior that damages a child's normal psychological development (e.g., permitting drug abuse in the home, having the child witness domestic violence).

Risk factors

The greatest risk factor for abuse is being young. In 2007, almost 32% of victims of maltreatment were under age four while another 24% were between ages four and seven. The **death** rate from abuse is skewed even more heavily toward the young with 42.2% of deaths in 2007 occurring in children under one year old and 33.5% in children between the ages of one and three years.

Children who are handicapped and those who are nonrhythmic (that is, with unpredictable eating and sleeping patterns), are more likely to be abused. Similarly, children who are distractible, impulsive, or who have high activity levels are more likely to experience physical abuse.

Causes and symptoms

Sociocultural factors contributing to abuse

Poverty is the sociocultural factor most strongly linked to abuse. Although physical abuse occurs at all income levels, it happens more often in very poor families. It is true that in middle-class families, child injuries are treated by a sympathetic personal physician who may be less likely to diagnose and report abuse-related injuries than the physician in the emergency room who is more likely to treat poor families. Even with such reporting bias, however, poverty seems strongly linked to abuse. It seems that the frustrating effects of poverty on parents are instrumental in creating situations for parents' abuse.

Physical crowding, more likely to occur in poverty, is also associated with abuse. If too many people share a small living space, severe punishment of children as a means of maintaining control is more likely.

Job loss and dissatisfaction are often associated with child abuse. Higher rates of abuse exist in military compared to non-military families. It is generally felt that the link between these environmental stressors and abuse is strengthened by the absence of social support networks that might otherwise buffer the family against adversity. Having no one to assist with child care and no one to question the use of severe discipline increase the chance that a parent may injure a child.

Pedophiles exist in all economic and cultural groups. Psychologically, however, they share certain traits. Pedophiles often have a history of being abused themselves, and abusing other children seems to be triggered by increased life stressors, such as marital problems, job layoffs, or abuse of drugs.

Caregiver factors

Parents who were themselves abused as children are more likely to abuse their own children. However, not every parent who was abused becomes an abuser;

some parents go to great lengths to insure that they never harm their children.

Parents who abuse their children are likely to be younger than the average parent. They are more likely to be single parents. Having mental illness, such as depression, or abusing drugs or alcohol also makes a parent more likely to abuse a child.

Abusive parents socialize differently from nonabusive parents. Nonabusive parents tend to use ignoring or time-out procedure, whereas abusive parents tend to shout, threaten, and spank. Some forms of child abuse escalate over time, with the parent spanking harder and more frequently to get the same effect or resorting to abuse to get results. Female caregivers inflict more soft tissue injuries, broken bones, and internal injuries than male caregivers. Severe injuries from a single, explosive incident in which the child is shaken, thrown, or struck are more likely to involve male caregivers.

Abusive parents often expect the child to perform behaviors he or she is not yet capable of performing. Parents who abuse their young children expect them to be able to control their impulses, recall and obey complex parental rules, and perform mature chains of behavior such a getting up, washing, and getting dressed by themselves. Nonabusive parents recognize that toddlers and preschool children are incapable of such behaviors. Understanding the limitations of a young child's memory, ability to be controlled by words, impulse control, and attention span is essential to developing reasonable expectations for the child. Parents who expect behavior the child cannot deliver are apt to progressively increase their control techniques in order to get the child to comply.

Abusive discipline is often the result of the belief that the young child is capable of better behavior and that he or she is deliberately misbehaving to cause the parent difficulty. Such parents often claim that their 18-month-old could stay clean if she wanted to but she dirties her pants just to make more work for the mother. Abusive parents who believe a child has chosen to misbehave inflict more punishment on their children than parents who accurately recognize when a child's behavior is not intentional.

Such abusive parents also often believe that effective parenting involves maintaining tight control over the child. A mother who can toilet train her child early and keep the child in line at the grocery store is viewed by abusive parents as a "good" mother. Closely tied to beliefs about the importance of control are aphorisms such as "spare the rod, spoil the child" and "respect comes through fear," which indicate that children learn best through the application of force.

Another belief abusive parents often hold is that their children should engage in reciprocal parenting. They believe that if they sometimes comfort, wait on, and take care of the child, the child should do the same for them. Such beliefs fit with abusive parents' lack of awareness of children's developmental capabilities and may also stem from the parents' own immaturity and lack of support from other adults. Regardless of the source, when such expectations are not met by the child, the parent often responds with anger and hostility.

Emotion

Anger is the most frequent trigger for parental abuse. Abusive parents appear to have a lower threshold for childish behaviors than average parents. Abusive parents are more upset by the same child cues than nonabusive parents. Thus, child behaviors that are merely irritating to average parents are infuriating to abusive parents. Finally, abusive parents may have less control over their anger than nonabusive parents, either because they are unaware of their level of anger, because they are chronically angry, or because they lack anger management skills.

When considering how emotion influences child abuse, it seems important to consider positive emotions as well. Abusive parents experience their children as less rewarding than nonabusive parents. In observation, abusive parents touch their children less, cuddle them less, less frequently call the affectionate names ("honey," "sweetheart"), and smile less at their children. Nonabusive parents respond flexibly to their children, letting the child lead the play interaction. Even in play, abusive parents have expectations that their children seem unable or unwilling to fulfill, making play a disagreeable chore rather than a rewarding endeavor. Abusive parents seem trapped by their own lack of skills, limited developmental understanding, inappropriate expectations, high negative emotion, and low enjoyment of the child.

Symptoms

Although these signs do not necessarily indicate that a child has been abused, they may help adults recognize that something is wrong. The possibility of abuse should be investigated if a child shows a number of these symptoms, or any of them to a marked degree:

Sexual Abuse

- Being overly affectionate or knowledgeable in a sexual way inappropriate to the child's age

- Medical problems such as chronic itching, pain in the genitals, venereal diseases
- Other extreme reactions, such as depression, self-mutilation, suicide attempts, running away, overdoses, anorexia
- Personality changes such as becoming insecure or clingy
- Regressing to younger behavior patterns such as thumb sucking or bringing out discarded cuddly toys
- Sudden loss of appetite or compulsive eating
- Being isolated or becoming withdrawn
- Inability to concentrate
- Lack of trust or fear someone they know well, such as not wanting to be alone with a babysitter or specific family member
- Starting to wet bed again, day or night/nightmares
- Become worried about clothing being removed
- Suddenly starting to draw sexually explicit pictures
- Trying to be "ultra-good" or perfect; overreacting to criticism

Physical Abuse

- Unexplained recurrent injuries or burns
- Improbable excuses or refusal to explain injuries
- Wearing clothes to cover injuries, even in hot weather
- Refusal to undress for gym
- Bald patches
- Chronic running away
- Fear of medical help or examination
- Self-destructive tendencies
- Aggression toward others
- Fear of physical contact; shrinking back if touched
- Admitting that they are punished, but the punishment is excessive (such as a child being beaten every night to make him/her study)
- Fear of suspected abuser being contacted

Psychological Abuse

- Physical, mental, and psychological developmental lags
- Sudden speech disorders
- Continual self-depreciation (e.g.,"I'm stupid, ugly, worthless")
- Overreaction to mistakes
- Extreme fear of any new situation
- Inappropriate response to pain (e.g., "I deserve this")
- Neurotic behavior (e.g., rocking, hair twisting, self-mutilation)

- Extremes of passivity or aggression

  Neglect

- Constant hunger
- Poor personal hygiene
- No social relationships
- Constant tiredness
- Poor state of clothing
- Compulsive scavenging
- Emaciation
- Untreated medical problems
- Destructive tendencies

A child may be subjected to a combination of different kinds of abuse. It is also possible that a child may show no outward signs and hide what is happening from everyone.

Diagnosis

Doctors and many other professionals who work with children are required by law to report suspected abuse to their state's CPS agency. Abuse investigations often are a group effort involving medical personnel, social workers, police officers, and others. Some hospitals and communities maintain child protection teams that respond to cases of possible abuse. Careful questioning of the parents is crucial, as is interviewing the child (if he or she is capable of being interviewed). Trained investigators must ensure, however, that their questioning does not further traumatize the child and also that their style of questioning does not prompt the child to give the answers the child thinks the questioner wants rather than accurate answers. A **physical examination** for signs of physical or sexual abuse or of neglect is necessary and may include x rays, blood tests, and other procedures.

Treatment

Notification of the appropriate authorities, treatment of the child's injuries, and protecting the child from further harm are the immediate priorities in abuse cases. If the child does not require hospital treatment, protection often involves placing him or her with relatives, in a group home, or in foster care. Once the immediate concerns are dealt with, it becomes essential to determine how the child's long-term medical, psychological, educational, and other needs can best be met. This process involves evaluating not only the child's needs but also the needs of the family (e.g., drug abuse counseling, parental skills training, anger management training). The authorities also must determine whether other children living in the same household also have been abused. On investigation, signs of physical abuse are discovered in about 20% of other children living in the abused child's household.

Prognosis

Child abuse often has lifelong consequences. Research shows that abused children and adolescents are more likely to do poorly in school, experience depression, extreme anger, antisocial personality traits, and other psychiatric problems. They also are more likely to become promiscuous, abuse drugs and alcohol, run away, and attempt **suicide**. As adults they often have trouble establishing intimate relationships.

Most children who have been abused experience some symptoms of posttraumatic stress disorder (PTSD). PTSD in children and adolescents may be acute or delayed, that is, the child may experience symptoms immediately or after a period of time has passed, perhaps when the child feels safe. Symptoms may include re-experiencing the abusive episodes at some level, feeling emotionally numb, or becoming physiologically aroused (elevated heart rate, respiration, and so forth). Children may experience disassociation and appear to "space out" when reminded of the abuse or perpetrator. They may have physical symptoms. They may become enraged or feel guilt at having provoked the episodes or survived them. They may have invasive memories, repeated behaviors, or fears related to the abusive situations. They may act out some of their issues in play—punishing the bad guy or victimizing another character while playing with dolls or action figures. In severe cases of chronic trauma, the child may develop serious or prolonged disassociation or depression. Severe and chronic abuse has also been implicated in cases of **multiple personality disorder**.

Once the abuse has stopped, some of these symptoms can be treated with some form of counseling or therapy. Some have argued that full recovery is a life-long task. Adults who have been abused as children may have to face issues long after the abuse has stopped, when they enter into their own sexual relationships or when they raise their own children. Long-term therapy by a professional trained in working with abused children and adults offers the best chance of overcoming childhood abuse.

Prevention

There are many barriers to changing abusive parental behavior. Most parents' own history suggests that strong physical discipline is the preferred model of parenting. Further, most abusive parents live in families and neighborhoods in which violence is not only condoned but also viewed as a necessary vehicle for interpersonal influence. The stresses that are omnipresent in abusive parents' lives assist in maintaining high levels of anger and depression, which block the positive enjoyment of the child. When the parent responds with strong physical discipline, the child's misbehavior typically stops, for that moment at any rate. Thus, the parent is intermittently rewarded for responding abusively. Thus, changing abusive parenting is a challenging task.

It may be preferable to prevent the development of abusive parenting by early interventions to give skills, alter developmental knowledge, change unreasonable parenting expectations, and block the steady build-up of anger and extinguishing of affection for the child. Prevention programs now target teenagers before **pregnancy** as well as young mothers to try to break the cycle of abuse.

Government efforts to prevent abuse include home-visitor programs aimed at high-risk families and school-based efforts to teach children how to respond to attempted sexual abuse. Psychological abuse prevention has been promoted through the media.

When children reach age three, parents should begin teaching them about "bad touches" and about confiding in a suitable adult if they are touched or treated in a way that makes them uneasy. Parents also need to exercise caution in hiring babysitters and other caregivers. Anyone who suspects abuse should report those suspicions to the police or his or her local CPS agency. Prevent Child Abuse America (listed in references) is an excellent source of information on the many support groups and other organizations that help abused and at-risk children and their families. One of these organizations, Parents Anonymous, sponsors local self-help groups throughout the United States, Canada, and Europe.

Resources

AMERICAN HELP HOTLINES

Childhelp National Child Abuse Hotline 1-800-4-A-CHILD. TDD for the Deaf 1-800-2-A-Child. Help for children who are being abused or adults who are concerned that a child they know is being abused or neglected.

Rape, Abuse and Incest National Network (RAINN) Online hotline http://www.rainn.org/get-help/national-sexual-assault-online-hotline or telephone: 1-800-656-HOPE. Online counseling and referral to local rape crisis centers using anonymous instant messaging or telephone counseling and referrals to local crisis center.

OTHER

"Child Abuse." *MedlinePlus, National Institutes of Health.* July 30, 2009 [August 20, 2009]. http://www.nlm.nih.gov/medlineplus/childabuse.html.
"Child Welfare Information Gateway." *United States Department of Health and Human Services.* July 22, 2009 [August 20, 2009]. http://www.childwelfare.gov.

ORGANIZATIONS

Parents Anonymous, 675 W. Foothill Blvd., Suite 220, Claremont, CA, 91711-3475, (909) 621-6184, (909) 625-6304, http://www.parentsanonymous.org.
Prevent Child Abuse America, 500 North Michigan Avenue, Suite 200, Chicago, IL, 60611-3703, (312) 663-3520, 1-800-CHILDREN, (312) 939-8962, mailbox@preventchildabuse.org, http://www.preventchildabuse.org/index.shtml.

Tish Davidson, A.M.

Child development *see* **Children's health**
Child safety *see* **Children's health**

Childbirth

Definition

Childbirth includes both labor (the process of birth) and delivery (the birth itself); it refers to the entire process as an infant makes its way from the womb down the birth canal to the outside world.

Description

Childbirth usually begins spontaneously, about 280 days after conception, but it may be started by artificial means if the **pregnancy** continues past 42 weeks gestation. The average length of labor is about 14 hours for a first pregnancy and about eight hours in subsequent pregnancies. However, many women experience a much longer or shorter labor.

Labor can be described in terms of a series of phases.

First stage of labor

During the first phase of labor, the cervix dilates (opens) from 0–10 cm. This phase has an early, or latent,

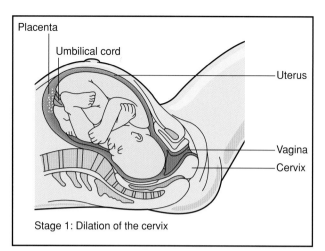

Stage 1: Dilation of the cervix

Stage 1: Dilation of the cervix. *(Illustration by Hans & Cassady, Inc. Reproduced by permission of Gale, a part of Cengage Learning.)*

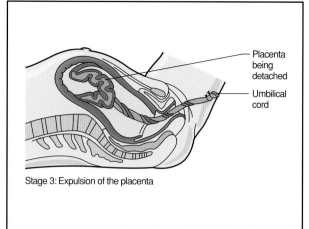

Stage 3: Expulsion of the placenta

Stage 3: Expulsion of the placenta. *(Illustration by Hans & Cassady, Inc. Reproduced by permission of Gale, a part of Cengage Learning.)*

phase and an active phase. During the latent phase, progress is usually very slow. It may take quite a while and many contractions before the cervix dilates the first few centimeters. Contractions increase in strength as labor progresses. Most women are relatively comfortable during the latent phase and walking around is encouraged, since it naturally stimulates the process.

As labor begins, the muscular wall of the uterus begins to contract as the cervix relaxes and expands. As a portion of the amniotic sac surrounding the baby is pushed into the opening, it bursts under the pressure, releasing amniotic fluid. This is called "breaking the bag of waters."

During a contraction, the infant experiences intense pressure that pushes it against the cervix,

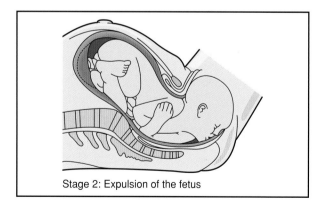

Stage 2: Expulsion of the fetus

Stage 2: Expulsion of the fetus. *(Illustration by Hans & Cassady, Inc. Reproduced by permission of Gale, a part of Cengage Learning.)*

eventually forcing the cervix to stretch open. At the same time, the contractions cause the cervix to thin. During this first stage, a woman's contractions occur more and more often and last longer and longer. The doctor or nurse will do a periodic **pelvic exam** to determine how the mother is progressing. If the contractions aren't forceful enough to open the cervix, a drug may be given to make the uterus contract.

As **pain** and discomfort increase, women may be tempted to request pain medication. If possible, though, administration of pain medication or anesthetics should be delayed until the active phase of labor begins—at which point the medication will not act to slow down or stop the labor.

The active stage of labor is faster and more efficient than the latent phase. In this phase, contractions are longer and more regular, usually occurring about every two minutes. These stronger contractions are also more painful. Women who use the breathing exercises learned in childbirth classes find that these can help cope with the pain experienced during this phase. Many women also receive some pain medication at this point—either a short-term medication, such as Nubain or Numorphan, or an epidural anesthesia.

As the cervix dilates to 8–9 cm, the phase called the transition begins. This refers to the transition from the first phase (during which the cervix dilates from 0–10 cm) and the second phase (during which the baby is pushed out through the birth canal). As the baby's head begins to descend, women begin to feel the urge to "push" or bear down. Active pushing by the mother should not begin until the second phase, since pushing too early can cause the cervix to swell or to tear and bleed. The attending healthcare practitioner should counsel the mother on when to begin to push.

Second stage of labor

As the mother enters the second stage of labor, her baby's head appears at the top of the cervix. Uterine contractions get stronger. The infant passes down the vagina, helped along by contractions of the abdominal muscles and the mother's pushing. Active pushing by the mother is very important during this phase of labor. If an epidural anesthetic is being used, many practitioners recommend decreasing the amount administered during this phase of labor so that the mother has better control over her abdominal muscles

When the top of the baby's head appears at the opening of the vagina, the birth is nearing completion. First the head passes under the pubic bone. It fills the lower vagina and stretches the perineum (the tissues between the vagina and the rectum). This position is called "crowning," since only the crown of the head is visible. When the entire head is out, the shoulders follow. The attending practitioner suctions the baby's mouth and nose to ease the baby's first breath. The rest of the baby usually slips out easily, and the umbilical cord is cut.

Episiotomy

As the baby's head appears, the perineum may stretch so tight that the baby's progress is slowed down. If there is risk of tearing the mother's skin, the doctor may choose to make a small incision into the perineum to enlarge the vaginal opening. This is called an **episiotomy**. If the woman has not had an epidural or pudendal block, she will get a local anesthetic to numb the area. Once the episiotomy is made, the baby is born with a few pushes.

Third stage

In the final stage of labor, the placenta is pushed out of the vagina by the continuing uterine contractions. The placenta is pancake shaped and about 10 inches in diameter. It has been attached to the wall of the uterus and has served to convey nourishment from the mother to the fetus throughout the pregnancy. Continuing uterine contractions cause it to separate from the uterus at this point. It is important that all of the placenta be removed from the uterus. If it is not, the uterine bleeding that is normal after delivery may be much heavier.

Breech presentation

Approximately 4% of babies are in what is called the "breech" position when labor begins. In breech presentation, the baby's head is not the part pressing against the cervix. Instead the baby's bottom or legs are positioned to enter the birth canal instead of the head. An obstetrician may attempt to turn the baby to a head down position using a technique called version. This is only successful approximately half the time.

The risks of vaginal delivery with breech presentation are much higher than with a head-first presentation. The mother and attending practitioner will need to weigh the risks and make a decision on whether to deliver via a **cesarean section** or attempt a vaginal birth. The extent of the risk depends to a great extent on the type of breech presentation, of which there are three. Frank breech (the baby's legs are folded up against its body) is the most common and the safest for vaginal delivery. The other types are complete breech (in which the baby's legs are crossed under and in front of the body) and footling breech (in which one leg or both legs are positioned to enter the birth canal). These are not considered safe to attempt vaginal delivery.

Even in complete breech, other factors should be met before considering a vaginal birth. An ultrasound examination should be done to be sure the baby does not have an unusually large head and that the head is tilted forward (flexed) rather than back (hyperextended). Fetal monitoring and close observation of the progress of labor are also important. A slowing of labor or any indication of difficulty in the body passing through the pelvis should be an indication that it is safer to consider a cesarean section.

Forceps delivery

If the labor is not progressing as it should or if the baby appears to be in distress, the doctor may opt for a forceps delivery. A forceps is a spoon-shaped device that resembles a set of salad tongs. It is placed around the baby's head so the doctor can pull the baby gently out of the vagina.

Forceps can be used after the cervix is fully dilated, and they might be required if:

- the umbilical has dropped down in front of the baby into the birth canal
- the baby is too large to pass through the birth canal unaided
- the baby shows signs of stress
- the mother is too exhausted to push

Before placing the forceps around the baby's head, pain medication or anesthesia may be given to the mother. The doctor may use a catheter to empty the mother's bladder, and may clean the perineal area with soapy water. Often an episiotomy is done before a forceps birth, although tears can still occur.

The obstetrician slides half of the forceps at a time into the vagina and around the side of the baby's head to gently grasp the head. When both "tongs" are in place, the doctor pulls on the forceps to help the baby through the birth canal as the uterus contracts. Sometimes the baby can be delivered this way after the very next contraction.

The frequency of forceps delivery varies from one hospital to the next, depending on the experience of staff and the types of anesthesia offered at the hospital. Some obstetricians accept the need for a forceps delivery as a way to avoid cesarean birth. However, other obstetrical services do not use forceps at all.

Complications from forceps deliveries can occur. Sometimes they may cause nerve damage or temporary **bruises** to the baby's face. When used by an experienced physician, forceps can save the life of a baby in distress.

Vacuum-assisted birth

This method of helping a baby out of the birth canal was developed as a gentler alternative to forceps. Vacuum-assisted birth can only be used after the cervix is fully dilated (expanded), and the head of the fetus has begun to descend through the pelvis. In this procedure, the doctor uses a device called a vacuum extractor, placing a large rubber or plastic cup against the baby's head. A pump creates suction that gently pulls on the cup to ease the baby down the birth canal. The force of the suction may cause a bruise on the baby's head, but it fades away in a day or so.

The vacuum extractor is not as likely as forceps to injure the mother, and it leaves more room for the baby to pass through the pelvis. However, there may be problems in maintaining the suction during the vacuum-assisted birth, so forceps may be a better choice if it is important to remove the baby quickly.

Cesarean sections

A cesarean section, also called a c-section, is a surgical procedure in which incisions are made through a woman's abdomen and uterus to deliver her baby.

Cesarean sections are performed whenever abnormal conditions complicate labor and vaginal delivery, threatening the life or health of the mother

or the baby. In 2002, just over 26% of babies were born by c-section, an increase of 7% from the previous year. The procedure may be used in cases where the mother has had a previous c-section and the area of the incision has been weakened. Dystocia, or difficult labor, is the another common reason for performing a c-section.

Difficult labor is commonly caused by one of the three following conditions: abnormalities in the mother's birth canal; abnormalities in the position of the fetus; abnormalities in the labor, including weak or infrequent contractions.

Another major factor is fetal distress, a condition where the fetus is not getting enough oxygen. Fetal brain damage can result from oxygen deprivation. Fetal distress is often related to abnormalities in the position of the fetus, or abnormalities in the birth canal, causing reduced blood flow through the placenta.

Other conditions also can make c-section advisable, such as vaginal herpes, **hypertension** (high blood pressure), and diabetes in the mother. Some parents choose to have a c-section because they fear the pain or unpredictability of labor or they want to avoid pelvic damage.

Causes and symptoms

One of the first signs of approaching childbirth may be a "bloody show," the appearance of a small amount of blood-tinged mucus released from the cervix as it begins to dilate. This is called the "mucus plug."

The most common sign of the onset of labor is contractions. Sometimes women have trouble telling the difference between true and false labor pains.

True labor pains:

• develop a regular pattern, with contractions coming closer together
• last from 15–30 seconds at the onset and get progressively stronger and longer (up to 60 seconds)
• may get stronger with physical activity
• occur high up on the abdomen, radiating throughout the abdomen and lower back

Another sign that labor is beginning is the breaking of the "bag of waters," the amniotic sac which had cushioned the baby during the pregnancy. When it breaks, it releases water in a trickle or a gush. Only about 10% of women actually experience this water flow in the beginning of labor, however. Most of the time, the rupture occurs sometime later in labor. If the amniotic sac doesn't rupture on its own, the doctor will break it during labor.

Some women have **diarrhea** or **nausea** as labor begins. Others notice a sudden surge of energy and the urge to clean or arrange things right before labor begins; this is known as "nesting."

Diagnosis

The onset of labor can be determined by measuring how much the cervix has dilated. The degree of dilation is estimated by feeling the opening cervix during a pelvic exam. Dilation is measured in centimeters, from zero to 10. Contractions that cause the cervix to dilate are the sign of true labor.

Fetal monitoring

Fetal monitoring is a process in which the baby's heart rate is monitored for indicators of **stress** during labor and birth. There are several types of fetal monitoring.

A special stethoscope called a fetoscope may be used. This is a simple and non-invasive method.

The Doppler method uses ultrasound; it involves a handheld listening device that transmits the sounds of the heart rate through a speaker or into an attached ear piece. It can usually pick up the heart sounds 12 weeks after conception. This method offers intermittent monitoring. It allows the mother freedom to move about and is also useful during contractions.

Electronic fetal monitoring uses ultrasound and provides a view of the heartbeat in relationship to the mother's contractions. It can be used either continuously or intermittently. It is often used in high risk pregnancies, and is not often recommended for low risk ones because it renders the mother immobile and requires interpretation.

Internal monitoring does not use ultrasound, is more accurate than electronic monitoring and provides continuous monitoring for the high risk mother. This requires the mother's water to be broken and that she be two to three centimeters dilated. It is used in high-risk situations only.

Telemetry monitoring is the newest type of monitoring. It uses radio waves transmitted from an instrument on the mother's thigh. The mother is able to remain mobile. It provides continuous monitoring and is used in high-risk situations.

Treatment

Most women choose some type of pain relief during childbirth, ranging from relaxation and imagery to drugs. The specific choice may depend on what's available, the woman's preferences, her doctor's recommendations, and how the labor is proceeding. All drugs have some risks and some advantages.

Regional anesthetics

Regional anesthetics include epidurals and spinals. In this technique, medication is injected into the space around the spinal nerves. Depending on the type of medications used, this type of anesthesia can block nerve signals, causing temporary pain relief, or a loss of sensation from the waist down. An epidural or spinal block can provide complete pain relief during cesarean birth.

An epidural is placed with the woman lying on her side or sitting up in bed with the back rounded to allow more space between the vertebrae. Her back is scrubbed with antiseptic, and a local anesthetic is injected in the skin to numb the site. The needle is inserted between two vertebrae and through the tough tissue in front of the spinal column. A catheter is put in place that allows continuous doses of anesthetic to be given.

This type of anesthesia provides complete pain relief, and can help conserve a woman's energy, since she can relax or even sleep during labor. This type of anesthesia requires an IV and fetal monitor. It may be harder for a woman to bear down when it comes time to push, although the amount of anesthesia can be adjusted as this stage nears.

Spinal anesthesia operates on the same principle as epidural anesthesia, and is used primarily in cases of c-section delivery. It is administered in the same way as an epidural, but the catheter is not left in place. The amount of anesthetic injected is large, since it must be injected at one time. Because of the anesthetic's effect on motor nerves, most women using it cannot push during delivery. This is a disadvantage in labor, but not an issue during a c-section. Spinals provide quick and strong anesthesia and allow for major abdominal surgery with almost no pain.

Narcotics

Short-acting **narcotics** can ease pain and do not interfere with a woman's ability to push. However, they can cause **sedation**, **dizziness**, nausea, and **vomiting**. Narcotics cross the placenta and may slow down

KEY TERMS

Amniotic sac—The membranous sac that surrounds the embryo and fills with watery fluid as pregnancy advances.

Breech birth—Birth of a baby bottom-first, instead of the usual head first delivery. This can add to labor and delivery problems because the baby's bottom doesn't mold a passage through the birth canal as well as does the head.

Cervix—A small cylindrical organ about an inch or so long and less than an inch around that makes up the lower part and neck of the uterus. The cervix separates the body and cavity of the uterus from the vagina.

Embryo—The unborn child during the first eight weeks of its development following conception.

Gestation—The period from conception to birth, during which the developing fetus is carried in the uterus.

Perineum—The area between the thighs that lies behind the genital organs and in front of the anus.

Placenta—The organ that develops in the uterus during pregnancy and that links the blood supplies of mother and baby.

a baby's breathing; they can't be given too close to the time of delivery.

Natural childbirth and preparation for childbirth

There are several methods to prepare for childbirth. The one selected often depends on what is available through the healthcare provider. Overall, family involvement is receiving increased attention by the healthcare systems, and many hospitals now offer birthing rooms and maternity centers to help the entire family. There are several choices available for childbirth preparation.

Lamaze, or Lamaze-Pavlov, is the most common in the United States today. It was the first popular natural childbirth method, becoming popular in the 1960s. Breathing exercises and concentration on a focal point are practiced to allow mothers to control pain while maintaining consciousness. This allows the flow of oxygen to the baby and to the muscles in the uterus to be maintained. A partner coaches the mother throughout the birthing process.

The Read method, named for Dick Read, is a technique of breathing that was originated in the 1930s to help mothers deal with apprehension and tension associated with childbirth. This natural childbirth method uses different breathing for the different stages of childbirth.

The LeBoyer method stresses a relaxed delivery in a quiet, dim room. It attempts to avoid overstimulation of the baby and to foster mother-child bonding by placing the baby on the mother's abdomen and having the mother massage him or her immediately after the birth. Then the father washes the baby in a warm bath.

The Bradley method is called father-coached childbirth, because it focuses on the father serving as coach throughout the process. It encourages normal activities during the first stages of labor.

Resources

PERIODICALS

Stevens, Laura Roe. "Gimme a C: Is Choosing a Cesarean Section for a Nonmedical Reason Wise?" *Fit Pregnancy* April–May 2004: 40–42.

ORGANIZATIONS

American Academy of Husband-Coached Childbirth, P.O. Box 5224, Sherman Oaks, CA, 91413, (800) 422-4784, (800) 423-2397.
American Society for Prophylaxis in Obstetrics/LAMAZE (ASPO/LAMAZE), 1840 Wilson Blvd., Ste. 204, Arlington, VA, 22201, (800) 368-4404.
Childbirth Education Foundation, P.O. Box 5, Richboro, PA, 18954, (215) 357-2792.
International Association of Parents and Professionals for Safe Alternatives in Childbirth, Rte. 1, Box 646, Marble Hill, MO, 63764, (314) 238-2010.
International Childbirth Education Association, P.O. Box 20048, Minneapolis, MN, 55420, (612) 854-8660.
Postpartum Support International, 927 North Kellogg Ave., Santa Barbara, CA, 93111, (805) 967-7636.

Carol A. Turkington
Teresa G. Odle

Childhood disintegrative disorder *see*
Pervasive developmental disorders

Childhood obesity

Definition

Childhood **obesity** is an excess percentage of body weight due to fat in children over age two, putting them at risk for a variety of health problems.

Demographics

Childhood obesity is a rapidly growing public health problem in the United States. Although childhood obesity is increasing throughout most of the developed world, the problem is growing fastest in the United States. Over the past two decades the number of obese children has doubled and the number of obese adolescents has tripled. According to the National Health and **Nutrition** Examination Survey of 2003–2006, 31.9% of children and teens were overweight and 16.3% were obese. Thus more than 12 million American children are overweight or obese. Other surveys have found a total obesity rate among children and adolescents of 21–24%. Among American adults 32% are obese and 66% are either overweight or obese.

Significant differences exist in obesity rates among children of different races and ethnic groups, mirroring differences in the adult population. Significantly more Mexican American boys are overweight than non-Hispanic American black or white boys. Significantly more Mexican American girls and non-Hispanic American black girls are overweight compared with non-Hispanic white girls. Native Americans and Hawaiians also have higher rates of obesity than whites.

Description

Obesity in children over age two is assessed by the body mass index (BMI), which uses weight and height to calculate a healthy weight range. For most children and teens the BMI is an accurate indicator of body fat. It is age- and sex-specific and is often referred to as BMI-for-age. Children between the ages of 2 and 19 are assigned to a percentile based on their BMI. The percentile is a comparison of their weights with those of other children of the same age and gender. For example, if a boy is in the 65th percentile for his age group, 65 out of every 100 children his age weigh less than he does and 35 weigh more. Adult BMIs are interpreted differently.

The BMI weight categories for children are:

- underweight: below the 5th percentile
- healthy weight: 5th percentile to below the 85th percentile
- overweight: 85th percentile to below the 95th percentile
- obese: 95th percentile and above. Children in the top 15 percentiles are considered to be at risk for developing health problems because of their weight.

Risk factors

Risk factors for childhood obesity include:

- inherited tendency toward weight gain
- having at least one obese parent
- eating in response to stress, boredom, or loneliness
- poor sleeping habits
- binge-eating disorders
- mental illness

Causes and symptoms

Obesity is caused by taking in more calories than the body uses. This difference is called the "energy gap." A 2006 study done by the Harvard School of Public Health and published in the journal *Pediatrics* found that, on average, American children consume between 110 and 165 more calories than they use every day. Over a 10-year period these extra calories add 10 pounds to their weight. Teens who are already overweight consume an average of 700–1,000 extra calories every day, resulting in a 10-year average of 58 extra pounds.

The causes of this energy gap are related to both increased food intake and decreased energy usage. Causes of increasing food intake include:

- increased consumption of sugary beverages, accompanied by decreased consumption of milk
- more meals eaten away from home
- more super-sized portions, with portions in some fast-food restaurants having almost tripled since the 1970s
- more use of prepared foods in the home
- increased snacking between meals and fewer family meals
- fewer children taking their lunches from home to school
- increasingly poor eating habits such as skipping breakfast and snacking on high-fat, sugary foods
- increased advertising for high-sugar, high-fat foods directed at children

There are various causes of decreased energy output:

- Children spend more time watching television or at computers than in the past.
- School physical-education requirements have decreased. According to the Centers for Disease Control only 8% of elementary schools, 6.4% of middle schools, and 5.8% of high schools require daily physical-education classes.

KEY TERMS

Body mass index (BMI)—A measure of body fat: the ratio of body weight in kilograms to the square of body height in meters.

Cognitive-behavioral therapy (CBT)—A psychotherapeutic approach that emphasizes correcting distorted thinking patterns and changing one's behaviors accordingly.

Hypothyroidism—Deficient thyroid gland activity, resulting in a lowered metabolic rate.

Prader-Willi syndrome—An uncommon genetic disorder that causes a constant feeling of hunger.

Saturated fat—Solid fats such as cheese, meat, butter, ice cream, palm and coconut oils, as well as whole-fat milk and cream; linked to coronary heart disease.

Trans fat—Fat that is produced by hydrogenation during food processing; trans fats increase bad cholesterol and decrease good cholesterol.

• Fewer children walk to school. In 1969 half of all U.S. school children walked or biked to school, including 87% of children living within 1 mile of their school. By 2003 only 15% of children walked or biked to school.

• Elementary schools have eliminated recesses. More than 28% of schools do not provide a regularly scheduled recess for grades 1–5.

• Increasing fear of crime limits children's outdoor activities.

• Growing affluence has increased teenage access to cars over the past 30 years.

In rare cases medical or genetic disorders can cause childhood obesity. For example Prader-Willi syndrome is a genetic disorder that causes an uncontrollable urge to eat. The only way to prevent a child with Prader-Willi disorder from constantly eating is to maintain an environment with no open access to food. Hormonal disorders such as **hypothyroidism** also can cause obesity. Certain medications such as cortisone and **tricyclic antidepressants** may cause weight gain as well. However these are exceptions. Most obese children eat too much and/or **exercise** too little.

The most obvious symptom of obesity is an accumulation of body fat. Other symptoms involve changes in body chemistry. Some of these changes cause disease in children and others put children at risk for developing health problems later in life.

Diagnosis

Examination

A diagnosis of obesity is usually made based on the child's BMI. The examination will include a family history, medical history, and a complete **physical examination**.

Tests

Tests will include standard blood and urine tests. A thyroid hormone test may be performed to rule out hypothyroidism as the cause of the obesity.

Procedures

Based on the physician's findings, other tests and procedures may be performed to rule out medical causes of the obesity.

Treatment

Traditional

Nutrition education usually involves the entire family. Obese children and their parents are typically referred to a registered dietician or nutritionist who can help them develop a plan for eliminating empty calories and increasing the amounts of nutrient-rich, low-calorie foods in their **diets**. A nutritionist or dietitian can help families understand how much and what kinds of food are appropriate for their child's age, weight, and activity level. Children may be asked to keep a food diary to record everything that they eat, in order to determine necessary changes in behavior and diet. Obese children are typically encouraged to increase their level of exercise rather than to drastically reduce their caloric intake.

Children who are overweight often have psychological and social problems that can be helped by **psychotherapy**. Cognitive-behavioral therapy (CBT) is designed to confront and change thoughts and feelings about one's body and behaviors toward food. CBT is relatively short-term and does not address the origins of those thoughts or feelings. CBT may include strategies to maintain self-control with regard to food. **Family therapy** may help children who overeat for emotional reasons related to conflicts within the family. Family therapy teaches strategies for reducing conflict, disorder, and **stress** that may be factors in triggering emotional eating.

Drugs

Weight-loss drugs or surgeries are used very rarely in children—only in the most extreme cases of health-threatening obesity after other methods of weight control have failed. However many overweight children suffer from **anxiety** and depression. Drug therapy to treat these conditions may help children better deal with their obesity and become more involved in physical activities and weight-loss strategies.

Alternative

Obese teenagers may benefit from structured weight-loss programs such as Weight Watchers or Jenny Craig, with the approval of their physician.

Home remedies

Treatment for childhood obesity begins and ends in the home. Families must make a commitment to following healthy nutritional guidelines, eliminating junk food, sugary drinks, and treats from the home, limiting sedentary activities, and increasing exercise.

The American Heart Association adapted the following dietary suggestions for children over age 2 from the federal *Dietary Guidelines for Americans*:

- Children aged 2–3 should obtain no more than 35% of their total calories from fats.
- Children over age 3 should limit their fat intake to about 30% of their total calories. These fats should be monounsaturated or polyunsaturated. Saturated fats and trans fats should be avoided.
- Fruit and vegetable intake should be increased, but fruit juice should be limited.
- At least half of all grains consumed should be whole grains.
- Sugary drinks, such as carbonated soft drinks, should be severely restricted.
- Dairy products should be low-fat or fat-free for children over age 2. Before age 2 children need milk fats for proper growth and development of the nervous system.
- Children should be offered a variety of foods, including fish and shellfish.
- Overfeeding children or making them "clean their plates" should be avoided.

It is often difficult for parents to determine how much food their child should eat at a particular age. However parents tend to overestimate the amount of food that small children require. Active children need more calories and slightly larger amounts of food. The American Heart Association guidelines for daily amounts of some common foods for children of different ages are based on children who are sedentary or physically inactive:

- children aged 2–3 years: total daily calories, 1,000; milk, 2 cups; lean meat or beans, 2 ounces; fruits, 1 cup; vegetables, 1 cup; grains, 3 ounces
- girls aged 4–8 years: total daily calories, 1,200; milk, 2 cups; lean meat or beans, 3 ounces; fruits, 1.5 cups; vegetables, 1 cup; grains, 4 ounces
- boys aged 4–8 years: total daily calories, 1,400; milk, 2 cups; lean meat or beans, 4 ounces; fruits, 1.5 cups; vegetables, 1.5 cups; grains, 5 ounces
- girls aged 9–13 years: total daily calories, 1,600; milk, 3 cups; lean meat or beans, 5 ounces; fruits, 1.5 cups; vegetables, 2 cups; grains, 5 ounces
- boys aged 9–13 years: total daily calories, 1,800; milk, 3 cups; lean meat or beans, 5 ounces; fruits, 1.5 cups; vegetables, 2.5 cups; grains, 6 ounces
- girls aged 14–18 years: total daily calories, 1,800; milk, 3 cups; lean meat or beans, 5 ounces; fruits, 1.5 cups; vegetables, 2.5 cups; grains, 6 ounces
- boys aged 14–18 years: total daily calories, 2,200; milk, 3 cups; lean meat or beans, 6 ounces; fruits, 2 cups; vegetables, 3 cups; grains, 7 ounces

Parents must be very careful in the ways that they approach weight loss with their children. Critical comments about weight from parents or excess zeal in enforcing a rigorous diet can trigger **eating disorders** such as **anorexia nervosa** or **bulimia nervosa** in some children, especially adolescent girls.

Prognosis

The younger that obese children are when they begin treatment, the better the chances that they will be able to maintain a normal weight. Obese children have an advantage over obese adults in that they are continuing to grow. Obese children that can maintain their weight without gaining may grow into a normal weight as they become taller.

Obese children are at increased risk for:

- type 2 diabetes, which was once seen primarily in older adults but is now being diagnosed in children and young adults at an alarmingly high rate
- high blood pressure (hypertension)
- fat accumulation in the liver (fatty liver/liver disease)
- sleep apnea
- early puberty
- eating disorders
- joint pain
- depression
- anxiety and stress
- low self-esteem
- social prejudice and discrimination

Children who remain obese have a much greater likelihood of becoming obese adults with concomitant health problems. Studies have found that 26–41% of obese preschoolers become obese adults. Among obese school-aged children, 42–63% become obese adults. The greater the degree of obesity, the higher the likelihood that it will continue into adulthood.

Prevention

Beginning at age two, children and adolescents should have their BMI calculated at each routine physical examination.

Parents must take the lead in preventing childhood obesity. Teaching children to eat a healthy diet sets the framework for lifetime eating habits. Parents should:

- Serve a healthy variety of foods.
- Keep healthy snacks on hand.
- Use low-fat cooking methods such as broiling or baking.
- Eliminate junk snack food and sugary beverages from the home. This removes temptation and eliminates the need to nag about what not to eat.
- Eat meals together as a family, rather than grabbing food on the run.
- Limit visits to fast-food restaurants.
- Avoid using food as a reward.
- Pack healthy homemade school lunches.
- Encourage school officials to eliminate campus soda machines, bake sales, and fundraisers with candy and cookies.
- Limit television and computer time.
- Plan family activities that involve physical exercise, such as hiking, biking, or swimming.
- Encourage children to become more active in small ways, such as walking to school, biking to friends' houses, or perfoming chores such as walking the dog or mowing the lawn.
- Set realistic goals for weight control and reward children's efforts.
- Model the eating behaviors and active lifestyle that they would like their child to adopt.

Resources

BOOKS

Fletcher, Anne M. *Weight Loss Confidential: How Teens Lose Weight and Keep It Off—And What They Wish Parents Knew.* Boston: Houghton Mifflin Co., 2006.

Hassink, Sandra, ed. *A Parent's Guide to Childhood Obesity: A Road Map to Health.* Elk Grove Village, IL: American Academy of Pediatrics, 2006.

Schumacher, Donald. *Overcoming Obesity in Childhood and Adolescence: A Guide For School Leaders.* Thousand Oaks, CA: Corwin Press, 2007.

World Health Organization. *WHO Child Growth Standards: Length/Height-for-Age, Weight-for-Age, Weight-for-Length, Weight-for-Height and Body Mass Index-for-Age: Methods and Development.* Geneva: World Health Organization, 2006.

PERIODICALS

Ogden, C., et al. "High Body Mass Index for Age Among US Children and Adolescents, 2003–2006." *Journal of the American Medical Association* 299 (2008): 2401–2405.

Rice, J., et al. "Successes and Barriers for a Youth Weight-Management Program." *Clinical Pediatrics* 47, no.2 (March 1, 2008): 143–147.

Terre, L. "Behavioral Medicine Review: Promoting Healthy Lifestyles in Pediatric Populations." *American Journal of Lifestyle Medicine* 2, no.1 (February 1, 2008): 37–39.

Yang, Y. C., et al. "Estimating the Energy Gap Among U.S. Children: A Counterfactual Approach." *Pediatrics* 118, no.6 (December 2006):1721–1733.

OTHER

AHA. "Dietary Guidelines for Healthy Children." *American Heart Association.* http://www.american-heart.org/presenter. jhtml?identifier = 4575

AHA Scientific Statement. "Dietary Recommendations for Children and Adolescents." *Circulation.* http://circ. ahajournals.org/cgi/content/full/112/13/2061

AAP. "Prevention and Treatment of Childhood Overweight and Obesity." *American Academy of Pediatrics.* http://www.aap.org/obesity/index.html

CDC. "About BMI for Children and Teens." *Centers for Disease Control and Prevention.* http://www.cdc.gov/nccdphp/dnpa/bmi/childrens_BMI/about_childrens_BMI.htm

CDC. "BMI Percentile Calculator for Child and Teen." *Centers for Disease Control and Prevention.* http://apps.nccd.cdc.gov/dnpabmi/Calculator.aspx

U.S. Department of Health & Human Services and Department of Agriculture. "Dietary Guidelines for Americans." *U.S. Department of Health & Human Services.* http://www.health.gov/dietaryguidelines/

ORGANIZATIONS

American Academy of Pediatrics, 141 Northwest Point Blvd., Elk Grove Village, IL, 60007-1098, (874) 434-4000, (874) 434-8000, kidsdocs@aap.org, http://www. aap.org.

American Heart Association, 7272 Greenville Avenue, Dallas, TX, 75231, (800) 242-8721, http://www. americanheart.org.

Centers for Disease Control and Prevention, 1600 Clifton Road, Atlanta, GA, 30333, (888) 232-6348, (301) 563-6595, cdcinfor@cdc.gov, http://www.cdc.gov.

The Obesity Society, 8630 Fenton St., Suite 814, Silver Spring, MD, 20910, (301) 563-6526, (301) 563-6595, http://www.obesity.org.

Weight-Control Information Network (WIN), 1 WIN Way, Bethesda, MD, 20892-3665, (888) 232-6348, (202) 828-1028, win@info.niddk.nih.gov, http://win.niddk.nih.gov.

Tish Davidson, AM
Margaret Alic, PhD

Children's health

Definition

Children's health encompasses the physical, mental, emotional, and social well-being of children from infancy through adolescence.

Description

All children should have regular well-child check-ups according to the schedule recommended by their physician or pediatrician. The American Academy of Pediatrics (AAP) advises that children be seen for well-baby checks at two weeks, two months, four months, six months, nine months, twelve months, fifteen months, and eighteen months. Well-child visits are recommended at ages two, three, four, five, six, eight, 10, and annually thereafter through age 21. Well-baby and well-child check-ups assess the child physically, behaviorally, developmentally, and

emotionally and are important in spotting developmental delays or behavioral abnormalities early. Well-child check-ups usually include reviewing medical history, measuring height, weight, blood pressure, and temperature, vision, hearing, reflex screening, a developmental/behavioral assessment, **physical examination**, immunizations, guidance about developmental milestones, **nutrition**, injury prevention, and referrals as needed to a pediatric dentist or other pediatric specialists. In 2004, it was estimated from interviews with parents that 87% of children in the United States with health insurance had seen a physician for a well-child check up within the past year, while only 66% of children without health insurance had been seen.

Immunization to protect against specific diseases is an important part of a child's healthcare program. Vaccines must be administered within certain time limits. When multiple doses are needed, a certain amount of time must elapse between each dose. As of 2009, the American Association of Pediatrics (AAP) and the Centers for Disease Control and Prevention (CDC) recommended these childhood immunizations:

- Hepatitis B vaccine. Three doses, beginning at birth and completed no later than 18 months with at least four weeks between doses.

- Rotavirus vaccine. Two or three doses depending on vaccine with the first dose given beginning no earlier than 6 weeks and no later than 14 weeks and the final dose completed no later than eight months.

- Diphtheria, Tetanus, and Pertussis (DTaP) vaccine. Doses at two and six months with a final dose between four and six years of age. A booster is given at 11–12 years of age.

- *Haemophilus influenzae* type b (Hib) vaccine. Three doses beginning no earlier than two months with a booster at 12–15 months.

- Pneumococcal conjugate vaccine. Doses at 2, 4, 6, and 12–15 months. High risk children may require additional doses of related vaccine.

- Inactivated Polio vaccine. Doses at 2, 4, 6–18 months and 4–6 years.

- Influenza vaccine. Two doses every year for children under age nine. Single dose every year through adulthood.

- Measles, Mumps, Rubella (MMR) vaccine. Two doses, the first no earlier than one year, the second between ages four and six years.

- Varicella (chickenpox) vaccine. Two doses, the first no earlier than one year, the second usually between ages four and six years.

Common childhood infections

Infection	Symptom(s)
Common cold	Runny nose, sneezing, cough, congestion
Conjunctivitis (pink eye)	Redness of the eye, pus-like discharge
Head lice	Intense itching, possible swelling of neck glands
Influenza	Fever, cough, chills, headache, fatigue, general discomfort
Mononucleosis	Weakness, fatigue, sore throat, fever, swollen lymph nodes
Otitis media (middle ear infection)	Fever, ear pulling, complaints of ear pain or fullness
Strep throat	Sore throat, fever, fatigue, swollen tonsils
Varicella (chickenpox)	Itchy, red, blistery rash; fever

(Table by PreMediaGlobal. Reproduced by permission of Gale, a part of Cengage Learning.)

- Hepatitis A vaccine. Two doses, the first no earlier than one year, the second six months later. High risk children may require additional doses during adolescence.
- Meningococcal vaccine. One dose between the ages of 11 and 18 years. High risk children only may require dose between the ages of two and 10 years.
- Human papillomavirus (HPV) vaccine. Girls only, three doses beginning at age 11. Older unvaccinated females may be vaccinated up to age 26.

Mental health

Children who have difficulty in areas of language acquisition, cognitive (mental) development, and behavior control may have a mental health disorder. Mental health problems that arise in children include:

- Attention deficit hyperactivity disorder (ADHD). ADHD is estimated to affect 3–7% of school-age children in the United States and is 3–5 times more common in boys than in girls. It is a disorder characterized by excessive motor activity, distractibility, and poor impulse control.
- Learning disorders. Learning disabilities affect one in 10 school children in the United States.
- Depression, anxiety, and bipolar disorder. Affective, or mood, disorders are now more commonly recognized in children than in the past.
- Eating disorders. Anorexia nervosa, bulimia nervosa, and binge eating disorder frequently occur in adolescent girls. It is estimated that one out of every 100–200 adolescent girls meets all the diagnostic criteria for anorexia.
- Schizophrenia. A disorder characterized by bizarre thoughts and behaviors, paranoia, impaired sense of reality, and psychosis may be diagnosed in childhood or adolescence.
- Obsessive-compulsive disorder (OCD). Symptoms often begin in childhood or adolescence.
- Autism and pervasive developmental disorder. Severe developmental disabilities that cause a child to become withdrawn and unresponsive.
- Mental retardation. Children under age 18 with an IQ of 70 or below and impairments in adaptive functioning are considered mentally retarded.

Emotional and social health

Children take their first significant steps toward socialization and peer interaction when they begin to engage in cooperative play at around age four. Their social development progresses throughout childhood and adolescence as they expand their social contacts, develop friendships, start to be influenced by their peers, and begin to show interest in the opposite sex. In adolescence, there is a strong, but normal, trend away from involvement with family and toward establishing their own identity and values.

Several factors may have a negative impact on the emotional and social well-being of children:

- Violence. Bullying can cause serious damage to a child's sense of self-esteem and personal safety, as can experiences with community violence.
- Family turmoil. Divorce, domestic abuse, death of a family member, and other life-changing events that alter the family dynamic can have a serious impact on a child. Even a positive event such as the birth of a sibling or a move to a new city and school can put emotional strain on a child.
- Stress. The pressure to perform well academically and in extracurricular activities such as sports can be overwhelming to some children. Emphasis on physical appearance also creates stress that can lead to eating disorders.
- Peer pressure. Although it can have a positive impact, peer pressure is often a source of significant stress for children. This is particularly true in adolescence when "fitting in" is important to most teens.
- Drugs and alcohol. Curiosity is intrinsic to childhood, and more than 30% of children have experimented with alcohol by age 13. Open communication with children that sets forth parental expectations about drug and alcohol use is essential.
- Negative sexual experiences. Sexual abuse and assault can emotionally scar a child and instill negative feelings about sexuality and relationships. Early and/or indiscriminate sexual relationships can cause emotional harm and increase the likelihood of pregnancy and sexually transmitted diseases.

Causes and symptoms

Childhood health problems may be congenital (i.e., present at birth) or acquired through infection, immune system deficiency, or another disease process. They may also be caused by physical trauma (e.g., a car accident or a playground fall), exposure to a toxic substance (e.g., drug allergy, or exposure to poisonous chemical), or triggered by a genetic factor (e.g., **celiac disease**, sickle cell anemia) or environmental factors (e.g., dust mite **allergies**, pollen allergies).

Physical and mental health problems in childhood can cause a wide spectrum of symptoms. The following behaviors suggest a larger emotional, social, or mental disturbance that may need to be evaluated by a health care professional.

- signs of alcohol and drug use
- suddenly falling grades or school avoidance
- lack of interest in activities that were previously enjoyable
- excessive anxiety
- persistent, prolonged depression
- withdrawal from friends and family
- involvement with violence or vandalism
- extreme or irrational perfectionism
- repeated, aggressive confrontations with authority figures
- age-inappropriate temper tantrums or inappropriate displays of anger
- self-inflicted injury
- bizarre behavior and/or speech
- trouble with the police
- sexual promiscuity
- prolonged, unexplained fatigue
- suicide threats or attempts

The causes of developmental disorders and delays and learning disabilities are not always fully understood. Pervasive developmental disorder (PDD) and autistic spectrum disorder (more commonly known as **autism**) are characterized by unresponsiveness and severe impairments in one or more of these areas:

- Social interaction. Autistic children often have difficulty interpreting social cues and are unaware of acceptable social behavior. They tend to be withdrawn and socially isolated. They frequently reject physical contact.
- Communication and language. A child with autism or PDD may not speak or may display limited or immature language skills.
- Behavior. Autistic or PDD children may have difficulty dealing with anger, can be self-injurious, and may display obsessive behavior.

Autism is associated with brain abnormalities, but the exact mechanisms that trigger the disorder are yet to be determined. Research suggests that it may be linked to certain congenital conditions such as **neurofibromatosis**, **fragile X syndrome**, and **phenylketonuria** (PKU). Despite much speculation, no well-designed, controlled studies have shown any link between autism and childhood vaccinations.

Diagnosis

Physical, intellectual, emotional, and social maturation are all-important markers of a child's overall health and well being. When evaluating children, pediatricians and child-care specialists assess related skill sets,

KEY TERMS

Bipolar disorder—Formerly called manic-depressive disorder. A mood disorder characterized by alternating periods of overconfidence and activity (manic highs) and depressive lows.

Child development—The process of physical, intellectual, emotional, and social growth that occurs from infancy through adolescence. Erik Erikson, Margaret Mahler, Sigmund Freud, and Jean Piaget are among the most well-known child development theorists.

Immunization—Administering a vaccine that stimulates the body to create antibodies to a specific disease (immunity) without causing symptoms of the disease.

Learning disabilities—An impairment of the cognitive processes of understanding and using spoken and written language that results in difficulties with one or more academic skill sets (e.g., reading, writing, mathematics).

Motor skills—Controlled movement of muscle groups. Fine motor skills involve tasks that require dexterity of small muscles, such as buttoning a shirt. Tasks such as walking or throwing a ball involve the use of gross motor skills.

Obsessive-compulsive disorder (OCD)—An anxiety disorder in which a person cannot prevent himself from dwelling on unwanted thoughts, acting on urges, or performing repetitious rituals, such as washing his hands or checking to make sure he turned off the lights.

Psychological tests—Written, verbal, or visual tasks that assess psychological functioning, intelligence, and/or personality traits.

Type 1 diabetes—A chronic immune system disorder in which the pancreas does not produce sufficient amounts of insulin, a hormone that enables cells to use glucose for energy. Also called juvenile diabetes, it must be treated with insulin injections.

such as a child's acquisition and use of language, fine and gross motor skills, cognitive growth, socialization, and achievement of certain milestones in these areas. A developmental milestone is a task or skill set that a child is expected to reach at a certain age or stage of life. For example, by age one, most children have achieved the physical milestone of walking with the assistance of an adult. Developmental disorders may be identified and/

DR. BENJAMIN SPOCK (1903–1998)

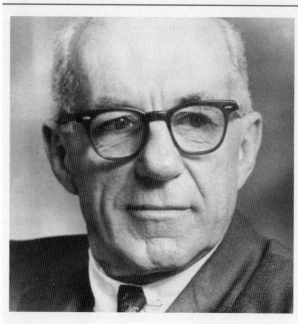

(The Library of Congress.)

Benjamin Spock, pediatrician and political activist, was most noted for his authorship of *Baby and Child Care*, which significantly changed predominant attitudes toward the raising of infants and children. He began medical school at Yale University in 1925, and transferred to Columbia University's College of Physicians and Surgeons in 1927. Spock had decided well before starting his medical studies that he would "work with children, who have their whole lives ahead of them" and so, upon taking his M.D. degree in 1929 and serving his general internship at the prestigious Presbyterian Hospital, he specialized in pediatrics at a small hospital crowded with children in New York's Hell's Kitchen area.

On a summer vacation in 1943 he began to write his most famous book and he continued to work on it from 1944 to 1946 while serving as a medical officer in the Navy. The book sharply broke with the authoritarian tone and rigorous instructions found in earlier generations of baby-care books, most of which said to feed infants on a strict schedule and not to pick them up when they cried. Spock, who spent ten years trying to reconcile his psychoanalytic training with what mothers were telling him about their children, told his readers, "You know more than you think you do.... Don't be afraid to trust your own common sense.... Take it easy, trust your own instincts, and follow the directions that your doctor gives you." The response was overwhelming. *Baby and Child Care* rapidly became America's all-time best-seller except for Shakespeare and the Bible; by 1976 it had also eclipsed Shakespeare.

Spock prided himself in keeping up with the times, a fact that's reflected in the many revisions of *Baby and Child Care* in which he incorporated the latest medical developments and dealt with emerging social issues such as working mothers, daycare centers, and single parenthood.

or diagnosed by physicians, teachers, child psychologists, therapists, counselors, and other professionals who interact with children on a regular basis.

It is important to remember that all children are unique, and develop at different paces within this broad framework. Reaching a milestone early or late does not necessarily indicate a developmental problem. However, if a child is consistently lagging in achieving milestones or has a significant deficit in one developmental area, he or she may be experiencing developmental delays that warrant professional evaluation.

Pediatricians and other medical professionals typically diagnose physical illness and disease in children as well as provide preventative health care. In cases of illness and injury, children will undergo a thorough physical examination and patient history. Diagnostic tests may be performed as appropriate. In cases of mental or emotional disorders, a psychologist or psychiatrist will meet with the patient to conduct an interview and take a detailed social and medical history.

Interviews with a parent or guardian and teacher may also be part of the diagnostic process. The physician may also administer one or more **psychological tests** (also called clinical inventories, scales, or assessments).

Treatment

Medications may be prescribed to treat certain childhood illnesses. Proper dosage is particularly important with infants and children, as medications such as **acetaminophen** can be toxic in excessive amounts. Parents and caregivers should always follow the instructions for use that accompany medications, and inform the child's pediatrician if the child is taking any other drugs or **vitamins** to prevent potentially negative **drug interactions**. Any side effects or adverse reactions to medication should be reported to the child's physician. If **antibiotics** are prescribed, the full course should always be taken. Parents should be especially careful when using herbal medicine or dietary supplements, as the pediatric doses for these treatments often have not been established.

Other treatments for childhood illness and/or injuries include, but are not limited to, nutritional therapy, **physical therapy**, respiratory therapy, medical devices (e.g., **hearing aids**, glasses, braces), and in some cases, surgery.

Counseling is typically a first treatment for psychological disorders. Therapy approaches include **psychotherapy**, cognitive therapy, behavioral therapy, family counseling, and **group therapy**. Therapy or counseling may be administered by social workers, nurses, licensed counselors and therapists, psychologists, or psychiatrists. Psychoactive medication may be prescribed by a psychiatrist for symptom relief in children and adolescents with mental disorders.

Support groups may provide emotional support for children with chronic illnesses or mental disorders. This approach, which allows individuals to seek advice and counsel from others in similar circumstances, can be extremely effective, especially in older children who look toward their peers for guidance and support. Support groups for family members often help adults and siblings cope with a chronically ill child.

Speech therapy may help children with developmental delays in language acquisition. Children with **learning disorders** can benefit from special education classes and accommodations arrived at through professional evaluation and the creation of an individualized educational plan (IEP).

Alternative

Therapeutic approaches that encourage self-discovery and empowerment may be useful in treating some childhood emotional traumas and mental disorders. **Art therapy**, the use of the creative process to express and understand emotion, encompasses a broad range of humanistic disciplines, including visual arts, dance, drama, music, film, writing, literature, and other artistic genres. It can be particularly effective in children who may have difficulty gaining insight to emotions and thoughts they are otherwise incapable of expressing.

Certain mild herbal remedies may also be safely used with children, such as ginger (*Zingiber officinale*) tea for **nausea** and aloe vera salve for **burns**. Parents and caregivers should always consult their healthcare provider before administering herbs to children, as certain herbs may affect children differently than adults.

Prognosis

The prognosis for childhood health problems varies widely. In general, early detection and proper treatment can greatly improve the odds of recovery from many childhood illnesses and disabilities. Early intervention is key in helping a child with disabilities reach his or her full potential.

Some learning disabilities and mild developmental disorders can be overcome or greatly improved through appropriate therapies. As of 2009, there were no known medical treatments or pharmacological therapies that eliminate all of the symptoms associated with pervasive developmental disorder (PDD), autism spectrum disorder, and **mental retardation**. Mental illnesses such as **schizophrenia** and **bipolar disorder** are chronic, lifelong disorders, although their symptoms can often be controlled with medication.

Prevention

Parents can take precautions to ensure the safety of their children. Childproofing the home, following a recommended immunization schedule, educating children on safety, learning **first aid**, and taking children for regular well-child check-ups can help to protect against physical harm. In addition, encouraging open communication with children can help them grow both emotionally and socially. Providing a loving and supportive home environment can help to nurture an emotionally healthy child who is independent, self-confident, socially skilled, insightful, and empathetic toward others.

Because they are still developing motor skills, children may be particularly accident prone. Observing the following safety guidelines may help protect children from injury:

- Helmets and padding. Children should always wear a properly fitted helmet and appropriate protective gear when riding a bike, scooter, or similar equipment or participating in sports. They should ride on designated bike paths whenever possible, and learn bicycle safety rules (i.e., ride with traffic, use hand signals).

- Playground safety. Swing sets and other outdoor play equipment should be well-maintained, have at least 12 in (30 cm) of loose fill materials (e.g., sand, wood chips) underneath to cushion falls, and children should be properly supervised at play.

- Staying apprised of recalls. Children's toys, play equipment, and care products are frequently involved in product recalls. The U.S. Consumer Safety Products

Commission (CSPC) is the agency responsible for tracking these recalls.

- Staying safe in the car. Up to 85% of children's car seats are improperly installed and/or used. Infants should always be in a rear-facing car seat until they are over 12 months of age and weigh more than 20 lb (9 kg). An infant or car seat should never be put in a front passenger seat that has an air bag. Once they outgrow their forward facing car seats, children between the ages of four and eight who weigh between 40–80 lb (18–36 kg) should ride in a booster seat. Every child who rides in a car over this age and weight should use a properly fitted lap and shoulder belt.

- Teaching children pedestrian safety. Young children should never be allowed to cross the street by themselves. Older children should know to follow traffic signs and signals, cross the street at the corner, and look both ways before stepping off the curb.

- Teaching children about personal safety. Children should know what to do in case they get lost or are approached by a stranger. It is also imperative that parents talk openly with their children about their body and sexuality, and what behavior is inappropriate, to protect them against sexual predators.

Childproofing the household is an important step toward keeping children healthy. To make a house a safe home, parents and caregivers should:

- Keep guns away from children. Accidental shootings in the home injure an estimated 1,500 children under age 14 each year. If a gun must be in the home, it should be securely locked in a tamper proof gun safe with the ammunition kept locked in a separate place.

- Keep matches, lighters, and flammable materials properly stored and out of the reach of children.

- Make sure hot water heaters are set to 120°F (49°C) or below to prevent scalding injuries.

- Equip the home with working fire extinguishers and smoke alarms; teach children what to do in case of fire.

- Secure all medications (including vitamins, herbs, and supplements), hazardous chemicals, and poisonous substances (including alcohol and tobacco) in ways that they cannot be accessed by children.

- Do not smoke. Aside from causing cancer and other health problems in smokers, second-hand smoke is hazardous to a child's health (e.g., increases their risk of developing allergies).

- Keep small children away from poisonous plants outdoors; remove any indoor plants that are toxic.

- Post the phone numbers of poison control and the pediatrician near the phone; teach children how to dial 9-1-1 and report an emergency.

- Children under age five should never be left alone in the bathtub, wading pool, or near any standing water source (including an open toilet). Fence all swimming pools and install a self-latching gate. Drowning is the leading cause of death by injury for children between the ages of one and four in the United States.

- Remove lead paint. Lead is a serious health hazard for children and can cause cognitive retardation. Houses built before 1978 should be tested for lead paint. If lead is found, the paint should be removed using the appropriate safety precautions.

- Be alert to coins, small play pieces, and similar items that are choking hazards for small children.

Resources

BOOKS

Brynie, Faith Hickman. *ADHD: Attention-Deficit Hyperactivity Disorder*. Minneapolis: Twenty-First Century Books, 2008.

Dietary Guidelines for Americans 2005. Washington, DC: U.S. Department of Health and Human Services, U.S. Department of Agriculture, 2005.

Larson Duyff, R. *ADA Complete Food and Nutrition Guide*. 3rd ed. Chicago: American Dietetic Association, 2006.

Robertson, Cathie. *Safety, Nutrition and Health in Early Education*. 4th ed. Florence, KY: Wadsworth Publishing, 2009.

Weight Watchers. *Weight Watchers Eat! Move! Play!: A Parent's Guide for Raising Healthy, Happy Kids*. Hoboken, NJ: Wiley, 2010.

ORGANIZATIONS

American Academy of Child and Adolescent Psychiatry, 3615 Wisconsin Avenue, NW, Washington, DC, 20016-3007, (202) 966-7300, (202) 966-2891, http://www.aacap.org.

American Academy of Family Physicians, P.O. Box 11210, Shawnee Mission, KS, 66207, (913) 906-6000, (800) 274-2237, (913) 906-6075, http://www.aafp.org.

American Academy of Pediatrics, 141 Northwest Point Boulevard, Elk Grove Village, IL, 60007-1098, (847) 434-4000, http://www.aap.org.

American Dietetic Association, 120 South Riverside Plaza, Suite 2000, Chicago, IL, 60605, (800) 877-1600, http://www.eatright.org.

National Eating Disorders Association, 603 Stewart St., No. 803, Seattle, WA, 98101, (206) 382-3587, http://www.nationaleatingdisorders.org.

National Institute of Child Health and Human Development (NICHD) , P.O. Box 3006, Rockville, MD, 30847, (800) 370-2943, TTY: (800) 320-6942, (866)

760-5947, NICHDInformationResourceCenter@
mail.nih.gov, http://www.nichd.nih.gov.
Project EAT, Eating Among Teens, University of Minnesota, 1300 S. Second St., Suite 300, Minneapolis, MN,
55454, (612) 624-1818, http://www.epi.umn.edu/
research/eat/index.shtm.

Tish Davidson, AM
Paula Anne Ford-Martin
Teresa G. Odle
Laura Jean Cataldo, RN, EdD

Chinese traditional herbal medicine *see*
Traditional Chinese herbalism

Chinese traditional medicine *see* **Traditional
Chinese medicine**

Chiropractic

Definition

Chiropractic is from Greek words meaning done
by hand. It is grounded in the principle that the body
can heal itself when the skeletal system is correctly
aligned and the nervous system is functioning properly. To achieve this, the practitioner uses his or her
hands or an adjusting tool to perform specific manipulations of the vertebrae. When these bones of the
spine are not correctly articulated, resulting in a condition known as subluxation, the theory is that nerve
transmission is disrupted and causes **pain** in the back,
as well as other areas of the body.

Chiropractic is one of the most popular alternative therapies currently available. Some would say it
now qualifies as mainstream treatment as opposed to
complementary medicine. Chiropractic treatment is
covered by many insurance plans and in 2004, the
U.S. Department of Veterans Affairs announced full
inclusion of chiropractic care for veterans. It has
become well-accepted treatment for acute pain and
problems of the spine, including lower back pain and
whiplash. Applications beyond that scope are not supported by current evidence, although there are ongoing
studies into the usefulness of chiropractic for such problems as ear infections, **dysmenorrhea**, infant **colic**,
migraine headaches, and other conditions.

Purpose

Most people will experience back pain at some time
in their lives. Injuries due to overexertion and poor
posture are among the most common. Depending
on the cause and severity of the condition, options

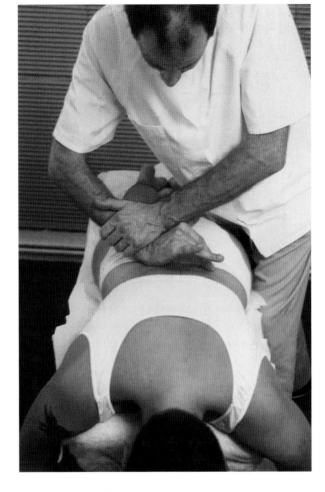

An example of a McTimoney chiropractic technique on
patient's lumbar vertebra. The McTimoney chiropractic is a
system of adjustment by hand of displacements of the spinal
column and bones. It can also be applied to animals. *(Custom
Medical Stock Photo, Inc. Reproduced by permission.)*

for treatment may include **physical therapy**, rest, medications, surgery, or chiropractic care. Chiropractic
treatment carries none of the risks of surgical or
pharmacologic treatment. Practitioners use a holistic
approach to health. The goal is not merely to relieve
the present ailment, but to analyze the cause and recommend appropriate changes of lifestyle to prevent the
problem from occurring again. They believe in a risk/
benefit analysis before use of any intervention. The
odds of an adverse outcome are extremely low. Chiropractic has proven in several studies to be less expensive
than many more traditional routes such as outpatient
physical therapy. Relief from some neuromuscular
problems is immediate, although a series of treatments
is likely to be required to maintain the improvement.
Spinal manipulation is an excellent option for acute
lower back pain, and may also relieve neck pain as

well as other musculoskeletal pain. Although most back pain will subside eventually with no treatment at all, chiropractic treatment can significantly shorten the time it takes to get relief. Some types of **headache** can also be successfully treated by chiropractic.

Description

Origins

Spinal manipulation has a long history in many cultures but Daniel D. Palmer is the founder of modern chiropractic theory, dating back to the 1890s. A grocer and magnetic healer, he applied his knowledge of the nervous system and manual therapies in an unusual situation. One renowned story concerns Harvey Lillard, a janitor in the office where Palmer worked. The man had been deaf for 17 years, ever since he had sustained an injury to his upper spine. Palmer performed an adjustment on a painful vertebra in the region of the injury and Lillard's hearing was reputedly restored. Palmer theorized that all communication from the brain to the rest of the body passes through the spinal canal, and areas that are poorly aligned or under **stress** can cause physical symptoms both in the spine and in other areas of the body. Thus the body has the innate intelligence to heal itself when unencumbered by spinal irregularities causing nerve interference. After his success with Lillard, other patients began coming to him for care, and responded well to adjustments. This resulted in Palmer's further study of the relationship between an optimally functional spine and normal health.

Palmer founded the first chiropractic college in 1897. His son, B. J. Palmer, continued to develop chiropractic philosophy and practice after his father's **death**. B. J. and other faculty members were divided over the role of subluxation in disease. B. J. saw it as the cause of all disease. The others disagreed and sought a more rational way of thinking, thus broadening the base of chiropractic education. From 1910 to 1920, many other chiropractic colleges were established. Other innovators, including John Howard, Carl Cleveland, Earl Homewood, Joseph Janse, Herbert Lee, and Claude Watkins, also helped to advance the profession.

The theories of the Palmers receive somewhat broader interpretation today. Many chiropractors believe that back pain can be relieved and health restored through chiropractic treatment even in patients who do not have demonstrable **subluxations**. Scientific development and research of chiropractic is gaining momentum. The twenty-first century will likely see the metaphysical concepts such as innate intelligence give way to more scientific proofs and reform.

Many people besides the Palmers have contributed to the development of chiropractic theory and technique. Some have gone on to create a variety of procedures and related types of therapy that have their roots in chiropractic, including McTimoney-Corley chiropractic, craniosacral manipulation, naprapathy, and **applied kinesiology**. **Osteopathy** is another related holistic discipline that utilizes spinal and musculoskeletal manipulation as a part of treatment, but osteopathic training is more similar in scope to that of an M.D.

Initial visit

An initial chiropractic exam will most often include a history and a physical. The patient should be asked about the current complaint, whether there are chronic health problems, family history of disease, dietary habits, medical care received, and any medications currently being taken. Further, the current complaint should be described in terms of how long it has been a problem, how it has progressed, and whether it is the result of an injury or occurred spontaneously. Details of how an injury occurred should be given. The physical exam should evaluate by observation and palpation whether the painful area has evidence of inflammation or poor alignment. Range of motion may also be assessed. In the spine, either hypomobility (fixation) or hypermobility may be a problem. Laboratory analysis is helpful in some cases to rule out serious infection or other health issues that may require referral for another type of treatment. Many practitioners also insist on x rays during the initial evaluation

Manipulation

When spinal manipulation is employed, it is generally done with the hands, although some practitioners may use an adjusting tool. A classic adjustment involves a high velocity, low amplitude thrust that produces a usually painless popping noise, and improves the range of motion of the joint that was treated. The patient may lie on a specially designed, padded table that helps the practitioner to achieve the proper positions for treatment. Some adjustments involve manipulating the entire spine, or large portions of it, as a unit; others are small movements designed to affect a single joint. Stretching, **traction**, and slow manipulation are other techniques that can be employed to restore structural integrity and relieve nerve interference.

A new use of technology with traditional chiropractic care has been introduced. Using a hand-held device that is pressed to the spine or joints, a chiropractor may soon be able to detect and manipulate the skeleton not only with his or her hands but with the computer-linked device that uses harmonic frequencies to detect a misalignment in the spine. The new technology was not widely accepted in 2004, however.

Length of treatment

The number of chiropractic treatments required will vary depending on several factors. Generally longer-term treatment is needed for conditions that are chronic, severe, or occur in conjunction with another health problem. Patients who are not in overall good health may also have longer healing times. Some injuries will inherently require more treatments than others in order to get relief. Care is given in three stages. Initially appointments are more frequent with the goal of relieving immediate pain. Next, the patient moves into a rehabilitative stage to continue the healing process and help to prevent a relapse. Finally, the patient may elect periodic maintenance, or wellness treatments, along with lifestyle changes if needed to stay in good health.

Follow-up care

Discharge and follow-up therapy are important. If an injury occurred as a result of poor fitness or health, a program of **exercise** or **nutrition** should be prescribed. Home therapy may also be recommended, involving such things as anti-inflammatory medication and applications of heat or ice packs. Conscious attention to posture may help some patients avoid sustaining a similar injury in the future, and the chiropractor should be able to discern what poor postural habits require correction. A sedentary lifestyle, particularly with a lot of time spent sitting, is likely to contribute to poor posture and may predispose a person to back pain and injury.

Types of practitioners

Some practitioners use spinal manipulation to the exclusion of all other modalities, and are known as straight chiropractors. Others integrate various types of therapy such as massage, nutritional intervention, or treatment with **vitamins**, herbs, or homeopathic remedies. They also embrace ideas from other health care traditions. This group is known as mixers. The vast majority of chiropractors, perhaps 85%, fall in this latter category.

DANIEL PALMER (1845–1913)

Chiropractic inventor, Daniel David Palmer, was born on March 7, 1845, in Toronto, Ontario. He was one of five siblings, the children of a shoemaker and his wife, Thomas and Katherine Palmer. Daniel Palmer and his older brother fell victim to wanderlust and left Canada with a tiny cash reserve in April 1865. They immigrated to the United States on foot, walking for 30 days before arriving in Buffalo, New York. They traveled by boat through the St. Lawrence Seaway to Detroit, Michigan. There they survived by working odd jobs and sleeping on the dock. Daniel Palmer settled in What Cheer, Iowa, where he supported himself and his first wife as a grocer and fish peddler in the early 1880s. He later moved to Davenport, Iowa, where he raised three daughters and one son.

Palmer was a man of high curiosity. He investigated a variety of disciplines of medical science during his lifetime, many of which were in their infancy. He was intrigued by phrenology and assorted spiritual cults, and for nine years he investigated the relationship between magnetism and disease. Palmer felt that there was one thing that caused disease. He was intent upon discovering this one thing, or as he called it: the great secret.

In September 1895, Palmer purported to have cured a deaf man by placing pressure on the man's displaced vertebra. Shortly afterward Palmer claimed to cure another patient of heart trouble, again by adjusting a displaced vertebra. The double coincidence led Palmer to theorize that human disease might be the result of dislocated or luxated bones, as Palmer called them. That same year he established the Palmer School of Chiropractic where he taught a three-month course in the simple fundamentals of medicine and spinal adjustment.

Palmer, who was married six times during his life, died in California in 1913; he was destitute. His son, Bartlett Joshua Palmer, successfully commercialized the practice of chiropractic.

Preparations

Patients should enter the chiropractic clinic with an open mind. This will help to achieve maximum results.

Precautions

Chiropractic is not an appropriate therapy for diseases that are severely degenerative and may require medication or surgery. Many conditions of the spine are amenable to manipulative treatment, but this does not include **fractures**. The practitioner should be informed in advance if the patient is on anticoagulants, or has **osteoporosis** or any other condition that may weaken the bones. Other circumstances might suggest the patient should not have chiropractic care. These should be detected in the history or physical exam. In addition to fractures, **Down syndrome**, some congenital defects, and some types of **cancer** are a few of the things that may preclude spinal manipulation. On rare occasions, a fracture or dislocation may occur. There is also a very slim possibility of experiencing a **stroke** as a result of spinal manipulation, but estimates are that it is no more frequent than 2.5 occurrences per one million treatments.

Patients should be wary of chiropractors who insist on costly x rays and repeated visits with no end in sight. Extensive use is not scientifically justifiable, especially in most cases of lower back pain. There are some circumstances when x rays are indicated, including acute or possibly severe injuries such as those that might result from a car accident.

Side effects

It is not uncommon to have local discomfort in the form of aches, pains, or spasms for a few days following a chiropractic treatment. Some patients may also experience mild headache or **fatigue** that resolves quickly.

Research and general acceptance

As recently as the 1970s, the American Medical Association (a national group of medical doctors) was quite hostile to chiropractic. AMA members were advised that it was unethical to be associated with chiropractors. Fortunately that has changed, and many allopathic or traditionally trained physicians enjoy cordial referral relationships with chiropractors. The public is strongly in favor of chiropractic treatment. Chiropractors see the lion's share of all patients who seek medical help for back problems, and chiropractic treatment is the most widely used of all alternative medical treatments.

Research has also supported the use of spinal manipulation for acute **low back pain**. There is some anecdotal evidence recommending chiropractic treatment for ailments unrelated to musculoskeletal problems, but there is not enough research-based data to support this. On the other hand, a chiropractor may be able to treat problems and diseases unrelated to the skeletal structure by employing therapies other than spinal manipulation.

Although many chiropractors limit their practice to spine and joint problems, others claim to treat disorders that are not closely related to the back or

---

KEY TERMS

Adjustment—A specific type of manipulation of the spine designed to return it to proper structural and functional form.

Allopathic—Conventional practice of medicine generally associated with M.D. physicians.

Dysmenorrhea—Painful menstruation.

Osteoporosis—A condition of decreased bone density, causing increased bone fragility, that is most common in elderly women.

Subluxation—Misalignment between vertebrae that structurally and functionally impairs nerve function.

---

musculoskeletal system. These include **asthma**, bed-wetting, **bronchitis**, coughs, **dizziness**, dysmenorrhea, earache, **fainting**, headache, hyperactivity, **indigestion**, **infertility**, migraine, **pneumonia**, and issues related to **pregnancy**. There are at least three explanations for the possible effectiveness for these conditions. One is that the problem could be linked to a nerve impingement, as may be possible with bed-wetting, dizziness, fainting, and headache. In a second group, chiropractic treatment may offer some relief from complicating pain and spasms caused by the disease process, as with asthma, bronchitis, coughs, and pneumonia. The discomforts of pregnancy may also be relieved with gentle chiropractic therapy. A third possibility is that manipulation or use of soft-tissue techniques may directly promote improvement of some conditions. One particular procedure, known as the endonasal technique, is thought to help the eustachian tube to open and thus improve drainage of the middle ear. The tube is sometimes blocked off due to exudates or inflammatory processes. This can offer significant relief from earaches. Some headaches also fall in this category, as skilled use of soft tissue techniques and adjustment may relieve the muscle tension that may initiate some headaches.

Dysmenorrhea, hyperactivity, indigestion, and infertility are said to be relieved as a result of improved flow of blood and nerve energy following treatment. Evidence for this is anecdotal at best, but manipulation is unlikely to be harmful if causes treatable by other modalities have been ruled out.

For conditions such as cancer, fractures, infectious diseases, neurologic disease processes, and anything that may cause increased orthopedic fragility, chiropractic treatment alone is not an effective therapy, and may even be harmful in some cases. Those who have known circulatory problems, especially with a history of thrombosis, should not have spinal manipulation.

Resources

PERIODICALS

"Technology Takes Tiny Steps in Hands-on Chiropractic Industry." *Medical Letter on the CDC & FDA* June 20, 2004: 17.

"VA Includes Chiropractic Care for Veterans." *Managed Care Weekly* May 3, 2004: 23.

ORGANIZATIONS

American Chiropractic Association, 1701 Clarendon Boulevard, Arlington, VA, 22209, (703) 276-8800, (703) 243-2593, memberinfo@acatoday.org, http://www.acatoday.org.

Judith Turner
Teresa G. Odle

Chlamydial infections *see* **Chlamydial pneumonia; Epididymitis; Nongonococcal urethritis; Sexually transmitted diseases**

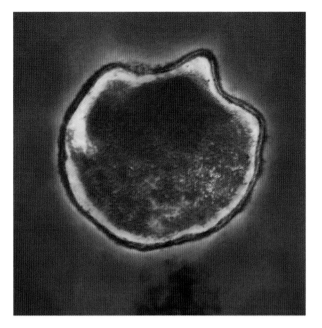

A transmission electron microscopy (TEM) of a sectioned *Chlamydia pneumonia* **bacterium.** *(Custom Medical Stock Photo, Inc. Reproduced by permission.)*

Chlamydial pneumonia

Definition

Chlamydial **pneumonia** refers to one of several types of pneumonia that can be caused by various types of the bacteria known as *Chlamydia*.

Description

Pneumonia is an infection of the lungs. The air sacs (alveoli) and/or the tissues of the lungs become swollen, and the alveoli may fill with pus or fluid. This prevents the lungs from taking in sufficient oxygen, which deprives the blood and the rest of the body's tissues of oxygen.

There are three major types of *Chlamydia*: *Chlamydia psittaci*, *Chlamydia pneumoniae*, and *Chlamydia trachomatis*. Each of these has the potential to cause a type of pneumonia.

Causes and symptoms

Chlamydia trachomatis is a major cause of **sexually transmitted diseases** (called **nongonococcal urethritis** and **pelvic inflammatory disease**). When a woman with an active chlamydial infection gives birth to a baby, the baby may aspirate (suck into his or her lungs) some of the mother's bacteria-laden secretions while passing through the birth canal. This can cause a form of relatively mild pneumonia in the newborn, occurring about two to six weeks after delivery.

Chlamydia psittaci is a bacteria carried by many types of birds, including pigeons, canaries, parakeets, parrots, and some gulls. Humans acquire the bacteria through contact with dust from bird feathers, bird droppings, or from the bite of a bird carrying the bacteria. People who keep birds as pets or who work where birds are kept have the highest risk for this type of pneumonia. This pneumonia, called psittacosis, causes **fever, cough**, and the production of sputum containing pus. This type of pneumonia may be quite severe, and is usually more serious in older patients. The illness can last several weeks.

Chlamydia pneumoniae usually causes a type of relatively mild "walking pneumonia." Patients experience fever and cough. This type of pneumonia is called a "community-acquired pneumonia" because it is easily passed from one member of the community to another.

Diagnosis

Laboratory tests indicating the presence of one of the strains of *Chlamydia* are sophisticated, expensive, and performed in only a few laboratories across the country. For this reason, doctors diagnose most cases of chlamydial pneumonia by performing a **physical examination** of the patient, and noting the presence of certain factors. For instance, if the mother of a baby sick with pneumonia is positive for a sexually transmitted disease caused by *Chlamydia trachomatis*, the diagnosis is obvious. History of exposure to birds in a patient sick with pneumonia suggests that *Chlamydia psittaci* may be the culprit. A mild pneumonia in an otherwise healthy person is likely to be a community-acquired walking pneumonia, such as that caused by *Chlamydia pneumoniae*.

Treatment

Treatment varies depending on the specific type of *Chlamydia* causing the infection. A newborn with *Chlamydia trachomatis* improves rapidly with erythromycin. *Chlamydia psittaci* infection is treated with tetracycline, bed rest, oxygen supplementation, and codeine-containing cough preparations. *Chlamydia pneumoniae* infection is treated with erythromycin.

Prognosis

The prognosis is generally excellent for the newborn with *Chlamydia trachomatis* pneumonia. *Chlamydia psittaci* may linger, and severe cases have a **death** rate of as high as 30%. The elderly are hardest hit by this type of pneumonia. A young, healthy person with *Chlamydia pneumoniae* has an excellent prognosis. In the elderly, however, there is a 5–10% death rate from this infection.

Prevention

Prevention of *Chlamydia trachomatis* pneumonia involves recognizing the symptoms of genital infection in the mother and treating her prior to delivery of her baby.

Chlamydia psittaci can be prevented by warning people who have birds as pets, or who work around birds, to be careful to avoid contact with the dust and droppings of these birds. Sick birds can be treated with an antibiotic in their feed. Because people can contract psittacosis from each other, a person sick with this infection should be kept in **isolation**, so as not to infect other people.

Chlamydia pneumoniae is difficult to prevent because it is spread by respiratory droplets from other sick people. Because people with this type of pneumonia do not always feel very sick, they often continue to attend school, go to work, and go to other public places. They then spread the bacteria in the tiny droplets that are released into the air during coughing. Therefore, this pneumonia is very difficult to prevent and often occurs in outbreaks within communities.

ORGANIZATIONS

American Lung Association, 1301 Pennsylvania Ave. NW, Suite 800, Washington, DC, 20001, (202) 758-3355, (202) 452-1805, (800) 548-8252, info@lungusa.org, http://www.lungusa.org/.

Rosalyn Carson-DeWitt, MD

Chlorhexidine *see* **Antibiotics, topical**

Chloroquine *see* **Antimalarial drugs**

Chlorzoxazone *see* **Muscle relaxants**

Choking

Definition

Choking is the inability to breathe because the trachea is blocked, constricted, or swollen shut.

Description

Choking is a medical emergency. When a person is choking, air cannot reach the lungs. If the airways cannot be cleared, **death** follows rapidly.

Anyone can choke, but choking is more common in children than in adults. Choking is a common cause of accidental death in young children who are apt to put toys or coins in their mouths, then unintentionally inhale them. About 3,000 adults die each year from choking on food.

People also choke because infection causes the throat tissue to swell shut. It is believed that this is what caused George Washington's death. Allergic reactions can also cause the throat to swell shut. Acute allergic reactions are called anaphylactic reactions and may be fatal. Strangulation puts external pressure on the trachea causing another form of choking.

Finally, people can choke from obstructive **sleep apnea**. This is a condition where tissues of the body obstruct the airways during sleep. Sleep apnea is most common in obese men who sleep on their backs. **Smoking**, heavy alcohol use, lung diseases such as **emphysema**, and an inherited tendency toward a narrowed airway and throat all increase the risk of choking during sleep.

Causes and symptoms

There are three reasons why people choke. These are:

- mechanical obstruction
- tissue swelling
- crushing of the trachea

Regardless of the cause, choking cuts off the air supply to the lungs. Indications that a person's airway is blocked include:

- the person cannot speak or cry out
- the person's face turns blue from lack of oxygen
- the person desperately grabs at his or her throat
- the person has a weak cough and labored breathing that produces a high-pitched noise
- the person has all of the symptoms previously mentioned, then becomes unconscious
- during sleep, the person has episodes of gasping, pauses in breathing, and sudden awakenings

Diagnosis

Diagnosing choking due to mechanical obstruction is straightforward, since the symptoms are obvious even to an untrained person. In choking due to infection, the person, usually a child, will have a **fever** and signs of illness before labored breathing begins. If choking is due to an allergic reaction to medication or insect **bites**, the person's earlobes and face will swell, giving an external sign that internal swelling is also occurring.

Choking due to sleep apnea is usually diagnosed on reports of symptoms by the person's sleep partner. There are also alarm devices to detect the occurrence of sleep apnea. Eventually sleep may be interrupted so frequently that daytime drowsiness becomes a problem.

KEY TERMS

Trachea—The windpipe. A tube extending from below the voice box into the chest where it splits into two branches, the bronchi, that go to each lung.

Tracheotomy—The surgical creation of an opening in the trachea that functions as an alternative airway so that the patient may breathe.

Treatment

Choking, except during sleep apnea, is a medical emergency. If choking is due to allergic reaction or infection, people should summon emergency help or go immediately to an emergency room. If choking is due to obstructed airways, the **Heimlich maneuver** (an emergency procedure in which a person is grasped from behind in order to forcefully expel the obstruction) should be performed immediately. In severe cases a **tracheotomy** (an incision into the trachea through the neck below the larynx) must be performed.

Patients who suffer airway obstruction during sleep can be treated with a device similar to an oxygen mask that creates positive airway pressure and delivers a mixture of oxygen and air.

Prognosis

Many people are treated successfully for choking with no permanent effects. However, if treatment is unsuccessful, the person dies from lack of oxygen. In cases where the airway is restored after the critical period passes, there may be permanent brain damage.

Prevention

Watching children carefully to keep them from putting **foreign objects** in their mouth and avoiding giving young children food like raisins, round slices of hot dogs, and grapes can reduce the chance of choking in children. Adults should avoid heavy alcohol consumption when eating and avoid talking and laughing with food in their mouths. The risk of obstructive sleep apnea choking can be reduced by avoiding alcohol, tobacco smoking, tranquilizers, and sedatives before bed.

ORGANIZATIONS

American Heart Association National Center, 7272 Greenville Avenue, Dallas, TX, 75231, (800) 242-8721, Review.personal.info@heart.org.

Tish Davidson, A.M.

Cholangitis

Definition

The term cholangitis means inflammation of the bile ducts. The term applies to inflammation of any portion of the bile ducts, which carry bile from the liver to the gallbladder and intestine. The inflammation is produced by bacterial infection or sometimes other causes.

Description

Bile, which is needed for digestion, is produced in the liver and then enters the common bile duct (CBD) through the hepatic ducts. Bile enters the gallbladder between meals, when the muscle or sphincter that controls flow of bile between the CBD and intestine is closed. During this period, bile accumulates in the CBD; the pressure in the CBD rises, as would a pipe closed off at one end. The increase in pressure eventually causes the bile to flow into the gallbladder. During meals, the gallbladder contracts and the sphincter between the gallbladder and intestine relaxes, permitting bile to flow into the intestine and take part in digestion.

Bile that has just been produced by the liver is sterile (free of bacteria). This is partly due to its antibacterial properties; these are produced by the immunoglobulins (antibodies) secreted in bile, the bile acids which inhibit bacterial growth themselves, and mucus.

A small number of bacteria may be present in the bile ducts and gallbladder, getting there by moving backward from the intestine, which unlike the bile ducts, contains large numbers of bacteria. The normal flow of bile out of the ducts and into the intestine also helps keep too many organisms from multiplying. Bacteria also reach the bile ducts from the lymph tissue or from the blood stream.

When the passage of bile out of the ducts is blocked, the few bacteria that are there rapidly reproduce. A partial blockage to the flow of bile can occur when a stone from the gallbladder blocks the duct, and also allows bacteria to flow back into the CBD, and creates ideal conditions for their growth. Tumors, on the other hand, cause a more complete blockage of bile flow, both in and out, so fewer infections occur. The reproducing organisms are often able to enter the bloodstream and infect multiple organs such as the liver and heart valves.

Another source of inflammation of the bile ducts occurs in diseases of altered immunity, known as "autoimmune diseases." In these diseases, the body fails to recognize certain cells as part of its normal composition. The body thinks these cells are foreign and produces antibodies to fight them off, just as it fights against bacteria and viruses. Primary sclerosing cholangitis is a typical example of an autoimmune disease involving the bile ducts.

Causes and symptoms

As noted previously, the two things that are needed for cholangitis to occur are: 1) obstruction to bile flow, and 2) presence of bacteria within the bile ducts. The most common cause of cholangitis is infection of the bile ducts due to blockage by a gallstone. Strictures (portions of ducts that have become narrow) also function in the same way. Strictures may be due to congenital (birth) abnormalities of the bile ducts, form as a result of injury to the bile duct (such as surgery, trauma), or result from inflammation that leads to scar tissue and narrowing.

The bacterium most commonly associated with infection of the bile ducts is *Escherichia coli (E. coli)* which is a normal inhabitant of the intestine. In some cases, more than one type of bacteria is involved. Patients with **AIDS** can develop infection of narrowed bile ducts with unusual organisms such as *Cryptosporidium* and others.

The three symptoms present in about 70% of patients with cholangitis are abdominal **pain**, **fever**, and **jaundice**. Some patients only have chills and fever with minimal abdominal symptoms. Jaundice or yellow discoloration of the skin and eyes occurs in about 80% of patients. The color change is due to bile pigments that accumulate in the blood and eventually in the skin and eyes.

Inflammation due to the autoimmune disease primary sclerosing cholangitis leads to multiple areas of narrowing and eventual infection. Tumors can block the bile duct and also cause cholangitis, but as noted, infection is relatively infrequent; in fact cholangitis occurs in only about one in six patients with tumors.

Another type of bile duct infection occurs mainly in Southeast Asia and is known as recurrent pyogenic cholangitis or Oriental cholangitis. It has also been identified in Asians immigrating to North America. Most patients have stones in the bile ducts and/or gallbladder, and many cases are associated with the presence of parasites within the ducts. The role of parasites in causing infection is not clear. Many researchers believe that they are just coincidental, and have nothing to do with the stones or infection.

Antibiotic—A medication that is designed to kill or weaken bacteria.

Bilirubin—A pigment produced by the liver that is excreted in bile which causes a yellow discoloration of the skin and eyes when it accumulates in those organs. Bilirubin levels can be measured by blood tests, and are most often elevated in patients with liver disease or a blockage to bile flow.

Computed tomography scan (CT scan)—A specialized x-ray procedure in which cross-sections of the area in question can be examined in detail. In evaluating the bile ducts, iodine-based dye is often injected intravenously. The procedure is of greatest value in diagnosing the complications of gallstones (such as abscesses, pancreatitis) rather than documenting the presence of a stone.

Endoscope—An endoscope as used in the field of gastroenterology is a thin flexible tube which uses a lens or miniature camera to view various areas of the gastrointestinal tract. When the procedure is performed to examine certain organs such as the bile ducts or pancreas, the organs are not viewed directly, but rather indirectly through the injection of x-ray dye into the bile duct.

Endoscopy—The performance of an exam using an endoscope is referred by the general term endoscopy.

Diagnosis through biopsies or other means and therapeutic procedures can be done with these instruments.

Primary sclerosing cholangitis—A chronic disease in which it is believed that the immune system fails to recognize the cells that compose the bile ducts as part of the same body, and attempts to destroy them. It is not clear what exactly causes the disease, but it is frequently associated with another inflammatory disease of the digestive tract, ulcerative colitis. The inflammation of the ducts eventually produces formation of scar tissue, causing multiple areas of narrowing (strictures) that block bile flow and lead to bacterial infection. Liver transplant gives the best chance for long-term survival.

Ultrasound—A non-invasive procedure based on changes in sound waves of a frequency that cannot be heard, but respond to changes in tissue composition. It requires no preparation and no radiation occurs. It has become the "gold standard" for diagnosis of stones in the gallbladder, but is less accurate in diagnosing stones in the bile ducts. Gallstones as small as 2 mm can be identified. The procedure can now also be done through an endoscope, greatly improving investigation of the bile ducts.

Diagnosis

The symptoms mentioned previously are alone very suggestive of cholangitis; however, it is important to determine the exact cause and site of possible obstruction. This is because attacks are likely to recur, and different causes require different treatments. For example, the treatment of cholangitis due to a stone in the CBD is different from that due to bile duct strictures. An elevated white blood count suggests infection, but may be normal in 20% of patients. Abnormal or elevated tests of liver function, such as bilirubin and others are also frequently present. The specific bacteria is sometimes identified from blood cultures.

X-ray techniques

A number of x-ray techniques can assist in confirming the diagnosis of bile duct obstruction; these include ultrasound and **computed tomography scans** (CT scans). However, ultrasound often cannot tell if an obstruction is due to a stricture or stone, missing a

stone in about half the cases. CT scans have an even poorer record of stone detection.

Another method of diagnosing and sometimes treating the cause of bile duct obstruction or narrowing is called **percutaneous transhepatic cholangiography**. In this procedure, dye is injected into the ducts by means of a needle placed into the liver. It is also used to drain bile and relieve an obstruction.

A newer imaging technique, magnetic resonance cholangiopancreatograpy (MRCP), may be used to determine the presence of CBD stones when other imaging techniques are inconclusive.

ENDOSCOPIC TECHNIQUES. An endoscope is a thin flexible tube that uses a lens or mirror to look at various parts of the gastrointestinal tract. **Endoscopic retrograde cholangiopancreatography** (ERCP) can accurately determine the cause and site of blockage. It also has the advantage of being able to treat the cause of obstruction, by removing stones and dilating (stretching) strictures. ERCP involves the injection of x-ray dye into the bile ducts through an endoscope. Endoscopic ultrasound is another endoscopic alternative, but is not as available as ERCP and is not therapeutic.

Treatment

The first aim is to control the bacterial infection. Broad-spectrum **antibiotics** are usually administered. Eighty % of patients respond promptly to conservative treatment with antibiotic therapy. If the infection does not come under control promptly (usually within 24 hours), as noted by decrease in fever and pain, then other methods to relieve the obstruction and infection will be needed. Either way, definitive treatment of the cause of bile duct infection is the next step, and this has undergone revolutionary changes in the past decade. Endoscopic, radiographic and other techniques have made it possible to successfully remove stones and dilate strictures that previously required surgical intervention, often with high morbidity and mortality.

Radiologic and endoscopic techniques

Just as with diagnosis, treatment of cholangitis involves a number of similar procedures that differ mainly in the way the bile ducts are entered. The aims of these techniques are immediate relief of obstruction and infection as well as correction of any abnormalities that have caused them. It is important to realize that even with **endoscopy**, x-ray dye is injected into the ducts and therefore the radiologist plays a role in both types of procedures. When endoscopy is used, the muscle between the intestine and bile duct is widened, to allow stones to pass. This is called a sphincterotomy and is often enough to relieve any obstruction and help clear infection. The widening of the muscle is needed if other procedures involving the bile duct are going to be performed. **Endoscopic sphincterotomy** with extraction of **gallstones** and/or insertion of a stent is now the treatment of choice for re-establishing biliary drainage in acute cholangitis. Common bile duct stones can be removed in most patients (up to 95% of patients) after the obstruction is removed with sphincterotomy.

The techniques mentioned previously can be summarized as follows:

- Insertion of a catheter or thin flexible tube to drain bile and relieve obstruction. When performed by insertion of a needle into the liver the technique is called percutaneous transhepatic biliary drainage (PTBD); when

performed endoscopically the catheter exits through the nose and is called a nasobiliary drain.
- Balloons can be inserted into the ducts with either method to dilate strictures.
- Insertion of a prosthesis which is a rigid or flexible tube designed to keep a narrowed area open; it is usually placed after a stricture is dilated with a balloon.

Surgical treatment

Fortunately, with recent advances in the methods mentioned previously, this is a last option. Nonetheless, about 5–10% of patients will need to undergo surgical exploration of the bile ducts.

In some instances, the bile duct is so narrowed due to prior inflammation or tumor, that it needs connection to a different area of the intestinal tract to drain. This is rather complicated surgery and carries a mortality rate of 2%.

Prognosis

The outlook for those with cholangitis has markedly improved in the last several years due in large part to the development of the techniques described previously. For those patients whose episode of infection is caused by something other than a simple stone, the future is not as bright, but still often responsive to treatment. Some patients with autoimmune disease will need **liver transplantation**.

Prevention

This involves eliminating those factors that increase the risk of infection of the bile ducts, mainly stones and strictures. If it is medically possible, patients who have their gallbladder and suffer a bout of cholangitis should undergo surgical removal of the gallbladder and removal of any stones.

For other patients, a variety of therapies as outlined previously, including dissolving small stones with bile acids are also available. A combination of several of these methods is needed in some patients. Patients should discuss the risks and alternatives of these treatments with their physicians.

Resources

PERIODICALS

Lee, C.-C., Chang, I.-J., Lai, Y.-C., Chen, S.-Y., and Chen, S.-C. "Epidemiology and Prognostic Determinants of Patients with Bacteremic Cholecystitis or Cholangitis." *American Journal of Gastroenterology*.(2007);102(3); 536–569.

Lee, J.G. "Diagnosis and Management of Acute Cholangitis."*Nat Rev Gastroenterol Hepatol.*(Aug 4, 2009).

OTHER

"Cholangitis."*eMedicine.*November 16, 2009 [cited June 27, 2010]. http:www.emedicine.medscape.com/article/184043-overview.

"Gallstones." *National Institute of Diabetes and Digestive and Kidney Disease.* July 2007 [cited June 27, 2010] http://www.digestive.niddk.nih.gov/diseases/pubs/gallstones.

"Primary Sclerosing Cholangitis." *National Institute of Diabetes and Digestive and Kidney Disease.* June 2008 [cited June 27, 2010] http://www.digestive.niddk.nih.gov/diseases/pubs/primarysclerosingcholangitis.

"Therapeutic Endoscopic Retrograde Cholangiopancreatography (ERCP)." *American Society for Gastrointestinal Endoscopy.*http://www.asge.org.

"Your Digestive System and How It Works." *National Institute of Diabetes and Digestive and Kidney Disease.* April 2008 [cited June 27, 2010] http://www.digestive.niddk.nih.gov/diseases/pubs/yrdd.

David Kaminstein, MD
Melinda Granger Oberleitner
RN, DNS, APRN, CNS

Cholecystectomy

Definition

A cholecystectomy is the surgical removal of the gallbladder. The two basic types of this procedure are open cholecystectomy and the laparoscopic approach. It is estimated that the laparoscopic procedure is currently used for approximately 80% of cases.

Purpose

A cholecystectomy is performed to treat cholelithiasis and **cholecystitis**. In cholelithiasis, **gallstones** of varying shapes and sizes form from the solid components of bile. The presence of stones, often referred to as gallbladder disease, may produce symptoms of excruciating right upper abdominal **pain** radiating to the right shoulder. The gallbladder may become the site of acute infection and inflammation, resulting in symptoms of upper right abdominal pain, **nausea and vomiting**. This condition is referred to as cholecystitis. The surgical removal of the gallbladder can provide relief of these symptoms.

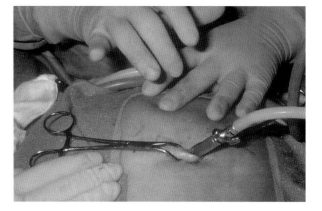

A surgeon performs a laparoscopic cholecystectomy on a patient. *(Custom Medical Stock Photo, Inc. Reproduced by permission.)*

Precautions

Although the laparoscopic procedure requires **general anesthesia** for about the same length of time as the open procedure, **laparoscopy** generally produces less postoperative pain, and a shorter recovery period. The laparoscopic procedure would not be preferred in cases where the gallbladder is so inflamed that it could rupture, or when **adhesions** (additional fibrous bands of tissue) are present.

Description

The laparoscopic cholecystectomy involves the insertion of a long narrow cylindrical tube with a camera on the end, through an approximately 1 cm incision in the abdomen, which allows visualization of the internal organs and projection of this image onto a video monitor. Three smaller incisions allow for insertion of other instruments to perform the surgical procedure. A laser may be used for the incision and cautery (burning unwanted tissue to stop bleeding), in which case the procedure may be called laser laparoscopic cholecystectomy.

In a conventional or open cholecystectomy, the gallbladder is removed through a surgical incision high in the right abdomen, just beneath the ribs. A drain may be inserted to prevent accumulation of fluid at the surgical site.

Preparation

As with any surgical procedure, the patient will be required to sign a consent form after the procedure is explained thoroughly. Food and fluids will be prohibited after midnight before the procedure. **Enemas** may be ordered to clean out the bowel. If **nausea** or

vomiting are present, a suction tube to empty the stomach may be used, and for laparoscopic procedures, a urinary drainage catheter will also be used to decrease the risk of accidental puncture of the stomach or bladder with insertion of the trocar (a sharp-pointed instrument).

Aftercare

Post-operative care for the patient who has had an open cholecystectomy, as with those who have had any major surgery, involves monitoring of blood pressure, pulse, respiration and temperature. Breathing tends to be shallow because of the effect of anesthesia, and the patient's reluctance to breathe deeply due to the pain caused by the proximity of the incision to the muscles used for respiration. The patient is shown how to support the operative site when breathing deeply and coughing, and given pain medication as necessary. Fluid intake and output is measured, and the operative site is observed for color and amount of wound drainage. Fluids are given intravenously for 24–48 hours, until the patient's diet is gradually advanced as bowel activity resumes. The patient is generally encouraged to walk 8 hours after surgery and discharged from the hospital within three to five days, with return to work approximately four to six weeks after the procedure.

Care received immediately after laparoscopic cholecystectomy is similar to that of any patient undergoing surgery with general anesthesia. A unique post-operative pain may be experienced in the right shoulder related to pressure from carbon dioxide used through the laparoscopic tubes. This pain may be relieved by laying on the left side with right knee and thigh drawn up to the chest. Walking will also help increase the body's reabsorption of the gas. The patient is usually discharged the day after surgery, and allowed to shower on the second postoperative day. The patient is advised to gradually resume normal activities over a three day period, while avoiding heavy lifting for about 10 days.

Risks

Potential problems associated with open cholecystectomy include respiratory problems related to location of the incision, wound infection, or **abscess** formation. Possible complications of laparoscopic cholecystectomy include accidental puncture of the bowel or bladder and uncontrolled bleeding. Incomplete reabsorption of the carbon dioxide gas could irritate the muscles used in respiration and cause respiratory distress.

Resources

OTHER

"Patient Information Documents on Digestive Diseases." *National Institute of Diabetes and Digestive and Kidney Disease.* http://www.niddk.nih.gov.

Kathleen D. Wright, RN

Cholecystitis

Definition

Cholecystitis refers to a painful inflammation of the gallbladder's wall. The disorder can occur a single time (acute), or can recur multiple times (chronic).

Description

The gallbladder is a small, pear-shaped organ in the upper right hand corner of the abdomen. It is connected by a series of ducts (tube-like channels) to the liver, pancreas, and duodenum (first part of the small intestine). To aid in digestion, the liver produces a substance called bile, which is passed into the gallbladder. The gallbladder concentrates this bile, meaning that it reabsorbs some of the fluid from the bile to make it more potent. After a meal, bile is squeezed out of the gallbladder by strong muscular contractions, and passes through a duct into the duodenum. Due to the chemical makeup of bile, the contents of the duodenum are kept at an optimal pH level for

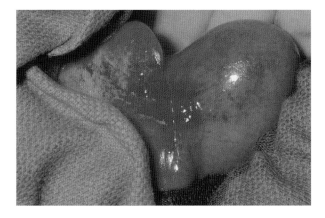

A close-up view of an inflamed gallbladder. *(Custom Medical Stock Photo, Inc. Reproduced by permission.)*

digestion. The bile also plays an important part in allowing fats within the small intestine to be absorbed.

Demographics

Gallstone formation is seen in twice as many women as men, particularly those between the ages of 20 and 60. Pregnant women or those on birth control pills or estrogen replacement therapy have a greater risk of **gallstones**, as do Native Americans and Mexican Americans.

Risk factors

People who are overweight, or who lose a large amount of weight quickly, are at greater risk for developing gallstones. Not all individuals with gallstones go on to have cholecystitis, since many people never have any symptoms from their gallstones and never know they exist. However, the vast majority of people with cholecystitis are found to have gallstones. Rare causes of cholecystitis include severe **burns** or injury, massive systemic infection, severe illness, diabetes, obstruction by a tumor of the duct leaving the gallbladder, and certain uncommon infections of the gallbladder (including bacteria and worms).

Causes and symptoms

In about 95% of all cases of cholecystitis, the gallbladder contains gallstones. Gallstones are solid accumulations of the components of bile, particularly cholesterol, bile pigments, and **calcium**. These solids may occur when the components of bile are not in the correct proportion to each other. If the bile becomes overly concentrated, or if too much of one component is present, stones may form. When these stones block the duct leaving the gallbladder, bile accumulates

within the gallbladder. The gallbladder continues to contract, but the bile cannot pass out of the gallbladder in the normal way. Back pressure on the gallbladder, chemical changes from the stagnating bile trapped within the gallbladder, and occasionally bacterial infection result in damage to the gallbladder wall. As the gallbladder becomes swollen, some areas of the wall do not receive adequate blood flow, and lack of oxygen causes cells to die.

When the stone blocks the flow of bile from the liver, certain normal byproducts of the liver's processing of red blood cells (called bilirubin) build up. The bilirubin is reabsorbed into the bloodstream, and over time this bilirubin is deposited in the skin and in the whites of the eyes. Because bilirubin contains a yellowish color, it causes a yellowish cast to the skin and eyes that is called **jaundice**.

Although there are rare reports of patients with chronic cholecystitis who never experience any **pain**, nearly 100% of the time cholecystitis is diagnosed after a patient has experienced a bout of severe pain in the region of the gallbladder and liver. The pain may be crampy and episodic, or it may be constant. The pain is often described as pushing through to the right upper back and shoulder. Because deep breathing increases the pain, breathing becomes shallow. **Fever** is often present, and **nausea and vomiting** are nearly universal. Jaundice occurs when the duct leaving the liver is also obstructed, although it may take a number of days for it to become apparent. When bacterial infection sets in, the patient may begin to experience higher fever and shaking chills.

Diagnosis

Examination

Diagnosis of cholecystitis involves a careful abdominal examination. The enlarged, tender gallbladder may be felt through the abdominal wall. Pressure in the upper right corner of the abdomen may cause the patient to stop breathing in, due to an increase in pain. This is called Murphy's sign. **Physical examination** may also reveal an increased heart rate and an increased rate of breathing.

Tests

Blood tests will show an increase in the white blood count and bilirubin. Ultrasound is used to look for gallstones and to measure the thickness of the gallbladder wall (a marker of inflammation and scarring). A scan of the liver and gallbladder, with careful attention to the system of ducts throughout

KEY TERMS

Bile—A substance produced by the liver, and concentrated and stored in the gallbladder. Bile contains many different substances, including bile salts, cholesterol, and bilirubin. After a meal, the gallbladder pumps bile into the duodenum (the first part of the small intestine) to keep the intestine's contents at the appropriate pH for digestion, and to help break down fats.

Bilirubin—Produced when red blood cells break down. It is a yellowish color and when levels are abnormally high, it causes the yellowish tint to eyes and skin known as jaundice.

Cholecystectomy—An operation to remove the gallbladder.

Cholecystotomy—An operation during which the gallbladder is opened, gallstones are removed, and excess bile is drained. The gallbladder is not removed.

Duct—A tube through which various substances can pass. These substances can travel through ducts to another organ or into the bloodstream.

(called the biliary tree) is used to demonstrate obstruction of ducts.

Rare complications of cholecystitis include:

- massive infection of the gallbladder, in which the gallbladder becomes filled with pus (called empyema)
- perforation of the gallbladder, in which the build-up of material within the gallbladder becomes so great that the wall of the organ bursts, with a resulting abdominal infection called peritonitis
- formation of abnormal connections between the gallbladder and other organs (the duodenum, large intestine, stomach), called fistulas
- obstruction of the intestine by a very large gallstone (called gallstone ileus)
- emphysema of the gallbladder, in which certain bacteria that produce gas infect the gallbladder, resulting in stretching of the gallbladder and disruption of its wall by gas

Treatment

Traditional

Initial treatment of cholecystitis usually requires hospitalization. The patient is given fluids, salts, and sugars through a needle placed in a vein (intravenous or IV). No food or drink is given by mouth. A tube, called a nasogastric or NG tube, may need to be passed through the nose and down into the stomach to drain out the excess fluids. Medications for pain and IV administration of broad spectrum **antibiotics** are initiated.

Treatment almost always involves removal of the gallbladder, a surgery called **cholecystectomy**. It is not usually recommended that the patient have surgery while acutely ill, however, patients with complications may require emergency surgery (immediately following diagnosis) because the **death** rate increases in these cases. Similarly, patients who have cholecystitis with no gallstones have a 50% chance of death if the gallbladder is not quickly removed. Most patients do best if surgery is performed after they have been stabilized with fluids, possibly an NG tube, and administration of antibiotics. Results of recent research indicate that early operation (laparoscopic cholecystectomy) by an experienced surgeon within 72 hours of admission results in the best outcomes for the patient. In patients who have other serious medical problems that may increase the risks of gallbladder removal surgery, the surgeon may decide to leave the gallbladder in place. In this case, the operation may involve removing obstructing gallstones and draining infected bile (called cholecystotomy).

Both cholecystectomy and cholecystotomy may be performed via the classical open abdominal operation (laparotomy). Tiny, "keyhole" incisions, a flexible scope, and a laser device that shatters the stones (a laparoscopic laser) can be used to destroy the gallstones. The laparoscopic procedure can also be used to remove the gallbladder through one of the small incisions. Because of the smaller incisions, laparoscopic cholecystectomy is a procedure that is less painful and promotes faster healing.

Prognosis

Hospital management of cholecystitis ends the symptoms for about 75% of all patients. Of these patients, 25% will have another attack of cholecystitis within a year, and 60% will have another attack within six years. Each attack of cholecystitis increases a patient's risk of developing life-threatening complications, requiring emergency surgery. Therefore, early removal of the gallbladder, rather than a "wait-and-see" approach, is usually recommended. Cure is complete in those patients who undergo cholecystectomy.

Prevention

Prevention of cholecystitis is best attempted by maintaining a reasonable ideal weight. Some studies have suggested that eating a diet high in fiber, vegetables, and fruit is also protective.

Resources

PERIODICALS

Huffman, J.L., and S. Schenker. "Acute Acalculous Cholecystitis—A Review." *Clinical Gastroenterology and Hepatology* (September 9, 2009).
Wilson, E., K. Gurusamy, C. Gluud, and B.R. Davidson. "Cost-Utility and Value-of-Information Analysis of Early versus Delayed Laparoscopic Cholecystectomy for Acute Cholecystitis." *British Journal of Surgery* 97, no. 2 (February 2010): 210–19.

ORGANIZATIONS

Digestive Disease National Coalition, 507 Capitol Court NE, Suite 200, Washington, DC, 20002, (202) 544-7497, http://www.ddnc.org.
National Digestive Diseases Information Clearinghouse, 2 Information Way, Bethesda, MD, 20892-3570, (800) 891-5389, http://www.digestive.niddk.nih.gov.

Rosalyn Carson-DeWitt, MD
Melinda Granger Oberleitner, RN, DNS, APRN, CNS

Cholecystography *see* **Gallbladder x rays**
Choledocholithiasis *see* **Gallstones**
Cholelithiasis *see* **Gallstones**
Cholelithotomy *see* **Gallstone removal**

Cholera

Definition

Cholera is a serious, acute, **infectious disease** characterized by watery **diarrhea** that is caused by the bacterium *Vibrio cholerae*, first identified by Robert Koch in 1883 during a cholera outbreak in Egypt. The name of the disease comes from a Greek word meaning "flow of bile."

Demographics

Although cholera was a public health problem in the United States and Europe a hundred years ago, modern sanitation and the treatment of drinking water have virtually eliminated the disease in developed countries. In 2005, the World Health Organization

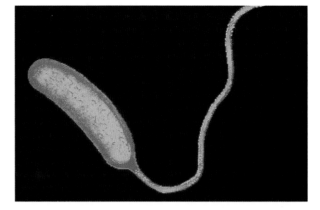

A false color transmission electron micrograph (TEM) of *Vibrio cholerae bacterium* magnified 6,000 times its original size. *(Custom Medical Stock Photo, Inc. Reproduced by permission.)*

(WHO) reported that there were 12 cases of cholera in the United States. Of these, eight were brought in by travelers and four were attributed to improperly cooked seafood in Louisiana following hurricanes Katrina and Rita.

Internationally, cholera outbreaks continue to occur in less developed countries, particularly following such natural disasters such as hurricanes and tsunamis during which water supplies become contaminated. In 2007, WHO reported that cholera occurred in 53 countries. A total of 177,693 cases and 4,031 cholera deaths were reported that year. However, WHO estimates that the number of reported cases represents only five to 10 percent of actual cases. In areas where cholera occurs, it is the most feared epidemic diarrheal disease because people can die from **dehydration** that results from severe diarrhea within hours of infection.

Cholera often occurs in major outbreaks or epidemics; seven pandemics (countrywide or worldwide epidemics) of cholera were recorded between 1817 and 2010. WHO estimates that during any cholera epidemic, approximately 0.2–1% of the local population will contract the disease.

Anyone can get cholera, but infants, children, pregnant women, and the elderly are more likely to die from the disease because they become dehydrated faster than adults. There is no particular season in which cholera is more likely to occur.

Description

Cholera is spread by eating food or drinking water that has been contaminated with *V. cholerae*. Contamination usually occurs when human feces from a person who has the disease seeps into a community water supply. Fruits and vegetables also can be contaminated in areas where crops are fertilized with human feces. Cholera bacteria live in warm, brackish water and can infect persons who eat raw or undercooked seafood obtained from such waters. Cholera is rarely transmitted directly from one person to another.

Because of an extensive system of sewage and water treatment in the United States, Canada, Europe, Japan, and Australia, cholera is not a concern for visitors and residents of these countries. However, people visiting or living in other parts of the world, particularly the Indian subcontinent and in parts of Africa and South America, should be aware of the potential for contracting cholera and practice prevention. Fortunately, the disease is both preventable and treatable. Deaths usually occur in developing countries because of lack of access to hospitals and treatment.

Causes and symptoms

Cholera is caused by the bacterium *V. cholerae*. This bacterium is a gram–negative aerobic bacillus, or rod–shaped bacterium. It has two major biotypes: classic and El Tor. El Tor is the biotype responsible for most of the cholera outbreaks reported from 1961 through the 2000s.

Because *V. cholerae* is sensitive to acid, most cholera–causing bacteria die in the acidic environment of the stomach. However, when a person has ingested food or water containing large amounts of cholera bacteria, some will survive to infect the intestines. As would be expected, antacid usage or the use of any medication that blocks or reduces acid production in the stomach allows more bacteria to survive and cause infection.

In the small intestine, the rapidly multiplying bacteria produce a toxin that causes a large volume of water and electrolytes to be secreted into the bowels and then to be abruptly eliminated in the form of watery diarrhea. **Vomiting** may also occur. Symptoms begin to appear between one and three days after contaminated food or water has been ingested.

Most cases of cholera are mild, but about one in 20 patients experience severe, potentially life–threatening symptoms. In severe cases, fluids can be lost through diarrhea and **vomiting** at the rate of one quart per hour. This loss of fluid can produce a dangerous state of dehydration unless the lost fluids and electrolytes are rapidly replaced.

Signs of dehydration include intense thirst, little or no urine output, dry skin and mouth, an absence of tears, glassy or sunken eyes, **muscle cramps**, weakness, and rapid heart rate. The fontanelle (soft spot on an infant's head) will appear to be sunken or drawn

in. Dehydration occurs most rapidly in the very young and the very old because they have fewer fluid reserves. A doctor should be consulted immediately any time signs of severe dehydration occur. Immediate replacement of lost fluids and electrolytes is necessary to prevent kidney failure, **coma**, and **death**.

Risk factors

Some people are at greater risk of having a severe case of cholera if they become infected. These risk factors include:

- People taking proton pump inhibitors, histamine (H2) blockers, or antacids to control acid indigestion. As noted earlier, *V. cholerae* is sensitive to stomach acid.
- People who have had chronic gastritis caused by infection with *Helicobacter pylori*.
- People who have had a partial gastrectomy (surgical removal of a portion of the stomach).

Diagnosis

Tests

Rapid diagnosis of cholera can be made by examining a fresh stool sample under the microscope for the presence of *V. cholerae* bacteria. Cholera can also be diagnosed by culturing a stool sample in the laboratory to isolate the cholera–causing bacteria. In addition, a blood test may reveal the presence of antibodies against the cholera bacteria. Because of the speed at which life–threatening dehydration can occur, in areas where cholera occurs often, however, patients are usually treated for diarrhea and vomiting symptoms as if they had cholera without laboratory confirmation.

Treatment

Traditional

The key to treating cholera lies in preventing dehydration by replacing fluids and electrolytes lost through diarrhea and vomiting. The discovery that rehydration can be accomplished orally revolutionized the treatment of cholera and other, similar diseases by making this simple, cost–effective treatment widely available throughout the world. WHO has developed an inexpensive oral replacement fluid containing appropriate amounts of water, sugar, and salts that is used worldwide. In cases of severe dehydration, replacement fluids must be given intravenously. Patients should be encouraged to drink when they can keep liquids down and eat when their appetite returns. Recovery generally takes three to six days.

Drugs

Adults may be given the antibiotic tetracycline to shorten the duration of the illness and reduce fluid loss. WHO recommends this antibiotic treatment only in cases of severe dehydration. If **antibiotics** are overused, the cholera bacteria may develop resistance to the drug, making the antibiotic ineffective in treating even severe cases of cholera. Tetracycline is not given to children whose permanent teeth have not come in because it can cause the teeth to become permanently discolored.

Other antibiotics that may be given to speed up the clearance of *V. cholerae* from the body include azithromycin (Zithromax), Doxycycline (Bio–Tab, Doryx, Vibramycin), ciprofloxacin (Cipro), and erythromycin.

Alternative

A possible complementary or alternative treatment for fluid loss caused by cholera is a plant–derived compound, an extract made from the tree bark of *Croton lechleri*, the Sangre de grado tree found in the South American rain forest. Researchers at a hospital research institute in California report that the extract appears to work by preventing the loss of chloride and other electrolytes from the body.

Prognosis

Cholera is a very treatable disease so long as resources are available for rehydration. Patients with milder cases of cholera usually recover on their own in three to six days without additional complications. They may eliminate the bacteria in their feces for up to two weeks. Chronic carriers of the disease are rare. With prompt fluid and electrolyte replacement, the death rate in patients with severe cholera is less than one percent. Untreated, the death rate can be greater than 50%. The difficulty in treating severe cholera does not lie in not knowing how to treat it but rather in getting medical care to the sick in developing areas of the world where medical resources are limited.

Prevention

The best form of cholera prevention is to establish good sanitation and waste treatment systems. In the absence of adequate sewage treatment, the following guidelines should be followed to reduce the possibility of infection:

- Boil water. Drink and brush teeth only with water that has been boiled or treated with chlorine or iodine tablets. Safe drinks include coffee and tea made with boiling water or carbonated bottled water and carbonated soft drinks.

- Cook foods. Eat only thoroughly cooked foods, and eat them while they are still hot. Avoid eating food from street vendors.

- Peel foods. Eat only fruit or nuts with a thick intact skin or shell that is removed immediately before eating.

- Avoid raw foods. Do not eat raw foods such as oysters or ceviche. Avoid salads and raw vegetables. Do not use untreated ice cubes in otherwise safe drinks.

- Avoid polluted water. Do not swim or fish in polluted water.

Preventive measures following natural disasters include guaranteeing the purity of community drinking water, either by large–scale chlorination and boiling, or by bringing in bottled or purified water from the outside. Other important preventive measures at the community level include provision for the safe disposal of human feces and good food hygiene.

Because cholera is one of the few infectious diseases that can be spread by human remains (through fecal matter leaking from corpses into the water supply), during natural disasters, emergency workers who handle human remains are at increased risk of infection. It is considered preferable to bury corpses rather than to cremate them, however, and to allow survivors time to conduct appropriate burial ceremonies or rituals. The remains should be disinfected prior to burial, and buried at least 90 feet (30 m) away from sources of drinking water.

A cholera vaccines exists that can be given to travelers and residents of areas where cholera is known to be active, but the vaccine is not highly effective. It provides only 25–50% immunity, and then only for a period of about six months. The vaccine is never given to infants under six months of age. The Centers for Disease Control and Prevention (CDC) does not currently recommend cholera **vaccination** for travelers. Residents of cholera–plagued areas should discuss the value of the vaccine with their doctor.

In 2006 another cholera vaccine known as WC/rBS was approved for use in the United States. It is also available in Sweden. This vaccine is designed to stimulate the formation of antibodies against both the cholera bacteria and the cholera toxin. It is more effective than previous vaccines but provides protection for only a limited time. The prevention strategies listed previously are still necessary precautions.

Resources

BOOKS

Hamlin, Christopher. *Cholera: The Biography*. New York: Oxford University Press, 2009.

Hempel, Sandra. *The Strange Case of the Broad Street Pump: John Snow and the Mystery of Cholera*. Berkeley, CA: University of California Press, 2007.

OTHER

"Cholera." World Health Organization. 2010. http://www.who.int/topics/cholera/en (accessed September 17, 2010).

Handa, Sajeev. "Cholera." eMedicine.com (February 26, 2010). http://emedicine.medscape.com/article/214911-overview (accessed September 17, 2010).

ORGANIZATIONS

Centers for Disease Control and Prevention (CDC), 1600 Clifton Rd., Atlanta, GA, 30333, (404) 639–3534, (800) CDC–INFO ((800) 232–4636). TTY: (888) 232–6348, inquiry@cdc.gov, http://www.cdc.gov.

World Health Organization (WHO), Avenue Appia 20, 1211 Geneva 27, Switzerland, + 22 41 791 21 11, + 22 41 791 31 11, info@who.int, http://www.who.int.

Tish Davidson, A.M.
Rebecca J. Frey, PhD
Tish Davidson, A.M.

Cholestasis

Definition

Cholestasis is a condition caused by rapidly developing (acute) or long-term (chronic) interruption in the excretion of bile (a digestive fluid that helps the body process fat). The term is taken from the Greek *chole*, bile, and *stasis*, standing still.

Description

Cholestasis is caused by obstruction within the liver (intrahepatic) or outside the liver (extrahepatic). The obstruction causes bile salts, the bile pigment bilirubin, and fats (lipids) to accumulate in the bloodstream instead of being eliminated normally.

Intrahepatic cholestasis is characterized by widespread blockage of small ducts or by disorders such as hepatitis that impair the body's ability to eliminate bile. Extrahepatic cholestasis can occur as a side effect of many medications. It can also occur as a complication of surgery, serious injury, tissue-destroying infection, or intravenous feeding. Extrahepatic cholestasis can be caused by conditions such as tumors and **gallstones** that block the flow of bile from the gallbladder to the first part of the small intestine (duodenum).

Pregnancy increases the sensitivity of the bile ducts to estrogen, and cholestasis often develops during the second and third trimesters of pregnancy. This condition is the second most common cause of **jaundice** during pregnancy, but generalized **itching** (pruritus gravidarum) is the only symptom most women experience. Cholestasis of pregnancy tends to run in families. Symptoms usually disappear within two to four weeks after the baby's birth but may reappear if the woman becomes pregnant again.

A similar condition affects some women who take birth control pills. Symptoms disappear after the woman stops using **oral contraceptives**. This condition does not lead to chronic **liver disease**. A woman who develops cholestasis from either of these causes (pregnancy or birth control hormones) has an increased risk of developing cholestasis from the other.

Benign familial recurrent cholestasis is a rare condition characterized by brief, repeated episodes of itching and jaundice. Symptoms often disappear. This condition does not cause **cirrhosis**.

Drug-induced cholestasis may be a complication of **chemotherapy** or other medications. The two major types of drug-induced cholestasis are direct toxic injury and reactions unique to an individual (idiosyncratic reactions). In direct toxic injury, the severity of symptoms parallels the amount of medication involved. This condition develops a short time after treatment begins, follows a predictable pattern, and usually causes liver damage.

Direct toxic reactions develop in 1% of all patients who take chlorpromazine (Thorazine), a tranquilizer and antinausea drug. Idiosyncratic reactions may occur at the onset of treatment or at a later time. Allergic responses are varied and are not related to the amount of medication being taken.

Newborns and infants are particularly susceptible to the development of cholestasis as a consequence of immaturity of the liver.

Causes and symptoms

Intrahepatic cholestasis is usually caused by hepatitis or by medications that can produce symptoms resembling hepatitis. Phenothiazine-derivative drugs, including chlorpromazine, can cause sudden **fever** and inflammation. Symptoms usually disappear after use of the drug(s) is stopped. In rare cases, a condition resembling chronic biliary cirrhosis (a progressive disease characterized by destruction of small bile ducts) persists even after the medication is stopped. Some patients experience a similar reaction in response to **tricyclic antidepressants** (amitriptyline, imipramine), phenylbutazone (Butazolidin), erythromycin estolate (Estomycin, Purmycin), and other drugs. Intrahepatic cholestasis may also be caused by alcoholic liver disease, **primary biliary cirrhosis**, **cancer** that has spread (metastasized) from another part of the body, and a number of rare disorders.

Extrahepatic cholestasis is most often caused by a stone obstructing the passage through which bile travels from the gallbladder to the small intestine (common bile duct) or by pancreatic cancer. Less often, the condition occurs as a result of non-cancerous narrowing of the common duct (strictures), ductal carcinoma, or disorders of the pancreas.

Cholestasis caused by the use of **steroids** causes little, if any, inflammation. Symptoms develop gradually and usually disappear after the drug is discontinued. Other drugs that can cause cholestasis are:

- allopurinol (Zyloprim)
- amitriptyline (Elavil)
- azathioprine (Imuran)
- benoxaprofen (Oraflex)
- capotril (Capoten)
- carbamazepine (Tegretol)
- cimetidine (Tagamet)

- hydralazine hydrochloride (Apresoline Hydrochloride)
- imipramine (Tofranil)
- penicillin
- quinidine sulfate (Quinidex)
- ranitidine (Zantac)
- sulfonamides (Apo-Sulfatrim, sulfamethoxazole)
- sulindac (Clinoril, Saldac)

Symptoms of both intrahepatic and extrahepatic cholestasis include a yellow discoloration of the skin (jaundice), dark urine, and pale stools. Itching over the skin may be severe if the condition is advanced.

Symptoms of chronic cholestasis include:

- skin discoloration
- scars or skin injuries caused by scratching
- bone pain
- yellowish fat deposits beneath the surface of the skin (xanthoma) or around the eyes (xanthelasma)

Patients with advanced cholestasis feel ill, tire easily, and are often nauseated. Abdominal **pain** and such systemic symptoms as anorexia, **vomiting**, and fever are usually due to the underlying condition that causes cholestasis.

Diagnosis

Examination and tests

Determining whether obstruction exists inside or outside the liver is the essential part of diagnosis. A history of hepatitis or heavy drinking, recent use of certain drugs, and symptoms like **ascites** (abnormal abdominal swelling) and splenomegaly (enlarged spleen) suggest intrahepatic cholestasis. Pain or rigidity in the gallbladder or pancreas suggest an extrahepatic form.

Blood tests and **liver function tests** can reveal the pattern and extent of liver injury, indicate functional abnormalities, and establish the cause of the condition. Most misdiagnoses occur when physicians rely more on laboratory analysis than on detailed medical history and the results of a thorough **physical examination**. Blood tests that may be ordered include measurement of serum bilirubin, serum bile salts, serum cholesterol, serum lipoprotein-X, serum 5-nucleotidase, and serum gamma-glutamyl transferase levels. Fecal fat levels may also be elevated in cholestasis. Special attention should be paid to liver function tests including levels of alkaline phosphatase (ALP). ALP levels more than three times greater than normal indicate cholestasis.

KEY TERMS

Bile—A bitter yellow-green substance produced by the liver. Bile breaks down fats in the small intestine so that they can be used by the body. It is stored in the gallbladder and passes from the gallbladder through the common bile duct to the top of the small intestine (duodenum) as needed to digest fat.

Biliary—Of bile or of the gallbladder and bile ducts that transport bile and make up the biliary system or tract.

Computed tomography scans (CT)—An imaging technique in which cross-sectional x rays of the body are compiled to create a three-dimensional image of the body's internal structures.

Endoscopic retrograde cholangiopancreatography—A diagnostic procedure for mapping the pancreatic and common bile ducts. A flexible tube with a light transmitter (fiberoptics) is placed in the duct. A contrast dye is instilled directly into the duct and a series of x-ray images are taken.

Hepatic—Of the liver, from the Greek word *hepar.*

Liver function tests—Tests used to evaluate liver metabolism, storage, filtration, and excretion. The tests include alkaline phosphatase and serum alanine aminotransferase and aspartate aminotransferase.

Magnetic resonance imaging (MRI)—An imaging technique that uses a large circular magnet and radio waves to generate signals from atoms in the body. These signals are used to construct images of internal structures.

Percutaneous transhepatic cholangiography—An x-ray examination of the bile ducts. A needle is passed through the skin (percutaneous) across or over the liver (transhepatic) and directly into a bile duct to inject a contrast dye. The dye enhances the x-ray image mapping the system of bile ducts (cholangiography).

Phenothiazine-derivative drugs—A large family of drugs derived from phenothiazine, a compound that in itself is too poisonous for human consumption. Phenothiazine derivatives include tranquilizers, medications that prevent vomiting, antihistamines, and drugs used to enhance the effectiveness of anesthesia.

Ultrasonography—A test using sound waves to measure blood flow. Gel is applied to a hand-held transducer that is pressed against the patient's body. Images are displayed on a monitor.

Once the disease pattern has been established, ultrasound may be performed to determine whether obstruction of the large duct has caused widening of small ducts located close to it. **Computed tomography scans** (CT) and **magnetic resonance imaging** (MRI) can provide more detailed information about the source of the obstruction.

Procedures

If these imaging procedures do not provide the information a physician, internist, or gastroenterologist needs to make a diagnosis of cholestasis, one of these procedures may be performed:

- direct cholangiography, an x-ray map of the bile ducts, enhanced by the use of contrast dye
- percutaneous transhepatic cholangiography, used to identify obstructions that impede the flow of bile from the liver to the digestive system, takes x-ray images of the bile ducts after a contrast dye has been injected by a needle passed directly into a hepatic duct
- endoscopic retrograde cholangiopancreatography (ERCP), which uses a special dye to outline the

pancreatic and common bile ducts and highlight the position of any obstruction; a special tube with a light transmitter is inserted into the duct and a series of x-ray images is taken

A doctor who thinks a physical obstruction is responsible for progressive deterioration of a patient's condition may consider an exploratory surgical procedure (diagnostic laparotomy). **Liver biopsy** is sometimes performed if imaging tests do not indicate why a duct is enlarged, but results of a single biopsy may not represent the status of the entire organ.

Treatment

Traditional

The goal of treatment is to eliminate or control the patient's symptoms. Discontinuing the use of certain drugs can restore normal liver function, but surgery may be needed to drain or remove obstructions or to widen affected ducts. A liver transplant may become necessary if complications occur.

Drugs

Rifampin (Rifadin, Rimactane), an antibacterial drug; Phenobarbital (Luminol), a barbiturate anticonvulsant that decreases serum bilirubin levels by increasing hepatic enzyme metabolims; and other drugs including urosodeoxycholic acid (Actigall, Urosol), and bile salt resins are sometimes prescribed to cleanse the system and eliminate bile salts and other toxic compounds.

Home remedies

Patients who have chronic cholestasis and have trouble digesting fat may have to restrict the amount of fat in their diet and take **calcium** and water-soluble vitamin supplements.

Prognosis

Symptoms almost always disappear after the underlying condition is controlled.

Some patients who have cholestasis experience symptoms only after infection develops, but chronic bile-duct obstruction always leads to cirrhosis. It may also cause **osteoporosis** (fragile bones) or osteomalacia (soft bones).

Emergency care is not required unless inflammation of the bile ducts (**cholangitis**) develops. Cancer should be considered when an adult suddenly develops cholestasis after the age of 50.

Resources

PERIODICALS

Festi, D., et al. "Clinical Efficacy and Effectiveness of Ursodeoxycholic Acid in Cholestatic Liver Diseases." *Current Clinical Pharmacology* 2, no. 2 (May 2007): 155–77.

Haber, B., et al. "Cholestasis: Current Issues and Plans for the Future." *Journal of Pediatric Gastroenterology and Nutrition* 47, no. 2 (August 2009): 220–4.

OTHER

"Cholestasis." *eMedicine.* March 9, 2010. http://emedicine.medscape.com/article/927624-overview (accessed October 3, 2010).

ORGANIZATIONS

American Liver Foundation, 75 Maiden Lane, Suite 603, New York, NY, 10038, (212) 668-1000, http://www.iverfoundation.org.

Maureen Haggerty
Melinda Granger Oberleitner, RN,
DNS, APRN, CNS

Cholesterol test

Definition

The cholesterol test is a quantitative analysis of the cholesterol levels in a sample of the patient's blood. Total serum cholesterol (TC) is the measurement routinely taken. Doctors sometimes order a complete lipoprotein profile to better evaluate the risk for **atherosclerosis** (**coronary artery disease**, or CAD). The full lipoprotein profile also includes measurements of triglyceride levels (a chemical compound that forms 95% of the fats and oils stored in animal or vegetable cells) and lipoproteins (high density and low density). Blood fats also are called "lipids." It is estimated that more than 200 million cholesterol tests are performed each year in the United States.

The type of cholesterol in the blood is as important as the total quantity. Cholesterol is a fatty substance and cannot be dissolved in water. It must combine with a protein molecule called a lipoprotein in order to be transported in the blood. There are five major types of lipoproteins in the human body; they differ in the amount of cholesterol that they carry in comparison to other fats and fatty acids, and in their functions in the body. Lipoproteins are classified, as follows, according to their density:

- Chylomicrons. These are normally found in the blood only after a person has eaten foods containing fats. They contain about 7% cholesterol. Chylomicrons transport fats and cholesterol from the intestine into the liver, then into the bloodstream. They are metabolized in the process of carrying food energy to muscle and fat cells.

- Very low-density lipoproteins (VLDL). These lipoproteins carry mostly triglycerides, but they also contain 16–22% cholesterol. VLDLs are made in the liver and eventually become IDL particles after they have lost their triglyceride content.

- Intermediate-density lipoproteins (IDL). IDLs are short-lived lipoproteins containing about 30% cholesterol that are converted in the liver to low-density lipoproteins (LDLs).

- Low-density lipoproteins (LDL). LDL molecules carry cholesterol from the liver to other body tissues. They contain about 50% cholesterol. Extra LDLs are absorbed by the liver and their cholesterol is excreted into the bile. LDL particles are involved in the formation of plaques (abnormal deposits of cholesterol) in the walls of the coronary arteries. LDL is known as "bad cholesterol."

- High-density lipoproteins (HDL). HDL molecules are made in the intestines and the liver. HDLs are about 50% protein and 19% cholesterol. They help to remove cholesterol from artery walls. Lifestyle changes, including exercising, keeping weight within recommended limits, and giving up smoking can increase the body's levels of HDL cholesterol. HDL is known as "good cholesterol."
- Lipoprotein subclasses. By identifying levels of multiple subclasses of lipid abnormalities, physicians can do a better job of prescribing lipid-lowering therapies, particularly in high-risk patients such as those with type 2 diabetes.

Because of the difference in density and cholesterol content of lipoproteins, two patients with the same total cholesterol level can have very different lipid profiles and different risk for CAD. The critical factor is the level of HDL cholesterol in the blood serum. Some doctors use the ratio of the total cholesterol level to HDL cholesterol when assessing the patient's degree of risk. A low TC/HDL ratio is associated with a lower degree of risk.

Purpose

The purpose of the TC test is to measure the levels of cholesterol in the patient's blood. The patient's cholesterol also can be fractionated (separated into different portions) in order to determine the TC/HDL ratio. The results help the doctor assess the patient's risk for coronary artery disease (CAD). High LDL levels are associated with increased risk of CAD whereas high HDL levels are associated with relatively lower risk.

In addition, the results of the cholesterol test can assist the doctor in evaluating the patient's metabolism of fat, or in diagnosing inflammation of the pancreas, **liver disease**, or disorders of the thyroid gland.

The frequency of cholesterol testing depends on the patient's degree of risk for CAD. People with low cholesterol levels may need to be tested once every five years. People with high levels of blood cholesterol should be tested more frequently, according to their doctor's advice. The doctor may recommend a detailed evaluation of the different types of lipids in the patient's blood. It is ideal to check the HDL and **triglycerides** as well as the cholesterol and LDL. In addition, the National Cholesterol Education Program (NCEP) suggests further evaluation if the patient has any of the symptoms of CAD or if she or he has two or more of the following risk factors for CAD:

- high blood pressure
- smoking
- diabetes
- low HDL levels
- family history of CAD before age 55

The necessity of widespread cholesterol screening is a topic with varying responses. In 2003, a report demonstrated that measuring the cholesterol of everyone at age 50 years was a simple and efficient way to identify those most at risk for heart disease from among the general population.

Precautions

Patients who are seriously ill or hospitalized for surgery should not be given cholesterol tests because the results will not indicate the patient's normal cholesterol level. Acute illness, high **fever**, **starvation**, or recent surgery lowers blood cholesterol levels.

Description

A pharmaceutical corporation announced in the spring of 2004 that it had received an application to patent a device that could use saliva to determine cholesterol levels. If the test becomes available, it could make screening much more convenient and accessible.

The cholesterol test requires a sample of the patient's blood. **Fasting** before the test is required to get an accurate triglyceride and LDL level. The blood is withdrawn by the usual vacuum tube technique from one of the patient's veins. The blood test takes between three and five minutes.

Preparation

Patients who are scheduled for a lipid profile test should fast (except for water) for 12–14 hours before the blood sample is drawn. If the patient's cholesterol is to be fractionated, he or she also should avoid alcohol for 24 hours before the test.

Patients also should stop taking any medications that may affect the accuracy of the test results. These include **corticosteroids**, estrogen or androgens, **oral contraceptives**, some **diuretics**, haloperidol, some **antibiotics**, and niacin. Antilipemics are drugs that lower the concentration of fatty substances in the blood. When these are taken by the patient, blood testing may be done frequently to evaluate the liver function as well as lipids. The patient's doctor will give the patient a list of specific medications to be discontinued before the test.

Aftercare

Aftercare includes routine care of the skin around the needle puncture. Most patients have no aftereffects, but some may have a small bruise or swelling. A washcloth soaked in warm water usually relieves discomfort. In addition, the patient should resume taking any prescription medications that were discontinued before the test.

Risks

The primary risk to the patient is a mild stinging or burning sensation during the venipuncture, with minor swelling or bruising afterward.

Normal results

The "normal" values for serum lipids depend on the patient's age, sex, and race. Normal values for people in Western countries were once presumed to be 140–220 mg/dL in adults, although as many as 5% of the population has TC higher than 300 mg/dL. Among Asians, the figures are about 20% lower. As a rule, both TC and LDL levels rise as people get older. However, in 2001, the NCEP released stricter guidelines for LDL and total cholesterol.

Some doctors prefer to speak of "desired" rather than "normal" cholesterol values, on the grounds that "normal" refers to statistically average levels that may still be too high for good health. The NCEP has outlined the levels according to desirable and risk:

- Optimal LDL cholesterol: less than 100 mg/dL and total cholesterol less than 160 mg/dL
- Desirable LDL cholesterol: 100–129 mg/dL; total cholesterol 160–199 mg/dL
- Borderline high risk: LDL cholesterol 130–159 mg/dL; total cholesterol 200–239 mg/dL
- High risk: LDL cholesterol greater than 160 mg/dL; total cholesterol greater than or at 240 mg/dL.

Abnormal results

It is possible for blood cholesterol levels to be too low as well as too high.

Abnormally low levels

TC levels less than 160 mg/dL are associated with higher mortality rates from **cancer**, liver disease, respiratory disorders, and injuries. The connection between unusually low cholesterol and increased mortality is not clear, although some researchers think

that the low level is a secondary sign of the underlying disease and not the cause of disease or **death**.

Low levels of serum cholesterol are also associated with **malnutrition** or **hyperthyroidism**. Further diagnostic testing may be necessary in order to locate the cause.

Abnormally high levels

Prior to 1980, **hypercholesterolemia** (an abnormally high TC level) was defined as any value above the 95th percentile for the population. These figures ranged from 210 mg/dL in persons younger than 20 to more than 280 mg/dL in persons older than 60. It is now known, however, that TC levels over 200 mg/dL are associated with significantly higher risk of CAD. Levels of 280 mg/dL or more are considered elevated. Treatment with diet and medication has proven to successfully lower risk of **heart attack** and **stroke**.

Elevated cholesterol levels also may result from hepatitis, blockage of the bile ducts, disorders of lipid metabolism, **nephrotic syndrome**, inflammation of the pancreas, or **hypothyroidism**.

Resources

PERIODICALS

Capriotti, Teri. "Stricter Cholesterol Guidelines Broaden Implications for the 'Statin' Drugs." *MedSurg Nursing* February 2003: 51–57.

"Cholesterol Test at Age 50 Spots Those in Greatest Danger." *Heart Disease Weekly* July 27, 2003: 3.

"Company Wins U.S. Patent for Saliva Cholesterol Test." *Heart Disease Weekly* May 23, 2004: 66.

"Study Shows Expanded Cholesterol Test Sparked Use of Lipid-lowering Therapy." *Heart Disease Weekly* July 13, 2003: 20.

Rebecca J. Frey, PhD
Teresa G. Odle

Cholesterol, high

Definition

Cholesterol is a waxy substance made by the liver and also acquired through diet. It is found in the blood and in all cells in the body. The body uses cholesterol to produce bile, some hormones, vitamin D, cell membranes, and myelin (the material that surrounds nerves). A high level of cholesterol in the blood is called **hypercholesterolemia**. High levels of blood cholesterol have been linked to heart disease.

Description

Cholesterol in small quantities is necessary for the body to function properly, but the liver is able to synthesize about 1,000 mg of cholesterol a day, which is all the body needs. However, because cholesterol is found in animal products— meat, fish, shellfish, egg yolks, and dairy products—people also get cholesterol through their diet, and too much cholesterol can be harmful.

Cholesterol does not dissolve in blood. Instead it moves through the circulatory system in combination with carrier substances called lipoproteins. There are

Cholesterol levels

Total cholesterol

<200 mg/dL	Desirable (lowers the risk of developing coronary heart disease)
200 to 239 mg/dL	Borderline high
≥240 mg/dL	High (more than doubles the risk of developing coronary heart disease)

HDL ("good") cholesterol

Men: <40 mg/dL	
Women: <50 mg/dL	Low (major risk factor for heart disease)
≥60 mg/dL	High (considered protective against heart disease)

LDL ("bad") cholesterol

<100 mg/dL	Optimal
100 to 129 mg/dL	Near optimal
130 to 159 mg/dL	Borderline high
160 to 189 mg/dL	High
≥190 mg/dL	Very high

Triglycerides

<150 mg/dL	Normal
150 to 199 mg/dL	Borderline high
200 to 499 mg/dL	High
≥ 500 mg/dL	Very high

SOURCE: American Heart Association, "What Your Cholesterol Levels Mean." Available online at: http://www.heart.org/HEARTORG/Conditions/Cholesterol/AboutCholesterol/What-Your-Cholesterol-Levels-Mean_UCM_305562_Article.jsp (accessed August 12, 2010).

(Table by PreMediaGlobal. Reproduced by permission of Gale, a part of Cengage Learning.)

two carrier-cholesterol combinations, low-density lipoprotein (LDL) or "bad" cholesterol and high-density lipoprotein or "good" cholesterol.

Most of the cholesterol in the body is LDL cholesterol. An excessive amount of LDL cholesterol is a major contributing factor to the development of heart disease. LDL picks up cholesterol in the liver and carries it through the circulatory system. When too much LDL cholesterol is present, it begins to drop out of the blood and stick to the walls of the arteries. The sticky material on artery walls is called plaque. (It is different from dental plaque that accumulates on teeth.) Plaque can reduce the amount of blood flowing through the arteries, and when bits of plaque break open, they can stimulate the formation of **blood clots**. If plaque or a blood clot block the coronary arteries that carry blood to the heart, **heart attack** (myocardial infarction) can occur. A **stroke** occurs if arteries carrying blood to the brain are blocked. In adults, a desirable LDL reading is less than 100 mg/dL.

High-density lipoprotein (HDL) or "good" cholesterol appears to carry excess LDL cholesterol away from the walls of the arteries to the liver where it can be processed and removed from the body. High levels of HDL cholesterol are helpful; they seem to help protect the body from heart disease and heart attack. Low levels seem to increase the risk of heart disease. In adults, a desirable level of HDL is greater than 60 mg/dL.

A desirable total cholesterol level (LDL + HDL) is less than 200 mg/dL. According to the United States Centers for Disease Control and Prevention (CDC), the average total cholesterol level in American adults is 203 mg/dL, and 17% of Americans over age 20 have total cholesterol levels of 240 mg/dL or higher. This percentage has decreased from a high of 33% in 1960 as people have become more aware of the connection between high cholesterol levels and heart disease.

Specific risk factors include a high-fat, high-calorie diet, family history of high cholesterol, **obesity**, **alcoholism**, and lack of regular **exercise**. Because cholesterol also is produced naturally in the liver, overproduction may occur in even in people who limit their intake of high-cholesterol food. The chance of developing high cholesterol increases after the age of 45, ans women are at higher risk of for developing high cholesterol levels than men. Both genetic inheritance and lifestyle factors affect cholesterol level.

Causes and symptoms

There are no readily apparent symptoms that indicate high LDL or low HDL cholesterol levels. The only way to determine cholesterol levels is through a simple blood test. According to the CDC, almost 75% of Americans reported in 2005 that they had had their cholesterol level checked within the previous five years.

Diagnosis

High cholesterol often is diagnosed from blood tests that are part of a routine **physical examination**. The condition usually is treated by general practitioners or family practice physicians unless other conditions concerns complicate the patient's health status. Total cholesterol, LDL, HDL, and **triglycerides** (another type of blood fat that plays a role in heart disease) are measured by a blood test called a lipid panel. The cost of a lipid panel is moderate and routinely is covered by health insurance and HMO plans, including Medicare. Home cholesterol testing kits are sold over the counter (without prescription), but these test only for total cholesterol. The results of a home test should be used only as a guide, and if the total cholesterol level is high, a physician should perform a lipid panel. The generally recommended levels of LDL, HDL, and total cholesterol are listed in the

previous table. However, physician recommendations for individuals may vary depending on the individual's risk factors such as **hypertension** (high blood pressure), a family history of heart disease, current heart disease, diabetes, age, alcoholism, and **smoking**.

Treatment

Treatment normally begins with lifestyle changes unless the individual already has heart disease and/or has high cholesterol and additional risk factors. In such situations drug therapy may begin at the same time lifestyle changes are implemented. Drug therapy is not a substitute for lifestyle changes; the two must be used together to effectively reduce blood cholesterol levels.

Lifestyle changes

The main lifestyle changes used to treat high cholesterol are diet, exercise, weight loss, and stopping smoking. The National Heart, Lung, and Blood Institute has developed a diet called the Therapeutic Lifestyle Changes (TLC) diet designed to help lower cholesterol and control weight. TLC diet recommendations include the following:

- Fewer than 7% of daily total calories should come from saturated fat.
- No more than 25–35% of total daily calories should come from any type of fat.
- Daily intake of cholesterol should be no more than 200 mg. (In 2007, the average American man ate 337 mg of cholesterol daily and the average woman ate 217 mg daily.)
- Daily sodium intake should be no more than 2,400 mg.
- Daily total calories should be limited to what will maintain or reduce weight.

In addition to reducing cholesterol and fat, increasing the amount of fiber in the diet helps lower total blood cholesterol. High-fiber foods include products made with whole wheat (e.g., pasta, bread), brown rice, lentils, dried beans, and raw vegetables (e.g., celery, carrots, apples, pears). In the United States, food labels are required to list in the **nutrition** information panel calories, calories from fat, total fat, saturated fat, *trans* fat, cholesterol, **sodium**, total carbohydrates, dietary fiber, sugars, protein, vitamin A, vitamin C, **calcium**, and iron. In addition, the following words have specific legal meanings on food labels.

- Cholesterol-free: Less than 2 mg of cholesterol and 2 g of saturated fat per serving.
- Low cholesterol: no more than 20 mg of cholesterol and 2 grams of saturated fat per serving.

- Fat-free: less than 0.5 grams of fat per serving.
- Low fat: no more than 3 grams or less of fat per serving.
- Less fat: A minimum of 25% less fat than the comparison food.
- Light (fat): A minimum of 50% less fat than the comparison food.

A calculator that factors in height, weight, age, and activity level to determine an individualized daily calorie and fats level can be found at http://www.nhlbisupport.com/cgi-bin/chd1/step2intro.cgi.

A vegetarian or vegan diet also may be effective in lowering cholesterol, since most cholesterol comes from eating cholesterol-containing animal products, which are reduced (vegetarian) or eliminated (vegan) in these **diets**. Vegetarians typically get up to 100% more fiber and up to 50% less cholesterol from food than non-vegetarians. The vegetarian low-cholesterol diet consists of at least six servings of whole grain foods, three or more servings of green leafy vegetables, two to four servings of fruit, two to four servings of legumes, and one or two servings of non-fat dairy products daily.

Exercise also is an important part of lowering LDL cholesterol and raising HDL cholesterol. Ideally, exercise should consist of 20–30 minutes of vigorous aerobic exercise (e.g., fast walking, bicycling, jogging, roller skating, swimming, walking up stairs) at least three times a week. Nevertheless, any regular exercise is helpful, especially for overweight individuals. Individuals should not avoid exercising simply because they cannot meet the ideal exercise regimen. Instead, they should make gentle exercise a part of their regular daily routine, gradually working up to more vigorous, sustained exercising.

Drug therapy

A variety of drugs may be prescrived to reduce cholesterol levels. All of these drugs have side effects that may make them unsuitable for certain individuals. Cholesterol-lowering medications include:

- Statins. These are the most frequently prescribed cholesterol-lowering class of drugs. Statins are effective in lowering LDL (bad) cholesterol by slowing the production of cholesterol in the body. However, some statins have been shown to cause a rare type of serious muscle damage (rhabdomyolysis). Other research suggests that statins benefit only to those at high risk for heart attack and not people at low to moderate risk. Examples of statins include atorvastatin (Lipitor), fluvastatin (Lescol), lovastatin (Altocor, Mevacor), pravastatin (Pravachol), and simvastatin (Zocor).

- Bile acid sequestrants, also called resins. These drugs increase the amount of bile excreted in feces. This forces the liver to make more bile, and since cholesterol is used in making bile, more cholesterol is used and less enters the bloodstream, thus lowering cholesterol levels. Bile acid sequestrants are prescribed along with other cholesterol-lowering drugs such as statins. Examples include acid sequestrants include cholestyramine (Prevalite, Questran), colesevelam (Welchol), and colestipol (Colestid).

- Niacin (nicotinic acid.) A dietary supplement that should be used only under supervision of a physician. It helps to lower LDL cholesterol.

- Cholesterol absorption inhibitors. These drugs reduce the amount or cholesterol in food that is absorbed by the intestines. Examples include Ezetimibe (Zetia) and a combination of ezetimibe and the statin simvastatin (Vytorin).

- Fibrates also called fibric acid derivatives. These mainly lower triglycerides, but also may raise HDL (good) cholesterol. They rarely used alone to treat high cholesterol. Examples include gemfibrozil (Loprid), clofibrate (Atromid-S), and fenofibrate (Tricor).

Alternative treatment

Alternative practitioners also recommend diet and exercise as first-line treatment to lower high cholesterol levels. Some herbal supplements are also recommended by alternative practitioners to reduce cholesterol levels. Individuals using any herbal remedy or alternative therapy should discuss its use with a physician. Harmful interactions between herbal remedies and conventional medicines are possible. The following are some of the alternative therapies that have been investigated.

- Garlic. As of 2009, the National Center for Complementary and Alternative Medicine (NCCAM) reported several studies that have shown short term (up to 3 months) reduction in total blood cholesterol levels when garlic (standardized dehydrated tablets, aged garlic extract, oil macerates, distillates, raw garlic) was compared to placebo treatments, but these reductions were not found in longer (6 month) studies. Research is ongoing to clarify these results.

- Soy. According to NCCAM, research suggests that soy may slightly lower levels of LDL cholesterol.

- Green tea. Some alternative practitioners suggest that green tea can lower LDL cholesterol. NCCAM finds that there is not yet enough reliable data to evaluate this claim.

- Red clover, grape seed extract, flaxseed oil, blue-green algae. Although these may be recommended by alternative practitioners, there is little evidence that they affect cholesterol levels.

- Cholestin (red yeast rice). This dietary supplement is a processed form of red yeast fermented with rice. It is a remedy used for centuries in traditional Chinese medicine. Cholestin is not approved or regulated by the United States Food and Drug Administration (FDA). It may reduce LDL cholesterol and increase HDL cholesterol, but should not be taken in place of prescription cholesterol-lowering drugs. Before using, discuss this supplement cholestrin with a physician.

Prognosis

High cholesterol is a major risk factor for heart disease. Left untreated, too much LDL cholesterol may clog the blood vessels, leading to chest **pain (angina)**, blood clots, and heart attacks. By reducing LDL and total cholesterol levels, people with heart disease may prevent further heart attacks and strokes, prolong and improve their quality of life, and slow or reverse cholesterol build up in the arteries. In people without heart disease, lowering cholesterol levels may decrease the risk of a first heart attack or stroke.

Prevention

The habit of eating a low-fat, low-cholesterol, high-fiber diet and regular exercise is the healthiest and least expensive way control cholesterol levels and reduce the risk of heart disease. Other preventative measures include not smoking, limiting alcohol consumption, and maintaining an optimal weight. In a small 2003 Canadian study, people who ate a low-fat vegetarian diet consisting of foods that are found to help lower cholesterol dropped their levels of LDL cholesterol as much as some individuals taking statin drugs. For people with high risk factors for heart disease or pre-existing heart disease, such as a family history of heart disease, diabetes, and being over the age of 45, cholesterol-lowering medication may be effective. However, as of 2009, there was some question about whether these drugs had a preventative

---

KEY TERMS

Dietary supplement—A product, such as a vitamin, mineral, herb, amino acid, or enzyme, that is intended to be consumed in addition to an individual's diet with the expectation that it will improve health.

Feces—The solid waste that is left after digestion. Feces form in the intestines and leave the body through the anus.

Fiber—Also known as roughage or bulk. Insoluble fiber moves through the digestive system almost undigested and gives bulk to stools. Soluble fiber dissolves in water and helps keep stools soft.

Hypertension—Abnormally high blood pressure in the arteries.

Placebo—A pill or liquid given during the study of a drug or dietary supplement that contains no medication or active ingredient. Usually study participants do not know if they are receiving a pill containing the drug or an identical-appearing placebo.

Triglycerides—A type of fat found in the blood. High levels of triglycerides can increase the risk of coronary artery disease.

---

effect in individuals with no pre-existing heart disease and low to moderate risk.

Resources

BOOKS

American Heart Association.*American Heart Association Low–Fat, Low–Cholesterol Cookbook: Delicious Recipes to Help Lower Your Cholesterol*. 3rd ed. New York: Clarkson Potter, 2004.

OTHER

"Cholesterol." *MedlinePlus*. February 3, 2009 [cited February 6, 2009]. http://www.nlm.nih.gov/medlineplus/cholesterol. html

"High Blood Cholesterol." *National Heart, Lung, and Blood Institute*. September 2008 [cited February 6, 2009]. http://www.nhlbi.nih.gov/health/dci/Diseases/Hbc/HBC_WhatIs.html

"Introducing the TLC Diet." *national Heart, Lung, and Blood Institute*. [cited February 9, 2009]. http://www.nhlbisupport.com/cgi-bin/chd1/step2intro.cgi

"Nutrition Fact Sheet: Dietary Cholesterol." *Northwestern University Feinberg School of Medicine*. July 28, 2007 [cited February 6, 2009]. http://www.feinberg.northwestern.edu/nutrition/factsheets/cholesterol.html

ORGANIZATIONS

American Dietetic Association, 120 S. Riverside Plaza, Suite 2000, Chicago, IL, 60606-6995, (312) 899-0040, 800 877-1600, http://www.eatright.org/.

American Heart Association National Center, 7272 Greenville Avenue, Dallas, TX, 75231, (800) 242-8721, Review.personal.info@heart.org.

National Cholesterol Education Program. National Heart, Lung, and Blood Information Center, P.O. Box 30105, Bethesda, MD, 30105, (301) 592-8573, (240) 629-3246, nhlbiinfo@nhlbi.nih.gov, http://www.nhlbi.nih.gov/about/ncep.

Ken R. Wells
Teresa G. Odle
Tish Davidson, A.M.

Cholesterol-reducing drugs

Definition

Cholesterol-reducing drugs belong to a group of medicines that reduce the amount of cholesterol (a fat-like substance) in the blood.

Purpose

Drugs in this group are used as part of a comprehensive treatment program of cholesterol management that includes diet, physical activity, and weight control to reduce the risks of heart attacks and strokes.

Description

There are four classes of cholesterol lowering drugs: bile acid sequesterants, HMG-CoA inhibitors, fibric acid derivatives, and miscellaneous.

Examples of bile acid sequesterants include cholestyramine (Questran); colestipol (Colestid); and colesevalam (Welchol). These drugs act by binding with bile in the intestine to block the digestion of fats and increase the excretion of cholesterol in the stool.

HMG-CoA inhibitors are called statins. Examples include atorvastatin (Lipitor), cerivastatin (Baycol), fluvastatin (Lescol), lovastatin (Mevacor), pravastatin (Pravachol), simvastatin (Zocor), and rosuvastatin (Crestor). These drugs block a liver enzyme involved in producing cholesterol.

The class of fibric acid derivatives includes clofibrate (Atromid-S); gemfibrozil (Lopid); and fenofibrate (Tricor). These drugs may act by reducing the ability of the liver to make cholesterol.

Niacin, vitamin B_3, is a miscellaneous cholesterol reducing drug. It reduces the ability of the liver to make cholesterol. Exetimibe (Zetia) is also a miscellaneous drug. It acts by blocking the absorption of cholesterol from the intestine.

Sometimes drugs are combined together from more than one class.

Recommended dosage

The dose of drug depends on the type of drug used. The prescribing physician or the pharmacist who filled the prescription can advise about the correct dosage.

Precautions

Periodic blood tests are usually done to check cholesterol and liver enzyme levels.

Drugs in this group are part of a comprehensive treatment program for managing cholesterol and the risk of **heart attack** and **stroke**, including diet, physical activity and weight management.

People over 60 years of age may be more sensitive to the side/adverse effects of some cholesterol-reducing drugs.

Anyone taking statins should notify health care professionals before having surgery or receiving emergency treatment in order to reduce the risk of side/adverse effects from additional drugs used at those times.

ALLERGIES. Anyone who has had unusual reactions to cholesterol-reducing drugs in the past should inform prescribing physicians before taking the drugs again. Prescribers should be told about **allergies** to foods, dyes, preservatives or other substances.

PREGNANCY. Statins should not be taken by women who are pregnant as they may interfere with normal fetal development.

Bile sequesterants may interfere with the ability of pregnant women to absorb fat soluble **vitamins** necessary for normal fetal growth and development.

BREASTFEEDING. Because Questran, Welchol and Colestid interfere with the absorption of vitamins, women who use these drugs while **breastfeeding** should ask their physicians about taking vitamin supplements.

Women who are breastfeeding should talk to their physicians before using Lopid. Whether this drug passes into breast milk is not known. But because animal studies suggest that it may increase the risk of some types of **cancer**, women should carefully consider the safety of using it while breastfeeding.

Statins enter breast milk and should not be used by women who are breastfeeding their babies.

OTHER MEDICAL CONDITIONS. Cholesterol-reducing drugs may make some medical problems worse. Before using these drugs, people with any of these medical conditions should make sure their physicians are aware of their conditions:

- stomach or liver problems, including stomach ulcer
- constipation
- hemorrhoids
- gallstones or gallbladder disease
- bleeding problems
- underactive thyroid

People with kidney or **liver disease** may be more likely to have blood problems or other side effects when they take certain cholesterol-reducing drugs. Some drugs of this type may actually raise cholesterol levels in people with liver disease.

Patients with any of the following medical conditions may develop problems that could lead to kidney failure if they take statins:

- organ transplant anti rejection medications
- recent major surgery
- seizures (convulsions) that are not well controlled

People with **phenylketonuria** (PKU) should be aware that sugar-free formulations of some cholesterol-reducing drugs contain phenylalanine.

USE OF CERTAIN MEDICINES. Cholesterol-reducing drugs may change the effects of other medicines. Patients should not take any other medicine that has not been prescribed or approved by a physician who knows they are taking cholesterol-reducing drugs.

Side effects

Lopid, Tricor, and Clofibrate

Adverse effects from these drugs include upset stomach, **nausea, vomiting** or **diarrhea, constipation, headache, fatigue, dizziness**, and skin rash.

Statins

Adverse effects from these drugs include headache; chest, back, and leg **pain**, cramps and weakness; swollen legs and feet; upset stomach, abdominal pain, and diarrhea or constipation.

Questran, Welchol, and Colestid

Adverse effects from these drugs include **heartburn**, upset stomach, nausea, **vomiting**, constipation, headache.

Zetia

Adverse effects from Zetia include fatigue and back and leg cramps, weakness and pain.

Niacin

Adverse effects from niacin include **palpitations**, irregular heart beat, flushed feeling of the skin, and dizziness.

Interactions

Lopid, Tricor, and Clofibrate

These drugs increase the blood thinning effects of warfarin (Coumadin).

These drugs increase the weakness and muscle damage, adverse effects, of statins. They should not be taken together.

statins

Antifungal drugs, Diflucan, Sporanoz and Nizoral increase the adverse effects of statins on muscles.

Lopid, Triccor, and Clofibrate decrease the effectiveness of statins and increase the risk of adverse muscle effects.

The antiseizure medicine Tegretol reduces the effectiveness of statins.

Cyclosporine, used to prevent organ rejection, increases the effectiveness and risk of adverse muscle effects of statins.

Diltiazem (Cardizem) increases the effects and risks of adverse muscle effects of statins.

Grapefruit juice increases the effects and risks of adverse muscle effects of statins.

The erythromycin family of **antibiotics** increases the risks of adverse muscle effects of statins.

Antiretroviral drugs used to treat **AIDS** may increase the risks of adverse muscle effects of statins.

Drugs used to treat **tuberculosis** may reduce the effectiveness of statins

Verapamil (Calan) may increase the effects and risks of adverse muscle effects of statins

Questran, Welchol, and Colestid

These drugs decrease the effectiveness of cortisone drugs.

These drugs decrease the effectiveness of statins.

Taking some cholesterol-reducing drugs with blood thinners (anticoagulants) may increase the chance of bleeding.

Combining statins with gemfibrozil, cyclosporine (Sandimmune) or niacin may cause or worsen problems with the kidneys or muscles.

James Waun, MD, RPh

Cholinergic drugs

Definition

Cholinergic drugs are medications that mimic the effects of acetylcholine, the naturally occurring neurotransmitter, on the parasympathetic nervous system.

Purpose

Cholinergic drugs produce the same effects as acetylcholine by stimulating smooth muscle contractions in the intestinal tract and bladder, dilating blood vessels, constricting bronchioles (breathing tubes), increasing production of saliva, mucus, sweat, and tears, and constricting the pupils in the eyes.

Cholinergic blockers (described elsewhere) are drugs that indirectly produce similar effects as cholinergic drugs by inhibiting the action of the naturally occurring enzyme, acetylcholinesterase, that inactivates acetylcholine.

Some cholinergic drugs, including edrophonium (Tensilon), neostigmine (Prostigmine), and piridogstimina (Mestinon) are used to improve muscle function in diagnosing and treating **myasthenia gravis**, a disease causing skeletal muscular weakness.

Pilocarpine (Isopto, Salagen, Pilopine) is a cholinergic drug that is used as an eye drop to constrict the pupil of the eye(s) to help control glaucoma, a disease caused by increased pressure inside the eye. As a tablet, it is used to counteract **dry mouth** from X-Ray treatments for cancers of the head and neck.

Bethanachol (Urecholine) is a cholinergic drug used to treat non-obstructive urinary retention after surgery and in **neurogenic bladder**.

Description

These drugs are available as capsules, tablets, injections, and eye drops.

KEY TERMS

Cholinergic nerves—Nerves that are stimulated by acetylcholine.

Glaucoma—A disease of the eye with increased pressure that can produce blindness.

Myasthenia gravis—A disease with progressive weakness of skeletal, voluntary muscles.

Parasympathetic nervous system—The part of the nervous system responsible for secretions, skeletal and smooth muscle tone, and slowing heart rate.

Recommended dosage

Physicians prescribe dosage of these drugs depending on the circumstances of individual cases.

Precautions

These drugs should not be used if there is obstruction or weakness in the muscles in the urinary or digestive tracts.

Cholinergic drugs may aggravate **asthma**, peptic ulcer disease, or slow heart beat.

These drugs may aggravate **hyperthyroidism**, parkinsonism, **coronary artery disease**, or low blood pressure.

Adverse effects

Possible adverse effects of cholinergic drugs include:

- slow heart beat and low blood pressure, possibly leading to cardiac arrest.
- flushing of the skin
- muscle cramps, and pain
- nausea, abdominal cramps, and pain
- headache, convulsions
- difficulty breathing
- increased stomach acid and saliva
- urinary urgency

Resources

PERIODICALS

"Classic Papers in Glaucoma." *Archives of Ophthalmology* March 2001.

Samuel D. Uretsky, PharmD
James Waun, MD, RPh

Chondromalacia patellae

Definition

Chondromalacia patellae refers to the progressive erosion of the articular cartilage of the knee joint, that is the cartilage underlying the kneecap (patella) that articulates with the knee joint.

Description

Chondromalacia patellae (CMP), also known as patello-femoral **pain** syndrome or patello-femoral **stress** syndrome, is a syndrome that causes pain/discomfort at the front of the knee. It is associated with irritation or wear on the underside of the kneecap, or patella. In a normal knee, the articular cartilage is smooth and elastic and glides smoothly over the surface of the thighbone, or femur, when the knee is bent. Erosion of the cartilage roughens the surface and prevents this smooth action.

CMP is most common in adolescent females, although older people may also develop it. An average of two out of 10,000 people develop this condition, many of them runners or other athletes.

Causes and symptoms

CMP is the result of the normal **aging** process, overuse, injury, or uneven pressures exerted on the knee joint. In teens, CMP may be caused by uneven growth or uneven strength in the thigh muscles. Growth spurts, common in teens, may result in a mildly abnormal alignment of the patella, which increases the angle formed by the thigh and the patellar tendon (Q-angle). This condition adds to the damage. Symptoms include pain, normally around the kneecap, and a grinding sensation felt when extending the leg. The pain may radiate to the back of the knee, or it may be intermittent and brought on by squatting, kneeling, going up or down stairs, especially down, or by repeated bending of the joint.

Diagnosis

Diagnosis is established during a **physical examination** performed by a general practitioner or an orthopedist, and is based on frequency of symptoms and confirmed by x rays of the knee. The CMP erosion can also be seen on an MRI, although this type of scan is not routinely performed for this purpose. The patient should inform the doctor about any previous injuries to the joint.

Treatment

Initial treatment may consist of resting the knee using crutches, along with **aspirin**, Tylenol, or a nonsteroidal anti-inflammatory drug (NSAID) such as Motrin for seven to 10 days. The person should limit sports activity until the joint is healed and may use ice followed by heat to decrease inflammation. When the doctor allows the patient to resume sports, a knee brace may be prescribed in the form of a stabilizer with a hole at the kneecap.

Treatment also includes low impact exercises to strengthen the quadriceps muscles which help stabilize the knee joint. **Physical therapy** may be suggested at the start of this program so as to help the patient learn the correct method of performing the exercises.

Approximately 85% of people do well with conservative CMP treatment. The remainder still have severe pain and may require **arthroscopic surgery** to repair the tissues inside the knee joint. In more severe cases, open surgery may be required to realign the kneecap and perhaps other corrections.

Alternative treatments

Physical therapy offers treatments that may help CMP patients. Aqua therapy has the benefit of exercising the knee without putting stress on it and it also strengthens the thigh muscles. **Biofeedback** can be used to learn tensing and relaxing specific muscles to relieve pain. These techniques have the benefit of no side effects. **Massage therapy** might be beneficial as well. **Calcium**, **minerals**, and **vitamins** as part of a balanced diet will aid healing and help prevent further problems.

Prognosis

In most teens with CMP, the prognosis is excellent since the damage is reversible when treatment starts before the cartilage begins to break down. With proper treatment and preventive techniques, teenagers will complete their growth without permanent damage to the joint. Only about 15% of patients require surgical intervention. Older people may go on to develop **osteoarthritis** in the knee.

Prevention

Proper exercises are the best preventive measure. Since tightness of thigh muscles is a risk factor, warming up before athletic activities is recommended, as well as participating in a variety of sports rather than just one. Stretching exercises increase flexibility of the quadriceps, hip flexors, and hamstrings. Strengthening exercises such as short arc leg extensions, straight leg raises, quadriceps isometric exercises, and stationary bicycling are also recommended.

Resources

OTHER

Chondromalacia patellae. http://my.webmd.com/content/asset/adam_disease_chondromalacia_patellae.

Chondromalacia Patellae. http://www.orthoseek.com/articles/chondromp.html.

Questions and Answers About Knee Problems. http://www.cbshealthwatch.com/cx/viewarticle/202777.

Questions and Answers About Knee Problems. http://www.nih.gov/niams/healthinfo/kneeprobs/kneeqa.htm.

"What is CAM?" http://nccam.nih.gov/health/whatiscam/overview.htm.

Barbara J. Mitchell

Chorea *see* **Movement disorders**

Choriocarcinoma

Definition

A choriocarcinoma is type of germ cell **cancer** containing trophoblast cells.

Demographics

Choriocarcinoma is a rare tumor type which, in women, develops in one out of every 40 hydatidiform **moles** and in one out of 20,000-40,0000 pregnancies in the United States. The incidence of choriocarcinoma is more prevalent in countries such as India (incidence rate of one in every 500-600 pregnancies), Mexico, Paraguay, and Sweden. African American women have the highest incidence rates of choriocarcinoma and have the lowest survival rates once diagnosed with this cancer. This type of cancer is 5-15 times more likely to be diagnosed in women over the age of 40 than in women under 40 years of age.

Choriocarcinoma that develops in men usually develops as a type of testicular tumor. Choriocarcinoma of the testes is a rare cancer in men. However, this tumor type, which is primarily diagnosed in younger men, is the most common cancer diagnosed in men between the ages of 15-35 years. This cancer affects white males more than males of other racial/ethnic groups.

Description

Choriocarcinomas are cancers that develop from germ cells, cells that ordinarily turn into sperm or eggs. Choriocarcinomas resemble the cells that surround an embryo in the uterus. Most of these cancers form inside the reproductive organs. Some originate in the testes or ovaries, especially in young adults. Others develop in the uterus after a **pregnancy** or miscarriage—particularly following the presence of a **hydatidiform mole**. A few choriocarcinomas arise in sites outside the reproductive organs.

Choriocarcinomas are one of the most dangerous germ cell cancers. They usually grow quickly and spread widely. Occasionally, this cancer grows so fast that the original tumor outgrows its blood supply and dies, leaving behind only a small scar.

Causes and symptoms

Choriocarcinomas result from genetic damage to a germ cell. Males with **Klinefelter syndrome** are especially likely to develop extragonadal **germ cell tumors**.

The symptoms of a choriocarcinoma vary, depending on where the tumor originates and where it spreads. In the uterus, the most common symptom is bleeding. Other symptoms associated with tumors that have metastasized include purple or blue/black nodules on the lower genital tract tissues, abdominal tenderness, and **jaundice** if the tumor has spread to the liver. Cancers in the ovary often have only subtle signs such as widening of the waistline or **pain**.

In the testes, choriocarcinomas can often be felt as small painless lumps.

Choriocarcinomas that spread to other organs may reveal their presence by bleeding. In the brain, this bleeding can cause a **stroke**.

Diagnosis

Examination

Choriocarcinomas are usually referred to an oncologist, a doctor who specializes in cancer treatment. To

KEY TERMS

Biopsy—A sample of an organ taken to look for abnormalities. Also, the technique used to take such samples.

Chemotherapy—The treatment of cancer with drugs.

Computed tomography (CT) scan—A special x-ray technique that produces a cross sectional image of the organs inside the body.

Extragonadal—In a location other than the reproductive organs.

Germ cell—One of the cells that ordinarily develops into eggs or sperm (also sperm and eggs).

Gonads—The ovaries or testes.

Hydatidiform mole—Also called a molar pregnancy. A mass of abnormal, partially developed tissues inside the uterus (womb). Moles develop during a pregnancy that begins with an abnormal fertilization. The mass may or may not be cancerous.

Klinefelter syndrome—A condition caused by extra X chromosome(s) in a male, that results in small testes and infertility together with increased height, decreased facial hair, and sometimes breast enlargement.

Magnetic resonance imaging—A type of study that uses changes induced by magnets to see cells and tissues inside the body.

Ovaries—The female sex organs that make eggs and female hormones.

Remission—The disappearance of the symptoms of cancer, although all of the cancer cells may not be gone.

Reproductive organs—The group of organs (including the testes, ovaries, and uterus) whose purpose is to produce a new individual and continue the species.

Testes—The male sex organs that make sperm and male hormones.

Testicular cancer—A cancer that originates in the testes.

Trophoblast—The tissues that surround an embryo and attach it to the uterus.

Tumor—A lump made up of abnormal cells.

Uterus—The organ where a child develops (womb).

diagnose this tumor, the doctor will do a **physical examination** and examine the internal organs with x rays or ultrasound studies.

Tests

Spreading of the cancer is detected with x rays, ultrasound studies, computed tomography (CT), or **magnetic resonance imaging** (MRI) scans.

Most choriocarcinomas make human chorionic gonadotropin (beta-hCG), a hormone normally found only during pregnancy. The presence of hCG in the blood can help diagnose this cancer and monitor the success of treatment.

Procedures

Choriocarcinomas are not always biopsied before being treated, because they tend to bleed heavily.

Treatment

Women diagnosed with choriocarcinomas that have not metastasized or who are diagnosed with tumors that are of low risk for metastasis are usually treated with the **chemotherapy** agent methotrexate. Another chemotherapy drug, actinomycin D, may be used if the patient has been diagnosed with liver

dysfunction. Beta-hCG levels are monitored to determine response to therapy.

Women diagnosed with metastatic disease are divided into two groups based on whether or not they are at high risk for treatment failure. Patients who are at lower risk are treated with methotrexate or actinomycin and are typically cured with chemotherapy. Women deemed to be at higher risk are treated with combination chemotherapy. Patients with metastasis to the brain also receive whole brain **radiation therapy**. Other patients with brain involvement may be treated with stereotactic radiotherapy. A **hysterectomy** may be required for women who experience vaginal bleeding that cannot be controlled by nonsurgical means.

Currently, there is no consensus as to the best treatment for testicular choriocarinomas. Some chemotherapy agents that may be used include a combination of the drugs bleomycin, etoposide, and cisplatin for four cycles and/or the drugs vinblastine and ifosfamide. However, most choriocarcinomas of the testicles respond poorly to chemotherapy.

Surgery is typically recommended to remove a testicle (or both testicles if cancer has been detected in both) utilizing a surgical procedure termed radical inguinal orchiectomy.

Prognosis

The prognosis for choriocarcinomas in the uterus is very good. Although these tumors often spread throughout the body, chemotherapy results in a cure or remission in 75–100% of cases. The probability of a recurrence of choriocarcinoma in women who have been in remission with normal beta-hCG levels for at least one year is very small, typically less than 1%. Women who have had choriocarcinomas often go on to have normal pregnancies and deliveries.

Choriocarcinomas in other sites have a poorer prognosis. These tumors tend to spread quickly and do not respond well to chemotherapy. Although treatment can be effective, the outcome depends on how widely the cancer has metastasized. The prognosis is worse if the cancer can be found in the liver or brain, if hCG levels are high, or if the original tumor developed outside the gonads.

Choriocarcinomas of the testes metastasize early and typically do not respond to chemotherapy or radiation therapy. These cancers have a dismal prognosis with high mortality rates despite aggressive treatment.

Prevention

There is no known means of prevention. Early detection of the symptoms and prompt medical treatment can improve the odds of survival.

Resources

PERIODICALS

Berney, D.M., et al. "Malignant Germ Cell Tumors in the Elderly: A Histopathological Review of 50 Cases in Men Aged 60 and Over." *Modern Pathology* 21, no. 1 (January 2008): 54–9.

Cole, L.A. "New Discoveries on the Biology and Detection of Human Chorionic Gonadotropin." *Reproductive Biology and Endocrinology* 7 (2009): 8.

Kenny, L., and M.J. Seckl. "Treatments for Gestational Trophoblastic Disease." *Expert Review of Obstetrics and Gynecology* 5, no. 2 (2010): 215–225.

Osborne, R., et al. "A Randomized Phase III Trial Comparing Weekly Parenteral Methotrexate and Pulsed Dactinomycin as Primary Management for Low-risk Gestational Trophoblastic Neoplasia: A Gynecologic Oncology Group Study." *Gynecology and Oncology* 108 (2008): S2–S3.

Smith, H.O., E. Kohorn, and L.A. Cole. "Choriocarcinoma and Gestational Trophoblastic Disease." *Obstetrics and Gynecology Clinics of North America* 32, no. 4 (December 2005): 661–684.

Soper, J.T. "Gestational Trophoblastic Disease." *Obstetrics and Gynecology* 108 (July 2006): 176–87.

OTHER

Hernandez, Enrique. "Gestational Trophoblastic Neoplasia." *eMedicine*. March 16, 2010. http://emedicine.medscape.com/article/279116-overview (accessed October 3, 2010).

Williams, Michael B., Paul Schellhammer, and John W. Davis. "Testicular Choriocarcinoma." *eMedicine*. May 21, 2009. http://emedicine.medscape.com/article/435577-overview (accessed October 3, 2010).

Anna Rovid Spickler, DVM, PhD
Melinda Granger Oberleitner, RN, DNS, APRN, CNS

Chorionic gonadotropin test *see* **Human chorionic gonadotropin pregnancy test**

Chorionic villus sampling

Definition

Chorionic villus sampling (CVS), also known as chorionic villus biopsy, is a prenatal test that can detect genetic and chromosomal abnormalities of a fetus.

Purpose

Chorionic villus sampling is performed on pregnant women who are at risk for carrying a fetus with a genetic or chromosomal defect. Although it carries a slightly higher risk, CVS may be used in place of **amniocentesis** for women who have one or more of the following risk factors:

- women age 35 and older. The chance of having a child with Down syndrome increases with maternal age. For instance, the chance of having a baby with Down syndrome is one in 378 for a 35-year-old woman and increases to one in 30 for a 45-year-old woman.
- a history of miscarriages or children born with birth defects.
- a family history of genetic disease. Prenatal genetic testing is recommended if either the mother or father of the unborn baby has a family history of genetic disease or is known to be a carrier of a genetic disease.

Analysis of the cells from the chorionic villus enables the detection of over 200 diseases and disorders such as **Down syndrome**, **Tay-Sachs disease**, and **cystic fibrosis**. Gross rearrangements of the chromosomes and chromosome additions or losses are detected.

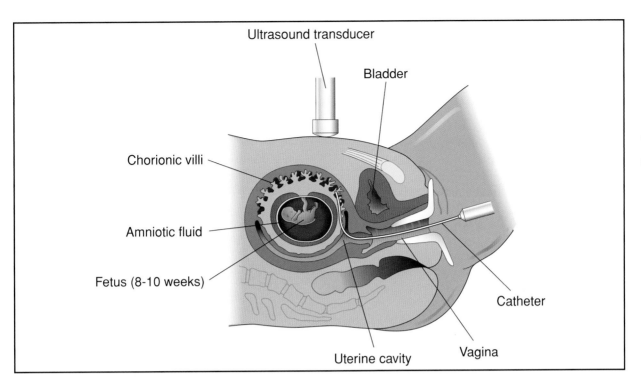

Chorionic villus sampling is performed on pregnant women who are at risk for carrying a fetus with a genetic or chromosomal defect. This procedure can be performed through the vagina and the cervix (transcervically) or through the abdomen (transabdominally). In the transcervical procedure, as depicted above, the physician uses ultrasound to help guide a catheter through the cervix into the uterus. By applying suction from the syringe attached to the other end of the catheter, a small sample of the chorionic villi is obtained. *(Illustration by Electronic Illustrators Group. Reproduced by permission of Gale, a part of Cengage Learning.)*

Description

Chorionic villus sampling has been in use since the 1980s. This prenatal testing procedure involves taking a sample of the chorion frondosum—that part of the chorionic membrane containing the villi—for laboratory analysis. The chorionic membrane is the outer sac that surrounds the developing fetus. Chorionic villi are microscopic, finger-like projections that emerge from the chorionic membrane and eventually form the placenta. The cells that make up the chorionic villi are of fetal origin so laboratory analysis can identify any genetic, chromosomal, or biochemical diseases of the fetus.

Chorionic villus sampling is best performed between 10 and 12 weeks of **pregnancy**. The procedure is performed either through the vagina and the cervix (transcervically) or through the abdomen (transabdominally) depending upon the preferences of the patient or the doctor. In some cases, the location of the placenta dictates which method the doctor uses. Both methods are equally safe and effective. Following the preparation time, both procedures take only about five minutes. Women undergoing chorionic villus

sampling may experience no **pain** at all or feel cramping or pinching. Occasionally, a second sampling procedure must be performed if insufficient villus material was obtained.

For the transcervical procedure, the woman lies on an examining table on her back with her feet in stirrups. The woman's vaginal area is thoroughly cleansed with an antiseptic, a sterile speculum is inserted into her vagina and opened, and the cervix is cleansed with an antiseptic. Using ultrasound as a guide, the doctor inserts a thin, plastic tube called a catheter through the cervix and into the uterus. The passage of the catheter through the cervix may cause cramping. The doctor carefully watches the image produced by the ultrasound and advances the catheter to the chorionic villi. By applying suction from the syringe attached to the other end of the catheter, a small sample of the chorionic villi are obtained. A cramping or pinching feeling may be felt as the sample is being taken. The catheter is then easily withdrawn.

For the transabdominal method, the woman lies on her back on an examining table. Ultrasound enables the doctor to locate the placenta. The specific area on the woman's abdomen is cleansed thoroughly with an antiseptic and a local anesthetic may be injected to numb the area. With ultrasound guidance, a long needle is inserted through the woman's abdominal wall, through the uterine wall and to the chorionic villi. The sample is obtained by applying suction from the syringe.

The chorionic villus sample is immediately placed into nutrient medium and sent to the laboratory. At the laboratory, the sample is examined under the microscope and any contaminating cells or material is carefully removed. The villi can be analyzed immediately, or incubated for a day or more to allow for cell division. The cells are stopped in the midst of cell division and spread onto a microscope slide. Cells with clearly separated chromosomes are photographed so that the type and number of chromosomes can be analyzed. Chromosomes are strings of DNA that have been tightly compressed. Humans have 23 pairs of chromosomes including the sex chromosomes. Rearrangements of the chromosomes or the presence of additional or fewer chromosomes can be identified by examination of the photograph. Down syndrome, for instance, is caused by an extra copy of chromosome 21. In addition to the chromosomal analysis, specialized tests can be performed as needed to look for specific diseases such as Tay-Sachs disease. Depending upon which tests are performed, results may be available as early as two days or up to eight days after the procedure.

Alternate procedures

There are alternate procedures for diagnosing genetic and chromosomal disorders of the fetus. Amniocentesis is commonly used and involves inserting a needle through the pregnant woman's abdomen to obtain a sample of amniotic fluid. Amniocentesis is usually performed in the second trimester at approximately 16 weeks gestation and the laboratory analysis may take two to three weeks. The two advantages of chorionic villus sampling are that it is performed during the first trimester and the results are available in about one week. The risk of **miscarriage** after amniocentesis is 0.5–1% (one to two women out of 200) which is lower than that for chorionic villus sampling (1–3%).

A noninvasive alternative is the maternal blood test called triple marker screening or multiple marker screening. A sample of the pregnant woman's blood is analyzed for three different markers: alphafetoprotein (AFP), human chorionic gonadotropin, and unconjugated estriol. The levels of these three markers in the

mother's blood can identify unborn babies who are at risk for certain genetic or chromosomal defects. This screening test determines the chance that the fetus has the defect, but it cannot diagnose specific defects. A negative test result does not necessarily mean the unborn baby does not have a birth defect. For instance, this screening test can only predict 60–70% of the fetuses with Down syndrome. Pregnant women who have a positive triple marker screen are encouraged to undergo a diagnostic test, such as amniocentesis (by the time an AFP is done, it is too late to perform a CVS).

Benefits

Chorionic villi sampling allows parents of fetuses found to have a genetic defect to determine at an early stage whether to continue or terminate the pregnancy. Should the decision be made to continue the pregnancy, parents will have time to prepare, both physically and psychologically, for parenting a child with disabilities related to a genetic defect.

Precautions

Chorionic villus sampling is not recommended for women who have vaginal bleeding or spotting during the pregnancy. It is not typically recommended for women who have Rh sensitization from a previous pregnancy.

Preparation

Prior to the chorionic villus sampling procedure the woman needs to drink fluids and refrain from urinating to ensure her bladder is full. These preparations create a better ultrasound picture.

Aftercare

It is generally recommended that women undergoing chorionic villus sampling have someone drive them home and have no plans for the rest of the day. Women with Rh negative blood must receive a Rho (D) immune globulin injection following the procedure. Women should call their doctor if they experience excessive bleeding, vaginal discharge, **fever**, or abdominal pain after the procedure.

Risks

Of women who undergo transcervical chorionic villus sampling, one third experience minimal vaginal spotting and 7–10% experience vaginal bleeding. One out of five women experience cramping following the procedure. Two to three women out of 100 (or 2–3%) will miscarry following chorionic villus sampling. The

KEY TERMS

Chorionic villi—Microscopic, finger-like projections that emerge from the outer sac which surrounds the developing baby. Chorionic villi are of fetal origin and eventually form the placenta.

Chromosomes—Human cells carry DNA in tightly compressed rod-like structures called chromosomes. Humans have 23 pairs of chromosomes including the sex chromosomes.

Down syndrome—A chromosomal disorder caused by an extra copy or a rearrangement of chromosome 21. Children with Down syndrome have varying degrees of mental retardation and may have heart defects.

Fetus—Term for an unborn baby after the eighth week of pregnancy. Prior to seven weeks, it is called an embryo.

Rh sensitization—A woman with a negative blood type (Rh negative) who has produced antibodies against her fetus with a positive blood type (Rh positive). The mother's body considered the fetal blood cells a foreign object and mounted an immune attack on it.

Ultrasound—A safe, painless procedure which uses sound waves to visualize internal organs. A wand that transmits and receives the sound waves is moved over the woman's abdomen and internal organs can be seen on a video screen.

risk of infection is very low. Rupture of the amniotic membranes is a rare complication. Women with Rh negative blood may be at an increased risk for developing Rh incompatibility following chorionic villus sampling.

There have been reports of limb defects in babies following chorionic villus sampling. However, in 1996 the World Health Organization reported that the incidence of babies born with limb defects from 138,966 women who had undergone chorionic villus sampling was the same as for women who had not. Therefore, this study found no connection between chorionic villus sampling and limb defects.

Resources

OTHER

Chorionic Villus Sampling. MedicineNet.com. December 13, 2007. http://www.medicinenet.com/chorionic_villus_sampling/article.htm
Chorionic Villus Sampling (CVS). WebMD. May 13, 2008. http://www.webmd.com/baby/chorionic-villus-sampling-cvs
Chorionic Villus Sampling. Mayo Foundation for Medical Education and Research. May 15, 2010. http://www.mayoclinic.com/health/chorionic-villus-sampling/my00154

ORGANIZATIONS

American College of Obstetricians and Gynecologists, P.O. Box 96920, Washington, DC, 20090-6920, (202) 638-5577, http://www.acog.org.
March of Dimes Foundation, 1275 Mamaroneck Avenue, White Plains, NY, 10605, (914) 997-4488, askus@marchofdimes.com, http://www.marchofdimes.com.
National Society of Genetic Counselors, 401 N. Michigan Avenue, Chicago, IL, 60611, (312) 321-6834, (312) 673-6972, nsgc@nsgc.org, http://www.nsgc.org.

Belinda Rowland, PhD
Brenda W. Lerner
Tish Davidson, AM

Choroiditis *see* **Uveitis**

Choroiretinitis *see* **Uveitis**

Chromosome studies *see* **Genetic testing**

Chronic arthritis of childhood *see* **Juvenile arthritis**

Chronic constrictive pericarditis *see* **Pericarditis**

Chronic Epstein-Barr virus *see* **Chronic fatigue syndrome**

Chronic fatigue syndrome

Definition

Chronic **fatigue** syndrome (CFS) is a condition that causes extreme tiredness. People with CFS have debilitating fatigue that lasts for six months or longer. They also have many other symptoms. Some of these are **pain** in the joints and muscles, **headache**, and **sore throat**. CFS does not have a known cause, but appears to result from a combination of factors.

Description

CFS is the most common name for this disorder, but it also has been called chronic fatigue and immune disorder (CFIDS), myalgic encephalomyelitis, low natural killer cell disease, post-viral syndrome, Epstein-Barr disease, and Yuppie flu. CFS has so many names because researchers have been unable to find out exactly what causes it and because there are many similar, overlapping conditions. Reports of a CFS-like syndrome called neurasthenia date back to 1869. Later, people with similar symptoms were said to have fibromyalgia because one of the main symptoms is myalgia, or muscle pain. Because of the similarity of symptoms, fibromyalgia and CFS are considered to be overlapping syndromes.

In the early to mid-1980s, there were outbreaks of CFS in some areas of the United States. Doctors found that many people with CFS had high levels of antibodies to the **Epstein-Barr virus** (EBV), which causes mononucleosis, in their blood. For a while they thought they had found the culprit, but it turned out that many healthy people also had high EBV antibodies. Scientists have also found high levels of other viral antibodies in the blood of people with CFS. These findings have led many scientists to believe that a virus or combination of viruses may trigger CFS.

CFS was sometimes referred to as Yuppie flu because it seemed to often affect young, middle-class professionals. In fact, CFS can affect people of any gender, age, race, or socioeconomic group. Although anyone can get CFS, most patients diagnosed with CFS are 25–45 years old, and about 80% of cases are in women. Estimates of how many people are afflicted with CFS vary due to the similarity of CFS symptoms to other diseases and the difficulty in identifying it. The Centers for Disease Control and Prevention (CDC) has estimated that four to 10 people per 100,000 in the United States have CFS. According to the CFIDS Foundation, about 500,000 adults in the United States (0.3% of the population) have CFS. This probably is a low estimate since these figures do not include children and are based on the CDC definition of CFS, which is very strict for research purposes.

Causes and symptoms

There is no single known cause for CFS. Studies have pointed to several different conditions that might be responsible. These include:

- viral infections
- chemical toxins
- allergies
- immune abnormalities
- psychological disorders

Although the cause is still controversial, many doctors and researchers now think that CFS may not be a single illness. Instead, they think CFS may be a group of symptoms caused by several conditions. One

theory is that a microorganism, such as a virus, or a chemical injures the body and damages the immune system, allowing dormant viruses to become active. About 90% of all people have a virus in the herpes family dormant (not actively growing or reproducing) in their bodies since childhood. When these viruses start growing again, the immune system may overreact and produce chemicals called cytokines that can cause flu-like symptoms. Immune abnormalities have been found in studies of people with CFS, although the same abnormalities are also found in people with **allergies**, autoimmune diseases, **cancer**, and other disorders.

The role of psychological problems in CFS is very controversial. Because many people with CFS are diagnosed with depression and other psychiatric disorders, some experts conclude that the symptoms of CFS are psychological. However, many people with CFS did not have psychological disorders before getting the illness. Many doctors think that patients become depressed or anxious because of the effects of the symptoms of their CFS. One recent study concluded that depression was the result of CFS and was not its cause.

Having CFS is not just a matter of being tired. People with CFS have severe fatigue that keeps them from performing their normal daily activities. They find it difficult or impossible to work, attend school, or even to take part in social activities. They may have sleep disturbances that keep them from getting enough rest or they may sleep too much. Many people with CFS feel just as tired after a full night's sleep as before they went to bed. When they **exercise** or try to be active in spite of their fatigue, people with CFS experience what some patients call "payback"–debilitating exhaustion that can confine them to bed for days.

Other symptoms of CFS include:

- muscle pain (myalgia)
- joint pain (arthralgia)
- sore throat
- headache
- fever and chills
- tender lymph nodes
- trouble concentrating
- memory loss

A recent study at Johns Hopkins University found an abnormality in blood pressure regulation in 22 of 23 patients with CFS. This abnormality, called neurally mediated **hypotension**, causes a sudden drop in blood pressure when a person has been standing, exercising, or exposed to heat for a while. When this occurs, patients feel lightheaded and may faint. They often are exhausted for hours to days after one of these episodes. When treated with salt and medications to stabilize blood pressure, many patients in the study had marked improvements in their CFS symptoms.

Diagnosis

CFS is diagnosed by evaluating symptoms and eliminating other causes of fatigue. Doctors carefully question patients about their symptoms, any other illnesses they have had, and medications they are taking. They also conduct a **physical examination**, neurological examination, and laboratory tests to identify any underlying disorders or other diseases that cause fatigue. In the United States, many doctors use the CDC case definition to determine if a patient has CFS.

To be diagnosed with CFS, patients must meet both of the following criteria:

- Unexplained continuing or recurring chronic fatigue for at least six months that is of new or definite onset, is not the result of ongoing exertion, and is not mainly relieved by rest, and causes occupational, educational, social, or personal activities to be greatly reduced.
- Four or more of the following symptoms: loss of short-term memory or ability to concentrate; sore throat; tender lymph nodes; muscle pain; multi-joint pain without swelling or redness; headaches of a new type, pattern, or severity; unrefreshing sleep; and post-exertional malaise (a vague feeling of discomfort or tiredness following exercise or other physical or mental activity) lasting more than 24 hours. These symptoms must have continued or recurred during six or more consecutive months of illness and must not have started before the fatigue began.

Treatment

There is no cure for CFS, but many treatments are available to help relieve the symptoms. Treatments usually are individualized to each person's particular symptoms and needs. The first treatment most doctors recommend is a combination of rest, exercise, and a balanced diet. Prioritizing activities, avoiding overexertion, and resting when needed are key to maintaining existing energy reserves. A program of moderate exercise helps to keep patients from losing physical conditioning, but too much exercise can worsen fatigue and other CFS symptoms. Counseling and **stress reduction** techniques also may help some people with CFS.

Many medications, **nutritional supplements**, and herbal preparations have been used to treat CFS. While many of these are unproven, others seem to provide some people with relief. People with CFS should discuss their treatment plan with their doctors, and carefully weigh the benefits and risks of each therapy before making a decision.

Drugs

Nonsteroidal anti-inflammatory drugs (NSAIDs), such as ibuprofen and naproxen, may be used to relieve pain and reduce **fever**. Another medication that is prescribed to relieve pain and **muscle spasms** is cyclobenzaprine (sold as Flexeril).

Many doctors prescribe low dosages of antidepressants for their sedative effects and to relieve symptoms of depression. **Antianxiety drugs**, such as **benzodiazepines** or buspirone may be prescribed for excessive anxiety that has lasted for at least six months.

Other medications that have been tested or are being tested for treatment of CFS are:

- Fludrocortisone (Florinef), a synthetic steroid, which is currently being tested for treatment of people with CFS. It causes the body to retain salt, thereby increasing blood pressure. It has helped some people with CFS who have neurally mediated hypotension.
- Beta-adrenergic blocking drugs, often prescribed for high blood pressure. Such drugs, including atenolol (Tenoretic, Tenormin) and propranolol (Inderal), are sometimes prescribed for neurally mediated hypotension.
- Gamma globulin, which contains human antibodies to a variety of organisms that cause infection. It has been used experimentally to boost immune function in people with CFS.
- Ampligen, a drug which stimulates the immune system and has antiviral activity. In one small study, ampligen improved mental function in people with CFS.

Alternative treatment

A variety of nutritional supplements are used for treatment of CFS. Among these are vitamin C, vitamin B_{12}, vitamin A, vitamin E, and various dietary **minerals**. These supplements may help improve immune and mental functions. Several herbs have been shown to improve immune function and have other beneficial effects. Some that are used for CFS are astragalus (*Astragalus membranaceus*), **echinacea** (*Echinacea* spp.), garlic (*Allium sativum*), **ginseng** (*Panax ginseng*), gingko (*Gingko biloba*), evening primrose oil (*Oenothera biennis*), shiitake

KEY TERMS

Arthralgia—Joint pain.

Cytokines—Proteins produced by certain types of lymphocytes. They are important controllers of immune functions.

Depression—A psychological condition, with feelings of sadness, sleep disturbance, fatigue, and inability to concentrate.

Epstein-Barr virus (EBV)—A virus in the herpes family that causes mononucleosis.

Fibromyalgia—A disorder closely related to CFS. Symptoms include pain, tenderness, and muscle stiffness.

Lymph node—Small immune organs containing lymphocytes. They are found in the neck, armpits, groin, and other locations in the body.

Lymphocytes—White blood cells that are responsible for the actions of the immune system.

Mononucleosis—A flu-like illness caused by the Epstein-Barr virus.

Myalgia—Muscle pain.

Myalgic encephalomyelitis—An older name for chronic fatigue syndrome; encephalomyelitis refers to inflammation of the brain and spinal cord.

Natural killer (NK) cell—A lymphocyte that acts as a primary immune defense against infection.

Neurally mediated hypotension—A rapid fall in blood pressure that causes dizziness, blurred vision, and fainting, and is often followed by prolonged fatigue.

Neurasthenia—Nervous exhaustion–a disorder with symptoms of irritability and weakness, commonly diagnosed in the late 1800s.

mushroom extract (*Lentinus edodes*), borage seed oil, and quercetin.

Many people have enhanced their healing process for CFS with the use of a treatment program inclusive of one or more alternative therapies. **Stress** reduction techniques such as **biofeedback**, **meditation**, **acupuncture**, and **yoga** may help people with sleep disturbances relax and get more rest. They also help some people reduce depression and anxiety caused by CFS.

Prognosis

The course of CFS varies widely for different people. Some people get progressively worse over time, while others gradually improve. Some individuals have periods of illness that alternate with periods of good health. While many people with CFS never fully regain their health, they find relief from symptoms and adapt to the demands of the disorder by carefully following a treatment plan combining adequate rest, **nutrition**, exercise, and other therapies.

Prevention

Because the cause of CFS is not known, there currently are no recommendations for preventing the disorder.

Resources

OTHER

"Chronic Fatigue Syndrome." *National Institutes of Health.* http://www.nih.gov.

"The Facts about Chronic Fatigue Syndrome." *Centers for Disease Control.* http://www.cdc.gov/ncidod/diseases/cfs/facts1.htm.

ORGANIZATIONS

National CFIDS Foundation, 103 Aletha Road, Needham, MA, 02492, (781) 449-3535, (781) 449-8606, info@ncf net. org, http://www.ncf-net.org/contact.

National Chronic Fatigue Syndrome and Fibromyalgia Association, PO Box 18426, Kansas City, MO, 64133, (816) 737-1343, http://www.ncfsfa.org.

The CFIDS Association of America, PO Box 220398, Charlotte, NC, 28222-0398, (704) 365-2343, cfids@ cfids.org, http://www.cfids.org.

Toni Rizzo

Chronic granulomatous disease

Definition

Chronic granulomatous disease (CGD) is an inherited disorder in which white blood cells lose their ability to destroy certain bacteria and fungi.

Description

CGD is an X-linked genetic disease, meaning the defective gene is carried on the X chromosome (one of the sex chromosomes). Females have two copies of the

X chromosome, whereas males have one X and one Y. CGD also is a recessive defect meaning that both copies of the chromosome must have the defect before it can be expressed. Females who have one X chromosome without the defect do not get this disease. Males, since they only have one X chromosome, get the disease if the defect is present. Thus, CGD affects mostly males.

CGD is an **immunodeficiency** disorder. Patients with immunodeficiency disorders suffer frequent infections. This happens because part of their immune system isn't working properly and the infectious microorganisms are not killed as rapidly as is normal. In CGD there is a defect in the ability of the white blood cells to kill bacteria and fungi. The white blood cells affected are phagocytic cells. They are part of the non-specific immune system and move via the blood to all parts of the body where they ingest and destroy microbes. Phagocytic cells are the first line of defense against microorganisms. In this disease, the decreased ability to kill microbes that they have ingested leads to a failure to effectively combat infectious diseases. Patients with CGD are subject to certain types of recurring infection, especially those of the skin, lungs, mouth, nose, intestines, and lymph nodes. With the exception of the lymph nodes, all of these areas are considered external tissues that come into contact with microorganisms from the environment. The lymph system drains all areas of the body to eliminate destroyed microorganisms and to assist the immune system in attacking microorganisms. Infections occur in the lymph nodes as a consequence of the normal draining function.

Causes and symptoms

The genetic defect that causes CGD reduces the amount of hydrogen peroxide and superoxide that white blood cells can make. These chemicals are important for killing bacteria and fungi. Without them the white blood cells ingest the microorganisms, but cannot kill them. In some cases, the microbes then replicate inside the white blood cell eventually causing its **death**.

Symptoms of the disease usually appear by age two. Frequent, recurrent infections of the skin, lungs (e.g. **pneumonia**), mouth (e.g. gingivitis), nose, intestines and lymph nodes are a hallmark of this disease. Patients may also develop multiple, recurrent liver abscesses and bone infections (**osteomyelitis**).

Diagnosis

Diagnosis is made based on the observation of a pattern of recurrent infections. Blood tests of lymphocyte

and antibody functions will be normal. Tests of phagocytic cells will show normal ingestion, but a greatly decreased ability to kill bacteria.

Treatment

Early, aggressive treatment of all infections is critical to the successful management of CGD. Patients are treated with **antibiotics** and immune serum. Antibiotics are used at the first sign of infection. Immune serum is a source of antibodies that help fight infections. Interferon gamma is an experimental treatment for CGD that has shown promising results. There is no cure for the underlying cause of chronic granulomatous disease

Prognosis

Although antibiotics can treat most infections and may help prevent others, premature death may result, typically due to repeated lung infections.

Prevention

Since CGD is a hereditary disorder, it cannot currently be prevented. Patients and their families may benefit from **genetic counseling**. Preventive (prophylactic) antibiotics may help keep some infections from occurring, and good hygiene, especially rigorous skin and mouth care, can help prevent infections in these areas. Avoiding crowds or other people who have infections are also effective preventive measures.

ORGANIZATIONS

Chronic Granulomatous Disease Association, 616 Monterey Road, San Marin, CA, 91108-1646, (626) 441-4118, cgda@socal.rr.com, http://www.cgd association.org.

National Organization for Rare Disorders, P.O. Box 8923, New Fairfield, CT, 06812-8923, (800) 999-6673, http://www.rarediseases.org.

John T. Lohr, PhD

Chronic kidney failure

Definition

Chronic kidney failure occurs when disease or disorder damages the kidneys so that they are no longer capable of adequately removing fluids and wastes from the body or of maintaining the proper level of certain kidney-regulated chemicals in the bloodstream.

Description

Chronic kidney failure, also known as chronic renal failure, affects over 250,000 Americans annually. It is caused by a number of diseases and inherited disorders, but the progression of chronic kidney failure is always the same. The kidneys, which serve as the body's natural filtration system, gradually lose their ability to remove fluids and waste products (urea) from the bloodstream. They also fail to regulate certain chemicals in the bloodstream, and deposit protein into the urine. Chronic kidney failure is irreversible, and will eventually lead to total kidney failure, also known as end-stage renal disease (ESRD). Without proper treatment intervention to remove wastes and fluids from the bloodstream, ESRD is fatal.

Causes and symptoms

Kidney failure is triggered by disease or a hereditary disorder in the kidneys. Both kidneys are typically affected. The four most common causes of chronic kidney failure include:

- Diabetes. Diabetes mellitus (DM), both insulin dependant (IDDM) and non-insulin dependant (NIDDM), occurs when the body cannot produce and/or use insulin, the hormone necessary for the body to process glucose. Long-term diabetes may cause the glomeruli, the filtering units located in the nephrons of the kidneys, to gradually lose functioning.
- Glomerulonephritis. Glomerulonephritis is a chronic inflammation of the glomeruli, or filtering units of the kidney. Certain types of glomerulonephritis are treatable, and may only cause a temporary disruption of kidney functioning.
- Hypertension. High blood pressure is unique in that it is both a cause and a major symptom of kidney failure. The kidneys can become stressed and ultimately sustain permanent damage from blood pushing through them at an excessive level of pressure over a long period of time.

- Polycystic kidney disease. Polycystic kidney disease is an inherited disorder that causes cysts to be formed on the nephrons, or functioning units, of the kidneys. The cysts hamper the regular functioning of the kidney.

Other possible causes of chronic kidney failure include **kidney cancer**, obstructions such as **kidney stones**, **pyelonephritis**, reflux nephropathy, **systemic lupus erythematosus**, **amyloidosis**, sickle cell anemia, **Alport syndrome**, and oxalosis.

Initially, symptoms of chronic kidney failure develop slowly. Even individuals with mild to moderate kidney failure may show few symtpoms in spite of increased urea in their blood. Among the symptoms that may be present at this point are frequent urination during the night and high blood pressure.

Most symptoms of chronic kidney failure are not apparent until **kidney disease** has progressed significantly. Common symptoms include:

- Anemia. The kidneys are responsible for the production of erythropoietin (EPO), a hormone which stimulates red cell production. If kidney disease causes shrinking of the kidney, this red blood cell production is hampered.
- Bad breath or a bad taste in mouth. Urea, or waste products, in the saliva may cause an ammonia-like taste in the mouth.
- Bone and joint problems. The kidneys produce vitamin D, which aids in the absorption of calcium and keeps bones strong. For patients with kidney failure, bones may become brittle, and in the case of children, normal growth may be stunted. Joint pain may also occur as a result of unchecked phosphate levels in the blood.
- Edema. Puffiness or swelling around the eyes, arms, hands, and feet.
- Frequent urination.
- Foamy or bloody urine. Protein in the urine may cause it to foam significantly. Blood in the urine may indicate bleeding from diseased or obstructed kidneys, bladder, or ureters.
- Headaches. High blood pressure may trigger headaches.
- Hypertension, or high blood pressure. The retention of fluids and wastes causes blood volume to increase, which in turn, causes blood pressure to rise.
- Increased fatigue. Toxic substances in the blood and the presence of anemia may cause feelings of exhaustion.
- Itching. Phosphorus, which is typically eliminated in the urine, accumulates in the blood of patients with

kidney failure. This heightened phosphorus level may cause itching of the skin.

- Lower back pain. Pain where the kidneys are located, in the small of the back below the ribs.
- Nausea, loss of appetite, and vomiting. Urea in the gastric juices may cause upset stomach. This can lead to malnutrition and weight loss.

Diagnosis

Kidney failure is typically diagnosed and treated by a nephrologist, a doctor that specializes in treating the kidneys. The patient that is suspected of having chronic kidney failure will undergo an extensive blood work-up. A blood test will assess the levels of creatinine, blood urea nitrogen (BUN), uric acid, phosphate, **sodium**, and potassium in the blood. Urine samples will also be collected, usually over a 24-hour period, to assess protein loss.

Uncovering the cause of kidney failure is critical to proper treatment. A full assessment of the kidneys is necessary to determine if the underlying disease is treatable and if the kidney failure is chronic or acute. An x ray, MRI, computed tomography scan, ultrasound, renal biopsy, and/or arteriogram of the kidneys may be employed to determine the cause of kidney failure and level of remaining kidney function. X rays and ultrasound of the bladder and/or ureters may also be taken.

Treatment

Chronic kidney failure is an irreversible condition. Hemodialysis, peritoneal dialysis, or **kidney transplantation** must be employed to replace the lost function of the kidneys. In addition, dietary changes and treatment to relieve specific symptoms such as anemia and high blood pressure are critical to the treatment process.

Hemodialysis

Hemodialysis is the most frequently prescribed type of dialysis treatment in the United States. Most hemodialysis patients require treatment three times a week, for an average of three to four hours per dialysis "run" depending on the type of dialyzer used and their current physical condition. The treatment involves circulating the patient's blood outside of the body through an extracorporeal circuit (ECC), or dialysis circuit. The dialysis circuit consists of plastic blood tubing, a two-compartment filter known as a dialyzer, or artificial kidney, and a dialysis machine that monitors and maintains blood flow and administers dialysate, a chemical bath used to draw waste products out of the blood. The patient's blood leaves and enters the body through two needles inserted into the patient's vein, called an access site, and is pushed through the blood compartment of the dialyzer. Once inside of the dialyzer, excess fluids and toxins are pulled out of the bloodstream and into the dialysate compartment, where they are carried out of the body. At the same time, electrolytes and other chemicals in the dialysate solution move from the dialysate into the bloodstream. The purified, chemically-balanced blood is then returned to the body.

Peritoneal dialysis

In peritoneal dialysis (PD), the patient's peritoneum, or lining of the abdomen, acts as a blood filter. A catheter is surgically inserted into the patient's abdomen. During treatment, the catheter is used to fill the abdominal cavity with dialysate. Waste products and excess fluids move from the patient's bloodstream into the dialysate solution. After a waiting period of six to 24 hours, depending on the treatment method used, the waste-filled dialysate is drained from the abdomen, and replaced with clean dialysate. There are three types of peritoneal dialysis, which vary by treatment time and administration method: Continuous Ambulatory Peritoneal Dialysis (CAPD), Continuous Cyclic Peritoneal Dialysis (CCPD), and Intermittent Peritoneal Dialysis (IPD).

Kidney transplantation

Kidney transplantation involves surgically attaching a functioning kidney, or graft, from a brain dead organ donor (a cadaver transplant), or from a living donor, to a patient with ESRD. Patients with chronic renal disease who need a transplant and don't have a living donor register with UNOS (United Network for Organ Sharing), the federal organ procurement agency, to be placed on a waiting list for a cadaver kidney transplant. Kidney availability is based on the patient's health status. When the new kidney is transplanted, the patient's existing, diseased kidneys may or may not be removed, depending on the circumstances surrounding the kidney failure. A regimen of immunosuppressive, or anti-rejection medication, is required after transplantation surgery.

Dietary management

A diet low in sodium, potassium, and phosphorous, three substances that the kidneys regulate, is critical in managing kidney disease. Other dietary restrictions, such as a reduction in protein, may be prescribed depending on the cause of kidney failure and the type of dialysis treatment employed. Patients with chronic kidney failure also need to limit their fluid intake.

Medications and dietary supplements

Kidney failure patients with **hypertension** typically take medication to control their high blood pressure. Epoetin alfa, or EPO (Epogen), a hormone therapy, and intravenous or oral iron supplements are used to manage anemia. A multivitamin may be prescribed to replace **vitamins** lost during dialysis treatments. Vitamin D, which promotes the absorption of **calcium**, along with calcium supplements, may also be prescribed.

Since 1973, Medicare has picked up 80% of ESRD treatment costs, including the costs of dialysis and transplantation and of some medications. To qualify for benefits, a patient must be insured or eligible for benefits under Social Security, or be a spouse or child of an eligible American. Private insurance and state Medicaid programs often cover the remaining 20% of treatment costs.

Prognosis

Early diagnosis and treatment of kidney failure is critical to improving length and quality of life in chronic kidney failure patients. Patient outcome varies by the cause of chronic kidney failure and the method chosen to treat it. Overall, patients with chronic kidney disease leading to ESRD have a shortened lifespan. According to the United States Renal Data System (USRDS), the lifespan of an ESRD patient is 18–47% of the lifespan of the age-sex-race matched general population. ESRD patients on dialysis have a lifespan that is 16–37% of the general population.

The demand for kidneys to transplant continues to exceed supply. In 1996, over 34,000 Americans were on the UNOS waiting list for a kidney transplant, but only 11,330 living donor and cadaver transplants were actually performed. Cadaver kidney transplants have a 50% chance of functioning nine years, and living donor kidneys that have two matching antigen pairs have a 50% chance of functioning for 24 years. However, some transplant grafts have functioned for over 30 years.

ORGANIZATIONS

American Association of Kidney Patients, 3505 E. Frontage Road, Suite 315, Tampa, FL, 33607, (813) 636-8122, (800) 749-2257, info@aakp.org, http://www.aakp.org.

American Kidney Fund (AKF), 6110 Executive Boulevard, Suite 1010, Rockville, MD, 20852, (800) 638-8299, http://www.kidneyfund.org.

National Kidney Foundation, Inc. , 30 East 33rd Street, New York, NY, 10016, (212) 889-2210, (212) 689-9261, (800) 622-9010, http://www.kidney.org/.

United States Renal Data System (USRDS), 914 South 8th Street, Suite S-206, Minneapolis, MN, 55404, (612) 347-7776, (888) 997-7737, usrds@usrds.org, http://www.usrds.org/.

Paula Anne Ford-Martin

Chronic leukemias *see* **Leukemias, chronic**

Chronic obstructive pulmonary disease

Definition

Chronic obstructive pulmonary disease (COPD) refers to two related, progressive diseases of the respiratory system, chronic **bronchitis** and **emphysema**. Emphysema is the enlargement and destruction of the air sacs (alveoli) of the lungs. Chronic bronchitis is ongoing inflammation that eventual results in narrowing of the airways. These are gradually progressive and permanent disease conditions in which there is persistent difficulty in expelling (exhaling) air from the lungs resulting in loss of lung function. Because **smoking** is the major cause of both diseases, chronic bronchitis and emphysema often occur together in the same individual.

Demographics

Almost all people with COPD are over age 40, and the highest rate of the disease is among those age 65 and older. More men than women have COPD, but at least in the United States the difference in rates between genders is narrowing.

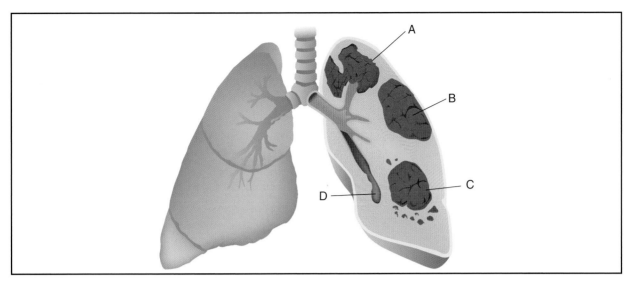

A. Lung cancer. B. Pneumonia. C. Emphysema. D. Phlegm from chronic bronchitis. *(Illustration by Argosy, Inc. Reproduced by permission of Gale, a part of Cengage Learning.)*

The exact prevalence of COPD in the United States is unknown, although it is estimated to be about 10% of the population, and some experts believe that that is an underestimate because many cases go unreported. According to the United States Centers for Disease Control and Prevention (CDC), COPD was the fourth leading cause of **death** in the United States in 2008. Internationally, COPD was the fifth leading cause of death. International prevalence estimates vary from a high of about 20% in South Africa to a low of about 5% in parts of Germany. Chronic bronchitis is about four times more common than emphysema.

Description

The lungs are the site where oxygen enters the blood and carbon dioxide is removed from the blood. Healthy lungs perform this process, known as gas exchange, efficiently. When air is inhaled through the nose or mouth, it moves through the windpipe (trachea) to large bronchial tubes (bronchi) then through smaller tubes (bronchioles). At the ends of the bronchioles are small air sacs (alveoli). In healthy lungs, the alveoli and the bronchi are springy and elastic. Much like a balloon, the alveoli can fill up with inhaled air and deflate when air is exhaled. In people with COPD, the alveoli lose their elasticity and shape so that a smaller volume of air moves in or out with each breath. COPD develops slowly over many years. Once it develops, COPD is irreversible (permanent); the damage done to the lungs, airways, and walls of the airways cannot be repaired by the body.

Chronic bronchitis

In chronic bronchitis, prolonged exposure to irritants such as smoke or airborne chemicals cause airways to lose their elasticity and narrow. Inflammation also causes glands that line the bronchi to produce excessive amounts of mucus, further narrowing the airways and blocking airflow. The result is often a chronic **cough** that produces sputum (mainly mucus) and **shortness of breath**. Cigarette smoke and other irritants also damage the cilia, small hair-like projections that move bacteria and foreign particles out of the airways. When the cilia are damaged, there is an increased the risk of lung infections.

Emphysema

Emphysema is a disease in which cigarette smoke causes an overproduction of the enzyme elastase, one of the immune system's infection-fighting biochemicals. This results in irreversible destruction of a protein in the lung called elastin. Elastin is essential in maintaining the structure of the walls of the alveoli, the terminal small air sacs of the respiratory system where gas exchange takes place. As the walls of the alveoli rupture, the number of alveoli is reduced and many of those remaining are enlarged. This reduces the surface area for gas exchange and makes the lungs of the patient with emphysema less elastic and over-inflated. Because higher pressure inside the chest that must be developed to force air out of the less-elastic lungs, the bronchioles, small air tubes of the respiratory system, tend to collapse during exhalation, blocking air flow. Stale air gets trapped in the air sacs and less fresh air can be inhaled.

Risk factors

Cigarette smoking is the greatest risk factor for developing COPD and accounts for about 80% of all cases. Cigar and pipe smoking also can cause COPD. Exposure to airborne pollutants (e.g., chemicals, industrial dust) in the work place also increases risk. Coal mining, cotton textile manufacturing, and gold mining are among the occupations where risk is increased, but the effects of these occupational exposures are lower than the effects of cigarette smoke. There is some debate about the role of exposure to air pollution in the development of COPD, but it is agreed to be a less important as a risk factor than cigarette smoking.

Causes and symptoms

The primary cause of COPD is cigarette smoking, along with the smoking of pipes and cigars. Secondary (passive) exposure to cigarette smoke is also a contributing factor to COPD. Occupational chemicals, dusts, and airborne particulates in the workplace also have been documented to be factors that can lead to the disease, as have air pollutants in the home. Outdoor air pollution has not been documented to be a significant factor to COPD, although such pollution is never good to anyone's lungs, especially those at risk for developing COPD.

Genetic and hereditary factors are also a consideration in developing COPD. One form of emphysema is known to run in families. People with this type of emphysema have a hereditary deficiency of a blood component, an enzyme inhibitor called alpha-1-antitrypsin (AAT). This type of emphysema is sometimes called early onset emphysema because it can appear when a person is as young as 30–40 years old. This type of emphysema is estimated to account for only 1–3% of all cases of emphysema. The risk of developing emphysema for an AAT-deficient individual who also smokes is much greater than for others.

The symptoms of COPD develop gradually, usually over years. The most common symptoms of chronic bronchitis are cough, production of sputum, and shortness of breath, especially with **exercise**. People with COPD also may experience **wheezing** and tightness in the chest. In emphysema, shortness of breath on exertion is the predominant early symptom. Coughing is usually minor, and there is little sputum. As emphysema progresses, shortness of breath occurs with less exertion, and eventually may be present even

---

KEY TERMS

Alveoli—Terminal air sacs of the respiratory system, where gas (oxygen and carbon dioxide) exchange occurs.

Bronchi—Large air tubes of the respiratory system.

Bronchioles—Small air tubes of the respiratory system.

Bronchodilators—Drugs that open wider the bronchial tubes of the respiratory system.

Corticosteroids—A group of hormones that are used as drugs to block inflammation.

Forced expiratory volume (FEV1)—The maximum amount of air expired in one second.

Spirometer—An instrument used by a doctor to perform a breathing test.

Vital capacity (VC)—The largest amount of air expelled after one's deepest inhalation.

---

when at rest. At this point, a sputum-producing cough may also occur. Either chronic bronchitis or emphysema can lead to **respiratory failure**, a condition in which there occurs a dangerously low level of oxygen or a serious excess of carbon dioxide in the blood.

Diagnosis

A history of heavy smoking is not enough to diagnose COPD. The first step in making a diagnosis is a good medical evaluation, including a medical history and a **physical examination** of the chest using a stethoscope. This may be followed by a variety of tests to evaluate lung function.

Tests

A pulmonary function test is a measure of how much air is passing into and out of the lungs. Using a spirometer, an instrument that measures the air taken into and exhaled from the lungs, the doctor will determine two important values: (1) vital capacity (VC), the largest amount of air expelled after the deepest inhalation, and (2) forced expiratory volume (FEV1), the maximum amount of air expired in one second. The pulmonary function test can be performed in the doctor's office. A person with chronic cough and sputum production but normal **spirometry** results may simply be at risk for COPD. With mild COPD, the test usually shows mild airflow limitation, and the patient may not be aware that airflow in the lungs is reduced. With moderate COPD, the pulmonary

---

function test shows that airflow limitation is worsening. The patient may have noticed that shortness of breath has worsened, particularly when walking fast or doing physical activity. Patients with severe or very severe COPD will have low volume readings.

Other tests used to diagnose COPD include diffusion studies, which determine how well oxygen in the air moves from the lungs into the blood. A blood sample may be taken to determine arterial blood gas. This test measures the amount of oxygen and carbon dioxide in the blood to see if these gases are being exchanged correctly. Low oxygen and high carbon dioxide levels are often indicative of chronic bronchitis, but not always of emphysema.

Chest x rays can detect only about half of the cases of emphysema. Chest x rays are rarely useful for diagnosing chronic bronchitis.

If infection is present, blood and sputum tests may be done to determine the cause of infection.

Many patients with lung disease also develop heart problems. An electrocardiogram (ECG) identifies signs of heart disease.

Treatment

Treatment for COPD is based on relieving symptoms, preventing complications, and improving a patient's overall health. The treatment varies depending on a patient's symptoms and stage of COPD. Treatment also may change over time and if a patient experiences complications or sudden onset of more severe symptoms.

Traditional

Only two treatments have been found to help people with COPD breathe more easily. Quitting smoking helps ease symptoms and slow the progress of the disease. Physicians will urge all patients with COPD who smoke to quit smoking. Quitting will not reverses the COPD, but will make the decline in lung function slower.

Supplemental oxygen is the only therapy that has been demonstrated to reduce the number of deaths in patients with COPD. The treatment usually is reserved for patients who are unable to get adequate oxygen on their own. The oxygen may be delivered by a portable tank that allows the patient to be mobile outside the home, through a concentrator unit placed in the home, or through some combination. Some patients will receive oxygen some of the time, such as when short of breath. Others may receive it only at night. Using

extra oxygen more than 15 hours a day helps people perform activities with less shortness of breath, remain more alert during the day, and protects the heart and other organs from damage.

Drugs

Medications frequently prescribed for COPD patients include:

• Bronchodilators. These agents open narrowed airways and offer significant symptomatic relief for many, but not all, people with COPD. There are three types of bronchodilators: Beta2 agonists, anticholinergic agents, and theophylline and its derivatives. Depending on the specific drug, a bronchodilator may be inhaled, injected, or taken orally.

• Corticosteroids. Corticosteroids, usually inhaled, block inflammation and are most useful for patients with chronic bronchitis with or without emphysema. Steroids are generally not useful in patients who have emphysema.

• Antibiotics. Antibiotics are frequently given at the first sign of a respiratory infection, such as increased sputum production or a change in color of sputum from clear to yellow or green.

• Vaccines. To prevent pulmonary infection from viruses and bacteria, people with COPD should be vaccinated against influenza each year at least six weeks before flu season and have a one-time pneumococcal (pneumonia) vaccine.

• Expectorants. These agents help loosen and expel mucus secretions from the airways.

• Diuretics. These drugs are given to prevent excess water retention in patients with associated right heart failure.

• Augmentation therapy (for emphysema due to AAT-deficiency only). Replacement AAT (Prolastin), derived from human blood which has been screened for viruses, is injected weekly or bimonthly for life.

Pulmonary rehabilitation

A structured, outpatient pulmonary **rehabilitation** program improves functional capacity in certain patients with COPD. Services may include general exercise training, administration of oxygen and **nutritional supplements**, intermittent mechanical ventilator support, continuous positive airway pressure, relaxation techniques, breathing exercises and techniques (such as pursed lip breathing), and methods for mobilizing and removing secretions.

Surgery

Surgical procedures for emphysema are very rare. They are expensive and often not covered by insurance. The great majority of patients cannot be helped by surgery, and no single procedure is ideal for those who can be helped.

Lung transplantation has been successfully employed in some patients with end-stage COPD. In the hands of an experienced team, the one-year survival rate is over 70% Lung transplantation is most often reserved for younger patients.

Lung volume reduction. These procedures remove 20–30% of severely diseased lung tissue; the remaining parts of the lung are joined together. Mortality rates can be as high as 15% and complication rates are even higher. When the operation is successful, patients report significant improvement in symptoms.

Alternative treatment

For both chronic bronchitis and emphysema, alternative practitioners recommend diet and nutritional supplements, a variety of herbal medicines, **hydrotherapy**, **acupressure** and **acupuncture**, **aromatherapy**, homeopathy, and **yoga**.

Home remedies

People with COPD may have more trouble breathing if they eat large meals because the stomach pushes on the diaphragm, the muscle that helps in breathing. Individuals with COPD also need to eat well-balanced **diets** because good **nutrition** helps fight infection. In the more severe stages of COPD, patients may experience weight loss and decreased muscle tissue, so these patients may need to eat high-calorie foods. Most people with COPD are encouraged to drink extra fluids to keep mucus thin and easier to cough up. Some have heart conditions and fluid retention and require fluid restriction.

Prognosis

COPD is a disease that can be treated and controlled, but not cured. Survival of patients with COPD is clearly related to the degree of their lung function when they are diagnosed and the rate at which they lose this function. Overall, the median survival is about 10 years for patients with COPD who have lost approximately two-thirds of their lung function at diagnosis.

Prevention

The most effective way to prevent COPD is to never smoke. Lifestyle modifications that can help prevent COPD, or improve function in COPD patients, include: quitting smoking, avoiding respiratory irritants and infections, avoiding allergens, maintaining good nutrition, drinking lots of fluids, avoiding excessively low or high temperatures and very high altitudes, maintaining proper weight, and exercising to increase muscle tone.

Resources

BOOKS

Kon, O. M., T. T. Hansel, and P. Barnes, eds. *Chronic Obstructive Pulmonary Disease (COPD)* New York: Oxford University Press, 2009.

OTHER

"COPD (Chronic Obstructive Pulmonary Disease)." MedlinePlus. August 4, 2009 [August 27, 2009] http://www.nlm.nih.gov/medlineplus/copdchronicobstructivepulmonarydisease.html

Torpy, Janet M. Alison E. Burk and Richard M. Glass. "Chronic Obstructive Pulmonary Disease." *JAMA* Patient Page. November 26, 2008 [August 27, 2009] http://jama.ama-assn.org/cgi/reprint/300/20/2448.pdf

ORGANIZATIONS

American Lung Association, 1301 Pennsylvania Ave., NW Suite 800, Washington, DC, 20004, (212) 315-8700, (800) LUNG-USA [(800) 548-8252], http://www.lungusa.org.

Global Alliance Against Chronic Respiratory Diseases (GARD), World Health Organization, Department of Chronic Diseases and Health Promotion, 20 Avenue Appia, CH-1211 27, Geneva, Switzerland., http://www.who.int/gard/en/index.html.

National Heart Lung and Blood Institute Health Information Center, P.O. Box 30105, Bethesda, MD, 20824-0105, (301) 592-8573; TTY: (240) 629-3255, (240) 629-3246, nhlbiinfo@nhlbi.nih.gov, http://www.nhlbi.nih.gov.

Harry W. Golden,
Tish Davidson, A.M.

Churg-Strauss syndrome *see* **Vasculitis**

Cingulotomy *see* **Psychosurgery**

Ciprofloxacin *see* **Fluoroquinolones**

Circadian rhythm sleep disorders *see* **Jet lag**

Circumcision

Definition

The surgical removal of the foreskin of the penis or prepuce.

Purpose

In the United States, circumcision in infant boys is performed for social, medical, or cultural/religious reasons. Once a routine operation urged by pediatricians and obstetricians for newborns in the middle of the twentieth century, circumcision has become an elective option that parents make for their sons on an individual basis. Families who practice Judaism or Islam may select to have their sons circumcised as a religious practice. Others choose circumcision for medical benefits.

Female circumcision (also known as **female genital mutilation**) is usually performed for cultural and social reasons by family members and others who are not members of the medical profession, with no anesthesia. Not only is the prepuce removed but often the vaginal opening is sewn to make it smaller. This practice is supposed to ensure the virginity of a bride on her wedding day. It also prevents the woman from achieving sexual pleasure during coitus. This practice is not universally approved by the medical profession and is considered by some as a human rights violation.

Though the incidence of male circumcision has decreased from 90% in 1979 to 60% in 1996, it is still the most common surgical operation in the United States. Circumcision rates are much lower for the rest of the industrialized world. In Britain, it is only done for religious practices or to correct a specific medical condition of the penis.

Some of the medical reasons parents choose circumcision are to protect against infections of the urinary tract and the foreskin, prevent **cancer**, lower the risk of getting **sexually transmitted diseases**, and prevent **phimosis** (a tightening of the foreskin that may close the opening of the penis). Though studies indicate that uncircumcised boys under the age of five are 20 times more likely than circumcised boys to have urinary tract infections (UTIs), the rate of incidence of UTIs is quite low. There are also indications that circumcised men are less likely to suffer from **penile cancer**, inflammation of the penis, or have many sexually transmitted diseases. Here again, the rate of incidence is low. Good hygiene usually prevents most infections of the penis. Phimosis and penile cancer are very rare, even in men who have not been circumcised. Education and good safe sex practices can prevent sexually transmitted diseases in ways that a surgical procedure cannot because these are diseases acquired through risky behaviors.

With these factors in mind, the American Academy of Pediatrics has issued a policy statement that

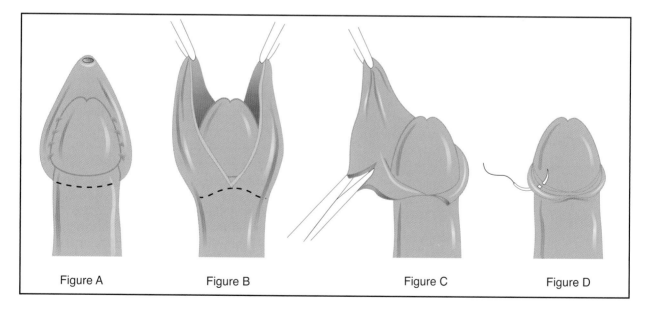

| Figure A | Figure B | Figure C | Figure D |

A typical circumcision procedure involves the following steps: **Figure A:** The surgeon makes an incision around the foreskin. **Figure B:** The foreskin is then freed from the skin covering the penile shaft. **Figure C:** The surgeon cuts the foreskin to the initial incision, lifting the foreskin from the mucous membrane. **Figure D:** The surgeon sutures the top edge of the skin that covers the penile shaft and the mucous membrane. *(Illustration by Electronic Illustrators Group. Reproduced by permission of Gale, a part of Cengage Learning.)*

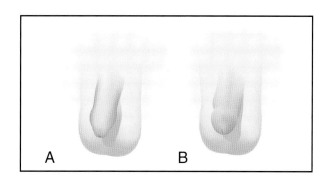

An uncircumcised penis (A) and a circumcised penis (B).
(Illustration by Argosy, Inc. Reproduced by permission of Gale, a part of Cengage Learning.)

states though there is existing scientific evidence that indicates the medical benefits of circumcision, the benefits are not strong enough to recommended circumcision as a routine practice.

Precautions

Circumcision should not be performed on infants with certain deformities of the penis that may require a portion of the foreskin for repair. The most common condition for surgery using the foreskin is **hypospadias**, a congenital deformity of the penis where the urinary tract opening is not at the tip of the glans. Also, infants with a large hydrocoele or **hernia** may suffer important complications through circumcision. Premature infants and infants with serious infections are also poor candidates to be circumcised, as are infants with **hemophilia**, other bleeding disorders, or whose mothers had taken **anticoagulant drugs**. In older boys or men, circumcision is a minor procedure. Therefore, it can be performed in virtually anyone without a serious illness or unusual deformity.

Description

The foreskin of the penis protects the sensitivity of the glans and shields it from irritation by urine, feces, and foreign materials. It also protects the urinary opening against infection and incidental injury.

In circumcision of infants, the foreskin is pulled tightly into a specially designed clamp, and the foreskin pulls away from the broadened tip of the penis. Pressure from the clamp stops bleeding from blood vessels that supplied the foreskin. In older boys or adults, an incision is made around the base of the foreskin, the foreskin is pulled back, and then it is cut away from the tip of the penis. Stitches are usually used to close the skin edges.

Preparation

Despite a long-standing belief that infants do not experience serious **pain** from circumcision, most authorities now believe that some form of **local anesthesia** is necessary. The physician injects local anesthesia at the base of the penis or under the skin around the penis (subcutaneous ring block). Both anesthetics block key nerves. EMLA cream, a topical formula of several anesthetics, can also be used.

Aftercare

After circumcision, the wound should be washed daily. An antibiotic ointment or petroleum jelly may be applied to the site. If there is an incision, a wound dressing will be present and should be changed each time the diaper is changed. Sometimes a plastic ring is used instead of a bandage. The ring will usually fall off in five to eight days. The penis will heal in seven to 10 days.

Infants who undergo circumcision may be fussy for some hours afterward, so parents should be prepared for crying, feeding problems, and sleep problems. Generally these go away within a day. In older boys, the penis may be painful, but this will go away gradually. A topical anesthetic ointment or spray may be used to relieve this temporary discomfort. There may also be a "bruise" on the penis, which typically goes away with no particular attention.

Risks

Complications following newborn circumcision appear in one out of every 500 procedures. Most complications are minor. Bleeding occurs in half of the complications and is usually easy to control. Infections are rare and present with **fever** and signs of inflammation.

There may be injuries to the penis itself, and these may be difficult to repair. In 2000, there were reports that the surgical clamps used in circumcision were at fault in over 100 injuries reported between July 1996 and January 2000. In nearly all cases, the clamps were assumed to be in working order but had been repaired with replacement parts that were not of the manufacturer's specifications. Physicians were urged to inspect the clamps before use and ensure that their dimensions fit their infant patients.

Resources

BOOKS

Glick, Leonard B. *Marked in Your Flesh: circumcision from Ancient Judea to Modern America.* Oxford, UK; New York: Oxford University Press, 2005.

OTHER

American Academy of Pediatrics. *New AAP Circumcision Policy Release (Press Release).* March 1, 1999. http://aappolicy.aappublications.org/cgi/content/full/pediatrics;103/3/686.

Janie F. Franz

Cirrhosis

Definition

Cirrhosis is a chronic degenerative disease in which normal liver cells are damaged and are then replaced by scar tissue.

Demographics

Cirrhosis is the seventh leading cause of disease-related **death** in the United States. It is the third most common cause of death in adults between the ages of 45 and 65. It is twice as common in men as in women. The disease occurs in more than half of all malnourished chronic alcoholics, and kills about 25,000 people a year. In Asia and Africa, however, most deaths from cirrhosis are due to chronic **hepatitis B**.

Description

Cirrhosis changes the structure of the liver and the blood vessels that nourish it. The disease reduces the liver's ability to manufacture proteins and process hormones, nutrients, medications, and poisons.

Cirrhosis gets worse over time and can become potentially life threatening. This disease can cause:

- excessive bleeding (hemorrhage)
- impotence
- liver cancer
- coma due to accumulated ammonia and body wastes (liver failure)
- sepsis (blood poisoning)
- death

Types of cirrhosis

Portal or nutritional cirrhosis is the form of the disease most common in the United States. About 30–50% of all cases of cirrhosis are this type. Nine out of every ten people who have nutritional cirrhosis have a history of **alcoholism**. Portal or nutritional cirrhosis is also called Laënnec's cirrhosis.

Biliary cirrhosis is caused by intrahepatic bile-duct diseases that impede bile flow. Bile is formed in the liver and is carried by ducts to the intestines. Bile then helps digest fats in the intestines. Biliary cirrhosis can scar or block these ducts. It represents 15–20% of all cirrhosis.

Various types of chronic hepatitis, especially hepatitis B and **hepatitis C**, can cause postnecrotic cirrhosis. This form of the disease affects up to 40% of all patients who have cirrhosis.

Disorders like the inability to metabolize iron and similar disorders may cause pigment cirrhosis (**hemochromatosis**), which accounts for 5–10% of all instances of the disease.

Risk factors

Most risk factors for cirrhosis can be prevented or avoided. The primary risk factors are alcohol and chronic liver infections, such as hepatitis B and C. People at high risk of contracting hepatitis B include those exposed to the virus through contact with blood and body fluids. This includes healthcare workers and intravenous (IV) drug users. In the past, people have contracted hepatitis C through blood transfusions. **Obesity** and poor **nutrition** are also significant risk factors.

Certain hereditary diseases can increase an individual's risk for cirrhosis. In most cases, these cannot be prevented or avoided but risk may be reduced with proper treatment of the disease or disorder.

Causes and symptoms

Long-term alcoholism is the primary cause of cirrhosis in the United States. Men and women respond

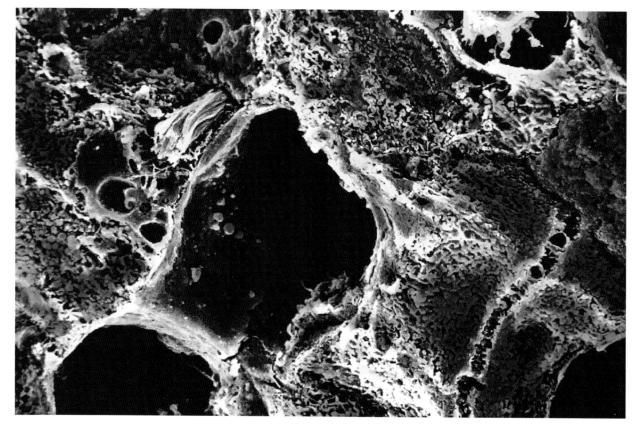

A micrograph of a human liver showing tissue damaged by cirrhosis. *(Professor P. Motta/Photo Researchers, Inc.)*

differently to alcohol. Although most men can safely consume two to five drinks a day, one or two drinks a day can cause liver damage in women. Individual tolerance to alcohol varies, but people who drink more and drink more often have a higher risk of developing cirrhosis. In some people, one drink a day can cause liver scarring.

Chronic liver infections, such as hepatitis B and particularly hepatitis C, are commonly linked to cirrhosis. Cirrhosis resulting from chronic hepatitis has emerged as a leading cause of death among HIV-positive patients; in Europe, about 30% of HIV-positive patients are co-infected with a hepatitis virus.

Liver injury, reactions to prescription medications, exposure to toxic substances, and repeated episodes of **heart failure** with liver congestion can cause cirrhosis. The disorder can also be a result of diseases that run in families (inherited diseases) like:

• a lack of a specific liver enzyme (alpha$_1$-antitrypsin deficiency)

• the absence of a milk-digesting enzyme (galactosemia)

• an inability to convert sugars to energy (glycogen storage disease)

• an absorption deficit in which excess iron is deposited in the liver, pancreas, heart, and other organs (hemochromatosis)

• a disorder characterized by accumulations of copper in the liver, brain, kidneys, and corneas (Wilson's disease)

Obesity has recently been recognized as a risk factor in nonalcoholic hepatitis and cirrhosis. Some surgeons recommend that patients scheduled for weight-reduction surgery have a **liver biopsy** to evaluate the possibility of liver damage.

Poor nutrition increases a person's risk of developing cirrhosis. In about 10 out of every 100 patients, the cause of cirrhosis cannot be determined. Many people who have cirrhosis do not have any symptoms (often called compensated cirrhosis). Their disease is detected during a routine physical or when tests for an unrelated medical problem are performed. This type of cirrhosis can also be detected when complications occur (decompensated cirrhosis).

Symptoms of cirrhosis are usually caused by the loss of functioning liver cells or organ swelling due to scarring. The liver enlarges during the early stages of illness. The palms of the hands turn red and patients may experience:

- constipation
- diarrhea
- dull abdominal pain
- fatigue
- indigestion
- loss of appetite
- nausea
- vomiting
- weakness
- weight loss

As the disease progresses, the spleen enlarges and fluid collects in the abdomen (**ascites**) and legs (**edema**). Spider-like blood vessels appear on the chest and shoulders, and bruising becomes common. Men sometimes lose chest hair. Their breasts may grow and their testicles may shrink. Women may have menstrual irregularities.

Cirrhosis can cause extremely dry skin and intense **itching**. The whites of the eyes and the skin may turn yellow (**jaundice**), and urine may be dark yellow or brown. Stools may be black or bloody. Sometimes the patient develops persistent high blood pressure due to the scarring (portal **hypertension**). This type of hypertension can be life threatening. It can cause veins to enlarge in the stomach and in the tube leading from the mouth to the stomach (esophagus). These enlarged veins are called varices, and they can rupture and bleed massively.

Other symptoms of cirrhosis include:

- anemia
- bleeding gums
- decreased interest in sex
- fever
- fluid in the lungs
- hallucinations
- lethargy
- lightheadedness
- muscle weakness
- musty breath
- painful nerve inflammation (neuritis)
- slurred speech
- tremors

KEY TERMS

Biopsy—The removal of cells or tissue for examination from a surface or organ for examination under a microscope. A needle biopsy uses a long needle and syringe device to aspirate (remove by suction) a sample of the target tissue.

Computed tomography (CT) scan—A series of detailed images of areas inside the body taken at various angles; the images are created on a computer linked to an x-ray machine.

Jaundice—Yellowing of the skin and whites of the eyes when pigments normally eliminated by the liver collect in high amounts in the blood.

If the liver loses its ability to remove toxins from the brain, the patient may have additional symptoms. The patient may become forgetful and unresponsive, neglect personal care, have trouble concentrating, and acquire new sleeping habits. These symptoms are related to ammonia intoxication and the failure of the liver to convert ammonia to urea. High protein intake in these patients can also lead to these symptoms.

Diagnosis

Examination

A patient's medical history can reveal illnesses or lifestyles likely to lead to cirrhosis. Liver changes can be seen during a **physical examination**. A doctor who suspects cirrhosis may order blood and urine tests to measure liver function. Because only a small number of healthy cells are needed to carry out essential liver functions, test results may be normal even when cirrhosis is present.

Tests

Computed tomography scans (CT), ultrasound, and other imaging techniques can be used during diagnosis. They can help determine the size of the liver, indicate healthy and scarred areas of the organ, and detect **gallstones**.

Procedures

Cirrhosis is sometimes diagnosed during surgery or by examining the liver with a laparoscope. This viewing device is inserted into the patient's body through a tiny incision in the abdomen.

Liver biopsy is usually needed to confirm a diagnosis of cirrhosis. In this procedure, a tissue sample is removed from the liver and is examined under a microscope in order to learn more about the organ.

A newer and less invasive test involves the measurement of hyaluronic acid in the patient's blood serum. The serum hyaluronic acid test is most useful in monitoring the progress of **liver disease**; it is unlikely to completely replace liver biopsy in the diagnosis of cirrhosis.

Treatment

The goal of treatment is to cure or reduce the condition causing cirrhosis, prevent or delay disease progression, and prevent or treat complications.

Traditional

Salt and fluid intake are often limited, and activity is encouraged. A diet high in calories and moderately high in protein can benefit some patients. **Tube feedings** or vitamin supplements may be prescribed if the liver continues to deteriorate. Patients are asked not to consume alcohol.

Drugs

Iron supplements, **diuretics**, and **antibiotics** may be used for anemia, fluid retention, and ammonia accumulation associated with cirrhosis. Vasoconstrictors are sometimes needed to stop internal bleeding and antiemetics may be prescribed to control nausea.

Laxatives help the body absorb toxins and accelerate their removal from the digestive tract. **Beta blockers** may be prescribed to control cirrhosis-induced portal hypertension. Because the diseased liver can no longer efficiently neutralize harmful substances, medications must be given with caution. Interferon medicines may be used by patients with chronic hepatitis B and hepatitis C to prevent post-hepatic cirrhosis.

Surgery

Medication that causes scarring can be injected directly into veins to control bleeding from varices in the stomach or esophagus. Varices may require a special surgical procedure called balloon tamponade ligation to stop the bleeding. Surgery may be required to repair disease-related throat damage. It is sometimes necessary to remove diseased portions of the spleen and other organs.

Liver transplants can benefit patients with advanced cirrhosis. However, the new liver will eventually become diseased unless the underlying cause of cirrhosis is removed. Patients with alcoholic cirrhosis must demonstrate a willingness to stop drinking before being considered suitable transplant candidates.

The incidence of **liver cancer** related to cirrhosis in the United States has increased 75% since the early 1990s. Partial surgical removal of the liver in patients with early-stage **cancer** of the liver appears to be as successful as transplantation, in terms of the 5-year survival rate.

Alternative

Alternative treatments for cirrhosis are aimed at promoting the function of healthy liver cells and relieving the symptoms associated with the disease. Several herbal remedies may be helpful to cirrhosis patients. Dandelion (*Taraxacum officinale*) and rock-poppy (*Chelidonium majus*) may help improve the efficiency of liver cells. Milk thistle extract (*Silybum marianum*) may slow disease progression and significantly improve survival rates in alcoholics and other cirrhosis patients. Practitioners of homeopathy and **traditional Chinese medicine** can also prescribe treatments that support healthy liver function.

Home remedies

A balanced diet promotes regeneration of healthy liver cells. Eating five or six small meals throughout the day should prevent the sick or bloated feeling patients with cirrhosis often have after eating. Alcohol and **caffeine**, which destroy liver cells, should be avoided. So should any foods that upset the stomach. Patients with brain disease associated with cirrhosis should avoid excessive amounts of protein in the diet.

A patient can keep a food diary that describes what was eaten, when it was eaten, and how the patient felt afterwards. This diary can be useful in identifying foods that are hard to digest and in scheduling meals to coincide with the times the patient is most hungry.

Patients who have cirrhosis should weigh themselves every day and notify their doctor of a sudden gain of 5 lb (2.3 kg) or more. A doctor should also be notified if symptoms of cirrhosis appear in anyone who has not been diagnosed with the disease. A doctor should also be notified if a patient diagnosed with cirrhosis:

- vomits blood
- passes black stools
- seems confused or unresponsive
- shows signs of infection (redness, swelling, tenderness, pain)

Prognosis

Cirrhosis-related liver damage cannot be reversed, but further damage can be prevented by patients who:

- eat properly
- get enough rest
- do not consume alcohol
- remain free of infection

If the underlying cause of cirrhosis cannot be corrected or removed, scarring will continue. The liver will fail, and the patient will probably die within five years. Patients who stop drinking after being diagnosed with cirrhosis can increase their likelihood of living more than a few years from 40% up to 70%.

Prevention

Eliminating alcohol **abuse** could prevent 75–80% of all cases of cirrhosis.

Other preventive measures include:

- obtaining counseling or other treatment for alcoholism
- taking precautions (practicing safe sex, avoiding dirty needles) to prevent hepatitis
- getting immunizations against hepatitis if a person is in a high-risk group
- receiving appropriate medical treatment quickly when diagnosed with hepatitis B or hepatitis C
- having blood drawn at regular intervals to rid the body of excess iron from hemochromatosis
- using medicines (chelating agents) to rid the body of excess copper from Wilson's disease
- wearing protective clothing and following product directions when using toxic chemicals at work, at home, or in the garden

In 2001, research scientists identified the protein segment and method in which excess tissue grows in diseases like cirrhosis. With further study, the discovery might one day result in an oral or inhalable peptide for those with cirrhosis.

Resources

BOOKS

Hanson, Dirk. *The Chemical Carousel: What Science Tells Us About Beating Addiction.* Charleston, SC: BookSurge Publishing, 2009.

KMS Publishing.com. *Living with Alcoholism: Your Guide to Dealing with Alcohol Abuse and Addiction While Getting the Alcoholism Treatment You Need.* Charleston, SC: CreateSpace, 2010.

Younossi, Zobair M. *Practical Management of Liver Diseases.* New York: Cambridge University Press, 2008.

Zein, Nizar, and Kevin M. Edwards. *The Cleveland Clinic Guide to Liver Disorders.* New York: Kaplan Publishing, 2009.

PERIODICALS

Cha, C. H., et al. "Resection of Hepatocellular Carcinoma in Patients Otherwise Eligible for Transplantation." *Annals of Surgery* 238 (September 2003): 315–321.

Foreman, M. G., D. M. Mannino, and M. Moss. "Cirrhosis as a Risk Factor for Sepsis and Death: Analysis of the National Hospital Discharge Survey." *Chest* 124 (September 2003): 1016–1020.

Higuchi, H., and G. J. Gores. "Mechanisms of Liver Injury: An Overview." *Current Molecular Medicine* 3 (September 2003): 483–490.

Kamath, B. M., and D. A. Piccoli. "Heritable Disorders of the Bile Ducts." *Gastroenterology Clinics of North America* 32 (September 2003): 857–875.

"Management of Alcoholic Hepatitis." *Drug Therapy Bulletin* 41 (July 2003): 49–52.

Moretto, M., et al. "Hepatic Steatosis in Patients Undergoing Bariatric Surgery and Its Relationship to Body Mass Index and Co-Morbidities." *Obesity Surgery* 13 (August 2003): 622–624.

Phillips, M. G., V. R. Preedy, and R. D. Hughes. "Assessment of Prognosis in Alcoholic Liver Disease: Can Serum Hyaluronate Replace Liver Biopsy?" *European Journal of Gastroenterology and Hepatology* 15 (September 2003): 941–944.

Ristig, M., et al. "Management of Chronic Hepatitis B in an HIV-Positive Patient with 3TC-Resistant Hepatitis B Virus." *AIDS Patient Care and STDs* 17 (September 2003): 439–442.

OTHER

"Cirrhosis of the Liver." National Institute of Diabetes and Digestive and Kidney Diseases (NIDDK). December 2008. NIH Publication No. 09-1134. http://www.niddk.nih.gov/health/digest/pubs/cirrhosi/cirrhosi.htm accessed August 4, 2010.

"Your Digestive System and How It Works." National Institute of Diabetes and Digestive and Kidney Disease. April 2008. NIH Publication No. 08-2681. http://digestive.niddk.nih.gov/ddiseases/pubs/yrdd/ accessed August 4, 2010.

ORGANIZATIONS

American Liver Foundation, 75 Maiden Lane, Suite 603, New York, NY, (212) 668-1000, http://www.liverfoundation.org.

National Institutes of Health (NIH), 9000 Rockville Pike, Bethesda, MD, 20892, (301) 496-4000, http://www.nih.gov.

United Network for Organ Sharing, P.O. Box 2484, Richmond, VA, 23218, (804) 782-4800, http://www.unos.org.

Maureen Haggert
Rebecca J. Frey, PhD
Laura Jean Cataldo, RN, EdD

Cisapride *see* **Antigastroesophageal reflux drugs**

CK test *see* **Creatine kinase test**

Clap *see* **Gonorrhea**

Clarithromycin *see* **Erythromycins**

Cleft lip and palate

Definition

A cleft is a birth defect that occurs when the tissues of the lip and/or palate of the fetus do not fuse very early in **pregnancy**. A cleft lip, sometimes referred to as a harelip, is an opening in the upper lip that can extend into the base of the nostril. A cleft palate is an opening in the roof of the mouth.

Description

Babies born with cleft lips will have an opening involving the upper lip. The length of the opening ranges from a small notch, to a cleft that extends into the base of the nostril. Cleft lips may involve one or both sides of the lip.

Babies born with cleft palates have openings in the palate, which is the roof of the mouth. The size and position of the opening varies. The cleft may be only in

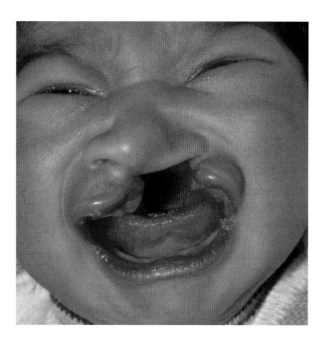

This infant has a unilateral cleft lip and palate. *(Custom Medical Stock Photo, Inc. Reproduced by permission.)*

the hard palate, the bony portion of the roof of the mouth, opening into the floor of the nose. It may be only in the soft palate, the soft portion of the roof of the mouth. The cleft palate may involve both the hard and soft palate and may occur on both sides of the center of the palate.

Babies may have cleft lips with or without cleft palates. Cleft palates may also occur without cleft lips.

The incidence of cleft lip and palate not associated with a syndrome is one in 700 newborns. Native Americans have an incidence of 3.6 in 1,000 newborns. The incidence among Japanese newborns is 2.1 in 1,000. The incidence among whites is one in 1,000 newborns. African Americans have an incidence of 0.3 in 1,000 newborns.

Causes and symptoms

Cleft lips and palates not associated with a syndrome are caused by a combination of genetic and environmental factors. Inheritance caused by such a combination is called multifactorial. The embryo inherits genes that increase the risk for cleft lip and/or palate. When an embryo with such genes is exposed to certain environmental factors the embryo develops a cleft.

The risk of a baby being born with a cleft lip or palate increases with the number of affected relatives and the number of relatives that have more severe clefts.

Environmental factors that increase the risk of cleft lip and palate include cigarette and alcohol use during pregnancy. Some drugs, such as phenytoin, **sodium** valproate, and methotrexate, also increase the incidence of clefting. The pregnant mother's **nutrition** may affect the incidence of clefting as well.

Babies born with a cleft lip will be seen to have an elongated opening in the upper lip. The size of this opening may range from a small notch in the upper lip to an opening that extends into the base of the nostril. The cleft lip may be below the right or left nostril or below both nostrils.

Babies born with a cleft palate will be seen to have an opening into the roof of the mouth. The size and position of the cleft varies and it may involve only the hard palate, or only the soft palate and may occur on both sides of the center of the palate.

In some cases the cleft palate will be covered with the normal lining of the mouth and can only be felt by the examiner.

Babies with cleft lips and palates have feeding difficulties, which are more severe in babies with cleft palates. The difficulty in feeding is due to the baby being unable to achieve complete suction. In the case of clefts of the hard palate, liquids enter the nose from the mouth through the opening in the hard palate.

A cleft palate also affects a child's speech, since the palate is necessary for speech formation. The child's speech pattern may still be affected despite surgical repair.

Ear infections are more common in babies born with cleft palates. The infections occur because the muscles of the palate do not open the Eustachian tubes that drain the middle ear. This allows fluid to collect and increases the risk of infection and **hearing loss**.

Teeth may also erupt misaligned.

Diagnosis

Cleft lip and palate can be diagnosed before birth by ultrasound. **Magnetic resonance imaging** (MRI) offers more accuracy for detecting cleft lip and palate, as it is a more detailed imaging method. It is particularly helpful in showing soft palate defects. In 2004, researchers reported discovery of a gene test for isolated cleft lip and cleft palate to help predict if parents who have one child with the isolated form of cleft lip or palate were likely to have a second child with the same defect. After birth, cleft lip and palate are diagnosed by physical exam.

Treatment

If cleft lip and/or palate are diagnosed by ultrasound before birth, further testing may be required to diagnose associated abnormalities if present. Referral to a cleft team is essential. A cleft team consists of specialists in the management of babies with clefts and includes surgeons as well as nurses and speech therapists. Members of the team inform the parents of all aspects of management. Feeding methods are also discussed, since feeding is the first problem that must be dealt with. It may be possible to breastfeed a baby born with only a cleft lip, but babies born with cleft palates usually have more problems with feeding and frequently require special bottles and teats. A palatal obturator is a device that fits into the roof of the mouth, thus blocking the cleft opening and allowing easier suckling.

Surgery to repair cleft lips is sometimes performed after orthodontic treatment to narrow the gap in the upper lip. The orthodontic treatment can involve acrylic splints with or without screws or may involve the use of adhesive tape placed across the gap in the lip. The orthodontic treatment for cleft lip should be started within the first three weeks of life and continue until the cleft lip is repaired.

The timing of surgical cleft lip repair depends on the judgment of the surgeon who will perform the operation. The procedure is usually performed between one and three months of age. The goals of the operation are to close the gap in the upper lip, place **scars** in the natural skin curves and to repair muscle so that the lip appears normal during movement. The closure is done in the three layers (skin, muscle, and mucosa) that line the inside of the lip. At the time of the procedure, if the nose is shaped abnormally due to the cleft lip, it is also corrected. Sometimes further surgery may be needed on the lip and/or nose to refine the result.

The goals of the surgeon repairing a cleft palate are normal speech, normal facial growth, and hearing for the affected infant. The repair of the cleft palate is usually performed between three and 18 months of age. The timing may extend beyond this and varies with the type of cleft palate and center where the procedure is being performed. Depending of the type of cleft palate, more than one operation may be needed to close the cleft and improve speech.

Nonsurgical treatment of a cleft palate is available for patients who are at high risk for surgery and consists of a prosthetic appliance worn to block the opening in the palate.

Babies born with cleft palates are vulnerable to ear infections. Their Eustachian tubes do not effectively drain fluid from the middle ear so fluid accumulates and infection sets in. This may lead to hearing loss. These children require drainage tubes to be inserted to prevent fluid accumulation.

Babies born with clefts usually require orthodontic treatment between 13 and 18 years of age. They also require **speech therapy**.

Prognosis

Babies born with cleft lip and palate have a good prognosis, and approximately 80% will develop normal speech. There is no known means of preventing clefting. Good prenatal care is essential and avoiding harmful substances appear to reduce the risk.

Resources

PERIODICALS

"MRI More Accurate for Detecting Prenatal Cleft Lip and Palate than Sonography." *Medical Devices & Surgical Technology Week* July 25, 2004: 160.

"Researchers Report New Gene Test for Isolated Cleft Lip and Palate." *Science Letter* September 28, 2004: 518.

ORGANIZATIONS

Cleft Palate Foundation, Cleft Palate Foundation, Chapel Hill, NC, 27514-2820, (919) 933-9044, (919) 933-9604, info@cleftline.org, http://www.cleftline.org.

Farris Farid Gulli, M.D.
Teresa G. Odle

Cleft palate *see* **Cleft lip and palate**

Clenched fist injury

Definition

A clenched fist injury (CFI) is a bite wound on the hand, caused when a person's closed fist strikes the teeth of another person, usually in the course of a fight. CFIs are sometimes referred to as closed fist injuries or fight bites.

Description

Clenched fist injuries are most common over the metacarpo phalangeal joint. Their appearance is deceptive because they do not bleed heavily and the underlying injury is hidden by soft tissue when the patient opens his hand and straightens the injured finger. CFIs can, however, have serious consequences, including infection, **cellulitis**, inflammation of the bone or bone marrow (**osteomyelitis**), septic arthritis, and inflammation of the sheaths covering the tendons of the hand (tenosynovitis). These may lead to permanent loss of function or **amputation**.

Most CFIs result in tissue injury due to the force of impact, ragged-edged tears in the skin resulting from contact with the teeth, and contamination of the wound by the bacteria in human saliva. As the patient opens his hand, the skin of the finger is pulled backward over the deeper part of the wound, thus sealing bacteria within the injured tissue. This sealing of the wound by normal motions of the finger is the reason why clenched fist injuries have the highest rate of infection of any human bite. The rate of infection of clenched-fist injuries varies from 15–50%.

Causes and symptoms

The causes of CFIs include fighting and other forms of aggressive behavior, often combined with drug or alcohol consumption.

The symptoms of clenched-fist injury include **pain** in the affected part of the hand and some stiffness of the injured finger with limitation of movement. If the patient has delayed getting medical treatment, there may be evidence of infection, including swelling, redness, and suppuration (a discharge of pus). The skin around the wound will be warm to the touch and **fever** may be present.

Diagnosis

Diagnosis of clenched fist injuries is usually made on the basis of the location of the injury and x-ray findings. The most common finding in CFI x rays is soft tissue swelling, but the x rays may also reveal air pockets in deep tissues or the joint spaces, fragments of teeth, fracture lines in the bones, or small loose bone chips. Diagnosis is often complicated by the fact that the patient will be reluctant to admit how the injury happened. The treating physician must maintain a high level of suspicion and often ask directly.

Treatment

Treatment of clenched fist injuries is complicated by several factors. One factor is the anatomical structure of the human hand, which contains many small closed spaces that make it easy for infection to spread and persist. Another is the number of disease-causing bacteria transmitted by human bites; at least 42 different species have been identified. In addition, CFIs typically do not receive immediate treatment because the patient is concerned about legal consequences. The longer the delay, the higher the chances of infection and permanent damage to the hand. Patients who wait longer than 24 hours to seek treatment or have signs of infection or damage to the tendon, joint capsule, or bones are usually referred immediately to a doctor who specializes in hand surgery.

The first step in treatment of clenched fist injury is irrigation, a procedure by which the wound is flushed with a stream of water under high pressure or with an antiseptic solution. Incision and drainage of the wound (I&D) may be required as well as **debridement**, the surgical removal of dead tissue and **foreign objects** from a wound. Careful examination of the depth of the wound is essential to proper treatment. The surgeon may need to enlarge the sides of the wound in order to make an accurate evaluation. The patient will be asked to move the affected joint through its full range of motion so that the surgeon can determine whether the tendon or joint capsule has been damaged. Following these procedures, the surgeon will pack the wound and put the hand in a splint. Bite **wounds** are never sutured (sewn shut) because of the possibility of enclosing bacteria inside the injury. After 24 hours, the packing will be removed and the hand reexamined for signs of infection.

If the wound has become infected, the patient is usually hospitalized and given parenteral (injectable) **antibiotics**. The wound is irrigated and examined to determine the extent of the injury. Cultures are taken for both aerobic (requiring air or oxygen to live) and anaerobic (not requiring air or oxygen) species of bacteria. The cultures should be taken from areas deep in the wound rather than from the surface for greater accuracy. **Tetanus** toxoid should be given if the patient has not been immunized within the last 10 years. The patient should also receive treatment and follow-up for the rare possibility of HIV and hepatitis transmission. Although no well-documented cases of HIV transmission by human bites exist, the potential for transmission by this route is still present.

Infected clenched fist injuries usually contain several disease-causing bacteria, the most common being *Streptococcus pyogenes*, *Staphylococcus aureus*, *Bacteroides sp.*, *Peptostreptococcus sp.*, and *Eikenella corrodens*. Broad-spectrum antibiotics are usually given. Uninfected and relatively superficial CFIs may be treated with oral penicillin plus dicloxacillin or Augmentin. For infected CFIs, parenteral penicillin G is usually given together with nafcillin or cefuroxime. CFIs infected by drug-resistant strains of *S. aureus* may require treatment with vancomycin. While some human bite wounds do not require routine use of antibiotics, a 2004 study confirmed that puncture wounds, deeper lacerations and bites to the hand all have high infection rates which may be lowered by preventive use of antibiotics.

Prognosis

The prognosis depends on the patient's underlying state of health and compliance with treatment; depth of the wound; the involvement of the joint capsule or tendon; and the length of time before the wound is treated. The more superficial the wound and the faster the treatment, the better the prognosis.

Prevention

The best way to prevent clenched fist injuries is to avoid fist fights, intoxication, and association with people who practice these forms of behavior. If

---

KEY TERMS

Antibiotic—A chemical substance produced by a microorganism which can inhibit the growth of or kill other microorganisms.

Debridement—Surgical removal of damaged tissue and foreign objects from a wound.

I&D—Incision and drainage of a wound.

Irrigation—Cleansing a wound with large amounts of water and/or an antiseptic solution.

Parenteral—Administered inside the body but outside the digestive tract.

Tetanus toxoid—Tetanus toxoid is a vaccine used to prevent tetanus (also known as lockjaw).

---

involved in a fist fight, people should avoid directing punches at their opponent's mouth. The next best preventive measure is to get medical treatment at once for a clenched-fist injury.

Resources

BOOKS

McPhee, Stephen, and Maxine Papadakis. *Current Medical Diagnosis and Treatment, 2010*, 49th ed. New York: McGraw–Hill Medical, 2009.
Rakel, Robert E., Edward T. Bope, and Howard F. Conn. *Conn's Current Therapy 2004: Latest Approved Methods of Treatment for the Practicing Physician*. Philadelphia: Saunders, 2004.

PERIODICALS

"Do All Human Bite Wounds Need Antibiotics?" *Emergency Medicine Alert* June 2004: 3.

ORGANIZATIONS

Massachusetts College of Emergency Physicians, 860 Winter Street, Waltham, MA, 02451, (781) 890-4407, (781) 890-4109, http://www.macep.org.

Rebecca J. Frey, PhD
Teresa G. Odle

Club drugs

Definition

Club drugs are a diverse group of recreation-enhancing substances, used illegally, and usually consumed along with alcohol at raves, bars, clubs, concerts, or parties.

Description

Club drugs include Ecstasy (MDMA), GHB (gamma hydroxybutyrate, liquid ecstasy, soap), Rohypnol (flunitraxapam, roofies, a relative of Valium and Xanax), Ketamine (Special K, Vitamin K), **methamphetamine** (meth, speed, crystal, crank), and **LSD** (acid).

These drugs have separate, different actions. They are usually produced or imported illegally, so their strengths and purity are unknowable. Taken together, with alcohol, and consumed in intense social situations, their effects cannot be accurately predicted.

Ecstasy (XTC, X, E, MDMA), the most commonly used club drug, was patented in 1914 by Merck and not used for six decades. In the 1970s and 1980s, psychologists and therapists began experimenting with it for treating **anxiety**, depression, and post traumatic **stress** syndrome. Patients reported various effects, including an increasing sense of empathy for self and others, **hallucinations**, and euphoria or ecstasy. Its use subsequently spread to the recreational drug subculture.

Ecstasy can increase body temperature, heart rate, and blood pressure, and can change perceptions of time, place and person. It can blunt sensations of thirst, allowing people to become dehydrated under its influence. It increases the amount of serotonin in the brain, producing euphoria, and/or anxiety and **paranoia**. After the drug wears off, temporarily decreased serotonin levels may leave users feeling depressed for days or even weeks.

MDMA is generally taken in doses of 125 milligrams, although effects are observable with as little as 60 milligrams. It is generally taken as tablets or capsules. Effects begin about an hour after ingestion, peak in three or four hours, and fade after six hours. Some users take a second dose to prolong the effects.

Dangers associated with Ecstasy include increased body temperature, complicated by excess physical activities such as dancing or immersion in hot tubs or saunas. **Dehydration**, increased heart rate and blood pressure are common. Because of its effects on serotonin in the brain, long-term Ecstasy users may have decreased memory. Other dangers include mixing the drug with alcohol, methamphetamine, or **cocaine**. People with heart problems, high blood pressure, or psychological disorders are at greater risk from taking this drug.

LSD (lysergic acid, acid) is a potent mood-changing drug that produces unpredictable effects, depending on the amount taken and the personality of the user. Effects range from euphoria to panic with intense hallucinations. Dangers associated with long term use of this drug include flash backs and **psychosis**.

Rohypnol (flunitrazepam, roofie) is a powerful sedative that is related to the sedative-tranquilizers, Valium and Xanax. It has been termed a "date rape" drug because it can cause "anterograde amnesia": those taking the substance may lose memory of events occurring under its effects. It is particularly dangerous to take Rohypnol with alcohol or other sedatives.

GHB (gamma hydroxybutyrate) is a substance with euphoric and depressant effects. There is a narrow range between safe, recreational use of GHB, overdose, producing **coma** or seizures, and life-threatening toxic dose.

Ketamine (special K, Vitamin K) is legitimately used as an animal tranquilizer. It can be taken orally, inhaled through the nose, or given intravenously and creates a sense of mind-body separation that can be experienced either pleasantly or as panic.

Methamphetamine (meth, crystal, speed, crank) is a dangerously addictive stimulant. Taken orally, inhaled through the nose, or given intravenously, it produces an intense rush of euphoric stimulation followed by an overwhelming desire for more drug. It increases heart rate and blood pressure and may lead to **heart attack**, **heart failure**, and **death**. Research has shown that it damages brain cells that produce dopamine and serotonin, contributors to pleasure, memory and motivation. Prolonged or excessive use of methamphetamine can slow thinking, depress mood, and impair muscle strength and coordination. Emotional problems associated with the use of methamphetamine include **addiction**, paranoia, anxiety, and **insomnia**. Methamphetamine use has been growing in the United States throughout the 2000s.

Diagnosis

Substance abuse is defined by the *Diagnostic and Statistical Manual IV* as occurring when: users take a substance in larger amounts or over longer time periods than intended; a persistent and unsuccessful desire to cease usage; spending large quantities of time procuring the substance; reduction in other social activities; continued use of a substance despite physical or emotional problems caused by the substance; increased tolerance of the substance; withdrawal symptoms or increased use of a substance to avoid withdrawal symptoms.

Treatment

Treatment for problems associated with the use and **abuse** of club drugs include psychiatric, psychological, and substance abuse counseling, as well as emergency medical treatment for overdoses and complications.

Resources

BOOKS

Espejo, Roman. *Club Drugs*. Detroit, MI: Greenhaven Press, 2009.
Mann, John. *Turn on and Tune in: Psychedelics, Narcotics and Euphoriants*. Cambridge, UK: Royal Society of Chemistry, 2009.
Swarts, Katherine. *Club Drugs*. Farmington Hills, MI: Greenhaven Press, 2006.

ORGANIZATIONS

DanceSafe, 536 45th Ave., Oakland, CA, 94609, http://www.dancesafe.org.
Multidisciplinary Association for Psychedelic Studies, 309 Cedar Street No. 2323, Santa Cruz, CA, 95060, (831) 429-6362, (831) 429-6370, http://www.maps.org.
National Institute on Drug Abuse, 6001 Executive Blvd., Room 5213, Bethesda, MD, (301) 443-1124, information@ nida.nih.gov, http://drugabuse.gov.

Douglas Dupler
James E. Waun, MD,RPh

Clubfoot

Definition

Clubfoot is a condition in which one or both feet are twisted into an abnormal position at birth. The condition is also known as talipes or talipes equinovarus.

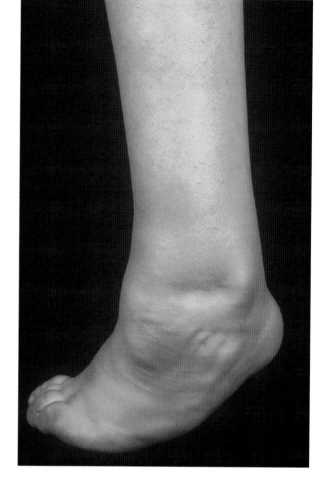

Person suffering from clubfoot. About one in every 1,000 newborns has some form of this birth defect. *(Photo Researchers, Inc.)*

Description

True clubfoot is characterized by abnormal bone formation in the foot. There are four variations of clubfoot, including talipes varus, talipes valgus, talipes equines, and talipes calcaneus. In talipes varus, the most common form of clubfoot, the foot generally turns inward so that the leg and foot look somewhat like the letter J. In talipes valgus, the foot rotates outward like the letter L. In talipes equinus, the foot points downward, similar to that of a toe dancer. In talipes calcaneus, the foot points upward, with the heel pointing down.

Clubfoot can affect one foot or both. Sometimes an infant's feet appear abnormal at birth because of the intrauterine position of the fetus birth. If there is no anatomic abnormality of the bone, this is not true clubfoot, and the problem can usually be corrected by applying special braces or casts to straighten the foot.

The ratio of males to females with clubfoot is 2.5 to 1. The incidence of clubfoot varies only slightly. In the United States, the incidence is approximately 1 in every 1,000 live births. A 1980 Danish study reported an overall incidence of 1.20 in every 1,000 children; by 1994, that number had doubled to 2.41 in every 1,000 live births. No reason was offered for the increase.

Causes and symptoms

Experts do not agree on the precise cause of clubfoot. The exact genetic mechanism of inheritance has been extensively investigated using family studies and other epidemiological methods. No definitive conclusions have been reached as of the early 2000s, although a Mendelian pattern of inheritance is suspected. This may be due to the interaction of several different inheritance patterns, different patterns of development appearing as the same condition, or a complex interaction between genetic and environmental factors. The MSX1 gene has been associated with clubfoot in animal studies. As of the early 2000s, however, these findings have not been replicated in humans.

A family history of clubfoot has been reported in 24.4% of families in a single study. These findings suggest the potential role of one or more genes being responsible for clubfoot.

Several environmental causes have been proposed for clubfoot. Obstetricians feel that intrauterine crowding causes clubfoot. This theory is supported by a significantly higher incidence of clubfoot among twins compared to singleton births. Intrauterine exposure to the drug misoprostol has been linked with clubfoot. Misoprostol is commonly used when trying, usually unsuccessfully, to induce abortion in Brazil and in other countries in South and Central America. Researchers in Norway have reported that males who are in the printing trades have significantly more offspring with clubfoot than men in other occupations. For unknown reasons, **amniocentesis**, a prenatal test, has also been associated with clubfoot. One international study published in 2004 reported that amniocentesis done at 13 weeks of gestation was associated with a fourfold increase in the risk of clubfoot. The infants of mothers who smoke during **pregnancy** have a greater chance of being born with clubfoot than are offspring of women who do not smoke.

True clubfoot is usually obvious at birth. The four most common varieties have been described. A clubfoot has a typical appearance of pointing downward and being twisted inwards. Since the condition starts in the first trimester of pregnancy, the abnormality is quite well established at birth, and the foot is often very rigid.

Uncorrected clubfoot in an adult causes only part of the foot, usually the outer edge, or the heel or the toes, to touch the ground. For a person with clubfoot, walking becomes difficult or impossible.

Diagnosis

True clubfoot is usually recognizable and obvious on **physical examination**. A routine x ray of the foot that shows the bones to be malformed or misaligned supplies a confirmed diagnosis of clubfoot. Ultrasonography is not always useful in diagnosing the presence of clubfoot prior to the birth of a child; however, ultrasound is increasingly used in the early 2000s to evaluate the severity of clubfoot after birth and monitor its response to treatment.

Treatment

Most orthopedic surgeons agree that the initial treatment of congenital (present at birth) clubfoot should be nonoperative. Nonsurgical treatment should begin in the first days of life to take advantage of the favorable fibroelastic properties of the foot's connective tissues, those forming the ligaments, joint capsules, and tendons. In a common treatment, a series of casts is applied over a period of months to reposition the foot into normal alignment. In mild cases, splinting and wearing braces at night may correct the abnormality.

Another treatment for clubfoot is the Ilizarov frame, named for the Russian physician who developed it in 1951. The Ilizarov frame has been used in the United States and Canada since 1981. It consists of two metal rings that encircle the leg to be corrected, wires that attach the rings to the bone, and metal rods between the rings that can be extended like a telescope. The frame must be applied by an orthopedic surgeon. After a week, the surgeon begins to lengthen the rods, usually at the rate of 1 mm per day. The frame must be kept in place for several months. Although the Ilizarov frame is somewhat cumbersome, it has been reported as giving satisfactory results in straightening clubfeet, particularly those untreated in infancy.

When clubfoot is severe enough to require surgery, the condition is usually not completely correctable, although significant improvement is possible. In the most severe cases, surgery may be required, especially when the Achilles tendon, which joins the muscles in the calf to the bone of the heel, needs to be lengthened. Because an early operation induces fibrosis, a scarring and stiffness of the tissue, surgery should be delayed until an affected child is at least three months old.

KEY TERMS

Enterovirus—Any of a group of viruses that primarily affect the gastrointestinal tract.

Ilizarov frame—A device invented by a Russian physician for correcting deformities of the legs and feet, consisting of rings to be attached to the bone and rods extending between the rings that stretch the affected limb.

Intrauterine—Situated or occuring in the uterus.

Orthopedist—A doctor specializing in treatment of the skeletal system and its associated muscles and joints.

Much of a clubfoot abnormality can be corrected by the use of manipulation and casting during the first three months of life. Proper manipulative techniques must be followed by applications of appropriately molded plaster casts to provide effective and safe correction of most varieties of clubfoot. Long-term care by an orthopedist is required after initial treatment to ensure that the correction of the abnormality is maintained. Exercises, corrective shoes, or nighttime splints may be needed until the child stops growing.

Prognosis

With prompt, expert treatment, clubfoot is usually correctable. One group of French researchers found that 77% of the children they followed over a period of 11 to 18 years had good results from non-surgical methods of treatment combined with **physical therapy**. Most individuals are able to wear regular shoes and lead active lives. If clubfoot is not appropriately treated, however, the abnormality may become fixed. This fixation affects the growth of the child's leg and foot, and some degree of permanent disability usually results.

Resources

BOOKS

Beers, Mark H., Robert S. Porter, and Thomas V. Jones, eds. *The Merck Manual of Diagnosis and Therapy*. 18th ed. Whitehouse Station, NJ: Merck Research Laboratories, 2006.

Cecil, Russell L., Lee Goldman, and D. A. Audiello. *Cecil Medicine*. 23rd ed, Philadelphia: Saunders Elsevier, 2008.

Kliegman, Robert M., and Waldo Emerson Nelson. *Nelson Textbook of Pediatrics*. 18th ed. Philadelphia: Saunders, Elsevier, 2007.

PERIODICALS

El Barbary H., H. Abdel Ghani, and M. Hegazy. "Correction of Relapsed or Neglected Clubfoot Using a Simple Ilizarov Frame." *International Orthopedics* 28 (June 2004): 183–186.

Gigante, C., E. Talente, and S. Turra. "Sonographic Assessment of Clubfoot." *Journal of Clinical Ultrasound* 32 (June 2004): 235–242.

Philip, J., R. K. Silver, R. D. Wilson, et al. "Late First-Trimester Invasive Prenatal Diagnosis: Results of an International Randomized Trial." *Obstetrics and Gynecology* 103 (June 2004): 1164–1173.

Souchet, P., H. Bensahel, C. Themar-Noel, et al. "Functional Treatment of Clubfoot: A New Series of 350 Idiopathic Clubfeet with Long-Term Follow-Up." *Journal of Pediatric Orthopaedics, Part B* 13 (May 2004): 189–196.

OTHER

Children's and Women's Health Centre of British Columbia. *The Ilizarov Apparatus*. http://www.bcchildrens.ca/NR/rdonlyres/42A7AAE8-A350-4FC0-8DB7-DA5896078EDB/11239/IlizarovApparatus.pdf.

"Clubfoot." *National Library of Medicine*. http://www.nlm.nih.gov/medlineplus/ency/article/001228.htm.

Clubfoot.net. http://www.clubfoot.net/treatment.php3.

ORGANIZATIONS

Easter Seals Disability Services, 233 South Wacker Drive, Suite 2400, Chicago, IL, 60606, (312) 726-6200, (312) 726-1494, (800) 221-6827, http://www.easterseals.com.

March of Dimes Birth Defects Foundation, 1275 Mamaroneck Ave., White Plains, NY, 10605, (914) 997-4488, http://www.modimes.org.

National Organization for Rare Disorders, P.O. Box 8923, New Fairfield, CT, 06812-8923, (800) 999-6673, http://www.rarediseases.org.

L. Fleming Fallon, Jr., MD, DrPH
Rebecca J. Frey, PhD

Cluster headache

Definition

Cluster headaches are characterized by an intense one-sided **pain** centered by the eye or temple. The pain lasts for one to two hours on average and may recur several times in a day.

Description

Cluster headaches have been known as histamine headaches, red migraines, and Horton's disease, among others. The constant factor is the pain, which transcends by far the distress of the more common tension-type **headache** or even that of a **migraine headache**.

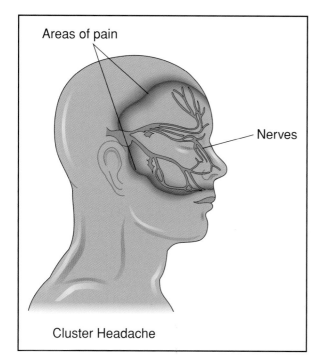

Areas of pain

Nerves

Cluster Headache

The primary cluster headache symptom is excruciating one-sided head pain located behind an eye or near the temple. Secondary symptoms include eye tearing, nasal congestion, and a runny nose. *(Illustration by Electronic Illustrators Group. Reproduced by permission of Gale, a part of Cengage Learning.)*

Cluster headaches afflict less than 0.5% of the population and predominantly affect men; approximately 80% of sufferers are male. Onset typically occurs in the late 20s, but there is no absolute age restriction. Approximately 80% of cluster headaches are classified as episodic; the remaining 20% are considered chronic. Both display the same symptoms. However, episodic cluster headaches occur during one- to five-month periods followed by 6- to 24-month attack-free, or remission, periods. There is no such reprieve for chronic cluster headache sufferers.

Causes and symptoms

Biochemical, hormonal, and vascular changes induce cluster headaches, but why these changes occur remains unclear. Episodic cluster headaches seem to be linked to changes in day length, possibly signaling a connection to the so-called biological clock. Alcohol, tobacco, histamine, or **stress** can trigger cluster headaches. Decreased blood oxygen levels (hypoxemia) can also act as a trigger, particularly during the night when an individual is sleeping. Interestingly, the triggers do not cause cluster headaches during remission periods.

The primary cluster headache symptom is excruciating one-sided head pain centered behind an eye or near the temple. This pain may radiate outward from the initial focus and encompass the mouth and teeth. For this reason, some cluster headache sufferers may mistakenly attribute their pain to a dental problem. Secondary symptoms, occurring on the same side as the pain, include eye tearing, nasal congestion followed by a runny nose, pupil contraction, and facial drooping or flushing.

Diagnosis

Cluster headache symptoms guide the diagnosis. A medical examination includes recording headache details, such as frequency and duration, when it occurs, pain intensity and location, possible triggers, and any prior symptoms. This history allows other potential problems to be discounted.

Treatment

Treatment for cluster headaches is composed of induction, maintenance, and symptomatic therapies. The first two therapies are prophylactic treatments, geared toward preventing headaches. Symptomatic therapy is meant to stop or shorten a headache.

Induction and maintenance therapies begin together. Induction therapy is intended to break the headache cycle with drugs such as **corticosteroids** (for example, prednisone) or dihydroergotamine. These drugs are not meant for long-term therapy, but rather as a jump-start for maintenance therapy. Maintenance therapy drugs include verapamil, lithium carbonate, ergotamine, and methysergide. These drugs have long-term effectiveness, but must be taken for at least a week before a response is observed. With long-term treatment, methysergide must be stopped for one month each year to avoid dangerous side effects (formation of fibrous tissue inside the abdominal artery, lungs, and heart valves).

Despite prophylactic treatment, headaches may still occur. Symptomatic therapy includes oxygen inhalation, sumatriptan injection, and application of local anesthetics inside the nose. Surgery is a last resort for chronic cluster headaches that fail to respond to therapy.

Alternative treatment

Since some cluster headaches are triggered by stress, **stress reduction** techniques, such as **yoga, meditation**, and regular **exercise**, may be effective. Some cluster headaches may be an allergic response triggered by food or environmental substances, therefore

KEY TERMS

Biological clock—A synonym for the body's circadian rhythm, the natural biological variations that occur over the course of a day.

Migraine headache—An intense throbbing pain that occurs on one or both sides of the head. The headache is usually accompanied by other symptoms, such as nausea, vomiting, and aversion to light.

Prophylactic—Referring to treatment that prevents symptoms from occurring.

Tension-type headache—A dull pain that seems to exert pressure on the head; the most common form of headache.

identifying and removing the allergen(s) may be key to resolution of the problem. Histamine is another suspected trigger of cluster headaches, and this response may be controlled with vitamin C and the bioflavonoids quercetin and bromelain (pineapple enzyme). Supplementation with essential fatty acids (EFA) will help decrease any inflammatory response.

Physical medicine therapies such as adjustments of the spine, craniosacral treatment, and massage at the temporomandibular joint (TMJ) can clear blockages, as can traditional Chinese medical therapies including **acupuncture**. Homeopathic treatment can also be beneficial. Nervous system relaxant herbs, used singly or in combination, can allow the central nervous system to relax as well as assist in peripheral nerve response. A few herbs to consider for relaxation are valerian (*Valeriana officinalis*), chamomile (*Matricaria recutita*), rosemary (*Rosemarinus officinalis*), and skullcap (*Scutellaria baicalensis*).

Prognosis

In general, drug therapy offers effective treatment.

Prevention

Avoiding triggers, adhering to medical treatment, and controlling stress can help ward off some cluster headaches.

ORGANIZATIONS

American Council for Headache Education (ACHE), 19 Mantua Road, Mount Royal, NJ, 08061, (856) 423-0043, (858) 423-0082, achehq@talley.com, http://www.achenet.org.

National Headache Foundation, 820 N. Orleans, Suite 217, Chicago, IL, 60610, (312), 274-2650, (888), NHF-5552, info@headaches.org, http://www.headaches.org.

Julia Barrett

CMV *see* **Cytomegalovirus infection**

CNS depressants *see* **Central nervous system depressants**

CNS stimulants *see* **Central nervous system stimulants**

Coagulation disorders

Definition

Coagulation disorders deal with disruption of the body's ability to control blood clotting. The most commonly known coagulation disorder is **hemophilia**, a condition in which patients bleed for long periods of time before clotting. There are other coagulation disorders with a variety of causes.

Description

Coagulation, or clotting, occurs as a complex process involving several components of the blood. Plasma, the fluid component of the blood, carries a number of proteins and coagulation factors that regulate bleeding. Platelets, small colorless fragments in the blood, initiate contraction of damaged blood vessels so that less blood is lost. They also help plug damaged blood vessels and work with plasma to accelerate blood clotting. A disorder affecting platelet production or one of the many steps in the entire process can disrupt clotting.

Coagulation disorders arise from different causes and produce different complications. Some common coagulation disorders are:

- Hemophilia, or hemophilia A (Factor VIII deficiency), an inherited coagulation disorder, affects about 20,000 Americans. This genetic disorder is carried by females but most often affects males.

- Christmas disease, also known as hemophilia B or Factor IX deficiency, is less common than hemophilia A with similar in symptoms.

- Disseminated intravascular coagulation disorder, also known as consumption coagulopathy, occurs as a result of other diseases and conditions. This disease accelerates clotting, which can actually cause hemorrhage.

- Thrombocytopenia is the most common cause of coagulation disorder. It is characterized by a lack of circulating platelets in the blood. This disease also includes idiopathic thrombocytopenia.
- Von Willebrand's disease is a hereditary disorder with prolonged bleeding time due to a clotting factor deficiency and impaired platelet function. It is the most common hereditary coagulation disorder.
- Hypoprothrombinemia is a congenital deficiency of clotting factors that can lead to hemorrhage.
- Other coagulation disorders include Factor XI deficiency, also known as hemophilia C, and Factor VII deficiency. Hemophilia C afflicts one in 100,000 people and is the second most common bleeding disorder among women. Factor VII is also called serum prothrombin conversion accelerator (SPCA) deficiency. One in 500,000 people may be afflicted with this disorder that is often diagnosed in newborns because of bleeding into the brain as a result of traumatic delivery.

Causes and symptoms

Some coagulation disorders present symptoms such as severe bruising. Others will show no apparent symptoms, but carry the threat of severe internal bleeding.

Hemophilia

Because of its hereditary nature, hemophilia A may be suspected before symptoms occur. Some signs of hemophilia A are numerous large, deep **bruises** and **pain** and swelling of joints caused by internal bleeding. Patients with hemophilia do not bleed faster, just longer. A person with mild hemophilia may first discover the disorder with prolonged bleeding following a surgical procedure. If there is bleeding into the neck, head, or digestive tract, or bleeding from an injury, emergency measures may be required.

Mild and severe hemophilia A are inherited through a complex genetic system that passes a recessive gene on the female chromosome. Women usually do not show signs of hemophilia but are carriers of the disease. Each male child of the carrier has a 50% chance of having hemophilia, and each female child has a 50% chance of passing the gene on.

Christmas disease

Christmas disease, or hemophilia B, is also hereditary but less common than hemophilia A. The severity of Christmas disease varies from mild to severe, although mild cases are more common. The severity depends on the degree of deficiency of the Factor IX (clotting factor). Hemophilia B symptoms are similar to those of hemophilia A, including numerous, large and deep bruises and prolonged bleeding. The more dangerous symptoms are those that represent possible internal bleeding, such as swelling of joints, or bleeding into internal organs upon trauma. Hemophilia most often occurs in families with a known history of the disease, but occasionally, new cases will occur in families with no apparent history.

Disseminated intravascular coagulation

The name of this disorder arises from the fact that malfunction of clotting factors cause platelets to clot in small blood vessels throughout the body. This action leads to a lack of clotting factors and platelets at a site of injury that requires clotting. Patients with disseminated intravascular coagulation (DIC) will bleed abnormally even though there is no history of coagulation abnormality. Symptoms may include minute spots of hemorrhage on the skin, and purple patches or hematomas caused by bleeding in the skin. A patient may bleed from surgery or intravenous injection (IV) sites. Related symptoms include **vomiting**, seizures, **coma**, **shortness of breath**, **shock**, and severe pain in the back, muscles, abdomen, or chest.

DIC is not a hereditary disorder or a common one. It is most commonly caused by complications during **pregnancy** or delivery, overwhelming infections, acute leukemia, metastatic **cancer**, extensive **burns** and trauma, and even snakebites. There are a number of other causes of DIC, and it is not commonly understood why or how these various disorders can lead to the coagulation problem. What the underlying causes of DIC have in common is some factor that affects proteins, platelets, or other clotting factors and processes. For example, uterine tissue can enter the mother's circulation during prolonged labor, introducing foreign proteins into the blood, or the venom of some exotic snakes can activate one of the clotting factors. Severe head trauma can expose blood to brain tissue. No matter the cause of DIC, the results are a malfunction of thrombin (an enzyme) and prothrombin (a glycoprotein), which activate the fibrinolytic system, releasing clotting factors in the blood. DIC can alternate from hemorrhage to thrombosis, and both can exist, which further complicates diagnosis and treatment.

Thrombocytopenia

Thrombocytopenia may be acquired or congenital. It represents a defective or decreased production of platelets. Symptoms include sudden onset of small spots of hemorrhage on the skin, or bleeding into mucous membranes (such as nosebleeds). The disorder may also be evident as blood in vomit or stools, bleeding during surgery, or heavy menstrual flow in women. Some patients show none of these symptoms, but complain of **fatigue** and general weakness. There are several causes of thrombocytopenia, which is more commonly acquired as a result of another disorder. Common underlying disorders include leukemia, drug toxicity, or **aplastic anemia**, all of which lead to decreased or defective production of platelets in the bone marrow. Other diseases may destroy platelets outside the marrow. These include severe infection, disseminated intravascular coagulation, and **cirrhosis** of the liver. The idiopathic form most commonly occurs in children, and is most likely the result of production of antibodies that cause destruction of platelets in the spleen and to a lesser extent the liver.

Von Willebrand's disease is caused by a defect in the Von Willebrand clotting factor, often accompanied by a deficiency of Factor VIII as well. It is a hereditary disorder that affects both males and females. In rare cases, it may be acquired. Symptoms include easy bruising, bleeding in small cuts that stops and starts, abnormal bleeding after surgery, and abnormally heavy menstrual bleeding. Nosebleeds and blood in the stool with a black, tarlike appearance are also signs of Von Willebrand's disease.

Hypoprothrombinemia

This disorder is a deficiency in prothrombin, or Factor II, a glycoprotein formed and stored in the liver. Prothrombin, under the right conditions, is converted to thrombin, which activates fibrin and begins the process of coagulation. Some patients may show no symptoms, and others will suffer severe hemorrhaging. Patients may experience easy bruising, profuse nosebleeds, postpartum hemorrhage, excessively prolonged or heavy menstrual bleeding, and postsurgical hemorrhage. Hypoprothrombinemia may also be acquired rather than inherited, and usually results from a **Vitamin K deficiency** caused by liver diseases, newborn hemorrhagic disease, or a number of other factors.

Other coagulation disorders

Factor XI deficiency, or hemophilia C, occurs more frequently among certain ethnic groups, with an incidence of about one in 10,000 among Ashkenazi Jews. Nearly 50% of patients with this disorder experience no symptoms, but others may notice blood in their urine, nosebleeds, or bruising. Although joint bleeding seldom occurs, some factor XI patients will experience bleeding long after an injury occurs. Some

women will experience prolonged bleeding after **childbirth**. Patients with factor VII deficiency vary greatly in their bleeding severity. Women may experience heavy menstrual bleeding, bleeding from the gums or nose, bleeding deep within the skin, and episodes of bleeding into the stomach, intestine, and urinary tract. Factor VII patients may also suffer bleeding into joints.

Diagnosis

Several blood tests can be used to detect various coagulation disorders. There are hundreds of different tests a doctor can order to look for indications of specific diseases. In addition to blood tests, physicians will complete a medical history and **physical examination**. In the case of acquired coagulation disorders, information such as prior or current diseases and medications will be important in determining the cause of the blood disorder.

- Hemohilia A will be diagnosed with laboratory tests detecting presence of clotting factor VIII, factor IX, and others, as well as the presence or absence of clotting factor inhibitors.

- Christmas disease will be checked against normal bleeding and clotting time, as well as for abnormal serum reagents in factor IX deficiency. Other tests of prothrombin time and thromboplastic generation may also be ordered.

- There is no one test or group of tests that can always make (or exclude) a diagnosis of DIC. DIC can be diagnosed through a number of laboratory tests that measure concentration of platelets and fibrinogen in the blood with normal counts and prolonged prothrombin time. Other supportive data include diminished levels of factors V, fibrinogen, and VIII, decreased hemoglobin, and others. Since many of the test results also indicate other disorders, the physician may have to put together several results to reach a diagnosis of DIC. Serial tests may also be recommended, because a single examination at one moment in time may not reveal the process that is occurring.

- Tests for thrombocytopenia include coagulation tests revealing a decreased platelet count, prolonged bleeding time, and other measurements. If these tests indicate that platelet destruction is causing the disorder, the physician may order bone marrow examination.

- Von Willebrand's disease will be diagnosed with the assistance of laboratory tests which show prolonged bleeding time, absent or reduced levels of factor VIII, normal platelet count, and others.

- Hypothrombinemia is diagnosed with history information and the use of tests that measure vitamin K deficiency, deficiency of prothrombin, and clotting factors V, VII, IX, and X.
- Factor XI deficiency is diagnosed most often after injury-related bleeding. Blood tests can help pinpoint factor VII deficiency.

Treatment

In mild cases, treatment may involve the use of drugs that stimulate the release of deficient clotting factors. In severe cases, bleeding may only stop if the clotting factor that is missing is replaced through infusion of donated human blood in the form of fresh frozen plasma or cryoprecipitate.

- Hemophilia A in mild episodes may require infusion of a drug called desmopressin or DDAVP. Severe bleeding episodes will require transfusions of human blood clotting factors. Hemophiliacs are encouraged to receive physical therapy to help damaged joints and to exercise in non-contact sports such as swimming, bicycle riding, or walking.
- Christmas disease patients are treated similarly to hemophilia A patients. There are commercial products and human blood products available to provide coagulation. Cryoprecipitate was invented in 1965 to replace the need for whole plasma transfusions, which introduced more volume than needed. By the 1970s, people were able to infuse themselves with freeze-dried clotting factor. Superficial wounds can be cleaned and bandaged. Parents of hemophiliac children receiving immunizations should inform the vaccination provider in advance to decrease the possibility of bleeding problems. These children should probably not receive injections that go into the muscle.
- Treatment for disseminated intravascular coagulation patients is complicated by the large variety of underlying causes of the disorder. If at all possible, the physician will first treat this underlying disorder. If the patient is not already bleeding, this supportive treatment may eliminate the DIC. However, if bleeding is occurring, the patient may need blood, platelets, fresh frozen plasma, or other blood products. Heparin has been controversial in treating DIC, but it is often used as a last resort to stop hemorrhage. Heparin has not proven useful in treating patients with DIC resulting from heat stroke, exotic snakebites, trauma, mismatched transfusions, and acute problems resulting from obstetrical complications.
- Secondary acquired thrombocytopenia is best alleviated by treating the underlying cause or disorder. The specific treatment may depend on the underlying cause. Sometimes, corticosteroids or immune globulin may be given to improve platelet production.
- Von Willebrand's disease is treated by several methods to reduce bleeding time and to replace factor VIII, which consequently will replace the Von Willebrand factor. This may include infusion of cryoprecipitate or fresh frozen plasma. Desmopressin may also help raise levels of the Von Willebrand factor.
- Hypoprothrombinemia may be treated with concentrates of prothrombin. Vitamin K may also be produced, and in bleeding episodes, the patient may receive fresh plasma products.
- Factor XI (hemophilia C) is most often treated with plasma, since there are no commercially available concentrates of factor XI in the United States. Factor VII patients may be treated with prothrombin complex concentrates. As of early 1998, factor VII concentrate was not licensed in the United States and could only be used with special permission.

Alternative treatment

This can be a very severe condition and should be managed by a practitioner of alternative medicine in conjunction with a medical doctor; this condition should not be self managed. For patients known to suffer from hemophilia A or B and other bleeding disorders, avoidance of activities that can cause severe injury should be practiced. Comprehensive care addresses the whole person by helping to deal with the psychosocial aspects of the disease.

Prognosis

The prognosis for patients with mild forms of coagulation disorders is normally good. Many people can lead a normal life and maintain a normal life expectancy. Without treatment of bleeding episodes, severe muscle and joint pain, and, eventually, damage can occur. Any incident that causes blood to collect in the head, neck, or digestive system can be very serious and requires immediate attention. DIC can be severe enough to cause clots to form and a **stroke** could occur. DIC is also serious enough to cause **gangrene** in the fingers, nose, or genitals. The prognosis depends on early intervention and treatment of the underlying condition. Hemorrhage from a coagulation disorder, particularly into the brain or digestive track, can prove fatal. In the past, patients who received regular transfusions of human blood products were subject to increased risk of **AIDS** and other diseases. However, efforts have been made since the early 1990s to ensure the safety of the blood supply.

KEY TERMS

Clotting factor—Also known as coagulation factors. Proteins in the plasma that serve to activate various parts of the blood clotting process by being transformed from inactive to active form.

Enzyme—A substance that causes a chemical reaction, usually a protein. Enzymes are secreted by cells.

Hemorrhage—Abnormal bleeding from the blood vessels.

Heparin—An anticoagulant, or blood clot "dissolver."

Idiopathic—Refers to a disease of unknown cause, and sometimes to a primary disease.

Metastatic—The term used to describe a secondary cancer, or one that has spread from one area of the body to another.

Serum reagents—Serum is fluid, or the fluid portion of the blood retained after removal of the blood cells and fibrin clot. Reagents are substances added to the serum to produce a chemical reaction.

Thrombosis—Formation of a clot in the blood that either blocks, or partially blocks a blood vessel. The thrombus may lead to infarction, or death of tissue, due to a blocked blood supply.

Prevention

Prevention of coagulation disorders varies. Acquired disorders may only be prevented by preventing onset of the underlying disorder (such as cirrhosis). Hereditary disorders can be predicted with prenatal testing and **genetic counseling**. Prevention of severe bleeding episodes may be accomplished by refraining from activities that could cause injury, such as contact sports. Open communication with healthcare providers prior to procedures or tests that could cause bleeding may prevent a severe bleeding incident.

ORGANIZATIONS

National Heart Lung and Blood Institute Health Information Center, P.O. Box 30105, Bethesda, MD, 20824-0105, (301) 592-8573, (240) 629-3246, http://www.nhlbi.nih.gov.

National Hemophilia Foundation, 116 West 32nd St., 11th Floor, New York, NY, 10001, (212) 328-3700, (212) 328-3777, http://www.hemophilia.org.

Teresa Odle

Coagulopathies *see* **Coagulation disorders**
Coal miner's disease *see* **Black lung disease**
Coal worker's pneumoconiosis *see* **Black lung disease**

Coarctation of the aorta

Definition

Coarctation of the aorta (CoA) is a defect that develops in the fetus in which there is a narrowing of the aortic arch, the main artery that delivers blood from the left ventricle of the heart to the rest of the body. The word *coarctation* by itself means a narrowing or constriction. Coarctation of the aorta is diagnosed in both newborns and adults.

Demographics

Coarctation of the aorta is a relatively common congenital heart defect; it is found in 6–8% of infants with **congenital heart disease**. It is more common in boys, the male:female ratio being 2:1. Although researchers are still studying data related to race and ethnicity, there is some evidence that Asian babies are 2% less likely to have CoA than babies born in Europe, North America, or South America. In the United States, Native Americans have a lower rate of CoA than other racial and ethnic groups. The reason for these differences is not known as of 2010.

Description

In humans, blood leaves the heart by way of the left ventricle and is distributed to the body by arteries. The aortic arch is the first artery to carry blood as it leaves the heart. Other arteries to the head and arms branch off the aortic arch. A narrowing of the aorta at any spot produces resistance to the flow of blood. This causes high blood pressure before the narrowing and low pressure below the narrowing (downstream). Parts of the body supplied by arteries that branch off the aortic arch before the narrowing have high blood pressure, while most of the lower body does not receive enough blood supply. Thus people with CoA have **hypertension** in their arms but low blood pressure in the legs and ankles. To compensate for the coarctation, the heart works harder, and the blood pressure rises.

KEY TERMS

Anastomosis—A type of surgical procedure in which the surgeon joins together two parts of a hollow organ (such as a blood vessel or portion of the intestine) after a diseased or damaged section has been removed.

Aorta—The largest artery in the body, arising from the left ventricle (lower chamber) of the heart and extending down into the abdomen.

Coarctation—The medical term for a constriction or narrowing.

Congenital—Present at birth.

Ductus arteriosus—A blood vessel in the human fetus that connects the aortic arch to the pulmonary artery before birth and normally closes shortly after birth in healthy newborns.

Dyspnea—Difficulty in breathing. Usually associated with heart or lung diseases.

Electrocardiogram—A graph of the heart's beating produced by an instrument that detects the electrical signals made by the heart.

Gallop rhythm—An abnormal heart rhythm in which the doctor can hear three (sometimes four) sounds instead of the usual two, resembling the rhythm of a horse's gallop.

Hypertension—High blood pressure.

Notching—A deformity of the surface of the ribs that is often associated with coarctation of the aorta.

Turner syndrome—A genetic disorder that affects only females, in which one of the two X chromosomes that determine female sex is missing or otherwise abnormal.

Ventricular septal defect (VSD)—A defect or opening in the ventricular septum, the wall of tissue that separates the two lower chambers of the heart.

There are three basic forms of CoA, defined by the location of the constriction or narrowing with regard to the ductus arteriosus, a blood vessel that connects the aortic arch and the pulmonary artery in the developing fetus. The purpose of this vessel is to bypass the lungs in the fetus, which are still filled with fluid. The ductus arteriosus normally closes shortly after birth when the newborn begins to breathe. Coarctation of the aorta may occur at the point where the ductus arteriosus enters the aorta (ductal); before that point (preductal); or below that point (postductal):

- Ductal coarctation: This form of CoA usually first appears when the ductus arteriosus closes after birth.
- Preductal: This form of CoA is potentially life-threatening, as closure of the ductus arteriosus after birth may close off blood flow to the lower body.
- Postductal: This is the form of CoA most often seen in adults. It is associated with notching of the ribs, high blood pressure in the arms, and weak pulses in the legs.

The internal appearance of the narrowed part of the aorta varies somewhat from patient to patient. In some, the coarctation is localized whereas in others the narrowing involves a longer section of the aorta. The coarctation may look like a shelf of tissue partially closing off the aorta, or it may resemble a curtain or membrane with an irregular opening in the middle.

Risk factors

There are two major risk factors for coarctation of the aorta:

- The presence of one or more other heart defects, particularly ventricular septal defect, patent ductus arteriosus, or abnormalities of the bicuspid, mitral, or aortic valves in the heart.

- In females, Turner syndrome. Turner syndrome is a genetic disorder in which a girl or woman has only one of the two X chromosomes that determine female sex.

Causes and symptoms

In newborns with congenital heart disease, coarctation of the aorta develops while the baby is in the womb. The exact cause or trigger of the abnormal development is not completely understood as of 2010. In rare cases, CoA can develop in adolescents or adults as a result of severe trauma, severe hardening of the arteries, or a rare disorder causing inflammation of the arteries known as Takayasu's arteritis.

Among the consequences of coarctation of the aorta is ventricular hypertrophy, an enlarging of the left ventricle in response to the increased back pressure of the blood and the demand for more blood by the body. Symptoms in infants include **shortness of breath** (dyspnea), difficulty in feeding, pale skin, heavy sweating, and poor weight gain. Older children may develop measurable hypertension; they may also display **fatigue**, shortness of breath, cold feet, headaches, nosebleeds, or a feeling of lameness in their legs.

Diagnosis

Children or adults with any of the following symptoms should see a doctor at once. Although these symptoms may have causes other than CoA, it is best to be checked, because early detection of CoA can be life-saving:

• Fainting

• Severe pains in the chest

• Shortness of breath

• Unexplained high blood pressure.

The initial diagnosis of CoA is often made by the infant or child's pediatrician, but in most cases the child will be referred to a pediatric cardiologist (heart specialist) for further evaluation. Approximately half of all infants with coarctation of the aorta are diagnosed within the first two months of life; however, the diagnosis is often missed during the first year. One study found that the average age of children referred to a pediatric cardiologist for treatment of CoA was 5 years. Frequently, there are other congenital cardiac complications present. The most common defects associated with coarctation of the aorta are **patent ductus arteriosus** (a ductus arteriosus that fails to close) and **ventricular septal defect** (VSD). In general, the younger the infant at the time of diagnosis, the greater the risk that he or she has other heart defects. Female infants with **Turner syndrome** have a 10% rate of also having coarctation. There is evidence that some cases of coarctation may be inherited.

Examination

Abnormal blood pressure readings can be detected during a **physical examination** in the doctor's office, as can abnormal heart rhythms. Infants with CoA usually have an abnormal "gallop" heart rhythm and may also have **heart murmurs**. Sometimes excessive arterial pulses can be seen in the carotid and suprasternal notch arteries, indicating increased pressure in these arteries, while the femoral pulse is weak or cannot be detected. The systolic pressure is higher in the arms than in the legs. Similar symptoms are seen in older children and adults. A 10 mm Hg (mercury) pressure difference between the upper and lower extremities is diagnostic for coarctation of the aorta. For some patients, the systolic pressure difference is observed only during **exercise**. Infants frequently have an abnormal electrocardiogram (ECG) that indicates that the right or both ventricles are enlarged, while in older children the ECG may be normal or show that the left ventricle is enlarged.

Tests

The doctor may also order imaging tests to evaluate any structural abnormalities in the heart and aorta. Enlargement of the heart can be seen in x rays. The coarctation may also be detected in echocardiographic examination or **magnetic resonance imaging** (MRI).

Procedures

In some cases the doctor may recommend **cardiac catheterization**. This is a procedure in which a long thin flexible tube called a catheter is threaded upward through an artery or vein in the leg until it reaches the heart. A dye is injected into the catheter in order to make the abnormalities in the aorta visible on x-ray. Cardiac catheterization helps doctors evaluate the location and severity of the CoA.

Treatment

Traditional

Drugs can be used to treat hypertension and **heart failure** while the patient is being evaluated for surgery. Surgery is recommended for infants with other associated cardiac defects and for those infants not responding to drug therapy. Surgery is indicated for infants that don't require immediate surgery, but who develop severe hypertension during the first several months of life. Patients are advised to avoid vigorous exercise prior to surgical correction of the coarctation. Recoarctation can occur in some patients even if they have had surgery; however, recoarctation can also be corrected by surgery.

Surgery

The first successful surgical correction of CoA was performed by a Swedish surgeon named Clarence Crafoord (1899–1983) in 1944. As of 2010, there are four major types of open-heart procedures used to repair CoAs in children:

• Resection and anastomosis. The surgeon removes the narrowed section of the aorta and reconnects the two ends of the blood vessel.

• Patch aortoplasty. The surgeon cuts across the narrowed section of the aorta and attaches a patch of synthetic material to widen the blood vessel.

• Flap angioplasty. The surgeon removes a portion of the left subclavian artery (the artery that carries blood to the left arm) and uses it to widen the narrowed portion of the aorta.

- Bypass graft. The surgeon inserts a plastic tube called a graft between the normal portions of the aorta, bypassing the coarctation.

Drugs

Medication cannot be used to treat CoA, but it can be used to control the patient's blood pressure before surgery. Some people may also have to take blood pressure drugs after corrective surgery.

Infants with severe CoA may be given a drug called prostaglandin E to keep the ductus arteriosus open. The open ductus arteriosus will act like a bypass around the coarctation until the CoA can be repaired surgically.

Prognosis

Approximately half of all infants diagnosed with coarctation of the aorta have no other cardiac defects and will respond well to medical management. Most of these children will eventually outgrow the condition after several years of life. Although their hypertension may increase for several months early in life, it will eventually decrease as the circulatory system develops.

The average life span of adults who have untreated coarctation of the aorta is 34 years of age; 90% of such untreated patients die by age 50. The most common complications for children who have not had surgery are hypertension, aortic rupture, intracranial bleeding, congestive heart failure, and kidney or liver failure. Women who have an uncorrected coarctation of the aorta have a mortality rate of 10% during **pregnancy** and a 90% rate of complications.

Prevention

There is no known way to prevent coarctation of the aorta as of 2010 because the condition is present at birth in most cases. However, prompt evaluation of children with known heart defects or Turner syndrome for CoA can help in preventing complications of the condition. Surgeons recommend correcting the defect before age 10 if possible in order to prevent **death** in early adulthood; if coarctation is repaired before the age of 14 years, the 20-year survival rate is 91%. If the coarctation is repaired after age 14, the 20-year survival rate drops to 79%.

Resources

BOOKS

Allen, Hugh D., et al., eds. *Moss and Adams' Heart Disease in Infants, Children, and Adolescents: Including the Fetus and Young Adult*, 7th ed. Philadelphia: Wolters Kluwer Health/Lippincott Williams and Wilkins, 2008.

Drose, Julia, ed. *Fetal Echocardiography*, 2nd ed. St. Louis, MO: Saunders, 2010.

Warnes, Carol A., ed. *Adult Congenital Heart Disease.* Hoboken, NJ: Wiley-Blackwell, 2009.

PERIODICALS

Abadir, S., et al. "Advances in Paediatric Interventional Cardiology Since 2000." *Archives of Cardiovascular Diseases* 102 (June–July 2009): 569–82.

Egan, M., and R.J. Holzer. "Comparing Balloon Angioplasty, Stenting and Surgery in the Treatment of Aortic Coarctation." *Expert Review of Cardiovascular Therapy* 7 (November 2009): 1401–12.

Hager, A. "Hypertension in Aortic Coarctation." *Minerva Cardioangiologica* 57 (December 2009): 733–42.

Kische, S., et al. "Technique of Interventional Repair in Adult Aortic Coarctation." *Journal of Vascular Surgery* 51 (June 2010): 1550–59.

Mortensen, K.H., et al. "Abnormalities of the Major Intrathoracic Arteries in Turner Syndrome as Revealed by Magnetic Resonance Imaging." *Cardiology in the Young* 20 (April 2010): 191–200.

Silversides, C.K., et al. "Canadian Cardiovascular Society 2009 Consensus Conference on the Management of Adults with Congenital Heart Disease: Outflow Tract Obstruction, Coarctation of the Aorta, Tetralogy of Fallot, Ebstein Anomaly and Marfan's Syndrome." *Canadian Journal of Cardiology* 26 (March 2010): e80–97.

Tanous, D., et al. "Coarctation of the Aorta: Evaluation and Management." *Current Opinion in Cardiology* 24 (November 2009): 509–15.

OTHER

Mayo Clinic. *Coarctation of the Aorta.* http://www.mayo-clinic.com/health/coarctation-of-the-aorta/DS00616

MedlinePlus Encyclopedia. *Coarctation of the Aorta.* http://www.nlm.nih.gov/medlineplus/ency/article/000191.htm

National Heart, Lung, and Blood Institute (NHLBI). *Congenital Heart Defects.* http://www.nhlbi.nih.gov/health/dci/Diseases/chd/chd_what.html

Rao, P. S., and Paul M. Seib. "Coarctation of the Aorta." *eMedicine*, July 20, 2009. http://emedicine.medscape.com/article/895502-overview

Shah, Sandy M., and Dawn N. Calderon. "Aortic Coarctation." *eMedicine*, October 2, 2008. http://emedicine.medscape.com/article/150369-overview

ORGANIZATIONS

American College of Cardiology (ACC), Heart House, 2400 N Street NW, Washington, DC, 20037, (202) 375-6000, (202) 375-7000, http://www.acc.org/.

American Heart Association, 7272 Greenville Avenue, Dallas, TX, 75231, (301) 592-8573, (800) 242-8721, (301) 592-8563, www.americanheart.org.

Center for Adults with Congenital Heart Disease, University of Chicago Medical Center, 5841 S. Maryland Avenue, Chicago, IL, 60637, (888) UCH-0200, http://www.

uchospitals.edu/specialties/heart/services/adult-congenital-heart/.

National Heart, Lung, and Blood Institute (NHLBI), Health Information Center, P.O. Box 30105, Bethesda, MD, 20824-0105, (301) 592-8573, 240-629-3246, nhlbiinfo@nhlbi.nih.gov, http://www.nhlbi.nih.gov/.

John T. Lohr, PhD
Rebecca J. Frey, PhD

Cocaine

Definition

Cocaine is a highly addictive central nervous system stimulant found in the leaves of the coca plant, *Erythroxylon coca*.

Description

Pure cocaine is a white crystalline powder.

Though most cocaine is used recreationally and illegally, it has legitimate medical uses as a potent local, topical anesthetic for the eye, ear drum, and mucous membranes of the nose, mouth, and respiratory system.

Forms of the drug

Street names for powdered cocaine include: "coke," "blow," "C," "flake," "snow" "nose candy," "basa," "smack," "powder," and "toot."

Cocaine can be sniffed or "snorted." through the nose, dissolved in water and injected intravenously, and smoked in a pipe and inhaled through the lungs.

Crack cocaine is the form that is smoked. Crack gets its name from the crackling sound made as cocaine powder is cooked with baking soda. The off-white, cooked product is broken into small pieces called "rocks," or "kibbles & bits."

Both cocaine and crack are sometimes mixed with other substances, like methcathinone, or "cat." A mixture of crack and **marijuana** is known as a "woolah." Either cocaine or crack, used together with heroin, is called a "speedball." Alcohol, frequently used together with cocaine, is the most common fatal two-drug combination.

Cocaine's effects include loss of **fatigue**, mental alertness, and increased energy. Their intensity and duration depend on how the drug is used. The more rapidly it reaches the brain, the faster its effects are felt and the quicker they dissipate. Intravenous injection and **smoking** produce faster and more intense effects.

History

Coca leaves were chewed by the Incas and other inhabitants of the Andean region of South America for thousands of years as a stimulant, to combat **altitude sickness**, and to suppress appetite.

Late in the nineteenth century, cocaine hydrochloride, coca's psychoactive ingredient, was extracted from the leaves and soon found its way into many patent medicines and other popular products, like colas. The drug's negative effects soon became apparent and in 1914, the Harrison Act banned the use of cocaine in non-prescription products. Its use subsequently declined substantially.

The drug culture of the 1960s sparked renewed interest in cocaine and, with the advent of crack cocaine in the 1980s, cocaine **abuse** once again become a national problem. Its use declined in the early 1990s, but remains a significant problem in certain age groups and geographic areas. A mid-1990s government report stated that Americans spend more money on cocaine than on all other illegal drugs combined.

Causes and symptoms

Like other addictions, cocaine abuse results from complex combinations of factors like genetic predisposition, family history, **stress**, and other environmental issues. As many as three to four million people are estimated to be chronic cocaine users.

How cocaine affects the brain

Cocaine increases the brain's levels of dopamine by preventing its being recycled back into brain cells. Dopamine is responsible for feelings of pleasure; the higher the dopamine levels, the greater the sensations of pleasure. With repeated drug use, tolerance develops and more frequent use produces diminishing sensations of pleasure.

Short-term effects of use

The short-term effects of cocaine can include:

- rapid heartbeat
- constricted blood vessels
- dilated pupils
- increased temperature
- increased energy
- reduced appetite
- increased sense of alertness

- euphoria
- sudden death due to overdose, heart attack, or stroke

Long-term effects of use

The long-term effects of cocaine and crack use include:

- dependence, addiction
- paranoia
- anxiety
- irritability
- mood swings
- restlessness
- weight loss and malnutrition
- auditory hallucinations
- loss of sense of smell
- nosebleeds
- ruptured nasal septum
- chronic runny nose
- hoarse voice
- bowel gangrene
- increased risk of contracting HIV and other blood-borne diseases

Cocaine use and pregnancy

The rise in the use of cocaine and crack in the 1980s raised fears about their effects on developing fetuses. But researchers have not been able to conclusively demonstrate consistent, adverse effects. Experts nowadays believe that the lack of good prenatal care, along with alcohol and tobacco use in cocaine users who are pregnant, are more important factors in premature delivery, low birth weight, and fetal and neonatal **death**.

The Center for Disease Control and Prevention (CDC), however, reports that mothers who use cocaine early in **pregnancy** are five times more likely to have babies with malformed urinary tracts than mothers who do not use the drug.

Thus, cocaine use, especially in the early weeks of pregnancy, is inadvisable.

Discouraging pregnant women from using cocaine, tobacco, and alcohol are important tasks for all health caregivers.

Diagnosis

Diagnosing cocaine **addiction** can be difficult. Many of the signs of short-term cocaine use are not obvious. Since cocaine users often also use other drugs, it may not be easy to distinguish the effects of one drug from another.

Cocaine use has been documented in significant numbers of eighth graders as well as older teens. Over all age groups, more men than women use the drug. The highest rate of cocaine use is found among adults 18 to 25 years old.

Medical complications

Cocaine has been linked to several serious health problems, including:

- arrhythmia
- heart attacks
- chest pain
- respiratory failure
- strokes
- seizures

Other complications may vary depending on how the drug is administered. Prolonged snorting, for example, can irritate the nasal septum, producing nosebleeds, chronic runny nose and ruptured nasal septum, and other problems. Intravenous users face an increased risk of infectious diseases such as HIV/AIDS and hepatitis.

Testing

Urine testing for cocaine can be useful in diagnosing cocaine abuse and monitoring adherence to drug-abuse treatment programs.

Treatment

The last two decades have seen a dramatic rise in the number of cocaine addicts seeking treatment. There are no specific, targeted treatments for cocaine abuse or addiction. Most programs combine **cognitive-behavioral therapy** with social support.

Pharmacological treatments

There are no specific medications for treating cocaine addiction.

Behavioral approaches

A wide range of behavioral interventions have successfully treated cocaine addiction. Approaches must be tailored to individuals' specific needs and available resources. Tailored programs with negotiated contingency rewards for drug avoidance, confirmed by urine testing, can work.

In cognitive-behavioral therapy, users learn to recognize, manage and avoid situations most likely to lead to cocaine use and develop healthy ways to cope with stressful situations.

Residential programs/therapeutic communities may also be helpful, particularly in more severe cases. Patients typically spend 6 to 12 months in such programs, which may also include vocational retraining.

Alternative treatment

Various alternative or complementary approaches, often combined with conventional therapies, have been used in treating cocaine addiction. In Japan, the herb acorus has been traditionally used both to assist early-stage cocaine withdrawal and in later recovery stages. Other herbs sometimes used to treat drug addictions of various kinds include kola nut, guarana seed and yohimbe (to boost short-term energy), and valerian root, hops leaf, scullcap leaf, and chamomile (to calm the patient). The amino acids phenylalanine and tyrosine have been used to reduce cocaine addicts' craving for the drug. Vitamin therapy may be used to help strengthen the patient. Gentle massage has been used to help infants born with congenital cocaine addiction. Other techniques, such as **acupuncture**, EEG **biofeedback**, and visualization, may also be useful in treating addiction.

Prognosis

Addiction is a complex disorder, and prospects for individual addicts vary widely. A 2004 study found that recovering drug addicts continue to crave the high and rush that they initially received from using the drug. However, research also has consistently shown that treatment can significantly reduce both drug abuse and subsequent criminal activity. The comprehensive Services Research Outcomes Study (1998) found a 45% drop in cocaine use five years after treatment, compared to use during the five years before treatment. The study also found that females generally respond better to treatment than males, and older patients tend to reduce their drug use more than younger patients.

Research supports the ability of twelve step programs, along with other approaches, to improve addiction treatment outcomes. One study in outpatient drug-treatment programs found that participation in a 12-step program nearly doubled the chances of remaining drug-free.

Prevention

Despite significant variation over time, cocaine addiction has proven to be a persistent public health problem. Interdiction and source control are expensive and have failed to eliminate the problem. Some law enforcement officials recommend more emphasis

---

KEY TERMS

Apoxia—Apoxia refers to altitude sickness.

Arrhythmia—Irregular heartbeat.

Central nervous system—Part of the nervous system consisting of the brain, cranial nerves, and spinal cord. The brain is the center of higher processes, such as thought and emotion and is responsible for the coordination and control of bodily activities and the interpretation of information from the senses. The cranial nerves and spinal cord link the brain to the peripheral nervous system, that is the nerves present in the rest of body.

Nasal septum—The membrane that separates the nostrils.

Neurotransmitter—A chemical that carries nerve impulses across a synapse.

Synapse—The gap between two nerve cells.

---

on demand reduction through education and other measures to address the causes of cocaine addiction.

Resources

PERIODICALS

"Craving for Cocaine May Last for Years after Recovery." *Health & Medicine Week* April 19, 2004: 846.

"Treating Cocaine Addiction with Viruses." *Ascribe Health News Service* June 21, 2004.

ORGANIZATIONS

Cocaine Anonymous, 21720 S. Wilmington Ave., Ste. 304, Long Beach, CA, 90810-1641, (310) 559-5833, (310) 559-2554, cawso@ca.org, http://www.ca.org/.

Nar-Anon Family Group Headquarters, 22527 Crenshaw Blvd., Suite 200B, Torrance, CA, 90505, (310) 534-8188, (800) 477-6291, naranonwso@nar-anon.org, http://www.nar-anon.org/Nar-Anon.

Peter Gregutt
Teresa G. Odle
James Waun, MD, RPh

Coccidioidomycosis

Definition

Coccidioidomycosis is an infection caused by inhaling the microscopic spores of the fungus *Coccidioides immitis*. Spores are the tiny, thick-walled structures that fungi use to reproduce. Coccidioidomycosis exists in three forms. The acute form produces flu-like symptoms. The chronic form can develop as many as 20 years after initial infection and, in the lungs, can produce inflamed, injured areas that can fill with pus (abscesses). Disseminated coccidioidomycosis describes the type of coccidioidomycosis that spreads throughout the body affecting many organ systems and is often fatal.

Description

Coccidioidomycosis is an airborne infection. The fungus that causes the disease is found in the dry desert soil of the southwestern United States, Mexico, and Central and South America. Coccidioidomycosis is sometimes called San Joaquin **fever**, valley fever, or desert fever because of its prevalence in the farming valleys of California. Although commonly acquired, overt coccidioidomycosis is a rare disease. Chronic infections occur in only one out of every 100,000 people.

Although anyone can get coccidioidomycosis, farm laborers, construction workers, and archaeologists who work where it is dusty are at greater risk to become infected. People of any age can get coccidioidomycosis, but the disease most commonly occurs in the 25–55 age group. In its acute form, coccidioidomycosis infects men and women equally.

Chronic and disseminated forms of coccidioidomycosis occur more frequently in men and pregnant women. Although it is not clear why, people of color are 10–20 times more likely to develop the disseminated form of the disease than caucasians. People who have a weakened immune system (immunocompromised), either from diseases such as **AIDS** or leukemia, or as the result of medications that suppressed the immune system (**corticosteroids**, **chemotherapy**), are more likely to develop disseminated coccidioidomycosis.

Causes and symptoms

When the spores of *C. immitis* are inhaled, they can become lodged in the lungs, divide, and cause localized inflammation. This is known as acute or primary coccidioidomycosis. The disease is not spread from one person to another. Approximately 60% of people who are infected exhibit no symptoms (asymptomatic). In the other 40%, symptoms appear 10–30 days after exposure. These symptoms include a fever which can reach 104°F (39.5°C), dry **cough**, chest pains, joint and muscle aches, **headache**, and weight loss. About two weeks after the start of the fever, some people develop a painful red rash or lumps on the lower legs. Symptoms usually disappear without treatment in about one month. People who have been infected gain partial immunity to reinfection.

The chronic form of coccidioidomycosis normally occurs after a long latent period of 20 or more years during which the patient experiences no symptoms of the disease. In the chronic phase, coccidioidomycosis causes lung abscesses that rupture, spilling pus and fluid into the lungs, and causing serious damage to the lungs. The patient experiences difficulty breathing and has a fever, chest **pain**, and other signs of **pneumonia**. Medical treatment is essential for recovery.

In its disseminated form, coccidioidomycosis spreads to other parts of the body including the liver, bones, skin, brain, heart, and lining around the heart (pericardium). Symptoms include fever, joint pain, loss of appetite, weight loss, night sweats, **skin lesions**, and difficulty breathing. Also, in 30–50% of patients with disseminated coccidioidomycosis, the tissue coverings of the brain and spinal cord become inflamed (**meningitis**).

Diagnosis

Many cases of coccidioidomycosis go undiagnosed because the symptoms resemble those of common viral diseases. However, a skin test similar to that for **tuberculosis** will determine whether a person has been infected. The test is simple and accurate, but it does not indicate whether the disease was limited to its acute form or if it has progressed to its chronic form.

Diagnosis of chronic or disseminated coccidioidomycosis is made by culturing a sample of sputum or other body fluids in the laboratory to isolate the fungus. A blood serum test is used to detect the presence of an antibody produced in response to *C. immitis* infection. Chest x rays are often used to assess lung damage, but alone cannot lead to a definitive diagnosis of coccidioidomycosis because other diseases can produce similar results on the x ray.

Treatment

In most cases of acute coccidioidomycosis, the body's own immune system is adequate to bring about recovery without medical intervention. Fever and pain can be treated with non-prescription drugs.

Chronic and disseminated coccidioidomycosis, however, are serious diseases that require treatment with prescription drugs. Patients with intact immune systems who develop chronic coccidioidomycosis are treated with the drug ketoconazole (Nizoral) or amphotericin B (Fungizone). Patients with suppressed

KEY TERMS

Abscess—An area of inflamed and injured body tissue that fills with pus.

Acidophilus—The bacteria *Lactobacillus acidophilus* that usually found in yogurt.

Antibody—A specific protein produced by the immune system in response to a specific foreign protein or particle called an antigen.

Antigen—A foreign protein to which the body reacts by making antibodies.

Asymptomatic—Persons who carry a disease but who do not exhibit symptoms of the disease are said to be asymptomatic.

Bifidobacteria—A group of bacteria normally present in the intestine. Commercial supplements containing these bacteria are available.

Corticosteroids—A group of hormones produced naturally by the adrenal gland or manufactured synthetically. They are often used to treat inflammation. Examples include cortisone and prednisone.

Immunocompromised—A state in which the immune system is suppressed or not functioning properly.

Meningitis—An inflammation of the membranes surrounding the brain or spinal cord.

Pericardium—The tissue sac around the heart.

immune systems are treated with amphotericin B (Fungizone). Amphotericin B is a powerful fungistatic drug with potentially toxic side effects. As a result, hospitalization is required in order to monitor patients. The patient may also receive other drugs to minimize the side effects of the amphotericin B.

Patients with AIDS must continue to take itraconazole (Sporonox) or fluconazole (Diflucan) orally or receive weekly intravenous doses of amphotericin B for the rest of their lives in order to prevent a relapse. Because of the high cost of fluconazole, Pfizer, the manufacturer of the drug, has established a financial assistance plan to make the drug available at lower cost to those who meet certain criteria. Patients needing this drug should ask their doctors about this program.

Alternative treatment

Alternative treatment for fungal infections focuses on creating an internal environment where the fungus cannot survive. This is accomplished by eating a diet low in dairy products, sugars, including honey and fruit juice, and foods like beer that contain yeast. This is complemented by a diet consisting, in large part, of uncooked and unprocessed foods. Supplements of **vitamins** C, E, A-plus, and B complex may also be useful. *Lactobacillus acidophilus* and *Bifidobacterium* will replenish the good bacteria in the intestines. Antifungal herbs, like garlic (*Allium sativum*), can be consumed in relatively large does and for an extended period of time in order to increase effectiveness.

Prognosis

Most people who are infected with coccidiodomycosis only suffer from the mild, acute form of the disease and recover without further complications. Patients who suffer from chronic coccidiodomycosis and who have no underlying lung or immune system diseases also stand a good change of recovery, although they must be alert to a relapse.

The picture for patients with the disseminated form of the disease, many of whom have AIDS, is less positive. Untreated disseminated coccidiodomycosis is almost always fatal within a short time. With treatment, chance of survival increases, but the **death** rate remains high when meningitis or diffuse lung (pulmonary) disease is present. AIDS patients must constantly guard against relapse.

Prevention

Because the fungus that causes coccidioidomycosis is airborne and microscopic, the only method of prevention is to avoid visiting areas where it is found in the soil. Unfortunately, for many people this is impractical. Maintaining general good health and avoiding HIV infection will limit coccidioidomycosis to the acute and relatively mild form in most people.

ORGANIZATIONS

American Lung Association, 1301 Pennsylvania Ave. NW, Suite 800, Washington, DC, 20001, (202) 758-3355, (202), 452-1805, (800) 548-8252, info@lungusa.org, http://www.lungusa.org/.

Canadian AIDS Treatment Information Exchange, 555 Richmond Street West, Suite 505, Toronto, Canada, Ontario, M5V 3B1, (426) 203-8242, (800) 263-1638, info@catie.ca, http://www.catie.ca.

Centers for Disease Control and Prevention (CDC), 1600 Clifton Road, Atlanta, GA, 30333, (800), 232-4636, cdcinfo@cdc.gov, http://www.cdc.gov.

National AIDS Hotline, CDC, 1600 Clifton Road, Atlanta, GA, 30333, (800), 232-4636, cdcinfo@cdc.gov, http://www.cdc.gov/hiv.

Project Inform, 1375 Mission Street, San Francisco, CA, 94103-2621, (415), 558-8669, (415), 558-0684, http://www.projinf.org.

Tish Davidson, A.M.

Coccyx injuries

Definition

The coccyx—or tailbone—is the last bone of the vertebral column, and usually consists of three to five fused vertebrae that connect with the sacrum, a part of the pelvis.

Description

The coccyx consists of fused vertebrae, which are not flexible like the other vertebrae of the vertebral column which are all interspaced by intervertebral disks and joined together by elastic ligaments. Since the spinal cord ends just before the coccyx begins, coccygeal vertebrae also lack a central foramen (hole). In the coccyx, the vertebrae generally fuse together in early adulthood and may also fuse with the sacrum, the bone located between the fifth lumbar vertebra and the coccyx, as a person ages. In males, the coccyx curves downward, and in females, it is straighter to allow a baby to pass through the birth canal without impediment.

Pain in or around the coccyx is called coccydynia or coccygodynia. Coccydynia presents a range of symptoms associated to a variety of underlying causes and conditions.

Causes and symptoms

Causes

Coccydynia can be caused by a number of factors. Usually, patients report pain after a fall onto their buttocks, as occurs when going down stairs or while skating. Others have pain during **pregnancy** or after **childbirth**. Some experience repetitive strain from rowing or cycling, and some cite anal intercourse as the cause of pain. In many cases, pain derives from a malformation of the coccyx itself. Sometimes bony spurs appear on the coccyx, but only seem to be painful in thin patients who do not have the padding to protect the region from the spur.

Other causes of coccydynia include **cancer** or damage to the sacrum that generates referred pain, meaning pain that appears in one region but originates from another. Muscle strain or tension, pinched nerves or damaged nerves, or dislocation of the coccyx due to gross **obesity** are other causes.

Symptoms

The most common symptom of coccydynia, irrespective of the cause of the condition, is pain when sitting, or when rising from a sitting position. If the condition lasts long enough, the patient may even experience pain when standing or lying down. Sometimes, **numbness** occurs in the lower part of the spine. Some patients will experience pain during bowel movements, sexual intercourse, or menstruation.

Secondary symptoms include back pain from sitting in odd positions in order to relieve pain, and painful feet from standing too much, because patients avoid sitting. Sometimes the entire buttocks experience pain. Rarely, exhaustion, depression, and lack of sleep may occur.

Diagnosis

Diagnosis of fracture is usually made by inserting a gloved finger in the rectum and pressing on the coccyx. X rays and **magnetic resonance imaging** (MRI) are also often used. Since coccyx pain may be the result of other factors like cancer, these must be ruled out through a variety of tests before treatment can begin.

Treatment

Treatment exists to either control the pain or eliminate the cause. Pain control may be dangerous if an underlying condition exists of which the pain is a warning sign. Nerve blocks and a variety of drugs are other options to control pain.

Elimination of the root cause of the pain is ideal. This is done through careful diagnosis and the application of manual treatments, corticosteroid injections into the coccyx vertebrae, or surgery. Injections into the fourth and fifth sacral nerves and coccygeal nerves often bring relief, but are considered more as a pain control measure than as curative treatment. Manual treatments have not been found to be effective. Surgery is a radical procedure whose indications are inconsistent and dependent on the subjectivity of the physician.

Prognosis

With current treatment, prognosis is good and patients usually are able to live pain free.

Prevention

There probably is no real prevention, expect weight control. Some women may choose to give birth through ceasarian section instead of vaginally after an episode of coccyx pain from a previous delivery.

Resources

OTHER

Maigne, Jean-Yves. "Treatment Strategies for Coccydynia." May 7, 2001. http://www.coccyx.org/whatisit.htm.

"Treatments for Coccydynia." May 7, 2001. http://www.coccyx.org/treatment.htm.

"What is Coccydynia?" May 7, 2001. http://www.coccyx.org/whatisit.htm.

Janie F. Franz

Cochlear implants

Definition

A cochlear implant is a surgical treatment for **hearing loss** that works like an artificial human cochlea in the inner ear, helping to send sound from the ear to the brain. It is different from a hearing aid, which simply amplifies sound.

Purpose

A cochlear implant bypasses damaged hair cells and helps establish some degree of hearing by stimulating the hearing (auditory) nerve directly.

Precautions

Because the implants are controversial, very expensive, and have uncertain results, the U.S. Food and Drug Administration (FDA) has limited the implants to people:

- who get no significant benefit from hearing aids
- who are at least two years old (the age at which specialists can verify severity of deafness)
- with severe to profound hearing loss

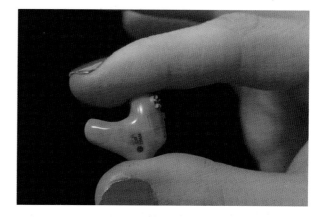

A close-up view of a cochlear implant. *(Custom Medical Stock Photo, Inc. Reproduced by permission.)*

Description

Hearing loss is caused by a number of different problems that occur either in the hearing nerve or parts of the middle or inner ear. The most common type of deafness is caused by damaged hair cells in the cochlea, the hearing part of the inner ear. Normally, hair cells stimulate the hearing nerve, which transmits sound signals to the brain. When hair cells stop functioning, the hearing nerve remains unstimulated, and the person cannot hear. Hair cells can be destroyed by many things, including infection, trauma, loud noise, **aging**, or **birth defects**.

All cochlear implants consist of a microphone worn behind the ear that picks up sound and sends it along a wire to a speech processor, which is worn in a small shoulder pouch, pocket, or belt. The processor boosts the sound, filters out background noise, and turns sound into digital signals before sending it to a transmitter worn behind the ear. A magnet holds the transmitter in place through its attraction to the receiver-stimulator, a part of the device that is surgically attached beneath the skin in the skull. The receiver picks up digital signs forwarded by the transmitter, and converts them into electrical impulses. These electrical impulses flow through electrodes contained in a narrow, flexible tube that has been threaded into the cochlea.

As many as 24 electrodes (depending on the type of implant) carry the impulses that stimulate the hearing nerve. The brain then interprets the signals as specific sounds.

Despite the benefits that the implant appears to offer, some hearing specialists and members of the deaf community still believe that the benefits may not outweigh the risks and limitations of the device. Because the device must be surgically implanted, it carries some surgical risk. Also, manufacturers cannot promise how well a person will hear with an implant. Moreover, after getting an implant, some people say they feel alienated from the deaf community, while at the same time not feeling fully a part of the hearing world.

The sounds heard through an implant are different from the normal hearing sounds, and have been described as artificial or "robotlike." This is because the implant's handful of electrodes cannot hope to match the complexity of a person's 15,000 hair cells.

Surgical procedure

During the procedure, the surgeon makes an incision behind the ear and opens the mastoid bone (the ridge on the skull behind the ear) leading into the middle ear. The surgeon then places the receiver-stimulator in the bone, and gently threads the electrodes into the cochlea. This operation takes between one and one-half to five hours.

Preparation

Before a person gets an implant, specialists at an implant clinic conduct a careful evaluation, including extensive hearing tests to determine how well the candidate can hear.

Unfortunately, it is not possible to predict who will benefit from an implant. In general, the later in life a person becomes deaf, and the shorter the duration of deafness, the better the person is likely to understand speech with an implant. Likewise, someone with a healthy hearing nerve will do better than someone with a damaged nerve.

First, candidates undergo a trial with a powerful hearing aid. If the aid cannot improve hearing enough, a physician then performs a physical exam and orders a scan of the inner ear (some patients with a scarred cochlea are not good candidates). A doctor may also order a psychological exam to better understand the person's expectations. Patients need to be highly motivated, and have a realistic understanding of what an implant can and cannot do.

Aftercare

The patient remains in the hospital for a day or two after the surgery. After a month, the surgical **wounds** will have healed and the patient returns to the implant clinic to be fitted with the external parts of the device (the speech processor, microphone, and transmitter). A clinicican tunes the speech processor and sets levels of stimulation for each electrode, from soft to loud.

The patient is then trained in how to interpret the sounds heard through the device. The length of the training varies from days to years, depending on how well the person can interpret the sounds heard through the device.

Risks

As with all operations, there are a few risks of surgery. These include:

- dizziness
- facial paralysis (rarely)
- infection at the incision site

296-5700, (301) 296-8580, (800) 638-8255, actioncenter@
asha.org, http://asha.org/.
Cochlear Implant Club International, 5335 Wisconsin Ave. NW,
Suite 440, Washington, DC, 20015-2052, (202) 895-2781.
National Association of the Deaf, 8630 Fenton St, #820,
Silver Spring, MD, 20910, (301) 587-1788, (301) 587-
1791, http://www.nad.org.

Carol A. Turkington

KEY TERMS

Cochlea—The hearing part of the inner ear. This snail-shaped structure contains fluid and thousands of microscopic hair cells tuned to various frequencies.

Hair cells—Sensory receptors in the inner ear that transform sound vibrations into messages that travel to the brain.

Inner ear—The interior section of the ear, where sound vibrations and information about balance are translated into nerve impulses.

Middle ear—The small cavity between the eardrum and the oval window that houses the three tiny bones of hearing.

Scientists are not sure about the long-term effects of electrical stimulation on the nervous system. It is also possible to damage the implant's internal components by a blow to the head, which will render the device unworkable.

Normal results

Most profoundly, deaf patients who receive an implant are able to discern medium and loud sounds, including speech, at comfortable listening levels. Many use sound clues from the implant, together with speech reading and other facial cues. Almost all adults improve their communication skills when combining the implant with speech reading (lip reading), and some can understand spoken words without speech reading. More than half of adults who lost hearing after they learned to speak can understand some speech without speech reading. About 30% can understand spoken sounds well enough to use the phone.

Children who were born deaf or who lost their hearing before they could speak have the most difficulty in learning to use the implant. Research suggests, however, that most of these children are able to learn spoken language and understand speech using the implant.

ORGANIZATIONS

Alexander Graham Bell Association for the Deaf and Hard of Hearing, 3417 Volta Place NW, Washington, DC, 20007, (202) 337-5220, (202) 337-8314, info@agbell. org, http://www.agbell.org.
American Speech Language Hearing Association, 2200 Research Boulevard , Rockville, MD, 20850-3289, (301)

Cognitive-behavioral therapy

Definition

Cognitive-behavioral therapy is an action-oriented form of psychosocial therapy that assumes that maladaptive, or faulty, thinking patterns cause maladaptive behavior and "negative" emotions. (Maladaptive behavior is behavior that is counter-productive or interferes with everyday living.) The treatment focuses on changing an individual's thoughts (cognitive patterns) in order to change his or her behavior and emotional state.

Purpose

Theoretically, cognitive-behavioral therapy can be employed in any situation in which there is a pattern of unwanted behavior accompanied by distress and impairment. It is a recommended treatment option for a number of mental disorders, including affective (mood) disorders, **personality disorders**, social phobia, **obsessive-compulsive disorder** (OCD), **eating disorders**, **substance abuse**, **anxiety** or **panic disorder**, **agoraphobia**, **post-traumatic stress disorder** (PTSD), and attention-deficit/hyperactivity disorder (**ADHD**). It is also frequently used as a tool to deal with chronic **pain** for patients with illnesses such as **rheumatoid arthritis**, back problems, and **cancer**. Patients with **sleep disorders** may also find cognitive-behavioral therapy a useful treatment for **insomnia**.

Precautions

Cognitive-behavioral therapy may not be suitable for some patients. Those who do not have a specific behavioral issue they wish to address and whose goals for therapy are to gain insight into the past may be better served by psychodynamic therapy. Patients must also be willing to take a very active role in the treatment process.

Cognitive-behavioral intervention may be inappropriate for some severely psychotic patients and for cognitively impaired patients (for example, patients with organic brain disease or a traumatic brain injury), depending on their level of functioning.

Description

Cognitive-behavioral therapy combines the individual goals of cognitive therapy and behavioral therapy.

Pioneered by psychologists Aaron Beck and Albert Ellis in the 1960s, cognitive therapy assumes that maladaptive behaviors and disturbed mood or emotions are the result of inappropriate or irrational thinking patterns, called *automatic thoughts*. Instead of reacting to the reality of a situation, an individual reacts to his or her own distorted viewpoint of the situation. For example, a person may conclude that he is "worthless" simply because he failed an exam or did not get a date. Cognitive therapists attempt to make their patients aware of these distorted thinking patterns, or cognitive distortions, and change them (a process termed cognitive restructuring).

Behavioral therapy, or behavior modification, trains individuals to replace undesirable behaviors with healthier behavioral patterns. Unlike psychodynamic therapies, it does not focus on uncovering or understanding the unconscious motivations that may be behind the maladaptive behavior. In other words, strictly behavioral therapists do not try to find out why their patients behave the way they do, they just teach them to change the behavior.

Cognitive-behavioral therapy integrates the cognitive restructuring approach of cognitive therapy with the behavioral modification techniques of behavioral therapy. The therapist works with the patient to identify both the thoughts and the behaviors that are causing distress, and to change those thoughts in order to readjust the behavior. In some cases, the patient may have certain fundamental core beliefs, called schemas, which are flawed and require modification. For example, a patient suffering from depression may be avoiding social contact with others, and suffering considerable emotional distress because of his isolation. When questioned why, the patient reveals to his therapist that he is afraid of rejection, of what others may do or say to him. Upon further exploration with his therapist, they discover that his real fear is not rejection, but the belief that he is hopelessly uninteresting and unlovable. His therapist then tests the reality of that assertion by having the patient name friends and family who love him and enjoy his company. By showing the patient that others value him, the therapist both exposes the irrationality of the patient's belief and provides him with a new model of thought to change his old behavior pattern. In this case, the person learns to think, "I am an interesting and lovable person; therefore I should not have difficulty making new friends in social situations." If enough "irrational cognitions" are changed, this patient may experience considerable relief from his depression.

A number of different techniques may be employed in cognitive-behavioral therapy to help patients uncover and examine their thoughts and change their behaviors. They include:

- Behavioral homework assignments. Cognitive-behavioral therapists frequently request that their patients complete homework assignments between therapy sessions. These may consist of real-life "behavioral experiments" where patients are encouraged to try out new responses to situations discussed in therapy sessions.

- Cognitive rehearsal. The patient imagines a difficult situation and the therapist guides him through the step-by-step process of facing and successfully dealing with it. The patient then works on practicing, or rehearsing, these steps mentally. Ideally, when the situation arises in real life, the patient will draw on the rehearsed behavior to address it.

- Journal. Patients are asked to keep a detailed diary recounting their thoughts, feelings, and actions when specific situations arise. The journal helps to make the patient aware of his or her maladaptive thoughts and to show their consequences on behavior. In later stages of therapy, it may serve to demonstrate and reinforce positive behaviors.

- Modeling. The therapist and patient engage in role-playing exercises in which the therapist acts out appropriate behaviors or responses to situations.

- Conditioning. The therapist uses reinforcement to encourage a particular behavior. For example, a child with ADHD gets a gold star every time he stays focused on tasks and accomplishes certain daily chores. The gold star reinforces and increases the desired behavior by identifying it with something positive. Reinforcement can also be used to extinguish unwanted behaviors by imposing negative consequences.

- Systematic desensitization. Patients imagine a situation they fear, while the therapist employs techniques to help the patient relax, helping the person cope with their fear reaction and eventually eliminate the anxiety altogether. For example, a patient in treatment for agoraphobia, or fear of open or public places, will relax and then picture herself on the sidewalk outside of her house. In her next session, she may relax herself and then imagine a visit to a crowded shopping mall. The imagery of the anxiety-producing situations gets progressively more intense until, eventually, the therapist and patient approach the anxiety-causing situation in real-life (a "graded exposure"), perhaps by visiting a mall. Exposure may be increased to the point of "flooding," providing maximum exposure to the real situation. By repeatedly pairing a desired response (relaxation) with a fear-producing situation (open, public spaces), the patient gradually becomes desensitized to the old response of fear and learns to react with feelings of relaxation.

- Validity testing. Patients are asked to test the validity of the automatic thoughts and schemas they encounter. The therapist may ask the patient to defend or produce evidence that a schema is true. If the patient is unable to meet the challenge, the faulty nature of the schema is exposed.

Initial treatment sessions are typically spent explaining the basic tenets of cognitive-behavioral therapy to the patient and establishing a positive working relationship between therapist and patient. Cognitive-behavioral therapy is a collaborative, action-oriented therapy effort. As such, it empowers the patient by giving him an active role in the therapy process and discourages any overdependence on the therapist that may occur in other therapeutic relationships. Therapy is typically administered in an outpatient setting in either an individual or group session. Therapists include psychologists (Ph.D., Psy.D., Ed.D. or M.A. degree), clinical social workers (M.S.W., D.S.W., or L.S.W. degree), counselors (M.A. or M.S. degree), or psychiatrists (M.D. with specialization in psychiatry) and should be trained in cognitive-behavioral techniques, although some brief cognitive-behavioral interventions may be suggested by a primary physician/caregiver. Treatment is relatively short in comparison to some other forms of **psychotherapy**, usually lasting no longer than 16 weeks. Many insurance plans provide reimbursement for cognitive-behavioral therapy services. Because coverage is dependent on the disorder or illness the therapy is treating, patients should check with their individual plans.

Rational-emotive behavior therapy

Rational-emotive behavior therapy (REBT) is a popular variation of cognitive-behavioral therapy developed in 1955 by psychologist Albert Ellis. REBT is based on the belief that a person's past experiences shape their belief system and thinking patterns. People form illogical, irrational thinking patterns that become the cause of both their negative emotions and of further irrational ideas. REBT focuses on helping patients discover these irrational beliefs that guide their behavior and replace them with rational beliefs and thoughts in order to relieve their emotional distress.

There are 10 basic irrational assumptions that trigger maladaptive emotions and behaviors:

- It is a necessity for an adult to be loved and approved of by almost everyone for virtually everything.
- A person must be thoroughly competent, adequate, and successful in all respects.
- Certain people are bad, wicked, or villainous, and should be punished for their sins.
- It is catastrophic when things are not going the way one would like.
- Human unhappiness is externally caused. People have little or no ability to control their sorrows or to rid themselves of negative feelings.
- It is right to be terribly preoccupied with and upset about something that may be dangerous or fearsome.
- It is easier to avoid facing many of life's difficulties and responsibilities than it is to undertake more rewarding forms of self-discipline.
- The past is all-important. Because something once strongly affected someone's life, it should continue to do so indefinitely.
- People and things should be different from the way they are. It is catastrophic if perfect solutions to the grim realities of life are not immediately found.
- Maximal human happiness can be achieved by inertia and inaction or by living passively and without commitment.

Meichenbaum's self-instructional approach

Psychologist Donald Meichenbaum pioneered the self-instructional, or "self-talk," approach to cognitive-behavioral therapy in the 1970s. This approach focuses on changing what people say to themselves, both internally and out loud. It is based on the belief that an individual's actions follow directly from this self-talk. This type of therapy emphasizes teaching patients coping skills that they can use in a variety of situations to help themselves. The technique used to accomplish this is self-instructional inner dialogue, a method of talking through a problem or situation as it occurs.

Preparation

Patients may seek therapy independently, or be referred for treatment by a primary physician,

KEY TERMS

Automatic thoughts—Thoughts that automatically come to mind when a particular situation occurs. Cognitive-behavioral therapy seeks to challenge automatic thoughts.

Cognitive restructuring—The process of replacing maladaptive thought patterns with constructive thoughts and beliefs.

Maladaptive—Unsuitable or counterproductive; for example, maladaptive behavior is behavior that is inappropriate to a given situation.

Psychodynamic therapy—A therapeutic approach that assumes dysfunctional or unwanted behavior is caused by unconscious, internal conflicts and focuses on gaining insight into these motivations.

Relaxation technique—A technique used to relieve stress. Exercise, biofeedback, hypnosis, and meditation are all effective relaxation tools. Relaxation techniques are used in cognitive-behavioral therapy to teach patients new ways of coping with stressful situations.

Schemas—Fundamental core beliefs or assumptions that are part of the perceptual filter people use to view the world. Cognitive-behavioral therapy seeks to change maladaptive schemas.

---

psychologist, or psychiatrist. Because the patient and therapist work closely together to achieve specific therapeutic objectives, it is important that their working relationship is comfortable and their goals are compatible. Prior to beginning treatment, the patient and therapist should meet for a consultation session, or mutual interview. The consultation gives the therapist the opportunity to make an initial assessment of the patient and recommend a course of treatment and goals for therapy. It also gives the patient an opportunity to find out important details about the therapist's approach to treatment, professional credentials, and any other issues of interest.

In some managed-care clinical settings, an intake interview or evaluation is required before a patient begins therapy. The intake interview is used to evaluate the patient and assign him or her to a therapist. It may be conducted by a psychiatric nurse, counselor, or social worker.

Normal results

Many patients who undergo cognitive-behavioral therapy successfully learn how to replace their maladaptive thoughts and behaviors with positive ones that facilitate individual growth and happiness. Cognitive-behavioral therapy may be used in conjunction with pharmaceutical and other treatment interventions, so overall success rates are difficult to gauge. However, success rates of 65% or more have been reported with cognitive-behavioral therapy alone as a treatment for panic attacks and agoraphobia. Relapse has been reported in some patient populations, perhaps due to the brief nature of the therapy, but follow-up sessions can put patients back on track.

ORGANIZATIONS

Albert Ellis Institute, 45 East 65th St., New York, NY, 10021, (800) 323-4738, http://www.rebt.org.

Beck Institute, GSB Building, City Line and Belmont Avenues, Suite 700, Bala Cynwyd, PA, 19004-1610, (610) 664-3020, http://www.beckinstitute.org.

National Association of Cognitive-Behavioral Therapists, P.O. Box 2195, Weirton, WV, 26062, (800) 853-1135, http://www.nacbt.org.

Paula Anne Ford-Martin
Brenda W. Lerner

Colchicine see **Gout drugs**

COLD see **Chronic obstructive pulmonary disease**

Cold agglutinins test

Definition

The cold agglutinins test is performed to detect the presence of antibodies in blood that are sensitive to temperature changes. Antibodies are proteins produced by the immune system in response to specific disease agents; autoantibodies are antibodies that the body produces against one of its own substances. Cold agglutinins are autoantibodies that cause red blood cells to clump, but only when the blood is cooled below the normal body temperature of 98.6°F (37°C). The clumping is most pronounced at temperatures below 78°F (25.6°C).

Agglutinin—An antibody that causes red blood cells to stick or clump together.

Antibody—A protein molecule produced by the immune system that is specific to a disease agent, such as *Mycoplasma pneumoniae*. The antibody combines with the organism and disables it.

Autoantibody—An antibody produced by the body in reaction to any of its own cells or cell products.

Cold agglutinins—Antibodies that cause clumping of red blood cells when the blood temperature falls below normal body temperature (98.6°F/ 37°C).

Hemolytic anemia—Oxygen deficiency in the blood, caused by shortened survival of red blood cells.

Mycoplasma—A type of free-living microorganism that has no cell wall. Mycoplasmas cause some varieties of pneumonia and urinary tract infections that stimulate the body to produce cold agglutinins.

Titer—The concentration of a substance in a given sample of blood or other tissue fluid.

Purpose

The cold agglutinins test is used to confirm the diagnosis of certain diseases that stimulate the body to produce cold agglutinins. The disease most commonly diagnosed by this test is mycoplasmal **pneumonia**, but mononucleosis, **mumps**, **measles**, **scarlet fever**, some parasitic infections, **cirrhosis** of the liver, and some types of **hemolytic anemia** can also cause the formation of cold agglutinins. Hemolytic **anemias** are conditions in which the blood is low in oxygen because the red blood cells are breaking down at a faster rate than their normal life expectancy of 120 days. In addition to these illnesses, some people have a benign condition called chronic cold agglutinin disease, in which exposure to cold causes temporary clumping of red blood cells and consequent **numbness** in ears, fingers, and toes.

Description

Since cold agglutinins cause red blood cells to clump only at temperatures lower than 98.6°F (37°C), the test consists of chilling a sample of the patient's blood. There is a bedside version of the test in which the doctor collects four or five drops of blood in a small tube, cools the tube in ice water for 30–60 seconds, and looks for clumping of red blood cells. If the cells clump after chilling and unclump as they rewarm, a cold agglutinin titer (concentration) greater than 1:64 is present. Bedside test results, however, should be confirmed by a laboratory. The laboratory test measures the clumping of red blood cells in different dilutions of the patient's blood serum at 39.2°F (4°C).

Normal results

The results of the cold agglutinins test require a doctor's interpretation. In general, however, a normal value is lower than 1:32.

Abnormal results

Any value higher than 1:32 suggests a diagnosis of mycoplasmal pneumonia or one of the other viral infections or disease conditions indicated by this test.

Resources

BOOKS

Kjeldsberg, Carl R. *Practical Diagnosis of Hematologic Disorders*. 4th ed. Chicago: ASCP Press, 2006.

Rebecca J. Frey, PhD

Cold sensitivity antibodies test *see*
Cryoglobulin test

Cold sores

Definition

Cold sores are the popular name for mouth sores caused by a type of herpes simplex virus (HSV) known as HSV-1. They are also sometimes referred to as **fever** blisters, herpes labialis, or oral herpes.

Demographics

Cold sores are a commonplace health problem around the world. According to the National Institutes of Health (NIH), about 80% of people in the United States are infected with HSV-1; other estimates give a figure of 90% of all adults worldwide. Most acquire the infection as children from contact with oral fluids from an infected person. Infection with the virus is thought to be equally common in both sexes and all races and ethnic groups. Although

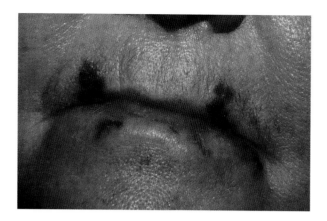

A close-up view of a patient's mouth with gingivostomatitis cold sores. *(Custom Medical Stock Photo, Inc. Reproduced by permission.)*

infection with HSV-1 is common, only about 10% of infected people actually develop cold sores.

Description

Cold sores are small blisters that form around the outside of the mouth; they should be distinguished from **canker sores**, which form inside the mouth and are not contagious. Caused by a virus known as herpes simplex type 1, cold sores are contagious; direct contact with an infected person may result in contracting the virus. The virus that causes cold sores is related to the herpes simplex virus type 2, HSV-2, that causes **genital herpes**.

Risk factors

People with weakened immune systems, such as patients who have had an organ transplant or are being treated for **cancer** or HIV infection, are at increased risk of getting cold sores if they are exposed to HSV-1.

Causes and symptoms

Causes

The cause of cold sores is HSV-1. The virus enters the body through tiny breaks in the tissues lining the mouth, which is one reason it can easily be spread by kissing or by sharing drinking glasses and other food utensils. The first time a person is infected by the virus, they may simply run a fever without having cold sores. HSV-1 then lies dormant in the cells of the nervous system until it is activated by emotional **stress**, an upper respiratory infection, sun exposure, or some other trigger. It then travels back down the nerves to

the skin surface. About 35% of people who get cold sores get them in the same area of skin each time.

Symptoms

Most people who become infected with HSV-1 develop cold sores within 20 days of infection, although symptoms may develop sooner. In most cases, the first eruption of the blisters is preceded by a prodrome, or period of warning symptoms before the main phase of the illness. The prodrome of cold sores usually consists of a **tingling**, **itching**, or burning sensation that starts one or two days before the blisters appear. The area of skin where the blisters will erupt may swell up, turn red, and be sore to the touch.

The sores themselves last about 7–10 days after they erupt. They appear most commonly on the lips or the area of skin between the upper lip and the nose, but may also appear on the cheeks. Cold sores sometimes appear inside the mouth. Some people may develop a **sore throat**, swelling of the lymph nodes in the neck, or have difficulty swallowing during an outbreak of cold sores.

The blisters associated with cold sores are small and thin-walled, filled with a clear fluid that may ooze out of the sores. HSV-1 is shed in the fluid from the sores and can be transmitted to other people if they come in contact with the blisters. This is the stage in the development of cold sores when the infection is most contagious. After a few days, the blisters break and form a yellow crust that eventually drops off, leaving an area of pinkish skin underneath. There is no permanent scar from a cold sore. Most people who get cold sores have one or two recurrences per year, although some have an outbreak every month.

Diagnosis

Most people can tell whether they have cold sores by the way they feel and where the sores appear. If necessary, the patient's doctor can run a blood test to tell whether the person is infected with HSV-1. This type of test is important if the person is HIV-positive or is being treated with **chemotherapy** for cancer.

Examination

In most cases, people do not need to visit the doctor or dentist for ordinary cold sores. They should make an appointment if they have any of the following symptoms or conditions:

- HIV or any other illness that weakens the immune system
- the cold sores do not heal on their own by the end of two weeks
- the patient's eyes feel sore or irritated
- the cold sores recur frequently
- the blisters are unusually large or painful

Tests

Testing is rarely needed to confirm a diagnosis of cold sores, as the doctor or dentist can usually tell by examining the patient in the office and noting the location of the blisters.

Treatment

Traditional

There is no permanent cure for HSV-1 infection. After a person is infected with the virus, it hides within nerve cells, making it difficult for the immune system to find and destroy it. HSV-1 remains in the body, so that cold sores can reappear at any time. Recurrences of oral herpes can be triggered by a number of factors, including getting the flu or a cold, not getting enough sleep, having dental work or oral surgery, getting traveler's **diarrhea**, menstruation (in women), emotional stress, an injury to the mouth or lips, or exposure to the sun for long periods of time. The connection between colds and flu in reactivating HSV-1 is the main reason why oral herpes is commonly known as cold sores or fever blisters.

Drugs

There are some medications that can be used to treat cold sores. The best time to start treating them is during the prodromal stage before the blisters appear. The doctor or dentist can prescribe an antiviral medication to shorten the length of the outbreak and reduce discomfort; the **antiviral drugs** most often prescribed for cold sores are acyclovir (Zovirax), famciclovir (Famvir), and valacyclovir (Valtrex). Some of these drugs are taken by mouth while others can be applied to the sores as gels or creams. A topical cream containing 10% docosanol, an antiviral drug available

without a prescription, has been shown to be an effective treatment for recurrent cold sores. Other treatments that can be used are topical anesthetics applied directly to the sores; and **aspirin**, Advil, or Tylenol to bring down fever.

Therapies for cold sores that are considered experimental as of 2010 include **photodynamic therapy** (PDT) and a medication taken by mouth made from vitamin C combined with a chemical compound derived from pine cones. One group of researchers reported that photodynamic therapy done with lasers reduced the size and swelling of the patients' cold sores but did not reduce the **pain** level or the frequency of recurrences, while a small study of four patients treated with laser PDT reported that all patients experienced at least some pain relief and found that their blisters healed more rapidly. Most observers think that PDT with lasers is a promising form of therapy for recurrent cold sores but needs further research.

Home remedies

Some people find that ice applied to cold sore blisters helps to relieve discomfort, while others are helped by warm compresses. An over-the-counter remedy that works for some people is zinc oxide cream.

Prognosis

Most cases of cold sores heal without any long-term problems, as the disease is considered self-limited; however, HSV-1 can cause an eye infection that may lead to permanent blindness if fluid from the sores gets into the eyes. For this reason it is important for people with cold sores to avoid scratching or squeezing the blisters.

Prevention

The National Institutes of Health (NIH) recommends the following measures to lower the risk of spreading HSV-1 to other parts of the body or to other people, and to lower the frequency of recurrences.

- Avoid kissing or close contact with others while the blisters are present.
- Avoid sharing items that touch the mouth. These include towels, washcloths, lipsticks, lip balms, razors, and toothbrushes as well as drinking glasses and food utensils.
- Keep the hands clean. Wash them frequently and avoid touching the eyes or genital area during an outbreak.
- Avoid putting the fingers in the mouth or biting fingernails.
- Try to avoid such common triggers of cold sores as colds or flu, high stress levels, or being short on sleep.

- Avoid contact sports (football, wrestling, etc.) during an outbreak.
- Use sunblock on the lips and face when outdoors for long periods of time.

Some people with frequent recurrences of cold sores benefit from an over-the-counter dietary supplement called lysine, which is an amino acid (one of the building blocks of proteins). Patients should check with their doctor to see whether lysine might be helpful for them.

People who develop significant related illnesses during cold sore outbreaks, are frequently exposed to sunlight or other known triggers, or have frequent outbreaks of cold sores may wish to ask their doctor or dentist for an antiviral drug to help prevent recurrent outbreaks.

Resources

BOOKS

Feigin, Ralph D., et al., eds. *Feigin and Cherry's Textbook of Pediatric Infectious Diseases*. 6th ed. Philadelphia: Saunders/Elsevier, 2009.

Frankel, David H., ed. *Field Guide to Clinical Dermatology*. 2nd ed. Philadelphia: Lippincott Williams and Wilkins, c. 2006.

Studahl, Marie, Paola Cinque, and Tomas Bergstroöm, eds. *Herpes Simplex Viruses*. Boca Raton, FL: Taylor and Francis, 2006.

PERIODICALS

de Carvalho, R.R., et al. "Effect of Laser Phototherapy on Recurring Herpes Labialis Prevention: An In Vivo Study." *Lasers in Medical Science* 25 (May 2010): 397–402.

Lopez, B.S., et al. "A Clinical Pilot Study of Lignin-Ascorbic Acid Combination Treatment of Herpes Simplex Virus." *In Vivo* 23 (November-December 2009): 1011–1016.

Marotti, J., et al. "High-intensity Laser and Photodynamic Therapy as a Treatment for Recurrent Herpes Labialis." *Photomedicine and Laser Surgery* 28 (June 2010): 439–44.

Sperandio, F.F., et al. "Photodynamic Therapy for the Treatment of Recurrent Herpes Labialis: Preliminary Results." *General Dentistry* 57 (July-August 2009): 415–19.

St. Pierre, S.A., et al. "Practical Management Measures for Patients with Recurrent Herpes Labialis." *Skin Therapy Letter* 14 (November-December 2009): 1–3.

Treister, N.S., and S.B. Woo. "Topical N-docosanol for Management of Recurrent Herpes Labialis." *Expert Opinion on Pharmacotherapy* 11 (April 2010): 853–60.

OTHER

American Academy of Dermatology (AAD). "Herpes Simplex." November 2003. http://www.aad.org/public/ publications/pamphlets/viral_herpes_simplex.html (accessed September 18, 2010).

American Dental Association (ADA). "Canker Sores, Cold Sores and Common Mouth Sores." http://www. ada.org/2610.aspx?currentTab = 2 (accessed September 18, 2010).

"Cold Sore." *MayoClinic.com*. March 13, 2010. http:// www.mayoclinic.com/health/cold-sore/DS00358 (accessed September 18, 2010).

Opstelten, W., et al. "Treatment and Prevention of Herpes Labialis." *Canadian Family Physician* 54 (December 2008): 1683–87. http://www.cfp.ca/cgi/content/full/54/ 12/1683 (accessed September 18, 2010).

Torres, Gisela, et al. "Herpes Simplex." *eMedicine*. August 25, 2009. http://emedicine.medscape.com/ article/1132351-overview (accessed September 18, 2010).

ORGANIZATIONS

American Academy of Dermatology (AAD), P.O. Box 4014, Schaumburg, IL, 60168, (847) 330-0230, (866) 503-SKIN, (847) 240-1859, http://www. aad.org.

American Dental Association (ADA), 211 East Chicago Ave., Chicago, IL, 60611, (312) 440-2500, http:// www.ada.org.

Rebecca J. Frey, PhD

Cold spot myocardial imaging *see* **Thallium heart scan**

Colds *see* **Common cold**

Colic

Definition

Colic is persistent, unexplained crying in a healthy baby between two weeks and five months of age.

Demographics

Colic affects between 10–30% of babies. It occurs equally in male and female babies and is independent of race or ethnicity.

Description

Colic is not a disease. Symptoms of colic usually appear when a baby is 14–21 days old, reach a crescendo at the age of three months, and disappear within the next eight weeks. Episodes occur frequently, but intermittently, and usually begin with prolonged periods of crying in the late afternoon or evening. Crying can last for a few minutes or continue for several hours.

Gastroesophageal reflux—A condition in which the stomach contents back up into the esophagus. Because the stomach contents are highly acidic, this can cause irritation and heartburn.

Some babies who have colic are simply fussy. Others cry so hard that their faces turn red, then pale.

Causes and symptoms

No one knows what causes colic or why some babies are colicky and others are not. The condition may be the result of swallowing large amounts of air, which becomes trapped in the digestive tract and causes bloating and severe abdominal **pain**.

Other possible causes of colic include:

- digestive tract immaturity
- food intolerances
- hunger or overfeeding
- gastroesophageal reflux
- overheated milk or formula
- overstimulation resulting from noise, light, or activity

During a colicky episode, babies' bellies often look swollen, feel hard, and make a rumbling sound. Crying intensifies, tapers off, and then gets louder. Many babies grow rigid, clench their fists, curl their toes, and draw their legs toward their body. A burp or a bowel movement can end an attack. Most babies who have colic do not seem to be in pain between attacks.

Diagnosis

Pediatricians and family physicians suspect colic in an infant who:

- has cried loudly for at least three hours a day at least three times a week for three weeks or longer
- is not hungry but cries for several hours between dinnertime and midnight
- demonstrates the clenched fists, rigidity, and other physical traits associated with colic

The baby's medical history and a parent's description of eating, sleeping, and crying patterns are used to confirm a diagnosis of colic. Studies have shown that colic crying is different from regular crying in that it is higher pitched, more turbulent, and more urgent than regular crying. **Physical examination** and laboratory tests are used to rule out infection, intestinal blockage, and other conditions that can cause abdominal pain and other colic-like symptoms.

Treatment

Home remedies

Medications do not cure colic. Doctors sometimes recommend simethicone (Mylicon Drops) to relieve gas pain, but generally advise parents to take a practical approach to the problem.

Gently massaging the baby's back can release a trapped gas bubble, and holding the baby in a sitting position can help prevent air from being swallowed during feedings. Bottle-fed babies can swallow air if nipple holes are either too large or too small.

Nipple-hole size can be checked by filling a bottle with cold formula, turning it upside down, and counting the number of drops released when it is shaken or squeezed. A nipple hole that is the right size will release about one drop of formula every second.

Babies should not be fed every time they cry, but feeding and burping a baby more often may alleviate symptoms of colic. A bottle-fed baby should be burped after every ounce, and a baby who is **breastfeeding** should be burped every five minutes.

When cow's milk is the source of the symptoms, bottle-fed babies should be switched to a soymilk hydrolyzed protein formula. A woman whose baby is breastfeeding should eliminate dairy products from her diet for seven days, then gradually reintroduce them unless the baby's symptoms reappear.

Since intolerance to foods other than cow's milk may also lead to symptoms of colic, breastfeeding women may also relieve their babies' colic by eliminating from their diet:

- coffee
- tea
- cocoa
- citrus
- peanuts
- wheat
- broccoli and other vegetables belonging to the cabbage family

Rocking a baby in a quiet, darkened room can prevent overstimulation, and a baby usually calms down when cuddled in a warm, soft blanket.

Colicky babies cry less when they are soothed by the motion of a wind-up swing, a car ride, or being carried in a parent's arms. Pacifiers can soothe babies who are upset, but a pacifier should never be attached to a string.

Alternative treatment

Applying gentle pressure to the webbed area between the thumb and index finger of either hand can calm a crying child. So can gently massaging the area directly above the child's navel and the corresponding spot on the spine. Applying warm compresses or holding your hand firmly over the child's abdomen can relieve cramping.

Teas made with chamomile (*Matricaria recutita*), lemon balm (*Melissa officinalis*), peppermint (*Mentha piperita*), or dill (*Anethum graveolens*) can lessen bowel inflammation and reduce gas. A homeopathic combination called "colic" may be effective, and constitutional homeopathic treatment can help strengthen the child's entire constitution.

A doctor should be notified if a baby who has been diagnosed with colic:

- develops a rectal fever higher than 101°F (38.3 °C)
- cries for more than four hours
- vomits
- has diarrhea or stools that are black or bloody
- loses weight
- eats less than normal

Prognosis

Colic is distressing, but it is not dangerous. Symptoms almost always disappear before a child is six months old.

Prevention

Many doctors believe that colic cannot be prevented. Some alternative practitioners, however, feel that colic can be prevented by an awareness of food intolerances and their impact.

Resources

BOOKS

Vartabedian, Bryan. *Colic Solved: The Essential Guide to Infant Reflux, and the Care of Your Screaming, Spitting, Congested, Hiccupping, Sleepless, Difficult-to-Feed Baby.* New York : Ballantine Books, 2007.

OTHER

"Colic." Mayo Foundation for Medical Education and Research. April 14, 2009. http://www.mayoclinic.com/health/colic/ds00058

Colic and Crying. MedlinePlus Encyclopedia. August 2, 2009. http://www.nlm.nih.gov/medlineplus/ency/article/000978.htm

Deshpande, Prashant G. Colic. eMedicine.com October 7, 2009. http://emedicine.medscape.com/article/927760-overview

ORGANIZATIONS

American Academy of Family Physicians, P. O. Box 11210, Shawnee Mission, KS, 66207, (913) 906-6000, (800) 274-2237, (913) 906-6075, http://familydoctor.org.

American Academy of Pediatrics, 141 Northwest Point Boulevard, Elk Grove Village, IL, 60007-1098, (847) 434-4000, (847) 434-8000, http://www.aap.org.

Maureen Haggerty
Tish Davidson, A.M.

Colitis

Definition

Colitis, also called ulcerative colitis, is an inflammatory bowel disease closely related to **Crohn's disease**. In individuals with colitis, the lining of the colon (large intestine) becomes inflamed, cells lining the wall die, and ulcers form on the colon wall.

Demographics

In the United States, the prevalence rate of ulcerative colitis is estimated at between 35 and 100 individuals per 100,000 population. This means that more than 2 million Americans have ulcerative colitis, which is a lifelong disease. The disease develops most often before the individual reaches age 30, although it can develop as late as age 60. People of Jewish ethnicity appear to be more likely to develop ulcerative colitis, and women are slightly more likely to develop colitis than men. The disease is less common in South America, Asia, and Africa than in the United States.

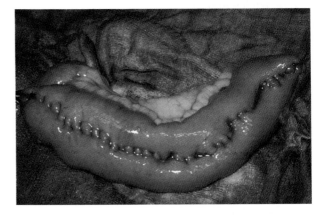

A specimen of a colon indicating ulcerative colitis. *(Photo Researchers, Inc.)*

KEY TERMS

Colonoscopy—A procedure in which the colon is cleansed and the a lighted fiber optic instrument is inserted through the anus to allow the physician to view the entire length of the colon and detect abnormalities in the colon lining, including polyps and ulcers.

Electrolyte—Ions in the body that participate in metabolic reactions. The major human electrolytes are sodium ($Na+$), potassium ($K+$), calcium ($Ca\ 2+$), magnesium ($Mg2+$), chloride ($Cl-$), phosphate ($HPO4\ 2-$), bicarbonate ($HCO3-$), and sulfate ($SO4\ 2-$).

Rectum—The last few inches of the large intestine that store waste until it is eliminated from the body through the anus.

Steroid—A family of compounds that share a similar chemical structure. This family includes estrogen and testosterone, vitamin D, cholesterol, and the drugs cortisone and prednisone.

Description

Colitis is an inflammatory bowel disease of uncertain origin. In this disease, the lining of the colon and rectum become inflamed and develop sores (ulcers) that produce pus and mucus. In mild cases, only the lining of the intestine is affected, but in severe cases, these ulcers may penetrate deeper layers of the colon or even perforate (break through) the colon wall. In ulcerative colitis, the inflamed area is continuous and develops only in the rectum and colon. This condition contrasts with Crohn's disease (a related inflammatory bowel disease), in which the inflamed area develops in patches and can occur in multiple places in the digestive system from the mouth to the rectum. There is no cure for ulcerative colitis, although treatment can bring symptoms under control or cause them to go into remission (disappear) for long periods.

Causes and symptoms

The cause of colitis is unclear. As of 2010, scientists believed that people who develop colitis carry an inherited susceptibility to developing the disease. Research has shown that people who have a parent or sibling with colitis are more likely to also develop colitis, and if one identical twins is affected, it is highly likely the other will also have the disease. However, inheritance does not completely predict who will develop colitis. Researchers believe that when a person with an inherited susceptibility to the disease is exposed to an outside agent, an inappropriate autoimmune reaction is triggered. As a result, the immune system attacks the body's own cells lining the intestine. No single outside trigger agent has been isolated. Suspect agents include bacteria, viruses, and environmental toxins. In the past, it was thought that **food allergies** could trigger colitis. Practitioners of conventional medicine subsequently determined that this was not the cause, although some alternative medical practitioners continued to accept the food allergy theory.

Symptoms associated with colitis include abdominal **pain** and cramps; frequent, urgent bowel movements; **diarrhea** with blood, pus, and mucus in the stool; and **fever**. Other signs of colitis occur because the disease interferes with the ability of the digestive system to absorb nutrients. These symptoms include **fatigue**, loss of appetite, weight loss, **dehydration**, and in severe cases, electrolyte imbalance. Because the immune system responds inappropriately, other parts of the body may be affected. The individual may develop joint pain, liver, kidney, and eye problems, and skin **rashes**. Although colitis is not caused by **stress** or food **allergies**, stress and certain foods (e.g., milk) tend to worsen symptoms.

Diagnosis

Symptoms of colitis mimic those of several other bowel diseases. Colitis is often diagnosed after extensive testing has ruled out other causes. After a health history and **physical examination**, the physician will order additional tests, including blood tests and a stool sample. The stool sample is examined for blood and parasites. Imaging tests include a **barium enema** and x rays of the intestine. By cleansing the intestine and filling it with barium, a white, chalky, non-toxic substance, abnormalities of the bowel are more easily seen on the x-ray film. Ultrasound and computed tomography, two non-invasive imaging techniques, may also be done. A definitive diagnosis usually is obtained by a **colonoscopy**, an invasive procedure that allows the physician to examine the colon lining for the entire length of the colon.

Treatment

The goal of colitis treatment is to control symptoms and improve quality of life. As of 2010, there was no cure for the disease. Conventional medicine treats the symptoms of ulcerative colitis primarily with drugs, although conventional practitioners also may recommend some complementary therapies suggested in the following text. Treatment is individualized and depends on the severity of the disease and the specific symptoms of the individual.

Drugs

Drug treatment depends on the severity of symptoms and whether ulcerative colitis is active or in remission. Anti-inflammatory drugs are at the heart of drug treatment for ulcerative colitis. Sulfasalazine (Azulfidine, EN-Tabs)is the most common anti-inflammatory drug used to treat mild to moderate ulcerative colitis because patients can safely take it for long maintenance periods, and it can be given with other drugs. Other anti-inflammatory drugs include mesalamine (Pentasa, Asacol, Rowasa, Canasa) and Balsalazide (Colazal). If these drugs do not provide adequate symptom relief, patients may be given **corticosteroids** such as prednisone and methylprednisolone. Corticosteroid drugs have substantial side effects and can be taken only for a short time during symptom flare-ups.

Medications used to treat diarrhea symptoms include diphenoxylate (Lomotil, Lofene), and loperamide (Imodium, Kaopectate). Anticholinergic drugs, which block the communication between nerves and muscles and thus reduce contraction of the intestine, include hyoscyamine (Anaspaz Cystospaz), and dicyclomine (Bentyl).

People with severe symptoms and complications beyond the digestive system may be hospitalized and given intravenous (IV) steroid drugs or drugs that suppress the immune system. These include the tumor necrosis factor inhibitor drug infliximab (Remicade), azathioprine (Imuran), cyclosporine (Neoral, Sandimmune), and 6-mercaptopurine (Purinethol). Since colitis is suspected of being caused by an inappropriate immune system response, suppressing the activity of the immune system may reduce symptoms. Once a flare-up is controlled, the individual continues on a maintenance dose of some combination of diarrhea-control, anti-inflammatory, and **immunosuppressant drugs**.

Surgery

Between 25% and 40% of people with ulcerative colitis develop symptoms so severe that they eventually need surgery (a colectomy) to remove their colon. When the colon is removed, the final portion of the small intestine is connected to a hole (stoma) in the abdomen. The individual wears a bag outside the body to collect waste. The bag must be emptied at regular intervals. Alternately, if part of the rectum is left intact the small intestine may be connected directly to the rectum after the colon is removed. Waste leaves the body through the anus in the regular manner. Bowel movements are more frequent and watery, as fluid that would normally be absorbed in the colon now passes out of the body.

Diet

Certain foods seem to worsen symptoms of colitis in many people. Individuals must determine their own problem foods and learn to avoid them. General suggestions for dietary changes that help many people include the following:

- Drink 8–10 glasses of water or clear fluids daily to prevent dehydration, which is especially important for people who have frequent watery bowel movements.
- Avoid high fiber foods. If symptoms are under control, some high-fiber foods may gradually be added back into the diet.
- Experiment with whether dairy products worsen symptoms; many people find that milk and cheese seem to exacerbate their symptoms.
- Avoid caffeine because it stimulates the digestive tract.
- Avoid drinking alcohol.
- Eat a low-fat diet.
- Eat smaller, more frequent meals.

Alternative and Complementary Therapies

HERBS. Certain herbal remedies have been shown to improve symptoms for some people. These include the following:

- Psyllium. Recommended by both alternative and conventional physicians, psyllium absorbs water and adds bulk to the stool.
- Boswellia resin (*Boswellia sacra.*) is thought to have anti-inflammatory properties. In a small study, when taken with sulfasalazine (a pharmaceutical drug), it increased the number of patients whose symptoms went into remission.
- Aloe (*Aloe vera*) juice or oral gel is thought to improve the chance of remission.
- Turmeric *Curcuma longa* is thought to have useful anti-inflammatory properties.

SUPPLEMENTS. Many people with moderate to severe symptoms develop vitamin and mineral deficiencies that need to be corrected with supplements and/or a multivitamin. Alternative practitioners also recommend a wide range of supplements that have shown mixed results in small trials. Some of these are:

- Probiotics. Probiotics are beneficial living organisms, usually bacteria that supplement the beneficial bacteria normally found in the intestines. Some studies have found that a non-disease producing strain of *Escherichia coli* helps some people with ulcerative colitis remain in remission. Probiotics and their effects on digestive diseases were active areas of research in 2010. Several Food and Drug Administration approved clinical trials of probiotics are being conducted in the United States for people with colitis. Information on trials enrolling participants is available at http://www.clinicaltrials.gov.

- Fish oil. Some studies have found that fish oil supplements increased weight gain and decreased the need for anti-inflammatory drugs, while others found fish oil was ineffective in patients with ulcerative colitis.

- Folic acid (Vitamin B_9). Sulfasalazine inhibits the absorption of folic acid, so people taking this drug may need supplementation. However, taking folic acid supplements can mask a vitamin B_{12} deficiency, so people taking folic acid may also need to take B_{12}. A physician should be consulted before taking these vitamins.

- Dehydroepiandrosterone (DHEA). This natural steroid hormone is produced in small amounts by the body. In studies, improvement was seen only with large supplement doses with a high likelihood of undesirable side effects.

- Iron. People who have a lot of blood in their stool are at risk of becoming iron deficient (anemic).

HOME REMEDIES. Although stress does not cause colitis, it often worsens symptoms, so **stress reduction** techniques such as the following should be incorporated into the daily routine.

- Mild to moderate exercise can help stabilize bowel function and improve mood.

- Yoga helps to relax the body and relieve tension.

- Meditation calms the body and mind.

- Biofeedback training helps individuals have more control over their body and allows individuals to consciously enter a relaxed state.

- Support groups allow people to share tips and frustrations in an atmosphere of mutual understanding.

Prognosis

Colitis cannot be cured. Most people go though periods of remission followed by periods of flare-ups when symptoms worsen. Remission can last from months to years depending on the individual.

Prevention

Ulcerative colitis cannot be prevented. About 5% of people who have ulcerative colitis later develop **colon cancer**. Regular yearly colonoscopies can detect colon **cancer** early when it can be easily treated.

Resources

BOOKS

Sklar, Jill. *Crohn's Disease and Ulcerative Colitis: An Essential Guide for the Newly Diagnosed,* 2nd ed. New York: Marlowe and Co., 2007.

OTHER

Ulcerative Colitis. Mayo Foundation for Medical Education and Research. August 15, 2009. http://www.mayoclinic.com/health/ulcerative-colitis/DS00598.

Ulcerative Colitis. MedlinePlus. January 15, 2010.http://www.nlm.nih.gov/medlineplus/ulcerativecolitis.html.

Wedro, Benjamin C. and Melissa Conrad Stoppler. Colitis. eMedicineHealth.com. December 5, 2008. http://www.emedicinehealth.com/colitis/article_em.htm.

ORGANIZATIONS

Alternative Medicine Foundation., PO Box 60016, Potomac, MD, 20859, (301) 340-1960, (301) 340-1936, http://www.amfoundation.org.

Crohn's & Colitis Foundation of America., 386 Park Avenue South, 17th Floor, New York, NY, 10016, (800) 932-2423, info@ccfa.org, http://www.ccfa.org.

National Digestive Diseases Information Clearinghouse (NDDIC)., 2 Information Way, Bethesda, MD, 20892-3570, (800) 891-5389; TTY (866) 569-1162 , (703) 738-4929, info@niddk.nih.gov, http://digestive.niddk.nih.gov.

Tish Davidson, A.M.

Collapsed lung *see* **Pneumothorax**
Colloidal bath *see* **Therapeutic baths**

Colon cancer

Definition

Cancer of the colon is a disease characterized by the development of malignant cells in the lining or epithelium of the large intestine. Malignant cells have lost normal control mechanisms governing growth. These cells may invade surrounding local tissue or they may spread throughout the body and invade other organ systems.

Synonyms for the colon include the large bowel or the large intestine. The rectum is the continuation of the large intestine into the pelvis that terminates in the anus.

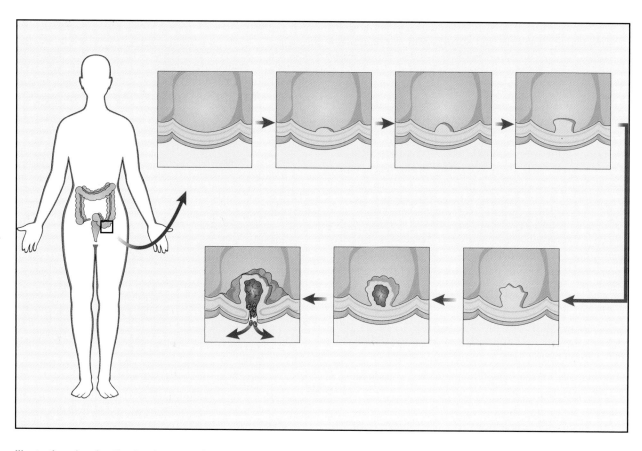

Illustration showing the development of a cancerous tumor within the colon. *(Illustration by Argosy, Inc. Reproduced by permission of Gale, a part of Cengage Learning.)*

Demographics

There are at least 100,000 new cases of colon cancer diagnosed per year in the United States. Excluding skin cancers, colorectal cancer is the 4th most commonly diagnosed cancer in both men and women in the United States. Colorectal cancer is the second leading cause of deaths from cancer. The **death** rate from colon cancer has been declining for the last 30 years. The decline in the death rate is attributed to more accurate screening procedures, which find and make possible the removal of problematic polyps before they convert to cancer. Screening also facilitates finding cancer in earlier, more treatable stages. In addition, treatment methodologies for colon cancer have improved dramatically over the last decade.

There are over one million colon cancer survivors in the United States alone.

Approximately one-third of colon cancer cases are associated with familial clustering. First degree relatives of patients with newly diagnosed colorectal adenomas or invasive colorectal cancer are considered to be at high risk for the development of the disease and should be screened for the presence of colorectal cancer.

Description

Risk factors

Several risk factors are related to the development of colon cancer including:

- increasing age; most cases of colon cancer are diagnosed after age 50

- personal history of colon polyps or colorectal cancer

- personal history of inflammatory bowel disease such as ulcerative colitis or Crohn's disease

- family history of colorectal cancer, especially in a first degree relative (parent of sibling)

- presence of an inherited syndrome such as familial adenomatous polyposis (FAP) and hereditary non–polyposis colorectal cancer (HNPCC). Between 5 and 10% of people have an inherited gene that causes colorectal cancer. The two most common types of these syndromes are FAP and HNPCC.

- African American race
- Jews of Eastern European descent (Ashkenazi Jews). Members of this ethnic group have some of the highest rates of colorectal cancer in the world.
- consuming a diet high in red meats, processed meats, and cooking foods at high temperatures
- physical inactivity
- obesity
- history of smoking
- history of heavy alcohol use
- personal history of type II diabetes

The colon is a tubular organ beginning in the right lower abdomen. It ascends on the right side of the abdomen, traverses from right to left in the upper abdomen, descends vertically down the left side, takes an S–shaped curve in the lower left abdomen, and then flows into the rectum as it leaves the abdomen for the pelvis. These portions of the colon are named separately although they are part of the same organ.

- cecum, the beginning of the colon
- ascending colon, the right vertical ascent of the colon
- transverse colon, the portion traversing from right to left
- descending colon, the left vertical descent of the colon
- sigmoid colon, the S–shaped segment of colon above the pelvis

These portions of the colon are recognized anatomically based on the arterial blood supply and venous and lymphatic drainage of these segments of the colon. Lymph, a protein–rich fluid that bathes the cells of the body, is transported in small channels known as lymphatics that run alongside the veins of the colon. Lymph nodes are small filters through which the lymph travels on its way back to the bloodstream. Cancer can spread elsewhere in the body by invading the lymph and vascular systems. Therefore, these anatomic considerations become very important in the treatment of colon cancer.

The small intestine is the continuation of the upper gastrointestinal tract responsible for carrying ingested nutrients into the body. The waste left after the small intestine has completed absorption of nutrients amounts to about a quart (a few liters), of material per day and is directly delivered to the colon, (at the cecum), for processing. The colon is responsible for the preservation of fluid and electrolytes as it propels the increasingly solid waste toward the rectum and anus for excretion.

When cells lining the colon become malignant, they first grow locally and may invade partially or totally through the wall of the bowel and even into adjacent structures and organs. In the process, the tumor can penetrate and invade the lymphatics or the capillaries locally and gain access to the circulation. As the malignant cells work their way to other areas of the body, they again become locally invasive in the new area to which they have spread. These tumor deposits, originating from the colon primary tumor, are then known as metastases. If metastases are found in the regional lymph nodes from the primary, they are known as regional metastases, or regional nodal metastases. If they are distant from the primary tumor, they are known as distant metastases. The patient with distant metastases has systemic disease. Thus the cancer originating in the colon begins locally and, given time, can become systemic.

In most cases, colon cancer develops slowly over several years. Prior to a cancer's developing, a non–cancerous polyp may appear on the inner lining of the colon. A polyp typically begins as a benign (non–cancerous) growth of tissue. Over time, some polyps can convert into cancerous tumors.

There are two major types of polyps, adenomatous polyps (adenomas) and hyperplastic and inflammatory polyps. Adenomatous polyps are considered pre–cancerous lesions while hyperplastic and inflammatory polyps are generally not pre–cancerous.

Some individuals may have evidence of dysplasia (cells look abnormal) in the lining of the colon. These abnormal–looking cells may transform to cancerous cells over time. Individuals with a history of Crohn's disease or ulcerative **colitis** may show evidence of dysplasia in the colon.

More than 95% of colorectal cancers are classified as adenocarcinomas. This type of cancer originates from glands that secrete mucus which lubricates the lining of the colon.

Causes and symptoms

Causes

Carcinogenesis is the process by which agents in the environment may induce mutation. It is caused by agents known as **carcinogens** (cancer–causing agents). Specific carcinogens related to the development of colon cancer have been difficult to identify; however, dietary factors seem to be involved.

KEY TERMS

Adenocarcinoma—Type of cancer beginning in glandular epithelium.

Adjuvant therapy—Treatment involving radiation, chemotherapy (drug treatment), or hormone therapy, or a combination of all three given after the primary treatment for the possibility of residual microscopic disease.

Anastomosis—Surgical reconnection of the ends of the bowel after removal of a portion of the bowel.

Anemia—The condition caused by too few circulating red blood cells, often manifested in part by fatigue.

Carcinogens—Substances in the environment that cause cancer, presumably by inducing mutations, with prolonged exposure.

Electolytes—Salts, such as sodium and chloride.

Epithelium—Cells composing the lining of an organ.

Lymph nodes—Cellular filters through which lymphatics flow.

Lymphatics—Channels that are conduits for lymph.

Malignant—Cells that have been altered such that they have lost normal control mechanisms and are capable of local invasion and spread to other areas of the body.

Metastasis—Site of invasive tumor growth that originated from a malignancy elsewhere in the body.

Mutation—A change in the genetic makeup of a cell that may occur spontaneously or be environmentally induced.

Occult blood—Presence of blood that cannot be seen with the naked eye.

Polyps—Localized growths of the epithelium that can be benign, precancerous, or harbor malignancy.

Radical resection—Surgical resection that takes the blood supply and lymph system supplying the organ along with the organ.

Resect—To remove surgically.

Sacrum—Posterior bony wall of the pelvis.

Systemic—Throughout the body.

Colon cancer is more common in industrialized nations. **Diets** high in fat, red meat, total calories, and alcohol seem to predispose people to the disease. Diets high in fiber appear to decrease risk. High–fiber diets may help lessen exposure of the colon lining to carcinogens from the environment, as the transit time through the bowel is faster with a high–fiber diet than it is with a low fiber diet.

Age plays a definite role in the predisposition to colon cancer. Two-thirds of all cases occur after age 50 and the average age for those who develop the disease is 62.

There is also a increased risk for colon cancer in the individual who smokes.

Patients who suffer from inflammatory diseases of the colon known as ulcerative colitis and Crohn's colitis are also at increased risk.

Researchers know there is a genetic link to many cases of colon cancer, those called familial cases. This type of colon cancer tends to run in families. In late 2003, a team of researchers identified the specific location on a human chromosome by analyzing blood samples from 53 families in which at least one member had a colon cancer or precancerous colon polyp.

The development of polyps of the colon almost always precedes the development of colon cancer by five or more years. Polyps are benign growths of the colon lining. They can be unrelated to cancer, precancerous, or malignant. Polyps, when identified, are removed for diagnosis. If the polyps are benign, the patient should undergo careful surveillance for the development of more polyps or the development of colon cancer.

Symptoms

Colon cancer causes symptoms related to its local presence in the large bowel or by its effect on other organs if it has spread. These symptoms may occur alone or in combination:

- a change in bowel habit
- blood in the stool
- bloating, persistent abdominal distention
- constipation
- a feeling of fullness even after having a bowel movement
- narrowing of the stool—so–called ribbon stools
- persistent, chronic fatigue
- abdominal discomfort
- unexplained weight loss
- (very rarely) nausea and vomiting

Most of these symptoms are caused by the physical presence of the tumor mass in the colon. Similar symptoms can be caused by other processes; they are not absolutely specific to colon cancer. The key is recognizing that the persistence of these symptoms without ready explanation should prompt the individual to seek medical evaluation.

If a tumor develops in the colon, it will begin to cause symptoms as it reaches a certain size. The symptoms are caused by the tumor blocking the opening in the colon. In addition, the tumor commonly oozes blood that is lost in the stool. (Often, this blood is not visible.) This condition results in anemia and chronic **fatigue**. Weight loss is a late symptom, often implying substantial obstruction or the presence of systemic disease.

Diagnosis

In all other cancers (breast and prostate, for example), screening tests look for small, malignant lesions. Screening for colorectal cancers, however, involves the search for pre–malignant, benign polyps. This screening can be close to 100% effective in preventing cancer development, not just in detecting small cancers.

Screening involves physical exam, simple laboratory tests, and the visualization of the lining of the colon. To visualize the colon epithelium, clinicians use x rays (indirect visualization) and **endoscopy** (direct visualization).

Examination

The **physical examination** involves the performance of a digital rectal exam (DRE). The DRE includes manual examination of the rectum, anus and the prostate. During this examination, the physician examines the anus and the surrounding skin for **hemorrhoids**, abscesses, and other irregularities. After lubricating the gloved finger and anus, the examiner gently slides the finger into the anus and follows the contours of the rectum. The examiner notes the tone of the anus and feels the walls and the edges for texture, tenderness, and masses as far as the examining finger can reach. At the time of this exam, the physician checks the stool on the examining glove with a chemical to see if any occult (invisible), blood is present. At home, after having a bowel movement, the patient is asked to swipe a sample of stool obtained with a small stick on a card. After three such specimens are on the card, the card is then easily chemically tested for occult blood also. (The stool analysis mentioned here is known as a **fecal occult blood test**, or FOBT, and, while it can be helpful, it is not 100% accurate. Only about 50% of cancers are FOBT–positive.) These exams are accomplished as an easy part of a routine yearly physical exam.

Tests

Proteins are sometimes produced by cancers and these may be elevated in the patient's blood. When this occurs, the protein produced is known as a tumor marker. There is a tumor marker for some cancers of the colon; it is known as carcinoembryonic antigen, or CEA. Unfortunately, this protein may be made by other adenocarcinomas as well, or it may not be produced by a particular colon cancer. Therefore, screening by chemical analysis for CEA has not been helpful. CEA has been helpful when used in a follow–up role for patients treated for colon cancer if their tumor makes the protein.

Procedures

Indirect visualization of the colon may be accomplished by inserting a compound of barium into the rectum and filling the colon with this compound. Barium compounds produce a white contrast image of the lining of the colon on x ray and thus the contour of the lining of the colon may be seen. Detail can be increased if the barium utilized is thinned and air also introduced. These studies are known as the **barium enema** (BE), and the double contrast barium enema (DCBE).

Direct visualization of the colon lining is accomplished using a scope or endoscope. The physician introduces the instrument through the rectum. Older, shorter scopes were rigid. Today, utilizing fiberoptic technology, the scopes are flexible and can reach into the colon much farther. If the left colon only is visualized, it is called flexible **sigmoidoscopy**. When the entire colon is visualized, the procedure is known as **colonoscopy**.

A procedure called virtual colonoscopy has been developed but debate continues on whether or not it is effective as colonoscopy. Virtual colonoscopy refers to the use of imaging, usually with computed tomography (CT) scans or **magnetic resonance imaging** (MRI) to produce images of the colon. Studies have shown that virtual colonoscopy is as effective as colonoscopy for screening purposes and it offers the advantage of being less invasive and less risky. However, many physicians are unwilling to accept it as a replacement for colonoscopy, particularly since some patients might still require the regular colonoscopy as a follow–up to the virtual procedure if a polyp or abnormality is found that requires biopsy.

Unlike the indirect visualizations of the colon (the BE and the DCBE), endoscopic screenings allow a physician to remove polyps and to biopsy suspicious tissue. (A biopsy is a removal of tissue for examination by a pathologist.) For this reason, many physicians prefer endoscopic screening. All of the visualizations, the BE, DCBE, and each type of endoscopy, require pre–procedure preparation (evacuation) of the colon.

If patients have symptoms that could possibly be related to colon cancer, the entire colon will be examined. The combination of a flexible sigmoidoscopy and DCBE may be performed, but the preferred evaluation of the entire colon and rectum is a complete colonoscopy. Colonoscopy allows direct visualization, photography, and the opportunity to obtain a biopsy of any abnormality visualized. If, for technical reasons, the entire colon is not visualized endoscopically, a DCBE should complement the colonoscopy.

The diagnosis of colon cancer is actually made by the performance of a biopsy of any abnormal lesion in the colon. When a tumor growth is identified, it could be either a benign polyp (or lesion) or a cancer; the biopsy resolves the issue. The endoscopist may take many samples to exclude any sampling errors.

If the patient has advanced disease at the time of diagnosis, areas where the tumor has spread (such as the liver) may be amenable to biopsy. Such biopsies are usually obtained using a special needle under **local anesthesia**.

Once a diagnosis of colon cancer has been established by biopsy, in addition to the physical exam, studies will be performed to assess the extent of the disease. Blood studies include a **complete blood count**, **liver function tests**, and a CEA. Imaging studies will include a CT scan (computed tomography scan) of the chest, abdomen, and pelvis. The scans will determine if the cancer has spread to the lung, will evaluate potential spread to the liver, and can determine whether any local spread of the primary tumor has occurred. If the patient has any neurologic symptoms, a CT scan of the brain will be performed, and if the patient is experiencing bone **pain**, a **bone scan** also will be performed.

Treatments

Once the diagnosis has been confirmed by biopsy, the clinical stage of the cancer is assigned. Stage is determined based on the characteristics of the primary tumor, its depth of penetration through the bowel, and the presence or absence of regional or distant metastases. Often, the depth of penetration through the bowel or the presence of regional lymph nodes can not be assigned before surgery.

Colon cancer is assigned stages I through IV, based on the following general criteria:

- Stage I: The tumor is confined to the epithelium or has not penetrated through the first layer of muscle in the bowel wall.
- Stage II: The tumor has penetrated through to the outer wall of the colon or has gone through it, possibly invading other local tissue.
- Stage III: The tumor has developed to include regional lymph node involvement.
- Stage IV: The cancer has spread to at least one distant organ (such as the liver or lungs) or lymph nodes, or has spread to a distant part of the peritoneum.

With many cancers other than colon cancer, staging plays an important role to best determine treatment options. Colon cancers are also graded based on how closely the cancer cells resemble normal cells. The grading scale is G1 to G4 with cells graded as G1 looking the most normal and cells graded as G4 looking the most abnormal. Low grade tumors (G1) tend to grow more slowly and are less likely to metastasize to distant organs which may result in a better prognosis.

Traditional

SURGERY. Almost all colon cancers are treated with surgery first, regardless of stage. Colon cancers through Stage III, and even some Stage IV colon cancers, are treated with surgery first, before any other treatments are considered.

Surgical removal of the involved segment of colon (colectomy) along with its blood supply and regional lymph nodes is the primary therapy for colon cancer. Usually, the partial colectomies are separated into right, left, transverse, or sigmoid sections based on the blood supply. The removal of the blood supply at its origin along with the regional lymph nodes that accompany it ensures an adequate margin of normal colon on either side of the primary tumor. When the cancer lies in a position such that the blood supply and lymph drainage between two of the major vessels, both vessels are taken to assure complete radical resection or removal (extended radical right or left colectomy). If the primary tumor penetrates through the bowel wall, any tissue adjacent to the tumor extension is also taken, if feasible.

Surgery is used as primary therapy for stages I through III colon cancer unless there are signs that local invasion will not permit complete removal of the tumor, as may occur in advanced stage III tumors. However, this circumstance is rare, occurring in less than 2% of all colon cancer cases.

After the resection is completed, the ends of the remaining colon are reconstructed; the reattachment is called an anastomosis. Once healing has occurred, there may be a slight increase in the frequency of bowel movements. This effect usually lasts only for several weeks. Most patients go on to develop completely normal bowel function.

Occasionally, the anastomosis is risky and cannot be performed. When the anastomosis cannot be performed, a **colostomy** is performed instead. A colostomy is performed by bringing the end of the colon through the abdominal wall and sewing it to the skin. The patient will have to wear an appliance (a bag) to manage the stool. The colostomy may be temporary and the patient may undergo a reattachment at a later, safer date, or the colostomy may be permanent. In most cases, emergent colostomies are not reversed and are permanent.

RADIATION. **Radiation therapy** is used as an adjunct to surgery if there is concern about potential for local recurrence post–operatively and the area of concern will tolerate the radiation. For instance, if the tumor invaded muscle of the abdominal wall but was not completely removed, this area would be considered for radiation. Radiation may also be given in combination with **chemotherapy** prior to surgery (neoadjuvant therapy) to shrink the size of the tumor. Radiation has significant dose limits when residual bowel is exposed to it because the small and large intestine do not tolerate radiation well.

CHEMOTHERAPY. Chemotherapy is useful for patients who have had all identifiable tumor removed and are at risk for recurrence (adjuvant chemotherapy). The FOLFOX chemotherapy regimen is a common regimen administered as adjuvant therapy in the treatment of colon cancer. This regimen includes the drugs oxaliplatin, 5–FU, and leucovorin. The drugs 5–FU and leucovorin given in combination or the drug capcetibine given alone may also be used. Adjuvant chemotherapy administered after surgery may be continued for a total of six months of chemotherapy.

TARGETED THERAPIES. Targeted therapies work in ways that are different from the way chemotherapy works. Targeted therapies, as the name implies, target specific proteins on the cellular structures of cancer cells in an attempt to kill the cancer cells. The advantage of targeted therapy is that normal cells which do not contain the abnormal proteins the cancer cells contain are usually not affected by the targeted therapy. Therefore, side effects of these drugs are often less pronounced than the side effects from chemotherapy.

Targeted therapy drugs used to treat colon cancer include bevacizumab (Avastin), cetuximab (Erbitux), and panitumumab (Vectibix).

Prognosis

Prognosis is the long–term outlook or survival after therapy. As expected, the survival rates are dependent upon the stage of the cancer at the time of diagnosis, making early detection crucial.

Colon cancer is highly treatable and often curable if detected when the cancer is localized in the bowel. Surgery is the primary treatment choice for most cases of colon cancer and results in a cure for about 50% of patients.

Five year survival rates for colon cancer range from 74% in patients diagnosed with Stage I disease to 6% for patients diagnosed in Stage IV.

Prevention

There is not an absolute method for preventing colon cancer. Still, there are steps an individual can take to dramatically lessen the risk or to identify the precursors of colon cancer so that it does not manifest itself. The patient with a familial history can enter screening and surveillance programs earlier than the general population. High–fiber diets and **vitamins**, avoiding **obesity**, and staying active lessen the risk. Avoiding cigarettes and alcohol may be helpful. By controlling these environmental factors, an individual can lessen risk and to this degree prevent the disease.

People who turn age 50, and all of those with a history of colon cancer in their families (even if younger than age 50), should speak with their physicians about the most recent screening recommendations from physician and cancer organizations. They should watch for symptoms and attend all recommended screenings to increase the likelihood of catching colon cancer early.

Resources

BOOKS

Compton, C., et al. "Colon Cancer." In Abelhoff, Martin, et al. *Clinical Oncology Library*. Philadelphia: Elsevier, 2008: 1535–1568.

PERIODICALS

Buunen, M., et al. "Survival After Laparoscopic Surgery Versus Open Surgery for Colon Cancer: Long-Term Outcome of a Randomized Clinical Trial." *Lancet Oncology* 10 (2009):44–52.

Levin, B., et al. "Screening and Surveillance for the Early Detection of Colorectal Cancer and Adenomatous Polyps, 2008. A Joint Guideline from the American

Cancer Society, the U.S. Multi-Society Task Force on Colorectal Cancer, and the American College of Radiology." *CA: A Cancer Journal for Clinicians.* 134 (2008):1570–1595.

Sargent, D., et al. "Evidence for Cure by Adjuvant Therapy in Colon Cancer: Observation Based on Individual Patient Data form 20,898 Patients in 18 Randomized Trials." *Journal of Clinical Oncology* 27 (2009):872–877.

ORGANIZATIONS

American Cancer Society, (800) ACS–2345, http://www.cancer.org.

Cancer Information Service of the NCI, 9000 Rockville Pike, Bethesda, MD, 20892, (800) 4–CANCER, NIHinfo@od.nih.gov, http://www.cancer.gov.

Colon Cancer Alliance, 1200 G Street, NW, Suite 800, Washington, DC, 20005, (202) 434–8980, (877) 422–2030, (866) 304–9075, aspiegel@ccalliance.org, www.ccalliance.org.

National Cancer Institute Cancer Trials, 6116 Executive Boulevard, Suite 300, Bethesda, MD, 20892–8322, (800) 422–6237, cancergovstaff@mail.nih.gov, http://www.cancer.gov.

Richard A. McCartney, M.D.
Melinda Granger Oberleitner, RN,
DNS, APRN, CNS

Colon therapy *see* **Colonic irrigation**

Colonic irrigation

Definition

Colonic irrigation is also known as **hydrotherapy** of the colon, high colonic, entero-lavage, or simply colonic. It is the process of cleansing the colon by passing several gallons of water through it with the use of special equipment. It is similar to an enema but treats the whole colon, not just the lower bowel. This has the effect of flushing out impacted fecal matter, toxins, mucous, and even parasites, that often build up over the passage of time. It is a procedure that should only be undertaken by a qualified practitioner.

Demographics

Colon and bowel **cancer** are two of the leading causes of **death** in the United States, and alternative practitioners insist that it can be prevented by efficient hygiene procedures. Providing that care is taken to replace the natural organisms that flourish in the bowel, many health benefits can be expected from colonic irrigation. In general, alternative practitioners maintain that an ill-functioning bowel is the source of all disease, and therefore keeping it clean will be an effective protection against this.

The cost of colonic irrigation treatments varies, but is generally $35–70 per session, which may last from 45 minutes to one hour. The cost of the machine itself is $4,000–12,000, but again, it should be noted that only qualified therapists should conduct sessions.

Purpose

Anyone suffering from gas, bloating, cramping pains, **acne** and other skin complaints, arthritis, and a list of bowel complaints such as **diverticulitis** and irritable bowel etc., may benefit from colonic irrigation. In particular, cancer patients are often advised to undertake a course of colonic irrigation sessions as an essential part of their treatment. When a biological cancer therapy begins to enable the body to breakdown a cancerous mass, it is essential that speedy and effective elimination of the resulting toxins is achieved.

Removing large amounts of toxic matter relieves the patient and can lead to the alleviation of symptoms such as arthritis, **chronic fatigue syndrome**, **candidiasis**, and a host of other illnesses. Properly executed, colonic irrigation can help restore normal peristaltic action to a sluggish bowel, thus reducing the need for more hydrotherapy treatments over time. In addition, removing the layer of fecal matter which coats the intestines in many individuals allows improved assimilation of the nutrients from foods and can alleviate symptoms of vitamin and other nutrient deficiencies. Many alternative health practitioners consider some form of hydrotherapy for the bowel to be essential in the treatment of degenerative diseases.

Description

Origins

Cleansing the colon with the use of hydrotherapy is not a new concept. Forms of colonic irrigation have been used successfully for decades to relieve chronic toxicity and even acute cases of toxemia.

Over time, many people develop a thick layer of fecal matter that coats their colon. It hardens and becomes impacted, reducing the efficiency of the bowel, and in some cases, completely obstructing normal elimination of waste matter from the body. It is quite common for people to have only one bowel movement per day, and some as few as one or two per week.

Alternative practitioners advise that we probably should have one bowel movement for every meal that we eat. If not, then we are not eliminating wastes completely, and if input exceeds output, then we will surely suffer the consequences at some point.

Incomplete elimination of body wastes may result in the following, depending on where the deposits end up:

- sluggish system
- joint pain and arthritis
- irritable bowel syndrome
- diverticulitis
- Crohn's disease
- leaky gut syndrome
- heart problem
- migraine
- allergies
- bad breath
- acne and other skin problems such as psoriasis
- asthma
- early senility and Alzheimer's disease
- chronic fatigue syndrome
- cancer, particularly of the bowel
- multiple sclerosis

During colonic irrigation, a small speculum is passed into the patient's bowel through the rectum. This is attached to a tube, which leads to a machine that pumps temperature-controlled water into the colon at a controlled rate (to be controlled by either the practitioner or the patient). The temperature of the water should ideally be kept as close to body temperature as possible.

The patient will temporarily be filled with water up to the level of the entire colon. Patients say they can feel the water up under their ribs but that the process, although sometimes uncomfortable, is not painful. The amount of water will vary but will generally be in the region of between two and six liters (or quarts) at any one time. This triggers peristaltic action and the patient will begin to expel the water along with fecal matter back through the tube and into the machine.

The fecal matter is flushed out through a viewing tube, so that what is eliminated may be monitored. Quite often, unsuspected parasites are expelled, along with very old fecal material, very dark in color, which may have been in the colon for years. Some therapists comment that it looks like **aging** rubber.

During the treatment, the therapist will gently massage the patient's abdomen to help dislodge impacted fecal matter. In addition to massage, sometimes **acupressure**, **reflexology**, or lymphatic drainage techniques may be used to loosen deposits and stimulate the bowel. It is important that the right amount of water is used, as too much will cause discomfort and too little will be ineffective. If correctly done, colonic irrigation is not painful at all and some patients claim to sleep through their treatment.

Sanitation is vital to this process. The tubes and speculums used are generally disposable, but other parts of the machine, such as the viewing tube, must be sterilized after each patient.

Normally, a series of treatments will be required to achieve desired results regarding the elimination of impacted, decaying matter, and restoration of bowel regularity. Initially only gas and recent fecal matter may be expelled. The residue attached to the colon wall is usually the result of years of neglect, and therapists say that one cannot expect complete relief in only one session.

Impacted fecal matter can cause an imbalance of the natural organisms that normally populate the bowel, causing what is known as dysbiosis. Under ideal conditions, the bowel is populated by a variety of naturally occurring organisms. It seems that the enzymes occurring in fresh fruit and vegetables encourage these beneficial organisms. One of the results of eating processed denatured foods is that this natural balance is upset, and food may begin to rot in the bowel instead of being processed.

Decomposing matter can cause a toxic condition and may lead to many health problems, as **constipation** causes backed up pollution of the body cells. The process of repair and elimination of wastes enters a downward spiral which at best will cause **fatigue**, lack of energy and premature aging, and, at worst, can cause degenerative diseases, among them **allergies**, and even cancer and **Alzheimer's disease**.

Preparations

Most practitioners prefer that distilled or purified water is used for colonic irrigation, but others use sterilized tap water.

Precautions

It may be advisable to use a probiotic pessary after colonic irrigation, to ensure replacement of desirable natural flora. There are certain conditions that either partly or completely preclude the use of colonic irrigation, such as an active attack of **Crohn's disease**, bleeding ulcers, and hyperacidosis. If in doubt, a qualified practitioner should be consulted. Anyone suffering from these conditions should always notify the practitioner when receiving colonic irrigation treatments.

Side effects

Some allopathic practitioners claim that colonic irrigation flushes out essential electrolytes and friendly bacteria from the bowel and that it can be dangerous. Practitioners counter that this can easily be remedied with the use of probiotics, and that in any case, these possible disadvantages are easily offset by the benefits of having large amounts of putrefying matter, harmful organisms, and parasites removed from the system.

Research and general acceptance

Although many alternative health care practitioners swear by colonic irrigation, there is a large allopathic lobby that claims that there are no benefits to be had, and that there are dangers involved. However, there are many decades of records and research from the alternative health care community that indicate that this therapy may have a valuable place in the treatment of degenerative diseases and toxic conditions.

Resources

PERIODICALS

Norlela S, Izham C, Khalid BA. Colonic Irrigation-Induced Hyponatremia. *Malays J Pathol.* 2004 Dec;26(2):117-8.

ORGANIZATIONS

California Colon Hygienist Society, 333 Miller Ave., Suite 1, Mill Valley, CA, 94941, (415) 383-7224.

Patricia Skinner
Karl Finley

Colonoscopy

Definition

Colonoscopy is an endoscopic medical procedure that uses a colonoscope, a long, flexible, thin, lighted tube-like instrument containing a tiny video camera, that allows a visual examination of the lining of the colon (large intestine) and rectum.

Purpose

A colonoscopy is generally recommended when the patient complains of rectal bleeding, has a change in bowel habits, and/or has other unexplained abdominal symptoms. The test is frequently used to look for colorectal **cancer**, especially when polyps or tumor-like growths have been detected by a **barium enema** examination and other diagnostic imaging tests. Polyps can be removed through the colonoscope, and samples of tissue (biopsies) can be taken to detect the presence of cancerous cells. In addition, colonoscopy can also be used to remove foreign bodies from the colon, control hemorrhaging, and excise tumors.

A colonoscopy allows the physician to visualize the lining of the entire colon and, therefore, it also enables physicians to check for bowel diseases such as ulcerative **colitis** and **Crohn's disease**. Colonoscopy is being used increasingly as a screening tool in asymptomatic patients. It is recommended as a screening test in all people 50 years or older and is an essential tool for monitoring patients who have a past history of polyps or **colon cancer**.

Description

Colonoscopy can be performed either in a physician's office or in an endoscopic procedure room of a hospital or freestanding clinic. For otherwise healthy patients, colonoscopy is usually performed by a gastroenterologist or surgeon in an office or clinic setting. When performed on patients with other medical conditions that could cause complications or that require hospitalization, it is usually performed in the **endoscopy** department of a hospital, where more intensive physiologic monitoring and/or **general anesthesia** can be better provided.

An intravenous line is usually inserted into a vein in the patient's arm to administer a sedative and a painkiller. During the colonoscopy, patients lie on their sides with their knees drawn up toward the abdomen. The doctor begins the procedure by inserting a lubricated, gloved finger into the anus to check for any abnormal masses or blockage. A thin, well-

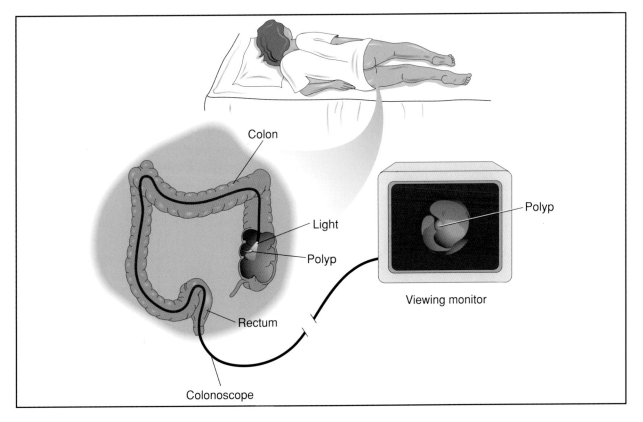

Colon

Light

Polyp

Rectum

Colonoscope

Polyp

Viewing monitor

Colonoscopy is a procedure where a long and flexible tubular instrument called a colonoscope is inserted into the patient's anus in order to view the lining of the colon and rectum. It is performed to test for colorectal cancer and other bowel diseases, and enables the physician to collect tissue samples for laboratory analysis. *(Illustration by Electronic Illustrators Group. Reproduced by permission of Gale, a part of Cengage Learning.)*

lubricated colonoscope is then inserted into the anus and gently advanced through the colon. The lining of the large intestine is examined through the colonoscope. The physician views images on a television monitor, and the procedure can be documented using a video recorder. Still images can be recorded and saved on a computer disk or printed. Occasionally, air may be pumped through the colonoscope to help clear the path or open the colon. If excessive secretions, stool, or blood obstructs the viewing, they are suctioned out through the scope. The doctor may press on the abdomen or ask the patient to change position in order to advance the scope through the colon.

The entire length of the large intestine can be examined in this manner. If suspicious growths are present, tiny biopsy forceps or brushes are inserted through the colon and tissue samples (biopsies) are obtained. Small polyps or inflamed tissue also can be removed using tiny instruments passed through the scope. For removing tumors or performing other types of surgery on the colon during colonoscopy, an electrosurgical device or laser system may be used in conjunction with the colonoscope. To stop bleeding in

the colon, a laser, heater probe, or electrical probe is used, or special medicines are injected through the scope. After the procedure, the colonoscope is slowly withdrawn and the instilled air is allowed to escape. The anal area is then cleansed with tissues. Tissue samples taken by biopsy are sent to a clinical laboratory, where they are analyzed by a pathologist.

The procedure may take anywhere from 30 minutes to two hours depending on how easy it is to advance the scope through the colon. Colonoscopy can be a long and uncomfortable procedure, and the bowel-cleansing preparation may be tiring and can produce **diarrhea** and cramping. During the colonoscopy, the sedative and the **pain** medications will keep the patient drowsy and relaxed. Some patients complain of minor discomfort and pressure from the colonoscope; however, the sedative and pain medication usually cause most patients to dose off during the procedure.

Preparation

Patients who regularly take **aspirin, nonsteroidal anti-inflammatory drugs** (NSAIDs), blood thinners,

Barium enema—An x-ray test of the bowel performed after giving the patient an enema of a white chalky substance (barium) that outlines the colon and the rectum.

Biopsy—A procedure in which a sample of suspicious tissue is removed and examined by a pathologist for cancer or other disease.

Colonoscope—A thin, flexible, hollow, lighted tube that is inserted through the anus and rectum to the colon to enable the physician to view the entire lining of the colon.

Computed tomography (CT) scan—A radiologic imaging technique that uses computer processing to generate an image of the tissue density; also called computerized axial tomography (CAT) and computerized transaxial tomography (CTAT).

Crohn's disease—A chronic inflammatory disease that generally starts in the gastrointestinal tract and causes the immune system to attack one's own body.

Diverticulosis—A condition that involves the development of sacs that bulge through the large intestine's muscular walls, but are not inflamed. It may cause bleeding, stomach distress, and excess gas.

Electrosurgical device—A medical device that uses electrical current to cauterize or coagulate tissue during surgical procedures; often used in conjunction with laparoscopy.

Magnetic resonance imaging (MRI)—A test that provides pictures of organs and structures inside the body using radio waves. In many cases, an MRI provides information that cannot be obtained from X-ray tests.

Pathologist—A doctor who specializes in the diagnosis of disease by studying cells and tissues under a microscope.

Polyps—An abnormal growth that develops on the inside of a hollow organ such as the colon.

Sigmoidoscopy—A process of passing a long, hollow tubular instrument through the anus in order to permit inspection, diagnosis, treatment, and imaging, especially of the sigmoid flexure.

Ulcerative colitis—A chronic condition in which recurrent ulcers are found in the colon. It is manifested clinically by abdominal cramping and rectal bleeding.

Virtual colonoscopy—Two new techniques that provide views of the colon to screen for colon polyps and cancer. The images are produced by computerized manipulations rather than direct observation through the colonoscope; one technique uses the x-ray images from a CT scan, and the other uses magnetic images from an MRI scan.

or insulin should be sure to inform the physician at the time the colonoscopy is scheduled. The physician also should be notified if the patient has **allergies** to any medications or anesthetics, bleeding problems, or is pregnant. The doctor should be informed of all the medications the patient is taking and if he or she has had a barium enema x-ray examination recently. If the patient has had heart valves replaced, the doctor should be informed so that appropriate **antibiotics** can be administered to prevent infection. Patients with severe active colitis, extremely dilated colon (toxic megacolon), or severely inflamed bowel may not be candidates for colonoscopy. Patients requiring continuous ambulatory peritoneal dialysis are generally not candidates for colonoscopy due to a higher risk of developing internal bleeding. The risks associated with the procedure are explained to the patient beforehand, and the patient is asked to sign a consent form.

The colon must be thoroughly cleansed before performing colonoscopy. Consequently, for about two days before the procedure, considerable preparation is necessary to clear the colon of all stool. The patient is asked to refrain from eating any solid food for 24–48 hours before the test. Only clear liquid such as juices, broth, and gelatin are allowed. Red or purple juices should be avoided, since they can cause coloring of the colon that may be misinterpreted as blood during the colonoscopy. The patient is advised to drink plenty of water to avoid **dehydration**. A day before the colonoscopy, the patient is prescribed liquid, tablet, and/or suppository **laxatives** by the physician. In addition, commercial **enemas** may be prescribed. The patient is given specific instructions on how and when to use the laxatives and/or enemas. This preparatory emptying of the colon assures that the colonoscope will not be obstructed and that the physician will be able to clearly see the colon lining.

On the morning of the colonoscopy, the patient is not to eat or drink anything. Unless otherwise instructed by the physician, the patient should continue to take all current medications. **Vitamins** with iron, iron supplements, or iron preparations should be discontinued for a few weeks before the colonoscopy because iron residue in the colon can inhibit viewing during the procedure. These preparatory procedures are extremely important to ensure a thoroughly clean colon for examination.

After the procedure, the patient is kept under observation until the medications' effects wear off. The patient has to be driven home and can generally resume a normal diet and usual activities unless otherwise instructed. The patient is advised to drink plenty of fluids to replace those lost by laxatives and **fasting**.

For a few hours after the procedure, the patient may feel groggy. There may be some abdominal cramping and a considerable amount of gas may be passed. If a biopsy was performed or a polyp was removed, there may be small amounts of blood in the stool for a few days. If the patient experiences severe abdominal pain or has persistent and heavy bleeding, this information should be brought to the physician's attention immediately.

Risks

The procedure is practically free of complications and risks. Rarely, (two in 1,000 cases) a perforation (hole) may occur in the intestinal wall. Heavy bleeding due to the removal of the polyp or from the biopsy site occurs infrequently (one in 1,000 cases). Some patients may have adverse reactions to the sedatives administered during the colonoscopy, but severe reactions are very rare. Infections due to a colonoscopy are also extremely rare. Patients with artificial or abnormal heart valves are usually given antibiotics before and after the procedure to prevent an infection.

Normal results

The results are normal if the lining of the colon is a pale reddish pink and there are no abnormal masses visible. In this case, the patient probably will not have to undergo another colonoscopy for several years.

Abnormal results indicate polyps or other suspicious masses in the lining of the colon. Many polyps can be removed during the procedure, and tissue samples can be taken by biopsy. If cancerous cells are detected in the tissue samples, then a diagnosis of colon cancer is made. A pathologist analyzes the tumor cells further to estimate the tumor's aggressiveness and the extent of the disease. This is crucial before deciding on the mode of treatment for the disease. Abnormal findings could also be due to inflammatory

bowel diseases such as ulcerative colitis or Crohn's disease. A condition called **diverticulosis**, which causes many small finger-like pouches to protrude from the colon wall, may also contribute to an abnormal result in the colonoscopy.

Morbidity and mortality rates

Colorectal cancer is the second leading cause of cancer deaths in the United States. In 2007, The American Cancer Society estimated that 52,180 people died from the disease. The World Health Organization (WHO) estimates that about 500,000 people worldwide die from colorectal cancer each year. Although colonoscopy screening can find precancerous growths (polyps), which lead to colorectal cancer, screening rates in the United States remain low. Removing polyps before they become cancerous can prevent the disease and potentially reduce deaths. Scientific evidence indicates that more than one-third of deaths from colorectal cancer could be avoided if people aged 50 years and older were screened regularly.

Alternatives

Individuals with a strong family history of colorectal cancer may wish to undergo genetic screening to detect a genetic alteration that may identify people who are more likely to develop the disease and who would benefit from earlier and more frequent screening. Only about 5% of colorectal cancers are inherited, so **genetic testing** provides limited benefits for most of the population.

Virtual colonoscopy is a new non-invasive technique for screening for colon polyps and cancer. The colon is cleaned out using potent laxatives just as it is for a standard colonoscopy. Instead of obtaining pictures through the insertion of a colonoscope, virtual colonoscopy uses X-ray images from a computerized tomography (CT) scan or **magnetic resonance imaging** (MRI) to create through computer manipulation two- and three-dimensional pictures of the colon.

Virtual colonoscopy offers several advantages. The procedure is non-invasive. It does not require patients to be sedated or put under anesthesia and is a good option for individuals who cannot or will not undergo standard colonoscopy. The procedure can be performed in less than one minute, compared with about 30–60 minutes plus recovery time required for standard colonoscopy. Another benefit of the CT scan is that it can find polyps that occasionally are missed by colonoscopy because the polyps lie behind folds within the colon.

Disadvantages of virtual colonoscopy include:

- It has difficulty finding small polyps (<0.2 in [5 mm] in size) that are easily seen in a colonoscopy.
- It is less able to find flat polyps compared to a colonoscopy.
- Small pieces of stool can look like polyps on the CT scan and lead to a diagnosis of polyp when there is none.
- It is not possible to remove suspect polyps or take a biopsy. If polyps are found by virtual colonoscopy, a standard colonoscopy must be done to remove the polyps. As a result, the individual must undergo two procedures.

Resources

BOOKS

Beers, Mark H., Robert S. Porter, and Thomas V. Jones, eds. *The Merck Manual*, 18th ed. Whitehouse Station, NJ: Merck, 2007.

Tierney, Lawrence M., Stephen J. McPhee, and Maxine A. Papadakis, eds. *Current Medical Diagnosis & Treatment 2003*. Stamford, CT: Appleton & Lange, 2002.

OTHER

"Colonoscopy." *Mayo Clinic*. June 29, 2007 [cited January 28, 2008]. http://www.mayoclinic.com/health/colonoscopy/CO00009.

"Patient Information from Your Surgeon & SAGES." *Society of American Gastrointestinal Endoscopic Surgeons*. March 2004 [cited January 28, 2008]. http://www.sages.org/sagespublication.php?doc=PI04.

"Screen for Life: National Colorectal Cancer Action Campaign." *Centers for Disease Control and Prevention*. March 10, 2008 [cited March 16, 2008]. http://www.cdc.gov/cancer/colorectal/sfl/.

"Virtual Colonoscopy." *National Digestive Diseases Information Clearinghouse*. May 2003 [cited January 28, 2008]. http://digestive.niddk.nih.gov/ddiseases/pubs/virtualcolonoscopy.

ORGANIZATIONS

American College of Gastroenterology, P.O. Box 342260, Bethesda, MD, 20827-2260, (301) 263-9000, http://www.acg.gi.org.

Colorectal Cancer Network (CCNetwork), P.O. Box 182, Kensington, MD, 20895-0182, (301) 879-1500, http://clickonium.com/colorectal-cancer.net/html/.

International Foundation for Functional Gastrointestinal Disorders (IFFGD), P.O. Box 170864, Milwaukee, WI, 53217, (414) 964-1799, (888) 964-2001, http://www.iffgd.org.

National Digestive Diseases Information Clearinghouse (NDDIC), 2 Information Way, Bethesda, MD, 20892-3570, (800) 891-5389, http://digestive.niddk.nih.gov.

Society of American Gastrointestinal Endoscopic Surgeons (SAGES), 11300 West Olympic Blvd., Suite 600, Los Angeles, CA, 90064, (310) 437-0544, http://www.sages.org.

Jennifer E. Sisk, M.A.
Crystal H. Kaczkowski, M.Sc.
Tish Davidson, A.M.
Brenda W. Lerner

Color blindness

Definition

Color blindness, also called color vision deficiency (CVD), is a group of conditions that affect the perception of color, characterized by the inability to clearly distinguish different colors of the spectrum. The difficulties range from mild to severe. Color blindness is a misleading term because people with color blindness are not blind. Rather, they tend to see colors in a limited range of hues; a rare few may not see colors at all.

Demographics

In the United States, red–green color vision defects are the most common form of color vision deficiency. This condition affects males more often than females. Some 10 million American men (7% of the male population) either cannot distinguish red from green, or see red and green differently from most people. This is the commonest form of color blindness, and it affects only 0.4% of women. Blue–yellow color vision defects affect males and females equally. This condition occurs in fewer than 1 in 10,000 people worldwide. Complete achromatopsia affects an estimated 1 in 30,000 people. The condition much more prevalent among Pingelapese islanders, who live on one of the Eastern Caroline Islands of Micronesia. Some 5–10% of this population have a total absence of color vision.

Description

Normal color vision requires the use of specialized receptor cells called cones, which are located in the retina of the eye. There are three types of cones, termed red, blue, and green. Each cone contains a special pigment, called a photopigment, that is most sensitive to a particular wavelength of light. The combined input from all three types of cones produces normal color vision. An abnormality, or deficiency, of any of the types of cones will result in abnormal color vision.

There are three basic variants of color blindness. Red–green color blindness is by far the most common deficiency. Affected persons cannot distinguish well between shades of red and green. They see these colors differently than most people and may experience difficulty naming different hues.

Blue–yellow color blindness is an inability to distinguish both blue and yellow, which are seen as white or gray. The condition is quite rare. Red–green and blue–yellow color vision deficiency disrupt the perception of color, but do not affect the sharpness of vision.

A total inability to distinguish colors (achromatopsia) is exceedingly rare. These affected individuals view the world in shades of gray. They frequently have poor visual acuity and are extremely sensitive to light (photophobia), which causes them to squint in ordinary light.

Risk factors

A family history of color blindness increases the risk since most color vision problems are inherited. Another risk factor for color vision deficiency is **aging**. The eye's lens can darken and yellow over time, which can impair the ability of older adults to see dark colors. Certain medications can also increase risk. For example, the drug hydroxychloroquine (Plaquenil), used to treat **rheumatoid arthritis**, can cause color blindness.

Causes and symptoms

As of 2009, mutations in the CNGA3, CNGB3, GNAT2, OPN1LW, OPN1MW, and OPN1SW genes are known to cause color vision deficiency. The OPN1LW gene makes pigments (L cones) that are more sensitive to light at the red end of the visible spectrum while the OPN1MW gene makes pigments (M cones) that are more sensitive to yellow–green light in the middle of the visible spectrum. As for the OPN1SW gene, it makes pigments (S cones) that are more sensitive to blue–violet light at the end of the visible spectrum. Genetic changes involving the OPN1LW and OPN1MW genes accordingly lead to an absence of L or M cones or the production of abnormal cones that affect red–green color vision. Mutations of the OPN1SW gene leads to the premature destruction of S cones or the production of defective cones which impairs perception of the color blue and makes it difficult to detect differences between

---

KEY TERMS

Achromatopsia—The inability to distinguish any colors.

Cones—Receptor cells that allow the perception of colors.

Photophobia—An extreme sensitivity to light.

Photopigment—Pigment that is most sensitive to a particular wavelength of light.

Retina—The light–sensitive layer of tissue in the back of the eye that receives and transmits visual signals to the brain through the optic nerve.

Rod—Photoreceptor that is highly sensitive to low levels of light and transmits images in shades of gray.

---

shades of blue and green. As for the CNGA3, CNGB3, and GNAT2 genes, their mutation is responsible for achromatopsia.

Color blindness is sometimes acquired. Chronic illnesses that can lead to color blindness include Alzheimer disease, **diabetes mellitus**, glaucoma, leukemia, **liver disease**, chronic **alcoholism**, **macular degeneration**, **multiple sclerosis**, **Parkinson disease**, sickle cell anemia, and **retinitis pigmentosa**. Accidents or strokes that damage the retina or affect particular areas of the brain can lead to color blindness. Some medications such as **antibiotics**, **barbiturates**, anti–tuberculosis drugs, high blood pressure medications, and several medications used to treat nervous disorders and psychological problems may cause color blindness. Industrial or environmental chemicals such as carbon monoxide, carbon disulfide, fertilizers, styrene, and some containing lead can cause loss of color vision. Occasionally, changes can occur in the affected person's capacity to see colors after age 60.

The inability to correctly identify colors is the only sign of color blindness. It is important to note that people with red/green or blue varieties of color blindness use other cues such as color saturation and object shape or location to distinguish colors. They can often distinguish red or green if they can visually compare the colors. However, most have difficulty accurately identifying colors without any other references. Most people with any impairment in color vision learn colors, as do other young children. These individuals often reach adolescence before their visual deficiency is identified.

Diagnosis

Tests

There are several tests available to identify problems associated with color vision. The most commonly used is the American Optical/Hardy, Rand, and Ritter Pseudoisochromatic test. It is composed of several discs filled with colored dots of different sizes and colors. A person with normal color vision looking at a test item sees a number that is clearly located somewhere in the center of a circle of variously colored dots. A color–blind person is not able to distinguish the number.

The Ishihara test is comprised of eight plates that are similar to the American Optical Pseudoisochromatic test plates. The individual being tested looks for numbers among the various colored dots on each test plate. Some plates distinguish between red/green and blue color blindness. Individuals with normal color vision perceive one number. Those with red/green color deficiency see a different number. Those with blue color vision see yet a different number.

A third analytical tool is the Titmus II Vision Tester Color Perception test. The subject looks into a stereoscopic machine. The test stimulus most often used in professional offices contains six different designs or numbers on a black background, framed in a yellow border. Titmus II can test one eye at a time. However, its value is limited because it can only identify red/green deficiencies and is not highly accurate.

Treatment

There is no treatment or cure for color blindness. Most color vision deficient persons compensate well for their abnormality and usually rely on color cues and details that are not consciously evident to persons with typical color vision.

Clinical trials

Clinical trials on color blindness and related conditions are currently sponsored by the National Institutes of Health (NIH) and other agencies. In 2009, NIH reported 15 on–going or recently completed studies on vision deficiency.

A few examples include:

- A study measuring color vision in patients with a blue light filtering lens implant in one eye and non–tinted implant in the other eye to determine whether blue light filtering lenses limit color vision. (NCT00403143)

- Evaluation of optical coherence tomography (OCT) scanners, instruments that use a beam of light to measure the thickness of the retina, the light–sensitive inner lining of the back of the eye. (NCT00069199)

- A genetic study of patients suffering from retinal dystrophies, conditions responsible for numerous cases of blindness. (NCT00422721)

Clinical trial information is constantly updated by NIH and the most recent information on blindness trials can be found at: http://clinicaltrials.gov.

Prognosis

In the case of some types of acquired color deficiency, if the cause of the problem is removed, the condition may improve with time. But for most people with acquired color blindness, the damage is usually permanent.

Prevention

Color blindness cannot be prevented.

Resources

BOOKS

Alexander, Sally Hobart. *Do You Remember the Color Blue? The Questions Children Ask About Blindness.* New York, NY: Puffin, 2002.

Jeffries, Benjamin J. *Color–Blindness; Its Dangers and Its Detection.* New York, NY: BiblioLife, 2008.

Jennings, John Ellis. *Color-Vision and Color-Blindness.* New York, NY: General Books LLC (Barnes & Noble), 2009.

Parker, Philip. *Color Vision Deficiency —A Bibliography and Dictionary for Physicians, Patients, and Genome Researchers.* San Diego, CA: ICON Health Publications, 2007.

PERIODICALS

Cole, B. L., and R. W. Harris. "Caution: coloured medication and the colour blind." *Lancet* 374, no. 9691 (August 2009): 720.

Cole, B. L., and J. D. Maddocks. "Color vision testing by Farnsworth lantern and ability to identify approach-path signal colors." *Aviation, Space, and Environmental Medicine* 79, no. 6 (June 2008): 585–590.

Fishman, G. A. "John Dalton: though in error, he still influenced our understanding of congenital color deficiency." *Ophthalmic Genetics* 29, no. 4 (December 2008): 162–165.

Shapley, R. "Vision: Gene therapy in colour." *Nature* 461, no. 7265 (October 2009): 737–739.

Stillman, J. A. "Psychophysical influences on the validity of anomaloscopic assessments of color vision." *Perception & Psychophysics* 70, no. 7 (October 2008): 1243–1247.

Waggoner, T. L. "What teachers, school nurses, and parents, should know about being colorblind." *School Nurse News* 26, no. 2 (March 2009): 35–36.

Yilmazbas T. P., et al. "Retinal nerve fiber layer thickness in congenital color vision deficiency." *European Journal of Ophthalmology* 18, no. 5 (2008): 845–847.

OTHER

"Color Blindness." *Medline Plus*. Health Topic. http://www.nlm.nih.gov/medlineplus/colorblindness.html (accessed November 9, 2009)

"Color Blindness Tests." *Medline Plus*. Encyclopedia. http://www.nlm.nih.gov/medlineplus/ency/imagepages/9962.htm (accessed November 9, 2009)

"Color Vision Deficiency." *Genetics Home Reference*. Information Page. http://ghr.nlm.nih.gov/condition = colorvisiondeficiency (accessed October 31, 2009)

"Color Vision Deficiency." *American Optometric Association*. Information Page. http://www.aoa.org/x4702.xml (accessed November 9, 2009)

"What's Color Blindness?" *Kids Health*. Information Page. http://kidshealth.org/kid/talk/qa/color_blind.html (accessed November 9, 2009)

ORGANIZATIONS

American Academy of Ophthalmology (AAO), PO Box 7424, San Francisco, CA, 94120-7424, (415) 561-8500, (415) 561-8533, patientinfo@aao.org, http://www.aao.org.

American Optometric Association (AOA), 243 N. Lindbergh Blvd., St. Louis, MO, 63141, (800) 365-2219, http://www.aoa.org.

National Eye Institute (NEI), 2020 Vision Place, Bethesda, MD, 20892-3655, (301) 496-5248, http://www.nei.nih.gov.

Prevent Blindness America, 211 West Wacker Drive, Suite 1700, Chicago, IL, 60606, (800) 331-2020, http://www.preventblindness.org.

L. Fleming Fallon, Jr., MD, MPH
Monique Laberge, PhD

Colorectal cancer *see* Colon cancer; Rectal cancer

Colostomy

Definition

A colostomy is a surgical procedure that brings a portion of the large intestine through the abdominal wall to carry feces out of the body.

Purpose

A colostomy is a means to treat various disorders of the large intestine, including **cancer**, obstruction, inflammatory bowel disease, ruptured diverticulum, **ischemia** (compromised blood supply), or traumatic injury. Temporary colostomies are created to divert stool from injured or diseased portions of the large intestine, allowing rest and healing. Permanent colostomies are performed when the distal bowel (at the farthest distance) must be removed or is blocked and inoperable. Although colorectal cancer is the most common indication for a permanent colostomy, only about 10–15% of patients with this diagnosis require a colostomy.

Demographics

Estimates of all ostomy surgeries (those involving any opening from the abdomen for the removal of either feces or urine) range from 42,000 to 65,000 each year; about half are temporary. Emergency surgeries for bowel obstruction and/or perforation comprise 10–15% of all colorectal surgeries; a portion of these result in colostomy.

Description

Surgery will result in one of three types of colostomies:

- End colostomy. The functioning end of the intestine (the section of bowel that remains connected to the upper gastrointestinal tract) is brought out onto the surface of the abdomen, forming the stoma (artificial opening) by cuffing the intestine back on itself and suturing the end to the skin. The surface of the stoma is actually the lining of the intestine, usually appearing moist and pink. The distal portion of bowel (now connected only to the rectum) may be removed, or sutured closed and left in the abdomen. An end colostomy is usually a permanent ostomy, resulting from trauma, cancer, or another pathological condition.

- Double-barrel colostomy. This involves the creation of two separate stomas on the abdominal wall. The proximal (nearest) stoma is the functional end that is connected to the upper gastrointestinal tract and will drain stool; the distal stoma, connected to the rectum and also called a mucous fistula, drains small amounts of mucus material. This is most often a temporary colostomy performed to rest an area of bowel, and to be later closed.

- Loop colostomy. This surgery brings a loop of bowel through an incision in the abdominal wall.

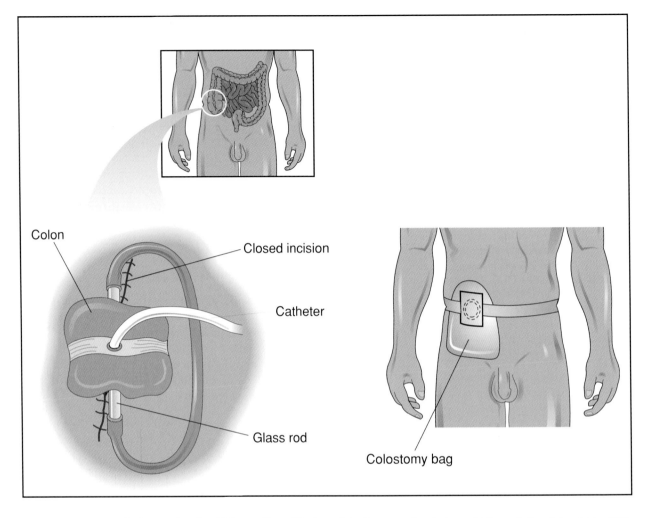

Colon

Closed incision

Catheter

Glass rod

Colostomy bag

A colostomy is a surgical procedure in which a portion of the large intestine, or colon, is brought through the abdominal wall to carry feces out of the body. There are three types of colostomies: end colostomy, double-barrel colostomy, and loop colostomy. The loop colostomy is featured in the illustration above. *(Illustration by Electronic Illustrators Group. Reproduced by permission of Gale, a part of Cengage Learning.)*

The loop is held in place outside the abdomen by a plastic rod slipped beneath it. An incision is made in the bowel to allow the passage of stool through the loop colostomy. The supporting rod is removed approximately 7 to 10 days after surgery, when healing has occurred that will prevent the loop of bowel from retracting into the abdomen. A loop colostomy is most often performed for creation of a temporary stoma to divert stool away from an area of intestine that has been blocked or ruptured.

Diagnosis/Preparation

A number of diseases and injuries may require a colostomy. Among the diseases are inflammatory bowel disease and colorectal cancer. Determining whether this surgery is necessary is a decision the physician makes based on a number of factors, including patient history, amount of **pain**, and the results of tests such as **colonoscopy** and lower G.I. (gastrointestinal) series. Due to lifestyle impact of the surgery, the decision is made after careful consultation with the patient. However, an immediate decision may be made in emergency situations involving injuries or puncture **wounds** in the abdomen or intestinal perforations related to diverticulear disease, ulcers, or life-threatening cancer.

As with any surgical procedure, the patient will be required to sign a consent form after the procedure is explained thoroughly. Blood and urine studies, along with various x rays and an electrocardiograph (EKG), may be ordered as the doctor deems necessary. If possible, the patient should visit an enterostomal therapist, who will mark an appropriate place on the

KEY TERMS

Diverticulum—Pouches that project off the wall of the intestine.

Embolism—Blockage of a blood vessel by any small piece of material traveling in the blood; the emboli may be caused by germs, air, blood clots, or fat.

Enema—Insertion of a tube into the rectum to infuse fluid into the bowel and encourage a bowel movement. Ordinary enemas contain tap water, mixtures of soap and water, glycerine and water, or other materials.

Intestine—Commonly called the bowels, divided into the small and large intestine. They extend from the stomach to the anus.

Ischemia—A compromise in blood supply delivered to body tissues that causes tissue damage or death.

Ostomy—A surgical procedure that creates an opening from the inside of the body to the outside, usually to remove body wastes (feces or urine).

abdomen for the stoma and offer preoperative education on ostomy management.

In order to empty and cleanse the bowel, the patient may be placed on a low-residue diet for several days prior to surgery. A liquid diet may be ordered for at least the day before surgery, with nothing by mouth after midnight. A series of **enemas** and/or oral preparations (GoLytely or Colyte) may be ordered to empty the bowel of stool. Oral anti-infectives (neomycin, erythromycin, or kanamycin sulfate) may be ordered to decrease bacteria in the intestine and help prevent postoperative infection. A nasogastric tube is inserted from the nose to the stomach on the day of surgery or during surgery to remove gastric secretions and prevent **nausea and vomiting**. A urinary catheter (a thin plastic tube) may also be inserted to keep the bladder empty during surgery, giving more space in the surgical field and decreasing chances of accidental injury.

Aftercare

Postoperative care for the patient with a new colostomy, as with those who have had any major surgery, involves monitoring of blood pressure, pulse, respirations, and temperature. Breathing tends to be shallow because of the effect of anesthesia and the patient's reluctance to breathe deeply and experience pain that is caused by the abdominal incision. The patient is instructed how to support the operative

site during deep breathing and coughing, and given pain medication as necessary. Fluid intake and output is measured, and the operative site is observed for color and amount of wound drainage. The nasogastric tube will remain in place, attached to low, intermittent suction until bowel activity resumes. For the first 24–48 hours after surgery, the colostomy will drain bloody mucus. Fluids and electrolytes are infused intravenously until the patient's diet can gradually be resumed, beginning with liquids. Usually within 72 hours, passage of gas and stool through the stoma begins. Initially, the stool is liquid, gradually thickening as the patient begins to take solid foods. The patient is usually out of bed in eight to 24 hours after surgery and discharged in two to four days.

A colostomy pouch will generally have been placed on the patient's abdomen around the stoma during surgery. During the hospital stay, the patient and his or her caregivers will be educated on how to care for the colostomy. Determination of appropriate pouching supplies and a schedule of how often to change the pouch should be established. Regular assessment and meticulous care of the skin surrounding the stoma is important to maintain an adequate surface on which to attach the pouch. Some patients with colostomies are able to routinely irrigate the stoma, resulting in regulation of bowel function; rather than needing to wear a pouch, these patients may only need a dressing or cap over their stoma. Often, an enterostomal therapist will visit the patient in the hospital or at home after discharge to help the patient with stoma care.

Dietary counseling will be necessary for the patient to maintain normal bowel function and to avoid **constipation**, impaction, and other discomforts.

Risks

Potential complications of colostomy surgery include:

- excessive bleeding
- surgical wound infection
- thrombophlebitis (inflammation and blood clot to veins in the legs)
- pneumonia
- pulmonary embolism (blood clot or air bubble in the lungs' blood supply)

Psychological complications may result from colostomy surgery because of the fear of the perceived social stigma attached to wearing a colostomy bag. Patients may also be depressed and have feelings of low self-worth because of the change in their lifestyle and their appearance. Some patients may feel ugly and sexually unattractive and may worry that their spouse or significant other will no longer find them appealing. Counseling and education regarding surgery and the inherent lifestyle changes are often necessary.

Normal results

Complete healing is expected without complications. The period of time required for recovery from the surgery may vary depending on the patient's overall health prior to surgery and the patient's willingness to participate in stoma care. The colostomy patient without other medical complications should be able to resume all daily activities once recovered from the surgery. Adjustments in diet and daily personal care will need to be made.

Morbidity and mortality rates

Complications after colostomy surgery can occur. The doctor should be made aware of any of the following problems after surgery:

- increased pain, swelling, redness, drainage, or bleeding in the surgical area
- headache, muscle aches, dizziness, or fever
- increased abdominal pain or swelling, constipation, nausea or vomiting, or black, tarry stools

Stomal complications can also occur. They include:

- Death (necrosis) of stomal tissue. Caused by inadequate blood supply, this complication is usually visible 12–24 hours after the operation and may require additional surgery.
- Retraction (stoma is flush with the abdomen surface or has moved below it). Caused by insufficient stomal length, this complication may be managed by use of special pouching supplies. Elective revision of the stoma is also an option.
- Prolapse (stoma increases length above the surface of the abdomen). Most often this results from an overly large opening in the abdominal wall or inadequate fixation of the bowel to the abdominal wall. Surgical correction is required when blood supply is compromised.
- Stenosis (narrowing at the opening of the stoma). Often this is associated with infection around the stoma or scarring. Mild stenosis can be removed under local anesthesia; severe stenosis may require surgery for reshaping the stoma.
- Parastomal hernia (bowel causing bulge in the abdominal wall next to the stoma). This occurs due to placement of the stoma where the abdominal wall is weak or an overly large opening in the abdominal wall was made. The use of an ostomy support belt and special pouching supplies may be adequate. If severe, the defect in the abdominal wall should be repaired and the stoma moved to another location.

Mortality rates for colostomy patients vary according to the patient's general health upon admittance to the hospital. Even among higher risk patients, mortality is about 16%. This rate is greatly reduced (between 0.8% and 3.8%) when the colostomy is performed by a board-certified colon and rectal surgeon.

Alternatives

When a colostomy is deemed necessary, there are usually few to no alternatives to the surgery, though there can be alternatives in the type of surgery involved and adjuvant therapies related to the disease. For example, laparoscopic surgery is being used with many diseases of the intestinal tract, including initial cancers. For this surgery, the colon and rectal surgeon inserts a laparoscope (an instrument that has a tiny video camera attached) through a small incision in the abdomen. Other small incisions are made for the surgeon to insert laparoscopic instruments to use in creating the colostomy. This surgery often results in a shorter stay in the hospital, less postoperative pain, a quicker return to normal activities, and far less scarring. It is not recommended for patients who have had extensive prior abdominal surgery, large tumors, previous cancer, or serious heart problems.

In some cases, rather than giving patients a colostomy for low rectal cancers, the surgeon creates a Colo-anal Pouch. The Colo-anal J Pouch operation has been developed in order to surgically recreate the back passage (rectum). In this operation the rectum is removed and the sphincter muscles and anal canal are left in place.

The surgeon needs to remove the rectum because of the disease affecting it. The rectum is where you store body waste until you wish to empty your bowel. The sphincter muscles surrounding the anus (back passage) are left intact. These muscles are important for bowel control. Surgeons will make a new rectum from a piece of your remaining bowel, and this new rectum is called a Colo-anal J Pouch, or simply a Pouch. It is stitched to your anal canal and this will eventually allow you to go to the toilet in the usual manner. A temporary loop ileostomy will probably be made in order to allow the pouch to heal. This is the first stage of the procedure and the operation takes between two to four hours.

Colostomy Irrigation

Colostomy irrigation is a way to regulate bowel movements by emptying the colon at a scheduled time. The process involves infusing water into the colon through the stoma. This stimulates the colon to empty. By repeating this process regularly, usually once per day or every other day, the colon is trained to empty with no spillage of waste in between irrigation. Colostomy irrigation also can help you avoid constipation. It is a personal decision patients should discuss with their doctors while still in the hospital after their surgery.

Resources

BOOKS

Cima RR, Pemberton JH. Ileostomy, Colostomy, and Pouches. In: Feldman M, Friedman LS, Brandt LJ, eds. *Sleisenger & Fordtran's Gastrointestinal and Liver Disease. 8th ed.* Philadelphia, Pa: Saunders Elsevier; 2006.

Fry RD, Mahmoud N, Maron DJ, et al. Colon and Rectum. In: Townsend CM, Beauchamp RD, Evers BM, Mattox KL, eds. *Sabiston Textbook of Surgery. 18th ed.* Philadelphia, Pa: Saunders Elsevier; 2008.

OTHER

National Digestive Diseases Information Clearinghouse. *Ileostomy, Colostomy, and Ileoanal Reservoir Surgery.* (February 1, 2000): 1.

ORGANIZATIONS

United Ostomy Association, Inc. (UOA), 19772 MacArthur Blvd., Suite 200, Irvine, CA, 92612-2405, (800) 826-0826, http://www.uoa.org.

Wound Ostomy and Continence Nurses Society, 2755 Bristol Street, Suite 110, Costa Mesa, CA, 92626, (714) 476-0268, http://www.wocn.org.

Janie F. Franz
Kathleen D. Wright, RN
Karl Finley
Brenda Lerner

Colposcopy

Definition

Colposcopy is a procedure that allows a physician to examine a woman's cervix and vagina using a special microscope called a colposcope. Colposcopy is used to check for precancerous or abnormal areas.

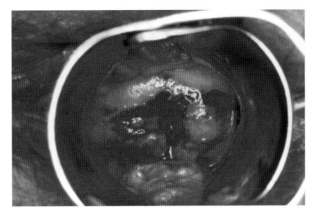

This colposcopic view of the cervix reveals CIN 2 dysplasia, or abnormal growth of cells. This is the second stage in the development of cervical cancer. *(Custom Medical Stock Photo, Inc. Reproduced by permission.)*

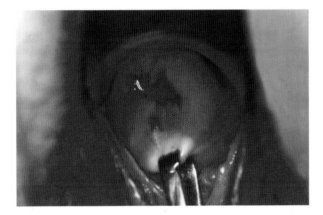

A colposcopy makes it possible for a physician to view this healthy cervix without surgery. *(Custom Medical Stock Photo, Inc. Reproduced by permission.)*

Purpose

Colposcopy is used to identify or rule out the existence of any precancerous conditions in the cervical tissue. If a Papanicolaou (Pap) test shows abnormal cell growth, colposcopy is usually the first follow-up test performed. The physician will attempt to find the area that produced the abnormal cells and remove a sample of it for further study (biopsy) and diagnosis.

Colposcopy may also be performed if the cervix looks abnormal during a routine examination. It may be suggested for women with **genital warts** and for diethylstilbestrol (DES) daughters (women whose mothers took the anti-miscarriage drug DES when pregnant with them). Colposcopy is used in the emergency department to examine victims of **sexual assault** and **abuse** and document any physical evidence of vaginal injury.

Biopsy—Removal of a sample of abnormal tissue for more extensive examination under a microscope.

Cervix—Narrow, lower end of the uterus forming the opening to the vagina.

Cryosurgery—Freezing and destroying abnormal cells.

Diathermy—Also called electrocautery, this is a procedure that heats and destroys abnormal cells.

Diethylstilbestrol (DES)—A synthetic form of estrogen that was widely prescribed to women from 1940 to 1970 to prevent complications during pregnancy, and linked to several serious birth defects and disorders of the reproductive system in daughters of women who took DES.

Dysplasia—Abnormal cellular changes that may become cancerous.

Human papillomavirus (HPV)—A family of viruses that cause common warts of the hands and feet, as

well as lesions in the genital and vaginal area. More than 50 types of HPV have been identified, some of which are linked to cancerous and precancerous conditions, including cancer of the cervix. A vaccine is now available against some of these viruses.

Loop electrosurgical excision (LEEP)—A procedure that can help diagnose and treat cervical abnormalities using a thin wire loop that emits a low-voltage high-frequency radio wave that can excise tissue.

Monsel's solution—A solution used to stop bleeding.

Pap test—The common term for the Papanicolaou test, a simple smear method of removing cervical cells to screen for abnormalities that indicate cancer or a precancerous condition.

Speculum—A retractor used to separate the walls of the vagina to make visual examination easier.

Demographics

Cervical cancer affects millions of women worldwide. In the United States, the routine use of Pap tests has substantially decreased the rate of this **cancer**. With the introduction of a vaccine against the family of viruses associated with cervical cancer, the rate in the developed world is expected to continue to fall. Cervical cancer continues to be a major health problem for women in the developing world. Even in the United States, it is estimated that about one-third of women fail to follow up with colposcopy after an abnormal **Pap test**. Minority women, teenagers, and those of low socioeconomic status are the least likely to follow up.

Description

Colposcopy is usually performed in a physician's office and is similar to a regular gynecologic exam. An instrument called a speculum is inserted to hold the vagina open, and the gynecologist looks at the cervix and vagina using a colposcope, a low-power microscope designed to magnify the cervix 10–40 times its normal size. Most colposcopes are connected to a video monitor that displays the area of interest. Photographs are taken during the examination to document abnormal areas.

The cervix and vagina are swabbed with dilute acetic acid (vinegar). The solution highlights abnormal areas by turning them white (instead of a normal

pink color). Abnormal areas can also be identified by looking for a characteristic pattern made by abnormal blood vessels.

If any abnormal areas are seen, the doctor takes a biopsy of the tissue, a common procedure that takes about 15 minutes. Several samples might be taken, depending on the size of the abnormal area. A biopsy may cause temporary discomfort and cramping, which usually go away within a few minutes. If the abnormal area appears to extend inside the cervical canal, a scraping of the canal may also be done. The biopsy results are usually available within a week.

If the tissue sample indicates abnormal growth (dysplasia) or is precancerous, and if the entire abnormal area can be seen, the doctor may destroy the tissue using one of several procedures, including ones that use high heat (diathermy), extreme cold (cryosurgery), or lasers. Another procedure, called loop electrosurgical excision (LEEP), uses low-voltage, high-frequency radio waves to excise tissue. If any of the abnormal tissue is within the cervical canal, a cone biopsy (removal of a conical section of the cervix for inspection) will be needed.

Diagnosis/Preparation

Women who are pregnant or who suspect that they are pregnant must tell their doctor before the procedure begins. Pregnant women may undergo colposcopy if they have an abnormal Pap test; special precautions, however, must be taken during biopsy of the cervix. Patients who are taking blood-thinning medications such as warfarin (Coumadin) should tell their doctor before the procedure.

Patients should be instructed not to douche, use tampons, or have sexual intercourse for 24 hours before colposcopy. Patients should empty their bladder and bowels before colposcopy for comfort. Colposcopy does not require any anesthetic medication because **pain** is minimal. If a biopsy is done, there may be mild cramps or a sharp pinching when the tissue is removed. To lessen this pain, the doctor may recommend ibuprofen (Motrin, Advil) taken the night before and the morning of the procedure (no later than 30 minutes before the appointment). Patients who are pregnant or allergic to **aspirin** or ibuprofen can instead take **acetaminophen** (Tylenol).

Aftercare

If a biopsy was done, there may be a dark vaginal discharge afterwards. After the sample is removed, the doctor applies Monsel's solution to the area to stop the bleeding. When this mixes with blood, it creates a black fluid that looks like coffee grounds. This fluid may be present for a several days after the procedure. It is also normal to have some blood spotting after colposcopy. Pain-relieving medication can be taken to lessen any post-procedural cramping.

Patients should not use tampons, douche, or have sex for at least a week after the procedure or until the doctor says it is safe because of the risk of infection.

Risks

Colposcopy is a very safe procedure. Patients may have bleeding or infection after biopsy. Bleeding is usually controlled with a topical medication prescribed by the physician or health care provider. If colposcopy is performed on a pregnant patient, there is a risk of **premature labor**.

A patient should call her doctor right away if she notices any of the following symptoms:

- heavy vaginal bleeding (more than one sanitary pad an hour);
- fever, chills, or an unpleasant vaginal odor; or
- lower abdominal pain.

Normal results

If visual inspection shows that the surface of the cervix is smooth and pink, this is considered normal.

Areas that look abnormal may actually be normal variations; a biopsy will indicate whether the tissue is normal or abnormal.

Abnormal conditions that can be detected using colposcopy and biopsy include precancerous tissue changes (cervical dysplasia), cancer, and cervical **warts** caused by human papillomavirus.

Morbidity and mortality rates

Complications associated with colposcopy are extremely rare. There is a risk that the procedure will miss precancerous or cancerous tissues and thus prolong treatment until the cancer has become advanced. The American Cancer Society estimated that 11,270 new cases of cervical cancer were diagnosed in 2009 and 4,070 deaths could be attributed to the disease.

Alternatives

While the Pap test is an effective screening test for abnormal cell growth of the cervix, it is an inadequate diagnostic alternative to colposcopy because of the potential for false negative results (10–50%). In some instances, a repeat Pap test may be recommended before performing colposcopy (e.g., in the case of inflammation or no previous abnormal Pap test).

Resources

OTHER

"Colposcopy (Position Paper)." *American Academy of Family Physicians.* 2004 [cited February 12, 2008]. http://www.aafp.org/online/en/home/policy/policies/c/colposcopypositionpaper.html.

"Colposcopy." *MedlinePlus.* [cited February 12, 2008]. http://www.nlm.nih.gov/medlineplus/tutorials/colposcopy/htm/index.htm.

Garcia, Agustin A. "Cervical Cancer." *eMedicine.com.* December 12, 2007 [cited February 12, 2008]. http://www.emedicine.com/med/topic324.htm.

Pattan, Charles, Alissa Zuellig, Bophal Hong, Shironda Stewart, and Michael P. Grossman. "Colposcopy." *eMedicine.com.* July 22, 2005 [cited February 12, 2008]. http://www.emedicine.com/med/topic3298.htm.

ORGANIZATIONS

American College of Obstetricians and Gynecologists, 409 12th St., SW, P.O. Box 96920, Washington, DC, 20090-6920, (202) 638-5577, http://www.acog.org.

American Society for Colposcopy and Cervical Pathology, 152 West Washington Street, Hagerstown, MD, 21740, (301) 733-3640, (800) 787-7227, http://www.asccp.org.

Association of Women's Health, Obstetric, and Neonatal Nurses, 2000 L St., NW, Suite 740, Washington, DC,

20036, (202) 261-2400, (800) 673-8499, http://www.
awhonn.org.

DES Action USA, 158 S. Stanwood Rd., Columbus, OH,
43209, (800) 337-9288, http://www.desaction.org.

Society of Gynecologic Oncologists, 230 West Monroe
Street, Suite 710, Chicago, IL, 60606, (312) 235-4060,
http://www.sgo.org.

Jennifer E. Sisk, M.A.
Stephanie Dionne Sherk
Tish Davidson, A.M.
Brenda W. Lerner

Coma

Definition

Coma, from the Greek word "koma," meaning
deep sleep, is a state of extreme unresponsiveness, in
which an individual exhibits no voluntary movement
or behavior. Furthermore, in a deep coma, even painful stimuli (actions which, when performed on a
healthy individual, result in reactions) are unable to
affect any response, and normal reflexes may be lost.

Description

Coma lies on a spectrum with other alterations in
consciousness. The level of consciousness required by, for
example, someone reading this passage lies at one extreme
end of the spectrum, while complete brain **death** lies at the
other end of the spectrum. In between are such states as
obtundation, drowsiness, and stupor. All of these are
conditions which, unlike coma, still allow the individual
to respond to stimuli, although such a response may be
brief and require stimulus of greater than normal
intensity.

In order to understand the loss of function suffered by a comatose individual, it is necessary to first
understand the important characteristics of the conscious state. Consciousness is defined by two fundamental elements: awareness and arousal.

Awareness allows one to receive and process all the
information communicated by the five senses, and thus
relate to oneself and to the outside world. Awareness
has both psychological and physiological components.
The psychological component is governed by an individual's mind and mental processes. The physiological
component refers to the functioning of an individual's
brain, and therefore that brain's physical and chemical
condition. Awareness is regulated by cortical areas
within the cerebral hemispheres, the outermost layer
of the brain that separates humans from other animals
by allowing for greater intellectual functioning.

Arousal is regulated solely by physiological functioning and consists of more primitive responsiveness to
the world, as demonstrated by predictable reflex (involuntary) responses to stimuli. Arousal is maintained by
the reticular activating system (RAS). This is not an
anatomical area of the brain, but rather a network of
structures (including the brainstem, the medulla, and
the thalamus) and nerve pathways, which function
together to produce and maintain arousal.

Causes and symptoms

Coma, then, is the result of something that interferes with the functioning of the cerebral cortex and/or
the functioning of the structures which make up the
RAS. In fact, a huge and varied number of conditions
can result in coma. A good way of categorizing these
conditions is to consider the anatomic and the metabolic causes of coma. Anatomic causes of coma are
those conditions that disrupt the normal physical architecture of the brain structures responsible for consciousness, either at the level of the cerebal cortex or
the brainstem, while metabolic causes of coma consist
of those conditions that change the chemical environment of the brain, thereby adversely affecting function.

There are many metabolic causes of coma,
including:

- A decrease in the delivery to the brain of substances
  necessary for appropriate brain functioning, such as
  oxygen, glucose (sugar), and sodium.

- The presence of certain substances that disrupt the
  functioning of neurons. Drugs or alcohol in toxic quantities can result in neuronal dysfunction, as can substances normally found in the body, but that, due to some
  diseased state, accumulate at toxic levels. Accumulated
  substances that might cause coma include ammonia due
  to liver disease, ketones due to uncontrolled diabetes, or
  carbon dioxide due to a severe asthma attack.

- The changes in chemical levels in the brain due to the
  electrical derangements caused by seizures.

Diagnosis

As in any neurologic condition, history and examination form the cornerstone of diagnosis when the patient
is in a coma; however, history must be obtained from
family, friends, or EMS. The Glasgow Coma Scale is a
system of examining a comatose patient. It is helpful for
evaluating the depth of the coma, tracking the patient's
progress, and predicting (somewhat) the ultimate outcome of the coma. The Glasgow Coma Scale assigns a
different number of points for exam results in three

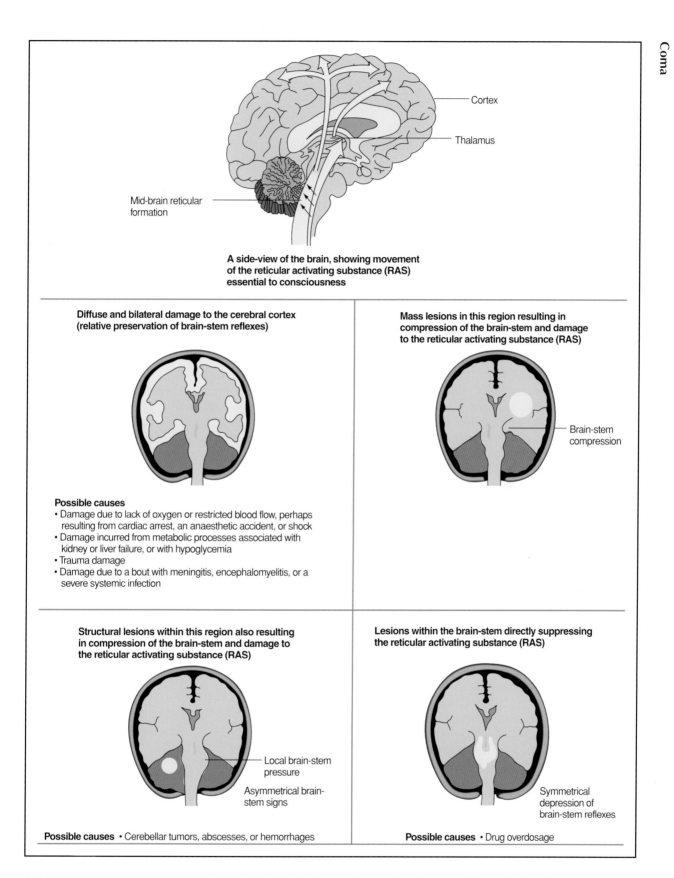

Cortex

Thalamus

Mid-brain reticular formation

A side-view of the brain, showing movement of the reticular activating substance (RAS) essential to consciousness

Diffuse and bilateral damage to the cerebral cortex (relative preservation of brain-stem reflexes)

Possible causes
• Damage due to lack of oxygen or restricted blood flow, perhaps resulting from cardiac arrest, an anaesthetic accident, or shock
• Damage incurred from metabolic processes associated with kidney or liver failure, or with hypoglycemia
• Trauma damage
• Damage due to a bout with meningitis, encephalomyelitis, or a severe systemic infection

Mass lesions in this region resulting in compression of the brain-stem and damage to the reticular activating substance (RAS)

Brain-stem compression

Structural lesions within this region also resulting in compression of the brain-stem and damage to the reticular activating substance (RAS)

Local brain-stem pressure

Asymmetrical brain-stem signs

Possible causes • Cerebellar tumors, abscesses, or hemorrhages

Lesions within the brain-stem directly suppressing the reticular activating substance (RAS)

Symmetrical depression of brain-stem reflexes

Possible causes • Drug overdosage

The four brain conditions that result in coma. *(Illustration by Hans & Cassady, Inc. Reproduced by permission of Gale, a part of Cengage Learning.)*

different categories: opening the eyes, verbal response (using words or voice to respond), and motor response (moving a part of the body). Fifteen is the largest possible number of total points, indicating the highest level of functioning. The highest level of functioning would be demonstrated by an individual who spontaneously opens his/her eyes, gives appropriate answers to questions about his/her situation, and can carry out a command (such as "move your leg" or "nod your head"). Three is the least possible number of total points and would be given to a patient for whom not even a painful stimulus is sufficient to provoke a response. In the middle are those patients who may be able to respond, but who require an intense or painful stimulus, and whose response may demonstrate some degree of brain malfunctioning (such as a person whose only response to **pain** in a limb is to bend that limb in toward the body). When performed as part of the admission examination, a Glasgow score of three to five points often suggests that the patient has likely suffered fatal brain damage, while eight or more points indicates that the patient's chances for recovery are good. Expansion of the pupils and respiratory pattern are also important. Metabolic causes of coma are diagnosed from blood work and **urinalysis** to evaluate blood chemistry, drug screen, and blood cell abnormalities that may indicate infection. Anatomic causes of coma are diagnosed from CT (computed tomography) or MRI (**magnetic resonance imaging**) scans.

Treatment

Coma is a medical emergency, and attention must first be directed to maintaining the patient's respiration and circulation, using intubation and ventilation, administration of intravenous fluids or blood as needed, and other supportive care. If head trama has not been excluded, the neck should be stablized in the event of fracture. It is obviously extremely important for a physician to determine quickly the cause of a coma, so that potentially reversible conditions are treated immediately. For example, an infection may be treated with **antibiotics**; a **brain tumor** may be removed; and brain swelling from an injury can be reduced with certain medications. Various metabolic disorders can be addressed by supplying the individual with the correct amount of oxygen, glucose, or **sodium**; by treating the underlying disease in **liver disease**, **asthma**, or diabetes; and by halting seizures with medication. Because of their low incidence of side effects and potential for prompt reversal of coma in certain conditions, glucose, the B-vitamin thiamine, and Narcan (to counteract any narcotic-type drugs) are routinely given.

Prognosis

Some conditions that cause coma can be completely reversed, restoring the individual to his or her original level of functioning. However, if areas of the brain have been sufficiently damaged due to the severity or duration of the condition which led to the coma, the individual may recover from the coma with permanent disabilities, or may even never regain consciousness. Take, for example, the situation of someone whose coma was caused by brain injury in a car accident. Such an injury can result in one of three outcomes. In the event of a less severe brain injury, with minimal swelling, an individual may indeed recover consciousness and regain all of his or her original abilities. In the event of a more severe brain injury, with swelling that resulted in further pressure on areas of the brain, an individual may regain consciousness, but may have some degree of impairment. The impairment may be physical (such as **paralysis** of a leg) or may even result in a change in the individual's intellectual functioning and/or personality. The most severe types of brain injury, short of death, result in states in which the individual loses all ability to function and remains deeply unresponsive. An individual who has suffered such a severe brain injury may remain in a coma indefinitely. This condition is termed persistent **vegetative state**.

Outcome from a coma is therefore quite variable and depends a great deal on the cause and duration of the coma. In the case of drug poisonings, extremely high rates of recovery can be expected following prompt medical attention. Patients who have suffered head injuries tend to do better than do patients whose coma was caused by other types of medical illnesses. Leaving out those people whose coma followed drug **poisoning**, only about 15% of patients who remain in a coma for more than just a few hours make a good recovery. Those adult patients who remain in a coma for greater than four weeks have almost no chance of eventually regaining their previous level of functioning. On the other hand, children and young adults have regained functioning even after two months in a coma.

ORGANIZATIONS

American Academy of Neurology, 1080 Montreal Ave., St. Paul, MN, 5516, (651) 695-2717, (651) 695-2791, (800) 879-1960, memberservices@aan.com, http://www.aan.com/.
Coma/Traumatic Brain Injury Recovery Association, 8300 Republic Airport Suite 106, Farmingdale, NY, 11735, (631) 756-1826, http://www.comarecovery.org.

Rosalyn Carson-DeWitt, MD

Combat neurosis *see* **Post-traumatic stress disorder**

Common cold

Definition

The common cold is a viral infection of the upper respiratory system, including the nose, throat, sinuses, eustachian tubes, trachea, larynx, and bronchial tubes. Although more than 200 different viruses can cause a cold, 30–50% are caused by a group known as rhinoviruses. Almost all colds clear up in less than two weeks without complications.

Common cold remedies and side effects

	Symptoms	Side effects
Antihistamines	Congestion Itchy eyes Runny nose Sneezing Stuffy nose	Drowsiness Dry mouth and eyes
Decongestants	Congestion Stuffy nose	Insomnia Rapid heartbeat Stimulation

(Table by PreMediaGlobal. Reproduced by permission of Gale, a part of Cengage Learning.)

Description

Colds, sometimes called rhinovirus or coronavirus infections, are the most common illness to strike any part of the body. It is estimated that the average person has more than 50 colds during a lifetime. Anyone can get a cold, although preschool and grade school children catch them more frequently than adolescents and adults. Repeated exposure to viruses causing colds creates partial immunity.

Although most colds resolve on their own without complications, they are a leading cause of visits to the doctor and of time lost from work and school. Treating symptoms of the common cold has given rise to a multi-million dollar industry in over-the-counter medications.

Cold season in the United States begins in early autumn and extends through early spring. Although it is not true that getting wet or being in a draft causes a cold (a person has to come in contact with the virus to catch a cold), certain conditions may lead to increased susceptibility. These include:

• fatigue and overwork

• emotional stress

• poor nutrition

• smoking

• living or working in crowded conditions

Colds make the upper respiratory system less resistant to bacterial infection. Secondary bacterial infection may lead to middle ear infection, **bronchitis**, **pneumonia**, sinus infection, or **strep throat**. People with chronic lung disease, **asthma**, diabetes, or a weakened immune system are more likely to develop these complications.

Causes and symptoms

Colds are caused by more than 200 different viruses. The most common groups are rhinoviruses and coronaviruses. Different groups of viruses are more infectious at different seasons of the year, but knowing the exact virus causing the cold is not important in treatment.

People with colds are contagious during the first two to four days of the infection. Colds pass from person to person in several ways. When an infected person coughs, sneezes, or speaks, tiny fluid droplets containing the virus are expelled. If these are breathed in by other people, the virus may establish itself in their noses and airways.

Colds may also be passed through direct contact. If a person with a cold touches his runny nose or watery eyes, then shakes hands with another person some of the virus is transferred to the uninfected person. If that person then touches his mouth, nose, or eyes, the virus is transferred to an environment where it can reproduce and cause a cold.

Finally, cold viruses can be spread through inanimate objects (door knobs, telephones, toys) that become contaminated with the virus. This is a common method of transmission in child care centers. If a child with a cold touches her runny nose, then plays with a toy, some of the virus may be transferred to the toy. When another child plays with the toy a short time later, he may pick up some of the virus on his hands. The second child then touches his contaminated hands to his eyes, nose, or mouth and transfers some of the cold virus to himself.

Once acquired, the cold virus attaches itself to the lining of the nasal passages and sinuses. This causes the infected cells to release a chemical called histamine. Histamine increases the blood flow to the infected cells, causing swelling, congestion, and increased mucus production. Within one to three days the infected person begins to show cold symptoms.

The first cold symptoms are a tickle in the throat, runny nose, and sneezing. The initial discharge from the nose is clear and thin. Later it changes to a thick yellow or greenish discharge. Most adults do not develop a **fever** when they catch a cold. Young children may develop a low fever of up to 102°F (38.9°C).

In addition to a runny nose and fever, signs of a cold include coughing, sneezing, nasal congestion, **headache**, muscle ache, chills, **sore throat**, hoarseness, watery eyes, tiredness, and lack of appetite. The **cough** that accompanies a cold is usually intermittent and dry.

Most people begin to feel better four to five days after their cold symptoms become noticeable. All symptoms are generally gone within ten days, except for a dry cough that may linger for up to three weeks.

Colds make people more susceptible to bacterial infections such as strep throat, middle ear infections, and sinus infections. A person whose cold does not begin to improve within a week; or who experiences chest **pain**, fever for more than a few days, difficulty breathing, bluish lips or fingernails, a cough that brings up greenish-yellow or grayish sputum, skin rash, **swollen glands**, or whitish spots on the tonsils or throat should consult a doctor to see if he or she has acquired a secondary bacterial infection that needs to be treated with an antibiotic.

People who have **emphysema**, chronic lung disease, diabetes, or a weakened immune system — either from diseases such as **AIDS** or leukemia, or as the result of medications, (**corticosteroids**, **chemotherapy** drugs)—should consult their doctor if they get a cold. People with these health problems are more likely to get a secondary infection.

Diagnosis

Colds are diagnosed by observing a person's symptoms. There are no laboratory tests readily available to detect the cold virus. However, a doctor may do a **throat culture** or blood test to rule out a secondary infection.

Influenza is sometimes confused with a cold, but flu causes much more severe symptoms and generally a fever. **Allergies** to molds or pollens also can make the nose run. Allergies are usually more persistent than the common cold. An allergist can do tests to determine if the cold-like symptoms are being caused by an allergic reaction. Also, some people get a runny nose when they go outside in winter and breathe cold air. This type of runny nose is not a symptom of a cold.

Treatment

There are no medicines that will cure the common cold. Given time, the body's immune system will make antibodies to fight the infection, and the cold will be resolved without any intervention. **Antibiotics** are useless against a cold. However, a great deal of money is spent by pharmaceutical companies in the United States promoting products designed to relieve cold symptoms. These products usually contain **antihistamines**, **decongestants**, and/or pain relievers.

Antihistamines block the action of the chemical histamine that is produced when the cold virus invades the cells lining the nasal passages. Histamine increases blood flow and causes the cells to swell. Antihistamines are taken to relieve the symptoms of sneezing, runny nose, itchy eyes, and congestion. Side effects are **dry mouth** and drowsiness, especially with the first few doses. Antihistamines should not be taken by people who are driving or operating dangerous equipment. Some people have allergic reactions to antihistamines. Common over-the-counter antihistamines include Chlor-Trimeton, Dimetapp, Tavist, and Actifed. The generic name for two common antihistamines are chlorpheniramine and diphenhydramine.

Decongestants work to constrict the blood flow to the vessels in the nose. This can shrink the tissue, reduce congestion, and open inflamed nasal passages, making breathing easier. Decongestants can make people feel jittery or keep them from sleeping. They should not be used by people with heart disease, high blood pressure, or glaucoma. Some common decongestants are Neo-Synepherine, Novafed, and Sudafed. The generic names of common decongestants include phenylephrine, phenylpropanolamine, pseudoephedrine, and in nasal sprays naphazoline, oxymetazoline, and xylometazoline.

Many over-the-counter medications are combinations of both antihistamines and decongestants; an ache and pain reliever, such as **acetaminophen** (Datril, Tylenol, Panadol) or ibuprofen (Advil, Nuprin, Motrin, Medipren); and a cough suppressant (dextromethorphan). Common combination medications include Tylenol Cold and Flu, Triaminic, Sudafed Plus, and Tavist D. **Aspirin** should not be given to children with a cold because of its association with a risk of **Reye's syndrome**, a serious disease.

Nasal sprays and nose drops are other products promoted for reducing nasal congestion. These usually contain a decongestant, but the decongestant can act more quickly and strongly than ones found in pills or liquids because it is applied directly in the nose. Congestion returns after a few hours.

People can become dependent on nasal sprays and nose drops. If used for a long time, users may suffer withdrawal symptoms when these products are discontinued. Nasal sprays and nose drops should not be used for more than a few days. The label lists recommendations on length and frequency of use.

Scientists reported in 2004 the possibility of a new oral drug for use in relieving common cold symptoms. Called pleconaril, it inhibited viral replication in at least 90% of rhinoviruses if taken within 24 hours of onset.

People react differently to different cold medications and may find some more helpful than others. A medication may be effective initially, then lose some of its effectiveness. Children sometimes react differently than adults. Over-the-counter cold remedies should not be given to infants without consulting a doctor first.

Care should be taken not to exceed the recommended dosages, especially when combination medications or nasal sprays are taken. Individuals should determine whether they wish to use any of these drugs. None of them shorten or cure a cold. At best they help a person feel more comfortable. People who are confused about the drugs in any over-the-counter cold remedies should ask their pharmacist for an explanation.

In addition to the optional use of over the counter cold remedies, there are some self-care steps that people can take to ease their discomfort. These include:

- drinking plenty of fluids, but avoiding acidic juices, which may irritate the throat
- gargling with warm salt water — made by adding one teaspoon of salt to 8 oz of water — for a sore throat
- not smoking
- getting plenty of rest
- using a cool-mist room humidifier to ease congestion and sore throat
- rubbing Vaseline or other lubricant under the nose to prevent irritation from frequent nose blowing
- for babies too young to blow their noses, the mucus should be suctioned gently with an infant nasal aspirator. It may be necessary to soften the mucus first with a few drops of salt water.

Alternative treatment

Alternative practitioners emphasize that people get colds because their immune systems are weak. They point out that everyone is exposed to cold viruses, but not everyone gets every cold. The difference seems to be in the ability of the immune system to fight infection. Prevention focuses on strengthening the immune system by eating a healthy diet low in sugars and high in fresh fruits and vegetables, practicing **meditation** to reduce **stress**, and getting regular moderate **exercise**.

Once cold symptoms appear, some naturopathic practitioners believe the symptoms should be allowed to run their course without interference. Others suggest the following:

- Inhaling a steaming mixture of lemon oil, thyme oil, eucalyptus, and tea tree oil (*Melaleuca* spp.). (Aromatherapy)
- Gargling with a mixture of water, salt, and turmeric powder or astringents such as alum, sumac, sage, and bayberry to ease a sore throat. (Ayurvedic medicine)
- Taking coneflower or goldenseal (*Hydrastis canadensis*). Other useful herbs to reduce symptoms include yarrow (*Achillea millefolium*), eyebright (*Euphrasia officinalis*), garlic (*Allium sativum*), and onions (*Allium cepa*). (Herbal)
- Microdoses of *Viscue album*, *Natrum muriaticum*, *Allium cepa*, or *Nux vomica*. (Homeopathy)
- Taking yin chiao (sometimes transliterated as yinquiao) tablets that contain honeysuckle and forsythia when symptoms appear. Natural herb loquat syrup for cough and sinus congestion and Chinese ephedra (*ma-huang*) for runny nose. (Chinese traditional medicine)

KEY TERMS

Bronchial tubes—The major airways to the lungs and their main branches.

Coronavirus—A genus of viruses that cause respiratory disease and gastroenteritis.

Corticosteroids—A group of hormones produced naturally by the adrenal gland or manufactured synthetically. They are often used to treat inflammation. Examples include cortisone and prednisone.

Eustachian tube—A thin tube between the middle ear and the pharynx. Its purpose is to equalize pressure on either side of the eardrum.

Rhinovirus—A virus that infects the upper respiratory system and causes the common cold.

• The use of zinc lozenges every two hours along with high doses of vitamin C is suggested. Some practitioners also suggest eliminating dairy products for the duration of the cold. (Nutritional therapy).

The use of zinc lozenges may be moving toward acceptance by practitioners of traditional medicine. In 1996 the Cleveland Clinic tested zinc gluconate lozenges and found using zinc in the first 24 hours after cold symptoms occurred shortened the duration of symptoms. The mechanism by which zinc worked was not clear, but additional studies are underway.

At one time, the herb (*Echinacea* spp.) was touted as a remedy to relieve cold symptoms. However, a study published in 2004 reported that the herb failed to relieve cold symptoms in 400 children taking it and caused skin **rashes** in some children.

Prognosis

Given time, the body will make antibodies to cure itself of a cold. Most colds last a week to 10 days. Most people start feeling better within four or five days. Occasionally a cold will lead to a secondary bacterial infection that causes strep throat, bronchitis, pneumonia, sinus infection, or a middle ear infection. These conditions usually clear up rapidly when treated with an antibiotic.

Prevention

It is not possible to prevent colds because the viruses that cause colds are common and highly

infectious. However, there are some steps individuals can take to reduce their spread. These include:

• washing hands well and frequently, especially after touching the nose or before handling food

• covering the mouth and nose when sneezing

• disposing of used tissues properly

• avoiding close contact with someone who has a cold during the first two to four days of their infection

• not sharing food, eating utensils, or cups with anyone

• avoiding crowded places where cold germs can spread

• eating a healthy diet and getting adequate sleep

Resources

PERIODICALS

"Study: Echinacea Is Ineffective." *Chain Drug Review* February 16, 2004: 25.

Zepf, Bill. "Pleconaril for Treatment of the Common Cold?" *American Family Physician* February 1, 2004: 703.

Tish Davidson, A.M.
Teresa G. Odle

Common variable immunodeficiency

Definition

Common variable **immunodeficiency** is an immunodeficiency disorder characterized by a low level of antibodies. Patients with this disease are subject to recurring infections.

Description

Immunodeficiency means that the immune system is deficient in one or more of its components and is unable to respond effectively. Common variable immunodeficiency is the most common of the immunodeficiency disorders. Patients with this disease have frequent infections, especially those caused by the same microorganism. Recurring infections are an indication that the immune system is not responding normally and developing immunity to reinfection. Patients with common variable immunodeficiency have a normal number of B cells, the lymphocytes that make antibodies. In approximately one-third of these patients, the number of B cells in the blood that have IgG antibodies on their

KEY TERMS

Antibodies—Molecules (immunoglobulins) produced by the immune system in response to the presence of a specific molecular trigger (antigen). Specific antibodies found in the blood or body tissues indicates that the corresponding antigen is present in the body.

Antigen—Part of an invading microorganism, which causes tissue damage and stimulates the body's immune system to produce antibodies.

Autoimmune disorder—A disorder in which the body's antibodies mistake the body's own tissues for foreign invaders. The immune system then attacks and causes damage to these tissues.

Immune globulin—A type of amino acid protein present in human serum.

Immune system—The system of the body responsible for producing various cells and chemicals that fight off infection by viruses, bacteria, fungi, and other foreign bodies. In autoimmune disease, these cells and chemicals are turned against the body itself.

surface is lower than normal, but there are normal numbers of B cells in their bone marrow. B cells with IgG antibodies on their surface are capable of responding to microorganisms. The lack of IgG on the surface of the B cells means that they are not prepared to fight infection. The T-cell lymphocytes, those cells responsible for cellular immunity, are usually normal, although some cell signal components may be lacking.

Causes and symptoms

The cause of common variable immunodeficiency is not known, although some forms seem to be hereditary. The main symptom is recurring infections that tend to be chronic rather than acute. Patients may develop **diarrhea** and, as a consequence of the diarrhea, do not absorb food efficiently. This can lead to malnourishment that can aggravate the disorder. Common variable immunodeficiency normally appears in children after the age of 10. **Autoimmune disorders** such as **rheumatoid arthritis**, **thyroiditis**, and **systemic lupus erythematosus** and certain cancers such as lymphomas and leukemias may be associated with common variable immunodeficiency.

Diagnosis

As is true of most immunodeficiency disorders, one of the first signs that the patient has the condition is recurrent infections. Patients with common variable immunodeficiency are subject to recurrent infections, especially those caused by microbes that do not normally cause disease.

Tests

The main diagnostic test that distinguishes common variable immunodeficiency from other immunodeficiency diseases is the low antibody level despite the normal number of B cells. Antibody levels are tested in the serum by a procedure called electrophoresis. This procedure both quantifies the amount of antibody present and identifies the various classes of antibodies. The main class of antibody for fighting infectious diseases is IgG.

Treatment

There is no treatment that will cure the disorder. Treatment for common variable immunodeficiency aims at boosting the body's immune response and preventing or controlling infections. Immune serum, obtained from donated blood, is given as a source of antibodies to boost the immune response. Immune serum is obtained from donated blood. It contains whatever antibodies the donors had in their blood. Consequently, it may not contain all the antibodies the patient needs and may lack antibodies specific for some of the recurring infections these patients develop. **Antibiotics** are used routinely at the first sign of an infection to help the patient eliminate infectious microorganisms.

Prognosis

With good medical care, people with common variable immunodeficiency usually have a normal life span.

Prevention

The disease itself cannot be prevented, but patients and their families can take precautions to prevent the recurrent infections commonly associated with it. For example, good hygiene and **nutrition** are important, as is avoiding crowds or other people who have active infections.

Resources

BOOKS

Coico, Richard, and Geoffrey Sunshine. *Immunology: A Short Course*. 6th ed. Hoboken, NJ: Wiley-Blackwell, 2009.

Dietert, Rodney R., and Janice Dietert. *Strategies for Protecting Your Child's Immune System: Tools for Parents and Parents-To-Be*. Hackensack, NJ: World Scientific, 2010.

ORGANIZATIONS

American Academy of Family Physicians, 114 Tomahawk Creek Parkway, Leawood, KS, 66211-2672, (800) 274-2237, (913) 906-6269, fp@aafp.org, www.familydoctor.org.

Centers for Disease Control and Prevention (CDC), 1600 Clifton Rd., Atlanta, GA, 30333, (800) 311-3435, http://www.cdc.gov.

National Institutes of Health (NIH), 9000 Rockville Pike, Bethesda, MD, 20892, (301) 496-4000, http://www.nih.gov.

U.S. National Library of Medicine, 8600 Rockville Pike, Bethesda, MD, 20894, http://www.nlm.nih.gov.

John T. Lohr, Ph.D.
Laura Jean Cataldo, RN, EdD

Complement deficiencies

Definition

Complement deficiencies are a group of disorders in which there is a reduced level of specific proteins, complement, involved in proper immune functioning.

Description

Complement plays several functions in immunity. It can poke holes in bacteria, kill bacteria that are first targeted by antibodies, or, working with antibodies, point out which bacteria need to be engulfed by white blood cells. Without sufficient complement, the body is prone to frequent infections, like **pneumonia** or **meningitis**, or other illnesses, including autoimmune diseases, like **systemic lupus erythematosus**. Since there are more than 20 different types of complement, the disease that results depends on the specific complement that is lacking.

Cause and symptoms

A defect in the complement system can be genetic, but a secondary complement deficiency can also result from ailments that involve a lot of protein loss, including serious **burns**, liver or **kidney disease**, and autoimmune diseases, like lupus. Symptoms vary depending on the specific complement deficiency and the disease that results. Some people remain healthy with no symptoms at all. Others, who suffer from frequent infections, may develop a high **fever**, **diarrhea**, headaches with a stiff neck, or a **cough** with chest **pain**. If an autoimmune disease develops, like lupus, the person may lose weight, suffer from a rash, and have joint pain. Other symptoms of complement deficiency diseases (like hereditary angioedema, paroxysmal nocturnal hemoglobinuria, or leukocyte adhesion deficiency syndrome) include abdominal and back pain, skin infections, **edema** or swelling of the face, and red bumps on the skin.

Diagnosis

There are blood tests which determine the activity of the complement system. The two most common screening tests, CH50 and APH50, tell the physician which group of complement components have a defect. More specific blood tests for the individual complement components (e.g., C3 or C4 complement) are then performed. Other specialized blood tests, including C1 esterase level, Ham test, and a white blood count, may also be performed.

Treatment

There is no way to treat the actual complement deficiency. However, **antibiotics** are used to treat infections and vaccinations are given to reduce the risk of disease. Often, the person is vaccinated against infections that include **influenza**, pneumonia, and meningitis. In some cases, (e.g. a specific disease called paroxysmal nocturnal hemoglobinuria [NH]) a bone marrow transplant may be recommended.

Alternative treatment

There is no alternative treatment for complement problems.

Prognosis

Since complement deficiencies include a wide range of disorders, the prognoses can also vary widely. Some patients remain healthy their entire life. Others are hospitalized frequently because of infections which, if not properly treated, can be

KEY TERMS

Autoimmune diseases—A group of diseases, like rheumatoid arthritis and systemic lupus erythematosus, in which immune cells turn on the body, attacking various tissues and organs.

Hereditary angioedema—A complement deficiency characterized by lymphatic vessel blockages that cause temporary swelling (edema) of areas of the skin, mucous membranes, and, sometimes, internal organs.

Leukocyte adhesion deficiency syndrome—A complement deficiency syndrome characterized by recurrent infections of the skin, mucous membranes, and gastrointestinal tract and the absence of pus formation. This disorder is sometimes apparent at birth when separation of the umbilical cord takes longer than normal.

Meningitis—An inflammation of the lining surrounding the brain and spinal cord.

Paroxysmal nocturnal hemoglobinuria (PNH)—A rare complement disorder characterized by episodes of red blood cell destruction (hemolysis) and blood in the urine (hemoglobinuria) that is worse at night.

Systemic lupus erythematosus—An autoimmune disease in which the immune system attacks the body's connective tissue. A butterfly-shaped facial rash is characteristic.

White blood cells—Cells that are key in immune defense. There are various types, including those that engulf and kill invading bacteria.

fatal. Those with autoimmune diseases could have a normal life expectancy. There are some complement deficiencies, that have a high mortality rate. In those cases, **death** may occur within 10 years after diagnosis.

Prevention

There is currently no way to prevent complement deficiencies.

Resources

OTHER

"The Clinical Presentation of the Primary Immunodeficiency Diseases." *International Patient Organization for Patients with Primary Immunodeficiences.* http://www.ipopi.org.

ORGANIZATIONS

Immune Deficiency Foundation, 40 West Chesapeake Avenue, Suite 308, Towson, MD, 21204, (800) 296-4433, http://www.primaryimmune.org/.

Jeanine Barone, Physiologist

Complete blood count

Definition

One of the most commonly ordered clinical laboratory tests, a complete blood count, also called a blood count (CBC), is a basic evaluation of the cells (red blood cells, white blood cells, and platelets)

suspended in the liquid part of the blood (plasma). It involves determining the numbers, concentrations, and conditions of the different types of blood cells.

Purpose

The purpose of a CBC is to help physicians to diagnose conditions related to abnormalities in the blood such as infections and anemia.

Description

A complete blood count usually includes the following elements:

- Red blood cell count (also called RBC or erythrocyte count)
- Red blood cell indices—mean corpuscular volume (MCV, mean corpuscular hemoglobin (MCH) and mean corpuscular hemoglobin concentration (MCHC)
- Hemoglobin (also called Hgb)
- Hematocrit (also called HCT)
- White blood cell count (also called WBC or leukocyte count)
- Platelet count (also called thrombocyte count)

Red blood cells (erythrocytes) transport oxygen between the lungs and cells throughout the rest of the body. They also transport carbon dioxide back to the lungs so it can be exhaled. A low red cell count may be due to anemia and cells in the body may not be getting the oxygen that they need. A red blood cell count that is abnormally high may be due to an uncommon condition called polycythemia.

White blood cells (leukocytes) protect the body against infection. When an infection develops, white blood cells attack and destroy the pathogen (bacteria, virus, or other organism) causing it. White blood cells are larger than red blood cells but fewer in number. When a person has a bacterial infection, the number of white cells increases very quickly. The number of white blood cells is sometimes used to pinpoint an infection or to see how the body is reacting to **cancer** treatment.

Platelets (thrombocytes) are the smallest type of blood cell. They are essential to the process of blood clotting. When bleeding occurs, platelets swell, clump together, and form a sticky plug that helps to stop the bleeding. If the **platelet count** is too low, uncontrolled bleeding may occur. If the platelet count is too high, there is a chance of a blood clot forming in a blood vessel. Platelets may contribute to the process of hardening of the arteries (**atherosclerosis**).

There are three **red blood cell indices**: mean corpuscular volume (MCV), mean corpuscular hemoglobin (MCH), and mean corpuscular hemoglobin concentration (MCHC). They are measured by a laboratory instrument machine that calculates their values from other measurements in a complete blood count. The mean corpuscular volume reflects the average size of red blood cells. The mean corpuscular hemoglobin value reflects the quantity of hemoglobin in an average red blood cell. The mean corpuscular hemoglobin concentration reflects the concentration of hemoglobin in an average red blood cell. These numbers are used in diagnosing different types of anemia.

The hemoglobin value reflects the amount of hemoglobin in blood and is a good measure of the ability of a person's blood stream to carry oxygen throughout the body. A hemoglobin molecule comprises much of he volume of red blood cells. It carries oxygen and gives red blood cells their normal color.

The **hematocrit** value reflects the amount of space (volume) that red blood cells occupy in the blood. The value is given as a percentage of red blood cells in a volume of blood. For example, a hematocrit of 46 means that 46% of the blood's volume is comprised of red blood cells. Males and females have different normal hematocrit values. The normal red blood cell count ranges from 4.2–5.4 million RBCs per microliter of blood for men and 3.6–5.0 million for women. Hemoglobin values range from 14–18 grams per deciliter of blood for men and 12–16 grams for women. The normal hematocrit is 42–54% for men and 36–48% for women. The normal number of white blood cells for both men and women is approximately 4,000–10,000 WBCs per microliter of blood.

Normal results

Normal values for the elements of a complete blood count include the following:

- Red blood cell (erythrocyte) count: 4.2–5.9 million
- White blood cell (leukocyte) count: 4,300–10,800
- Platelet (thrombocyte) count: 150,000–400,000
- Mean corpuscular volume (MCV): 86–98
- Mean corpuscular hemoglobin (MCH): 27–32
- Mean corpuscular hemoglobin concentration (MCHC): 32–36%
- Hemoglobin (Hgb): 13–18 for men and 12–16 for women
- Hematocrit (HCT): 45–52% for men and 37–48% for women

Abnormal results

Abnormal blood count results are seen in a variety of conditions. One of the most common is **anemias**, which are characterized by low RBC counts, hemoglobins, and hematocrits. Infections and leukemias are associated with increased numbers of WBCs.

A complete blood count can be ordered at any time.

Precautions

Precautions are generally not needed for a complete blood count.

At the time of drawing blood, the only precaution needed is to clean the venipuncture site with alcohol.

Side effects

The most common side effects of a complete blood count are minor bleeding (hematoma) or bruising at the site of venipuncture.

Interactions

There are no interactions for a complete blood count.

Resources

BOOKS

Fischbach, F. T., and M. B. Dunning. *A Manual of Laboratory and Diagnostic Tests.* 8th ed. Philadelphia: Lippincott Williams & Wilkins, 2008.

McGhee, M. *A Guide to Laboratory Investigations.* 5th ed. Oxford, UK: Radcliffe, 2008.

Price, C. P. *Evidence-Based Laboratory Medicine: Principles, Practice, and Outcomes.* 2nd ed. Washington, DC: AACC Press, 2007.

Scott, M.G., A. M. Gronowski, and C. S. Eby. *Tietz's Applied Laboratory Medicine.* 2nd ed. New York: Wiley-Liss, 2007.

Springhouse, A. M. *Diagnostic Tests Made Incredibly Easy!* 2nd ed. Philadelphia: Lippincott Williams & Wilkins, 2008.

PERIODICALS

Amati, L., M. Chiloiro, E. Jirillo, and V. Covelli. "Early pathogenesis of atherosclerosis: the childhood obesity." *Current Pharmaceutical Design* 13, no. 36 (2007): 3696–3700.

James, T. R., H. L. Reid, and A. M. Mullings. "Are published standards for haematological indices in pregnancy applicable across populations: an evaluation in healthy pregnant Jamaican women." *BMC Pregnancy and Childbirth* 8, no. 1 (2008): 8–19.

Liao, S. C., M. F. Yang, and I. N. Lee. "Transforming laboratory data to improve medical care for patients with chronic kidney disease." *Journal of Nephrology* 21, no. 1 (2008): 74–80.

Lippi, G., A. Bassi, G. P. Solero, G. L. Salvagno, and G. C. Guidi. "Prevalence and type of preanalytical errors on inpatient samples referred for complete blood count." *Clinical Laboratory* 53, no. 9-12 (2007): 555–556.

OTHER

American Clinical Laboratory Association. "Information about clinical chemistry." 2008 [cited February 24, 2008]. http://www.clinical-labs.org/.

Clinical Laboratory Management Association. "Information about clinical chemistry." 2008 [cited February 22, 2008]. http://www.clma.org/.

Lab Tests On Line. "Information about lab tests." 2008 [cited February 24, 2008]. http://www.labtestsonline.org/.

National Accreditation Agency for Clinical Laboratory Sciences. "Information about laboratory tests." 2008 [cited February 25, 2008]. http://www.naacls.org/.

ORGANIZATIONS

American Association for Clinical Chemistry, 1850 K Street NW, Suite 625, Washington, DC, 20006, (800) 892-1400, (202) 887-5093, http://www.aacc.org/AACC.

American Society for Clinical Laboratory Science, 6701 Democracy Boulevard, Suite 300, Bethesda, MD, 20817, (301) 657-2768, (301) 657-2909, http://www.ascls.org.

American Society of Clinical Pathologists, 33 West Monroe Street, Suite 1600, Chicago, IL, 60603, (312) 541-4999, (312) 541-4998, http://www.ascp.org.

College of American Pathologists, 325 Waukegan Road, Northfield, IL, 60093-2750, (847) 832-7000, (800) 323-4040, (800) 823-8000, www.cap.org/apps/cap.portal.

L. Fleming Fallon, Jr, MD, DrPH
Brenda W. Lerner

Computed tomography scans

Definition

Computed tomography (CT) scans are completed with the use of a 360-degree x-ray beam and computer production of images. These scans allow for cross-sectional views of body organs and tissues.

Purpose

CT scans are used to image a wide variety of body structures and internal organs. Since the 1990s, CT equipment has become more affordable and available. In some diagnoses, CT scans have become the first imaging exam of choice. Because the computerized image is so sharp, focused, and three-dimensional, many tissues can be better differentiated than on standard x rays. Common CT indications include:

- Sinus studies. The CT scan can show details of a sinusitis, and bone fractures. Physicians may order CT of the sinuses to provide an accurate map for surgery.

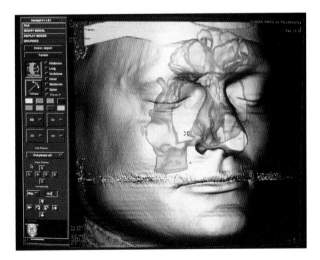

CT scan of facial sinuses. *(Pascal Goetgheluck/Photo Researchers, Inc.)*

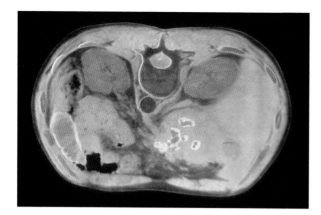

Colorized CT scan of human abdomen—aorta is dead center in red. *(SPL/Photo Researchers, Inc.)*

- Brain studies. Brain scans can detect hematomas, tumors, and strokes. The introduction of CT scanning, especially spiral CT, has helped reduce the need for more invasive procedures such as cerebral angiography.
- Body scans. CT scans of the body will often be used to observe abdominal organs, such as the liver, kidneys, adrenal glands, spleen, and lymph nodes, and extremities.
- Aorta scans. CT scans can focus on the thoracic or abdominal aorta to locate aneurysms and other possible aortic diseases.
- Chest scans. CT scans of the chest are useful in distinguishing tumors and in detailing accumulation of fluid in chest infections.

Precautions

Pregnant women or those who could possibly be pregnant should not have a CT scan unless the diagnostic benefits outweigh the risks. Pregnant patients should particularly avoid full body or abdominal scans. If the exam is necessary for obstetrics purposes, technologists are instructed not to repeat films if there are errors. Pregnant patients receiving CT or any x-ray exam away from the abdominal area may be protected by a lead apron; most radiation, known as scatter, travels through the body and is not blocked by the apron.

Contrast agents are often used in CT exams and the use of these agents should be discussed with the medical professional prior to the procedure. Patients should be asked to sign a consent form concerning the administration of contrast. One of the common contrast agents, iodine, can cause allergic reactions. Patients who are known to be allergic to iodine (or shellfish) should inform the physician prior to the CT scan.

Description

Computed tomography, also called CT scan, CAT scan, or computerized axial tomography, is a combination of focused x-ray beams and computerized production of an image. Introduced in the early 1970s, this radiologic procedure has advanced rapidly and is now widely used, sometimes in the place of standard x rays.

CT equipment

A CT scan may be performed in a hospital or outpatient imaging center. Although the equipment looks large and intimidating, it is very sophisticated and fairly comfortable. The patient is asked to lie on a gantry, or narrow table, that slides into the center of the scanner. The scanner looks like a doughnut and is round in the middle, which allows the x-ray beam to rotate around the patient. The scanner section may also be tilted slightly to allow for certain cross-sectional angles.

CT procedure

The patient will feel the gantry move very slightly as the precise adjustments for each sectional image are made. A technologist watches the procedure from a window and views the images on a computer screen.

It is essential that the patient lie very still during the procedure to prevent motion blurring. In some studies, such as chest CTs, the patient will be asked to hold his or her breath during image capture.

Following the procedure, films of the images are usually printed for the radiologist and referring physician to review. A radiologist can also interpret CT exams on a special computer screen. The procedure time will vary in length depending on the area being imaged. Average study times are from 30 to 60 minutes. Some patients may be concerned about claustrophobia, but the width of the "doughnut" portion of the scanner is such that many patients can be reassured of openness.

The CT image

While traditional x rays image organs in two dimensions, with the possibility that organs in the front of the body are superimposed over those in the back, CT scans allow for a more three-dimensional effect. Some have compared CT images to slices in a loaf of bread. Precise sections of the body can be located and imaged as cross-sectional views. The screen before the technologist shows a computer's analysis of each section detected by the x-ray beam. Thus, various densities of tissue can be easily distinguished.

Contrast agents

Contrast agents are often used in CT exams and in other radiology procedures to illuminate certain details of anatomy which may not be easily seen. Some contrasts are natural, such as air or water. Other times, a water-based contrast agent is administered for specific diagnostic purposes. Barium sulfate is commonly used in gastroenterology procedures. The patient may drink this contrast, or receive it in an enema. Oral and rectal contrast are usually given when examining the abdomen or cells, and not given when scanning the brain or chest. Iodine is the most widely used intravenous contrast agent and is given through an intravenous needle.

If contrast agents are used in the CT exam, these will be administered several minutes before the study begins. Abdominal CT patients may be asked to drink a contrast medium. Some patients may experience a salty taste, flushing of the face, warmth or slight **nausea**, or **hives** from an intravenous contrast injection. Technologists and radiologists have equipment and training to help patients through these minor reactions and to handle more severe reactions. Severe reactions to contrast are rare, but do occur.

Spiral CT

Spiral CT, also called helical CT, is a newer version of CT scanning which is continuous in motion and allows for three-dimensional recreation of images. For example, traditional CT allows the technologist to take slices at very small and precise intervals one after the other. Spiral CT allows for a continuous flow of images, without stopping the scanner to move to the next image slice. A major advantage of spiral CT is the ability to reconstruct images anywhere along the length of the study area. The procedure also speeds up the imaging process, meaning less time for the patient to lie still. The ability to image contrast more rapidly after it is injected, when it is at its highest level, is another advantage of spiral CT's high speed.

Some facilities will have both spiral and conventional CT available. Although spiral is more advantageous for many applications, conventional CT is still a superior and precise method for imaging many tissues and structures. The physician will evaluate which type of CT works best for the specific exam purpose.

Preparation

If a contrast medium is administered, the patient may be asked to fast from about four to six hours prior to the procedure. Patients will usually be given a gown (like a typical hospital gown) to be worn during the procedure. All metal and jewelry should be removed to avoid artifacts on the film.

Aftercare

No aftercare is generally required following a CT scan. Immediately following the exam, the technologist will continue to watch the patient for possible adverse contrast reactions. Patients are instructed to advise the technologist of any symptoms, particularly respiratory difficulty. The site of contrast injection will be bandaged and may feel tender following the exam. Hives may develop later and usually do not require treatment.

Risks

Radiation exposure from a CT scan is similar to, though higher than, that of a conventional x ray. Although this is a risk to pregnant women, the exposure to other adults is minimal and should produce no effects. Although severe contrast reactions are rare, they are a risk of many CT procedures.

Normal results

Normal findings on a CT exam show bone, the most dense tissue, as white areas. Tissues and fat will show as various shades of gray, and fluids will be gray or black. Air will also look black. Intravenous, oral, and rectal contrast appear as white areas. The radiologist can determine if tissues and organs appear normal by the sensitivity of the gray shadows. In CT, the images that can cut through a section of tissue or organ provide three-dimensional viewing for the radiologist and referring physician.

Abnormal results

Abnormal results may show different characteristics of tissues within organs. Accumulations of blood or other fluids where they do not belong may be detected. Radiologists can differentiate among types of tumors throughout the body by viewing details of their makeup.

Sinus studies

The increasing availability and lowered cost of CT scanning has led to its increased use in sinus studies, either as a replacement for a sinus x ray or as a follow-up to an abnormal sinus radiograph. The sensitivity of CT allows for location of areas of sinus infection, particularly chronic infection. CT scans can show the extent and location of tiny **fractures** to the sinus and nasal bones. Foreign bodies in the sinus and nasal area are also easily detected by CT. CT imaging of the sinuses is important in evaluating trauma or disease

KEY TERMS

Aneurysm—The bulging of the blood vessel wall. Aortic aneurysms are the most dangerous. Aneurysms can break and cause bleeding.

Contrast (agent, medium)—A substance injected into the body that illuminates certain structures that would otherwise be hard to see on the radiograph (film).

Gantry—A name for the couch or table used in a CT scan. The patient lies on the gantry while it slides into the x-ray scanner portion.

Hematoma—A collection of blood that has escaped from the vessels. It may clot and harden, causing pain to the patient.

Hydrocephalus—A collection of fluid on or around the brain. The pressure from the spinal fluid causes the ventricles to widen.

Metastasis—Secondary cancer, or cancer that has spread from one body organ or tissue to another.

Radiologist—A medical doctor specially trained in radiology (x ray) interpretation and its use in the diagnosis of disease and injury.

Spiral CT—Also referred to as helical CT, this method allows for continuous 360-degree x-ray image capture.

Thoracic—Refers to the chest area. The thorax runs between the abdomen and neck and is encased in the ribs.

of the sphenoid bone (the wedge shaped bone at the base of the skull). Sinus tumors will show as shades of gray indicating the difference in their density from that of normal tissues in the area.

Brain studies

The precise differences in density allowed by CT scan can clearly show tumors, strokes, or lesions in the brain area as altered densities. These lighter or darker areas on the image may indicate a tumor or hematoma within the brain and skull area. Different types of tumors can be identified by the presence of **edema**, by the tissue's density, or by studying blood vessel location and activity. The speed and convenience of CT often allows for detection of hemorrhage before symptoms even occur. Congenital abnormalities in children, such as **hydrocephalus**, may also be confirmed with CT. Hydrocephalus is suggested by enlargement of the fluid structures called ventricles of the brain.

Body scans

The body scan can identify abnormal body structures and organs. Throughout the body, a CT may indicate tumors or cysts, enlarged lymph nodes, abnormal collections of fluids, blood or fat, and metastasis of **cancer**. Tumors resulting from metastasis are different in makeup than primary tumors, or those that originate in the location of study. Fractures or damage to soft tissues and ligaments will be more easily seen on the sensitive images produced by CT scanning, though CT is not usually done for these. Liver conditions, such as **cirrhosis** or abscessed or **fatty liver**, may be observed on the body scan.

CT of the aorta

CT provides the ability to see and measure the thickness of the aortal wall, which is very helpful in diagnosing aortic aneurysms. The use of contrast will help see details within the aorta. In addition, density can identify calcification, and this helps differentiate between acute and chronic problems. An abnormal CT scan may indicate signs of aortic clots. Aortic rupture is suggested by signs such as a hematoma around the aorta or the escape of blood from its cavity.

Chest scans

In addition to those findings that may indicate aortic aneurysms, chest CT studies can show other problems in the heart and lungs, and distinguish between an **aortic aneurysm** and a tumor adjacent to the aorta. The computer will not only show differences between air, water, tissues, and bone, but will also assign numerical values to the various densities. Coin-sized lesions in the lungs may be indicative of **tuberculosis** or tumors. CT will help distinguish among the two. Enlarged lymph nodes in the chest area may indicate Hodgkin's disease. Spiral CT is particularly effective at identifying pulmonary emboli (clots in the lung's blood vessels).

Resources

PERIODICALS

Papatheofanis, Frank J. "Helical CT and Pulmonary Disease." *Decisions in Imaging Economics* (January-February 1997): 61–63.

ORGANIZATIONS
American College of Radiology, 1891 Preston White Drive, Reston, VA, 22091, (800) 227-5463, http://www.acr.org.

Teresa Odle
Brenda W. Lerner

Computerized axial tomography *see*
Computed tomography scans

Concussion

Definition

Concussion is a trauma-induced change in mental status, with confusion and **amnesia**, and with or without a brief loss of consciousness. Concussion is also called traumatic brain injury.

Demographics

The incidence of concussion is estimated to be 2 per 1,000 individuals per year in the United States.

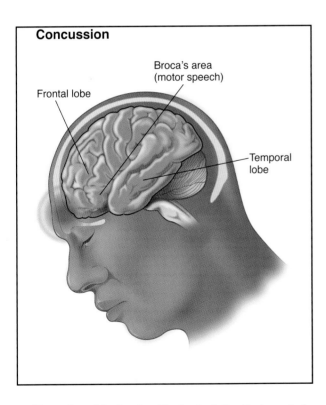

Concussion

Broca's area (motor speech)

Frontal lobe

Temporal lobe

An illustration of the head and brain, depicting the impact of a concussion on the parts of the brain. *(Illustration by Electronic Illustrators Group. Reproduced by permission of Gale, a part of Cengage Learning.)*

Most of these concussions are mild, but about 10% cause disability or **death**. Statistics collected by the Centers for Disease Control and Prevention (CDC) between 2002 and 2006 showed that on average 1.7 million people suffered a concussion annually. Of them, about 275,000 were hospitalized, and 52,000 died.

Description

A concussion occurs when the head hits or is hit by an object, or when the brain is jarred against the skull, with sufficient force to cause temporary loss of function in the higher centers of the brain. The injured person may remain conscious or lose consciousness briefly, and is disoriented for some minutes after the blow.

While concussion usually resolves on its own without lasting effect, it can set the stage for a much more serious condition. "Second impact syndrome" occurs when a person with a concussion, even a very mild one, suffers a second blow before fully recovering from the first. The brain swelling and increased intracranial pressure that can result is potentially fatal. More than 20 such cases have been reported since the syndrome was first described in 1984.

Causes and symptoms

Causes

Playing contact sports is a risk factors for experiencing one or more concussions. According to the CDC, approximately 300,000 people sustain mild to moderate sports-related brain injuries each year. However, sports-related concussions are widely thought to be under reported because athletes do not want to be medically disqualified from continuing to play their sport. Most sports-related brain injuries occur in young men between the ages of 16 and 25 years.

The risk of concussion from football is extremely high, especially at the high school level. Studies show that approximately one in five players suffer concussion or more serious brain injury during their brief high-school careers. The rate at the collegiate level is approximately one in 20. Rates for hockey players are not known as certainly, but are believed to be similar.

Concussion and lasting brain damage is an especially significant risk for boxers, since the goal of the sport is, in fact, to deliver a concussion to the opponent. For this reason, the American Academy of Neurology has called for a ban on boxing. Repeated concussions over months or years can cause cumulative **head injury**. The cumulative brain injuries suffered by most boxers can lead to permanent brain damage. Multiple blows to the head can cause "punch-drunk" syndrome or **dementia** pugilistica, as evidenced by Muhammaed Ali, whose parkinsonism is a result of his career in the ring.

Falls account for the greatest number of concussions in children ages 0–4 years and in people over age 65. Individuals over age 75 have the greatest rate of hospitalization and death from concussions.

Motor vehicle accident are most likely to cause concussions that result in death. The death rate from motor vehicle concussions is highest in males ages 20–24 years. In motor vehicle accidents, concussion can occur without an actual blow to the head. Instead, concussion occurs because the skull suddenly decelerates or stops, which causes the brain to be jarred against the skull.

Child abuse is, unfortunately, another common cause of concussion.

Symptoms

Symptoms of concussion include:

- headache
- disorientation as to time, date, or place
- confusion
- dizziness
- vacant stare or confused expression
- incoherent or incomprehensible speech
- incoordination or weakness
- amnesia for the events immediately preceding the blow
- nausea or vomiting
- double vision
- ringing in the ears

These symptoms may last from several minutes to several hours. More severe or longer-lasting symptoms may indicate more severe brain injury. The person with a concussion may or may not lose consciousness from the blow. More prolonged unconsciousness indicates more severe brain injury.

The severity of concussion is graded on a three-point scale, used as a basis for treatment decisions.

- Grade 1: no loss of consciousness, transient confusion, and other symptoms that resolve within 15 minutes.
- Grade 2: no loss of consciousness, transient confusion, and other symptoms that require more than 15 minutes to resolve.
- Grade 3: loss of consciousness for any period.

KEY TERMS

Amnesia—A loss of memory that may be caused by brain injury, such as concussion.

Parkinsonism—A neurological disorder that includes a fine tremor, muscular weakness and rigidity, and an altered way of walking.

Days or weeks after the accident, the person may show symptoms of a condition called "post-concussion syndrome." Signs of **post-concussion syndrome** include:

- headache
- poor attention and concentration
- memory difficulties
- anxiety
- depression
- sleep disturbances
- light and noise intolerance

Diagnosis

Examination

It is very important for those attending a person with concussion to pay close attention to the person's symptoms and progression immediately after the accident. The duration of unconsciousness and degree of confusion are important indicators of the severity of the injury and help guide the diagnostic process and treatment decisions.

A doctor, nurse, or emergency medical technician may make an immediate assessment based on the severity of the symptoms; a neurologic exam of the pupils, coordination, and sensation; and brief tests of orientation, memory, and concentration. Those with very mild concussions may not need to be hospitalized or have expensive diagnostic tests.

Tests

Questionable or more severe cases may require computed tomography scan (CT) or **magnetic resonance imaging** (MRI) scans to look for brain injury. More extensive neuropsychologic testing may be done, especially on athletes who are at risk for repeat concussions.

Treatment

The symptoms of concussion usually clear quickly and without lasting effect, if no further injury is sustained during the healing process. Guidelines for

---

returning to sports activities are based on the severity of the concussion.

Traditional

A grade 1 concussion can usually be treated with rest and continued observation alone. The person may return to sports activities that same day, but only after examination by a trained professional, and after all symptoms have completely resolved. If the person sustains a second concussion of any severity that same day, he or she should not be allowed to continue contact sports until he or she has been symptom-free, during both rest and activity, for one week.

A person with a grade 2 concussion must discontinue sports activity for the day, should be evaluated by a trained professional, and should be observed closely throughout the day to make sure that all symptoms have completely cleared. Worsening of symptoms, or continuation of any symptoms beyond one week, indicates the need for a CT or MRI scan. Return to contact sports should only occur after one week with no symptoms, both at rest and during activity, and following examination by a physician. Following a second grade 2 concussion, the person should remain symptom-free for two weeks before resuming contact sports.

A person with a grade 3 concussion (involving any loss of consciousness, no matter how brief) should be examined by a medical professional either on the scene or in an emergency room. More severe symptoms may warrant a CT or MRI scan, along with a thorough neurological and physical exam. The person should be hospitalized if any abnormalities are found or if confusion persists. Prolonged unconsciousness and worsening symptoms require urgent neurosurgical evaluation or transfer to a trauma center. Following discharge from professional care, the patient is closely monitored for neurological symptoms, which may arise or worsen. If headaches or other symptoms worsen or last longer than one week, a CT or MRI scan should be performed. Contact sports are avoided for one week following unconsciousness of only seconds, and for two weeks for unconsciousness of a minute or more.

For someone who has sustained a concussion of any severity, it is critically important that he or she avoid the possibility of another blow to the head until well after all symptoms have cleared to prevent second-impact syndrome. The previous guidelines were designed to minimize the risk of this syndrome. A person receiving a second grade 3 concussion should avoid contact sports for at least a month after all symptoms have cleared, and then only with the approval of a physician. If signs of brain swelling or bleeding are seen on a CT or MRI scan,

the athlete should not return to the sport for the rest of the season, or even indefinitely.

Prognosis

About 90% of concussions leave no lasting neurological problems. Nonetheless, symptoms of post-concussion syndrome may last for weeks or even months.

Studies of concussion in contact sports have shown that the risk of sustaining a second concussion is even greater than it was for the first if the person continues to engage in the sport.

Prevention

Many cases of concussion can be prevented by using appropriate protective equipment. This includes seat belts and air bags in automobiles, and helmets in all contact sports. Helmets should also be worn when bicycling, skiing, skateboarding, or horseback riding. Soccer players should avoid heading the ball when it is kicked at high velocity from close range. Playground equipment should be underlaid with soft material, either sand or special matting.

The value of high-contact sports such as boxing, football, or hockey should be weighed against the high risk of brain injury during a young person's participation in the sport. Steering a child's general enthusiasm for sports into activities less apt to produce head impacts may reduce the likelihood of brain injury.

Resources

OTHER

Benhardt, David T. Concussion. eMedicine.com August 6, 2009. http://emedicine.medscape.com/article/92095-overview

Concussion. MedlinePlus June 21, 2010. http://www.nlm.nih.gov/medlineplus/concussion.html

American Association of Neurological Surgeons. Concussion. NeurologyToday.org November 2005. http://www.neurosurgerytoday.org/what/patient_e/concussion.asp

ORGANIZATIONS

American Academy of Neurology, 1080 Montreal Avenue, St. Paul, MN, 55116, (651) 695-2717, (800) 879-1960, Fax: (651) 695-2791, http://www.aan.com.

Brain Injury Association of America, 1608 Spring Hill Road, Vienna, VA, 22182, (703) 761-0750, (800) 444-6443, (703) 761-0755, braininjuryinfo@biausa.org, http://www.biausa.org.

Richard Robinson
Tish Davidson, AM

Condoms

Definition

Condoms are a barrier method of **contraception** intended to block the entry of semen from the male into the cervix of the female uterus, thus preventing fertilization of the female ovum. Most condoms are male-controlled contraceptive devices that consist of a thin flexible sheath placed over the erect male penis prior to intercourse. There are also female condoms, first introduced in 1984, that consist of a pouch with flexible rings at each end.

The derivation of the term *condom* is unknown. There was an urban legend for many years that the name was derived from either a court physician named Dr. Condom or the Earl of Condom, supposedly a noble at the court of King Charles II of England (1630–1685). Charles was known as the "Merry Monarch" and his court was famous for its irresponsible pleasure-seeking; however, there are no records of anyone named Condom in the court circle, and condoms were in use in England for over a century before Charles became king in 1660. Most historians of medicine now state that the origin of the word *condom* cannot be traced.

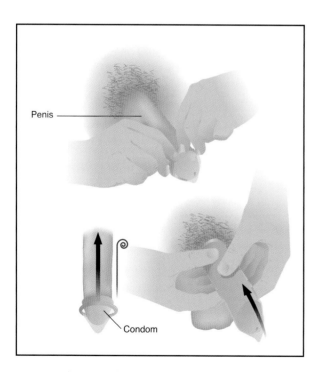

A condom is most effective when it is placed on the penis correctly without trapping air between the penis and the condom. *(Illustration by Argosy, Inc. Reproduced by permission of Gale, a part of Cengage Learning.)*

Penis ——————

Condom

Purpose

Both male and female condoms are used to prevent **pregnancy** and to protect against such **sexually transmitted diseases** (STDs) as human **immunodeficiency** virus (HIV), **gonorrhea**, chlamydia, and **syphilis**. To accomplish these goals, however, a condom must be applied and removed correctly. The Centers for Disease Control and Prevention (CDC) states, "To achieve the maximum protective effect, condoms must be used both consistently and correctly. Inconsistent use can lead to STD acquisition because transmission can occur with a single act of intercourse with an infected partner. Similarly, if condoms are not used correctly, the protective effect may be diminished even when they are used consistently."

In addition to standard condoms used for contraception and disease **prophylaxis**, there are also specialized condoms used to collect male semen for artificial insemination or sperm analysis as part of an **infertility** workup. Collection condoms are usually made of silicone or polyurethane rather than latex, as latex is harmful to sperm and may yield inaccurate results when the number and viability of the sperm are measured.

Demographics

Condoms have been the most widely used method of contraception and disease prevention worldwide since they were first mass manufactured in the late nineteenth century. After birth control pills were introduced in 1960, condoms became the second most common method of birth control in the developed countries. In Japan, however, 80% of married couples still prefer condoms to other methods of birth control, compared to 28% of couples in the United States and Canada. In Africa, only 8% of couples use condoms as a method of contraception.

Although exact statistics of the number of condoms manufactured each year worldwide are difficult to obtain, it is safe to assume that billions are produced, as the number purchased by the government of India alone for distribution in family planning clinics is 2 billion per year.

Description

Both male and female condoms collect the male semen at ejaculation, acting as a barrier to fertilization. Condoms serve as barriers to the exchange of bodily fluids and are subsequently an important tool in the prevention of sexually transmitted diseases (STDs).

Male condoms

Male condoms are thin sheaths of latex (rubber), polyurethane (plastic), or animal tissue that are rolled onto an erect penis immediately prior to intercourse. They are commonly called "safes," "rubbers," or "prophylactics," from their use in preventing disease. In England they are sometimes called "French letters."

Because many men and women are allergic to latex, the Food and Drug Administration (FDA) approved the use of Vytex for condoms sold in the United States in May 2009. Vytex is a form of latex that has been treated to remove 90% of the proteins that cause allergic reactions. A completely allergen-free condom made of polyisoprene, a synthetic latex, is also available. Polyisoprene is more expensive than standard latex but has the advantages of being as flexible and soft as latex without triggering allergic reactions.

Most condoms made of animal tissue as of 2010 are made from sheep intestines and are labeled as lambskin. They provide more sensation than latex and are also less likely to trigger allergic reactions. They are also significantly more expensive than latex condoms and offer less protection against STDs. The reason for this difference is that sheep intestine is a porous material whose pores are large enough to permit the HIV virus and other infectious organisms to pass through even though the pores are small enough to block sperm.

Male condoms may be purchased lubricated, ribbed, or studded on the outside. Studded condoms should not be used for anal intercourse, however, because they can irritate the tissues lining the rectum and increase the risk of HIV transmission. To be effective, condoms must be removed carefully so as not to "spill" the contents into the vaginal canal. Condoms that leak or break do not provide complete protection against pregnancy or disease, although they are more effective than completely unprotected intercourse.

Female condoms

Female condoms are made of polyurethane and are inserted into the vaginal canal before sexual relations. The open end covers the outside of the vagina, and the closed ring fits over the cervix (opening into the uterus). Newer female condoms are made of nitrile, a synthetic rubber that is also used to make disposable surgical gloves. Nitrile is as flexible as latex but is more resistant to puncture.

Origins

Male condoms made from animal tissue and linen have been in use for centuries. In Japan and China, upper-class men used condoms made from tortoise shell or animal horn. The first documented use of condoms in Europe dates from 1564, in a treatise on preventing syphilis. Syphilis, which first entered Europe in the 1490s, was an extremely virulent disease at that time and could cause **death** within a few months. The 1564 treatise described the use of linen sheaths soaked in some kind of chemical solution and dried before wearing. Condoms made from pig bladders or intestines were also used during the Renaissance. These devices were initially used in Europe to prevent STDs; the first reference to their use as contraceptives was published in 1605.

Latex condoms were introduced in the late 1800s and gained immediate popularity because they were inexpensive and effective. The German army was the first to recommend condoms to soldiers, beginning in the late nineteenth century. Although condoms were the first effective method of contraception that the poor could afford, a common complaint made then as now by many consumers is that condoms reduce penis sensitivity and impair satisfaction. In addition, both men and women may develop **allergies** to latex. Consumer interest in female condoms was relatively slight when it was first introduced; however, the fact that the female condom can be used by women whose partners refuse to use a male condom has increased its popularity in a number of countries.

Benefits

An important fact to keep in mind when reading statistics about condom effectiveness is the distinction between "perfect" or "method effectiveness" use rates and "actual" or "typical" use rates. Perfect or method effectiveness rates include only consumers who use condoms properly and consistently. Typical or actual use rates include all persons who use condoms, including those who use them incorrectly or do not use them during every act of intercourse. Thus while perfect use of condoms results in a pregnancy rate of 2% per year, typical users have a pregnancy rate of 10% to 18% per year.

With regard to disease transmission, in 2000 the National Institutes of Health (NIH) reported that correct and consistent use of latex condoms reduces the risk of HIV/AIDS transmission by approximately 85% relative to a person's risk when unprotected. In 2007 the World Health Organization (WHO) reported a similar risk reduction rate of 80% to 95%. The CDC states that "Latex condoms, when used consistently and correctly, are highly effective in preventing the sexual transmission of HIV, the virus that causes **AIDS**. In addition, consistent and correct use of latex

KEY TERMS

Carcinogen—Any substance or form of radiation that increases the risk of cancer or stimulates the growth of an existing cancer.

Contraception—The use of a device, sexual practice, or chemical intended to prevent conception; birth control.

Ejaculate—To expel semen.

Nonoxynol-9—The chemical name of the organic compound most commonly used in contraceptive creams, foams, and jellies. It was also used in the manufacture of spermicide-treated condoms until 2005, but the use of such condoms is now discouraged.

Perfect use—A measurement of the effectiveness of a contraceptive based only on those who use the method correctly and use it every time they have intercourse. It is also called the method effectiveness rate.

Prophylactic—A drug, medical device, or technique intended to prevent (rather than treat) disease. Condoms are sometimes called prophylactics.

Semen—The thick whitish liquid released from the penis during sexual intercourse. It contains sperm and other secretions.

Sperm or spermatozoa—The part of the semen that is generative—can cause fertilization of the female ovum.

Spermicide—An agent that is destructive to sperm.

Typical use—A measurement of the effectiveness of a contraceptive that counts all users, including those who use the method incorrectly or only occasionally.

Vagina—The genital canal in the female, leading from the vulva to the uterus.

condoms reduces the risk of other sexually transmitted diseases (STDs), including diseases transmitted by genital secretions, and to a lesser degree, genital ulcer diseases."

With regard to contraception, male condoms have an effectiveness rate of about 90% for preventing pregnancy when used correctly and consistently, but this rate can be increased to about 98% if used with a spermicide that is applied separately. (Several types of spermicides are available; they can be purchased in the form of contraceptive creams and jellies, foams, or films.) Benefits associated with this type of contraceptive device include easy availability (no prescription is required), convenience of use, and absence of serious side effects. The primary disadvantage is that sexual activity must be interrupted in order to put on the male condom.

Female condoms, when used correctly and at every instance of intercourse, were shown to prevent pregnancy in over 95% of women surveyed over the course of six months. When used inconsistently, the female condom was shown to have a failure rate of 21% in the same study. One benefit of the female condom is that it may be inserted immediately before sexual intercourse or up to eight hours prior, so that sexual activity does not need to be interrupted for its insertion. One study performed by a manufacturer of the female condom indicated that 50–75% of couples in numerous countries found the barrier acceptable for use.

Precautions

Before purchasing a condom, the user should check the expiration date. Prior to use, examine the condom for holes. If a lubricant is going to be used with a latex condom, it should be water-soluble because petroleum jellies, such as Vaseline, and other oil-based lubricants can weaken latex. It is also important to note that condoms made from animal tissue or plastic are not recommended as a protection against STDs.

Spermicide-treated condoms are no longer recommended because the spermicide used in them, a chemical called nonoxynol-9, was reported in 2003 to actually increase the risk of transmitting HIV because it causes tiny tears or breaks in the tissues lining the vagina or rectum. In addition, spermicide-treated condoms increase the risk of urinary tract infections in the female partner. After 2005, several major manufacturers of condoms stopped producing condoms treated with spermicide.

Preparation

A person intending to use a condom should avoid heavy drinking or drug use prior to having sex, because intoxication or a drug "high" can impair judgment and increase the risk of using the condom incorrectly.

A male condom should be removed carefully from its foil wrapper and placed on the tip of the erect penis. Leaving some space at the tip of the condom to collect the semen, the user then unrolls the condom downward toward the base of the penis.

To use a female condom, the woman inserts a flexible ring at the closed end of the sheath deep into the vagina; this ring holds the device in place. The flexible ring at the open end of the sheath remains outside the opening to the vagina and serves to guide the man's penis into the vagina.

Aftercare

To remove a male condom after use, the user should withdraw carefully, holding the condom around the base of the penis. To remove a female condom, the user should twist the outer ring shut and gently withdraw the condom from the vagina. Because most condoms are not biodegradable, they should not be flushed down toilets. Instead, they should be wrapped in toilet paper or a paper towel and discarded in a waste container.

Risks

In addition to the risks of pregnancy or disease transmission from incorrect or inconsistent use, condoms have been associated with risks from substances used in their manufacture. Nitrosamines, which are chemicals identified as carcinogenic in humans, are used by some manufacturers of latex condoms to increase the flexibility of the latex. One group of German researchers reported in 2005 that nitrosamines can migrate from rubber products into human sweat or tissue fluid.

Another risk of condom use is partner violence in some cultures and ethnic groups. Women in Africa and in some Latino subcultures in developed countries have reported threats of violence from their partners if they ask the men to use condoms as a form of contraception. In addition, there is a high correlation of alcohol **abuse**, condom non-use, and sexual assaults on women.

Research and general acceptance

Condoms are widely accepted as an effective method of contraception and disease prophylaxis. Research is ongoing, however, into improving the effective use of condoms among drug users and other high-risk populations, and into newer types of condoms. These newer types include:

- Rape-aXe. Rape-aXe is a female condom that has been produced since 2006. It consists of a latex sheath containing sharp barbs. The woman inserts the device like a tampon. If a male attacker attempts vaginal penetration, the device attaches itself to his penis and requires surgical removal, thus identifying the rapist.
- Spray-on condoms. As of 2010, several companies are working on developing a latex formula that could be sprayed on the penis and allowed to dry. The major difficulty is developing a compound that will dry in less time than 2–3 minutes.
- A so-called invisible condom. Developed by a university in Quebec, the invisible condom is a gel that hardens after insertion into the vagina or rectum, and then liquefies after several hours. It is still in the clinical trials phase as of 2010.
- Condoms containing lubricants intended to help the male partner maintain his erection, thus reducing the risk of condom slippage. These condoms are also still in clinical trials as of 2010.

Resources

BOOKS

Eddington, Patricia I, and Umberto V. Mastolli, eds. *Health Knowledge, Attitudes and Practices.* New York: Nova Biomedical Books, 2008.

Haerens, Margaret, ed. *Sexually Transmitted Diseases.* Detroit, MI: Greenhaven Press, 2006.

Lord, Alexandra M. *Condom Nation: The U.S. Government's Sex Education Campaign from World War I to the Internet.* Blatimore, MD: Johns Hopkins University Press, 2010.

PERIODICALS

Altkofer, W., et al. "Migration of Nitrosamines from Rubber Products—Are Balloons and Condoms Harmful to the Human Health?" *Molecular Nutrition and Food Research* 49 (March 2005): 235–38.

Davis, K.C., et al. "The Use of Alcohol and Condoms During Sexual Assault." *American Journal of Men's Health* 2 (September 2008): 281–90.

Hart, G.J., and J. Elford. "Sexual Risk Behaviour of Men Who Have Sex with Men: Emerging Patterns and New Challenges." *Current Opinion in Infectious Diseases* 23 (February 2010): 39–44.

Mathers, B.M., et al. "HIV Prevention, Treatment, and Care Services for People Who Inject Drugs: A Systematic Review of Global, Regional, and National Coverage." *Lancet* 375 (March 20, 2010): 1014–1028.

McDaid, L.M., and G.J. Hart. "Sexual Risk Behaviour for Transmission of HIV in Men Who Have Sex with Men: Recent Findings and Potential Interventions." *Current Opinion in HIV and AIDS* 5 (July 2010): 311–15.

Omar, R.F., et al. "Distribution of a Vaginal Gel (Invisible Condom) Before, During and After Simulated Sexual Intercourse and Its Persistence When Delivered by Two Different Vaginal Applicators: A Magnetic Resonance Imaging Study." *Contraception* 77 (June 2008): 447–55.

Peters, A., et al. "The Female Condom: The International Denial of a Strong Potential." *Reproductive Health Matters* 18 (May 2010): 119–28.

Sadeghi-Nejad, H., et al. "Sexually Transmitted Diseases and Sexual Function." *Journal of Sexual Medicine* 7 (January 2010): 389–413.

OTHER

American Social Health Association (ASHA). *How to Use a Condom.* Page includes a brief animation. http://www.ashastd.org/condom/condom_overview.cfm

AVERT. *The Female Condom.* Web page includes a 2-1/2-minute video explaining how to use the female condom correctly. http://www.avert.org/female-condom.htm

Centers for Disease Control and Prevention (CDC). *Condoms and STDs: Fact Sheet for Public Health Personnel.* http://www.cdc.gov/condomeffectiveness/latex.htm

Rape-aXe. *Introduction.* Page includes a video showing how the anti-rape female condom works. http://www.antirape.co.za/intro.htm

ORGANIZATIONS

American Congress of Obstetricians and Gynecologists (ACOG), 409 12th St., S.W., P.O. Box 96920, Washington, DC, 20090-6920, (202) 638-5577, resources@acog.org, http://www.acog.org/.

Centers for Disease Control and Prevention (CDC), 1600 Clifton Road, Atlanta, GA, 30333, (800) 232-4636, cdcinfo@cdc.gov, http://www.cdc.gov.

American Social Health Association (ASHA), P.O. Box 13827, Research Triangle Park, NC, 27709, (919) 361-8400, (919) 361-8425, http://www.ashastd.org/index.cfm.

National Institute of Allergy and Infectious Diseases (NIAID), 6610 Rockledge Drive, MSC 6612, Bethesda, MD, 20892-6612, (301) 496-5717, (866) 284-4107, (301) 402-3573, http://www3.niaid.nih.gov.

U.S. Food and Drug Administration (FDA), 10903 New Hampshire Ave., Silver Spring, MD, 20993, (888) 463-6332, http://www.fda.gov/.

AVERT, an International AIDS Charity, 4 Brighton Road, HorshamWest Sussex, United Kingdom, RH13 5BA, + 44 (0)1403 210202, http://www.avert.org/.

World Health Organization (WHO), Avenue Appia 20, 1211 Geneva 27, Switzerland, + 41 22 791 21 11, + 41 22 791 31 11, info@who.int, http://www.who.int/en/.

Stephanie Dionne
Rebecca J. Frey, PhD

Conduct disorder

Definition

Conduct disorder (CD) is a behavioral and emotional disorder of childhood and adolescence. Children with conduct disorder act inappropriately, infringe on the rights of others, and violate the behavioral expectations of others.

Description

CD is present in approximately 9% of boys and 2–9% of girls under the age of 18. Children with conduct disorder act out aggressively and express anger inappropriately. They engage in a variety of antisocial and destructive acts, including violence toward people and animals, destruction of property, lying, stealing, truancy, and running away from home. They often begin using and abusing drugs and alcohol, and having sex at an early age. Irritability, temper tantrums, and low self-esteem are common personality traits of children with CD.

Causes and symptoms

There are two sub-types of CD, one beginning in childhood and the other in adolescence. There is no known cause. Researchers and physicians suggest that this disease may be caused by the following:

- poor parent-child relationships
- dysfunctional families
- drug abuse
- physical abuse
- poor relationships with other children
- cognitive problems leading to school failures
- brain damage
- biological defects

Difficulty in school is an early sign of potential conduct disorder problems. While the patient's IQ tends to be in the normal range, they can have trouble with verbal and abstract reasoning skills and may lag behind their classmates, and consequently, feel as if they don't "fit in." The frustration and loss of self-esteem resulting from this academic and social inadequacy can trigger the development of CD.

A dysfunctional home environment can be another major contributor to CD. An emotionally, physically, or sexually abusive home environment, a family history of antisocial personality disorder, or parental **substance abuse** can damage a child's perceptions of himself and put him on a path toward negative behavior. Other less obvious environmental factors can also play a part in the development of conduct disorder. Long-term studies have shown that maternal **smoking** during **pregnancy** may be linked to the development of CD in boys. Animal and human studies point out that nicotine can have undesirable effects on babies. These include altered structure and function of their nervous systems, learning deficits, and behavioral problems. In a study of 177 boys ages 7 to 12 years, those with mothers who smoked over one-half a package of cigarettes daily while pregnant were more apt to have a CD than those with mothers who did not smoke.

Other conditions that may cause or co-exist with CD include **head injury**, substance abuse disorder, major depressive disorder, and **attention deficit hyperactivity disorder (ADHD)**. Thirty to 50 percent of children diagnosed with **ADHD**, a disorder characterized by a persistent pattern of inattention and/or hyperactivity, also have CD.

CD is defined as a repetitive behavioral pattern of violating the rights of others or societal norms. Three of the following criteria, or symptoms, are required over the previous 12 months for a diagnosis of CD (one of the three must have occurred in the past 6 months):

- bullies, threatens, or intimidates others
- picks fights
- has used a dangerous weapon
- has been physically cruel to people
- has been physically cruel to animals
- has stolen while confronting a victim (for example, mugging or extortion)
- has forced someone into sexual activity
- has deliberately set a fire with the intention of causing damage
- has deliberately destroyed property of others
- has broken into someone else's house or car
- frequently lies to get something or to avoid obligations
- has stolen without confronting a victim or breaking and entering (e.g., shoplifting or forgery)
- stays out at night; breaks curfew (beginning before 13 years of age)
- has run away from home overnight at least twice (or once for a lengthy period)
- is often truant from school (beginning before 13 years of age)

Diagnosis

CD is diagnosed and treated by a number of social workers, school counselors, psychiatrists, and psychologists. Genuine diagnosis may require psychiatric expertise to rule out such conditions as **bipolar disorder** or ADHD. A comprehensive evaluation of the child should ideally include interviews with the child and parents, a full social and medical history, a cognitive evaluation, and a psychiatric exam. One or more clinical inventories or scales may be used to assess the

---

KEY TERMS

ADHD—Attention deficit hyperactivity disorder; a disorder characterized by a persistent pattern of inattention and/or hyperactivity.

Major depressive disorder—A mood disorder characterized by profound feelings of sadness or despair.

---

child for conduct disorder—including the Youth Self-Report, the Overt Aggression Scale (OAS), Behavioral Assessment System for Children (BASC), Child Behavior Checklist (CBCL), and Diagnostic Interview Schedule for Children (DISC). The tests are verbal and/or written and are administered in both hospital and outpatient settings.

Treatment

Treating conduct disorder requires an approach that addresses both the child and his environment. Behavioral therapy and **psychotherapy** can help a child with CD to control his anger and develop new coping skills. Family **group therapy** may also be effective in some cases. Parents should be counseled on how to set appropriate limits with their child and be consistent and realistic when disciplining. If an abusive home life is at the root of the conduct problem, every effort should be made to move the child into a more supportive environment. Parent training programs are increasing in number.

For children with coexisting ADHD, substance abuse, depression, or **learning disorders**, treating these conditions first is preferred, and may result in a significant improvement to the CD condition. In all cases of CD, treatment should begin when symptoms first appear. Recent studies have shown Ritalin to be a useful drug for both ADHD and CD.

When aggressive behavior is severe, mood stabilizing medication, including lithium (Cibalith-S, Eskalith, Lithane, Lithobid, Lithonate, Lithotabs), carbamazepine (Tegretol, Atretol), and propranolol (Inderal), may be an appropriate option for treating the aggressive symptoms. However, placing the child into a structured setting or treatment program such as a psychiatric hospital may be just as beneficial for easing aggression as medication.

Prognosis

The prognosis for children with CD is not bright. Follow-up studies of conduct disordered children have

---

shown a high incidence of antisocial personality disorder, affective illnesses, and chronic criminal behavior later in life. However, proper treatment of co-existing disorders, early identification and intervention, and long-term support may improve the outlook significantly.

Prevention

A supportive, nurturing, and structured home environment is believed to be the best defense against CD. Children with learning disabilities and/or difficulties in school should get immediate and appropriate academic assistance. Addressing these problems when they first appear helps to prevent the frustration and low self-esteem that may lead to CD later on.

Resources

BOOKS

Liabø, Kristin, and Joanna Richardson.*Conduct Disorder and Offending Behaviour in Young People: Findings from Research.* Philadelphia: Jessica Kingsley Publishers, 2007.

ORGANIZATIONS

American Academy of Child and Adolescent Psychiatry (AACAP), 3615 Wisconsin Ave. NW, Washington, DC, 20013-3007, (202) 966-7300, (202) 966-2891, communications@aacap.org, http://www.aacap.org.

Paula Anne Ford-Martin

Conductive hearing loss *see* **Hearing loss**
Condylomata acuminata *see* **Genital warts**
Cone biopsy *see* **Cervical conization**

Congenital adrenal hyperplasia

Definition

Congenital adrenal hyperplasia (CAH) is a genetic disorder that affects the adrenal glands, a pair of walnut-sized organs located over the kidneys. It is characterized primarily by a deficiency in the steroid hormone group glucocorticoid (usually cortisol), and secondarily by deficient amounts of the steroid hormone group mineralocorticoid (usually aldosterone). Because these two hormones are produced in lower-than-normal amounts, CAH is also secondarily characterized by an over-production of the steroid hormone group androgen (such as testosterone). Due to it being hereditarily

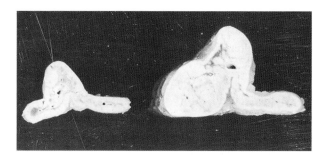

Adrenal cortical hyperplasia. The adrenal on the right is normal; the one on the left shows hyperplasia. *(© Biophoto Associates/Photo Researchers, Inc.)*

caused, CAH is present at birth. CAH affects the sexual development of children.

Demographics

CAH is a genetic disorder that interferes with the normal growth and development, especially the sexual development. It affects male and female children equally. According to the National Institutes of Health, about one child in 10,000 to 18,000 children in the United States are born with congenital adrenal hyperplasia. It also affects adults, men and women equally, in all populations of the world. It is especially common in Yupik Eskimos, where the incidence is about one in 400.

Congenital adrenal hyperplasia is the most common adrenal gland disorder found in infants and children, occurring in one in 10,000 total births worldwide. It is also called adrenogenital syndrome.

Description

Congenital adrenal hyperplasia (CAH) is a form of adrenal insufficiency in which the enzyme that produces two important adrenal steroid hormones, cortisol and aldosterone, is deficient. Cortisol and aldosterone play roles in maintaining the body's health. Therefore, a low concentration of cortisol makes it difficult for a body to regulate blood pressure, maintain blood sugar levels, and energy levels. In addition, low levels of aldosterone produce lower **sodium** levels and higher potassium levels, which when not in balance can adversely effect muscle and nerve control.

Because cortisol and aldosterone production is impeded, the adrenal gland instead overproduces androgens (male steroid hormones). Consequently, females with CAH are generally born with genitals that appear more like male than female, such as an enlarged clitoris (which is called ambiguous external genitalia). They may also develop other male characteristics. However, females will possess normal internal reproductive tract structures (such as ovaries, fallopian tubes, and uterus). Males usually have normal genitals at birth but may experience premature sexual development; however, in a small percentage of cases such male infants have an enlarged penis. CAH causes abnormal growth for both sexes; with patients being tall as children but short as adults.

In its most severe form, called salt-wasting CAH, a life-threatening adrenal crisis can occur if the disorder is untreated. This form, which occurs in newborns and very young children, is also called classic congenital adrenal hyperplasia. The adrenal crisis can cause **dehydration**, **shock**, and **death** within 14 days of birth. There is also a mild form of CAH, which occurs later in childhood or young adult life. This form of CAH, called non-classic congenital adrenal hyperplasia, causes patients to have a partial enzyme deficiency.

Risk factors

Because it is an hereditary disease, a child or fetus is at increased risk if both parent have CAH or if both parent are carriers of the disease. Some ethnic groups have a higher risk for getting congenital adrenal hyperplasia than others. Ashkenazi Jews, who have descended from along the Rhine River in Germany, are most likely to contract CAH. Others at high risk include Eskimos, Hispanics, Italians, and Yugoslavs (a small group of southern Slavic people originally found in the former Yugoslavia).

Causes and symptoms

CAH is an inherited disorder that occurs when one of many different enzymes, which are used by the adrenal glands to produce cortisol, is not produced in sufficient quantities. The most commonly enzyme associated with the disorder is 21-hydroxylase. Consequently, CAH is also sometimes called 21-hydroxylase deficiency. (Two other enzymes associated with CAH are 1-beta-hydroxylase and 17-alpha-hydroxylase.) Because varied amounts of 21-hydroxylase are produced within the human body, the degree that CAH affects people is different. Some people have severe cases of CAH, while others have only mild cases.

CAH is a recessive disease, which means that a child must inherit one copy of the defective gene from each parent who is a carrier; when two carriers have children, each **pregnancy** carries a 25% risk of producing an affected child.

The symptoms inherent within this condition are due to the fetus manufacturing lower-than-normal levels of cortisol and being exposed to abnormally high levels of male sex hormones (androgens). In females, CAH produces an enlarged clitoris at birth and masculinization of features as the child grows, such as deepening tone of voice, facial hair, excess facial and armpit hair, and failure to menstruate or abnormal periods at **puberty**. Females with severe CAH may be mistaken for males at birth. In males, the genitals are usually normal at birth, but the child becomes muscular, the penis enlarges while the testes remain small, pubic and armpit hair appears, and the voice deepens long before normal puberty, sometimes as early as two to three years of age.

In the severe salt-wasting form of CAH, newborns may develop symptoms shortly after birth, including **vomiting**, dehydration, weight loss (and inability to regain birth weight), electrolyte (a compound such as sodium or **calcium** that separates to form ions when dissolved in water) changes, and cardiac arrhythmia.

In the mild form of CAH, which first occurs in late childhood or early adulthood, symptoms include early and excessive development of body hair, **fatigue**, high blood cholesterol, low blood pressure, low bone density, **nausea**, **obesity**, reduced ability to cope with infections, and severe **acne**. Even though the older child grows rapidly, once adulthood is reached, the eventual height of the person is usually shorter than normal. In addition, most males and females with CAH are infertile as adults. Women also have unusually irregular menstrual cycles. However, sometimes symptoms are not present.

Diagnosis

CAH is diagnosed by a careful examination of the genitals and blood and urine tests that measure the hormones produced by the adrenal gland. Abnormal levels of cortisol, aldosterone, and androgen will confirm the diagnosis. A number of states in the United States perform a hormonal test (a heel prick blood test) for CAH and other inherited diseases within a few days of birth. In questionable cases, **genetic testing** can provide a definitive diagnosis. For some forms of CAH, prenatal diagnosis is possible through chronic villus sampling in the first trimester and by measuring certain hormones in the amniotic fluid (within the womb) during the second trimester; what is called **amniocentesis**. Such tests are performed when parents (or other family members) are known carriers or have the disease, or older siblings of the parents have CAH.

Treatment

The goal of treatment for CAH is to return the androgen levels to normal. This is usually accomplished

KEY TERMS

Adrenal glands—The two endocrine glands located above the kidney that secrete hormones and epinephrine.

Aldosterone—A hormone secreted by the adrenal glands that is important for maintaining salt and water balance in the body.

Androgens—Steroid hormones that cause masculinization.

Congenital—Present at birth.

Cortisol—A steroid hormone secreted by the adrenal cortex that is important for maintenance of body fluids, electrolytes, and blood sugar levels.

Hormone—A chemical messenger produced by the endocrine glands or certain other cells. Hormones are usually carried in the blood stream and regulate some metabolic activities.

Steroids—Hormones, including aldosterone, cortisol, and androgens, derived from cholesterol that share a four-ring structure.

through drug therapy, although surgery is an alternative. Lifelong treatment is required.

Drug therapy consists of one of a group of cortisol-like steroid medications called glucocorticoids. Oral hydrocortisone is prescribed for children, and prednisone or dexamethasone is prescribed for older patients. For patients with salt-wasting CAH, fludrocortisone, which acts like aldosterone (the missing hormone), is also prescribed. Infants and small children may also receive salt tablets, while older patients are told to eat salty foods. Medical therapy achieves hormonal balance most of the time, but CAH patients can have periods of fluctuating hormonal control that lead to increases in the dose of **steroids** prescribed. Side effects of steroids include stunted growth. Steroid therapy should not be suddenly stopped, since adrenal insufficiency results.

Patients with CAH should see a pediatric endocrinologist frequently. The endocrinologist will assess height, weight, and blood pressure, and order an annual x ray of the wrist (to assess bone age [bone mass]), as well as assess blood hormone levels. CAH patients with the milder form of the disorder are usually effectively treated with hydrocortisone or prednisone, if they need medical treatment at all.

Females with CAH who have masculine external genitalia require surgery to reconstruct the clitoris and/or vagina. This is usually performed between the ages of one and six months.

An experimental type of drug therapy—a three-drug combination, with an androgen blocking agent (flutamide), an aromatase inhibitor (testolactone), and low dose hydrocortisone—is currently being studied by physicians at the National Institutes of Health. Preliminary results are encouraging, but it

will be many years before the safety and effectiveness of this therapy is fully known.

Adrenalectomy, a surgical procedure to remove the adrenal glands, is a more radical treatment for CAH. It was widely used before the advent of steroids. Currently, it is recommended for CAH patients with little or no enzyme activity and can be accomplished by **laparoscopy**. This is a minimally invasive type of surgery done through one or more small 1 inch (2.5 cm) incisions and a laparoscope, an instrument with a fiber-optic light containing a tube with openings for surgical instruments. Adrenalectomy is followed by hormone therapy, but in lower doses than CAH patients not treated surgically receive.

Prenatal treatment is also possible to diagnose CAH in a fetus. If diagnosed within the fetus, the doctor can prescribe a cortisosteroid drug, such as dexamethasone, to the pregnant woman. The drug will enter the womb from the mother's placenta and help to bring the fetus' adrenal glands back to normal function. A stronger dose of dexamethasone is usually prescribed for female fetuses and a milder dose to males.

Prognosis

Although CAH can potentially cause death in those it affects, the disorder can be controlled and successfully treated in most patients as long as they remain on drug therapy. When drug therapy is successfully applied, CAH patients usually lead normal lives. People with congenital adrenal hyperplasia will usually be shorter in height than most people, and they often times have fertility problems throughout their adult lives. Women are more likely to experience various sexual problems later in life if they had corrective surgery on their genitals. People with CAH may need some counseling to deal with their problems, but in all likelihood should lead a healthy and long life with proper treatment and care by their physician.

Prevention

Prenatal therapy, in which a pregnant woman at risk for a second CAH child is given dexamethasone to decrease secretion of androgens by the adrenal glands of the female fetus, has been in use for over ten years. This therapy is started in the first trimester when fetal adrenal production of androgens begins, but before prenatal diagnosis is done that would provide definitive information about the sex of the fetus and its disease status. This means that a number of fetuses are exposed to unnecessary steroid treatment in order to prevent the development of male-like genitals in female fetuses with CAH. Several hundred children have undergone this treatment with no major adverse effects, but its long-term risks are unknown. Since there is very little data on the effectiveness and safety of prenatal therapy, it should only be offered to patients who clearly understand the risks and benefits and who are capable of complying with strict monitoring and follow-up throughout pregnancy and after the child is born.

Parents with a family history of CAH, including a child who has CAH, should seek **genetic counseling**. Genetic testing during pregnancy can provide information on the risk of having a child with CAH.

Resources

BOOKS

Chrousos, George P. and Constantine Tsigos. *Stress, Obesity, and Metabolic Syndrome*. Boston: Blackwell, 2006.

Hannigan, Steve, editor. *Inherited Metabolic Diseases: A Guide to 100 Conditions*. Oxford: Radcliffe, 2007.

Hsu, C. Y. *Congenital Adrenal Hyperplasia: A Parents' Guide*. Bloomington, IN: Author House, 2005.

Linos, Dimitrios, and Jon J. van Heerden, editors. *Adrenal Glands: Diagnostic Aspects and Surgical Therapy*. Berlin: Springer, 2005.

OTHER

Congenital Adrenal Hyperplasia. Mayo Clinic. (March 24, 2009), http://www.mayoclinic.com/health/congenital-adrenal-hyperplasia/DS00915 (accessed September 9, 2010).

Congenital Adrenal Hyperplasia. Medline Plus, National Library of Medicine and National Institutes of Health . (January 21, 2010), http://www.nlm.nih.gov/medlineplus/ency/article/000411.htm; (accessed September 9, 2010).

Congenital Adrenal Hyperplasia. eMedicine, WebMD. (April 19, 2010), http://emedicine.medscape.com/article/919218-overview; (accessed September 9, 2010).

Congenital Adrenal Hyperplasia Due to 21-Hydroxylase Deficiency. The Johns Hopkins Children's Center.

http://www.hopkinschildrens.org/cah/ (accessed September 9, 2010).

ORGANIZATIONS

American Academy of Pediatrics, 141 Northwest Point Boulevard, Elk Grove Village, IL, 60007-1098, (847) 434-4000, http://www.aap.org/.

MAGIC Foundation, 6645 West North Avenue, Oak Park, IL, 60302, (708) 383-0808, (800) 362-4423, http://www.magicfoundation.org/.

National Adrenal Diseases Foundation, 505 Northern Boulevard, Great Neck, NY, 11021, (516) 487-4992, nadf mail@aol.com, http://medhlp.netusa.net/www/nadf.htm.

Jennifer Sisk

Congenital amputation

Definition

Congenital **amputation** is the absence of a fetal limb or fetal part at birth. This condition may be the result of the constriction of fibrous bands within the membrane that surrounds the developing fetus (amniotic band syndrome) or the exposure to substances known to cause **birth defects** (teratogenic agents). Other factors, including genetics, may also play a role.

Description

An estimated one in 2000 babies are born with all or part of a limb missing, ranging from a missing part of a finger to the absence of both arms and both legs. Congenital amputation is the least common reason for amputation. However, there are occasional periods in history where the number of congenital amputations increased. For example, the thalidomide tragedy of the early 1960s occurred after pregnant mothers in western Europe were given a tranquilizer containing the drug. The result was a drastic increase in the number of babies born with deformed limbs. In this example, the birth defect usually presented itself as very small, deformed versions of normal limbs. More recently, birth defects as a result of radiation exposure near the site of the Chernobyl disaster in Russia have left numerous children with malformed or absent limbs.

Causes and symptoms

The exact cause of congenital amputations is unknown. However, according to the March of Dimes, most birth defects have one or more genetic factors and one or more environmental factors. It is also known that most birth defects occur in the first three months of **pregnancy**, when the organs of the fetus are forming. Within these crucial first weeks, frequently prior to when a woman is aware of the pregnancy, the developing fetus is most susceptible to substances that can cause birth defects (teratogens). Exposure to teratogens can cause congenital amputation. In other cases, tight amniotic bands may constrict the developing fetus, preventing a limb from forming properly if at all. It is estimated that this amniotic band syndrome occurs in between one in 12,000 and one in 15,000 live births.

An infant with congenital amputation may be missing an entire limb or just a portion of a limb. Congenital amputation resulting in the complete absence of a limb beyond a certain point (and leaving a stump) is called transverse deficiency or amelia. Longitudinal deficiencies occur when a specific part of a limb is missing; for example, when the fibula bone in the lower leg is missing, but the rest of the leg is intact. Phocomelia is the condition in which only a mid-portion of a limb is missing, as when the hands or feet are attached directly to the trunk.

Diagnosis

Many cases of congenital amputation are not diagnosed until the baby is born. Ultrasound examinations may reveal the absence of a limb in some developing fetuses, but routine ultrasounds may not pick up signs of more subtle defects. However, if a doctor suspects that the fetus is at risk for developing a limb deficiency (for example, if the mother has been exposed to radiation), a more detailed ultrasound examination may be performed.

Treatment

Successful treatment of a child with congenital amputation involves an entire medical team, including a pediatrician, an orthopedist, a psychiatrist or psychologist, a prosthetist (an expert in making prosthetics, or artificial limbs), a social worker, and occupational and physical therapists. The accepted method of treatment is to fit the child early with a functional prosthesis because this leads to normal development and less wasting away (atrophy) of the muscles of the limbs present. However, some parents and physicians believe that the child should be allowed to learn to play and perform tasks without a prosthesis, if possible. When the child is older, he or she can be involved in the decision of whether or not to be fitted for a prosthesis.

In the case of congenital amputation of the fingers, **plastic surgery** can sometimes be used to

---

KEY TERMS

Amniotic band—An abnormal condition of fetal development in which fibrous bands of tissue develop out of the amniotic sac. The bands encircle and constrict parts of the baby's body, interfering with normal development and sometimes causing congenital amputation.

Prosthesis—An artificial replacement for a missing part of the body.

Teratogen—Any substance, agent, or process that interferes with normal prenatal development, causing the formation of one or more developmental abnormalities of the fetus.

---

reconstruct the missing digits by transferring parts of the great and second toes to the hand. Some defects in the leg bones can be treated by removing the malformed bone, grafting bone from other parts of the child's body, and inserting a metal rod to strengthen the limb; this technique, however, is controversial as of the early 2000s.

There have been cases in which physicians have detected amniotic band constriction interfering with limb development fairly early in its course. In 1997, doctors at the Florida Institute for Fetal Diagnosis and Therapy reported two cases in which minimally invasive surgery freed constricting amniotic bands and preserved the affected limbs.

Alternative treatment

Prevention of birth defects begins with building the well-being of the mother before pregnancy. Prenatal care should be strong and educational so that the mother understands both her genetic risks and her environmental risks. Several disciplines in alternative therapy also recommend various supplements and **vitamins** that may reduce the chances of birth defects. If a surgical procedure is planned, naturopathic and homeopathic pre- and post-surgical therapies can speed recovery.

Prognosis

A congenital limb deficiency has a profound effect on the life of the child and parents. However, **occupational therapy** can help the child learn to accomplish many tasks. In addition, some experts believe that early fitting of a prosthesis will enhance acceptance of the prosthesis by the child and parents.

Prevention

Studies have suggested that a multivitamin including **folic acid** may reduce birth defects, including congenital abnormalities. **Smoking**, drinking alcohol, and eating a poor diet while pregnant may increase the risk of congenital abnormalities. Daily, heavy exposure to chemicals may be dangerous while pregnant.

Resources

BOOKS

Beers, Mark H., Robert S. Porter, and Thomas V. Jones, eds. *The Merck Manual of Diagnosis and Therapy*. 18th ed. Whitehouse Station, NJ: Merck Research Laboratories, 2006.

PERIODICALS

Dobbs, M. B., M. M. Rich, J. E. Gordon, et al. "Use of an Intramedullary Rod for Treatment of Congenital Pseudarthrosis of the Tibia. A Long-Term Follow-Up Study." *Journal of Bone and Joint Surgery, American Volume* 86-A (June 2004): 1186–1197.

Garcia Julve G., and G. Martinez Villen. "The Multiple Monoblock Toe-to-Hand Transfer in Digital Reconstruction. A Report of Ten Cases." *Journal of Hand Surgery* 29 (June 2004): 222–229.

ORGANIZATIONS

International Child Amputee Network (I-CAN), P.O. Box 514, Abilene, TX, 79604-0514, job525@att.net, http://www.child-amputee.net/.

March of Dimes Birth Defects Foundation, 1275 Mamaroneck Ave., White Plains, NY, 10605, (914) 997-4488, http://www.modimes.org.

National Organization for Rare Disorders, P.O. Box 8923, New Fairfield, CT, 06812-8923, (800) 999-6673, http://www.rarediseases.org.

Jeffrey P. Larson, RPT
Rebecca J. Frey, PhD

Congenital bladder anomalies

Definition

The two most common congenital bladder abnormalities are exstrophy and congenital diverticula. An exstrophic bladder is one that is open to the outside and turned inside-out, so that its inside is visible at birth, protruding from the lower abdomen. A diverticulum is an extension of a hollow organ, usually shaped like a pouch with a narrow opening.

Description

During fetal development, folds enclose tissues and organs and eventually fuse at the edges to form sealed compartments. Both in the front and the back, folds eventually become major body structures. In the back, the entire spinal column folds in like a pipe wrapped in a pillow. In the front, the entire lower urinary system is folded in.

- Exstrophy of the bladder represents a failure of this folding process to complete itself, so the organs form with more or less of their front side missing and open to the outside. At the same time, the front of the pelvic bone is widely separated. The abdominal wall is open, too. In fact, the defect often extends all the way to the penis in the male or splits the clitoris in the female.
- A congenital bladder diverticulum represents an area of weakness in the bladder wall through which extrudes some of the lining of the bladder. (A small balloon squeezed in a fist will create a diverticula-like effect between the fingers.) Bladder diverticula may be multiple, and they often occur at the ureterovesical junction—the entrance of the upper urinary system into the bladder. In this location, they may cause urine to reflux into the ureter and kidney, leading to infection and possible kidney damage.

Causes and symptoms

As with many **birth defects**, the causes are not well known. Lack of prenatal care and **nutrition** has been linked to many birth defects, however beyond the avoidance of known teratogens (anything that can cause a birth defect), there is little prevention possible. Exstrophy is rare, occurring in about one in 40,000 births. Diverticula are more common, but less serious.

If left untreated, the patient with bladder exstrophy will have no control over urination and is more likely to develop **bladder cancer**. Diverticula, particularly if it causes urine reflux, may lead to chronic infection and its subsequent consequences.

Diagnosis

A major consideration with congenital abnormalities is that they tend to be multiple. Further, each one is unique in its extent and severity. Exstrophy can involve the rectum and large bowel and coexist with hernias. The obvious bladder exstrophy seen at birth will prompt immediate action and a search for other anomalies.

Diverticula are not visible and will be detected only if they cause trouble. They are usually found in

KEY TERMS

Congenital—Present at birth.

Cystoscopy—Examination of the urinary bladder with a thin telescope-like instrument.

Exstrophy—Being turned inside out combined with being outside the body.

Diverticulum—A pouch extending from a hollow organ.

Radiologist—A physician who specializes in creating images of the internal organs of the body.

Teratogen—Any agent that can cause birth defects.

Ureter—The tube that transports urine from the kidney to the bladder.

Ureterovesical junction—The joining of the ureter to the bladder.

Urologist—A physician who specializes in diseases of the urinary system.

an examination for the cause of recurring urinary infections. X rays of the urinary system or a **cystoscopy** (examination with a telescope-like instrument) will identify them. Often, the two procedures are done together: a urologist will perform the cystoscopy, then a radiologist will instill a contrast agent into the bladder and take x rays.

Treatment

Surgery is necessary and can usually produce successful results. If possible, the surgery must be done within 48 hours of birth. Prior to surgery, the exposed organs must be protected and all related defects identified and managed. Delay in the surgery leads to the frequent need to divert the urine into the bowel because the partially repaired bladder cannot control the flow. After surgery, the likelihood of infection requires monitoring.

Alternative treatment

After surgery, ongoing precautions to reduce frequency of infection may need to be used. Cranberry juice has the ability to keep bacteria from adhering to the membranes and can help prevent infection whenever there is increased risk. There are botanical and homeopathic treatments available; however, consultation by a trained practitioner is recommended before treatment.

Prognosis

With immediate surgery, three-quarters of patients can be successfully repaired. They will have control of their urine and no long-term consequences. The rate of infection is greater for those with congenital bladder anomalies, since any abnormality in the urinary system predisposes it to invasion by bacteria.

Prevention

Birth defects often have no precisely identified cause, therefore, prevention is limited to general measures such as early and continuous prenatal care, appropriate nutrition, and a healthy lifestyle.

Resources

BOOKS

Tanagho, Emil A., Jack W McAninch, and Donald Ridgeway Smith. *Smith's General Urology*. New York: McGraw–Hill Medical, 2008.

J. Ricker Polsdorfer, MD

Congenital bladder diverticulum *see* **Congenital bladder anomalies**

Congenital brain defects

Definition

Congenital brain defects are a group of disorders involving deficiencies of brain development. People are born with such brain defects (damage); thus, they are called congenital, or existing at birth. (Those brain defects that result from trauma or other types of injuries are called acquired brain defects, or non-congenital brain defects.) Congenital brain detects develop during the growth and development of the fetus. They are caused by a variety of factors, such as genetic defects, infections, prenatal problems, and environmental toxins. The causal factors disrupt the development of the brains of these fetuses, which, for the most part, leads to physical and cognitive problems after birth. Many disorders can be grouped within congenital brain defects.

Demographics

Congenital brain defects can occur in any population of humans around the world. They primarily affect fetuses within the womb or, in some cases, infants who have just been born. They do not generally favor one particular race or gender, although some of the disorders within congenital brain defects may favor a particular race or gender.

Description

Brain development begins shortly after conception and continues throughout the growth of a fetus. A complex genetic program coordinates the formation, growth, and migration of billions of neurons, or nerve cells, and their development into discrete, interacting brain regions. Interruption of this program, especially early in development, can cause structural defects in the brain. In addition, normal brain formation requires proper development of the surrounding skull, and skull defects may lead to brain malformation. Congenital brain defects may be caused by inherited genetic defects, spontaneous mutations within the genes of the embryo, or effects on the embryo due to infection, trauma, drug use, or environmental factors from the mother.

Some of the disorders grouped within congenital brain defects are anencephaly, encephalocele, **spina bifida**, Dandy-Walker malformation, holoprosencephaly, lissencephaly, schizencephaly, schizencephaly, and megalencephaly. They are described in the following paragraphs.

Anencephaly

Early on in embryonic development, a flat strip of tissue along the back of the fetus rolls up to form a tube. This so-called "neural tube" develops into the spinal cord and, at one end, the brain. Closure of the tube is required for subsequent development of the tissue within. Anencephaly (literally "without brain"), results when the topmost portion of the tube fails to close, which results in the absence of most of the brain (primarily the cerebral hemispheres and cerebellum) and skull. Anencephaly is the most common severe malformation seen in stillborn births. According to the National Institutes of Health, it occurs in about one out of 10,000 births; however, the exact figure is unknown because many pregnancies end up as miscarriages. It is about four times more common in females than males. Anencephaly is sometimes seen to run in families, and for parents who have conceived one anencephalic fetus, the risk of a second is as high as 5%. Fewer than half of babies with anencephaly are born alive, and survival beyond the first month is rare, with most babies dying within the first few days of being born.

Encephalocele

Encephalocele is a rare type of neural tube defect (NTD) that results in a sac-like protrusion (or projection) of part of the brain through a defect in the skull. It happens during **pregnancy** when the neural tube does not close completely. The most common site for encephalocele is along the front-to-back midline of the skull, usually at the rear, although frontal encephaloceles (in an area between the forehead and the nose) are more common among Asians. Pressure within the skull pushes out cranial tissue. The protective layer over the brain, the meninges, grows to cover the protrusion, as does skin in some cases. Defects in skull closure are thought to cause some cases of encephalocele, while defects in neural tube closure may cause others. Encephaloceles may be small and contain little or no brain tissue, or may be quite large and contain a significant fraction of the brain. The Centers for Diseases Control and Prevention states that in any given year about 375 babies are born in the United States with encephalocele; that is, about one in 10,000 births involve babies with encephalocele.

Spina Bifida

Failure of neural-tube closure below the level of the brain prevents full development of the surrounding vertebral bones and leads to spina bifida, or a divided spinal column. The medical community usually classifies three types of spina bifida. In spina bifida occulta, only a small separation in one or more vertebral bones of the spinal column occurs. This mild form of spina bifida usually involves few if any symptoms because the nerves within the spine are not adversely affected. Most children grow up without any problems. The only sign that may occur is a small lump or tiny tuft of hair near the spine. The second type, called meningocele, is a rare form of the condition, one in which the membranes around the spinal cord (the meninges) are pushed out through an opening in the vertebrae. Since the spinal cord develops normally, surgeons can remove the problematic membranes with little risk of further complications to the spine. In the third type, incomplete closure of the neural tube causes a protrusion of the spinal cord and meninges. This type is called myelomeningocele (also called open spina bifida or spina bifida cystica), and is the most severe form of spina bifida. In fact, when spina bifida is mentioned in common usage people are usually discussing myelomeningocele. Some cases of spina bifida are accompanied by another defect at the base of the brain, known as the Arnold-Chiari malformation or Chiari II malformation. For reasons that are unclear, part of the cerebellum is displaced downward into the spinal column. Symptoms may be present at birth or delayed until early childhood.

Dandy-Walker Malformation

The Dandy-Walker malformation (DWM) is marked by incomplete formation, or absence of, the central section of the cerebellum, and the growth of cysts within the lowest of the brain's ventricles (the fourth ventricle). The cerebellum helps to coordinate movement for humans, along with assisting in behavior and cognition (learning). The ventricles are fluid-filled cavities within the brain, through which cerebrospinal fluid (CSF) normally circulates. The cysts may block the exit of the fluid, causing **hydrocephalus**. Symptoms may be present at birth or delayed until early childhood. DWM usually results in a size smaller than normal for the middle portion of the cerebellum, along with an abnormal position for it. The fourth ventricle is also enlarged, as is the base of the skull. Hydrocephalus sometimes also occurs with DWM. When this happens, spinal fluid is blocked from flowing. This results from excessive fluid in and around the brain. Neurological problems can occur when pressures increase inside the skull and the head swells.

Holoprosencephaly

Soon after closure of the neural tube, the embryonic forebrain (prosencephalon) divides into two halves, or cerebral hemispheres. Failure of division is termed holoprosencephaly (literally "whole forebrain"). Holoprosencephaly, in its most severe case called alobar, results in a single-lobed brain structure. It is almost always accompanied by severe facial and cranial deformities along the midline, including **cleft lip**, **cleft palate**, fused eye sockets and a single eye (cyclopia), and deformities of the limbs, heart, gastrointestinal tract, and other internal organs. Most infants are either stillborn or die soon after birth. In some intermediate cases of holoprosencephaly, the brain's hemispheres partially divide. This form is called semilobar holoprosencephaly. In a third case called lobar holoprosencephaly, the brain has considerable separation of the hemispheres. Survivors, those with less severe forms of the condition, suffer from neurological impairments and facial deformities, such as of the eyes, nose, and upper lip. In the least forms, the brain develops almost normally.

Lissencephaly

The normal ridges and valleys of the mature brain are formed after cells from the inside of the developing brain migrate to the outside and multiply. When these cells fail to migrate, the surface remains smooth, a rare, genetic condition called lissencephaly ("smooth brain"). Lissencephaly involves the cerebral cortex. Specifically, the normal folds (convolutions) of the cerebral cortex are not present. It causes the head to be abnormally small; what is called microcephaly. Lissencephaly occurs when the embryo does not develop normally due to defects in migration of nerve cells. It is often associated with facial abnormalities including a small jaw, a high forehead, a short nose, and low-set ears. The condition may also produce deformations in the fingers and hands, along with the toes. In addition, lissencephaly causes difficulties in swallowing, **muscle spasms**, seizures, and psychomotor retardation.

Schizencephaly

If damaged during growth, especially within the first 20 weeks, brain tissue may stop growing, while tissue around it continues to form. This causes an abnormal cleft or groove to appear on the surface of the brain, called schizencephaly (literally "split brain"). This cleft should not be confused with the normal wrinkled brain surface, nor should the name be mistaken for **schizophrenia**, a mental disorder. Generalized destruction of tissue or lack of brain development may lead to hydranencephaly, in which cerebrospinal fluid (CSF) fills much of the space normally occupied by the brain. Hydranencephaly is distinct from hydrocephalus, in which CSF accumulates within a normally formed brain, putting pressure on it and possibly causing skull expansion. Babies with schizencephaly usually have delays in learning skills such as language and speech. They normally have **mental retardation**, partial or complete **paralysis**, and a smaller-than-normal head. Some babies have unilateral clefts, in which clefts appear on only one hemisphere of the brain. They may be paralyzed on one side of their bodies; however, these babies may not have any degradation to their intelligence.

Megalencephaly

Excessive brain size is termed megalencephaly (literally "big brain"). Megalencephaly, is a condition described as an infant or child with an abnormally large, heavy head for his/her age and gender. It occurs more often in males than females. Megalencephaly is usually associated with brain that does not function properly. It is defined as any brain size above the 98th percentile (about two standard deviations) within the population. Some cases are familial (common among families, hereditary), and may be entirely benign. Others are due to metabolic or neurologic disease. Unilateral megalencephaly—sometimes also called hemimegalencephaly—is characterized by only one side of the brain being abnormally large. Megalencephaly is different from macrocephaly, which is also referred to as megacephaly or megalocephaly. Macrocephaly is a condition in which a large head does not necessarily mean is it considered "abnormally" large. Microcephaly, an opposite condition to macrocephaly, is considered a condition involving a smaller-than-average brain, but one that is not necessarily considered abnormal. It may be caused by failure of the brain to develop, or by intrauterine infection, drug toxicity, or brain trauma.

Causes and symptoms

Causes

Congenital brain defects may have genetic, infectious, toxic, or traumatic causes. In most cases, a certain cause cannot be identified.

GENETIC CAUSES. Some brain defects are caused by trisomy, the inclusion of a third copy of a chromosome normally occurring in pairs. Most trisomies occur because of improper division of the chromosomes during formation of eggs or sperm. Trisomy of chromosome 9 can cause some cases of Dandy-Walker and Chiari II malformation. Some cases of holoprosencephaly are caused by trisomy of chromosome 13, while others are due to abnormalities in chromosomes 7 or 18. Individual gene defects, either inherited or spontaneous, are responsible for other cases of congenital brain malformations.

DRUGS. Drugs known to cause congenital brain defects when used by the mother during critical developmental periods include:

- anticonvulsant drugs
- retinoic acid and tretinoin
- warfarin
- alcohol
- cocaine

OTHER. Other causes of congenital brain defects include:

- intrauterine infections, including cytomegalovirus, rubella, herpes simplex, and varicella zoster
- maternal diabetes mellitus
- maternal phenylketonuria
- fetal trauma

Symptoms

Besides the features listed previously, symptoms of congenital brain defects may include:

- Chiari II malformation: impaired swallowing and gag reflex, loss of the breathing reflex, facial paralysis, uncontrolled eye movements (nystagmus), impaired balance and gait.
- Dandy-Walker malformation: symptoms of hydrocephalus, lack of muscle tone or "floppiness," seizures, vomiting, spasticity, deafness, abnormal breathing patterns, irritability, visual impairment, deterioration of consciousness, paralysis.
- Lissencephaly: lack of muscle tone, irregular facial features, difficulty swallowing, seizures, developmental delay, spasticity, cerebral palsy.
- Hydranencephaly: visual impairment, deafness, blindness, paralysis, irritability, spasticity, seizures, temperature oscillations, lower-than-normal intelligence.
- Megalencephaly due to neurological or metabolic disease: mental retardation, seizures, brain cortex and spinal cord disfunction.

Diagnosis

Congenital brain defects are diagnosed either from direct **physical examination** or imaging studies including computed tomography (CT) scans and **magnetic resonance imaging** (MRI) scans. **Electroencephalography** (EEG) may be used to reveal characteristic abnormalities.

Prenatal diagnosis of neural tube defects causing anencephaly or meningomyelocele is possible through ultrasound examination and maternal blood testing for alpha-fetoprotein, which is almost always elevated. Ultrasound can also be used to diagnose Dandy-Walker and Chiari II malformations. **Amniocentesis** may reveal trisomies or other chromosomal abnormalities. Myelomeningocele is tested with a maternal serum alpha-fetoprotein (MSAFP) test, which tests the mother for alpha-fetoprotein (AFP), a protein that is produced by the fetus. Along with the MSAFP test, three other bloods tests may be used: human chorionic gonadotropin (HCG, a hormone produced by the placenta), Inhibin A (a hormone produced by the placenta), and Estriol (an estrogen produced by the fetus and placenta)

Treatment

Treatment generally varies depending on the type of defect. Meningomyelocele may be treated with surgery to close the open portion of the spinal cord. Surgery for encephalocele is possible only if there is a minimal amount of brain tissue protruding. Malformations associated with hydrocephalus (Dandy-Walker, Chiari II, and some cases of hydranencephaly) may be treated by installation of a drainage

KEY TERMS

Amniocentesis—Removal of fluid from the sac surrounding a fetus for purposes of diagnosis.

Cerebrospinal fluid—Fluid produced within the brain for nutrient transport and structural purposes. CSF circulates through the ventricles, open spaces within the brain, and drains through the membranes surrounding the brain.

Congenital—Defect present at birth.

Fetus—The unborn human, developing in a woman's uterus, from the eighth week after fertilization to birth.

shunt for cerebrospinal fluid. Drugs may be used to treat some symptoms of brain defects, including seizures and spasticity.

Treatment for lissencephaly is unlikely to be successful in the most severe cases of it. However, support and care can be provided to the patient, and medication should control seizures. Treatment for megalencephaly has yet to be standardized. Treatment primarily depends on the symptoms and disabilities present with the patient.

Prognosis

Most congenital brain defects carry a very poor prognosis. Surgical treatment of meningomyelocele and encephalocele may be successful, with lasting neurological deficiencies, which vary in severity. Early treatment of hydrocephalus may prevent more severe brain damage. Infants and children with megalencephaly have a varied prognosis depending on the underlying cause and the related neurological disorder. For children with hemimegalencephaly, the prognosis is generally poor.

Prevention

Some cases of congenital brain defects can be prevented with good maternal **nutrition**, including **folic acid** supplements. Folic acid is a vitamin that has been shown to reduce the incidence of neural tube defects, both before and during pregnancy. Pregnant women should avoid exposure to infection, especially during the first trimester. Abstention from drugs and alcohol during pregnancy may reduce risk. **Genetic counseling** is advisable for parents who

have had one child with anencephaly, since the likelihood of having another is increased.

Resources

BOOKS

David, Ronald B., et al., editors. *Clinical Pediatric Neurology.* New York: Demos Medical, 2009.

Ferretti, Patrizia, et al. *Embryos, Genes, and Birth Defects.* Chichester, UK: Wiley, 2006.

Levene, Malcolm L, and Frank A. Chervenak, editors. *Fetal and Neonatal Neurology and Neurosurgery.* Edinburgh, Scotland: Churchill Livingstone/Elsevier, 2009.

OTHER

Anencephaly. Medline Plus, National Library of Medicine and National Institutes of Health. (May 12, 2009), http://www.nlm.nih.gov/medlineplus/ency/article/001580.htm (accessed September 10, 2010).

Dandy Walker Malformation. WebMD. (February 21, 2010), http://children.webmd.com/dandy-walker-malformation (accessed September 10, 2010).

Encephalocele. Centers of Disease Control and Prevention. (October 28, 2009), http://www.cdc.gov/ncbddd/birth defects/Encephalocele.htm (accessed September 10, 2010).

Holoprosencephaly. National Institute of Neurological Disorders and Stroke. (February 13, 2007), http://www.ninds.nih.gov/disorders/holoprosencephaly/holopro sencephaly.htm (accessed September 10, 2010).

Lissencephaly. Cleveland Clinic. (March 9, 2009), http://my.clevelandclinic.org/disorders/lissencephaly/hic_lissencephaly.aspx (accessed September 10, 2010).

Megalencephaly. National Institute of Neurological Disorders and Stroke. (March 9, 2009), http://www.ninds.nih.gov/disorders/megalencephaly/megalencephaly.htm (accessed September 10, 2010).

Schizencephaly. National Institute of Neurological Disorders and Stroke. (May 5, 2010), http://www.ninds.nih.gov/disorders/schizencephaly/schizencephaly.htm (accessed September 10, 2010).

Spina Bifida. Mayo Clinic. (October 3, 2009), http://www.mayoclinic.com/health/spina-bifida/DS00417 (accessed September 10, 2010).

ORGANIZATIONS

American Academy of Pediatrics, 141 Northwest Point Boulevard, Elk Grove Village, IL, 60007-1098, (847) 434-4000, http://www.aap.org/.

National Institute of Neurological Disorders and Stroke, Post Office Box 5801, Bethesda, MD, 20824, (301) 496-5751, (800) 352-9424, (301) 402-2186, http://www.ninds.nih.gov/.

National Organization for Rare Disorders, Post Office Box 1968; 55 Kenosia Avenue, Danbury, CT, 06813-1968, (203) 744-0100, (800) 999-6673, (203) 798-2291, http://www.rarediseases.org.

March of Dimes Foundation, 1275 Mamaroneck Avenue, White Plains, NY, 10605, (914) 997-4488, http://www.marchofdimes.com/.

Office of Rare Diseases Research, 6100 Executive Boulevard, Bethesda, MD, 20892-7518, (301) 402-4336, (888) 205-2311, (301) 480-9655, ordr@od.nih.gov, http://rarediseases.info.nih.gov/Default.aspx.

Richard Robinson

Congenital defects *see* **Birth defects**

Congenital heart disease

Definition

Congenital heart disease, also called congenital heart defect, includes a variety of malformations of the heart and/or its major blood vessels that are present at birth.

Description

Congenital heart disease occurs when the heart or blood vessels entering or leaving the heart do not develop normally before birth. Some infants are born with mild types of congenital heart disease that do not become apparent until later in life, but others need surgery as newborns or infants in order to survive.

Congenital heart disease is the most common birth defect. About 35,000 infants are born each year with some form of congenital heart disease. About half of these cases require medical treatment; the rest either correct (resolve) spontaneously shortly after birth or are so mild as to need no treatment or to go undetected. More than 1.4 million people with congenital heart defects were living in the United States in 2007.

Anatomy of the heart

The heart has four compartments or chambers, a left and right atrium above a left and right ventricle. These chambers keep blood carrying oxygen (oxygenated blood) from mixing with blood that has already given up its oxygen to cells (deoxygenated blood). Blood moves through the heart in a specific pattern. Deoxygenated blood returning from the body enters the right atrium. It moves through a valve into the right ventricle. When the right ventricle contracts, blood is pumped through another valve and is carried to the lungs where it picks up oxygen. The newly oxygenated blood returns to heart and enters the left atrium. It flows through a valve into the left ventricle, and is then pumped through another valve to the aorta, a large artery. From the aorta, oxygenated blood is distributed to the rest of the body. Congenital heart disease causes a disruption or inefficiency in this pattern.

There are many types of congenital heart defects, but they fall into four major categories:

- defects that obstruct the flow of blood to the heart, lungs, or the nearby blood vessels. This can be caused by narrowed or malformed blood vessels or heart valves.
- defects that allow oxygenated and deoxygenated blood to mix. This can be caused by holes in the partitions (septa) between chambers or leaky valves that separate the chambers.
- arrhythmias, which are defects in the timing of contractions of the various chambers so that the chambers do not fill and empty completely; heartbeat may be too fast, too slow, or uncoordinated.
- major structural defects such as missing or underdeveloped heart chambers or incorrectly located blood vessels.

Obstruction defects

When heart valves, arteries, or veins are narrowed, they partly or completely block the flow of blood. The most common obstruction defects are **pulmonary valve stenosis**, **aortic valve stenosis**, and **coarctation of the aorta**. Bicuspid aortic valve and subaortic stenosis are less common.

Stenosis is a narrowing of the valves or arteries. In pulmonary stenosis, the pulmonary valve does not open properly, forcing the right ventricle to work harder. In aortic stenosis, the improperly formed aortic valve is narrowed. As the left ventricle works harder to pump blood through the body, it becomes enlarged. In coarctation of the aorta, the aorta is constricted, reducing the flow of blood to the lower part of the body and increasing blood pressure in the upper body.

A bicuspid aortic valve has only two flaps instead of three, which can lead to stenosis in adulthood. Subaortic stenosis is a narrowing of the left ventricle below the aortic valve that limits the flow of blood from the left ventricle.

Cyanotic defects

Heart defects that cause a decreased, inadequate amount of oxygen in blood pumped to the body are called cyanotic defects. When a baby is born with a hole in the septum (the wall separating the right and left sides of the heart), blood can leak from one chamber to another, allowing oxygenated and deoxygenated blood to mix. This causes less oxygen to be delivered to the body. Major leakage can lead to enlargement of the heart and failing circulation. The most common types of septal defects are **atrial septal defect**, an opening between the two upper heart chambers, and **ventricular septal defect**, an opening between the two lower heart chambers. Ventricular septal defect accounts for about 15% of all cases of congenital heart disease in the United States.

Patent ductus arteriosus refers to the opening of a temporary blood vessel (ductus) that carries blood from the heart to the aorta before birth, allowing blood to bypass the lungs, which are not yet functional. The ductus should close spontaneously in the first few hours or days after birth. When it does not close in the newborn, some of the blood that should flow through the aorta returns to the lungs. Patent ductus arteriosus is common in premature babies, but rare in full-term babies. It also has been associated with mothers who had German **measles (rubella)** while pregnant.

Ebstein's anomaly is a rare congenital syndrome that causes malformed tricuspid valve leaflets, which allow blood to leak between the right ventricle and the right atrium. It also may cause a hole in the wall between the left and right atrium. Treatment often involves repairing the tricuspid valve.

Other cyanotic defects, including truncus arteriosus, total anomalous pulmonary venous return, and **tetralogy of Fallot**, result in a blue discoloration of the skin due to low oxygen levels. About 10% of cases of congenital heart disease in the United States are tetralogy of Fallot, which includes four defects. The major defects are a large hole between the ventricles, which allows oxygen-poor blood to mix with oxygen-rich blood, and narrowing at or beneath the pulmonary valve. The other defects are an overly muscular right ventricle and an aorta that lies over the ventricular hole.

Major structural defects

In transposition (reversal of position) of the great arteries, the pulmonary artery and the aorta are reversed, causing oxygenated blood to recirculate to the lungs while deoxygenated blood goes to the rest of the body. In tricuspid atresia, the baby lacks a triscupid valve and blood cannot flow properly from the right atrium to the right ventricle.

Hypoplastic left heart syndrome, a condition in which the left side of the heart is underdeveloped, is rare, but it is the most serious type of congenital heart disease. With this condition, blood reaches the aorta only from the ductus, which then closes normally within a few days of birth. In hypoplastic left heart syndrome, the baby seems normal at birth, but as the ductus closes, blood cannot reach the aorta and circulation fails.

Infants born with DiGeorge sequence can have heart defects such as a malformed aortic arch and tetralogy of Fallot. Researchers believe DiGeorge sequence most often is caused by mutations in genes in the region 22q11.

Other defects

Brugada syndrome is another rare congenital heart defect that appears in adulthood and may cause sudden **death** if untreated. Symptoms, which include rapid, uneven heart beat, often appear at night. Scientists believe that Brugada syndrome is caused by mutations in the gene SCN5A, which involves cardiac **sodium** channels.

Marfan syndrome is a connective tissue disorder that causes tears in the aorta. Since the disease also causes excessive bone growth, most Marfan syndrome patients are over six feet tall. In athletes, and others, it can lead to sudden death. Researchers believe the defect responsible for Marfan's syndrome is found in gene FBN1, on chromosome 15.

Causes and symptoms

In most cases, the causes of congenital heart disease are unknown. Genetic, environmental, and lifestyle factors all can be involved. The likelihood of having a child with congenital heart disease increases if a parent or other close relative has congenital heart disease or if there is a family history of early **sudden cardiac death**. Congenital heart disease is common in children with other genetic disorders that affect many organ systems, such **Down syndrome**. In addition, as of 2008, researchers had identified about ten genetic changes (mutations) that caused some type of congenital heart disease, but no widespread symptoms.

During **pregnancy**, viral infections such as German measles can result in congenital heart disease in the newborn. Women with diabetes and **phenylketonuria** (PKU, an inherited liver disorder) also are at higher risk of having children with congenital heart defects. Some cases of congenital heart disease result from the mother's excessive use of alcohol or taking illegal street drugs, such as **cocaine** or methamphetamines, during pregnancy. The mother's use of certain anticonvulsant (anti-seizure) drugs or dermatologic drugs (e.g., isotretinon [Accutane and other brand names], thalidomide) during pregnancy also can cause congenital heart disease.

Symptoms of congenital heart disease in general include **shortness of breath**, difficulty feeding in infancy, excessive sweating, **cyanosis** (bluish discoloration of the skin), heart murmur, respiratory infections that recur excessively, stunted growth, and limbs and muscles that are underdeveloped.

Symptoms of specific types of congenital heart disease are as follows:

- Patent ductus arteriosus: quick tiring, slow growth, susceptibility to pneumonia, rapid breathing. If the ductus is small, there are no symptoms.
- Hypoplastic left heart syndrome: ashen color, rapid and difficult breathing, inability to eat.
- Obstruction defects: cyanosis (skin that is discolored blue), chest pain, tiring easily, dizziness or fainting, congestive heart failure, and high blood pressure.
- Septal defects: difficulty breathing, stunted growth. Sometimes there are no symptoms.
- Cyanotic defects: cyanosis, sudden rapid breathing or unconsciousness, and shortness of breath and fainting during exercise.

Diagnosis

Echocardiography and cardiac **magnetic resonance imaging** (MRI) commonly are used to confirm congenital heart disease when it is suggested by the symptoms and **physical examination**. These are noninvasive (nothing enters the body) tests. An echocardiograph displays an image of the heart that is formed by sound waves. It may detect valve and other heart problems. Fetal echocardiography is used to help diagnose congenital heart disease in utero, usually after 20 weeks of pregnancy. Between 10 and 14 weeks of pregnancy, physicians also may use an ultrasound to look for a thickness at the nuchal translucency, a pocket of fluid in back of the embryo's neck, which may indicate a cardiac defect. Cardiac MRI, a scanning method that uses magnetic fields and radio waves, can help physicians evaluate congenital heart disease, but is not always necessary. Physicians also may use a **chest x ray** to look at the size and location of the heart and lungs, or an electrocardiograph (ECG), which measures electrical impulses to create a graph of the heartbeat. After birth pulse oximetry is a noninvasive way to measure the amount of oxygen in the blood (a sensor is clipped on a finger or toe). **Cardiac catheterization**, an invasive test done under anesthesia, allows a dye to be inserted into the heart so that blood circulation through the heart can be seen on an x ray. Cardiac catheterization also can measure pressure in the heart chambers to determine if there is blood mixing or leakage between heart chambers.

Treatment

Congenital heart disease is treated with drugs and/or surgery. Drugs used include **diuretics**, which increase the excretion water and salts, and **digoxin**, which strengthens the contraction of the heart, slows the heartbeat, and removes fluid from tissues.

Surgical procedures seek to repair the defect as much as possible and restore circulation to as close to normal as possible. Sometimes, multiple surgical procedures are necessary. Surgical procedures include arterial switch, balloon atrial septostomy, **balloon valvuloplasty**, Damus-Kaye-Stansel procedure, Fontan procedure, pulmonary artery banding, Ross procedure, shunt procedure, and venous switch or intra-atrial baffle.

Arterial switch, to correct **transposition of the great arteries**, involves connecting the aorta to the left ventricle and connecting the pulmonary artery to the right ventricle. Balloon atrial septostomy, also done to correct transposition of the great arteries, enlarges the atrial opening during heart catheterization. Balloon valvuloplasty uses a balloon-tipped catheter to open a narrowed heart valve, improving the flow of blood in pulmonary stenosis. It is sometimes used in aortic stenosis. Transposition of the great arteries also can be corrected by the Damus-Kaye-Stansel procedure, in which the pulmonary artery is cut in two and connected to the ascending aorta and the farthest section of the right ventricle.

For tricuspid atresia and pulmonary atresia, the Fontan procedure connects the right atrium to the pulmonary artery directly or with a conduit, and the atrial defect is closed. Pulmonary artery banding, narrowing the pulmonary artery with a band to reduce blood flow and pressure in the lungs, is used for ventricular septal defect, atrioventricular canal defect, and tricuspid atresia. Later, the band can be removed and the defect corrected with open-heart surgery.

To correct aortic stenosis, the Ross procedure grafts the pulmonary artery to the aorta. For tetralogy of Fallot, tricuspid atresia, or pulmonary atresia, the shunt procedure creates a passage between blood vessels, sending blood into parts of the body that need it. For transposition of the great arteries, venous switch creates a tunnel inside the atria to redirect oxygen-rich

KEY TERMS

Aorta—The main artery located above the heart that pumps oxygenated blood out into the body. Many congenital heart defects affect the aorta.

Atrium (plural: atria)—The right or left upper chamber of the heart.

Cardiac catheterization—A diagnostic procedure (using a catheter inserted through a vein and threaded through the circulatory system to the heart) which does a comprehensive examination of how the heart and its blood vessels function.

Congenital—Refers to a disorder that is present at birth.

Cyanotic—Marked by bluish discoloration of the skin due to a lack of oxygen in the blood. It is one of the types of congenital heart disease.

Ductus—The blood vessel that joins the pulmonary artery and the aorta. When the ductus does not close at birth, it causes a type of congenital heart disease called patent ductus arteriosus.

Echocardiogram—A non-invasive imaging procedure used to create a picture of the heart's movement, valves, and chambers.

Electrocardiograph (ECG, EKG)—A test used to measure electrical impulses coming from the heart in order to gain information about its structure or function.

Endocarditis—Infection of the heart endocardium tissue, the inner most tissue and structures of the heart.

Hypoplastic—Incomplete or underdevelopment of a tissue or organ. Hypoplastic left heart syndrome is the most serious type of congenital heart disease.

Marfan syndrome—An inherited condition that affects connective tissue throughout the body including weakening the connective tissue found in arteries.

Neuchal translucency—A pocket of fluid at the back of an embryo's neck visible via ultrasound that, when thickened, may indicate the infant will be born with a congenital heart defect.

Septal—Relating to the septum, the thin muscle wall dividing the right and left sides of the heart. Holes in the septum are called septal defects.

Stenosis (plural: stenoses)—The narrowing or constriction of an opening or passageway in the body.

Ventricle—A lower pumping chambers of the heart. There are two ventricles, right and left. The right ventricle pumps oxygen-poor blood to the lungs to be re-oxygenated. The left ventricle pumps oxygen-rich blood to the body.

blood to the right ventricle and aorta and venous blood to the left ventricle and pulmonary artery.

When surgery is not a viable option to correct the problem, some patients undergo a heart transplant. Children with congenital heart disease require lifelong monitoring, even after successful surgery. The American Heart Association recommends regular dental check-ups and preventive use of **antibiotics** to protect patients from heart infection (**endocarditis**). However, a 2003 study reported that preventive antibiotics are underused in people with congenital heart disease. Many patients did not understand the risk of endocarditis. Since children with congenital heart disease often have slower growth, good **nutrition** is important. Physicians also may limit their athletic activity.

Prognosis

The outlook for children with congenital heart disease has improved markedly in the past two decades. Many types of congenital heart disease that would have been fatal now can be treated successfully.

Because many children with these defects survive into adulthood, they will require continued medical observation as they mature. Research on diagnosing heart defects when the fetus is in the womb may lead to future treatment to correct some defects before birth. Promising new prevention methods and treatments include genetic screening and the cultivation of cardiac tissue in the laboratory that might be useful in repairing some congenital heart defects. As scientists continue to advance the study of genetics, they also will better understand genetic causes of many congenital heart diseases.

Resources

BOOKS

Gerber, Max S. *My Heart vs. the Real World: Children with Heart Disease, In Photographs & Interviews.* Cold Spring Harbor, NY: Cold Spring Harbor Laboratory Press, 2008.

Hoffman, Julien I.E. *The Natural and Unnatural History of Congenital Heart Disease.* Chichester, UK; Hoboken, NJ: Wiley–Blackwell, 2009.

Warnes, Carole A. *Adult Congenital Heart Disease*. Chichester, UK; Hoboken, NJ: Wiley–Blackwell, 2009.

OTHER

"Congenital Heart Defects." *MedlinePlus*. February 11, 2009 [cited February 12, 2009]. http://www.nlm.nih.gov/medlineplus/congenitalheartdefects.html

"Fact Sheet: Congenital Heart Defects." *March of Dimes*. May 2008 [cited February 12, 2009]. http://www.marchofdimes.com/professionals/14332_1212.asp

National Heart, Lung, and Blood Institute. "Congenital Heart Defects." *Medicinenet.com*. May 12, 2008 [cited February 12, 2009]. http://www.medicinenet.com/congenital_heart_disease/article.htm

ORGANIZATIONS

American Heart Association National Center, 7272 Greenville Avenue, Dallas, TX, 75231, (800) 242-8721, Review.personal.info@heart.org.

Congenital Heart Information Network (C.H.I.N.), 101 N. Washington Ave., Suite 1A, Margate City, NJ, 08402-1195, (609) 882-1572, (609) 822-1574, mb@tchin.org, http://tchin.org/.

March of Dimes Birth Defects Foundation, 1275 Mamaroneck Ave., White Plains, NY, 10605, (914) 997-4488, http://www.modimes.org.

National Heart Lung and Blood Institute Health Information Center, P.O. Box 30105, Bethesda, MD, 20824-0105, (301) 592-8573, (240) 629-3246, http://www.nhlbi.nih.gov.

Melissa Knopper
Teresa G. Odle
Tish Davidson, A.M.

Congenital hip dysplasia

Definition

A condition of abnormal development of the hip, resulting in hip joint instability and potential dislocation of the thigh bone from the socket in the pelvis. This condition has been more recently termed developmental hip dysplasia, as it often develops over the first few weeks, months, or years of life.

Description

Congenital hip dysplasia is a disorder in children that is either present at birth or shortly thereafter. During gestation, the infant's hip should be developing with the head of the thigh bone (femur) sitting perfectly centered in its shallow socket (acetabulum).

The acetabulum should cover the head of the femur as if it were a ball sitting inside of a cup. In the event of congenital hip dysplasia, the development of the acetabulum in an infant allows the femoral head to ride upward out of the joint socket, especially when weight bearing begins.

Causes and symptoms

Clinical studies show a familial tendency toward hip dysplasia, with more females affected than males. This disorder is found in many cultures around the world. However, statistics show that the Native American population has a high incidence of hip dislocation. This has been documented to be due to the common practice of swaddling and using cradleboards for restraining the infants. This places the infant's hips into extreme adduction (brought together). The incidence of congenital hip dysplasia is also higher in infants born by caesarian and breech position births. Evidence also shows a greater chance of this hip abnormality in the first born compared to the second or third child. Hormonal changes within the mother during **pregnancy**, resulting in increased ligament laxity, is thought to possibly cross over to the placenta and cause the baby to have lax ligaments while still in the womb. Other symptoms of complete dislocation include a shortening of the leg and limited ability to abduct the leg.

Diagnosis

Because the abnormalities of this hip problem often vary, a thorough **physical examination** is necessary for an accurate diagnosis of congenital hip dysplasia. The hip disorder can be diagnosed by moving the hip to determine if the head of the femur is moving in and out of the hip joint. One specific method, called the Ortolani test, begins with each of the examiner's hands around the infant's knees, with the second and third fingers pointing down the child's thigh. With the legs abducted (moved apart), the examiner may be able to discern a distinct clicking sound with motion. If symptoms are present with a noted increase in abduction, the test is considered positive for hip joint instability. It is important to note this test is only valid a few weeks after birth.

The Barlow method is another test performed with the infant's hip brought together with knees in full bent position. The examiner's middle finger is placed over the outside of the hipbone while the thumb is placed on the inner side of the knee. The hip is abducted to where it can be felt if the hip is sliding out and then back in the joint. In older babies, if there is a lack of range of motion in one hip or even both hips, it is possible that the movement is blocked because the hip has dislocated and the muscles have contracted in that position. Also in older infants, hip dislocation is evident if one leg looks shorter than the other.

X-ray films can be helpful in detecting abnormal findings of the hip joint. X rays may also be helpful in finding the proper positioning of the hip joint for treatments of casting. Ultrasound has been noted as a safe and effective tool for the diagnosis of congenital hip dysplasia. Ultrasound has advantages over x rays, as several positions are noted during the ultrasound procedure. This is in contrast to only one position observed during the x ray.

Treatment

The objective of treatment is to replace the head of the femur into the acetabulum and, by applying constant pressure, to enlarge and deepen the socket. In the past, stabilization was achieved by placing rolled cotton diapers or a pillow between the thighs, thereby keeping the knees in a frog like position. More recently, the Pavlik harness and von Rosen splint are commonly used in infants up to the age of six months. A stiff shell cast may be used, which achieves the same purpose, spreading the legs apart and forcing the head of the femur into the acetabulum. In some cases, in older children between 6 to 18 months, surgery may be necessary to reposition the joint. Also at this age, the use of closed manipulation may be applied successfully, by moving the leg around manually to replace joint. Operations are not only performed to reduce the dislocation of the hip, but also to repair a defect in the acetabulum. A cast is applied after the operation to hold the head of the femur in the correct position. The use of a home **traction** program is now more common. However, after the age of eight years, surgical procedures are primarily done for **pain** reduction measures only. Total hip surgeries may be inevitable later in adulthood.

Alternative treatment

Nonsurgical treatments include **exercise** programs, orthosis (a force system, often involving braces), and medications. A physical therapist may develop a program that includes strengthening, range-of-motion exercises, pain control, and functional activities. **Chiropractic** medicine may be helpful, especially the procedures of closed manipulations, to reduce the dislocated hip joint.

Prognosis

Unless corrected soon after birth, abnormal stresses cause malformation of the developing femur, with a characteristic limp or waddling gait. If cases of congenital hip dysplasia go untreated, the child will have difficulty walking, which could result in life-long pain. In addition, if this condition goes untreated, the abnormal hip positioning will force the acetabulum to locate to another position to accommodate the displaced femur.

Prevention

Prevention includes proper prenatal care to determine the position of the baby in the womb. This may be helpful in preparing for possible breech births associated with hip problems. Avoiding excessive and prolonged infant hip adduction may help prevent strain on the hip joints. Early diagnosis remains an important part of prevention of congenital hip dysplasia.

ORGANIZATIONS

March of Dimes Birth Defects Foundation, 1275 Mamaroneck Ave., White Plains, NY, 10605, (914) 997-4488, http://www.modimes.org.

Jeffrey P. Larson, RPT

Congenital lobar emphysema

Definition

Congenital lobar **emphysema** is a chronic disease that causes respiratory distress in infants.

Description

Congenital lobar emphysema, also called infantile lobar emphysema, is a respiratory disease that occurs in infants when air enters the lungs but cannot leave easily. The lungs become over-inflated, causing respiratory function to decrease and air to leak out into the space around the lungs.

Half of the cases of congenital lobar emphysema occur in the first four weeks of life, and three-quarters occur in infants less than six months old. Congenital lobar emphysema is more common in boys than in girls.

Each person has two lungs, right and left. The right lung is divided into three sections, called lobes, and the left lung into two lobes. Congenital lobar emphysema usually affects only one lobe, and this is usually an upper lobe. It occurs most frequently in the left upper lobe, followed by the right middle lobe.

Causes and symptoms

The cause of congenital lobar emphysema often cannot be identified. The airway may be obstructed or the infant's lungs may not have developed properly. Congenital lobar emphysema is almost never of genetic origin.

Symptoms of congenital lobar emphysema include:

- shortness of breath
- wheezing
- lips and fingernail beds that have a bluish tinge

Diagnosis

Congenital lobar emphysema is usually identified within the first two weeks of the infant's life. It is diagnosed by respiratory symptoms and a **chest x ray**, which shows the over-inflation of the affected lobe and may show a blocked air passage.

Treatment

For infants with no, mild, or intermittent symptoms, no treatment is necessary. For more serious cases of congenital lobar emphysema, surgery is necessary, usually a **lobectomy** to remove the affected lung lobe.

Alternative treatment

Alternative treatments that may be helpful for congenital lobar emphysema are aimed at supporting and strengthening the patient's respiratory function. Vitamin and mineral supplementation may be recommended as may herbal remedies such as lobelia (*Lobelia inflata*) that strengthen the lungs and enhance their elasticity. Homeopathic constitutional care may also be beneficial for this condition.

KEY TERMS

Congenital—A disease or condition that is present at birth.

Emphysema—A condition in which the air sacs in the lungs become overinflated, causing a decrease in respiratory function.

Lobar—Relating to a lobe, a rounded projecting part of the lungs.

Prognosis

Surgery for congenital lobar emphysema has excellent results.

Prevention

Congenital lobar emphysema cannot be prevented.

ORGANIZATIONS

American Lung Association, 1301 Pennsylvania Ave. NW, Suite 800, Washington, DC, 20001, (202) 758-3355, (202) 452-1805, (800) 548-8252, info@lungusa.org, http://www.lungusa.org/.

National Heart Lung and Blood Institute Health Information Center, P.O. Box 30105, Bethesda, MD, 20824-0105, (301) 592-8573, (240) 629-3246, http://www.nhlbi.nih.gov.

Lori De Milto

Congenital megacolon *see* **Hirschsprung's disease**

Congenital thymic hypoplasia *see* **DiGeorge syndrome**

Congenital ureter anomalies

Definition

The ureter drains urine from the kidney into the bladder. It is not simply a tube but an active organ that propels urine forward by muscular action. It has a valve at its bottom end that prevents urine from flowing backward into the kidney. Normally there is one ureter on each side of the body for each kidney. However, among the many abnormalities of ureteral development, duplication is quite common. Ureters may also be malformed in a variety of ways–some harmful, others not.

Description

The urogenital system, for some reason, is more likely than any other to have **birth defects**, and they can occur in endless variety. Ureters can be duplicated completely or partially, they can be in the wrong place, they can be deformed, and they can end in the wrong place. The trouble these abnormalities bring is directly related to their effect on the flow of urine. As long as urine flows normally through them, and only in one direction, no harm is done.

- Duplication of ureters is quite common, either in part or completely. Kidneys are sometimes duplicated as well. Someone may have four kidneys and four ureters or two kidneys, half of each drained by a separate ureter, or a single kidney with two, three, or four ureters attached. As long as urine can flow easily in the correct direction, such malformations may never be detected. If, however, one of the ureters has a dead end, a stricture or stenosis (narrowing), or a leaky ureterovesical valve (valve between the ureter and bladder), infection is the likely result.

- Stricture or stenosis of a ureter prevents urine from flowing freely. Whenever flow is obstructed in the body–urine, bile, mucus, or any other liquid–infection follows. Ureters can be obstructed anywhere along their course, though the ureterovesical valve is the most common place.

- A ureter may have an ectopic (out of place) orifice (opening)–it may enter the bladder, or even another structure, where it does not belong and therefore without an adequate valve to control reflux.

- The primary ureter, or a duplicate, may not even reach the bladder, but rather terminate in a dead end. Urine will stagnate there and eventually cause infection.

- A ureter can be perfectly normal but in the wrong place, such as behind the vena cava (the large vein in the middle of the abdomen). A so-called retrocaval ureter may be pinched by the vena cava so that flow is hindered. Other aberrant locations may also lead to compression and impaired flow.

Besides infection, urine that backs up will cause the ureter and the kidney to dilate. Eventually, the kidney will stop functioning because of the back pressure. This condition is called hydronephrosis–a kidney swollen with urine.

Causes and symptoms

The causes of birth defects are multiple and often unknown. Furthermore, the precise cause of specific birth defects has only rarely been identified. Such is the case with congenital ureteral anomalies.

Practically the only symptom generated by ureteral abnormalities is **urinary tract infection**. A lower tract infection–in the bladder–is called **cystitis**. In children, it may cause **fever** and systemic symptoms, but in adults it causes only cloudy, burning, and frequent urine. Upper tract infections, on the other hand, can be serious for both adults and children, causing high fevers, back **pain**, severe generalized discomfort, and even leading to kidney failure or septicemia (infection spreading throughout the body by way of the blood stream).

In rare cases, urine from an ectopic ureter will bypass the bladder and dribble out of the bottom somewhere, through a natural orifice like the vagina or a completely separate unnatural opening.

Diagnosis

Serious or recurrent urinary infections will prompt a search for underlying abnormalities. **Cystoscopy** (looking into the bladder with a thin telescope-like instrument) and x rays with a contrast agent to illuminate the urinary system will usually identify the defect. **Computed tomography scans** (CT) and **Magnetic resonance imaging** (MRI) may provide additional information. Urine cultures to identify the infecting germs will be repeated frequently until the problem is corrected.

Treatment

Sometimes the recurring infections caused by flow abnormalities can be treated with repeated and changing courses of **antibiotics**. Over time, the infecting germs develop resistance to most treatments, especially the safer ones. If it can be done with acceptable risk, it is better to repair the defect surgically. Urologists have an arsenal of approaches to urine drainage that range from simply reimplanting a ureter into the bladder, in such a way that an effective valve is created, to building a new bladder out of a piece of bowel.

Alternative treatment

There are botanical and homeopathic treatments available for urinary tract infection. None can take the place of correcting a problem that is occurring because of a malformed or dysfunctional organ system. Once correction of the cause is addressed and there is unimpeded flow of urine, adequate fluid intake can contribute to prevention of future infections.

KEY TERMS

Congenital—Present at birth.

Contrast agent—A chemical or other substance placed in the body to show structures that would not otherwise be visible on x ray or other imaging studies.

Cystoscopy—Looking into the urinary bladder with a thin telescope-like instrument.

Ectopic—Out of place.

Septicemia—A serious whole body infection spreading through the blood stream.

Ureterovesical valve—A sphincter (an opening controlled by a circular muscle), located where the ureter enters the bladder, that keeps urine from flowing backward toward the kidney.

Urogenital—Both the urinary system and the sexual organs, which form together in the developing embryo.

Prognosis

As long as damage to the kidneys from infection or back pressure has not become significant, the surgical repair of troublesome ureteral defects produces excellent long-term results in the great majority of cases. Monitoring for recurrent infections is always a good idea, and occasional checking of kidney function will detect hidden ongoing damage.

Resources

BOOKS

Tanagho, Emil A., Jack W McAninch, and Donald Ridgeway Smith. *Smith's General Urology*. New York: McGraw–Hill Medical, 2008.

J. Ricker Polsdorfer, MD

Congestive cardiomyopathy

Definition

Cardiomyopathy is an ongoing disease process that damages the muscle wall of the lower chambers of the heart. Congestive cardiomyopathy is the most common form of cardiomyopathy. In congestive cardiomyopathy, also called dilated cardiomyopathy, the walls of the heart chambers stretch (dilate) to hold a greater volume of blood than normal. Congestive cardiomyopathy is the final stage of many heart diseases and the most common condition resulting in congestive **heart failure**.

Description

About 50,000 Americans develop cardiomyopathy each year. Of those, 87% have congestive cardiomyopathy. Primary cardiomyopathy accounts for only 1% of all deaths from heart disease.

When the heart muscle is damaged by a disease process, it cannot pump enough blood to meet the body's needs. Uninjured areas of the walls of the two lower heart chambers (called ventricles) stretch to make up for the lost pumping action. At first, the enlarged chambers allow more blood to be pumped with less force. The stretched muscle can also contract more forcefully. Over time, the heart muscle continues to stretch, ultimately becoming weaker. The heart is forced to work harder to pump blood by beating faster. Eventually it cannot keep up, and blood backs up into the veins, legs, and lungs. When this happens, the condition is called congestive heart failure.

Congestive cardiomyopathy usually affects both ventricles. Blood backed up into the lungs from the left ventricle causes fluid to congest the lung tissue. This is called **pulmonary edema**. When the right ventricle fails to pump enough blood, blood backs up into the veins causing **edema** in the legs, feet, ankles, and abdomen.

Causes and symptoms

Congestive cardiomyopathy may be caused by a number of conditions. Cardiomyopathy with a known cause is called secondary cardiomyopathy. When no cause can be identified, it is called primary cardiomyopathy or idiopathic cardiomyopathy. About 80% of all cases of cardiomyopathy do not have a known cause. Many heart specialists think that many cases of idiopathic congestive cardiomyopathy may be caused by a viral infection. Because cardiomyopathy may occur many years after a viral infection and viruses sometimes go undetected in laboratory tests, it is difficult to know if a virus is the cause. Some people have a weak heart from advanced **coronary artery disease** that causes heart muscle damage. This is sometimes called ischemic cardiomyopathy.

Conditions that can cause congestive cardiomyopathy are:

- coronary artery disease
- infections
- noninfectious inflammatory conditions
- alcohol and other drugs or toxins

- hypertension
- nutritional and metabolic disorders
- pregnancy

Coronary artery disease is one of the most common causes of congestive cardiomyopathy. In coronary artery disease, the arteries supplying blood to the heart become narrowed or blocked. When blood flow to an area of the heart is completely blocked, the person has a **heart attack**. The heart muscle suffers damage when its blood supply is reduced or blocked. Significant recurrent muscle damage can occur silently. This damage can lead to congestive cardiomyopathy.

Infections caused by bacteria, viruses, and other microorganisms can involve the heart, causing inflammation of the heart muscle (**myocarditis**). The inflammation may damage the heart muscle and cause congestive cardiomyopathy. In the United States, the coxsackievirus B is the most common cause of viral congestive cardiomyopathy.

Myocarditis can also be caused by noninfectious disorders. For example, the conditions **sarcoidosis**, granulomatous myocarditis, and **Wegener's granulomatosis** cause inflammation and tissue **death** in the heart muscle.

Years of drinking excessive amounts of alcohol can weaken the heart muscle, leading to congestive cardiomyopathy. Other drugs and toxins, such as **cocaine**, pesticides, and other chemicals, may have the same effect.

High blood pressure (**hypertension**) puts extra pressure on blood vessels and the heart. This increased pressure makes the heart work harder to pump blood, which may thicken and damage the chamber walls.

Severe nutritional deficiencies can weaken the heart muscle and affect its pumping ability. Certain disorders of metabolism, including **diabetes mellitus** and thyroid disorders, can also lead to congestive cardiomyopathy.

Occasionally, inflammation of the heart muscle and congestive cardiomyopathy may develop late in **pregnancy** or shortly after a woman gives birth. This type of congestive cardiomyopathy is called peripartum cardiomyopathy. The cause of congestive cardiomyopathy in pregnancy is not known.

Congestive cardiomyopathy usually is a chronic condition, developing gradually over time. Patients with early congestive cardiomyopathy may not have symptoms. The most common symptoms are **fatigue** and **shortness of breath** on exertion. Unfortunately, **sudden cardiac death** is not uncommon with this condition. It stems from irregular heart rhythms in the ventricles (ventricular **arrhythmias**).

Patients with more advanced congestive cardiomyopathy may also have chest or abdominal pains, extreme tiredness, **dizziness**, and swelling of the legs and ankles.

Diagnosis

Diagnosis of congestive cardiomyopathy is based on:

- symptoms
- medical history
- physical examination
- chest x ray
- electrocardiogram (ECG; also called EKG)
- echocardiogram
- cardiac catheterization

The diagnosis is based on the patient's symptoms, a complete **physical examination**, and tests that detect abnormalities of the heart chambers. The physician listens to the heart with a stethoscope to detect abnormal heart rhythms and heart sounds. A heart murmur might mean that the heart valves are not closing properly due to the ventricles being enlarged.

A **chest x ray** can show if the heart is enlarged and if there is fluid in the lungs. Abnormalities of heart valves and other structures may also be seen on a chest x ray.

An electrocardiogram provides a record of electrical changes in the heart muscle during the heartbeat. It gives information on the heart rhythm and can show if the heart chamber is enlarged. An ECG can detect damage to the heart muscle and the amount of damage.

Echocardiography uses sound waves to make images of the heart. These images can show if the heart wall or chambers are enlarged and if there are any abnormalities of the heart valves. Echocardiography can also evaluate the pumping efficiency of the ventricles.

Cardiac catheterization usually is only used if a diagnosis cannot be made with other methods. In cardiac catheterization, a small tube (called a catheter) is inserted into an artery and passed into the heart. It is used to measure pressure in the heart and the amount of blood pumped by the heart. A small tissue sample of the heart muscle can be removed through the catheter for examination under a microscope (biopsy). This biopsy can show the type and amount of damage to the heart muscle.

Angiotensin-converting enzyme (ACE) inhibitor—A drug that relaxes blood vessel walls and lowers blood pressure.

Atherosclerosis—Buildup of a fatty substance called a plaque inside blood vessels.

Cardiac catheterization—A diagnostic test for evaluating heart disease; a catheter is inserted into an artery and passed into the heart.

Cardiomyopathy—Disease of the heart muscle.

Congestive cardiomyopathy—Also called dilated cardiomyopathy; cardiomyopathy in which the walls of the heart chambers stretch, enlarging the heart ventricles so they can hold a greater volume of blood than normal.

Coxsackievirus B—A type of virus in the group Enterovirus that causes an infection similar to polio, but without paralysis.

Digitalis—A drug that helps the heart muscle to have stronger pumping action.

Dilated cardiomyopathy—Also called congestive cardiomyopathy; cardiomyopathy in which the walls of the heart chambers stretch, enlarging the heart ventricles so they can hold a greater volume of blood than normal.

Diuretic—A type of drug that helps the kidneys eliminate excess salt and water.

Edema—Swelling caused by fluid buildup in tissues.

Granulomatous myocarditis—Also called giant cell myocarditis, this noninfectious inflammation of the heart causes large areas of tissue death in the heart muscle, ventricular enlargement, and clots inside the heart chambers.

Idiopathic cardiomyopathy—Cardiomyopathy without a known cause.

Sarcoidosis—A chronic disease that causes formation of abnormal areas containing inflammatory cells, called granulomas, in any organ or tissue; in the heart, large areas of the heart muscle can be involved, causing cardiomyopathy.

Vasodilator—Any drug that relaxes blood vessel walls.

Ventricle—One of the two lower chambers of the heart.

Wegener's granulomatosis—A disease usually affecting males that causes the infiltration of inflammatory cells and tissue death in the lungs, kidneys, blood vessels, heart, and other tissues.

Treatment

When a patient is diagnosed with congestive cardiomyopathy, physicians try to find out the cause. If coronary artery disease is not the culprit, in most other cases a cause is not identified. When a condition responsible for the congestive cardiomyopathy is diagnosed, treatment is aimed at correcting the underlying condition. Congestive cardiomyopathy caused by drinking excess alcohol or by drugs or toxins can be treated by eliminating the alcohol or toxin completely. In some cases, the heart may recover after the toxic substance is removed from the body. Bacterial myocarditis is treated with an antibiotic to eliminate the bacteria.

There is no cure for idiopathic congestive cardiomyopathy. Medicines are given to reduce the workload of the heart and to relieve the symptoms.

One or more of the following types of medicines may be prescribed for congestive cardiomyopathy:

- digitalis
- diuretics
- vasodilators
- beta blockers
- angiotensin converting enzyme inhibitors (ACE inhibitors)
- angiotensin receptor blockers

Digitalis helps the heart muscle to have stronger pumping action. **Diuretics** help eliminate excess salt and water from the kidneys by making patients urinate more often. This helps reduce the swelling caused by fluid buildup in the tissues. **Vasodilators**, **beta blockers**, and ACE inhibitors lower blood pressure and expand the blood vessels so blood can move more easily through them. This action makes it easier for the heart to pump blood through the vessels.

Patients may also be given anticoagulant medications to prevent clots from forming due to pooling of blood in the heart chambers. Medicines to prevent abnormal heart rhythms (arrhythmias) may be given, but some of these drugs can also reduce the force of heart contractions. Automatic implantable cardioverter defibrillators

(AICDs) can treat life-threatening arrhythmias, which are relatively common in severe cardiomyopathy.

Certain lifestyle changes may help reduce the workload on the heart and relieve symptoms. Some patients may need to change their diet, stop drinking alcohol, begin a physician-supervised **exercise** program, and/or stop **smoking**.

Severe congestive cardiomyopathy usually causes heart failure. When the heart muscle is damaged so severely that medicines cannot help, a heart transplant may be the only remaining treatment to be considered.

Prognosis

The outlook for a patient with congestive cardiomyopathy depends on the severity of the disease and the person's health. Generally, congestive cardiomyopathy worsens over time and the prognosis is not good. About 50% of patients with congestive cardiomyopathy live for five years after the diagnosis. Twenty five percent of patients are alive 10 years after diagnosis. Women with congestive cardiomyopathy live twice as long as men with the disease. Many of the deaths are caused by sudden abnormal heart rhythms.

Prevention

Because idiopathic congestive cardiomyopathy does not have a known cause, there is no sure way to prevent it. The best way to prevent congestive cardiomyopathy is to avoid known causes such as drinking excess alcohol or taking toxic drugs. Eating a nutritious diet and getting regular exercise to improve overall fitness also can help the heart to stay healthy.

Congestive cardiomyopathy may also be prevented by identifying and treating any conditions that might damage the heart muscle. These include high blood pressure and coronary artery disease. Regular blood pressure checks and obtaining immediate medical care for hypertension and symptoms of coronary artery disease, such as chest **pain**, are important to keep the heart functioning properly.

Finally, diagnosing and treating congestive cardiomyopathy before the heart becomes severely damaged may improve the outlook.

Resources

BOOKS

Hosenpud, Jeffrey D., and Barry H. Greenberg. *Congestive Heart Failure.* New York: Lippincott Williams & Wilkins, 2006.

Silver, Marc A. *Success With Heart Failure: Help and Hope for Those Coping With Congestive Heart Failure.* New York: Perseus Books Group, 2006.

PERIODICALS

Bates, Betsy. "Obese Children May Face Heart Failure in Their 20s." *Skin & Allergy News* (April 2007): 51.

Chin-Peuckert, Lily. "From the Heart." *CMAJ: Canadian Medical Association Journal* (February 27, 2007): 661–672.

Elliott, William T. "Pharmacology Watch: Avandia, Risk of Congestive Heart Failure Significant Safety Risk." *Infectious Disease Alert* (July 1, 2007).

Grant, Judith. "Chronic Heart Failure and Depression." *Australian Nursing Journal* (May 2006): 35.

Satpathy, Chhabi, et al. "Diagnosis and Management of Diastolic Dysfunction and Heart Failure." *American Family Physician* (March 1, 2006): 841.

Sullivan, Michele G. "Ibuprofen Plus Aspirin Might Pose Risks for Some." *Family Practice News* (May 15, 2007): 12.

ORGANIZATIONS

American Heart Association National Center, 7272 Greenville Avenue, Dallas, TX, 75231, (800) 242-8721, Review.personal.info@heart.org.

Heart and Stroke Foundation of Canada, 222 Queen Street, Suite 1402, Ottawa, CanadaON, K1P 5V9, (613) 569-4361, (613) 569-3278, http://www.heartandstroke.com.

Heart Association of Australia, Level 3, 80 William Street, Sydney, Australia, NSW 2011, 02 02 9219 2444, reception.sydney@heartfoundation.org.au, http://www.heartfoundation.org.au.

National Heart Lung and Blood Institute Health Information Center, P.O. Box 30105, Bethesda, MD, 20824-0105, (301) 592-8573, (240) 629-3246, http://www.nhlbi.nih.gov.

Toni Rizzo
Ken R. Wells

Congestive heart failure

Definition

Congestive **heart failure** (CHF) is a chronic, progressive condition in which the heart gradually becomes unable to pump enough blood to meet the needs of the body. This can result in failure of other organs and **death**. CHF is the leading cause of hospitalizations of people over age 65.

Description

The heart is a muscle containing four compartments or chambers that separate oxygen-poor blood from oxygen-rich blood. The atria are the top chambers. They receive blood from the body. The ventricles are the bottom chambers. They pump blood out to the body. Oxygen-poor blood enters the right atrium, then moves through a valve to the right ventricle. It is then pumped out of the right ventricle to the lungs where it picks up oxygen. The oxygen-rich blood returns to the left atrium of the heart, flows through a valve to the left ventricle, and is then pumped out to the body. This sequence occurs with every heartbeat. The timing of the contraction of each chamber of the heart must be tightly coordinated in order for each chamber empty efficiently and completely.

In CHF, the heart fails to pump enough blood to meet the needs of other organs in the body. This failure occurs for one of two reasons. In systolic heart failure (systole is the period when the heart contracts), disease weakens the wall of the ventricles, so that they pump less forcefully. In response, the heart muscle stretches to create larger chambers in the ventricles. This compensates for the heart's reduced pumping ability, but over time, the heart wall thickens, the chambers narrow, and the heart pumps out less and less blood. The volume of blood pumped out of the ventricle is called the ejection fraction (EF). In a healthy heart, the EF is greater than 50%, while in people with CHF, it is less than 50% and can be as low as 30%. Systolic heart failure is the most common kind of CHF.

In diastolic heart failure (diastole is the period when the heart relaxes and refills with blood), the heart is not weakened, but it becomes stiff. After each contraction, it does not relax enough to fill completely. The EF is normal (over 50%), but with less blood in the ventricle, the absolute amount of blood pumped is decreased. Diastolic heart failure is most common among people over age 75.

When the left side of the heart begins to fail, fluids collect in the lungs causing lung congestion (**pulmonary edema**) and difficulty breathing. When the right side of the heart begins to fail, fluid collects in the feet and legs causing swelling. CHF is often complicated by other health problems such as **coronary artery disease**, diabetes, high blood pressure, **alcoholism**, **emphysema**, **chronic obstructive pulmonary disease** (COPD), and renal (kidney) disease.

Demographics

About 5 million Americans have CHF, with about 500,000 new cases diagnosed each year. Most people with CHF are elderly. Only 1% of people under age 50 are diagnosed with CHF, but it is found in about 5% of people over age 75 and 25% of people over age 80. Men ages 40–75 are more likely to have CHF than women, but after age 75, the percentage of men and women with CHF is about equal. African Americans are 1.5 times more likely to die of CHF than white Americans. The number of people with CHF is expected to increase as the American population ages.

Causes and symptoms

The end cause of CHF is failure of the heart to pump enough blood, but many other conditions can contribute to or accelerate this failure. These include heart damage caused by disease and lifestyle. Some common conditions contributing to CHF that make the heart work harder and can increase the risk of CHF include:

- coronary artery disease
- prolonged, uncontrolled high blood pressure (hypertension)
- previous heart attack (myocardial infarction)
- heart valve abnormalities
- prolonged heart arrhythmias
- infection of the heart muscle or surrounding tissue (endocarditis)
- damage to the heart muscle from alcohol, cocaine, or other substance abuse
- congenital (present at birth) heart defects
- obesity
- diabetes, particularly poorly controlled diabetes
- smoking

Symptoms of CHF usually begin gradually and initially may go unnoticed. The exception is after a **heart attack**, when moderate-to-severe symptoms can develop rather rapidly. CHF symptoms are similar to those caused by many diseases, making diagnosis more difficult. Often symptoms are complicated by other diseases in the elderly such as diabetes, emphysema or other lung diseases, and reduced kidney function.

The first symptom usually noticed is **shortness of breath** when performing normal activities such as walking, cleaning the house, or doing easy yard work, along with general **fatigue**. Symptoms then progress to include:

- shortness of breath and difficulty breathing even at rest
- fluid retention and swelling of the feet and legs
- weakness and extreme fatigue
- dizziness from not enough oxygen reaching the brain
- fast and/or irregular heartbeat

Diagnosis

Diagnosis begins with a complete **physical examination** and a health, medication, and lifestyle history.

The following tests are used to make a diagnosis of CHF:

- chest x ray: non-invasive test shows if fluid is building up in the lungs or if the heart is enlarged.
- electrocardiogram (ECG): non-invasive test helps detect abnormalities in heart rhythm and heart health by measuring the electrical activity of the heart
- blood tests: check for anemia (low iron) and chemical (electrolyte) imbalances in the blood.
- kidney function tests: help pinpoint the cause of fluid retention
- B-type natriuetic peptide (BNP) test: measures the hormone BNP, which is produced in greater quantity when the heart begins to fail
- echocardiogram: non-invasive imaging test that produces a picture of the heart in motion as it beats; extremely helpful in showing heart and valve damage.
- multiple-gated acquisition (MUGA) scan: imaging test that uses radioactive dye injected in the veins to produce a picture of blood circulation in the heart
- stress test: an electrocardiogram done while exercising or, for people who cannot exercise, while the heart is stimulated by medication

The degree or stage of CHF can be designated using several different scales. The two most common are the New York Heart Association (NYHA) scale that uses a numbered system (I-IV) that classifies CHF by symptoms and functional limits and the American College of Cardiology (ACC) scale that use a letter system (A-D) to designate risk factors for CHF.

Treatment

Treatment does not cure CHF, but it can slow its progression, extend life, and to some degree improve symptoms. Treatment of CHF falls into three categories: lifestyle changes, drug therapy, and surgery.

Lifestyle changes

Self-care lifestyle changes that help slow the progression of CHF include:

- reducing sodium (salt) in the diet
- eating a heart-healthy diet high in fresh fruits, fresh vegetables and whole grains, and low in fats, especially saturated (animal) fats.
- controlling calorie intake and losing weight if overweight or obese
- quitting smoking
- avoiding alcohol

- exercising moderately (e.g., walking) or joining a cardiac rehabilitation program
- treating any other health problems or underlying diseases
- elevating the feet when sitting to discourage fluid accumulation
- taking all medicines as prescribed
- weighing daily to check for sudden spikes in fluid retention
- scheduling regular examinations with a healthcare provider

Drug therapy

Many drugs are available to treat CHF. People with CHF often need more than one drug to control or slow symptoms. The development of new drugs to treat CHF is an area of active research because of the **aging** population of many developed countries.

Some common drugs used to treat CHF include:

- angiotensin converting enzyme (ACE) inhibitors. These drugs block the formation of angiotensin, a hormone that may adversely affect the heart. ACE inhibitors include captopril (Capoten), enalapril (Vasotec), lisinopril (Zestril, Prinvil), benazepril (Lotensin), and ramipril (Altace).
- angiotensin receptor blockers. These drugs also block the formation of angiotensin using a different mechanism than ACE inhibitors. They are generally less effective than ACE inhibitors and are given to people who do not tolerate ACE-inhibiting drugs. Examples include losartan (Cozzar), candesartan (Atacand), telmisartan (Micardis), valsartan (Diovan), and irbesartan (Avapro).
- beta-blockers. These drugs block the effect of stimulant hormones such as epinephrine (adrenalin) and norepinephrine (noradrenaline). Carvedilol (Coreg) is approved by the United Sates Food and Drug Administration (FDA) for this use, although other beta-blockers are sometimes prescribed as off-label use.
- digoxin (Lanoxin). This is one of the oldest treatments for CHF. It is a natural compound found in the plant foxglove *Digitalis purpurea*.
- diuretics. These drugs help rid the body of excess fluid by increasing urine production. Common diuretics include furosemide (Lasix), bumetanide (Bumex), torsemide (Demadex), metolazone (Zaroxolyn), spironolactone (Aldactone), and hydrochlorothiazide.
- hydralazine (Apresoline). A large study showed that this drug benefited African Americans but conferred

no benefit on people of other races. Research is ongoing.

There are also drugs that a CHF patient should avoid because they worsen CHF or interfere with treatment drugs. These include **nonsteroidal anti-inflammatory drugs** (e.g., Aleve, Motrin), **decongestants** (e.g., Sudafed), **calcium channel blockers**, anti-arrhythmia drugs, growth hormones, **antacids** that contain **sodium**, and salt substitutes. Patients with CHF should not take any herbal remedy or dietary supplement without first consulting their healthcare provider. In addition, some drugs used to treat underlying diseases may need to be adjusted because they interfere with drug therapy for CHF.

Surgery

Surgery does not cure CHF although it can prolong life and improve the quality of life. Surgery can be done to remedy a defect or condition that is contributing to CHF. Examples are **heart valve repair** and coronary artery surgery to improve blood flow in the heart. Complete heart **transplant surgery** to treat CHF is severely limited by the number of donor hearts available. It is normally done only on younger patients such as those with congenital heart defects.

Nutrition/Dietetic concerns

Sodium (Na) found in salt promotes water retention in the body. People with CHF need to severely restrict their intake of salt. Salt is found in many processed foods, so that even a "no salt added" diet provides between 4,000–6,000 mg of salt daily. People with CHF need to limit their salt intake to no more than 2,000 mg of salt per day. This requires careful reading of food labels (sodium content is listed in the **nutrition** panel) and for many, a major change in the foods they eat. Fluid intake is also a concern for people with CHF and is often limited to no more than 8 cups (2 L) of fluids daily from all sources combined.

Exercise therapy

Studies have found that limited, supervised **exercise** can benefit people with CHF. An individualized **cardiac rehabilitation** program can provide an appropriate type and level of exercise.

Prognosis

CHF is a progressive condition; it can be slowed but not cured. Between 30% and 40% of people with CHF are hospitalized every year, and it is a leading

cause of death among the elderly. About half the deaths among people with CHF are from progressive heart failure, and the other half are sudden deaths, most often due to severe heart **arrhythmias**. The average survival time from diagnosis is 3.2 years in men and 5.4 years in women. Nevertheless, survival times vary widely depending on the individual's general health, the treatment they receive, and how well they maintain their lifestyle and drug regimens.

Prevention

Prevention activities are the same as the lifestyle changes used to slow the progression of CHF, namely eating a heart-healthy diet, exercising regularly, maintaining a healthy weight, avoiding tobacco products, and limiting alcohol consumption. Treating or controlling any underlying diseases such as diabetes and high blood pressure also are important preventative steps.

Caregiver concerns

Staying on the prescribed drug regimen and making positive lifestyle changes is important in slowing the progression of CHF and improving patient symptoms. People with CHF often take multiple drugs several times a day. Care givers can help their charges achieve maximum benefits from their medications by familiarizing themselves with the required drug regimen and organizing a system that makes it easy for them and their charges to remember to take these medications. A medicine box with separate compartments for several times of day and all the days of the week is helpful. Another part of caring for a person with CHF is organizing a daily weighing in order to determine if fluid retention has suddenly increased. Finally, the care giver must understand and conform to the dietary needs of their charge, with special care paid to the amount of salt in the diet.

Resources

BOOKS

American Medical Association, Martin S. Lipsky, Marla Mendelson, and Stephen Havas. *American Medical Association Guide to Preventing and Treating Heart Disease: Essential Information You and Your Family Need to Know about Having a Healthy Heart.* Indianapolis, IN: Wiley, 2008.

Esselstyn, Caldwell B. *Prevent and Reverse Heart Disease: The Revolutionary, Scientifically Proven, Nutrition-Based Cure.* New York: Avery, 2008.

Hosenpud, Jeffrey D., and Barry H. Greenberg, eds. *Congestive Heart Failure,* 3rd ed. Philadelphia: Lippincott Williams & Wilkins, 2007.

Katzenstein, Larry. *An AARP Guide: Living With Heart Disease: Everything You Need to Know to Safeguard Your Health and Take Control of Your Life.* New York: Sterling, 2007.

Lipsky, Martin S, et al. *American Medical Association Guide to Preventing and Treating Heart Disease: Essential Information You and Your Family Need to Know About Having a Healthy Heart.* Hoboken, NJ: Wiley, 2008.

Quinn, Campion. *100 Questions & Answers About Congestive Heart Failure.* Sudbury, MA: Jones & Bartlett, 2006.

Silver, Marc A. *Success With Heart Failure: Help and Hope for Those Coping With Congestive Heart Failure.* Cambridge, MA: Perseus Book Group, 2006.

Sinatra, Stephen T., et al. *Reverse Heart Disease Now: Stop Deadly Cardiovascular Plaque Before It's Too Late.* Hoboken, NJ: Wiley, 2008.

PERIODICALS

Grant, Ruth Ann. "Study: Elderly Lacking Heart Attack Care." *McKnight's Long-Term Care News* (September 2007): 6.

Guthrie, Catherine. "Damage Control: The 6 Best Natural Supplements to Protect Against Heart Disease, Cholesterol, and High Blood Pressure." *Natural Health* (February 2008): 62(6).

Hanna, Ibrahim R., and Nanette K. Wenger. "Secondary Prevention of Coronary Heart Disease in Elderly Patients." *American Family Physician* (June 15, 2005): 2289.

Kuriyama, Shinichi, et al. "Green Tea Consumption and Mortality Due to Cardiovascular Disease, Cancer, and All Causes in Japan: The Ohsaki Study." *Journal of the American Medical Association)* 296, no. 10 (September 13, 2006): 1255–1265.

Lowry, Fran. "Gastric Bypass Also Cuts Cancer, Diabetes, Heart Disease Mortality" *Family Practice News* (February 1, 2008): 38.

Mast, Carlotta. "Go With the Flow: Support Your Circulatory System and Lower Your Risk of Stroke and Heart Disease With These Drug-Free Recommendations." *Delicious Living* (February 2008): 41(4).

Sherman, Carl. "Reducing the Risk of Heart Disease in Women: Incorporating New Research Findings, the American Heart Association's Updated Guidelines Make Several Changes in the Previous Recommendations." *Clinical Advisor* (January 2008): 49(3).

OTHER

"Congestive Heart Failure." *eMedicineHealth.* September 29, 2005. http://www.emedicinehealth.com/congestive_heart_failure/article_em.htm

"Congestive Heart Failure." *MedicineNet.com.* May 7, 2007. http://www.medicinenet.com/congestive_heart_failure/article.htm

Grossman, Shamai. "Congestive Heart Failure and Pulmonary Edema." *eMedicnie.com.* May 11, 2006. http://www.emedicine.com/emerg/topic108.htm

"Heart Failure." *MayoClinic.* January 3, 2008. http://www.mayoclinic.com/health/heartfailure/DS00061

"Hormone Therapy: Is It Right for You?" *MayoClinic.com* February 12, 2008. http://www.mayoclinic.com/health/hormone-therapy/WO00046

ORGANIZATIONS

Adult Congenital Heart Association, 6757 Greene St., Suite 335, Philadelphia, PA, 19119-3508, (215) 849-1260, (888) 921-2242, (215) 849-1261, info@achaheart.org, http://www.achaheart.org.

American Heart Association, 7272 Greenville Ave., Dallas, TX, 75231, (301) 223-2307, (800) 242-8721, http://www.americanheart.org.

Centers for Disease Control and Prevention, Division for Heart Disease and Stroke Prevention, 4770 Buford Hwy NE, Atlanta, GA, 30341-3717, (770) 488-2424, http://www.cdc.gov/cholesterol/faqs.htm.

European Society of Cardiology, The European Heart House, 2035 Route des Colles, B.P. 179-Les Templiers,

Sophia-Antipolis, France, 06903, 33 4 9294 7600, 33 4 9294 7601, http://www.escardio.org.

Heart Foundation, 80 William St., Level 3, Sydney NSW Australia, 2011, 02 9219 2444, 300 36 27 87, http://www.heartfoundation.org.au.

National Heart, Lung, and Blood Institute, P.O. Box 30105, Bethesda, MD, 20824-0105, (301) 592-8573, (204) 629-3246, nhlbiinfo@nhlbi.nih.gov, http://www.nhlbi.nih.gov.

Tish Davidson, AM
Laura Jean Cataldo, RN, Ed.D.

Congestive heart failure *see* **Heart failure**

Conjunctivitis

Definition

Conjuctivitis is an inflammation or redness of the lining of the white part of the eye and the underside of the eyelid (conjunctiva) that can be caused by bacterial or viral infection, allergic reaction, chemical irritants, or physical agents like infrared or ultraviolet light. Viral conjunctivitis is sometimes called pink eye or red eye because the tissues lining the affected eye often develop a bright pink color as well as being swollen.

Conjunctivitis in the newborn, sometimes called neonatal conjunctivitis or ophthalmia neonatorum, is

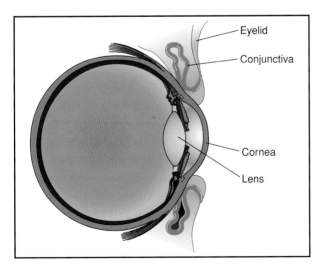

Conjunctivitis is the inflammation of the conjunctiva, a thin, delicate membrane that covers the eyeball and lines the eyelid. It may be caused by a viral infection, such as a cold or acute respiratory infection, or by such diseases as measles, herpes simplex, or herpes zoster. *(Illustration by Electronic Illustrators Group. Reproduced by permission of Gale, a part of Cengage Learning.)*

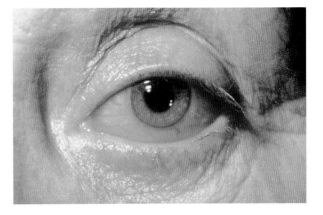

This person has severe conjunctivitis, most likely caused by an allergic reaction. *(Custom Medical Stock Photo, Inc. Reproduced by permission.)*

sometimes discussed as a distinctive type of conjunctivitis because it is caused by an infection passed from the mother to the child during delivery. If untreated, it can cause blindness.

Demographics

Conjunctivitis is a common eye disorder in all age groups worldwide, in part because it has so many possible causes. It is one of the most common nontraumatic eye disorders that are seen in hospital emergency rooms, accounting for about 1% of all ER visits in North America. The conjunctivae of the human eye are continually exposed to microorganisms and environmental agents that can cause infections or allergic reactions. Conjunctivitis can be acute or chronic depending upon how long the condition lasts, the severity of symptoms, and the type of organism or agent involved. It can also affect one or both eyes and, if caused by infection, can be very easily transmitted to others during close physical contact, particularly among children in a daycare center.

About 15% of people in the United States will have at least one episode of allergic conjunctivitis over a lifetime; rates in other countries are thought to be similar.

Viral conjunctivitis is most likely to affect people in the United States and Canada in the late fall and early spring. This type of conjunctivitis is equally common in males and females, and in members of all races and ethnic groups.

Between 1% and 2% of babies born in the United States are diagnosed with infectious neonatal conjunctivitis. The most common cause of this type of conjunctivitis is *Chlamydia trachomatis*, a parasite that lives within the tissues of an infected mother's cervix. The second most common cause is *Neisseria gonorrhoeae*, the gonococcus or bacterium that causes **gonorrhea**. Conjunctivitis caused by *N. gonorrhoeae* is potentially the most dangerous to newborns.

Description

The conjunctiva (plural, conjunctivae) in humans is a loose sheet of connective tissue that covers the eyeball and doubles back to form the inner lining of the eyelid. Some of the smaller tear glands that keep the eye lubricated are located within the conjunctivae. Because the conjunctivae are moist mucous membranes, **infectious disease** organisms can easily cling to them until they multiply and overwhelm the eye's defense mechanisms, producing redness, irritation, and sand-in-the-eye or itchy sensations, discharge, and sometimes photophobia (extreme sensitivity to light).

Conjunctivitis in newborns is typically characterized by swelling of the eyelid, tenderness of the eyeball, and a discharge. Depending on the organism causing the infection, the discharge may be either watery mucus or a liquid form of pus. In some cases the discharge may be thick enough to form a yellowish crust on the baby's eyelids.

Risk factors

The most common risk factors for conjunctivitis include:

- exposure to other children or family members with conjunctivitis
- exposure to allergens, most commonly grass or tree pollen
- recent history of an upper respiratory infection; this is a risk factor for viral conjunctivitis
- weakened immune system
- personal history of asthma or eczema; this is a risk factor for allergic conjunctivitis
- frequent use of eye cosmetics
- wearing contact lenses, particularly the extended-wear type

Causes and symptoms

The symptoms of conjunctivitis vary somewhat according to its cause. Conjunctivitis may be caused by a viral infection, such as a cold, acute respiratory infection, or disease such as **measles**, herpes simplex, or herpes zoster. Symptoms include mild to severe discomfort in one or both eyes, redness, swelling of the eyelids, and watery, yellow or green discharge. Symptoms may last anywhere from several days to two weeks. Infection with an adenovirus, may also cause a significant amount of pus-like discharge and a scratchy, foreign body-type of sensation in the eye. This may also be accompanied by swelling and tenderness of the lymph nodes near the ear.

Bacterial conjunctivitis can occur in adults and children and is caused by such organisms as *Staphylococcus*, *Streptococcus*, and *Hemophilus*. Symptoms of bacterial conjunctivitis include a pus-like discharge and crusty eyelids after awakening. Redness of the conjunctiva can be mild to severe and may be accompanied by swelling. Persons with symptoms of conjunctivitis who are sexually active may possibly be infected with the bacteria that cause either gonorrhea or chlamydia. There may be large amounts of pus-like discharge, and symptoms may include intolerance to light (photophobia), watery mucous discharge, and tenderness in the lymph nodes near the ear that may persist for up to three months.

Conjunctivitis may also be caused by such environmental hazards as wind, smoke, dust, and allergic reactions caused by pollen, dust, or grass. Symptoms range from **itching** and redness to a mucous discharge. Persons who wear **contact lenses** may develop allergic conjunctivitis caused by the various eye solutions and foreign proteins contained in them.

Other less common causes of conjunctivitis include exposure to sun lamps or the electrical arcs used during welding, and problems with inadequate drainage of the tear ducts.

In a few cases children can get conjunctivitis from accidental exposure to chemical irritants, such as strong detergents.

Diagnosis

The most important aspect of diagnosing conjunctivitis is to separate the cases with benign causes (the great majority) from the small group of cases with complications or more serious causes (particularly chemical injury). Conjunctivitis can be diagnosed by a primary care doctor, pediatrician, emergency room physician, or ophthalmologist (specialist in eye disorders); patients with severe inflammation or conjunctivitis caused by getting a strong chemical in the eye will usually be referred to an ophthalmologist.

Examination

An accurate diagnosis of conjunctivitis centers on taking a patient history to learn when symptoms began, the specific symptoms experienced, and other predisposing factors, such as upper respiratory

Adenovirus—A virus that affects the upper respiratory tract.

Chlamydia—The most common bacterial sexually transmitted disease in the United States that often accompanies gonorrhea and is known for its lack of evident symptoms in the majority of women.

Gonococcus (plural, gonococci)—The bacterium *Neisseria gonorrheae* that causes gonorrhea, a sexually transmitted infection of the genitals and urinary tract. Gonococci may occasionally affect the eye, causing blindness if not treated.

Herpes simplex virus—A virus that can cause fever and blistering on the skin, mucous membranes, or genitalia.

Herpes zoster virus—Acute inflammatory virus that attacks the nerve cells on the root of each spinal nerve with skin eruptions along a sensory nerve ending.

Neonatal—Referring to the period shortly after birth.

Ophthalmia neonatorum—The medical term for conjunctivitis in newborns.

Photophobia—Extreme sensitivity to light.

Staphylococcus—A bacterial organism, looking much like a cluster of grapes, that can infect various body systems.

Streptococcus—An organism that causes infections of either the upper respiratory or gastrointestinal tract.

complaints, **allergies**, **sexually transmitted diseases**, herpes simplex infections, and exposure to schoolmates or other persons with pink eye. It may be helpful to learn whether an aspect of an individual's occupation may be the cause.

After taking the history, the doctor will examine the patient's eye with a light to check the eyelid and conjunctiva for swelling, change in color, discharge, and any other abnormalities. The doctor may also collect a small sample of the discharge for culture if bacterial conjunctivitis is suspected.

Tests

Laboratory tests are usually not indicated in adults unless initial treatment fails (usually within 24–36 hours) or an infection with gonorrhea or chlamydia is suspected. In such cases, the discharge may be cultured and Gram-stained to determine the organism responsible for the condition. Cultures and smears are relatively painless procedures.

Cultures are usually taken when the patient is a newborn, has a weakened immune system, or is thought to have conjunctivitis caused by *N. gonorrhoeae*.

Treatment

Traditional

The treatment of conjunctivitis depends on what caused the condition. In all cases, warm compresses applied to the affected eye several times a day may help to reduce discomfort. Some treatment choices will be based on patient preference, convenience of use, and cost to the patient.

Conjunctivitis due to a viral infection, particularly those due to adenoviruses, are usually treated by applying warm compresses to the eye(s) and applying topical antibiotic ointments to prevent secondary bacterial infections. Viral conjunctivitis caused by herpes simplex should be referred to an ophthalmologist. Topical **steroids** are commonly prescribed in combination with antiviral therapy.

Allergic conjunctivitis can be treated by removing the allergic substance from a person's environment, if possible; by applying cool compresses to the eye; and by administering eye drops four to six times daily for four days. Oral **antihistamines** may help to relieve itchy eyes. However, many of these drugs also dry the eyes. Therefore, many physicians suggest a combination of antihistamines and lubricating drops or the use of nasal corticosteroid sprays to help relieve allergic conjunctivitis, particularly when it is combined with nasal symptoms. Non steroidal anti-inflammatory drugs (NSAIDs) can be used to reduce the itching associated with allergic conjunctivitis as well as to reduce inflammation.

Drugs

Medications of various types are used to treat conjunctivitis caused by bacteria. In cases of bacterial conjunctivitis, a physician may prescribe an antibiotic eye ointment or eye drops containing **sodium** sulfacetamide (Sulamyd) to be applied daily for 7 to 14 days. If, after 72 hours, the condition does not improve, a physician or primary care provider should be notified because the bacteria involved may be resistant to the antibiotic used or the cause may not be bacterial. In May 2009 the U.S. Food and Drug Administration (FDA) approved a new drug, besifloxacin (Besivance), for the treatment of bacterial conjunctivitis. The new drug is given as eye drops, can be safely used in patients older than 12 months, and has fewer side effects than other antibacterial eye drops.

For cases of conjunctivitis caused by *N. gonorrhoeae*, a physician may prescribe an intramuscular injection of ceftriaxone (Rocephin) and a topical antibiotic ointment containing erythromycin or bactracin to be applied four times daily for two to three weeks. Sexual partners should also be treated.

With accompanying chlamydia infection, a topical antibiotic ointment containing erythromycin (Ilotycin) may be prescribed to be applied one to two times daily. In addition, oral erythromycin or tetracycline therapy may be indicated for three to four weeks. Again, sexual partners should also be treated.

Conjunctivitis in the newborn is treated with a combination of eye drops or eye ointments containing erythromycin or tetracycline. Salt water drops may be used to wash away any sticky crust that has formed on the eyelids. Babies born to mothers with untreated gonorrhea may need intravenous or intramuscular injections of ceftriaxone, ciprofloxacin, or cefotaxime.

Alternative

Conjunctivitis caused by gonococcal and chlamydial infection usually requires conventional medical treatment. With bacterial, viral, and allergic conjunctivitis, however, alternative options can be helpful. Internal immune enhancement with supplementation can aid in the resolution of bacterial and viral conjunctivitis. Removal of the allergic agent is an essential step in treating allergic conjunctivitis. As with any of the recommended treatments, however, if no improvement is seen within 48–72 hours, a physician should be consulted.

There are a number of acute homeopathic remedies designed to treat conjunctivitis. These include *Pulsatilla* (windflower, *Pulsatilla nigricans*), *Belladonna*, and eyebright (*Euphrasia officinalis*). Eye drops prepared with homeopathic remedies and/or herbs can be a good substitute for pharmaceutical eye drops. Eye washes can also be made. Herbal eyewashes made with eyebright (1 tsp. dried herb steeped in 1 pint of boiling water) or chamomile (*Matricaria recutita*; 2–3 tsp. in 1 pint of boiling water) may be helpful. Eyewashes should be strained and cooled before use, and close attention should be paid to make sure that any solution put into the eye is sterile.

Home remedies

Several simple home remedies may help relieve the discomfort associated with conjunctivitis. A boric acid eyewash can be used to clean and soothe the eyes. A warm compress applied to the eyes for 5–10 minutes three times a day can help relieve the discomfort of bacterial and viral conjunctivitis. A cool compress or cool, damp tea bags placed on the eyes can ease the discomfort of allergic conjunctivitis.

Prognosis

If treated properly, the prognosis for conjunctivitis in adults and older children is good. Conjunctivitis caused by an allergic reaction should clear up once the allergen is removed. Allergic conjunctivitis will likely recur if the individual again comes into contact with the particular allergen. Conjunctivitis caused by bacteria or a virus, if treated properly, is usually resolved in 10–14 days. If there is no relief of symptoms in 48–72 hours, or there is moderate to severe eye **pain**, changes in vision, or the conjunctivitis is suspected to be caused by herpes simplex, a physician should be notified immediately. If untreated or if treatment fails and is not corrected, conjunctivitis may cause **visual impairment** by spreading to other parts of the eye, such as the cornea.

Untreated conjunctivitis in newborns caused by sexually transmitted diseases can lead to blindness. A century ago, as many as 24% of American children enrolled in schools for the blind had lost their sight as a result of gonorrheal conjunctivitis.

Prevention

The American Academy of Ophthalmology recommends the following preventive measures to lower the risk of conjunctivitis:

• Wash hands frequently using antiseptic soap, and use single-use towels during the disease to prevent spreading the infection. People with viral conjunctivitis can spread the disease to others for as long as two weeks after symptoms appear.

• Avoid chemical irritants and known allergens; handle strong detergents, drain cleaners, ammonia, chlorine bleach, and other household chemicals with care.

• If in an area where welding occurs, using the proper protective eye wear and screens to prevent damaging the eyes.

- Use a clean tissue to remove discharge from eyes.
- If medication is prescribed, finish the course of antibiotics as directed to make sure that the infection is cleared up and does not recur.
- Avoid such contact as vigorous physical activities with other persons until symptoms resolve; in particular, stay away from swimming pools.
- Women who use mascara and other eye cosmetics should replace them frequently and not share them with others.
- Avoid sharing pillowcases and bath towels.
- Clean contact lenses carefully and properly.

Chlamydial or bacterial conjunctivitis of the newborn can be avoided by treating the mother for sexually transmitted diseases before delivery; by delivering the baby by **cesarean section**; and by placing an antibiotic ointment in the baby's eyes as soon as possible after delivery.

Resources

BOOKS

Friedman, Neil J., and Peter K. Kaiser. *Essentials of Ophthalmology*. Philadelphia: Saunders Elsevier, 2007.

Pavan-Langston, Deborah. *Manual of Ocular Diagnosis and Therapy*. 6th ed. Philadelphia: Wolters Kluwer Health/ Lippincott Williams and Wilkins, 2008.

Wilson, M. Edward, et al., eds. *Pediatric Ophthalmology*. New York: Springer, 2008.

PERIODICALS

Bremond-Gignac, D., et al. "Efficacy and Safety of Azithromycin 1.5% Eye Drops for Purulent Bacterial Conjunctivitis in Pediatric Patients." *Pediatric Infectious Disease Journal* 29 (March 2010): 222–26.

Chigbu, D.I. "The Management of Allergic Eye Diseases in Primary Eye Care." *Contact Lens and Anterior Eye* 32 (December 2009): 260–72.

Comstock, T.L., et al. "Besifloxacin: A Novel Anti-infective for the Treatment of Bacterial Conjunctivitis." *Clinical Ophthalmology* 4 (April 26, 2010): 215–25.

Cronau, H., et al. "Diagnosis and Management of Red Eye in Primary Care." *American Family Physician* 81 (January 15, 2010): 137–44.

Origlieri, C., and L. Bielory. "Emerging Drugs for Conjunctivitis." *Expert Opinion on Emerging Drugs* 14 (September 2009): 523–36.

Visscher, K.L., et al. "Evidence-based Treatment of Acute Infective Conjunctivitis: Breaking the Cycle of Antibiotic Prescribing." *Canadian Family Physician* 55 (November 2009): 1071–75.

OTHER

American Academy of Ophthalmology (AAO). "Conjunctivitis." *eyeSmart*. March 2010. http://www.geteyesmart. org/eyesmart/diseases/conjunctivitis.cfm (accessed September 19, 2010).

Jatta, Kalpana K., et al. "Conjunctivitis, Neonatal." *eMedicine*. December 21, 2009. http://emedicine.medscape. com/article/1192190-overview (accessed September 19, 2010).

"Pink Eye (Conjunctivitis)." *MayoClinic.com*. May 22, 2010. http://www.mayoclinic.com/health/pink-eye/ DS00258 (accessed September 18, 2010).

"Conjunctivitis." *MedlinePlus*. November 10, 2008. http:// www.nlm.nih.gov/medlineplus/ency/article/001010. htm (accessed September 19, 2010).

"Facts about the Cornea and Corneal Disease." National Eye Institute (NEI). http://www.nei.nih.gov/health/ cornealdisease/#b (accessed September 19, 2010).

Silverman, Michael A., and Edward Bessman. "Conjunctivitis." *eMedicine*. April 27, 2010. http://emedicine. medscape.com/article/797874-overview (accessed September 19, 2010).

ORGANIZATIONS

American Academy of Ophthalmology, P.O. Box 7424, San Francisco, CA, 94120, (415) 561-8500, (415) 561-8533, eyesmart@aao.org, http://www.aao.org.

National Eye Institute (NEI), Information Office, 31 Center Drive MSC 2510, Bethesda, MD, 20892, (301) 496-5248, 2020@nei.nih.gov, http://www.nei.nih.gov.

Lisa Papp, RN
Teresa G. Odle
Rebecca J. Frey, PhD

Consciousness disorders *see* **Coma**

Constipation

Definition

Constipation is difficulty in producing a bowel movement or infrequent, hard, dry stools that are painful or difficult to pass.

Demographics

Constipation is one of the most common medical complaints in the United States. About 2% of Americans describe being constipated continuously or frequently. Internationally, the incidence of constipation varies, depending largely on dietary habits.

Constipation can occur at any age, and is more common among individuals who resist the urge to move their bowels at their body's signal. This often happens when children start school or enter daycare and feel shy about asking permission to use the

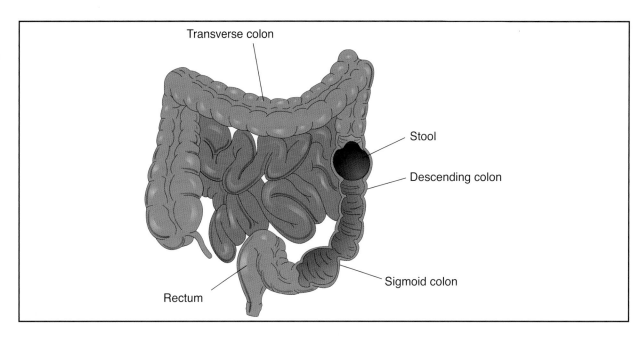

Transverse colon

Stool

Descending colon

Sigmoid colon

Rectum

Constipation is an acute or chronic condition in which bowel movements occur less often than usual or consist of hard, dry stools that are painful or difficult to pass. *(Illustration by Electronic Illustrators Group. Reproduced by permission of Gale, a part of Cengage Learning.)*

bathroom. It also can happen to adults who are in jobs where they cannot take bathroom breaks at will.

Constipation is more common in women than in men and is especially likely to occur during **pregnancy**. Age alone does not increase the frequency of constipation, but people over age 65, especially women, are more likely to experience constipation.

Description

Bowel habits vary, but an adult who has not had a bowel movement in three days or a child who has not had a bowel movement in four days is considered constipated.

Although constipation is rarely serious, it can lead to:

- bowel obstruction
- chronic constipation
- hemorrhoids (a mass of dilated veins in swollen tissue around the anus)
- hernia (a protrusion of an organ through a tear in the muscle wall)
- spastic colitis (irritable bowel syndrome, a condition characterized by alternating periods of diarrhea and constipation)
- laxative dependency

Chronic constipation may be a symptom of other diseases such as colorectal **cancer**, depression, diabetes, **diverticulosis** (small pouches in the muscles of the large intestine), **lead poisoning**, or Parkinson's disease.

In someone who is elderly or disabled, constipation may be a symptom of bowel impaction, a more serious condition in which feces are trapped in the lower part of the large intestine. A doctor should be called if an elderly or disabled person is constipated for a week or more or if a child seems to be constipated.

A doctor should be notified whenever constipation occurs after starting a new prescription, vitamin, or mineral supplement or herbal remedy or when constipation is accompanied by blood in the stools, changes in bowel patterns, **fever**, or abdominal **pain**.

Causes and symptoms

Constipation usually results from not getting enough **exercise**, not drinking enough water, or from a diet that does not include an adequate amount of fiber-rich foods such as dried beans, bran cereals, fruits, raw vegetables, rice, and whole-grain breads.

Other causes of constipation include anal fissure (a tear or crack in the lining of the anus); **chronic kidney failure**; colon or **rectal cancer**; depression; **hypercalcemia** (abnormally high levels of **calcium** in the blood); **hypothyroidism** (underactive thyroid gland); illness requiring complete bed rest; **irritable bowel syndrome**; and **stress**.

KEY TERMS

Beta blocker—An anti-hypertensive (blood pressure-lowering) drug that limits the activity of epinephrine, a hormone that increases blood pressure.

Calcium channel blocker—A drug that lowers blood pressure by regulating calcium-related electrical activity in the heart.

Diverticulitis—A condition of the diverticulum of the intestinal tract, especially in the colon, where inflammation may cause distended sacs extending from the colon and pain.

Constipation also can be a side effect of various medications including:

- aluminum salts in antacids
- antihistamines
- antipsychotic drugs
- aspirin
- belladonna (*Atopa belladonna,* source of atropine, a medication used to relieve spasms and dilate the pupils of the eye)
- beta blockers (medications used to stabilize irregular heartbeat, lower high blood pressure, reduce chest pain)
- blood pressure medications
- calcium channel blockers (medication prescribed to treat high blood pressure, chest pain, some types of irregular heartbeat and stroke, and some non-cardiac diseases)
- diuretics (drugs that promote the formation and secretion of urine)
- iron or calcium supplements
- narcotics (potentially addictive drugs that relieve pain and cause mood changes)
- tricyclic antidepressants (medications prescribed to treat chronic pain, depression, headaches, and other illnesses)

An adult who is constipated may feel bloated, have a **headache**, swollen abdomen, or pass rock-like feces; or strain, bleed, or feel pain during bowel movements. A constipated baby may strain, cry, draw the legs toward the abdomen, or arch the back when having a bowel movement.

Diagnosis

Everyone becomes constipated once in a while, but a doctor should be notified if significant changes in bowel patterns last for more than a week or if symptoms continue more than three weeks after increasing activity and fiber and fluid intake.

Examination

The patient's observations and medical history help a primary care physician diagnose constipation. The doctor uses his fingers to see if there is a hardened mass in the abdomen, and may perform a **rectal examination**.

Physical and psychological assessments and a detailed history of bowel habits are especially important when an elderly person complains of constipation.

Tests

Diagnostic procedures may include a **barium enema**, which reveals blockage inside the intestine; laboratory analysis of blood and stool samples for internal bleeding or other symptoms of systemic disease; and a **sigmoidoscopy** (examination of the sigmoid area of the colon with a flexible tube equipped with a magnifying lens).

Treatment

If changes in diet and activity fail to relieve occasional constipation, an over-the-counter laxative may be used for a few days. Preparations that soften stools or add bulk (bran, psyllium) work more slowly but are safer than Epsom salts and other harsh **laxatives** or herbal laxatives containing senna (*Cassia senna*) or buckthorn (*Rhamnus purshianna*), which can harm the nerves and lining of the colon.

Fiber supplements containing psyllium (*Plantago psyllium*) usually become effective within about 48 hours and can be used every day without causing dependency. Powdered flaxseed (*Linium usitatissimum*) works the same way. Insoluble fiber, like wheat or oat bran, is as effective as psyllium but may give the patient gas at first.

A woman who is pregnant should never use a laxative without consulting her doctor. Neither should anyone who is experiencing abdominal pain, **nausea**, or **vomiting**.

A warm-water or mineral oil enema can relieve constipation, and a non-digestible sugar (lactulose) or special electrolyte solution is recommended for adults and older children with stubborn symptoms.

If a patient has an impacted bowel, the doctor inserts a gloved finger into the rectum and gently dislodges the hardened feces.

Alternative treatment

Initially, alternative practitioners will suggest that the patient drink an adequate amount of water each day (six to eight glasses), exercise on a regular basis, and eat a diet high in soluble and insoluble fibers. Soluble fibers include pectin, flax, and gums; insoluble fibers include psyllium and brans from grains like wheat and oats. Fresh fruits and vegetables contain both soluble and insoluble fibers. Castor oil, applied topically to the abdomen and covered by a heat source (a heating pad or hot water bottle), can help relieve constipation when used nightly for 20–30 minutes.

ACUPRESSURE. This needleless form of **acupuncture** is said to relax the abdomen, ease discomfort, and stimulate regular bowel movements when diet and exercise fail to do so. After lying down, the patient closes his eyes and takes a deep breath. For two minutes, he applies gentle fingertip pressure to a point about two and one-half inches below the navel.

Acupressure can also be applied to the outer edges of one elbow crease and maintained for 30 seconds before pressing the crease of the other elbow. This should be done three times a day to relieve constipation.

AROMATHERAPY. Six drops of rosemary (*Rosmarinus officinalis*) and six drops of thyme (*Thymus* spp.) diluted by 1 oz of almond oil, olive oil, or another carrier oil can relieve constipation when used to massage the abdomen.

HERBAL THERAPY. A variety of herbal therapies can be useful in the treatment of constipation. Several herbs, including chamomile (*Matricaria recutita*), dandelion (*Taraxacum mongolicum*), and burdock (*Arctium lappa*), act as bitters, stimulating the movement of the digestive and excretory systems. There are also "laxative" herbs that assist with bowel movement. Two of these are senna (*Cassia senna*) and buckthorn (*Rhamnus purshiana*). These laxative-like herbs are stronger acting on elimination than bitters and can sometimes cause cramping (mixing them with a calming herb like fennel or caraway can help reduce cramping). Both senna and buckthorn are powerful herbs that are best used with direction from an experienced practitioner, since they can have adverse side effects and the patient may become dependent on them.

HOMEOPATHY. Homeopathy also can offer assistance with constipation. There are acute remedies for constipation that can be found in one of the many home remedy books on **homeopathic medicine**. A constitutional prescription can help rebalance someone who is struggling with constipation.

MASSAGE. Massaging the leg from knee to hip in the morning, at night, and before trying to move the bowels is said to relieve constipation. There is also a specific Swedish massage technique that can help relieve constipation.

YOGA. The knee-chest position, said to relieve gas and stimulate abdominal organs, involves:

- standing straight with arms at the sides
- lifting the right knee toward the chest
- grasping the right ankle with the left hand
- pulling the leg as close to the chest as possible
- holding the position for about eight seconds
- repeating these steps with the left leg

The cobra position, which can be repeated as many as four time a day, involves:

- lying on the stomach with legs together
- placing the palms just below the shoulders, holding elbows close to the body
- inhaling, then lifting the head (face forward) and chest off the floor
- keeping the navel in contact with the floor
- looking as far upward as possible
- holding this position for three to six seconds
- exhaling and lowering the chest

Prognosis

Changes in diet and exercise usually eliminate constipation.

Prevention

Most Americans consume between 11–18 g of fiber a day. Consumption of 35 g of fiber (an amount equal to five servings of fruits and vegetables, and a large bowl of high-fiber cereal) and between six and eight glasses of water each day can generally prevent constipation.

Daily use of 500 mg vitamin C and 400 mg magnesium may help to prevent constipation. Sitting on the toilet for 10 minutes at the same time every day, preferably after a meal, can induce regular bowel movements. This may not become effective for a few months, and it is important to defecate whenever necessary

Resources

BOOKS

Sauers, Joan, and Joanna McMillan-Price. *Get to Know Your Gut: Everything You Wanted to Know About Burping, Bloating, Candida, Constipation, Food Allergies, Farting, and Poo but Were Afraid to Ask.* New York: Marlowe, 2005.

OTHER

Basson, Marc D. "Constipation." *eMedicine.com.* January 28, 2010. http://emedicine.medscape.com/article/ 184704-overview (accessed September 19, 2010.

"Constipation." *MedlinePlus.* January 19, 2010. http://
www.nlm.nih.gov/medlineplus/constipation.html
(accessed September 18, 2010).

"Constipation." National Digestive Diseases Information
Clearinghouse. NIH Publication No. 07-2754. July
2007. http://digestive.niddk.nih.gov/ddiseases/pubs/
constipation (accessed September 18, 2010).

Levitt, Marc A., and Alberto Pena. "Constipation and
Bowel Management." *eMedicine.com.* February 19,
2010. http://emedicine.medscape.com/article/937030-
overview (accessed September 18, 2010).

ORGANIZATIONS

American Academy of Family Physicians, P.O. Box 11210,
Shawnee Mission, KS, 66207, (913) 906-6000, (800)
274-2237, (913) 906-6075, http://familydoctor.org.

American Gastroenterological Association (AGA), 4930
Del Ray Avenue, Bethesda, MD, 20814, (310) 654-
2055, (301) 654-5920, http://www.gastro.org.

International Foundation for Functional Gastrointestinal
Disorders, P.O. Box 170864, Milwaukee, WI 53217-
8076, (414) 964-1799, (888) 964-2001, (414) 964-7176,
iffgd@iffgd.org, http://www.iffgd.org.

National Institute of Diabetes and Digestive and Kidney
Diseases (NIDDK), 2 Information Way, Bethesda,
MD, 20892, (800) 891-5389. TTY: (866) 569-1162,
nddic@niddk.nih.gov, http://digestive.niddk.nih.gov.

Maureen Haggerty
Tish Davidson, AM

Constitutional homeopathic remedies *see*
**Homeopathic remedies, constitutional
prescribing**

Consumption *see* **Tuberculosis**

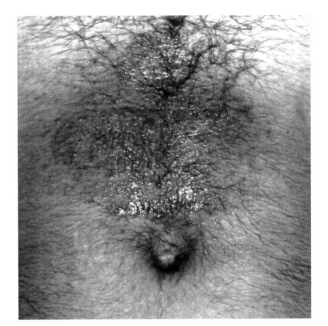

The abdomen of a male patient afflicted with contact
dermatitis, triggered by an allergic reaction to a nickel belt
buckle. *(Custom Medical Stock Photo, Inc. Reproduced by
permission.)*

Contact dermatitis

Definition

Contact **dermatitis** is the name for any skin
inflammation that occurs when the skin's surface
comes in contact with a substance originating outside
the body. There are two kinds of contact dermatitis,
irritant and allergic.

Demographics

At any given time in the United States, 2% of the
population will have contact dermatitis. This condition accounts for between 4% and 7% of all visits to
the dermatologist. Women are twice as likely as men to
develop contact dermatitis, and are at highest risk
immediately after giving birth.

Description

Contact dermatitis is a skin irritation that manifests as a rash. Thousands of natural and man-made
substances can cause contact dermatitis, which is
the most common skin condition requiring medical
attention and the foremost source of work-related
disease.

Risk factors

Florists, domestic workers, hairdressers, food
preparers, and employees in industry, construction,
and health care are the people most at risk of contracting work-related contact dermatitis.

Causes and symptoms

Irritant contact dermatitis (ICD) is the more commonly reported of the two kinds of contact dermatitis,
and is seen in about 80% of cases. It can be caused by
soaps, detergents, solvents, adhesives, fiberglass, and
other substances that are able to directly injure the
skin. Most attacks are slight and confined to the
hands and forearms, but can affect any part of the
body that comes in contact with an irritating substance. The symptoms can take many forms: redness,
itching, crusting, swelling, blistering, oozing, dryness,
scaliness, thickening of the skin, and a feeling of

KEY TERMS

Allergen—A foreign substance that causes an allergic reaction in some sensitive people but not in most others.

Antibiotics—Substances used against microorganisms that cause infection.

Corticosteroids—A group of anti-inflammatory substances often used to treat skin conditions.

Immune response—The protective reaction by the immune system against foreign antigens (substances that the body perceives as potentially dangerous). The immune system combats disease by neutralizing or destroying antigens.

warmth at the site of contact. In extreme cases, severe blistering can occur and open sores can form. Jobs that require frequent skin exposure to water, such as hairdressing and food preparation, can make the skin more susceptible to ICD.

Allergic contact dermatitis (ACD) results when repeated exposure to an allergen (an allergy-causing substance) triggers an immune response that inflames the skin. Tens of thousands of drugs, pesticides, cosmetics, food additives, commercial chemicals, and other substances have been identified as potential allergens. Fewer than 30, however, are responsible the majority of ACD cases. Common culprits include **poison ivy**, **poison oak**, and poison sumac; fragrances and preservatives in cosmetics and personal care products; latex items such as gloves and **condoms**; and formaldehyde. Many people find that they are allergic to the nickel in inexpensive jewelry. ACD is usually confined to the area of skin that comes in contact with the allergen, typically the hands or face. Symptoms range from mild to severe and resemble those of ICD; a patch test may be needed to determine which kind of contact dermatitis a person is experiencing.

Diagnosis

Examination

Diagnosis begins with a **physical examination** and asking the patient questions about his or her health and daily activities. When contact dermatitis is suspected, the doctor attempts to learn as much as possible about the patient's hobbies, workplace duties, use of medications and cosmetics, etc.–anything that might shed light on the source of the disease. In some cases, an examination of the home or workplace is

undertaken. If the dermatitis is mild, responds well to treatment, and does not recur, ordinarily the investigation is at an end. More difficult cases require patch testing to identify the allergen.

Tests

Patch testing is used to rule out ICD and determine which substances cause an allergic reaction. Most of the TRUE test is used, as it allows testing of multiple substances. A small amount of various diluted chemicals are applied to the skin and covered for two days. Forty-eight hours later, the covering is removed and the doctor examines the patch areas for a reaction. The area is examined again at 72 hours and in one week. Identifying the allergen may require repeated testing. If the TRUE test chemicals do not cause a reaction, additional specialized testing may be required. Patch testing works only with ACD, although it is considered an essential step in ruling out ICD.

Treatment

Traditional

The best treatment for contact dermatitis is to identify the allergen or irritating substance and avoid further contact with it. If the culprit is, for instance, a cosmetic, avoidance is a simple matter, but in some situations, such as an allergy to an essential workplace chemical for which no substitute can be found, avoidance may be impossible or force the sufferer to find new work or make other drastic changes in his or her life. Barrier creams and protective clothing such as gloves, masks, and long-sleeved shirts are ways of coping with contact dermatitis when avoidance is impossible, though they are not always effective.

For the symptoms themselves, treatments in mild cases include cool compresses and nonprescription lotions and ointments. When the symptoms are severe, **corticosteroids** applied to the skin or taken orally are used. Contact dermatitis that leads to a bacterial skin infection is treated with **antibiotics**.

Alternative treatment

Herbal remedies have been used for centuries to treat skin disorders including contact dermatitis. An experienced herbalist can recommend the remedies that will be most effective for an individual's condition. Among the herbs often recommended are:

- burdock (*Arctium lappa*) minimizes inflammation and boosts the immune system. It is taken internally as a tea or tincture (a concentrated herbal extract prepared with alcohol).

- calendula (*Calendula officinalis*) is a natural antiseptic and anti-inflammatory agent. It is applied topically in a lotion, ointment, or oil to the affected area.
- aloe (*Aloe barbadensis*) soothes skin irritations. The gel is applied topically to the affected area.

A homeopath treating a patient with contact dermatitis will do a thorough investigation of the individual's history and exposures before prescribing a remedy. One homeopathic remedy commonly prescribed to relieve the itching associated with contact dermatitis is *Rhus toxicodendron* taken internally three to four times daily.

Poison ivy, poison oak, and poison sumac are common culprits in cases of allergic contact dermatitis. Following exposure to these plants, rash development may be prevented by washing the area with soap and water within 15 minutes of exposure. The leaves of jewelweed (*Impatiens* spp.), which often grows near poison ivy, may neutralize the poison-ivy allergen if rubbed on the skin right after contact. Several topical remedies may help relieve the itching associated with allergic contact dermatitis, including the juice of plantain leaves (*Plantago major*); a paste made of equal parts of green clay and goldenseal root (*Hydrastis canadensis*); a paste made of salt, water, clay, and peppermint (*Mentha piperita*) oil; and calamine lotion.

Prognosis

If the offending substance is promptly identified and avoided, the chances of a quick and complete recovery are excellent. Otherwise, symptom management—not cure—is the best doctors can offer. For some people, contact dermatitis becomes a chronic and disabling condition that can have a profound effect on employability and quality of life.

Prevention

Avoidance of known or suspected allergens or irritating substances is the best prevention. If avoidance is difficult, barrier creams and protective clothing can be tried. Skin that comes in contact with an offending substance should be thoroughly washed as soon as possible.

Resources

OTHER

American Academy of Dermatology. Allergic Contact Rashes. 2005. http://www.aad.org/public/publications/pamphlets/skin_allergic.html
Mayo Foundation for Medical Education and Research. Contact Dermatitis. July 31, 2009. http://www.mayoclinic.com/health/contact-dermatitis/ds00985
Rashes. MedlinePlus. May 17, 2010. http://www.nlm.nih.gov/medlineplus/rashes.html
Shy, Bradley D. and David Todd Schwartz. Dermatitis, Contact. eMedicine.com September 22, 2009. http://emedicine.medscape.com/article/762139-overview

ORGANIZATIONS

American Academy of Dermatology, P. O. Box 4014, Schaumburg, IL, 60168-4014, (847) 330-0230, (866) 503-SKIN (7546), (847) 240-1859, MRC@aad.org, http://www.aad.org.

Howard Baker

Contact lenses *see* **Eye glasses and contact lenses**

Continent urinary diversion *see* **Urinary diversion surgery**

Continuous ambulatory electrocardiography *see* **Holter monitoring**

Continuous positive airway *see* **Inhalation therapies**

Contraception

Definition

Contraception (birth control) prevents **pregnancy** by interfering with the normal process of ovulation, fertilization, and implantation. There are different kinds of birth control that act at different points in the process.

Purpose

Every month, a woman's body begins the process that can potentially lead to pregnancy. An egg (ovum) matures, the mucus that is secreted by the cervix (a cylindrical-shaped organ at the lower end of the uterus) changes to be more inviting to sperm, and the lining of the uterus grows in preparation for receiving a fertilized egg. Any woman who wants to prevent pregnancy must use a reliable form of birth control.

Birth control (contraception) is designed to interfere with the normal process and prevent the pregnancy that could result. There are different kinds of birth control that act at different points in the process, from

Effectiveness of contraceptives: Percentage of women experiencing an unintended pregnancy within first year of typical[1] and perfect[2] contraceptive use

Form of birth control	Typical use	Perfect use
Birth control pills	8.0%	0.3%
Condom, female	21.0%	5.0%
Condom, male	15.0%	2.0%
Depo-Provera® (injection)	3.0%	0.3%
Diaphragm	16.0%	6.0%
Intrauterine devices (IUDs)	0.8%	0.6%
Spermicides	29.0%	18.0%

[1]Effectiveness based on average or typical usage.
[2]Effectiveness based on perfect or correct usage.

SOURCE: Centers for Disease Control and Prevention, "U.S. Medical Eligibility Criteria for Contraceptive Use, 2010," *Morbidity and Mortality Weekly Report*, vol. 59 (May 28, 2010). Available online at: http://www.cdc.gov/mmwr/pdf/rr/rr59e0528 .pdf (accessed August 18, 2010).

(Table by PreMediaGlobal. Reproduced by permission of Gale, a part of Cengage Learning.)

ovulation, through fertilization, to implantation. Each method has its own side effects and risks. Some methods are more reliable than others.

There are more different types of birth control available today than ever. They can be divided into a few groups based on how they work. These groups include:

- Hormonal methods—These use medications (hormones) to prevent ovulation. Hormonal methods include birth control pills (oral contraceptives), Depo Provera injections, and Norplant.

- Barrier methods—These methods work by preventing the sperm from getting to and fertilizing the egg. Barrier methods include the condom, diaphragm, and cervical cap. The condom is the only form of birth control that also protects against sexually transmitted diseases, including HIV (the virus that causes AIDS).

- Spermicides—These medications kill sperm on contact. Most spermicides contain nonoxynyl-9. Spermicides come in many different forms such as jelly, foam, tablets, and even a transparent film. All are placed in the vagina. Spermicides work best when they are used at the same time as a barrier method.

- Intrauterine devices—Intrauterine contraceptive devices (IUDs) are inserted into the uterus, where they stay from one to 10 years. An IUD prevents

the fertilized egg from implanting in the lining of the uterus, and may have other effects as well.

- Tubal sterilization—Tubal sterilization is a permanent form of contraception for women. Each fallopian tube is either tied or burned closed. The sperm cannot reach the egg, and the egg cannot travel to the uterus.

- Vasectomy—is the male form of sterilization, and should also be considered permanent. In vasectomy, the vas defrens, the tiny tubes that carry the sperm into the semen, are cut and tied off. Thus, no sperm can get into the semen.

- A newer and somewhat controversial form of birth control is emergency contraception. This type is used after unprotected intercourse and sometimes is referred to as the "morning-after pill."

Unfortunately, there is no perfect form of birth control. Only abstinence (not having sexual intercourse) can protect against unwanted pregnancy with 100% reliability. The failure rates, which means the rates of pregnancy, for most forms of birth control are quite low. However, some forms of birth control are more difficult or inconvenient to use than others. In actual practice, the birth control methods that are more difficult or inconvenient have much higher failure rates because they are not used regularly or as prescribed.

Description

Most forms of birth control have one thing in common. They are only effective if used faithfully. Birth control pills will work only if taken every day; the diaphragm is effective only if used during every episode of sexual intercourse. The same is true for **condoms** and the cervical cap. Some methods automatically work every day. These methods include Depo Provera, Norplant, the **IUD**, and tubal sterilization.

There are many different ways to use birth control. They can be divided into several groups:

- By mouth (oral)—Birth control pills must be taken by mouth every day.

- Injected—Depo Provera is a hormonal medication that is given by injection every three months.

- Implanted—Norplant is a long-acting hormonal form of birth control that is implanted under the skin of the upper arm.

- Vaginal—Spermicides and barrier methods work in the vagina.

- Intrauterine—The IUD is inserted into the uterus.

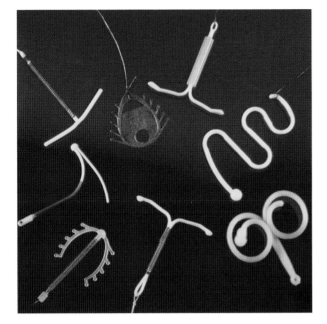

A variety of intrauterine contraceptive devices. The probability of a pregnancy for year of use is about 2 to 3%. IUDs made with copper coils should be replaced every 3 to 5 years. *(Photo Researchers, Inc.)*

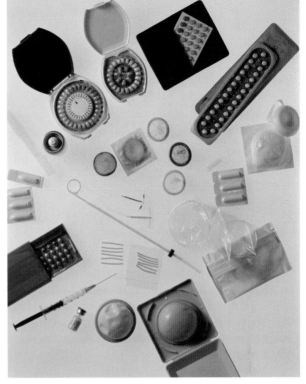

Various forms of contraception. *(Charles Thatcher/Stone/Getty Images.)*

- Surgical—Tubal sterilization is a form of surgery. A doctor must perform the procedure in a hospital or surgical clinic. Many women need general anesthesia.

The methods of birth control differ from each other in the timing of when they are used. Some methods of birth control must be used specifically at the time of sexual intercourse (condoms, diaphragm, cervical cap, spermicides). **Emergency contraception** must be started as soon as possible after intercourse and no more than 72 hours after. All other methods of birth control (hormonal methods, IUDs, tubal sterilization) must be working all the time to provide protection.

Precautions

There are risks associated with certain forms of birth control. Some of the risks of each method appear in the following list:

- Birth control pills—The hormone (estrogen) in birth control pills can increase the risk of heart attack in women over 35, particularly those who smoke. Certain women cannot use birth control pills.
- IUD—The IUD can increase the risk of serious pelvic infection. The IUD can also injure the uterus by poking into or through the uterine wall. Surgery might be needed to fix this.
- Tubal sterilization—"Tying the tubes" is a surgical procedure and has all the risks of any other surgery,

including those associated with anesthesia, as well as infection and bleeding.
- Emergency contraceptive pills should not be used regularly for birth control. They can interrupt the menstrual cycle and are not 100% effective. If the emergency contraception fails, an ectopic pregnancy can occur.

Preparation

No specific preparation is needed before using contraception. However, a woman must be sure that she is not already pregnant before using a hormonal method or having an IUD placed.

Aftercare

No aftercare is needed.

Risks

Many methods of birth control have side effects. Knowing the side effects can help a woman to determine which method of birth control is right for her.

- Hormonal methods—The hormones in birth control pills, Depo Provera, and Norplant can cause changes in menstrual periods, changes in mood, weight gain, acne, and headaches. In addition, it may take many months to begin ovulating again once a woman stops using Depo Provera or Norplant.

- Barrier methods—A woman must insert the diaphragm in just the right way to be sure that it works properly. Some women get more urinary tract infections if they use a diaphragm. This is because the diaphragm can press against the urethra, the tube that connects the bladder to the outside.

- Spermicides—Some women and men are allergic to spermicides or find them irritating to the skin.

- IUD—The IUD is a foreign body that stays inside the uterus, and the uterus tries to get it out. A woman may have heavier menstrual periods and more menstrual cramping with an IUD in place.

- Tubal sterilization—Some women report increased menstrual discomfort after tubal ligation. It is not known if this is related to the tubal ligation itself.

There is no perfect form of birth control. Every method has a small failure rate and side effects. Some methods carry additional risks. However, every method of birth control can be effective if used properly.

Resources

PERIODICALS

"Contraception; Overview." *NWHRC Health Center – Contraception.* March 9, 2004.

"Ectopic Pregnancy Is a Possibility When Emergency Contraception Fails." *Health & Medicine Week* March 15, 2004: 222.

Amy B. Tuteur, MD
Teresa G. Odle

Contractures

Definition

Contractures are the chronic loss of joint motion due to structural changes in non-bony tissue. These non-bony tissues include muscles, ligaments, and tendons.

Description

Contractures can occur at any joint of the body. This joint dysfunction may be a result of **immobilization** from injury or disease; nerve injury, such as spinal cord damage and **stroke**; or muscle, tendon, or ligament disease.

Causes and symptoms

There are a number of pathologies and diseases that can lead to joint contractures. The primary causes resulting in a joint contraction are muscle imbalance, **pain**, prolonged bed rest, and immobilization. Because of the frequency of **fractures** and surgery, immobilization is the most frequent cause of joint contractures. Symptoms include a significant loss of motion to any specific joint that results in immobility. If the contracture is of a significant degree, pain can result even without any voluntary joint movement.

Diagnosis

Manual testing of joint mobility by a healthcare professional skilled in joint mobilization techniques (e.g., a physical therapist) will identify indications of restricted structures within the joint. Measuring the motion of the joint with a device termed a "goniometer" can be useful if the decrease of motion can be shown to be a proven result of a joint contracture. X rays can be of some benefit in the diagnosis of contractures, because a visible decrease in joint space may indicate a tight, contracted joint. Most physicians will make the diagnosis after a thorough **physical examination** involving physical and manual testing of the joint motion.

Treatment

Manual techniques

Joint mobilization and stretching of soft tissues is a common technique used to increase joint elasticity. Structures are stretched in similar directions to those which take place upon normal joint motion. Some healthcare professionals may use some form of heat prior to the stretching and mobilization. If appropriate,

exercise may follow manual techniques to help maintain the additional motion achieved.

Mechanical techniques

Devices known as continuous passive motion machines are very popular, especially following surgery of joints. Continuous passive motion machines (CPM) are specifically adjusted to each individual's need. This method is administered within the first 24–72 hours after the injury or surgery. The joint is mechanically moved through the patient's tolerable motion. CPM machines have been proved to accelerate the return motion process, allowing patients more function in less time.

Casting or splinting

Casting or splinting techniques are used to provide a constant stretch to the soft tissues surrounding a joint. It is most effective when used to increase motion of a joint from prolonged immobilization. It is also popular for treating contractures resulting from an increase in muscle tone from nerve injury. After an initial holding cast is applied for 7 to 10 days, a series of positional casts are applied at weekly intervals. Before the application of each new cast, the joint is moved as much as can be tolerated by the patient, and measured by a goniometer. When as much motion as possible is obtained after stretching, another final cast is applied to maintain the newly acquired motion.

Surgery

In some cases, the contracture may be severe and not respond to conservative treatment. In this event, manipulation of the joint under a **general anesthesia** may be necessary.

Alternative treatment

In some areas of the body, **chiropractic** techniques have been found to be useful to improve motion. **Massage therapy** can be beneficial by promoting additional circulation to joint structures, causing better elasticity. **Yoga** can help prevent as well as rehabilitate a contracture and can facilitate the return of joint mobility.

Prognosis

Prognosis of contractures will depend upon the cause of the contracture. In general, the earlier the treatment for the contracture begins, the better the prognosis.

Prevention

Prevention of contractures and deformities from **spinal cord injury**, fracture, and immobilization is achieved through a program of positioning, splinting if appropriate, and range-of-motion exercises either manually or mechanically aided. These activities should be started as early as possible for optimal results.

ORGANIZATIONS

American College of Rheumatology, 2200 Lake Boulevard NE, Atlanta, GA, 30319, (404) 633-3777, (404) 633-1870, acr@rheumatology.org, http://www.rheumatology.org/.
American Physical Therapy Association, 1111 North Fairfax St., Alexandria, VA, 22314-1488, (703) 684-2782, (703) 684-7343, (800) 999-2782, http://www.apta.org/.

Jeffrey P. Larson, RPT

Conversion disorder *see* **Somatoform disorders**
Cooley's anemia *see* **Thalassemia**

Cooling treatments

Definition

Cooling treatments lower body temperature in order to relieve **pain**, swelling, constriction of blood vessels, and to decrease the likelihood of cellular damage by slowing the metabolism. Sponge baths, cold compresses, and cold packs are all wet cooling treatments. Dry treatments, such as ice bags and chemical cold packs, are also used to lower body temperature.

Purpose

The most common reason for cooling a body is **fever** or hyperthermia (extremely high fever). The body can sustain temperatures up to 104°F (40°C) with relative safety; however, when temperatures rise above 104°F (40°C), damage to the brain, muscles, blood, and kidneys is increasingly likely. Cooling treatments are also applied immediately following sprains, **bruises**, **burns**, eye injuries, and **muscle spasms** to help alleviate the resulting swelling, pain, and discoloration of the skin.

Cooling treatments slow chemical reactions within the body. For this reason, cooling tissues below normal temperature (98.6°F/37°C) can prevent injury from inadequate oxygen or **nutrition**. Cold water drowning victims suffering from **hypothermia** (cooling of the body below its normal temperature) have been successfully resuscitated after long periods underwater without medical complications because of this effect. For the past 40 years, heart surgeons have been experimenting with hypothermia to protect tissues from lack of blood circulation during an operation. Neurosurgeons are also working with hypothermia to protect the very sensitive brain tissues during periods of absent or reduced blood flow.

Description

Depending on the medical need, various cooling methods are used.

- Cold packs and ice bags are placed on a localized site and provide topical relief. These compresses should be covered with a waterproof material to protect the skin. Repeated treatments produce the desired pain and swelling relief.
- Cold treatments are placed on the groin and under the arms to treat hyperthermia. Treatments are refreshed periodically until the appropriate temperature is attained.
- A tepid sponge bath relieves fever without cooling the body too fast. Eighty degrees Fahrenheit is still 20°F below body temperature and yet warm enough not to drive blood from the skin, thereby preventing the cooling from getting to the body's core. Limbs are bathed first and then the chest, abdomen, back, and buttocks.
- Perfusion of isolated regions like the brain by using cooled blood is an experimental treatment, offering promising results for the treatment of stroke.

Preparation

Topical treatments are prepared with ice, cold water (59°F/15°C), and chemical cold packs. Tepid baths should be 80–93°F (26.7–34°C).

Risks

Small children, adults with circulation problems, and the elderly are all at risk of tissue damage. Rapid cooling causes chills, which in effect raise the body's temperature by raising its metabolism. **Blood clots** may form from thickened blood caused by the temperature change.

Resources

PERIODICALS

Plattner, O., et al. "Efficacy of Intraoperative Cooling Methods." *Anesthesiology* 87 (November 1997): 1089-1095.

J. Ricker Polsdorfer, MD

Coombs' tests

Definition

Coombs' tests are blood tests that identify the causes of anemia.

Purpose

Anemia, which literally means no blood, refers to blood with abnormally low oxygen-carrying capacity. The hemoglobin in red blood cells carries oxygen. One of the many causes of anemia is destruction of red blood cells, a process called hemolysis (*hemo* means blood and *lysis* means disintegration). A simple blood count detects anemia. Even the test done before a **blood donation** can identify anemia. To detect hemolysis requires other tests. The Coombs' tests are conducted in order to determine the cause of anemia.

One characteristic of hemolysis is the autoimmune response against the body's red blood cells. Instead of protecting the body from outside agents, the immune system attacks parts of its own body with a deluge of antibodies. Autoimmunity is thought to be the cause of many collagen-vascular diseases, including **rheumatoid arthritis** and **systemic lupus erythematosus**. It is also the cause of the autoimmune hemolytic **anemias**. The Coombs' tests detect the antibodies responsible for the destruction of the red blood cells.

Causes of autoimmune **hemolytic anemia** include:

- drugs such as penicillin, methyldopa (lowers blood pressure), and quinidine (treats heart rhythm disturbances)
- cancers of the lymph system–Hodgkin's disease and lymphomas
- virus infections
- collagen-vascular diseases
- mismatched blood transfusions
- Rh incompatibility between a mother and fetus. (erythroblastosis fetalis)

Many times the cause cannot be identified.

Anemia—Reduced oxygen-carrying capacity of the blood, due to too little hemoglobin or too few red blood cells.

Antibody—A protein made by the immune system and used as a weapon against foreign invaders in the body.

Antigen—The chemical that stimulates an immune response.

Collagen-vascular disease—Various diseases inflaming and destroying connective tissue.

Hematologist—Physician who specializes in diseases of the blood.

Hemoglobin—The red pigment in blood that carries oxygen.

Hemolysis—Breaking apart red blood cells.

Rh—A blood typing group, like the ABO system. When a mother is Rh negative and her baby is Rh positive, she may develop antibodies to the baby's blood that will cause it to hemolyze.

Description

There are two Coombs' tests. A direct Coombs' test detects the two different antigens that might induce hemolysis in the patient's red blood cells. An indirect Coombs' test looks for antibodies to someone else's red blood cells in the patient's serum (the blood without the cells). Combining the two tests gives clues to the origin of the hemolysis.

Preparation

No preparation is needed for this test. It will probably be among the second or third set of blood tests done after anemia is diagnosed and there is a suspicion that its cause is hemolysis.

Aftercare

Coombs' tests are done on blood that is drawn from the arm.

Risks

Taking blood for testing is the most common medical procedure performed. The worst complication is a bruise at the site of the puncture or punctures. It is extremely rare for the needle to injure an important structure such as an artery or a nerve.

Normal results

If the Coombs' tests are negative, the anemia is unlikely to be autoimmune, and the hematologist will have to search elsewhere for a cause.

Abnormal results

If the test is positive, the antigens that react will narrow the search for a cause. Coombs' tests are also done for blood **transfusion** reactions to determine why the transfused blood did not match, and when there is a chance a newborn may have an Rh problem.

Resources

BOOKS

Fauci, Anthony S., et al., eds. *Harrison's Principles of Internal Medicine.* 17th ed. New York: McGraw–Hill Professional, 2008.

J. Ricker Polsdorfer, MD

Coordination tests *see* **Balance and coordination tests**
COPD *see* **Emphysema; Chronic obstructive pulmonary disease**
Copper deficiency *see* **Mineral deficiency**
Copper excess *see* **Wilson's disease**

Cor pulmonale

Definition

Cor pulmonale is an increase in bulk of the right ventricle of the heart, generally caused by chronic diseases or malfunction of the lungs. This condition can lead to **heart failure**.

Description

Cor pulmonale, or pulmonary heart disease, occurs in 25% of patients with **chronic obstructive pulmonary disease** (COPD). In fact, about 85% of patients diagnosed with cor pulmonale have COPD. Chronic **bronchitis** and **emphysema** are types of COPD. High blood pressure in the blood vessels of the lungs (**pulmonary hypertension**) causes the enlargement of the right ventricle. In addition to COPD, cor pulmonale may also be caused by lung diseases, such as **cystic fibrosis**, **pulmonary embolism**, and pneumoconiosis. Loss of lung tissue after **lung surgery** or certain chest-wall disturbances can produce cor pulmonale, as can neuromuscular diseases, such as **muscular dystrophy**. A large pulmonary thromboembolism (blood clot) may lead to acute cor pulmonale.

Causes and symptoms

Any respiratory disease or malfunction that affects the circulatory system of the lungs may lead to cor pulmonale. These circulatory changes cause the right ventricle to compensate for the extra work required to pump blood through the lungs. The right ventricle has thin walls and is crescent-shaped. The resulting pressure causes the right ventricle to dilate and bulge, eventually leading to its failure.

Cor pulmonale should be expected in any patient with COPD and other respiratory or neuromuscular diseases. Initial symptoms of cor pulmonale may actually reflect those of the underlying disease. These may include chronic coughing, **wheezing**, weakness, **fatigue**, and **shortness of breath**. **Edema** (abnormal buildup of fluid), weakness, and discomfort in the upper chest may be evident in cor pulmonale.

Diagnosis

An electrocardiograph (EKG) will show signs such as frequent premature contractions in the atria or ventricles. Chest x rays may show enlargement of the right descending pulmonary artery. This sign, along with an enlarged main pulmonary artery, indicates pulmonary artery **hypertension** in patients with COPD. **Magnetic resonance imaging** (MRI) is often the preferred method of diagnosis for cor pulmonale because it can clearly show and measure volume of the pulmonary arteries. Other tests used to support a diagnosis of cor pulmonale may include arterial **blood gas analysis**, **pulmonary function tests**, and **hematocrit**.

Treatment

Treatment of cor pulmonale is aimed at increasing a patient's exercise tolerance and improving oxygen levels of the arterial blood. Treatment is also aimed at the underlying condition that is producing cor pulmonale. Common treatments include **antibiotics** for respiratory infection; anticoagulants to reduce the risk of thromboembolism; and digitalis, oxygen, and **phlebotomy** to reduce red blood cell count. A low-salt diet and restricted fluids are often prescribed.

Alternative treatment

Co-management of the patient with cor pulmonale should be coordinated between the medical doctor and the alternative practitioner. The first step in

---

KEY TERMS

Ventricle—A cavity, as in the brain or heart. The right ventricle of the heart drives blood from the heart into the pulmonary artery, which supplies blood to the lungs.

---

treatment is to determine the cause of the condition and to evaluate all organ systems of the body. Dietary considerations, for example, a low-salt diet and reduced fluid intake aimed at reducing the edema associated with cor pulmonale, can be supportive aspects of treatment.

Prognosis

The prognosis for cor pulmonale is poor, particularly because it occurs late in the process of serious disease.

Prevention

Cor pulmonale is best prevented by prevention of COPD and other irreversible diseases that lead to heart failure. **Smoking** cessation is critically important. Carefully following the recommended course of treatment for the underlying disease may help prevent cor pulmonale.

ORGANIZATIONS

American Heart Association National Center, 7272 Greenville Avenue, Dallas, TX, 75231, (800) 242-8721, Review.personal.info@heart.org.
National Heart Lung and Blood Institute Health Information Center, P.O. Box 30105, Bethesda, MD, 20824-0105, (301) 592-8573, (240) 629-3246, http://www.nhlbi.nih.gov.

Teresa Odle

Cori's disease see **Glycogen storage diseases**

Corkscrew esophagus see **Diffuse esophageal spasm**

Corneal abrasion

Definition

A corneal abrasion is a worn or scraped-off area of the outer, clear layer of the eye (cornea).

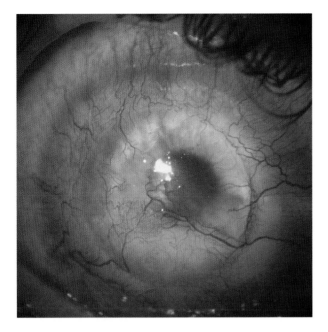

A close-up view of an abrasion on patient's cornea. *(Custom Medical Stock Photo, Inc. Reproduced by permission.)*

Demographics

The exact incidence of corneal abrasions is not known; many are work-related; many result in time lost from work. In work-related injuries, men in their twenties are most likely to experience a corneal abrasion.

Description

The cornea is the clear, dome-shaped outer area of the eye. It lies in front of the colored part of the eye (iris) and the black hole in the iris (pupil). The outermost layer of the eyeball consists of the cornea and the white part of the eye (sclera). A corneal abrasion is a superficial cut or scrape on the cornea. A corneal abrasion is not as serious as a corneal ulcer, which is generally deeper and more severe than an abrasion.

Causes and symptoms

A corneal abrasion is usually the result of direct injury to the eye, often from a fingernail scratch, makeup brushes, **contact lenses**, foreign body, or even twigs. Patients often complain of feeling a foreign body in their eye, and they may have **pain**, sensitivity to light, or tearing.

Diagnosis

Examination

Ophthalmologists and optometrists who treat eye disorders are well qualified to diagnose corneal

abrasions. The doctor will check the patient's vision (visual acuity) in both eyes with an eye chart. A patient history will also be taken, which may help to determine the cause of the abrasion. A slit lamp, which is basically a microscope and light source, will allow the doctor to see the abrasion. Fluorescein, a yellow dye, may be placed into the eye to determine the extent of the abrasion. The fluorescein will temporarily stain the affected area.

Treatment

The cornea has a remarkable ability to heal itself, so treatment is designed to minimize complications. If the abrasion is very small, the doctor might just suggest an eye lubricant and a follow-up visit the next day. A very small abrasion should heal in one to two days; others usually in one week. However, to avoid a possible infection, an antibiotic eye drop may be prescribed. Sometimes additional eye drops may make the eye feel more comfortable. Depending upon the extent of the abrasion, some doctors may patch the affected eye. It is important to go for the follow-up checkup to make sure an infection does not occur. Use of contact lenses should not be resumed without the doctor's approval.

Prognosis

In typical cases, the prognosis is good. The cornea will heal itself, usually within several days. A very deep abrasion may lead to scarring. If the abrasion does not heal properly, a recurrent corneal erosion (RCE) may result months or even years later. The symptoms are the same as for an abrasion (e.g., tearing, foreign body sensation, and blurred vision), but it will keep occurring. Similar or additional treatment for the RCE may be necessary.

Prevention

Everyone should wear eye protection whenever this is recommended. This should be standard practice when using power tools and playing certain sports. Goggles should even be worn when mowing the lawn, because a twig can be thrown upward toward the face. Contact lens wearers should be careful to follow their doctor's instructions on caring for and wearing their lenses. Ill-fitting or dirty lenses could lead to an abrasion, so patients should go for their prescribed checkups.

Resources

OTHER

American Academy of Family Physicians. Corneal Abrasions. FamilyDoctor.org November 2009. http://familydoctor.org/online/famdocen/home/healthy/firstaid/basics/205.html

Kanh, Feras H. and Mark Silverberg. Corneal Abrasion. eMedicine.com May 6, 2010.http://emedicine.medscape.com/article/799316-overview

Corneal Abrasion (Scratch): First Aid. Mayo Foundation for Medical Education and Research. December 23, 2009. http://www.mayoclinic.com/health/first-aid-corneal-abrasion/fa00037

ORGANIZATIONS

American Academy of Family Physicians, P. O. Box 11210, Shawnee Mission, KS, 66207, (913) 906-6000, (800) 274-2237, (913) 906-6075, http://familydoctor.org.

EyeCare America Foundation of the American Academy of Ophthalmology, P. O. Box 429098, San Francisco, CA, 94142-9098, (877) 887-6327, (800) 324-EYES (3937), (415) 561-8567, pubserv@aao.org, http://www.eyecareamerica.org.

National Eye Institute Information Office, 31 Center Drive MSC 2510, Bethesda, MD, 20892-2510, (301) 496-5248, 2020@nei.nih.gov, http://www.nei.nih.gov.

Richard H. Lampert
Tish Davidson, AM

Corneal infection *see* **Keratitis**

Corneal keratoplasty *see* **Corneal transplantation**

Corneal transplantation

Definition

In corneal transplant, also known as keratoplasty, a patient's damaged cornea is replaced by the cornea from the eye of a human cadaver. This is the single most common type of human **transplant surgery** and has the highest success rate. Eye banks acquire and

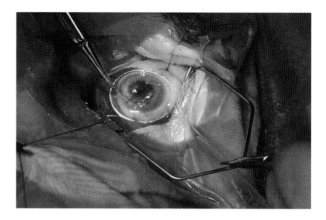

A corneal transplant in progress. *(© Chet Szymecki/Phototake. — All rights reserved.)*

store eyes from donor individuals largely to supply the need for transplant corneas.

Purpose

Corneal transplant is used when vision is lost in an eye because the cornea has been damaged by disease or traumatic injury. Some of the disease conditions that might require corneal transplant include the bulging outward of the cornea (keratoconus), a malfunction of the inner layer of the cornea (Fuchs' dystrophy), and painful swelling of the cornea (pseudophakic bullous keratopathy). Some of these conditions cause cloudiness of the cornea; others alter its natural curvature, which can also reduce the quality of vision.

Injury to the cornea can occur because of chemical **burns**, mechanical trauma, or infection by viruses, bacteria, fungi, or protozoa. The herpes virus produces one of the more common infections leading to corneal transplant.

Surgery would only be used when damage to the cornea is too severe to be treated with corrective lenses. Occasionally, corneal transplant is combined with other types of eye surgery (such as **cataract surgery**) to solve multiple eye problems in one procedure.

Precautions

Corneal transplant is a very safe procedure that can be performed on almost any patient who would benefit from it. Any active infection or inflammation of the eye usually needs to be brought under control before surgery can be performed.

Description

The cornea is the transparent layer of tissue at the very front of the eye. It is composed almost entirely of

KEY TERMS

Cadaver—The human body after death.

Cataract—A condition of cloudiness of the lens of the eye.

Cornea—The transparent layer of tissue at the very front of the eye.

Corticosteroids—Synthetic hormones widely used to fight inflammation.

Epikeratophakia—A procedure in which the donor cornea is attached directly onto the host cornea.

Epithelial cells—Cells that form a thin surface coating on the outside of a body structure.

Fibrous connective tissue—Dense tissue found in various parts of the body containing very few living cells.

Fuchs' dystrophy—A hereditary disease of the inner layer of the cornea. Treatment requires penetrating keratoplasty. The lens of the eye may also be affected and require surgical replacement at the same time as the cornea.

Glaucoma—A vision defect caused when excessive fluid pressure within the eye damages the optic nerve.

Histocompatibility antigens—Proteins scattered throughout body tissues that are unique for almost every individual.

Keratoconus—An eye condition in which the cornea bulges outward, interfering with normal vision. Usually both eyes are affected.

Pseudophakic bullous keratopathy—Painful swelling of the cornea occasionally occurring after surgery to implant an artificial lens in place of a lens affected by cataract.

Retinal detachment—A serious vision disorder in which the light-detecting layer of cells inside the eye (retina) is separated from its normal support tissue and no longer functions properly.

Trephine—A small surgical instrument that is rotated to cut a circular incision.

a special type of collagen. It normally contains no blood vessels, but because it contains nerve endings, damage to the cornea can be very painful.

In a corneal transplant, a disc of tissue is removed from the center of the eye and replaced by a corresponding disc from a donor eye. The circular incision is made using an instrument called a trephine. In one form of corneal transplant (penetrating keratoplasty), the disc removed is the entire thickness of the cornea and so is the replacement disc. Over 90% of all corneal transplants in the United States are of this type. In lamellar keratoplasty, on the other hand, only the outer layer of the cornea is removed and replaced.

The donor cornea is attached with extremely fine sutures. Surgery can be performed under anesthesia that is confined to one area of the body while the patient is awake (**local anesthesia**) or under anesthesia that places the entire body of the patient in a state of unconsciousness (**general anesthesia**). Surgery requires 30–90 minutes.

Over 40,000 corneal transplants are performed in the United States each year. Medicare reimbursement for a corneal transplant in one eye was about $1,200 in 1997.

A less common but related procedure called epikeratophakia involves suturing the donor cornea directly onto the surface of the existing host cornea. The only tissue removed from the host is the extremely thin epithelial cell layer on the outside of the host cornea. There is no permanent damage to the host cornea, and this procedure can be reversed. It is usually employed in children. In adults, the use of **contact lenses** can usually achieve the same goals.

Preparation

No special preparation for corneal transplant is needed. Some eye surgeons may request the patient have a complete **physical examination** before surgery. The patient may also be asked to skip breakfast on the day of surgery.

Aftercare

Corneal transplant is often performed on an outpatient basis, although some patients need brief hospitalization after surgery. The patient will wear an eye patch at least overnight. An eye shield or glasses must be worn to protect the eye until the surgical wound has healed. Eye drops will be prescribed for the patient to use for several weeks after surgery. These drops include **antibiotics** to prevent infection as well as

corticosteroids to reduce inflammation and prevent graft rejection.

For the first few days after surgery, the eye may feel scratchy and irritated. Vision will be somewhat blurry for as long as several months.

Sutures are often left in place for six months, and occasionally for as long as two years.

Risks

Corneal transplants are highly successful, with over 90% of operations in United States achieving restoration of sight. However, there is always some risk associated with any surgery. Complications that can occur include infection, glaucoma, **retinal detachment**, cataract formation, and rejection of the donor cornea.

Graft rejection occurs in 5–30% of patients, a complication possible with any procedure involving tissue transplantation from another person (allograft). Allograft rejection results from a reaction of the patient's immune system to the donor tissue. Cell surface proteins called histocompatibility antigens trigger this reaction. These antigens are often associated with vascular tissue (blood vessels) within the graft tissue. Since the cornea normally contains no blood vessels, it experiences a very low rate of rejection. Generally, **blood typing** and **tissue typing** are not needed in corneal transplants, and no close match between donor and recipient is required. Symptoms of rejection include persistent discomfort, sensitivity to light, redness, or a change in vision.

If a rejection reaction does occur, it can usually be blocked by steroid treatment. Rejection reactions may become noticeable within weeks after surgery, but may not occur until 10 or even 20 years after the transplant. When full rejection does occur, the surgery will usually need to be repeated.

Although the cornea is not normally vascular, some corneal diseases cause vascularization (the growth of blood vessels) into the cornea. In patients with these conditions, careful testing of both donor and recipient is performed just as in transplantation of other organs and tissues such as hearts, kidneys, and bone marrow. In such patients, repeated surgery is sometimes necessary in order to achieve a successful transplant.

Cornea donors are carefully screened. Individuals with infectious diseases are not accepted as donors.

ORGANIZATIONS

American Academy of Ophthalmology (AAO), P. O. Box 7424, San Francisco, CA, 94120-7424, (415) 561-8500, (415) 561-8500, http://www.aao.org.

Victor Leipzig, PhD

Corneal ulcers

Definition

The cornea, the clear front part of the eye through which light passes, is subject to many infections and to injury from exposure and from **foreign objects**. Infection and injury cause inflammation of the cornea–a condition called **keratitis**. Tissue loss because of inflammation produces an ulcer. The ulcer can either be centrally located, thus greatly affecting vision, or peripherally located. There are about 30,000 cases of bacterial corneal ulcers in the United States each year.

Description

The most common cause of corneal ulcers is germs, but most of them cannot invade a healthy cornea with adequate tears and a functioning eyelid. They gain access because injury has impaired these defense mechanisms. A direct injury from a foreign object inoculates germs directly through the outer layer of the cornea, just as it does to the skin. A caustic chemical can inflame the cornea by itself or so damage it that germs can invade. Improper use of **contact lenses** has become a common cause of corneal injury. Eyelid or tear function failure is

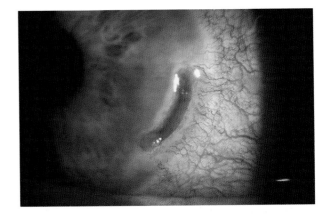

A close-up view of an ulcer on cornea. *(Custom Medical Stock Photo, Inc. Reproduced by permission.)*

the other way to make the eye vulnerable to infection. Tears and the eyelid together wash the eye and prevent foreign material from settling in. Tears contain enzymes and other substances to help protect against infection. Certain diseases dry up tear production, leaving the cornea dry and defenseless. Other diseases paralyze or weaken the eyelids so that they cannot effectively protect and cleanse the eyes.

Causes and symptoms

Viruses, bacteria, fungi, and a protozoan called *Acanthamoeba* can all invade the cornea and damage it under suitable conditions.

- Bacteria from a common conjunctivitis (pink eye) rarely spread to the cornea, but can if untreated.
- Fecal bacteria are more likely to be able to infect the cornea.
- A bacterium called *Pseudomonas aeruginosa*, which can contaminate eyedrops, is particularly able to cause corneal infection.
- A group of incomplete bacteria known as *Chlamydia* can be transmitted to the eye directly by flies or dirty hands. One form of chlamydial infection is the leading cause of blindness in developing countries and is known as Egyptian ophthalmia or trachoma. Another type of *Chlamydia* causes a sexually transmitted disease.
- Other sexually transmitted diseases–for example, syphilis–can affect the cornea.

The most common viruses to damage the cornea are adenoviruses and herpes viruses. Viral and fungal infections are often caused by improper use of topical **corticosteroids**. If topical corticosteroids are used in a patient with the herpes simplex keratitis, the ulcer can get much worse and blindness could result.

Symptoms are obvious. The cornea is intensely sensitive, so corneal ulcers normally produce severe **pain**. If the corneal ulcer is centrally located, vision is impaired or completely absent. Tearing is present and the eye is red. It hurts to look at bright lights.

Diagnosis

The doctor will take a case history to try to determine the cause of the ulcer. This can include improper use of contact lenses; injury, such as a scratch from a twig; or severe dry eye. An instrument called a slit lamp will be used to examine the cornea. The slit lamp is a microscope with a light source that magnifies the cornea, allowing the extent of the ulcer to be seen. Fluorescein, a yellow dye, may be used to illuminate further detail. If a germ is responsible for the ulcer, identification may require scraping samples directly

---

from the cornea, conjunctiva, and lids, and sending them to the laboratory.

Treatment

A corneal ulcer needs to be treated aggressively, as it can result in loss of vision. The first step is to eliminate infection. Broad spectrum **antibiotics** will be used before the lab results come back. Medications may then be changed to more specifically target the cause of the infection. A combination of medications may be necessary. Patients should return for their follow-up visits so that the doctor can monitor the healing process. The cornea can heal from many insults, but if it remains scarred, **corneal transplantation** may be necessary to restore vision. If the corneal ulcer is large, hospitalization may be necessary.

Prognosis

Treated early enough, corneal infections will usually resolve, perhaps even without the formation of an ulcer. However, left untreated, infections can lead to ulcers and the corneal ulcer can result in scarring or perforation of the cornea. Other problems may occur as well, including glaucoma. Patients with certain systemic diseases that impede healing (such as **diabetes mellitus** or **rheumatoid arthritis**) may need more aggressive treatment. The later the treatment, the more damage will be done and the more scarring will result. Corneal transplant is standard treatment with a high probability of success.

Prevention

Attentive care of contact lenses will greatly reduce the incidence of corneal damage and ulceration. Germs that cause no problems in the mouth or on the hands can damage the eye, so contact lens wearers must wash their hands before touching their lenses and must not use saliva to moisten them. Tap water should not be used to rinse the lenses. Contacts should be removed whenever there is irritation and left out until the eyes are back to normal. It is not advisable to wear contact lenses while swimming or in hot tubs. Daily wear contact lenses have been found to be less of a risk than contacts for overnight wear (extended wear). Organisms have been cultured from contact lens cases, so the cases should be rinsed in hot water and allowed to air dry. Cases should be replaced every three months. Patients should follow their doctors' schedules for replacement of the contacts.

Eye protection in the workplace, or wherever tiny particles are flying around, is essential. Ultra-violet (UV) coatings on glasses or sunglasses can help protect the eyes from the sun's rays. Goggles with UV protection should be worn when skiing or in suntanning salons to protect against UV rays. Prompt attention to any red eye should prevent progressive damage.

For people with inadequate tears, use of artificial tears eyedrops will prevent damage from drying. Eyelids that do not close adequately may temporarily have to be sewn shut to protect the eye until more lasting treatment can be instituted.

ORGANIZATIONS

American Academy of Ophthalmology (AAO), P. O. Box 7424, San Francisco, CA, 94120-7424, (415) 561-8500, (415) 561-8500, http://www.aao.org.

American Optometric Association, 243 North Lindbergh Blvd., St. Louis, MO, 63141, (314) 991-4100, (314) 991-4101, (800) 365-2219, http://www.aoa.org/.

Prevent Blindness America, 211 West Wacker Drive, Suite 1700, Chicago, IL, 60606, (800) 331-2020, http://www.preventblindness.org.

J. Ricker Polsdorfer, MD

Corns and calluses

Definition

A corn is a small, painful, raised bump on the outer skin layer. A callus is a rough, thickened patch of skin.

Description

Corns and calluses are one of the three major foot problems in the United States. The other two are foot infections and toenail problems. Corns and calluses affect about 5% of the population.

Corns usually appear on non-weight-bearing areas like the outside of the little toe or the tops of other toes. Women have corns more often than men,

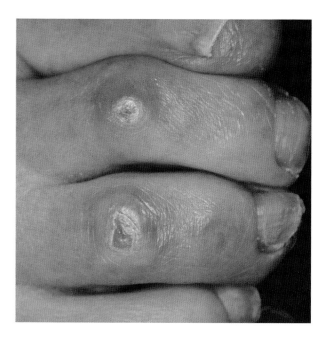

Corns on toes. *(Custom Medical Stock Photo, Inc. Reproduced by permission.)*

probably because women wear high-heeled shoes and other shoes that do not fit properly. Corns have hard cores shaped like inverted pyramids. Sharp **pain** occurs whenever downward pressure is applied, and a dull ache may be felt at other times.

Calluses occur most often on the heels and balls of the feet, the knees, and the palms of the hands. However, they can develop on any part of the body that is subject to repeated pressure or irritation. Calluses are usually more than an inch wide–larger than corns. They generally don't hurt unless pressure is applied.

Types of corns

A hard corn is a compact lump with a thick core. Hard corns usually form on the tops of the toes, on the outside of the little toe, or on the sole of the foot.

A soft corn is a small, inflamed patch of skin with a smooth center. Soft corns usually appear between the toes.

A seed corn is the least common type of corn. Occurring only on the heel or ball of the foot, a seed corn consists of a circle of stiff skin surrounding a plug of cholesterol.

Types of calluses

A plantar callus, a callus that occurs on the sole of the foot, has a white center. Hereditary calluses develop where there is no apparent friction, run in families, and occur most often in children.

Causes and symptoms

Corns and calluses form to prevent injury to skin that is repeatedly pinched, rubbed, or irritated. The most common causes are:

- shoes that are too tight or too loose, or have very high heels
- tight socks or stockings
- deformed toes
- walking down a long hill, or standing or walking on a hard surface for a long time

Jobs or hobbies that cause steady or recurring pressure on the same spot can also cause calluses.

Symptoms include hard growths on the skin in response to direct pressure. Corns may be extremely sore and surrounded by inflamed, swollen skin.

Diagnosis

Corns can be recognized on sight. A family physician or podiatrist may scrape skin off what seems to be a callus, but may actually be a wart. If the lesion is a wart, it will bleed. A callus will not bleed, but will reveal another layer of dead skin.

Treatment

Corns and calluses do not usually require medical attention unless the person who has them has **diabetes mellitus**, poor circulation, or other problems that make self-care difficult.

Treatment should begin as soon as an abnormality appears. The first step is to identify and eliminate the source of pressure. Placing moleskin pads over corns can relieve pressure, and large wads of cotton, lamb's wool, or moleskin can cushion calluses.

Using hydrocortisone creams or soaking feet in a solution of Epsom salts and very warm water for at least five minutes a day before rubbing the area with a pumice stone will remove part or all of some calluses. Rubbing corns just makes them hurt more.

Applying petroleum jelly or lanolin-enriched hand lotion helps keep skin soft, but corn-removing ointments that contain acid can damage healthy skin. They should never be used by pregnant women or by people who are diabetic or who have poor circulation.

It is important to see a doctor if the skin of a corn or callus is cut, because it may become infected. If a corn discharges pus or clear fluid, it is infected. A family physician, podiatrist, or orthopedist may:

- remove (debride) affected layers of skin
- prescribe oral antibiotics to eliminate infection
- drain pus from infected corns
- inject cortisone into the affected area to decrease pain or inflammation
- perform surgery to correct toe deformities or remove bits of bone

Alternative treatment

Standing and walking correctly can sometimes eliminate excess foot pressure. Several types of bodywork can help correct body imbalances. Bodywork is a term used for any of a number of systems, including **Aston-Patterning**, the **Feldenkrais method**, and **rolfing**, that manipulate the body through massage, movement education, or meditational techniques.

Aloe (*Aloe barbadensis*) cream is an effective skin softener, and two or three daily applications of calendula (*Calendula officinalis*) salve can soften skin and prevent inflammation. One teaspoon of lemon juice mixed with one teaspoon of dried chamomile (*Matricaria recutita*) tea and one crushed garlic clove dissolves thickened skin.

An ayurvedic practitioner may recommend the following treatment:

- apply each day a paste made by combining one teaspoon of aloe vera gel with half that amount of turmeric (*Circuma longa*)
- bandage overnight
- soak in warm water for 10 minutes every morning
- massage gently with mustard (*Brassica cruciferae*) oil

Prognosis

Most corns and calluses disappear about three weeks after the pressure that caused them is eliminated. They are apt to recur if the pressure returns.

Extreme pain can change the way a person stands or walks. Such changes can, in turn, cause pain in the ankle, back, hip, or knee.

Bursitis, a painful, inflamed fluid-filled sac, can develop beneath a corn. An ulcer or broken area within a corn can reach to the bone. Infection can have serious consequences for people who have diabetes or poor circulation.

Prevention

Corns and calluses can usually be prevented by avoiding friction-causing activities and wearing shoes that fit properly, are activity-appropriate, and are kept

KEY TERMS

Ayurveda—Ayurveda is a system of wholistic medicine from India that aims to bring the individual into harmony with nature. It provides guidance regarding food and lifestyle, so that healthy people can stay healthy and people with health challenges can improve their health.

Bursitis—Inflammation of a bursa, a fluid-filled cavity or sac. In the body, bursae are located at places where friction might otherwise develop.

in good repair. Soles and heels that wear unevenly may indicate a need for corrective footwear or special insoles. Socks and stockings should not cramp the toes. Gloves, kneepads, and other protective gear should also be worn as needed.

Feet should be measured, while standing, whenever buying new shoes. It is best to shop for shoes late in the day, when feet are likely to be swollen. It is also important to buy shoes with toe-wiggling room and to try new shoes on both feet.

Resources

OTHER

"Foot Disorders: Corns." *Calgary Foot Clinic* http://www.foottalk.com/d_corns.html.

ORGANIZATIONS

American Podiatric Medical Association, 9312 Old Georgetown Road, Bethesda, MD, 20814-1621, (301) 581-9200, http://www.apma.org.

Maureen Haggerty

Coronary artery bypass graft surgery

Definition

Coronary artery bypass graft surgery (CABG) is a procedure in which one or more blocked coronary arteries are bypassed by a blood vessel graft to restore normal blood flow to the heart. These grafts usually come from the patient's own arteries and veins located in the leg, arm, or chest.

Purpose

Coronary artery bypass graft surgery, also called coronary artery bypass surgery and bypass operation, is performed to restore blood flow to the heart. Doing so relieves chest **pain** and **ischemia**, improves the patient's quality of life, and, in some cases, prolongs the patient's life. The goals of the procedure are to relieve symptoms of **coronary artery disease**, enable the patient to resume a normal lifestyle, and lower the risk of a **heart attack** or other heart problems.

According to the American Heart Association, appropriate candidates for coronary artery bypass graft surgery include patients for whom the following applies:

- have blockages in at least two or three major coronary arteries, especially if the blockages are in arteries that feed the heart's left ventricle or are in the left anterior descending artery;
- have angina so severe that even mild exertion causes chest pain;
- have poor left ventricular function; and
- cannot tolerate percutaneous transluminal coronary angioplasty and do not respond well to drug therapy.

Demographics

The American Heart Association estimated that in the United States in 2005, 469,000 coronary artery bypass procedures were performed on 261,000 individual patients. More than twice as many of these surgeries were performed on men than women. Fifteen thousand of these procedures were performed on people between the ages of 15–44, 188,000 on people between ages 45 and 64, and the remainder on people age 65 and older.

Description

Coronary artery bypass graft surgery builds a detour around one or more blocked coronary arteries with a graft from a healthy vein or artery. The graft goes around the clogged artery (or arteries) to create new pathways for oxygen-rich blood to flow to the heart.

Procedure

After **general anesthesia** is administered, the surgeon removes the veins or prepares the arteries for grafting. The surgeon decides which grafts to use based on the location of the blockage, the amount of blockage, and the size of the patient's coronary arteries. If the saphenous vein is to be used for the

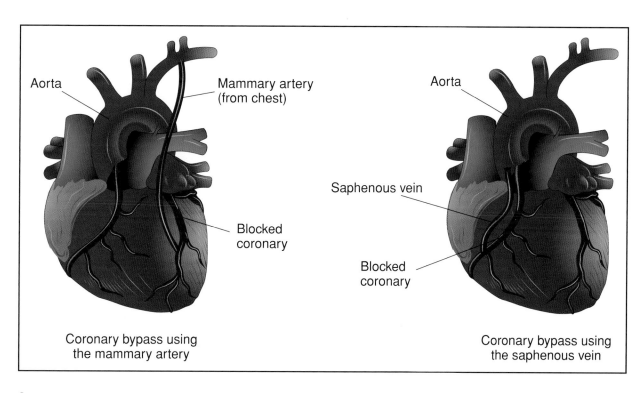

Aorta

Mammary artery (from chest)

Blocked coronary

Coronary bypass using the mammary artery

Aorta

Saphenous vein

Blocked coronary

Coronary bypass using the saphenous vein

Coronary artery bypass graft surgery builds a detour around one or more blocked coronary arteries with a graft from a healthy vein or artery. The graft goes around the clogged artery (or arteries) to create new pathways for oxygen-rich blood to flow to the heart. *(Illustration by Electronic Illustrators Group. Reproduced by permission of Gale, a part of Cengage Learning.)*

graft, a series of incisions are made in the patient's thigh or calf. If the radial artery is to be used for the graft, incisions are made in the patient's forearm. More commonly, a segment of the internal mammary artery is used for the graft, and the incisions are made in the chest wall. The internal mammary arteries are often used because they have shown the best long-term results. The removal of veins or arteries for grafting does not deprive the area from which they are removed of adequate blood flow.

In traditional coronary artery bypass surgery, the surgeon makes an incision down the center of the patient's chest, cuts through the breastbone, and retracts the rib cage open to expose the heart. The patient is connected to a heart-lung bypass machine, also called a cardiopulmonary bypass pump, that takes over for the heart and lungs during the surgery. During this "on-pump" procedure, the heart-lung machine removes carbon dioxide from the blood and replaces it with oxygen. A tube is inserted into the aorta to carry the oxygenated blood from the bypass machine to the aorta for circulation to the body. The heart-lung machine allows heart contractions to be stopped, so the surgeon can operate on a still heart. Aortic clamps are used to restrict blood flow to the area of the heart where grafts will be placed so the

heart is blood-free during the surgery. The clamps remain until the grafts are in place.

Some patients may be candidates for minimally invasive coronary artery bypass surgery or for off-pump bypass surgery. During minimally invasive surgery, smaller chest and graft removal incisions are used, promoting a quicker recovery and less risk of infection. Off-pump bypass surgery, also called beating heart surgery, is a surgical technique performed while the heart is still contracting (beating). The surgeon uses advanced equipment to stabilize portions of the heart and bypass the blocked artery while the rest of the heart keeps pumping and circulating blood through the body.

After the grafts are prepared, a small opening is made in the diseased coronary artery just below the blockage. Blood will be redirected through this opening once the graft is sewn in place. If a leg or arm vein is used, one end is connected to the coronary artery and the other to the aorta. If a mammary artery is used, one end is connected to the coronary artery while the other is already attached to the aorta and remains in place. The procedure is repeated on as many coronary arteries as necessary. On average, three or four coronary arteries are bypassed during surgery. Blood flow

KEY TERMS

Angina—Also called angina pectoris, chest pain or discomfort that occurs when diseased blood vessels restrict blood flow to the heart.

Angiotensin-converting enzyme (ACE) inhibitor—A drug that lowers blood pressure by interfering with the breakdown of a protein-like substance involved in blood pressure regulation.

Aorta—The main artery that carries blood from the heart to the rest of the body. The aorta is the largest artery in the body.

Artery—A vessel that carries oxygen-rich blood to the body.

Atherectomy—A non-surgical technique for treating diseased arteries with a rotating device that cuts or shaves away obstructing material inside the artery.

Atrium (plural Atria)—The right or left upper chamber of the heart.

Beta blocker—An anti-hypertensive drug that limits the activity of epinephrine, a hormone that increases blood pressure.

Brachytherapy—The use of radiation during angioplasty to prevent the artery from narrowing again (a process called restenosis).

Calcium channel blocker—A drug that lowers blood pressure by regulating calcium-related electrical activity in the heart.

Cardiac rehabilitation—A structured program of education and activity offered by hospitals and other organizations.

Coronary artery disease—Also called atherosclerosis, it is a build-up of fatty matter and debris in the coronary artery wall that causes narrowing of the artery.

Echocardiogram—An imaging procedure used to create a picture of the heart's movement, valves, and chambers.

Graft—To implant living tissue surgically.

Homocysteine—An amino acid normally found in small amounts in the blood.

Ischemia—Decreased blood flow to an organ, usually caused by constriction or obstruction of an artery.

Lipoproteins—Substances that carry fat through the blood vessels for use or storage in other parts of the body.

Mammary artery—A chest wall artery that descends from the aorta and is commonly used for bypass grafts.

Radial artery—An artery located in the arm and used for bypass grafts.

Rotoblation—A non-surgical technique for treating diseased arteries.

Saphenous vein—A long vein in the thigh or calf commonly used for bypass grafts.

Stent—A device made of expandable, metal mesh that is placed (by using a balloon catheter) at the site of a narrowing artery; the stent stays in place to keep the artery open.

Sternum—Also called the breastbone, the sternum is the bone in the chest that is separated during open heart surgery.

Stress test—A test used to determine how the heart responds to stress.

Vein—A blood vessel that returns oxygen-depleted blood from various parts of the body to the heart.

Ventricle—A lower pumping chambers of the heart. There are two ventricles, right and left. The right ventricle pumps oxygen-poor blood to the lungs to be re-oxygenated. The left ventricle pumps oxygen-rich blood to the body.

is checked to assure the graft supplies adequate blood to the heart.

If the procedure was done on-pump, electric shocks start the heart pumping again after the grafts have been completed. The heart-lung machine is turned off and the blood slowly returns to normal body temperature. After implanting pacing wires and inserting a chest tube to drain fluid, the surgeon closes the chest cavity. Sometimes a temporary pacemaker is attached to the pacing wires to regulate the heart rhythm until the patient's condition improves. After

surgery, the patient is transferred to an intensive care unit (ICU) for close monitoring.

Diagnosis/Preparation

Diagnosis

The diagnosis of coronary artery disease is made after the patient's medical history is carefully reviewed, a physical exam is performed, and the patient's symptoms are evaluated. Tests used to diagnose coronary artery disease include:

- electrocardiogram;
- stress tests;
- cardiac catheterization;
- imaging tests such as a chest x ray, echocardiography, or computed tomography (CT) scan; and
- blood tests to measure blood cholesterol, triglycerides, and other substances.

Preparation

The patient should quit **smoking** or using tobacco products before the surgery, and the patient needs to make the commitment to be a nonsmoker after the surgery. There are many smoking cessation programs available through hospital or community groups. A health care provider can provide more information about ways quit smoking.

Coronary artery bypass graft surgery should ideally be postponed for three months after a heart attack. Whenever possible, patients should be medically stable before the surgery. If the patient develops a cold, **fever**, or **sore throat** within a few days before the surgery, he or she should notify the surgeon's office.

During a preoperative appointment, usually scheduled one to two weeks before surgery, the patient will receive information about what to expect during the surgery and the recovery period. The patient will usually meet the cardiologist, anesthesiologist, nurse clinicians, and surgeon during this appointment or just before the procedure.

The evening before the surgery, the patient showers with antiseptic soap provided by the surgeon's office. After midnight, the patient should not eat or drink anything.

The patient is usually admitted to the hospital on the day the surgery is scheduled. The patient should bring a list of current medications, **allergies**, and appropriate medical records upon admission to the hospital.

Before the surgery, the patient is given a blood-thinning drug (usually heparin) that helps to prevent **blood clots**. A sedative is given the morning of surgery. The chest and the area from where the graft will be taken are shaved.

Coronary **angiography** will have been previously performed to show the surgeon where the arteries are blocked and where the grafts might best be positioned. Heart monitoring is initiated. The patient is given general anesthesia before the procedure.

The length of the procedure depends upon the number of arteries being bypassed, but it generally takes from three to five hours or sometimes longer.

Aftercare

Recovery in the hospital

The patient recovers in a surgical intensive care unit for one to two days after the surgery. The patient will be connected to chest and breathing tubes, a mechanical ventilator, a heart monitor, and other monitoring equipment. A urinary catheter will be in place to drain urine. The breathing tube and ventilator are usually removed about six hours after surgery, but the other tubes remain in place as long as the patient is in the intensive care unit.

Drugs are prescribed to control pain and infection and to prevent unwanted blood clotting. Daily doses of **aspirin** are started within 6–24 hours after the procedure.

The patient is closely monitored during the recovery period. Vital signs and other parameters such as heart sounds, oxygen, and carbon dioxide levels in arterial blood are checked frequently. The chest tube is checked to ensure that it is draining properly. The patient may be fed intravenously for the first day or two.

Chest physiotherapy is started after the ventilator and breathing tubes are removed. The therapy includes coughing, turning frequently, and taking deep breaths. Sometimes oxygen is delivered via a mask to help loosen and clear secretions from the lungs. Other exercises will be encouraged to improve the patient's circulation and prevent complications due to prolonged bed rest.

If there are no complications, the patient begins to resume a normal routine on the second day, including eating regular food, sitting up, and walking around a bit. Before being discharged from the hospital, the patient usually spends a few days under observation in a non-surgical unit. During this time, counseling is usually provided on eating right and starting a light **exercise** program to keep the heart healthy. The average hospital stay after coronary artery bypass graft surgery is five to seven days.

Recovery at home

INCISION AND SKIN CARE. The incision should be kept clean and dry. When the skin is healed, the incision should be washed with soapy water. The scar should not be bumped, scratched, or otherwise disturbed. Ointments, lotions, and **dressings** should not be applied to the incision unless specific instructions have been given to do so.

DISCOMFORT. While the incision scar heals, which takes one to two months, it may be sore. **Itching**, tightness, or **numbness** along the incision are common. Muscle or incision discomfort may occur in the chest during activity.

Swelling or aching may occur in the legs if the saphenous vein was used for the graft. Special support stockings may be needed to decrease leg swelling after surgery. While sitting, the patient should not cross the legs and the feet should be elevated. Walking daily, even if the legs are swollen, will help improve circulation and reduce swelling.

LIFESTYLE CHANGES. The patient needs to make several lifestyle changes after surgery, including:

- quitting smoking. Smoking causes damage to the bypass grafts and other blood vessels, increases the patient's blood pressure and heart rate, and decreases the amount of oxygen available in the blood.
- managing weight. Maintaining a healthy weight, by watching portion sizes and exercising, is important. Being overweight increases the work of the heart.
- participating in an exercise program. The exercise program is usually tailored for the patient, who will be encouraged to participate in a cardiac rehabilitation program supervised by exercise professionals.
- making dietary changes. Patients should eat a lot of fruits, vegetables, whole grains, and non-fat or low-fat dairy products, and reduce fat intake to less than 30% of all calories.
- taking medications as prescribed. Aspirin and other heart medications may be prescribed, and the patient may need to take these medications for life.
- following up with health care providers. The patient must schedule follow-up visits to determine how effective the surgery was, to confirm that progressive exercise is safe, and to monitor his or her recovery and control risk factors.

Risks

Coronary artery bypass graft surgery is major surgery and patients may experience any of the normal complications associated with major surgery and anesthesia, such as the risk of bleeding, **pneumonia**, or infection. Other possible complications include:

- graft closure or blockage;
- development of blockages in other arteries;
- damage to the aorta;
- long-term development of atherosclerotic disease of saphenous vein grafts;
- abnormal heart rhythms;
- high or low blood pressure;

- recurrence of angina;
- blood clots that can lead to a stroke or heart attack;
- kidney failure;
- depression or severe mood swings; and
- possible short-term memory loss, difficulty thinking clearly, and problems concentrating for long periods (these effects generally subside within six months after surgery).

There is a higher risk for complications in patients who:

- are heavy smokers;
- have a history of lung, kidney, or metabolic diseases;
- have diabetes;
- have had a recent heart attack; or
- have a history of angina, ventricular arrhythmias, congestive heart failure, cerebrovascular disease, or mitral regurgitation.

Normal results

Full recovery from coronary artery bypass graft surgery takes two to three months and is a gradual process. Upon release from the hospital, the patient will feel weak because of the extended bed rest in the hospital. Within a few weeks, the patient should begin to feel stronger.

Most patients are able to drive in three to eight weeks, after receiving approval from their physician. Sexual activity can generally be resumed in three to four weeks, depending on the patient's rate of recovery.

It takes about six to eight weeks for the sternum to heal. During this time, the patient should not perform activities that cause pressure or weight on the breastbone or tension on the arms and chest. Pushing and pulling heavy objects (as in mowing the lawn) should be avoided and lifting objects more than 20 lbs (9 kg) is not permitted. The patient should not hold his or her arms above shoulder level for a long period, such as when doing household chores. The patient should try not to stand in one place for longer than 15 minutes. Stair climbing is permitted unless other instructions have been given. Within four to six weeks, people with sedentary office jobs can return to work. People with physical jobs, such as construction work or jobs requiring heavy lifting, must wait longer (up to 12 weeks) or may have to change careers.

About 90% of patients experience significant improvements after coronary artery bypass graft surgery. Patients experience full relief from chest pain and resume their normal activities in about 70% of the cases; the remaining 20% experience partial relief.

Coronary artery bypass surgery does not prevent coronary artery disease from recurring. For most people, the graft remains open for about 10–15 years. Therefore, lifestyle changes are strongly recommended and medications are prescribed to reduce the risk for the return of coronary artery disease. About 40% of patients have a new blockage within 10 years after surgery and require a second bypass, change in medication, or an interventional procedure.

Morbidity and mortality rates

The risk of **death** while in the hospital during and after coronary artery bypass graft surgery is 1–2%, although the rate varies among individual hospitals and surgeons. In 5–10% of coronary artery bypass graft surgeries, the bypass graft stops supplying blood to the bypassed artery within one year. Younger people who are healthy except for the heart disease achieve good results with bypass surgery. Patients who have poorer results from coronary artery bypass graft surgery include those over the age of 70, those who have poor left ventricular function, are undergoing a repeat surgery or other procedures concurrently, and those who continue smoking, do not treat high cholesterol or other coronary risk factors, or have another debilitating disease.

Over the long term, symptoms recur in only about 3–4% of patients per year. Five years after coronary artery bypass graft surgery, survival expectancy is 90%, at 10 years it is about 85%, at 15 years it is about 55%, and at 20 years it is about 40%.

Angina recurs in about 40% of patients after 10 years. In most cases, it is less severe than before the surgery and can be controlled with drug therapy. In patients who have had vein grafts, 40% of the grafts are severely obstructed 10 years after the procedure. Repeat coronary artery bypass graft surgery may be necessary, and is usually less successful than the first surgery.

Alternatives

All patients with coronary artery disease can help improve their condition by making lifestyle changes such as quitting smoking, losing weight if they are overweight, eating healthy foods, reducing blood cholesterol, exercising regularly, and controlling diabetes and high blood pressure.

All patients with coronary artery disease should be prescribed medications to treat their condition. Antiplatelet medications such as aspirin or clopidogrel (Plavix) are usually recommended. Other medications used to treat angina may include **beta blockers**, nitrates, and angiotensin-converting enzyme (ACE) inhibitors. Medications may also be prescribed to lower lipoprotein levels, since elevated lipoprotein levels have been associated with an increased risk of cardiovascular problems.

Treatment with vitamin E is not recommended because it does not lower the rate of cardiovascular events in people with coronary artery disease. **Antioxidants** such as vitamin C and beta-carotene show some signs of helping reduce coronary artery disease, but not enough rigorously documented information about their effects is available and they are not recommended for routine use. Treatment with **folic acid** and **vitamins** B_6 and B_{12} lowers **homocysteine** levels (reducing the risk for cardiovascular problems), but more studies are needed to determine if lowered homocysteine levels correlate with a reduced rate of cardiovascular problems in treated patients.

Less invasive, nonsurgical interventional procedures, such as balloon **angioplasty**, stent placement, rotoblation, **atherectomy**, or brachytherapy, can be performed to open a blocked artery. These procedures may be the appropriate treatment for some patients before coronary artery bypass graft surgery is considered.

Enhanced external counterpulsation (EECP) may be a treatment option for patients who are not candidates for interventional procedures or coronary artery bypass graft surgery. During EECP, a set of cuffs is wrapped around the patient's calves, thighs, and buttocks. These cuffs gently but firmly compress the blood vessels in the lower limbs to increase blood flow to the heart. The inflation and deflation of the cuffs are electronically synchronized with the heartbeat and blood pressure using **electrocardiography** and blood pressure monitors. EECP may encourage blood vessels to open small channels to eventually bypass blocked vessels and improve blood flow to the heart. Not all patients are candidates for this procedure, and treatments, lasting one to two hours, must be repeated about five times a week for up to seven weeks.

Resources

BOOKS

Lichtenberg, Maggie. *The Open Heart Companion: Preparation and Guidance for Open-Heart Surgery Recovery.* Santa Fe, NM: Open Heart, 2006.

Sheridan, Brett C. *So You're Having Heart Bypass Surgery.* Hoboken, NJ: Wiley, 2003.

OTHER

"Coronary Artery Bypass Surgery." *Medline Plus.* January 24, 2008 [cited January 29, 2008]. http://www.nlm.nih.gov/medlineplus/coronaryarterybypasssurgery.html.

MyHeartCentral.com. [cited March 16, 2008]. http://www.healthcentral.com/heart-disease/.

Your Total Health: Heart Health. http://yourtotalhealth. ivillage.com/heart-health.

ORGANIZATIONS

American College of Cardiology, Heart House2400 N. Street NW, Washington, DC, 20037, (800) 253-4636, http://www.acc.org.

American Heart Association, 7272 Greenville Avenue, Dallas, TX, 75231, (800) 242-8721, http://www. americanheart.org.

Cleveland Clinic Heart & Vascular Institute, 9500 Euclid Avenue, F25, Cleveland, OH, 44195, (866) 289-6911, http://www.clevelandclinic.org/heartcenter.

National Heart, Lung, and Blood Institute, P.O. Box 30105, Bethesda, MD, 20824-0105, (301) 592-8573, http://www. nhlbi.nih.gov.

Texas Heart Institute, Heart Information Service, P.O. Box 20345, Houston, TX, 77225-0345, (800) 292-2221, http://www.texasheartinstitute.org.

Lori De Milto
Angela M. Costello
Tish Davidson, AM
Brenda W. Lerner

Coronary artery disease

Definition

Coronary artery disease is a narrowing or blockage of the arteries and vessels that provide oxygen and nutrients to the heart. It is caused by **atherosclerosis**, an accumulation of fatty materials on the inner linings of arteries. The resulting blockage restricts blood flow to the heart. When the blood flow is completely cut off, the result is a **heart attack**.

Description

Coronary artery disease, also called coronary heart disease or heart disease, is the leading cause of **death** for both men and women in the United States. According to the American Heart Association, deaths from coronary artery disease have declined some since about 1990, but more than 40,000 people still died from the disease in 2000. About 13 million Americans have active symptoms of coronary artery disease.

Coronary artery disease occurs when the coronary arteries become partially blocked or clogged. This blockage limits the flow of blood from the coronary arteries, which are the major arteries supplying oxygen-rich blood to the heart. The coronary arteries expand when the heart is working harder and needs more oxygen. Arteries expand, for example, when a person is climbing stairs, exercising, or having sex. If the arteries are unable to expand, the heart is deprived of oxygen (myocardial **ischemia**). When the blockage is limited, chest **pain** or pressure, called **angina**, may occur. When the blockage cuts off the flow of blood, the result is heart attack (myocardial infarction or heart muscle death).

Healthy coronary arteries are clean, smooth, and slick. The artery walls are flexible and can expand to let more blood through when the heart needs to work harder. The disease process in arteries is thought to begin with an injury to the linings and walls of the arteries. This injury makes them susceptible to atherosclerosis and **blood clots** (thrombosis).

Causes and symptoms

Coronary artery disease is usually caused by atherosclerosis. Cholesterol and other fatty substances accumulate on the inner wall of the arteries. They attract fibrous tissue, blood components, and **calcium**, and harden into artery-clogging plaques. Atherosclerotic plaques often form blood clots that also can block the coronary arteries (coronary thrombosis). Congenital defects and **muscle spasms** can also block blood flow. Recent research indicates that infection from organisms such as chlamydia bacteria may be responsible for some cases of coronary artery disease.

A number of major contributing factors increase the risk of developing coronary artery disease. Some of these can be changed and some cannot. People with more risk factors are more likely to develop coronary artery disease.

Major risk factors

Major risk factors significantly increase the chance of developing coronary artery disease. Those that cannot be changed are:

- Heredity–People whose parents have coronary artery disease are more likely to develop it. African Americans also are at increased risk because they experience a higher rate of severe hypertension than whites.

- Sex–Men are more likely to have heart attacks than women and to have them at a younger age. Over age 60, however, women have coronary artery disease at a rate equal to that of men.

- Age–Men who are 45 years of age and older and women who are 55 years of age and older are more likely to have coronary artery disease. Occasionally, coronary disease may strike a person in the 30s. Older people (those over 65) are more likely to die of a heart attack. Older women are twice as likely as older men to die within a few weeks of a heart attack.

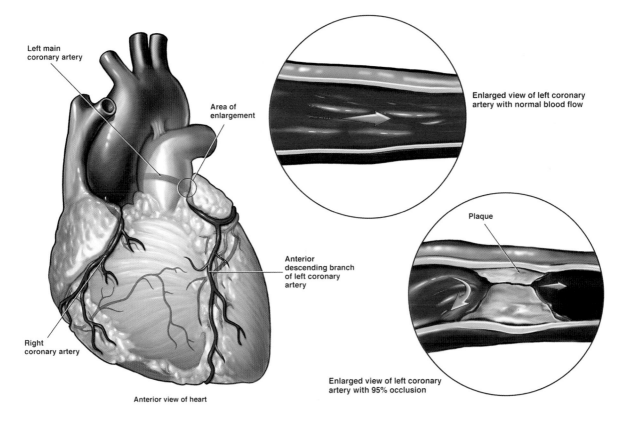

Normal blood flow through the coronary artery compared to blood flow blocked by an occlusion. (© *Nucleus Medical Art, Inc./ Alamy.*)

Major risk factors that can be changed are:

- Smoking–Smoking increases both the chance of developing coronary artery disease and the chance of dying from it. Smokers are two to four times more likely than are non-smokers to die of sudden heart attack. They are more than twice as likely as non-smokers to have a heart attack. They also are more likely to die within an hour of a heart attack. Second hand smoke also may increase risk.

- High cholesterol–Dietary sources of cholesterol are meat, eggs, and other animal products. The body also produces it. Age, sex, heredity, and diet affect one's blood cholesterol. Total blood cholesterol is considered high at levels above 240 mg/dL and borderline at 200-239 mg/dL. High-risk levels of low-density lipoprotein (LDL cholesterol) begin at 130-159 mg/dL, depending on other risk factors. Risk of developing coronary artery disease increases steadily as blood cholesterol levels increase above 160 mg/dL. When a person has other risk factors, the risk multiplies.

- High blood pressure–High blood pressure makes the heart work harder and weakens it over time. It increases the risk of heart attack, stroke, kidney failure, and congestive heart failure. A blood pressure of 140 over 90 or above is considered high. As the numbers rise, high blood pressure goes from Stage 1 (mild) to Stage 4 (very severe). In combination with obesity, smoking, high cholesterol, or diabetes, high blood pressure raises the risk of heart attack or stroke several times.

- Lack of physical activity–Lack of exercise increases the risk of coronary artery disease. Even modest physical activity, like walking, is beneficial if done regularly.

- Diabetes mellitus–The risk of developing coronary artery disease is seriously increased for diabetics. More than 80% of diabetics die of some type of heart or blood vessel disease.

Contributing risk factors

Contributing risk factors have been linked to coronary artery disease, but the degree of their significance is not known yet. Contributing risk factors are:

- Hormone replacement therapy–Evidence from a large trial called the Women's Health Initiative released in 2002 and 2003 found that hormone replacement therapy is a risk factor for coronary artery disease in postmenopausal women. The therapy was once thought to help protect women against heart disease, but in the trial, it was discovered that it was harmful to women with existing coronary artery disease.

• Obesity–Excess weight increases the strain on the heart and increases the risk of developing coronary artery disease even if no other risk factors are present. Obesity increases blood pressure and blood cholesterol and can lead to diabetes.

• Stress and anger–Some scientists believe that stress and anger can contribute to the development of coronary artery disease and increase the blood's tendency to form clots (thrombosis). Stress, the mental and physical reaction to life's irritations and challenges, increases the heart rate and blood pressure and can injure the lining of the arteries. Evidence shows that anger increases the risk of dying from heart disease. The risk of heart attack is more than double after an episode of anger.

Chest pain (angina) is the main symptom of coronary heart disease but it is not always present. Other symptoms include **shortness of breath**, and chest heaviness, tightness, pain, a burning sensation, squeezing, or pressure either behind the breastbone or in the arms, neck, or jaws. Many people have no symptoms of coronary artery disease before having a heart attack; 63% of women and 48% of men who died suddenly of coronary artery disease had no previous symptoms of the disease, according to the American Heart Association.

Diagnosis

Diagnosis begins with a visit to the physician, who will take a medical history, discuss symptoms, listen to the heart, and perform basic screening tests. These tests will measure weight, blood pressure, blood lipid levels, and **fasting** blood glucose levels. Other diagnostic tests include resting and exercise electrocardiogram, **echocardiography**, radionuclide scans, and coronary **angiography**. The treadmill exercise (**stress**) test is an appropriate screening test for those with high risk factors even when they feel well.

An electrocardiogram (ECG) shows the heart's activity and may reveal a lack of oxygen (ischemia). Electrodes covered with conducting jelly are placed on the patient's chest, arms, and legs. They send impulses of the heart's activity through an oscilloscope (a monitor) to a recorder that traces them on paper. The test takes about 10 minutes and is performed in a physician's office. A definite diagnosis cannot be made from **electrocardiography**. About 50% of patients with significant coronary artery disease have normal resting electrocardiograms. Another type of electrocardiogram, known as the exercise **stress test**, measures how the heart and blood vessels respond to exertion when the patient is exercising on a treadmill or a stationary bike. This test is performed in a physician's office or an exercise laboratory. It takes 15–30 minutes. It is not perfectly accurate. It sometimes gives a normal reading when the patient has a heart problem or an abnormal reading when the patient does not.

If the electrocardiogram reveals a problem or is inconclusive, the next step is exercise echocardiography or nuclear scanning (angiography). Echocardiography, cardiac ultrasound, uses sound waves to create an image of the heart's chambers and valves. A technologist applies gel to a hand-held transducer, then presses it against the patient's chest. The heart's sound waves are converted into an image that can be displayed on a monitor. It does not reveal the coronary arteries themselves, but can detect abnormalities in heart wall motion caused by coronary disease. Performed in a cardiology outpatient diagnostic laboratory, the test takes 30–60 minutes.

Radionuclide angiography enables physicians to see the blood flow of the coronary arteries. Nuclear scans are performed by injecting a small amount of radiopharmaceutical such as thallium into the bloodstream. A device that uses gamma rays to produce an image of the radioactive material (gamma camera) records pictures of the heart. Radionuclide scans are not dangerous. The radiation exposure is about the same as that in a **chest x ray**. The tiny amount of radioactive material used disappears from the body in a few days. Radionuclide scans cost about four times as much as exercise stress tests but provide more information.

In radionuclide angiography, a scanning camera passes back and forth over the patient who lies on a table. Radionuclide angiography is usually performed in a hospital's nuclear medicine department and takes 30–60 minutes. Thallium scanning usually is done in conjunction with an exercise stress test. When the stress test is finished, thallium or sestamibi is injected. The patient resumes exercise for one minute to absorb the thallium. For patients who cannot exercise, cardiac blood flow and heart rate may be increased by intravenous dipyridamole (Persantine) or adenosine. Thallium scanning is done twice, immediately after injecting the radiopharmaceutical and again four hours (and maybe 24 hours) later. It is usually performed in a hospital's nuclear medicine department. Each scan takes 30–60 minutes.

Coronary angiography is the most accurate method for making a diagnosis of coronary artery disease, but it also is the most invasive. It is a form of **cardiac catheterization** that shows the heart's chambers, great vessels, and coronary arteries using x-ray technology. During coronary angiography the patient is awake but sedated. ECG electrodes are placed on the patient's chest and an intravenous line is inserted. A local anesthetic is injected into the site where the catheter will be inserted. The cardiologist inserts a catheter into a blood vessel and guides it into the heart. A contrast dye is injected to make the heart visible on x-ray cinematography. Coronary angiography is performed in a cardiac catheterization laboratory either in an outpatient or inpatient surgery unit. It takes from 30 minutes to two hours.

Treatment

Coronary artery disease can be treated many ways. The choice of treatment depends on the severity of the disease. Treatments include lifestyle changes and drug therapy, percutaneous transluminal coronary **angioplasty**, and coronary artery bypass surgery. Coronary artery disease is a chronic disease requiring lifelong care. Angioplasty or bypass surgery is not a cure.

People with less severe coronary artery disease may gain adequate control through lifestyle changes and drug therapy. Many of the lifestyle changes that prevent disease progression–a low-fat, low-cholesterol diet, weight loss if needed, exercise, and not smoking– also help prevent the disease from developing.

Drugs such as nitrates, beta-blockers, and calcium-channel blockers relieve chest pain and complications of coronary artery disease, but they cannot clear blocked arteries. Nitrates (nitroglycerin) improve blood flow to the heart. Beta-blockers (acebutelol, propranolol) reduce the amount of oxygen required by the heart during stress. One type of calcium-channel blocker (verapamil, diltiazem hydrochloride) helps keep the arteries open and reduces blood pressure. **Aspirin** helps prevent blood clots from forming on plaques, reducing the likelihood of a heart attack. Cholesterol-lowering medications are also indicated in most cases.

Percutaneous transluminal coronary angioplasty and bypass surgery are procedures that enter the body (invasive procedures) to improve blood flow in the coronary arteries. Percutaneous transluminal coronary angioplasty, usually called coronary angioplasty, is a non-surgical procedure. A catheter tipped with a balloon is threaded from a blood vessel in the thigh into the blocked artery. The balloon is inflated, compressing the plaque to enlarge the blood vessel and open the blocked artery. The balloon is deflated, and the catheter is removed. Coronary angioplasty is performed in a hospital and generally requires a stay of one or two days. Coronary angioplasty is successful about 90% of the time, but for one-third of patients, the artery narrows again within six months. The procedure can be repeated. It is less invasive and less expensive than coronary artery bypass surgery.

In coronary artery bypass surgery, a healthy artery or vein from an arm, leg, or chest wall is used to build a detour around the coronary artery blockage. The healthy vessel then supplies oxygen-rich blood to the heart. Bypass surgery is major surgery. It is appropriate for those patients with blockages in two or three major coronary arteries, those with severely narrowed left main coronary arteries, and those who have not responded to other treatments. It is performed in a hospital under **general anesthesia**. A heart-lung machine is used to support the patient while the healthy vein or artery is attached past the blockage to the coronary artery. About 70% of patients who have bypass surgery experience full relief from angina; about 20% experience partial relief. Only about 3–4% of patients per year experience a return of symptoms. Survival rates after bypass surgery decrease over time. At five years after surgery, survival expectancy is 90%; at 10 years about 80%, at 15 years about 55%, and at 20 years about 40%.

Various semi-experimental surgical procedures for unblocking coronary arteries are currently being studied. **Atherectomy** is a procedure in which the surgeon shaves off and removes strips of plaque from the blocked artery. In laser angioplasty, a catheter with a laser tip is inserted into the affected artery to burn or break down the plaque. A metal coil called a stent can be implanted permanently to keep a blocked artery open. Stenting is becoming more common.

Alternative treatment

Natural therapies may reduce the risk of certain types of heart disease, but once symptoms appear, conventional medical attention is necessary. A healthy diet (including cold-water fish as a source of essential fatty acids) and exercise, important components of conventional prevention and treatment strategies, also are emphasized in alternative approaches to coronary artery disease. Herbal medicine offers a variety of remedies that may have a beneficial effect on coronary artery disease. For example, ginger (*Zingiber officinale*) may help reduce cholesterol. Garlic (*Allium sativum*), ginger, and hot red or chili peppers all are circulatory enhancers that can help prevent blood clots. **Yoga** and other bodywork, massage, relaxation therapies, and talking therapies also may help prevent coronary artery disease and stop, or even reverse, the progression of atherosclerosis. Vitamin and mineral therapy to reduce, reverse, or protect against coronary artery disease include chromium, calcium and magnesium, B-complex **vitamins**, the antioxidant vitamins C and E, selenium, and zinc. **Traditional Chinese medicine** may recommend herbal remedies, massage, **acupuncture**, and dietary modification. However, studies released in 2003 showed that vitamins C and E fell short of claims that they helped narrow blockage caused by coronary artery disease. In fact, high doses of the vitamins should be avoided.

Prognosis

In many cases, coronary artery disease can be successfully treated. Advances in medicine and healthier lifestyles have caused a substantial decline in death rates from coronary artery disease since the mid-1980s. New diagnostic techniques enable doctors to identify and treat coronary artery disease in its earliest stages. New technologies and surgical procedures have extended the lives of many patients who would otherwise have died. Research on coronary artery disease continues.

Prevention

A healthy lifestyle can help prevent coronary artery disease and help keep it from progressing. A heart-healthy lifestyle includes eating right, regular exercise, maintaining a healthy weight, no **smoking**, moderate drinking, no recreational drugs, controlling **hypertension**, and managing stress. **Cardiac rehabilitation** programs are excellent to help prevent recurring coronary problems for people who are at risk and who have had coronary events and procedures.

Eating right

A healthy diet includes a variety of foods that are low in fat, especially saturated fat, low in cholesterol, and high in fiber. It includes plenty of fruits and vegetables, nuts and whole grains, and limited **sodium**. Some foods are low in fat but high in cholesterol and some are low in cholesterol but high in fat. Saturated fat raises cholesterol and, in excessive amounts, increases the amount of the clot-forming proteins in blood. Polyunsaturated and monounsaturated fats are good for the heart. Fat should comprise no more than 30% of total daily calories.

Cholesterol, a waxy substance containing fats, is found in foods such as meat, eggs, and other animal products. It also is produced in the liver. Soluble fiber can help lower cholesterol. Dietary cholesterol should be limited to about 300 milligrams per day. Many popular lipid-lowering drugs can reduce LDL cholesterol by an average of 25–30% when used with a low-fat, low-cholesterol diet.

Fruits and vegetables are rich in fiber, vitamins, and **minerals**. They are low calorie and nearly fat free. Vitamin C and beta-carotene, found in many fruits and vegetables, keep LDL cholesterol from turning into a form that damages coronary arteries.

Excess sodium can increase the risk of high blood pressure. Many processed foods contain large amounts of sodium. Daily intake should be limited to about 2,400 milligrams, about the amount in a teaspoon of salt.

The "Food Guide" Pyramid developed by the U.S. Departments of Agriculture and Health and Human Services provides easy-to-follow guidelines for daily heart-healthy eating. It recommends 6 to 11 servings of bread, cereal, rice, and pasta; three to five servings of vegetables; two to four servings of fruit; two to three servings of milk, yogurt, and cheese; and two to three servings of meat, poultry, fish, dry beans, eggs, and nuts. Fats, oils, and sweets should be used sparingly. Canola and olive oil are better for the heart than other cooking oils. Coronary patients should be on a strict diet. In 2003, the American Heart Association advised a diet rish in fatty fish such as salmon, herring, trout, or sardines. If people cannot eat daily servings of these fish, the association recommends three fish oil capsules per day.

Regular exercise

Aerobic exercise can lower blood pressure, help control weight, and increase HDL ("good") cholesterol. It may keep the blood vessels more flexible. The Centers for Disease Control and Prevention and the American College of Sports Medicine recommend moderate to intense aerobic exercise lasting about 30 minutes four or more times per week for maximum heart health. Three 10-minute exercise periods also are beneficial. Aerobic exercise–activities such as walking, jogging, and cycling–uses the large muscle groups and forces the body to use oxygen more efficiently. It also can include everyday activities such as active gardening, climbing stairs, or brisk housework. People with coronary artery disease or risk factors should consult a doctor before beginning an exercise program.

Maintaining a desirable body weight

About one-fourth of all Americans are overweight and nearly one-tenth are obese, according to the

KEY TERMS

Atherosclerosis—A process in which the walls of the coronary arteries thicken due to the accumulation of plaque in the blood vessels. Atherosclerosis is the cause of coronary artery disease.

Angina—Chest pain that happens when diseased blood vessels restrict the flow of blood to the heart. Angina often is the first symptom of coronary artery disease.

Beta-blocker—A drug that blocks some of the effects of fight-or-flight hormone adrenaline (epinephrine and norepinephrine), slowing the heart rate and lowering the blood pressure.

Calcium-channel blocker—A drug that blocks the entry of calcium into the muscle cells of small blood vessels (arterioles) and keeps them from narrowing.

Coronary arteries—The main arteries that provide blood to the heart. The coronary arteries surround the heart like a crown, coming out of the aorta, arching down over the top of the heart, and dividing into two branches. These are the arteries in which coronary artery disease occurs.

HDL cholesterol—High-density lipoprotein cholesterol is a component of cholesterol that helps protect against heart disease. HDL is nicknamed "good" cholesterol.

LDL cholesterol—Low-density lipoprotein cholesterol is the primary cholesterol molecule. High levels of LDL increase the risk of coronary heart disease. LDL is nicknamed "bad" cholesterol.

Plaque—A deposit of fatty and other substances that accumulate in the lining of the artery wall.

Triglyceride—A fat that comes from food or is made from other energy sources in the body. Elevated triglyceride levels contribute to the development of atherosclerosis.

Surgeon General's Report on **Nutrition** and Health. People who are 20% or more over their ideal body weight have an increased risk of developing coronary artery disease. Losing weight can help reduce total and LDL cholesterol, reduce **triglycerides**, and boost HDL cholesterol. It also may reduce blood pressure. Eating right and exercising are two key components of losing weight.

Avoiding recreational drugs

Smoking has many adverse effects on the heart. It increases the heart rate, constricts major arteries, and can create irregular heartbeats. It raises blood pressure, contributes to the development of plaque, increases the formation of blood clots, and causes blood platelets to cluster and impede blood flow. Heart damage caused by smoking can be repaired by quitting. Even heavy smokers can return to heart health. Several studies have shown that ex-smokers face the same risk of heart disease as non-smokers within 5 to 10 years after quitting.

Drink in moderation. Modest consumption of alcohol may actually protect against coronary artery disease because alcohol appears to raise levels of HDL cholesterol. The American Heart Association defines moderate consumption as one ounce of alcohol per day, roughly one cocktail, one 8-ounce glass of wine, or two 12-ounce glasses of beer. However, even moderate drinking can increase risk factors for heart disease for some people (by raising blood pressure, for example). Excessive drinking always is bad for the heart. It usually raises blood pressure and can poison the heart and cause abnormal heart rhythms or even **heart failure**.

Do not use other recreational drugs. Commonly used recreational drugs, particularly **cocaine** and "crack," can seriously harm the heart and should never be used.

Seeking treatment for hypertension

High blood pressure, one of the most common and serious risk factors for coronary artery disease, can be controlled completely through lifestyle changes and medication. Moderate hypertension can be controlled by reducing dietary intake of sodium and fat, exercising regularly, managing stress, abstaining from smoking, and drinking alcohol in moderation. People for whom these changes do not work or people with severe hypertension may be helped by many categories of medication.

Managing stress

Everyone experiences stress. Stress sometimes can be avoided and when it is inevitable, it can be controlled. It is particularly important for those at risk for heart disease. A 2003 report showed that middle-aged men with high **anxiety** were less likely to adhere to heart healthy lifestyle practices. Techniques for controlling stress include: taking life more slowly, spending more time with family and friends, thinking positively, getting enough sleep, exercising, and practicing relaxation techniques.

Resources

BOOKS

Bybee, Kevin A., et al. *Cardiovascular Disease in Women Essentials 2011.* Sudbury, MA: Jones & Bartlett Learning, 2011.

Fuster, Valentin, Eric J. Topol, and Elizabeth G. Nabel. *Atherothrombosis and Coronary Artery Disease.* 2nd ed. Philadelphia: Lippincott, Williams, and Wilkins, 2005.

PERIODICALS

"For Fighting Heart Disease, Vitamins C and E Fall Short." *Tufts University Health and Nutrition Newsletter* January 2003: 2.

Jancin, Bruce. "High Anxiety Level Predicts Heart-unhealthy Lifestyle." *Internal Medicine News* March 15, 2003: 25.

"Optimal Diets for Prevention of CHD." *Clinical Cardiology Alert* February 2003.

Wellbery, Caroline. "No HRT or Antioxidants in Women with Coronary Disease." *American Family Physician* March 15, 2003: 1371.

Zoler, Michael L. "Heart Association Advocates Fish Oil Supplements." *Family Practice News* January 15, 2003: 6.

ORGANIZATIONS

American Heart Association National Center, 7272 Greenville Avenue, Dallas, TX, 75231, (800) 242-8721, Review. personal.info@heart.org.

National Heart Lung and Blood Institute Health Information Center, P.O. Box 30105, Bethesda, MD, 20824-0105, (301) 592-8573, (240) 629-3246, http://www.nhlbi.nih.gov.

Texas Heart Institute. Heart Information Service, MC 3-116, PO Box 20345, Houston, TX, 77225, (832) 355-4011, (800) 292-2221, http://www.texasheart.org.

Lori De Milto
Teresa G. Odle

Coronary disease *see* **Coronary artery disease**

Coronary heart disease *see* **Coronary artery disease**

Coronary stenting

Definition

A coronary stent is an artificial support device used in the coronary artery to keep the vessel open.

Purpose

The coronary stent is a relatively new tool used to keep coronary arteries expanded, usually following a balloon **angioplasty**. Balloon angioplasty is used in patients with **coronary artery disease**. In this disease, the blood vessels on the heart become narrow. When this happens, the oxygen supply is reduced to the heart muscle. The primary cause of coronary artery disease is fat deposits blocking the arteries (**atherosclerosis**). In many cases, balloon angioplasty is unsuccessful and the vessel closes after the procedure (restenosis). By forming a rigid support, the stent can prevent restenosis and reduce the need for coronary bypass surgery. The stent is usually a stainless steel mesh tube. Since the stent will be placed inside an artery, the device comes in various sizes to match the size of the artery.

Precautions

Any foreign object in the body, like a stent, will increase the risk of thrombosis. Anticlotting medication is given to prevent this complication.

Description

Coronary stenting usually follows balloon angioplasty, which requires inserting a balloon catheter into the femoral artery in the upper thigh. When this catheter is positioned at the location of the blockage in the coronary artery, it is slowly inflated to widen that artery, and is then removed. The stent catheter is then threaded into the artery and the stent is placed around a deflated balloon. When this is correctly positioned in the coronary artery, the balloon is inflated, expanding the stent against the walls of the coronary artery. The balloon catheter is removed, leaving the stent in place to hold the coronary artery open. A cardiac **angiography** will follow to insure that the stent is keeping the artery open.

Alternative procedures

Balloon angioplasty and coronary stenting are performed to relieve the symptoms of coronary artery disease. By the time coronary artery disease progresses and requires balloon angioplasty, there is no alternative to balloon angioplasty other than coronary

KEY TERMS

Balloon angioplasty—The use of a balloon attached to a catheter to widen an artery that has become narrowed. As the balloon is inflated, it opens the artery.

Cardiac angiography—A procedure used to visualize blood vessels of the heart. A catheter is used to inject a dye into the vessels; the vessels can then be seen by x ray.

Catheter—A long thin flexible tube that can be inserted into the body; in this case, it is threaded to the heart.

Restenosis—The narrowing of a blood vessel after it has been opened, usually by balloon angioplasty.

Thrombosis—The development of a blood clot in the vessels. This thrombosis may clog a blood vessel and stop the flow of blood.

bypass surgery. Coronary bypass surgery carries greater risks. However, since coronary artery disease can be related to high fat **diets**, **smoking**, and lack of **exercise**, changes in lifestyle may reduce the risk of developing the disease. Various medications for **cholesterol, high** blood pressure, and diabetes also can help treat or prevent coronary artery disease.

Preparation

Before the stent is inserted, the patient will probably be instructed to take **aspirin** for several days. Aspirin can help decrease the possibility of **blood clots** forming at the stent. Because anesthesia will be used during the procedure, the patient should not eat or drink after midnight of the previous day.

Aftercare

Following the procedure, blood thinners (anticoagulants) will be given through a needle in a vein for about 24 hours. The patient should remain flat and still for awhile to allow the femoral artery to heal from the insertion of the catheter. Medication to control blood clotting should be taken after the patient is discharged from the hospital. A special diet may also be recommended that is low in vitamin K and cholesterol. With time, the patient should begin light exercise, like walking. It is important that no **magnetic resonance imaging** (MRI) tests are given for six months because the magnetic field may move the stent.

Risks

Although coronary stents greatly reduce the risk of restenosis following balloon angioplasty, there is still some risk that the stented artery may close. Thrombosis, bleeding, and artery damage are also risks.

Resources

OTHER

AdvocateHealthCare. http://www.advocatehealth.com.

ORGANIZATIONS

American Heart Association National Center, 7272 Greenville Avenue, Dallas, TX, 75231, (800) 242-8721, Review.personal.info@heart.org.

Cindy L. A. Jones, PhD

Coronary thrombosis *see* **Heart attack**
Coronavirus infection *see* **Common cold**

Corticosteroids

Definition

Corticosteroids are group of natural and synthetic analogues of the hormones secreted by the hypothalamic-anterior pituitary-adrenocortical (HPA) axis, more commonly referred to as the pituitary gland. These include glucocorticoids, which are anti-inflammatory agents with a large number of other functions; mineralocorticoids, which control salt and water balance primarily through action on the kidneys; and corticotropins, which control secretion of hormones by the pituitary gland.

Purpose

Glucocorticoids have multiple effects, and are used for a large number of conditions. They affect glucose utilization, fat metabolism, and bone development, and are potent anti-inflammatory agents. They may be used for replacement of natural hormones in patients with pituitary deficiency (**Addison's disease**), as well as for a wide number of other conditions including, but not limited to, arthritis, **asthma**, anemia, various cancers, and skin inflammations. Additional uses include inhibition of **nausea and vomiting** after **chemotherapy**, treatment of **septic shock**, treatment of spinal cord injuries, and treatment of hirisutism (excessive hair growth). The choice of drug will vary with the condition. Cortisone and hydrocortisone, which have both glucocorticoid and mineralocorticoid effects, are the

KEY TERMS

Hallucination—A false or distorted perception of objects, sounds, or events that seems real. Hallucinations usually result from drugs or mental disorders.

Hormone—A substance that is produced in one part of the body, then travels through the bloodstream to another part of the body where it has its effect.

Inflammation—Pain, redness, swelling, and heat that usually develop in response to injury or illness.

Ointment—A thick, spreadable substance that contains medicine and is meant to be used on the outside of the body.

Pregnancy category— A system of classifying drugs according to their established risks for use during pregnancy. Category A: controlled human studies have demonstrated no fetal risk. Category B: animal studies indicate no fetal risk, but no human studies; or adverse effects in animals, but not in well-controlled human studies. Category C: no adequate human or animal studies; or adverse fetal effects in animal studies, but no available human data. Category D: evidence of fetal risk, but benefits outweigh risks. Category X: evidence of fetal risk. Risks outweigh any benefits.

drugs of choice for replacement therapy of natural hormone deficiency. Synthetic compounds, which have greater anti-inflammatory effects and less effect on salt and water balance, are usually preferred for other purposes. These compounds include dexamethasone, which is almost exclusively glucocorticoid in its actions, as well as prednisone, prednisolone, betamethasone, trimacinolone, and others. Glucocorticoids are formulated in oral dosage forms, topical creams and ointments, oral and nasal inhalations, rectal foams, and ear and eye drops.

Mineralocorticoids control the retention of **sodium** in the kidneys. In mineralocorticoid deficiency, there is excessive loss of sodium through the kidneys, with resulting water loss. Fludrocortisone (Florinef) is the only drug available for treatment of mineralocorticoid deficiency, and is available only in an oral dosage form.

Corticotropin (ACTH, adrenocorticotropic hormone) stimulates the pituitary gland to release cortisone. A deficiency of corticotropic hormone will have the same effects as a deficiency of cortisone. The hormone, which is available under the brand names Acthar and Actrel, is used for diagnostic testing, to determine the cause of a glucocorticoid deficiency, but is rarely used for replacement therapy since direct administration of glucocorticoids may be easier and offers better control over dosages.

Recommended dosage

The dosage of glucocorticoids varies with the drug, route of administration, condition being treated, and patient. Consult specific references.

Fludrocortisone, for use in replacement therapy, is normally dosed at 0.1 mg/day. Some patients require higher doses. It should normally be administered in conjunction with cortisone or hydrocortisone.

ACTH, when used for diagnostic purposes, is given as 10 to 25 units dissolved in 500 mL of 5% dextrose injection infused IV over eight hours. A long-acting form, which may be used for replacement therapy, is given by subcutaneous (SC) or intramuscular (IM) injection at a dose of 40 to 80 units every 24–72 hours.

Precautions

Glucocorticoids

The most significant risk associated with administration of glucocorticoids is suppression of natural corticosteroid secretion. When the hormones are administered, they suppress the secretion of ACTH, which in turn reduces the secretion of the natural hormones. The extent of suppression varies with dose, drug potency, duration of treatment, and individual patient response. While suppression is seen primarily with drugs administered systemically, it can also occur with topical drugs such as creams and ointments, or drugs administered by inhalation. Abrupt cessation of corticosteroids may result in acute adrenal crisis (Addisonian crisis) that is marked by **dehydration** with severe **vomiting** and **diarrhea**, **hypotension**, and loss of consciousness. Acute adrenal crisis is potentially fatal.

Chronic overdose of glucocorticoids leads to Cushingoid syndrome, which is clinically identical to **Cushing's syndrome** and differs only in that in Cushingoid the excessive **steroids** are from drug therapy rather than excessive glandular secretion. Symptoms vary, but most people have upper body **obesity**, rounded face, increased fat around the neck, and thinning arms and legs. In its later stages, this condition leads to weakening of bones and muscles with rib and spinal column **fractures**.

The short term adverse effects of corticosteroids are generally mild, and include **indigestion**, increased appetite, **insomnia**, and nervousness. There are also a very large number of infrequent adverse reactions, the most significant of which is drug-induced **paranoia**. **Delirium**, depression, menstrual irregularity, and increased hair growth are also possible. Consult detailed reviews for further information.

Long-term use of topical glucocorticoids can result in thinning of the skin. Oral steroid inhalations may cause fungal overgrowth in the oral cavity. Patients must be instructed to rinse their mouths carefully after each dose. Corticosteroids are **pregnancy** category C. The drugs have caused congenital malformations in animal studies, including **cleft palate**. **Breastfeeding** should be avoided.

Mineralocorticoids

Because fludrocortisone has glucocorticoid activity as well as mineralocorticoid action, the same hazards and precautions apply to fludrocortisone as to the glucocorticoids. Overdose of fludrocortisone may also cause **edema**, **hypertension** and congestive **heart failure**.

Corticotropin has all the same risks as the glucocorticoids. Prolonged use may cause reduced response to the stimulatory effects of corticotropin.

Warnings and contraindications

Use corticosteroids with caution in patients with the following conditions:

- osteoporosis or any other bone disease
- current or past tuberculosis
- glaucoma or cataracts
- infections of any type (virus, bacteria, fungus, amoeba)
- sores in the nose or recent nose surgery (if using nasal spray forms of corticosteroids)
- underactive or overactive thyroid
- liver disease
- stomach or intestine problems
- diabetes
- heart disease
- high blood pressure
- high cholesterol
- kidney disease or kidney stones
- myasthenia gravis

- systemic lupus erythematosus (SLE)
- emotional problems
- skin conditions that cause the skin to be thinner and bruise more easily

Interactions

Corticosteroids have many **drug interactions**. Consult specific references.

Resources

BOOKS

ICON Health Publications. *Corticosteroids.* San Diego: ICON Health Publications, 2004.

Katzung, Bertram G. *Basic & Clinical Pharmacology.* New York: McGraw–Hill Medical, 2006.

PERIODICALS

Al-Dhalimi, M.A., and N. Aljawahiry. "Misuses of Topical Corticosteroids: A Clinical Study in an Iraqi Hospital." *Eastern Mediterranean Health Journal* (November 2006): 847–852.

Kirn, Timothy F. "Corticosteroids Are Not for All Asthma Patients: Physicians Need to Be Careful about Greatly Raising the Dose When a Patient Fails to Achieve Control." *Pediatric News* (February 2007): 52.

Martinez, Fernando D. "Inhaled Corticosteroids and Asthma Prevention." *The Lancet* (August 26, 2006): 708–710.

Miller, Karl E. "Inhaled Corticosteroids Effective in Acute Asthma Attacks." *American Family Physician* (May 1, 2007): 1383.

Saunders, Cathy. "Reduced Lung Cancer Risk with Inhaled Corticosteroids." *Australian Doctor* (April 13, 2007): 1.

ORGANIZATIONS

American Academy of Allergy, Asthma & Immunology, 555 East Wells Street, Suite 1100, Milwaukee, WI, 53202-3823, (414) 272-6071, http://www.aaaai.org.

Asthma and Allergy Foundation of America, 8201 Corporate Drive, Suite 1000, Landover, MD, 20785, (800) 727-8462, info@aafa.org, http://www.aafa.org/.

National Heart Lung and Blood Institute Health Information Center, P.O. Box 30105, Bethesda, MD, 20824-0105, (301) 592-8573, (240) 629-3246, http://www.nhlbi. nih.gov.

Samuel D. Uretsky, PharmD
Ken R. Wells

Corticosteroids, dermatologic

Definition

Dermatologic **corticosteroids** are anti-inflammatory compounds formulated for application to the skin. They are intended for local effects only and are not meant for internal use.

KEY TERMS

Corticosteroids—Any of the steroid hormones produced by the adrenal cortex or their synthetic equivalents.

Dermatitis—A disease in which the skin is red and painful. This condition may have different causes. In contact dermatitis, the redness is a reaction to something touching the skin, such as a fabric dye or a metal. Atopic dermatitis is an intense reddening reaction, associated with allergies.

Eczema—A skin disease that causes redness, itching, and scaly or crusty sores. In asteatotic eczema the skin is dry and scaly. Stasis eczema is caused by reduced blood flow.

Lichen planus—An uncommon disorder involving a recurrent, itchy, inflammatory rash or lesion on the skin or in the mouth. The exact cause is unknown, but the disorder is likely to be related to an allergic or immune reaction. The skin lesions are distinct from other disorders.

Systemic—Affecting the entire body.

Topical—Pertaining to a particular surface area and affecting only the area to which it is applied.

Ulceration—Being eroded away, as by an ulcer.

Purpose

Dermatologic corticosteroids are used to treat skin conditions that involve inflammation, usually marked by redness or **itching**. These include **contact dermatitis**, **atopic dermatitis**, nummular **eczema**, stasis eczema, asteatotic eczema, **lichen planus**, **lichen simplex chronicus**, insect and arthropod bite reactions, and first- and second-degree localized **burns** and sunburns.

In addition, dermatologic corticosteroids may be used together with other drugs to treat the symptoms of other conditions which are marked by inflammation of the skin.

Description

All dermatologic **steroids** are based on the natural hormone hydrocortisone, but most have been subject to chemical modification to increase their effectiveness. While many chemical changes to the original molecule will increase the anti-inflammatory effects, the best known is halogenation, replacing one or more of the carbon atoms in the molecule with an atom of fluorine or, less often, chlorine. This change increases the anti-inflammatory effects of the steroid but also increases the risk of some adverse effects.

Topical steroids are usually classed by their potency, ranging from very high to low potency. The most powerful steroids include clobetasol propionate, diflorasone diacetate, and halobetasol propionate. The high and medium potency group includes betamethasone valerate, desoximetasone, fluocininide, halcinonide, and fluandrenolide. Low potency topical steroids include desonide, dexamethasone, fluocinolone acetate, and hydrocortisone.

Topical steroids are particularly affected by their vehicle, which can alter the potency of the product and is particularly important in view of the parts of the body being treated. Lotions are liquid at room temperature and are usually the best choice for application to hairy areas of the body since they can easily reach past the hair. Creams are semi-solid and appropriate for application to most areas. They are usually designed to disappear and leave no sticky residue. This feature makes them appropriate for areas such as the palms of the hands, the face, or areas that are in direct contact with clothing. Ointments are thicker than creams and tend to stay on the skin longer than creams. Pastes are particularly thick ointments, often containing a powder such as zinc oxide, and may be used where a protective effect is needed.

Because of variations in skin thickness, it is essential to match the potency of the steroid with the area being treated. Areas of thick skin may require a very potent steroid in order to penetrate the outer layer of skin. In areas where the skin is thin, a high potency steroid may increase the risk of serious adverse reactions.

Recommended dosage

Most topical steroids are applied twice a day, but applications as frequently as four times a day may be appropriate. In some cases, penetration through the skin may be increased by use of occlusion.

Precautions

Excessive use of topical corticosteroids may lead to systemic side effects. Patients using high potency steroids over large areas of the body for a prolonged period should have adrenal function tests.

Normally, areas covered by steroid creams should not be bandaged, since doing so increases the absorption of the steroid and may lead to increased adverse effects.

Some commercially available formulations of topical corticosteroids contain sulfites that may cause allergic reactions. Allergic reactions to other ingredients in topical formulations are very infrequent but have been reported.

Topical corticosteroids should not be used in patients with markedly impaired circulation since skin ulceration has occurred in these patients following use of the drugs.

Topical corticosteroids should be used with extreme caution in areas where the skin is infected and should never be used in infected areas unless the infection is being appropriately treated.

When used properly, these medicines have not been shown to cause problems in humans. Studies on **birth defects** have not been done in humans. However, studies in animals have shown that topical corticosteroids, when applied to the skin in large amounts or used for a long time, can cause birth defects. Maternal use of topical corticosteroids has not been reported to cause problems in nursing babies when used properly. However, corticosteroids should not be applied to the breasts before nursing.

Side effects

When dermatologic corticosteroids are used properly, adverse effects are very rare. Even so, the following effects have been reported:

- blood-containing blisters on skin
- burning and itching of skin
- increased skin sensitivity (for some brands of betamethasone lotion)
- lack of healing of skin condition
- numbness in fingers
- painful, red, or itchy, pus-containing blisters in hair follicles
- raised, dark red, wart-like spots on skin, especially when used on the face
- skin infection
- thinning of skin with easy bruising

Excessive use, either because of use of an inappropriately potent steroid, prolonged use, or inappropriate use of occlusion has been known to lead to more severe adverse effects. However, these reactions are very rare.

Interactions

When used properly, topical steroids have no **drug interactions** or interactions with foods because they do not reach significant levels in the body. Application of another ointment to the same area at the same time may dilute the corticosteroid ointment and result in lowered effectiveness.

Resources

BOOKS

Green, Steven M. *Tarascon Pocket Pharmacopoeia*. Lompoc, CA: Tarascon Publishing, 2005.
ICON Health Publications. *Corticosteroids*. San Diego: ICON Health Publications, 2004.
ICON Health Publications. *Hydrocortisone—A Medical Dictionary, Bibliography, and Annotated Research Guide to Internet References*. San Diego: ICON Health Publications, 2004.
Katzung, Bertram G. *Basic & Clinical Pharmacology*. New York: McGraw-Hill Medical, 2006.

PERIODICALS

Al-Dhalimi, M.A., and N. Aljawahiry. "Misuses of Topical Corticosteroids: A Clinical Study in an Iraqi Hospital." *Eastern Mediterranean Health Journal* (November 2006): 847–852.
Beer, Kenneth, and Jeanine Downie. "Sequelae from Inadvertent Long-Term Use of Potent Topical Steroids." *Journal of Drugs in Dermatology* (May 2007): 550–551.
Dawn, Aerlyn, and Gil Yosipovitch. "Treating Itch in Psoriasis."*Dermatology Nursing* (June 2006): 227–234.
Wendling, Patrice. "Tailor Acne Treatment to Teen's Needs, Expert Says."*Pediatric News* (June 2007): 39.

ORGANIZATIONS

American Academy of Dermatology, PO Box 4014, Schaumburg, IL, 60168-4014, (847) 240-1859, (866) 503-SKIN (7546), http://www.aad.org.
European Dermato-Epidemiology Network, Department of Dermatology University Medical Centre, Groningen, The Netherlands, 9700 RB, 003150, 3612520, 003150, 3619247, p.j.coenraads@med.umcg.nl, http://eden.dermis.net/

Samuel D. Uretsky, Pharm.D.
Ken R. Wells

Corticosteroids, inhaled

Definition

Inhaled **corticosteroids** are glucocorticoids (a class of steroid hormones that are synthesized by the adrenal cortex and have anti-inflammatory activity) formulated to be used in the respiratory tract and lungs.

Purpose

Inhaled corticosteroids are glucocorticoid compounds designed to be applied directly to the tissues of the respiratory tract. There are two types. The intranasal are deposited into the nasal passages and may be used to treat **nasal polyps**, perennial **allergic rhinitis**, seasonal allergic **rhinitis**, and recurrent chronic **sinusitis**.

The second type is used when the **steroids** are designed for deposition further into the respiratory tract. These are used for treatment of chronic **asthma** and prevention of asthmatic attacks.

Because they have anti-inflammatory effects, corticosteroids are invaluable in treatment of asthma and other respiratory conditions which are associated with an allergic reaction. In many cases, the corticosteroids are life saving. But **systemic corticosteroids** affect all parts of the body and may cause very severe adverse effects, particularly with long-term use. These reactions include inhibitions of the adrenal glands and weakening of bones. By administering these drugs by inhalation, it is possible to target the areas that require treatment and reduce the amount of drug that reaches other parts of the body. Some patients may be able to do without systemic steroids entirely, while others can reduce their doses of systemic steroids and thereby reduce the risk and severity of unwanted effects.

The drugs used as inhaled steroids are all anti-inflammatory corticosteroids and are very similar to each other in action and use. The way they are formulated, the size of the particles, the design of the inhaler, and whether the drugs are inhaled by the mouth or nose determine how far into the respiratory tract the steroids go. The formulations designed for nasal inhalation are only effective for nasal polyps or rhinitis because the steroid does not penetrate deeply into the respiratory tract. Oral inhalations, containing the same drug but in different particle size and inhaler design, deposit medication deeply into the lungs and are of value in treatment of asthma.

Description

As of 2007, there are eight corticosteroid medications designed for inhalation:

- beclomethasone dipropionate (Qvar, Vanceril, and Beclovent)
- budesonide (Pulmicort)
- flunisolide (AeroBID)
- fluticasone propionate (Flovent)
- triamcinolone acetonide (Azmacort)

Also, there is a combination drug of fluticasone propionate and salmeterol xinafoate (Advair Diskus)

available for children over 12 years old. Although the different products vary in potency and duration of action, once dose size and frequency have been adjusted to offer comparable results, there do not appear to be significant differences between the drugs. The design of the inhalers, their ease of use, and the training each patient receives in the proper use of the inhaler may be of greater significance than the drug itself.

Recommended dosage

Although the different products vary in milligram potency, for practical purposes, doses are measured in puffs on the inhaler. For example, beclomethasone will deliver 40 micrograms each time the inhaler is used, while triamcinolone delivers 100 micrograms with each inhalation. However, the effects are essentially equal.

The appropriate dose of inhaled corticosteroids depends on the severity of the case, and in some instances, on what treatment has been used prior to starting inhaled steroid therapy. The doses listed are typical of the inhaled steroids used for asthma therapy but do not represent all possible cases:

- beclomethasone: one to two puffs two times a day
- budesonide: one to two puffs two times a day
- flunisolide: two puffs two times a day
- fluticasone propionate: available in forms that deliver either 50 or 100 micrograms of fluticase in each puff; typical initial dose, 100 micrograms two times a day, representing either one puff of the 100 microgram product or two puffs of the 50 microgram product
- triamcinolone acetonide: two puffs three or four times a day or four puffs twice a day, not to exceed 16 puffs daily

Precautions

Particular care is essential for patients who are transferred from systemic corticosteroids to inhaled steroids. Because the long-term use of oral steroids lowers the output of these compounds from the adrenal gland and normal production does not recur for several months, patients who have their oral doses reduced are at risk of adrenal insufficiency. This condition may become particularly serious in the event of trauma, surgery, or infections. While inhaled steroids may provide adequate control of asthma during these periods, the inhaled drugs do not replace the systemic compounds. In the event of **stress** or a severe asthma attack, oral therapy must immediately begin. Regular testing for cortisol levels is essential until the normal levels have been resumed.

For patients who had been on systemic therapy and are being switched to corticosteroid inhalation, the immediate period during which the oral dose is reduced may cause symptoms, including joint or muscle **pain**, tiredness, and depression. Continuous monitoring is required until normal functions have been resumed.

It is essential that patients learn proper use of inhalers. If inhalers are not used properly, the corticosteroids may not reach their intended site of action. Instead, they may be left in the mouth or swallowed and be deposited in the digestive tract. This situation may increase the risk of adverse effects, while reducing the protection from asthmatic attacks.

Inhaled corticosteroids are not for treatment of acute asthmatic attacks or rapid relief of bronchospasm.

Inhaled corticosteroids are designated as **pregnancy** category C. This designation means one of two levels of knowledge concerning the drugs adverse effects. In one instance, studies on animals show adverse fetal effects but there are no controlled studies on women. In the other instance, no studies on animals and women are not available.

Side effects

It can be difficult to evaluate the side effects of inhaled corticosteroids because many of the reported adverse effects are closely associated with dose reduction or discontinuation of systemic steroids. Not all of the adverse reactions listed have been associated with all of the marketed inhaled steroids, but because of the similarities between these drugs, an adverse reaction reported with one must be considered possible for the others.

The most common severe problem is white patches in the mouth due to localized infection. Additional common side effects are:

- cough
- general aches and pains or general feeling of illness
- greenish-yellow mucus in nose
- headache
- hoarseness or other voice changes
- loss of appetite
- runny, sore, or stuffy nose
- unusual tiredness
- weakness

Very rare but severe adverse effects include the following:

- blindness, blurred vision, eye pain
- large hives
- bone fractures
- diabetes mellitus (increased hunger, thirst, or urination)

- excess facial hair in women
- fullness or roundness of face, neck, and trunk
- growth reduction in children or adolescents
- heart problems
- high blood pressure
- hives and skin rash
- impotence in males
- lack of menstrual periods
- muscle wasting
- numbness and weakness of hands and feet
- weakness
- swelling of face, lips, or eyelids
- tightness in chest, troubled breathing, or wheezing

Interactions

Because inhaled steroids do not reach therapeutic levels in the blood stream, there are no serious interactions. Ketoconazole (Nizoral), an antifungal agent, has been reported to increase blood levels of budesonide and fluticasone, but it is unclear whether this has any importance when the steroids are administered by inhalation.

Resources

BOOKS

Katzung, Bertram G. *Basic & Clinical Pharmacology*. New York: McGraw-Hill Medical, 2006.

PERIODICALS

Kirn, Timothy F. "Corticosteroids Are Not for All Asthma Patients: Physicians Need to Be Careful about Greatly Raising the Dose When a Patient Fails to Achieve Control."*Pediatric News* (February 2007): 52.

Martinez, Fernando D. "Inhaled Corticosteroids and Asthma Prevention."*The Lancet* (August 26, 2006): 708–710.

Miller, Karl E. "Inhaled Corticosteroids Effective in Acute Asthma Attacks."*American Family Physician* (May 1, 2007): 1383.

Saunders, Cathy. "Reduced Lung Cancer Risk with Inhaled Corticosteroids."*Australian Doctor* (April 13, 2007): 1.

ORGANIZATIONS

American Academy of Allergy, Asthma & Immunology, 555 East Wells Street, Suite 1100, Milwaukee, WI, 53202-3823, (414) 272-6071, http://www.aaaai.org.

Asthma and Allergy Foundation of America, 8201 Corporate Drive, Suite 1000, Landover, MD, 20785, (800) 727-8462, info@aafa.org, http://www.aafa.org/.

National Heart Lung and Blood Institute Health Information Center, P.O. Box 30105, Bethesda, MD, 20824-0105, (301) 592-8573, (240) 629-3246, http://www.nhlbi.nih.gov.

Samuel D. Uretsky, Pharm.D.
Ken R. Wells

Corticosteroids, systemic

Definition

Corticosteroids are a group of drugs which are chemically related to the hormones produced by the adrenal glands as a response to adrenocorticotropic hormone (ACTH), but excluding the sex hormones that are produced by this gland. The primary adrenal corticosteroids are cortisol and aldosterone. Cortisol is a glucocorticoid, responsible for influencing carbohydrate, fat, and protein metabolism. Aldosterone is a mineralocorticoid, responsible for regulating salt and water balance.

All corticosteroids, both natural ones and those which have been developed synthetically, share a similar chemical structure, which is based on the structure of cholesterol.

Purpose

The primary purpose of corticosteroids is replacement of naturally occurring hormones when the adrenal glands do not make enough of the natural hormones. Known as **Addison's disease**, this deficit is marked by low blood pressure, weight loss, loss of appetite, weakness, and a bronze-like **hyperpigmentation** of the skin. Addison's disease requires both glucocorticoid and mineralocorticoid treatment.

Because the glucocorticoids inhibit some portions of the immune response, they are used in treatment of a large number of diseases. The following list includes some of the established uses of systemic corticosteroids.

- acute, severe allergic reactions
- arthritis, osteoarthritis, rheumatoid arthritis, psoriatic arthritis, and gouty arthritis
- adrenocortical insufficiency
- allergic conjunctivitis
- allergic rhinitis
- anemia
- (acquired hemolytic and congenital hypoplastic)
- ankylosing spondylitis
- asthma
- beryliosis
- bursitis
- corneal ulcers
- Crohn's disease
- dermatitis (atopic, contact, exfoliative, and seborrheic)
- dermatomyositis
- erythema multiforme
- erythroblastopenia
- herpes zoster of the eye
- hypercalcemia secondary to cancer
- hypersensitivity reactions
- idiopathic thrombocytopenic purpura
- leukemia
- lupus erythematosis
- lymphoma
- multiple myeloma
- multiple sclerosis, acute exacerbations
- mycosis fungoides
- optic neuritis
- pemphigus
- pneumonitis (aspiration)
- rheumatic carditis
- Stevens-Johnson syndrome
- thrombocytopenia
- trichinosis with nerve or heart involvement
- tuberculosis, disseminated and fulminating
- tuberculous meningitis
- ulcerative colitis

Dexamethasone, a related corticosteroid, is widely used to prevent the **nausea and vomiting** associated with **cancer** therapy.

Glucocorticoid treatment is not a cure for any disease or condition, but it may be used as supportive therapy in addition to other treatments.

Description

Because they both have mineralocorticoid and glucocorticoid effects, cortisone and hydrocortisone are preferred for use in treating adrenal insufficiency. When glucocorticoids are used for their anti-inflammatory and immunosuppressant properties and their effects on blood and lymphatic systems, synthetic compounds, which have increased glucocorticoid effects and minimal mineralocorticoid effects, are generally preferred.

A number of systemic corticosteroid compounds are commercially available. Although they are generally similar, they vary in their potency, sodium-retaining effects, and duration of action.

Short acting

Cortisone has both glucocorticoid and mineralocorticoid effects. It has the lowest potency of the commercially available corticosteroids and a short duration of action. It is appropriate for replacement therapy in patients with adrenal insufficiency.

Hydrocortisone has both glucocorticoid and mineralocorticoid effects. It is more potent than cortisone and has a somewhat longer duration of action. Although hydrocortisone may be used for its systemic effects, it is most commonly used in skin preparations.

Intermediate acting

Prednisone is probably the most widely used of the systemic **steroids**. It has about half the sodium-retaining effects of hydrocortisone but several times the anti-inflammatory effects. Because of the low level of mineralocorticoid effects, however, prednisone is not suitable for treatment of adrenal insufficiency unless it is used in combination with a mineralocorticoid drug. Prednisolone is very similar to prednisone. In addition to oral dosage form, it is available for subcutaneous, intramuscular, and intravenous injection.

Triamcinolone is slightly more potent than prednisone or prednisolone but has no sodium-retaining effects. It is administered various ways, including inhalation for respiratory problems and as ointments and creams for skin conditions. Methylprednisolone, which is similar to triamcinolone, is most commonly given by injection.

Long acting

Dexamethasone is a very potent glucocorticoid, with no mineralocorticoid activity. It is used in various forms, including tablets, injection, ointments, and eye and eardrops. In cancer treatment, dexamethasone is used both for its corticosteroid properties and as an antinauseant, to help control the side effects of other drugs. Betamethasone is similar to dexamethasone. Although the drug is available for systemic use, it is more commonly used in the form of inhalations and ointments. Other corticosteroids are available but are most often used in inhalation form, for **asthma, allergic rhinitis**, or other respiratory conditions.

Recommended dosage

Dosages of corticosteroids must be individualized based on the drug selected, the condition being treated, and the response of the patient. In adrenal insufficiency, a dose equivalent to 25 mg of cortisone or 20 mg of hydrocortisone is normally appropriate. In other conditions, a pharmacologic dose (any dose in excess of the replacement dose) is called for. The equivalent doses of corticosteroids are as follows:

- cortisone: 25 mg
- hydrocortisone: 20 mg
- prednisolone: 5 mg
- prednisone: 5 mg
- methylprednisolone: 4 mg
- triamcinolone: 4 mg
- dexamethason: 0.75 mg
- betamethasone: 0.6 mg

For short-term use, corticosteroids are normally administered in two or three doses each day. In most cases, an initial dose equivalent to 5 to 60 milligrams of prednisone per day is appropriate. Usually, a response will be seen within ten days. Once a response has been observed, the dose should be carefully reduced to the lowest dose that will provide adequate control. If no response is seen after a reasonable period of time, an alternative method of treatment should be considered. On rare occasions, patients will respond better to one corticosteroid than to others.

In the case of acute exacerbations of **multiple sclerosis**, doses as high as 200 milligrams of prednisone or prednisolone for a week followed by 80 mg every other day for one month have been used.

Because administration of corticosteroids reduces the output of cortisone from the adrenal glands, dosing should be designed to minimize the effects of corticosteroid therapy on the adrenal glands. For patients who will be taking corticosteroids for a long time, a single dose of the corticosteroid is taken every other morning. This regimen provides benefits for most conditions, while minimizing many adverse effects of long-term steroid administration, including adrenal suppression and protein breakdown. Although alternate day treatment is the preferred dosing schedule, it is not suited for treatment of **rheumatoid arthritis** or ulcerative **colitis**, for which daily doses are essential. Only the shorter acting corticosteroids such as prednisone or prednisolone should be used for alternate-day dosing.

When corticosteroid treatment is being discontinued, it is frequently useful to reduce the dose gradually, over several days. Many of these tapering schedules have been described. In one tapering schedule glucocorticoid dosage is reduced by the equivalent of 2.5–5 mg of prednisone every three to seven days until the physiologic dose (e.g., 5 mg of prednisone or prednisolone, 0.75 mg of dexamethasone, or 20 mg of hydrocortisone) is reached. Other schedules may call for slower dose adjustments. The dose may have to be increased if there is a flare-up of the condition being treated while the dose is being reduced. Then, tapering may begin again, but at a slower rate.

Precautions

Because corticosteroids reduce the immune response, they should not be used in patients who have active fungal infections. Similarly, patients being treated with corticosteroids should avoid receiving live virus vaccines.

Corticosteroids may mask some signs of infection, and new infections may appear during their use. There may be decreased resistance and inability to localize infection. Any evidence of infection should be treated promptly with appropriate anti-infective therapy.

Corticosteroids may activate latent amebic infections. Therefore, it is recommended that latent or active **amebiasis** be ruled out before starting corticosteroid therapy in any patient who has spent time in the tropics or any patient with unexplained **diarrhea**.

Adequate human reproduction studies have not been done with corticosteroids. Use of these drugs in **pregnancy** or in women of childbearing potential requires that the anticipated benefits be weighed against the possible hazards to the mother and embryo or fetus. Infants born of mothers who have received substantial doses of corticosteroids during pregnancy should be carefully observed for signs of hypoadrenalism.

Corticosteroids have been associated with an increased risk of gastric ulcers, and patients are usually advised to take these drugs either with food or a drug which inhibits gastric acid. Those taking high dose steroids or on maintenance therapy should take the medication with meals or a gastric acid blocker to reduce the risk of gastric ulcers. However, these precautions are probably not needed for patients taking low doses for a short period of time.

Side effects

Corticosteroids are generally safe when used for a short period of time with appropriate monitoring. When used for longer periods, the frequency and severity of adverse effects increases dramatically. Many of these effects are the unavoidable results of the normal actions of the steroid drugs and must be considered when people decide on a course of long-term corticosteroid therapy.

Fluid and electrolyte disturbances

Sodium retention, fluid retention, congestive **heart failure** in susceptible patients, potassium loss, **calcium** loss, **hypertension** may result from long-term use.

Muscle and bone

Muscle weakness, loss of muscle mass, **osteoporosis**, compression **fractures** of the spine, aseptic necrosis of femoral and humeral heads, pathologic fracture of long bones, and tendon rupture are all possible effects from long-term use.

Gastrointestinal effects

Peptic ulcer with possible perforation and hemorrhage, perforation of the small and large bowel particularly in patients with inflammatory bowel disease, **pancreatitis**, abdominal distention, and ulcerative esophagitis can result from long-term use.

Skin reactions

Impaired wound healing, thin fragile skin, red spots, increased sweating, reduced reactions to skin tests, along with other reactions, including **rashes**, **itching** and swelling can all result from long-term use.

Crohn's disease—A chronic inflammatory disease of unknown cause, involving any part of the gastro-intestinal tract from mouth to anus, but commonly involving the large intestine, with scarring and thickening of the bowel wall. Crohn's disease frequently leads to intestinal obstruction and has a high rate of recurrence after treatment.

Erythema multiforme—A type of hypersensitivity (allergic) reaction that occurs in response to medications, infections, or illness. Medications associated with erythema multiforme include sulfonamides, penicillins, barbiturates, and phenytoin. Associated infections include herpes simplex and mycoplasma infections. In severe cases, the condition is called Stevens-Johnson syndrome.

Erythroblastopenia—A deficiency in the cells that create red blood cells. This condition may be severe and life-threatening, but there is a transient form, seen in young children, which resolves spontaneously and does not recur.

Hypercalcemia—An excessive amount of calcium in the blood. The most common cause an excess hormone secretion from the parathyroid gland, but hypercalcemia may also be seen in some cancers (lung, breast, multiple myeloma), as a side effect of some drugs, or from excess calcium in the diet.

Mycosis fungoides—The most common type of cutaneous T-cell lymphoma. This low-grade lymphoma primarily affects the skin. Generally, it has a slow course and often remains confined to the skin. Over time, in about 10% of cases, it can progress to the lymph nodes and internal organs.

Optic neuritis—Inflammation of the optic nerve (cranial nerve II) which connects to the retina of the eye. This variable condition can be present with any of the following symptoms: blurred vision, loss of visual acuity, loss of some or all color vision, complete or partial blindness, and pain behind the eye.

Pemphigus—An autoimmune disorder in which the immune system produces antibodies against specific proteins in the skin and mucous membrane. These antibodies produce a reaction that leads to a separation of skin cells.

Pneumonitis (aspiration)—Inflammation of the lung caused by inhaling a liquid, usually carbon based.

Stevens-Johnson syndrome—A severe form of erythema multiforme in which the systemic symptoms are severe and the lesions extensive, involving multiple body areas, especially the mucous membranes.

Trichinosis—A roundworm infection, usually contracted by eating raw or undercooked meat. Trichinosis is rare in the United States but a common infection in some parts of the world.

Ulcerative colitis—A chronic, episodic, inflammatory disease of the large intestine and rectum characterized by bloody diarrhea.

Nerves and central nervous system

Convulsions, increased intracranial pressure with **papilledema** (pseudotumor cerebri) usually after treatment, **dizziness** and loss of balance, **headache**, and emotional disturbances can result from long-term use.

Endocrine gland system

Menstrual irregularities, development of cushingoid state, suppression of growth in children, secondary adrenocortical and pituitary unresponsiveness (particularly in times of **stress**, as in trauma, surgery, or illness), decreased carbohydrate tolerance, manifestations of latent **diabetes mellitus**, hyperglycemia, increased requirements for insulin or oral hypoglycemic agents in diabetics, and increased hair growth can result from long-term use.

Eye problems

Cataracts, increased intraocular pressure, glaucoma, and bulging eyes can result from long-term use.

Other problems

Hypersensitivity, blood clotting problems, weight gain, increased appetite, **nausea**, and **hiccups** can result from long-term use.

In addition to this incomplete list of long-term effects, other serious effects have been associated with systemic corticosteroid treatment. The severity and likelihood of adverse effects increases both with dose and duration of treatment. Because of their greater effects on sodium and water, the natural corticosteroids, cortisone, and hydrocortisone are more likely to cause fluid and electrolyte problems than the pure glucocorticoids such as dexamethasone and betamethasone.

Interactions

Drugs that stimulate liver enzymes such as phenobarbital, phenytoin, and rifampin may increase the rate of elimination of corticosteroids and may require increases in corticosteroid dose to achieve the desired response.

Drugs such as troleandomycin and ketoconazole may reduce the rate of metabolism of corticosteroids and decrease the rate of elimination. Therefore, the dose of corticosteroid should be lowered to avoid steroid toxicity.

Corticosteroids may increase the rate of elimination of chronic high dose **aspirin**. This effect could lead to decreased salicylate serum levels or increase the risk of salicylate toxicity when corticosteroid is withdrawn.

The effects of corticosteroid treatment on anticoagulants vary. There have been reports of both increased anticoagulant activity and decreased anticoagulant activity. Careful monitoring is essential when corticosteroids are used together with anticoagulants.

Resources

BOOKS

ICON Health Publications.*Corticosteroids*. San Diego: ICON Health Publications, 2004.

Katzung, Bertram G.*Basic & Clinical Pharmacology*. New York: McGraw–Hill Medical, 2006.

PERIODICALS

Al-Dhalimi, M.A., and N. Aljawahiry. "Misuses of Topical Corticosteroids: A Clinical Study in An Iraqi Hospital."*Eastern Mediterranean Health Journal* (November 2006): 847–852.

Kirn, Timothy F. "Corticosteroids Are Not For All Asthma Patients: Physicians Need to Be Careful About Greatly Raising the Dose When a Patient Fails to Achieve Control."*Pediatric News* (February 2007): 52.

Martinez, Fernando D. "Inhaled Corticosteroids and Asthma Prevention."*The Lancet* (August 26, 2006): 708–710.

Miller, Karl E. "Inhaled Corticosteroids Effective in Acute Asthma Attacks."*American Family Physician* (May 1, 2007): 1383.

Saunders, Cathy. "Reduced Lung Cancer Risk With Inhaled Corticosteroids."*Australian Doctor* (April 13, 2007): 1.

ORGANIZATIONS

American Academy of Allergy, Asthma & Immunology, 555 East Wells Street, Suite 1100, Milwaukee, WI, 53202-3823, (414) 272-6071, http://www.aaaai.org.

American Academy of Dermatology, PO Box 4014, Schaumburg, IL, 60168-4014, (847) 240-1859, (866) 503-SKIN (7546), http://www.aad.org.

Arthritis National Research Foundation, 200 Oceangate, Suite 830, Long Beach, CA, 90802, (562) 983-1410, (800) 588-2873, http://www.curearthritis.org.

Asthma and Allergy Foundation of America, 8201 Corporate Drive, Suite 1000, Landover, MD, 20785, (800) 727-8462, info@aafa.org, http://www.aafa.org/.

European Dermato-Epidemiology Network, Department of Dermatology, University Medical Centre, Groningen, The Netherlands, 9700 RB, 003150 3612520, 003150 3619247, p.j.coenraads@med.umcg.nl, http://eden.dermis.net.

National Heart Lung and Blood Institute Health Information Center, P.O. Box 30105, Bethesda, MD, 20824-0105, (301) 592-8573, (240) 629-3246, http://www.nhlbi.nih.gov.

Samuel D. Uretsky, Pharm.D.
Ken R. Wells

Corticotropin test *see* **Adrenocorticotropic hormone test**

Cortisol tests

Definition

This test is a measure of serum cortisol (also known as hydrocortisone), or urine cortisol, (also known as urinary free cortisol), an important hormone produced by a pair of endocrine glands called the adrenal glands.

Purpose

This test is performed on patients who may have malfunctioning adrenal glands. Blood and urine cortisol, together with the determination of adrenocorticotropic hormone (ACTH), are the three most important tests in the investigation of **Cushing's syndrome** (caused by an overproduction of cortisol) and **Addison's disease** (caused by the underproduction of cortisol).

Precautions

Increased levels of cortisol are associated with **pregnancy**. Physical and emotional **stress** can also elevate cortisol levels. Drugs that may cause increased levels of cortisol include estrogen, **oral contraceptives**, amphetamines, cortisone, and spironolactone (Aldactone). Drugs that may cause

KEY TERMS

Addison's disease—A rare disorder in which symptoms are caused by a deficiency of hydrocortisone (cortisol) and aldosterone, two corticosteroid hormones normally produced by a part of the adrenal glands called the adrenal cortex. Symptoms include weakness, tiredness, vague abdominal pain, weight loss, skin pigmentation and low blood pressure.

Adrenal glands—A pair of endocrine glands (glands that secrete hormones directly into the bloodstream) that are located on top of the kidneys.

Adrenocorticotropic hormone (ACTH)—Also called corticotropin, this hormone is produced by the pituitary gland to stimulate the adrenal cortex to release various corticosteroid hormones.

Cushing's syndrome—A hormonal disorder caused by an abnormally high level of corticosteroid hormones that are produced by the adrenal glands. Corticosteroid hormones control the body's use of nutrients and the excretion of salts and water in the urine. Symptoms include high blood sugar levels, a moon face, weight gain, and increased blood pressure.

decreased levels include androgens, aminoglutethimide, betamethasone, and other steroid medications, danazol, lithium, levodopa, metyrapone and phenytoin (Dilantin).

Description

Cortisol is a potent hormone known as a glucocorticoid that affects the metabolism of carbohydrates, proteins, and fats, but especially glucose. Cortisol increases blood sugar levels by stimulating the release of glucose from glucose stores in cells. It also acts to inhibit insulin, thus affecting glucose transport into cells.

The hypothalamus (an area of the brain), the pituitary gland (sometimes called the "master gland"), and the adrenal glands coordinate the production of cortisol. After corticotropin-releasing hormone (CRH) is made in the hypothalamus, CRH stimulates the pituitary to produce adrenocorticotropic hormone (ACTH). The production of ACTH in turn stimulates a part of the adrenal glands known as the adrenal cortex to produce cortisol. Rising levels of cortisol act as a negative feedback to curtail further production of CRH and ACTH, thus completing an elaborate feedback mechanism.

There are two methods for evaluating cortisol: blood and urine. The most reliable index of cortisol secretion is the 24-hour urine sample collection, but when blood levels are required or requested by the physician, plasma cortisol should be measured in the morning and again in the afternoon. Cortisol levels normally rise and fall during the day in what is called a diurnal variation, so that cortisol is at its highest level between 6–8 a.m. and gradually falls, reaching its lowest point around midnight. One reason for ordering blood cortisol levels versus a 24-hour urine collection is that sometimes the earliest sign of adrenal malfunction is the loss of this diurnal variation, even though the cortisol levels are not yet elevated. For example, individuals with Cushing's syndrome often have upper normal plasma cortisol levels in the morning and exhibit no decline as the day progresses.

Preparation

When testing for cortisol levels through the blood, a blood specimen is usually collected at 8 a.m. and again at 4 p.m. It should be noted that normal values may be transposed in individuals who have worked during the night and slept during the day for long periods of time.

When testing for cortisol level through the urine, a 24-hour urine sample is collected, refrigerated, and sent to the reference laboratory for examination.

Risks

Risks for the blood test are minimal, but may include slight bleeding from the blood-drawing site, **fainting** or feeling lightheaded after venipuncture, or hematoma (blood accumulating under the puncture site).

Results

Reference ranges for cortisol vary from laboratory to laboratory but are usually within the following ranges for blood:

- adults (8 a.m.): 6–28 mg/dL; adults (4 p.m.): 2–12 mg/dL

- child one to six years (8 a.m.): 3–21 mg/dL; child one to six years (4 p.m.): 3–10 mg/dL
- newborn: 1/24 mg/dL

Reference ranges for cortisol vary from laboratory to laboratory, but are usually within the following ranges for 24-hour urine collection:

- adult: 10–100 mg/24 hours
- adolescent: 5–55 mg/24 hours
- child: 2–27 mg/24 hours

Abnormal results

Increased levels of cortisol are found in Cushing's syndrome, excess thyroid (**hyperthyroidism**), **obesity**, ACTH-producing tumors, and high levels of stress.

Decreased levels of cortisol are found in Addison's disease, conditions of low thyroid, and **hypopituitarism**, in which pituitary activity is diminished.

Resources

BOOKS

Pagana, Kathleen Deska, and Timothy J. Pagana.*Mosby's Manual of Diagnostic and Laboratory Tests*. 4th ed. St. Louis: Mosby, 2009.

Janis O. Flores

Cosmetic dentistry

Definition

Cosmetic dentistry includes a variety of dental treatments aimed at improving the appearance of the teeth.

Purpose

The purpose of cosmetic dentistry is to improve the appearance of the teeth using bleaching, bonding, veneers, reshaping, **orthodontics**, or implants.

Description

Bleaching is done to lighten teeth that are stained or discolored. It entails the use of a bleaching solution applied by a dentist or a gel in a tray that fits over the teeth used at home under a dentist's supervision. Bonding involves applying tooth-colored plastic putty, called composite resin, to the surface of chipped or broken teeth. This resin is also used to fill cavities in front teeth (giving a more natural-looking result) and to fill gaps between teeth. Veneers are thin, porcelain shells that cover the front of the teeth. They can improve the appearance of damaged, discolored, misshapen, or misaligned teeth. Reshaping involves the removal of enamel from a misshapen tooth so that it matches other teeth. Orthodontics uses braces to correct the position of crowded or misaligned teeth. Implants are artificial teeth which are attached directly to the jaw to replace missing teeth.

Preparation

Bleaching involves having a custom-made bleaching tray made by the dentist. This tray is worn at home for several hours each day or night. Teeth slowly become white over a period of one to six weeks. Bleaching can also be done in a dentist's office. A heat- or light-activated bleaching solution is applied to six to eight teeth per visit.

Bonding involves etching the surface of the tooth so composite resin can adhere. The dentist then contours the resin to the right shape, and smooths and polishes the resin after it is hard and dry.

To prepare for the application of a veneer, a thin layer of enamel is removed from the tooth (so that the finished tooth will be flush with surrounding teeth) and an impression of the tooth is taken from which the veneer will be created. Before a veneer is applied, the tooth is etched with an acid solution and an adhesive resin is painted on the tooth. The veneer is then applied, the resin is hardened with a bonding light, and the dentist polishes the veneer.

During cosmetic reshaping, some enamel is removed from the uneven tooth so it more closely matches other teeth.

Orthodontics involves applying braces to the teeth, and wires are threaded through the braces. These wires are adjusted to gradually move the teeth to the desired new positions. Over time, crowded or misaligned teeth are straightened.

Implants are more secure and natural looking than dentures or bridgework, but are much more expensive. First, an anchor for the implant is attached to the jaw bone. This surgery can take several hours. About six months later, after the bone around the anchor has healed, a post is attached to the anchor, and an artificial tooth is attached to the post. The whole process may take about nine months to complete.

Aftercare

Periodic touch-up may be needed to keep the teeth white if the teeth have been bleached or bonded.

Bleaching—Technique used to brighten stained teeth.

Bonding—Rebuilding, reshaping, and covering tooth defects using tooth-colored materials.

Composite resin—Plastic material matching natural tooth color used to replace missing parts of a tooth.

Also, the resin used in bonded teeth can be chipped by ice, popcorn kernels, or hard candy, requiring repair. Veneered teeth may need to be reveneered after five to 12 years. Once orthodontic braces are removed, regular visits to the orthodontist are advised because teeth can shift position. Implanted teeth require regular dental checkups to ensure that the anchor and post are stable.

Risks

After teeth are bleached, they may darken faster if exposed to staining products such as coffee or tobacco. Some patients experience increased sensitivity to cold while teeth are being bleached, but the sensitivity usually disappears shortly after completion of the treatment.

Bonded teeth, like bleached teeth, may also stain more easily than natural teeth. Bonding materials also chip easily.

Because cosmetic reshaping involves the removal of enamel, the process is irreversible because enamel cannot be replaced once it is removed.

The anchors of implanted teeth can loosen and cause **pain**; regular dental checkups are recommended.

Results

Cosmetic dentistry can improve the appearance of stained, chipped, misshapen, or crowded teeth.

ORGANIZATIONS

American Dental Association, 211 E. Chicago Ave., Chicago, IL, 60611-2678, (312) 440-2500, http://www.ada.org.

Joseph Knight, PA

Cosmetic surgery *see* **Plastic, cosmetic, and reconstructive surgery**

Costochondritis

Definition

Costochondritis is an inflammation and associated tenderness of the cartilage (i.e., the costochondral joints) that attaches the front of the ribs to the breastbone.

Description

Costochondritis causes **pain** in the lower rib area or upper breastbone. Some patients fear they are having a **heart attack**. The most severe pain is usually between the breast and the upper abdomen. The pain may be greater when in sitting or reclining positions. **Stress** may aggravate this condition. Generally the third or fourth ribs are affected. However, any of the seven costochondral junctions may be affected, and more often than not more than one site is involved. The inflammation can involve cartilage areas on both sides of the sternum, but usually is on one side only. Costochondritis should be distinguished from Tietze Syndrome, which is an inflammation involving the same area of the chest, but also includes swelling.

Causes and symptoms

The causes of costochondritis are not well-understood and may be difficult to establish. The most likely causes include injury, repetitive minor trauma, and unusual excessive physical activity.

The primary symptom of costochondritis is severe chest wall pain, which may vary in intensity. The pain becomes worse with trunk movement, deep breathing, and/or exertion, and better with decreased movement, quiet breathing, or changing of position. It is usually localized but may radiate extensively from the chest area. The pain has been described as sharp, nagging, aching, or pressure-like.

Diagnosis

Diagnosis is based on pain upon palpation (gentle pressing) of the affected joints. Swelling is not associated with costochondritis. Diagnosis is also dependent on the exclusion of other causes, including heart attack or bacterial or fungal infections found in IV drug users or postoperative **thoracic surgery** patients.

Treatment

The goals of treatment are to reduce inflammation and to control pain. To accomplish these goals, nonsteroidal anti-inflammatory agents (NSAIDs) are used, with ibuprofen usually selected as the drug of choice. Other NSAIDS options are flurbiprofen, mefenamic acid, ketoprofen, and naproxen. Additional treatment recommendations include the use of local heat, **biofeedback**, and gentle stretching of the pectoralis muscles two to three times a day.

For more difficult cases, where the patient continues to exhibit pain and discomfort, cortisone injections are used as therapy.

Alternative treatment

Supplements that are used to reduce inflammation have been used to treat costochondritis. Examples of such supplements include ginger root, evening primrose oil, bromelain, vitamin E, omega-3 oils, and white willow bark. Glucosamine/chondroitin sulfate, which may aid in the healing of cartilage, has also been used. Other alternative therapies include **acupuncture** and massages.

Prognosis

The prognosis for recovery from costochondritis is good. For most patients, the condition lessens in six months to a year. However, after one year, about one-half of patients continue with some discomfort, while about one-third still report tenderness with palpation.

Prevention

Though the causes of costochondritis are not well known, avoidance of activities that may strain (e.g., the repetitive misuse of muscles) or cause trauma to the rib cage is recommended to prevent the occurrence of costochondritis. Modification of improper posture or ergonomics of the home or work place may also deter the development of this condition.

Resources

OTHER

Day, C. *Costochondritis.* 2001. http://wwhttp://www.cfids-cab.org/cfs-inform/Ic/costomm.htm#Frequently Asked Questions.
Flowers, L. K., and B. D. Wippermann. "Costochondritis." *eMedicine Journal: Emergency Medicine/Rheumatology.* February 23, 2001. http://www.emedicine.com/emerg/topic116.htm.

Judith Sims

Cotrel-Dubousset spinal instrumentation *see* **Spinal instrumentation**

Cough

Definition

A cough is a forceful release of air from the lungs that can be heard. Coughing helps to protect the respiratory system by clearing it of irritants and secretions.

Demographics

Forty percent of Americans are estimated to experience a chronic cough, defined as a cough that persists for at least eight weeks, at some point during their lives.

Description

While people can generally cough voluntarily, a cough is usually a reflex triggered when an irritant stimulates one or more of the cough receptors found at different points in the respiratory system. These receptors then send a message to the cough center in the brain, which in turn tells the body to cough. A cough begins with a deep breath in, at which point the opening between the vocal cords at the upper part of the larynx (glottis) shuts, trapping the air in the lungs. As the diaphragm and other muscles involved in breathing press against the lungs, the glottis suddenly opens, producing an explosive outflow of air at speeds greater than 100 mi (160 km) per hour.

In normal situations, most people cough once or twice an hour during the day to clear the airway of irritants. However, when the level of irritants in the air is high or when the respiratory system becomes infected, coughing may become frequent and prolonged. It may interfere with **exercise** or sleep, and it may cause distress if accompanied by **dizziness**, chest **pain**, or breathlessness. In the majority cases, frequent coughing lasts one to two weeks and tapers off as the irritant or infection subsides. If a cough lasts more than eight weeks, it is considered a chronic cough, and physicians will try to determine a cause beyond an acute infection or irritant.

Coughs are generally described as either dry or productive. A dry cough does not bring up a mixture of mucus, irritants, and other substances from the lungs (sputum), while a productive cough does. In the case of a bacterial infection, the sputum brought up in a productive cough may be greenish, gray, or brown. In the case of an allergy or viral infection it may be clear or white. In the most serious conditions, the sputum may contain blood.

Causes and symptoms

In the majority of cases, coughs are caused by respiratory infections, including:

- colds or influenza, the most common causes of coughs
- bronchitis, an inflammation of the mucous membranes of the bronchial tubes
- croup, a viral inflammation of the larynx, windpipe, and bronchial passages that produces a bark-like cough in children
- whooping cough, a bacterial infection accompanied by the high-pitched cough for which it is named
- pneumonia, a potentially serious bacterial infection that produces discolored or bloody mucus
- tuberculosis, another serious bacterial infection that produces bloody sputum
- fungal infections, such as aspergillosis, histoplasmosis, and cryptococcoses

Environmental pollutants, such as cigarette smoke, dust, or smog, can also cause a cough. In the case of cigarette smokers, the nicotine present in the smoke paralyzes the hairs (cilia) that regularly flush mucus from the respiratory system. The mucus then builds up, forcing the body to remove it by coughing. Postnasal drip, the irritating trickle of mucus from the nasal passages into the throat caused by **allergies** or **sinusitis**, can also result in a cough. Some chronic conditions, such as **asthma**, chronic **bronchitis**, **emphysema**, and **cystic fibrosis**, are characterized in part by a cough. A condition in which stomach acid backs up into the esophagus (gastroesophageal reflux) can cause coughing, especially when a person is lying down. A cough can also be a side effect of medications that are administered via an inhaler. It can also be a side-effect of beta-blockers and ACE inhibitors, which are drugs used for treating high blood pressure.

Diagnosis

Examination

To determine the cause of a cough, a physician should take an exact medical history and perform an exam. Information regarding the duration of the cough, other symptoms may accompany it, and environmental factors that may influence it aid the doctor in his or her diagnosis. The appearance of the sputum will also help determine what type of infection, if any, may be involved. The doctor may even observe the sputum microscopically for the presence of bacteria and white blood cells.

Tests

Chest x rays may help indicate the presence and extent of such infections as **pneumonia** or **tuberculosis**. If these actions are not enough to determine the cause of the cough, a **bronchoscopy** or **laryngoscopy** may be ordered. These tests use slender tubular instruments to inspect the interior of the bronchi and larynx.

Treatment

Drugs

Treatment of a cough generally involves addressing the condition causing it. An acute infection such as pneumonia may require **antibiotics**, an asthma-induced cough may be treated with the use of **bronchodilators**, or an antihistamine may be administered in the case of an allergy. Physicians prefer not to suppress a productive cough, since it aids the body in clearing the respiratory system of infective agents and irritants. However, cough medicines may be given if the patient cannot rest because of the cough or if the cough is not productive, as is the case with most coughs associated with colds or flu. The two types of drugs used to treat coughs are antitussives and **expectorants**.

ANTITUSSIVES. Antitussives are drugs that suppress a cough. Narcotics—primarily codeine—are used as antitussives and work by depressing the cough center in the brain. However, they can cause such side effects as drowsiness, **nausea**, and **constipation**. Dextromethorphan, the primary ingredient in many over-the-counter cough remedies, also depresses the brain's cough center, but without the side effects associated with **narcotics**. Demulcents relieve coughing by coating irritated passageways.

EXPECTORANTS. Expectorants are drugs that make mucus easier to cough up by thinning it.

Guaifenesin and terpin hydrate are the primary ingredients in most over-the-counter expectorants. However, some studies have shown that in acute infections, simply increasing fluid intake has the same thinning effect as taking expectorants.

Alternative treatment

Coughs due to bacterial or viral upper respiratory infections may be effectively treated with botanical and homeopathic therapies. The choice of remedy will vary and be specific to the type of cough the patient has. Some combination over-the-counter herbal and homeopathic cough formulas can be very effective for cough relief. Lingering coughs or coughing up blood should be treated by a trained practitioner.

Many health practitioners advise increasing fluids and breathing in warm, humidified air as ways of loosening chest congestion. Others recommend hot tea flavored with honey as a temporary home remedy for coughs caused by colds or flu. Various **vitamins**, such as vitamin C, may be helpful in preventing or treating conditions (including colds and flu) that lead to coughs. Avoiding mucous-producing foods can be effective in healing a cough condition. These mucous-producing foods vary, based on individual intolerance, but dairy products are a major mucous-producing food for most people.

Prognosis

Because the majority of coughs are related to the **common cold** or **influenza**, most will end in seven to 21 days. The outcome of coughs due to a more serious underlying disease depends on the pathology of that disease.

Prevention

It is important to identify and treat the underlying disease and origin of the cough. Avoiding **smoking** and direct contact with people experiencing cold or flu symptoms is recommended. Washing hands frequently during episodes of upper-respiratory illnesses is advised. Parents should follow recommended **vaccination** schedules for pertussis (**whooping cough**) to help prevent the disease from occurring.

Resources

OTHER

American Academy of Family Physicians. Chronic Cough: Causes and Cures. FamilyDoctor.org December 2009. http://familydoctor.org/online/famdocen/home/articles/237.html

Chen, Harry H. and Bruce Jafek. Chronic Cough. eMedicine. com June 4,2010. http://emedicine.medscape.com/article/1048560-overview

Chronic Cough. Mayo Foundation for Medical Education and Research. May 8, 2009. http://www.mayoclinic.com/health/chronic-cough/ds00957

Cough. MedlinePlus June 24, 2010. http://www.nlm.nih.gov/medlineplus/cough.html

ORGANIZATIONS

American Lung Association, 1301 Pennsylvania Ave., NW Suite 800, Washington, DC, 20004, (212) 315-8700, (800)LUNG-USA [(800) 548-8252], http://www.lungusa.org.

National Heart Lung and Blood Institute Health Information Center, P.O. Box 30105, Bethesda, MD, 20824-0105, (301) 592-8573; TTY: (240) 629-3255, (240) 629-3246, nhlbiinfo@nhlbi.nih.gov, http://www.nhlbi.nih.gov.

Jeffrey P. Larson, RPT
Tish Davidson, AM

Cough suppressants

Definition

Cough suppressants, antitussives, are medicines that reduce or prevent coughing.

Purpose

These medicines are meant to be used to relieve dry, hacking coughs associated with minor conditions like colds and flu. They should not be used to treat coughs associated with coughs that are productive of phlegm or sputum, or from **smoking** or chronic lung conditions like **asthma** or **emphysema**.

Description

Benzonatate (Tessalon) is chemically related to local anesthetics and comes in liquid-filled capsules that are available only by prescription.

Codeine and hydrocodone are opoid drugs that are combined in cough medicines used to suppress coughs. They are available only by prescription

Dextromethorphan is available in over-the-counter cough preparations as liquids, capsules, liquid-filled capsules, lozenges and tablets.

Recommended dosage:

Consult with prescribers or pharmacists regarding dose of prescription cough suppressant medications.

Tessalon is usually taken in 100mg capsules every four hours or three times daily.

Read labels on over-the-counter dextramethorphan cough suppressant medications.

Precautions

Because of fears of overdose, dextromethorphan products should not be given to children under four years of age.

Do not take more than the recommended daily dosage of cough suppressants.

A lingering cough could be a sign of a more serious medical condition. Coughs that last more than seven days or are associated with **fever**, rash, **sore throat**, or lasting **headache** should have medical attention.

People with **phenylketonuria** should be aware that some cough suppressant products contain the artificial sweetener aspartame, which breaks down in the body to phenylalanine.

All cough suppressants can produce or accentuate drowsiness associated with other medicines.

Anyone who has asthma or **liver disease** should check with a physician before taking dextromethorphan.

Women who are pregnant or **breastfeeding** or who plan to become pregnant should check with their physicians before taking dextromethorphan.

The dye tartrazine is an ingredient in some cough suppressant products. This dye causes allergic reactions in some people, especially those who are allergic to **aspirin**.

Side effects

Side effects may include drowsiness, **dizziness**, upset stomach or **nausea and vomiting**.

Interactions

Taking dextromethorphan and **monoamine oxidase inhibitors** (MAOI) (Nardil, Marplan and Parnate) together can be deadly. The effects of MAOI last for up to two weeks after stopping the drugs.

Combining dextromethorphan and sibutramine (Meridia) can produce irritability, weakness and altered consciousness.

All cough suppressants can accentuate the sedative effects of sedative and tranquilizing medicines.

James Waun, MD, RPh

Coughing and deep-breathing exercises *see* **Chest physical therapy**

Couvade syndrome

Definition

Couvade syndrome, which is also known as sympathetic **pregnancy**, male pregnancy experience, or "pregnant dad syndrome," refers to a condition in which a father-to-be experiences some of the physical symptoms of pregnancy prior to the baby s birth. The term *couvade* comes from the French verb *couver*, meaning "to brood," in the sense of a bird protecting its eggs before they hatch.

Description

The term couvade was first used by the anthropologist E. B. Tylor in 1865 to describe certain fatherhood rituals performed by husbands while their wives were giving birth. These rituals were found in many different historical periods as well as various cultures around the world, ranging from ancient Greece and parts of the Roman Empire to Chinese Turkestan, the Basque regions of northern Spain, China, Thailand, Borneo, parts of Russia, and many Indian tribes in North as well as South America. In some cultures the expectant father avoids eating certain foods or handling knives or other sharp tools while the mother is in labor. In Papua New Guinea the father builds a hut apart from the rest of the village and goes to bed when his wife s **childbirth** begins. He then stays in bed and imitates the pains of childbirth until the baby is born. A similar custom is observed among the Basques. Couvade rituals are thought to have a number of possible purposes, depending on the specific culture:

- To draw the attention of evil spirits away from the mother to the father instead.

- To strengthen the emotional bond between father and child.

- To show that the man is the child's biological father.

- To relieve the father's anxiety while the mother is in labor.

- To strengthen the father's relationship with supernatural beings so that he can guide the child into the world.

Ritual couvade is no longer observed in most developed countries, but the term couvade syndrome has been applied to the physical symptoms that many men in these countries experience during a wife's pregnancy, ranging from mild **nausea** or backaches to weight gain or **toothache**. One group of Italian researchers reported that the number of men who experience couvade syndrome ranges between 11 and 65 percent, while others estimate that as many as 80 percent of expectant fathers develop these symptoms. It is thought that more men in Western societies experience couvade syndrome in the early 2000s than was the case with previous generations of fathers, due in part to changes in men s involvement with the birthing process. Some doctors think that the participation of fathers in the delivery room as "coaches" or comforters is one reason for the increased number of men who develop pregnancy symptoms.

Causes and symptoms

Causes

Several different types of explanation have been proposed for couvade syndrome:

- It is a psychiatric disorder. This type of explanation is more common among European than American physicians. Some attribute the symptoms of couvade syndrome to jealousy of the woman s ability to give birth, while others maintain that they result from male guilt over impregnating the woman or to sibling rivalry—that is, the husband regards the wife as a competitor that he must try to outperform.

- It results from real biological changes in the expectant father s body. A team of Canadian researchers reported that their sample of expectant fathers had higher levels of estradiol (a female hormone) and lower levels of testosterone (a male sex hormone) in their blood and saliva than a control group of childless men. The researchers have cautioned, however, that their findings should be checked by studying groups of men from other cultures.

- It is a reaction to a changed social role; that is, the syndrome is one way that some men "work through" their feelings about assuming the social expectations and responsibilities associated with fatherhood.

- It is a set of psychosomatic symptoms that is within the range of normal experience and does not indicate mental illness. Psychosomatic refers to physical symptoms that are caused or influenced by emotional factors, such as stress headaches or "butterflies in the stomach" before an examination.

Symptoms

Expectant fathers may experience one or more of the following:
- weight gain
- nausea and vomiting
- stomach cramps
- constipation or diarrhea
- loss of appetite
- sleep disturbances
- food cravings
- headaches
- toothache
- nosebleeds
- itchy skin

KEY TERMS

Anthropology—The study of the origins, biological characteristics, beliefs, and social customs of human beings.

Psychosomatic—Referring to physical symptoms that are caused or significantly influenced by emotional factors. Some doctors regard couvade syndrome as a psychosomatic condition.

Syndrome—A set of symptoms that occur together.

Only a few men, however, develop the more dramatic symptoms. Some studies report that couvade syndrome is most severe during the third or fourth month of the wife s pregnancy and again just before birth. Some researchers report that the syndrome is more common in first-time fathers, while others have found that it is equally likely to develop in men who already have children.

Diagnosis

Couvade syndrome is not listed as a diagnostic category in the most recent editions of the American *Diagnostic and Statistical Manual of Mental Disorders*, fourth edition, text revision (2000) or the World Health Organization's *International Classification of Diseases*, version 10 (1993). In addition, it is not described or discussed in most medical textbooks, although a few handbooks for doctors in family practice mention it in passing as a condition of unknown origin. Since most men with couvade syndrome have only mild symptoms, they are unlikely to consult a doctor about the condition by itself.

Treatment

There is no standard mainstream treatment recommended for couvade syndrome because it is not usually mentioned in medical textbooks. Anecdotal evidence, however, indicates that most fathers-to-be are helped by a simple explanation of the syndrome and reassurance that it is not uncommon among American and Canadian men.

Alternative treatment

Some expectant fathers report that **meditation** or such movement therapies as **yoga** and t'ai chi are calming and relaxing. Peppermint tea or ginger are herbal remedies that help to relieve nausea.

Prognosis

Couvade syndrome almost always goes away after the baby is born. While a few instances of the syndrome developing into full-blown **psychosis** (loss of contact with reality) have been reported in European medical journals, such cases are extremely rare.

Prevention

There is no known way to prevent couvade syndrome as doctors do not yet understand why some men develop it and others do not.

Resources

BOOKS

Reed, Richard K. *Birthing Fathers: The Transformation of Men in American Rites of Birth*. Piscataway, NJ: Rutgers University Press, 2005.

PERIODICALS

Budur, K., and M. Mathews. "Couvade Syndrome Equivalent?" *Psychosomatics* 46 (January 2005): 71–72.

OTHER

Polinski, Michael. "Feeling Her Pain: The Male Pregnancy Experience." *Pregnancy Today*, http://www.pregnancytoday.com/reference/articles/malepg.htm.

ORGANIZATIONS

American Academy of Family Physicians (AAFP), 11400 Tomahawk Creek Parkway, Leawood, KS, 66211-2680, (913) 906-6000, (913) 906-6075, (800) 271-2237, http://www.aafp.org/.

Rebecca Frey, PhD

Cox-2 inhibitors

Definition

Cox-2 inhibitors are **nonsteroidal anti-inflammatory drugs** (NSAIDs) that are used to relieve **pain** and reduce inflammation.

Purpose

By blocking the Cox-2 enzyme in the intestine, these drugs were expected to lower the risk of ulcers that is inherent in using most other NSAIDS, while relieving pain and inflammation.

Description

Celecoxib (Celebrex) is the only available Cox-2 inhibitor drug.

Celecoxib is used to treat rheumatoid and **osteo-arthritis**, acute pain, and the pain associated with primary **dysmenorrhea**. In the U.S., but not Canada, the drug is also approved to reduce the number of **intestinal polyps** in familial adenomatous polyposis (FAP).

Recommended dosage

For osteoarthritis, the usual dose is 200 mg/day administered as a single dose or as 100 mg twice/day.

For **rheumatoid arthritis**: 100–200 mg twice/day.

Acute pain and primary dysmenorrhea: 400 mg initially, followed by an additional 200 mg dose if needed on the first day. On subsequent days, the recommended dose is 200 mg twice daily as needed.

Precautions

Celebrex is chemically related to sulfa drugs and should not be used by patients with sulfa allergy.

This drug should not be used to treat post-operative pain in patients who have had **coronary artery bypass graft surgery** (CABG).

Celebrex should not be used by patients who have had sensitivity reactions to **aspirin** or other NSAIDS.

This drug should not be used in patients who have aspirin-associated **asthma**.

Celebrex should not be used late in **pregnancy** as it may cause heart problems for newborn babies.

This drug may aggravate active peptic ulcers, liver, kidney and/or heart diseases and intestinal bleeding.

Side effects

The most common side effects of Celebrex include:

- high blood pressure
- headache
- upset stomach, abdominal pain, diarrhea, gas or bloating
- rash and sometimes more serious skin conditions
- fatigue
- swelling of the feet and legs
- severe allergic reaction, including swelling of the face, throat, tongue, lips, eyes, hoarseness and difficulty swallowing, or breathing

Interactions

Because of its large number of possible side/adverse effects, the effects of other drugs may make it difficult to tell with certainty which adverse effects come from which drug. Drugs that Celebrex can interact with include:

- Taking aspirin and other NSAIDS with Celebrex increases the risk of ulcers and intestinal bleeding.
- Celebrex increases the blood thinning effects of warfarin (Coumadin)
- Celebrex increases the blood thinning effects of the injectable anticoagulants heparin, enoxaparin (Lovenox) and Dalteparin (Fragmin).
- Fluconazole (Diflucan) may increase the blood levels, and possibility of adverse effects, of Celebrex.
- Celebrex increases the blood levels, and possibility of toxicity of lithium (Eskalith).

Resources

BOOKS

Physicians' Desk Reference 2005. Montvale, NJ: Thomson Healthcare, 2004.

ORGANIZATIONS

Arthritis Foundation, P.O. Box 7669, Atlanta, GA, 30357-0669, (404) 872-7100, http://www.arthritis.org.

Arthritis National Research Foundation , 200 Oceangate, Suite 830, Long Beach, CA, 90802, (562) 983-1410, (800) 588-2873, http://www.curearthritis.org.

Samuel D. Uretsky, Pharm.D.
James Waun, MD, RPh

Craniopharyngioma

Definition

Craniopharyngiomas are benign tumors which affect the central nervous system. This type of **brain tumor** is diagnosed primarily in children but can occur at any age.

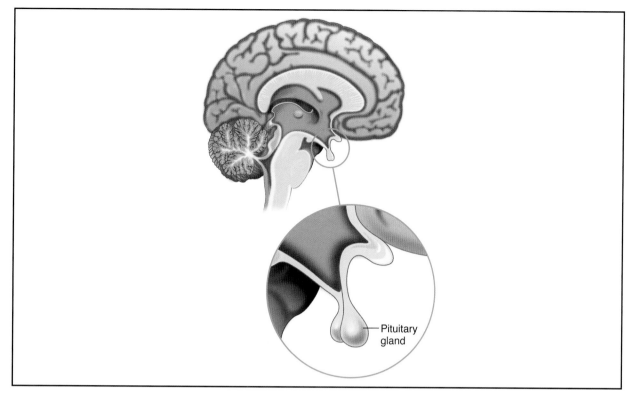

Craniopharyngiomas are a type of benign brain tumors that affect the functioning of the pituitary gland, which regulates the other endocrine glands in the body. *(Illustration by Electronic Illustrators Group. Reproduced by permission of Gale, a part of Cengage Learning.)*

Demographics

Craniopharyngiomas are a rare type of benign brain tumor. Approximately 300 new cases of craniopharyngioma are diagnosed in the United States each year. Higher incidence rates of craniopharyngioma have been reported in Asia, Africa and Japan.

About 100 of the 300 new cases that occur in the U.S. each year occur in children ages 0–14 years. One incidence peak of craniopharyngioma occurs between the ages of 5–14. A second incidence peak has been noted in individuals ages 50–74 years.

Description

Craniopharyngiomas develop from embryonic squamous cells located along the craniopharyngeal duct. These tumors frequently occur near critical structures in the brain and can grow to be quite large. As they grow in size they can impair vision, obstruct the flow of cerebrospinal fluid and can affect the normal functioning of the pituitary gland and the hypothalamus which can result in serious complications. Although the tumors are classified as benign tumors, they have a propensity to recur even after treatment. Because of their typical locations near vital structures, treatment is often associated with significant morbidity.

Differences have been noted between craniopharyngiomas that occur in children and adults. Craniopharyngiomas affecting pediatric patients is predominantly of the adamantinomatous cell type. The squamous papillary variant is diagnosed more frequently in adults.

Risk factors

Currently, there are no risk factors identified related to the development of craniopharyngioma.

Causes and symptoms

At this time the cause of craniopharyngioma is unknown. Craniopharygiomas that occur in pediatric patients are thought to arise from the remnants of an embryonic structure that forms a portion of the pituitary gland. These cellular remnants transform into a

KEY TERMS

Hypothalmus—An area of the brain located below the thalmus which regulates important functions such as body temperature, hunger and thirst.

Hypothyroidism—Insufficient production of thyroid hormone often resulting from an underactive thyroid gland. Can usually be treated with synthetic hormone replacement therapy.

Increased intracranial pressure—A rise in the normal pressure levels inside the brain.

Intracavitary—Inside a space or cavity within the body.

Morbidity—Adverse effects of treatment; a diseased condition or state; caused by disease; incidence of a particular disease.

Papilledema—Swelling which occurs at the level of the optic nerve. Presence of papilledema is indicative of increased intracranial pressure.

Pituitary gland—Often referred to as the master gland within the endocrine system. Produces hormones that control the functions of other glands within the endocrine system. Controls many body functions especially growth.

Projectile vomiting—Vomiting that occurs forcefully such that stomach contents may be ejected from the body in a way that propels expelled contents to a distance.

benign tumor by a process that is not yet fully understood. Researchers believe that a defect in the beta–catenin pathway at the cellular level may contribute to the development of craniopharyngioma. Beta-catenin is a component of the Wnt pathway which has a role in the regulation of cell development, cell differentiation, and cell growth.

The location of craniopharyngiomas in the brain leads to a variety of symptoms which result from compression of adjacent structures by the tumor. Symptoms associated with craniopharyngiomas include:

- Headache, a common presenting symptom, is present in up to 80% of cases and is a result of increasing intracranial pressure.
- Vomiting, which is often projectile in nature, commonly accompanies headaches in children. Projectile vomiting is also an indicator of increased intracranial pressure.
- Vision loss is another common symptom present at time of diagnosis. Vision loss varies in terms of pattern and severity of loss and ranges from blurred vision to complete visual field loss.
- Symptoms of growth hormone deficiency are present in up to 95% of cases. The most common clinical presentation is short stature.
- Symptoms of hypothyroidism including weight gain, tiredness and fatigue, dry skin and hair, intolerance to cold, anorexia and other related symptoms are often evident.
- Delayed puberty, which may occur in up to 100% of adolescents diagnosed with craniopharyngioma, is a common symptom.

- Mental changes, including seizures, are more commonly seen in adults but are rarely observed in children with craniopharyngioma.

Diagnosis

Examination

A thorough history will be elicited and a comprehensive **physical examination** will be conducted. The clinician's examination will focus on the presenting neurologic and endocrine signs and symptoms. The examination will include checks for **papilledema** and visual field problems which result from increased intracranial pressure. The clinician will also determine whether there is an enlarged head circumference. This finding combined with the presence of papilledema is highly suggestive of a mass within the brain.

The physician will also examine the child to determine whether growth has been compromised. Short stature and stunted growth that is not appropriate for age is a result of endocrine dysfunction and is commonly associated with craniopharyngioma.

Tests

Lab testing indicated for patients with craniopharyngioma includes testing to determine serum electrolyte levels, which may be impaired as a result of endocrine dysfunction. Other blood testing will include testing to determine levels of growth hormones, thyroid hormone, and follicle-stimulating and luteinizing hormones that may also be abnormal.

Radiology and imaging studies that may be performed include x-rays of the head and skull, computed tomography (CT) scans of the head, brain **magnetic resonance imaging** (MRI) and MRI/magnetic imaging **angiography** which is useful in preoperative planning. Tests to evaluate intellectual and psychological capabilities may also be conducted.

Treatment

Historically, the most common approach to treating craniopharyngioma was radical surgery which was used to remove as much of the tumor as possible in an effort to prevent recurrence. However, complications from radical surgical approaches often resulted in significant morbidity because of the location of the tumor and did not always prevent tumor recurrence with relapse of tumor occurring in as many as 60% of patients. In addition, the mortality rate from radical surgery although declining in recent years, can be as high as 10–25%.

Recent approaches to treating craniopharyngiomas include more conservative surgery followed by external beam **radiation therapy**. Outcomes from this treatment strategy include low rates of recurrence (5–20%) at 5–20 years with low long-term complications. However, radiation therapy may be not a viable treatment option for children less than 3 years of age because of the serious long-term side-effects associated with radiation therapy in this age group.

Patients with tumors that cannot be surgically removed, patients who are not candidates for treatment with radiation therapy, and those that relapse after treatment with surgery and radiation therapy may be candidates for **chemotherapy**. Systemic chemotherapy has not been effective in treating craniopharyngiomas however, some patients may respond to administration of intracavitary/intracystic administration of the chemotherapy agent bleomycin which is administered directly into the tumor cavity via a catheter.

Prognosis

Ten-year overall rates for patients whose tumors were able to be surgically resected range from 86–100%. Ten-year overall survival rates for patients whose tumors were not able to be completely surgically removed and for those whose tumors relapsed after treatment with surgery and radiation therapy range from 57–86%.

Patients require close monitoring of endocrine, ophthalmologic and neuropsychiatric function even after **tumor removal** and subsequent treatment. Assessment of growth and development, hormonal function, ophthalmologic function, and neuropsychiatric function is recommended. For example,

problems with the visual field may indicate relapse of tumor. In addition, long-term hormone supplementation is required for virtually all patients diagnosed with craniopharyngioma.

Prevention

As the cause of craniopharyngiomas is not known, there is currently no known way to prevent occurrence of these rare tumors.

Following treatment, patients diagnosed with craniopharyngioma continue to require close follow–up to detect potential recurrence. Current recommendations related to follow-up include screening with brain MRI every 3 months for 1 year, followed by MRI every 6 months for 1 year and then MRI once per year until the fifth year. For patients who received radiation therapy, the recommended follow-up is an MRI every year or every other year for life to screen for the occurrence of a second malignancy.

Resources

PERIODICALS

Garre, M.L., & Cama, A. "Craniopharyngioma: Modern Concepts in Pathogenesis and Treatment." *Curr Opin Pediatr.* (Aug 2007); 19(4):471–9.

Karavitaki, N., & Wass, J.A. "Craniopharyngiomas." *Endocriniol Metab Clin North Am.* (Mar 2008); 37(1): 173–93.

Kiehna, E.N., & Merchant, T.E. "Radiation Therapy for Pediatric Craniopharyngioma." *Neurosurg Focus.* (Apr 2010); 28(4).

Pettorini, B.L., Frassanito, P., Caldarelli, M., Tamburrini,G., Massimi, L., & DiRocco, C. "Molecular Pathogenesis of Craniopharyngioma: Switching from a Surgical Approach to a Biological One." *Neurosurg Focus.* (2010; 26(4).

Prabhu, V.C., & Brown, H.G. "The Pathogenesis of Craniopharyngiomas." *Childs Nerv Syst.* (Aug 2005); 21(8–9); 622–7.

Rodriguez, F.J., Scheithauer, B.W., Tsunoda, S, Kovacs, K., et al. "The Spectrum of Malignancy in Craniopharyngioma." *Am J Surg Pathol.* (Jul 2007); 31(7): 1020–8.

Yang, I., Sughrue, M.E., Rutkowski, M.J., Kaur, , R., et al. "Craniopharyngioma: A Comparison of Tumor Control with Various Treatment Strategies." *Neurosurg Focus.* (2010); 29(4).

OTHER

Lasky, J.L., Sakamoto, K.M., & Barker, L. "Craniopharyngioma." eMedicine. August 11, 2010 [cited August 28, 2010]. http://www.emedicine.medscape.com

ORGANIZATIONS

Childhood Brain Tumor Foundation, 20312 Watkins Meadow Drive, Germantown, Maryland, 20876, (310)

515-2900, (877) 217-4166, http://www.childhood braintumor.org.

Genetic and Rare Disease Information Center (GARD), P.O. Box 8126, Gaithersburg, Maryland, 20898-8126, (888) 205-2311, (301) 251-4911, http://www.rarediseases. info.nih.gov/GARD.

Melinda Granger Oberleitner
RN, DNS, APRN, CNS

Craniosacral therapy

Definition

Craniosacral therapy is a holistic healing practice that uses very light touching to balance the craniosacral system in the body, which includes the bones, nerves, fluids, and connective tissues of the cranium and spinal area.

Purpose

According to Dr. John Upledger, craniosacral therapy is ideally suited for attention-deficit hyperactivity disorder, headaches, chronic middle ear infection, **pain**, and general health maintenance. It is recommended for **autism**, fibromyalgia, heart disease, **osteoarthritis**, **pneumonia**, **rheumatoid arthritis**, chronic sinus infections, and **gastroenteritis** (inflammation of the lining of the stomach or small intestine). It is also used with other therapies to treat **chronic fatigue syndrome**, back pain, and menstrual irregularity. In addition, other craniosacral practitioners have reported benefits for eye dysfunction, **dyslexia**, depression, motor coordination difficulties, temporomandibular joint dysfunction (TMD), hyperactivity, **colic**, **asthma** in babies, floppy baby syndrome, **whiplash**, **cerebral palsy**, certain **birth defects**, and other central nervous system disorders.

Description

Origins

The first written reference to the movement of the spinal nerves and its importance in life, clarity, and "bringing quiet to the heart" is found in a 4,000-year-old text from China. Craniosacral work was referred to as "the art of listening." Bone setters in the Middle Ages also sensed the subtle movements of the body. They used these movements to help reset **fractures** and **dislocations** and to treat headaches.

In the early 1900s, the research of Dr. William Sutherland, an American osteopathic physician, detailed the movement of the cranium and pelvis. Before his research it was believed that the cranium was a solid immovable mass. Sutherland reported that the skull is actually made up of 22 separate and movable bones that are connected by layers of tissue. He called his work cranial **osteopathy**. Nephi Cotton, an American chiropractor and contemporary of Sutherland, called this approach craniology. The graduates of these two disciplines have refined and enhanced these original approaches and renamed their work as sacro-occipital technique, cranial **movement therapy**, or craniosacral therapy.

Dr. John Upledger, an osteopathic physician, and others at the Department of Biomechanics at Michigan State University, College of Osteopathic Medicine learned of Sutherland's research and developed it further. He researched the clinical observations of various osteopathic physicians. This research provided the basis for Upledger's work that he named craniosacral therapy.

Craniosacral therapy addresses the craniosacral system. This system includes the cranium, spine, and sacrum that are connected by a continuous membrane of connective tissue deep inside the body, called the dura mater. The dura mater also encloses the brain and the central nervous system. Sutherland noticed that cerebral spinal fluid rises and falls within the compartment of the dura mata. He called this movement the primary respiratory impulse; today it is known as the craniosacral rhythm (CSR) or the cranial wave.

Craniosacral therapists can most easily feel the CSR in the body by lightly touching the base of the skull or the sacrum. During a session, they feel for disturbances in the rate, amplitude, symmetry, and quality of flow of the CSR. A therapist uses very gentle touch to balance the flow of the CSR. Once the cerebrospinal fluid moves freely, the body's natural healing responses can function.

A craniosacral session generally lasts 30–90 minutes. The client remains fully clothed and lays down on a massage table while the therapist gently assesses the flow of the CSR. Upledger describes several techniques which may be used in a craniosacral therapy session. The first is energy cyst release. According to Upledger, "This technique is a hands-on method of releasing foreign or disruptive energies from the patient's body. Energy cysts may cause the disruption of the tissues and organs where they are

WILLIAM SUTHERLAND
(1873–1954)

William Garner Sutherland studied osteopathy under its founder, Andrew Taylor Still. Dr. Sutherland made his own important discovery while examining the sutures of cranial bones the skull bones that protect the brain. What he noticed is that the sutures were designed for motion. Sutherland termed this motion the *Breath of Life*. Through his experiments and research he determined that primary respiration was essential to all other physiological functions.

When Sutherland developed his techniques for craniosacral therapy, he wanted it to serve as a vehicle for listening to the body's rhythmic motions, and treat the patterns of inertia, when those motions become congested. He believed that the stresses—any physical or emotional trauma—created an imbalance in the body that needed correction to restore it to full health. The therapy is a hands-on method so that the therapist can feel the subtleties of the patterns of movement and inertia. Sutherland felt that this was the way to encourage self-healing and restoration of the body's own mechanisms, taking a holistic approach to creating optimal health.

The Craniosacral Therapy Educational Trust, based on Sutherland's pioneering work, is located at 10 Normington Close, Leigham Court Road, London SW16 2QS, United Kingdom. http://www.cranio.co.uk/

located." The therapist feels these cysts in the client's body and gently releases the blockage of energy.

Sutherland first wrote about a second practice called direction of energy. In this technique the therapist intends energy to pass from one of his hands, through the patient, into the other hand.

The third technique is called myofascial release. This is a manipulative form of bodywork that releases tension in the fascia or connective tissue of the body. This form of bodywork uses stronger touch.

Upledger's fourth technique is position of release. This involves following the client's body into the positions in which an injury occurred and holding it there. When the rhythm of the CSR suddenly stops the therapist knows that the trauma has been released.

The last technique is somatoemotional release. This technique was developed by Upledger and is an offshoot of craniosacral therapy. It is used to release the mind and body of the residual effects of trauma and injury that are "locked in the tissues."

The cost of a session varies due to the length of time needed and the qualifications of the therapist. The cost may be covered by insurance when the therapy is performed or prescribed by a licensed health care provider.

Precautions

This gentle approach is extremely safe in most cases. However, craniosacral therapy is not recommended in cases of acute systemic infections, recent skull fracture, intracranial hemorrhage or aneurysm, or herniation of the medulla oblongata (brain stem). Craniosacral therapy does not preclude the use of other medical approaches.

Side effects

Some people may experience mild discomfort after a treatment. This may be due to re-experiencing a trauma or injury or a previously numb area may come back to life and be more sensitive. These side effects are temporary.

Research and general acceptance

More than 40 scientific papers have been published that document the various effects of craniosacral therapy. There are also 10 authoritative textbooks on this therapy. The most notable scientific papers include Viola M. Fryman's work documenting the successful treatment of 1,250 newborn children with birth defects. Edna Lay and Stephen Blood showed the effects on TMD, and John Wood documented results with psychiatric disorders. The American Dental Association has found craniosacral therapy to be an effective adjunct to orthodontic work. However, the conventional medical community has not endorsed these techniques.

Resources

BOOKS

Upledger, John E., et al. *CranioSacral Therapy: What It Is, How It Works*. Berkeley, CA: North Atlantic Books, 2008.

OTHER

Milne, Hugh. *A Client's Introduction to Craniosacral Work*. Pamphlet. Milne Institute.

ORGANIZATIONS

Milne Institute Inc., P.O. Box 220, Big Sur, CA, 93920, (831) 667-2323, (831) 667-2525, infomilne@aol.com, http://www.milneinstitute.com/contact.

Upledger Institute, 11211 Prosperity Farms Rd., Suite D-325, Palm Beach Gardens, FL, 33410, (561) 622-4334, (561) 622-4771, (800) 233-5880, upledger@upledger.com, http://www.upledger.com/.

Linda Chrisman

Craniotomy

Definition

Surgical removal of part of the skull to expose the brain.

Purpose

A craniotomy is the most commonly performed surgery for brain **tumor removal**. It may also be done to remove a blood clot and control hemorrhage, inspect the brain, perform a biopsy, or relieve pressure inside the skull.

Precautions

Before the operation, the patient will have undergone diagnostic procedures such as **computed tomography scans** (CT) or **magnetic resonance imaging** (MRI) scans to determine the underlying problem that required the craniotomy and to get a better look at the brain's structure. Cerebral **angiography** may be used to study the blood supply to the tumor, aneurysm, or other brain lesion.

Description

There are two basic ways to open the skull:

- a curving incision from behind the hairline, in front of the ear, arching above the eye
- at the nape of the neck around the occipital lobe

The surgeon marks with a felt tip pen a large square flap on the scalp that covers the surgical area. Following this mark, the surgeon makes an incision into the skin as far as the thin membrane covering the skull bone. Because the scalp is well supplied with blood, the surgeon will have to seal many small

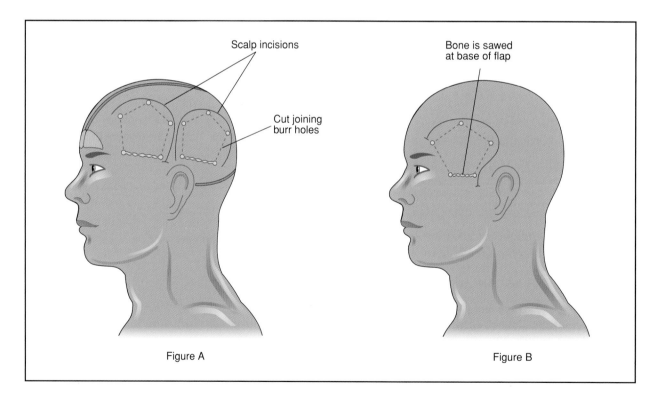

Scalp incisions

Cut joining burr holes

Bone is sawed at base of flap

Figure A

Figure B

A craniotomy is the most commonly performed surgery for brain tumor removal. There are two basic ways to open the skull: a curving incision from behind the hairline in front of the ear and at the nape of the neck (figure A). To reach the brain, the surgeon uses a hand drill to make holes in the skull, pushing a soft metal guide under the bone. The bone is sawed through until the bone flap can be removed to expose the brain (figure B). *(Illustration by Electronic Illustrators Group. Reproduced by permission of Gale, a part of Cengage Learning.)*

arteries. The surgeon then folds back a skin flap to expose the bone.

Using a high speed hand drill or an automatic craniotome, the surgeon makes a circle of holes in the skull, and pushes a soft metal guide under the bone from one hole to the next. A fine wire saw is then moved along the guide channel under the bone between adjacent holes. The surgeon saws through the bone until the bone flap can be removed to expose the brain.

After the surgery for the underlying cause is completed, the piece of skull is replaced and secured with pieces of fine, soft wire. Finally, the surgeon sutures the membrane, muscle, and skin of the scalp.

Preparation

Before the surgery, patients are usually given drugs to ease **anxiety**, and other medications to reduce the risk of swelling, seizures, and infection after the operation. Fluids may be restricted, and a diuretic may be given before and during surgery if the patient has a tendency to retain water. A catheter is inserted before the patient goes to the operating room.

The scalp is shaved in the operating room right before surgery; this is done so that any small nicks in the skin will not have a chance to become infected before the operation.

Aftercare

Oxygen, painkillers, and drugs to control swelling and seizures are given after the operation. Codeine may be given to relieve the **headache** that may occur as a result of stretching or irritation of the nerves of the scalp that happens during the craniotomy. Some type of drainage from the head may be in place, depending on the reason for the surgery.

Patients are usually out of bed within a day and out of the hospital within a week. Headache and **pain** from the scalp wound can be controlled with medications.

The bandage on the skull should be changed regularly. Sutures closing the scalp will be removed, but soft wires used to reattach the skull are permanent and require no further attention. The patient should avoid getting the scalp wet until all the sutures have been removed. A clean cap or scarf can be worn until the hair grows back.

Risks

Accessing the area of the brain that needs repair may damage other brain tissue. Therefore, the procedure carries with it some risk of brain damage that

---

KEY TERMS

Craniotome—A type of surgical drill used to operate on the skull. It has a self-controlled system that stops the drill when the bone is penetrated.

---

could leave the patient with some loss of brain function. The surgeon performing the operation can give the patient an assessment of the risk of his or her particular procedure.

Results

While every patient's experience is different depending on the reason for the surgery, age, and overall health, if the surgery has been successful, recovery is usually rapid because of the good supply of blood to the area.

Possible complications after craniotomy include:

- swelling of the brain
- excessive intracranial pressure
- infection
- seizures

Resources

BOOKS
Moore, Charles E., and Jeffrey J. Olson. *Skull Base Surgery: Basic Techniques*. San Diego: Plural, 2010.

Carol A. Turkington

Creatine kinase test

Definition

The creatine kinase test measures the blood levels of certain muscle and brain enzyme proteins.

Purpose

Creatine kinase (CK or CPK) is an enzyme (a type of protein) found in muscle and brain. Normally, very little CK is found circulating in the blood. Elevated levels indicate damage to either muscle or brain; possibly from a myocardial infarction (**heart attack**), muscle disease, or **stroke**.

There are three types, or isoforms, of CK:

- CK-I, or BB, is produced primarily by brain and smooth muscle.
- CK-II, or MB, is produced primarily by heart muscle.
- CK-III, or MM, is produced primarily by skeletal muscle.

Precautions

No special precautions are necessary, except in patients with a bleeding disorder.

Description

A small amount of blood is drawn and used for laboratory analysis.

Preparation

Physical activity may cause a rise in CK levels, especially the CK-III fraction. Therefore, patients should not engage in strenuous physical activity the day of the test. The patient should report any recent injections, falls, or **bruises** that have occurred, as these may elevate CK levels as well.

Aftercare

No aftercare is required, except to keep the puncture site clean while it heals.

Risks

There are no risks to this test beyond the very slight risk of infection at the puncture site.

Results

In females, total CK should be 10–79 units per liter (U/L). In males, total CK should be 17–148 U/L. CK levels are reduced in the first half of **pregnancy**, and increased in the second half. CK levels are elevated in newborns.

The distribution of isoenzymes should be:

- CK-I: 0%
- CK-II: 0–5%
- CK-III: 95–100%.

Abnormal results

Elevation of CK-I may be seen in stroke, extreme **shock**, or **brain tumor**.

Elevation of CK-II is seen after a myocardial infarction. It begins to rise three to six hours after the heart attack, and may peak within 24 hours. It should then return to normal. For this reason, it is a useful

marker for recent myocardial infarction, but not for one which occurred more than a day before the test.

Elevation of CK-III indicates skeletal muscle damage. This may occur from normal **exercise**, trauma, or muscle disease. CK levels may be very high early on in **muscular dystrophy**, but may fall to normal later as muscle tissue is lost. Elevated CK is also seen in **myositis**, myoglobinuria, **toxoplasmosis**, and **trichinosis**. **Hypothyroidism** may also cause elevated CK.

Resources

BOOKS

Corbett, Jane Vincent. *Laboratory Tests and Diagnostic Procedures with Nursing Diagnoses.* 6th ed. Upper Saddle River, NJ: Pearson/Prentice Hall, 2004.

Richard Robinson

Creatine phosphokinase test *see* **Creatine kinase test**

Creatinine test

Definition

Creatine is an important compound produced by the body. It combines with phosphorus to make a high–energy phosphate compound in the body. Creatine phosphate is used in skeletal muscle contraction.

Purpose

The creatinine test is used to diagnose impaired kidney function and to determine renal (kidney) damage.

Precautions

A diet high in meat content can cause transient elevations of serum creatinine. Some drugs that may increase creatinine values include gentamicin, cimetidine, heavy-metal chemotherapeutic agents (e.g., cisplatin), and other drugs toxic to the kidneys, such as the **cephalosporins**.

Description

The creatinine test is used to measure the amount of creatinine in the blood. Because creatinine is a non-protein end-product of creatine phosphate, which is used in skeletal muscle contraction, the daily production of creatine, and the following product, creatinine, depends on muscle mass, which fluctuates very little.

Creatinine is excreted entirely by the kidneys, and therefore is directly related to renal function. When the kidneys are functioning normally, the serum creatinine level should remain constant and normal. Slight increases in creatine levels can appear after meals, especially after ingestion of large quantities of meat, and some diurnal variation may occur, with a low point at 7 a.m. and a peak at 7 p.m. Serious renal disorders, such as **glomerulonephritis**, **pyelonephritis**, and urinary obstruction, will cause abnormal elevations.

The creatinine level is interpreted in conjunction with another kidney function test called the Blood Urea Nitrogen (BUN). The serum creatinine level has much the same significance as the BUN but tends to rise later. Because of this, determinations of creatinine help to chronicle a disease process. Generally, a doubling of creatinine suggests a 50% reduction in kidney filtration rate.

Preparation

The creatinine test requires a blood sample. It is recommended that the patient be **fasting** (nothing to eat or drink) for at least eight hours before the test. The physician may also require that ascorbic acid (vitamin C), **barbiturates**, and **diuretics** be withheld for 24 hours.

Risks

Risks for this test are minimal, but may include slight bleeding from the blood-drawing site, **fainting** or feeling lightheaded after venipuncture, or hematoma (blood accumulating under the puncture site).

Results

Normal values can vary from laboratory to laboratory, but are generally in the following ranges:

- adult female: 0.5–1.1 mg/dL
- adult male: 0.6–1.2 mg/dL
- adolescent: 0.5–1.0 mg/dL

KEY TERMS

Glomerulonephritis—Glomerulonephritis is an inflammation of the filtering units of the kidney (glomeruli). The condition hinders removal of waste products, salt, and water from the bloodstream, leading to serious complications. It is the most common cause of renal failure.

Pyelonephritis—Pyelonephritis is an inflammation of the kidney itself, usually caused by a bacterial infection. In its most serious form, complications can include high blood pressure (hypertension) and renal failure.

- child: 0.3–0.7 mg/dL
- infant: 0.2–0.4 mg/dL
- newborn: 0.3–1.2 mg/dL

Variations between sources for serum creatinine normal ranges are greater than for other important tests. For example, due to the greater amount of muscle mass generally present, males normally demonstrate higher creatinine levels than females. Also, because the kidney filtration rate normally increases in **pregnancy**, serum creatinine should be slightly less during such periods. In older patients, creatinine is reduced because of decreased muscle mass. Similarly, other patients may have creatinine levels in which muscle abnormalities must be taken into consideration, such as long-term corticosteroid therapy, high thyroid (**hyperthyroidism**), **muscular dystrophy**, or **paralysis**.

Abnormal results

Two to 4 mg/dL indicate the presence of impairment of renal function. Greater than 4 mg/dL indicates serious impairment in renal function.

Resources

BOOKS

Pagana, Kathleen Deska, and Timothy J. Pagana. *Mosby's Manual of Diagnostic and Laboratory Tests.* 4th ed. St. Louis: Mosby, 2009.

Janis O. Flores

Creeping eruption *see* **Cutaneous larva migrans**

CREST syndrome *see* **Scleroderma**

Cretinism *see* **Hypothyroidism**

Creutzfeldt-Jakob disease

Definition

Creutzfeldt-Jakob disease (CJD) is a transmissible, rapidly progressing, neurodegenerative disorder called a spongiform degeneration related to "mad cow disease."

Description

Before 1995, Creutzfeldt-Jakob disease was not well known outside the medical profession. Even within it, many practitioners did not know much about it. Most doctors had never seen a case. With the recognition of a so-called "new variant" form of CJD and the strong possibility that those with it became infected simply by eating contaminated beef, CJD has become one of the most talked-about diseases in the world. Additionally, the radical theory that the infectious agent is a normal protein that has been changed in its form also has sparked much interest.

First described in the early twentieth century independently by Creutzfeldt and Jakob, CJD is a neurodegenerative disease causing a rapidly progressing **dementia** ending in **death**, usually within eight months of symptom onset. It also is a very rare disease, affecting only about one in every million people throughout the world. In the United States, CJD is thought to affect about 250 people each year. CJD affects adults primarily between ages 50 and 75.

Spongiform encephalopathies

The most obvious pathologic feature of CJD is the formation of numerous fluid-filled spaces in the brain (vacuoles) resulting in a sponge-like appearance. CJD is one of several human "spongiform encephalopathies," diseases that produce this characteristic change in brain tissue. Others are kuru; Gerstmann-Straussler-Scheinker disease, a genetic disorder predominantly characterized by cerebellar ataxia (a kind of movement disorder); and fatal familial **insomnia**, with symptoms of progressive sleeplessness, weakness, and dysfunction of the nervous system that affects voluntary and involuntary movements and functions.

Kuru was prevalent among the Fore people in Papua, New Guinea, and spread from infected individuals after their deaths through the practice of ritual cannibalism, in which the relatives of the dead person honored him by consuming his organs, including the brain. Discovery of the infectious nature of kuru won the Nobel Prize for Carleton Gadjusek in 1976. The incubation period for kuru was between four to 30

years or more. While kuru has virtually disappeared since these cannibalistic practices stopped, several new cases continue to arise each year.

Cases of CJD have been grouped into three types: familial, iatrogenic, and sporadic.

- Familial CJD, representing 5–15% of cases, is inherited in an autosomal dominant manner, meaning that either parent may pass along the disease to a child, who then may develop CJD later in life.
- Iatrogenic CJD occurs when a person is infected during a medical procedure, such as organ donation, blood transfusion, or brain surgery. The rise in organ donation has increased this route of transmission; grafts of infected corneas and dura mater (the tissue covering the brain) have been shown to transmit CJD. Another source is hormones concentrated from the pituitary glands of cadavers, some of whom carried CJD, for use in people with growth hormone deficiencies. Iatrogenic infection from exposure to nerve-containing tissue represents a small fraction of all cases. The incubation period after exposure to the infectious agent is very long and is estimated to be from less than 10 to more than 30 years. It remains unlikely, but not impossible, that blood from patients with CJD is infectious to others by transfusion.
- Sporadic CJD represents at least 85% of all cases. Sporadic cases have no identifiable source of infection. Death usually follows first symptoms within eight months.

Animal forms and "mad cow disease"

Six forms of spongiform encephalopathies are known to occur in other mammals: scrapie in sheep, recognized for more than 200 years; chronic wasting disease in elk and mule deer in Wyoming and Colorado; transmissible mink encephalopathy; exotic ungulate encephalopathy in some types of zoo animals; feline spongiform encephalopathy in domestic cats; and bovine spongiform encephalopathy (BSE) in cows.

BSE was first recognized in Britain in 1986. Besides the spongiform changes in the brain, BSE causes dementia-like behavioral changes—hence the name "mad cow disease." BSE was thought to be an altered form of scrapie, transmitted to cows when they were fed sheep offal (slaughterhouse waste) as part of their feed, but researchers believe it is a primary cattle disease spread by contaminated feed.

The use of slaughterhouse offal in animal feed has been common in many countries and has been practiced for at least 50 years. The trigger for the BSE epidemic in

Great Britain seems to have come in the early 1980s, when the use of organic solvents for preparation of offal was altered there. It is possible that these solvents had been destroying the agent called a prion, thereby preventing infection, and that the change in preparation procedure opened the way for the agent to "jump species" and cause BSE in cows that consumed scrapie-infected meal. The slaughter of infected (but not yet visibly sick) cows at the end of their useful farm lives, and the use of their carcasses for feed, spread the infection rapidly and widely. For at least a year after BSE was first recognized in British herds, infected bovine remains continued to be incorporated into feed, spreading the disease still further. Although milk from infected cows never has been shown to pass the infectious agent, passage from infected mother to calf may have occurred through unknown means. Researchers also have tried to confirm how to stop infection of the human food chain once the disease spread among cows. In 2003, a study reported that it spread through nervous system tissue in processed meat and that proper temperature and pressure controls could help ensure safety of commercial beef.

Beginning in 1988, the British government took steps to stop the spread of BSE, banning the use of bovine offal in feed and other products and ordering the slaughter of infected cows. By then, the slow-acting agent had become epidemic in British herds. In 1992, it was diagnosed in more than 25,000 animals (1% of the British herd). By mid-1997, the cumulative number of BSE cases in the United Kingdom had risen to more than 170,000. The feeding ban stemmed the tide of the epidemic; however, the number of new cases each week fell from a peak of 1,000 in 1993 to less than 300 two years later.

The export of British feed and beef to member countries was banned by the European Union, but cases of BSE had developed in Europe by then as well; however, by mid-1997, only about 1,000 cases had been identified. In 1989, the United States banned import of British beef and began monitoring United States herds in 1990. In December 2003, the first case of BSE was discovered in the United States. This prompted recommendations of new safeguards to prevent further spread. Among these were regulations banning animal blood in cattle feed.

Variant CJD: The human equivalent of mad cow disease

From the beginning of the BSE epidemic, scientists and others in Britain feared that BSE might jump species again to infect humans who had consumed infected beef. This, however, had never occurred in scrapie from sheep, a disease known for hundreds of years. In 1996, the first report of this possibility occurred and the fear seemed to be realized with the first cases of a new variant of Creutzfeldt-Jacob disease, termed nvCJD, now just vCJD. Its victims are much younger than the 60–65 year old average for CJD, and the time from symptom onset to death has averaged 12 months or more instead of eight. The disease appears to cause more psychiatric symptoms early on. EEG abnormalities characteristic of CJD are not typically seen in vCJD.

By early 2004, CJD had claimed 143 victims in Great Britain and 10 in other countries. It is of major concern that the number of cases per year seems to be increasing by a factor of 1.35 each year. The only known case in the United States to date had been acquired while the person had been in Great Britain.

Evidence is growing stronger that vCJD is in fact caused by BSE:

- almost all of the cases so far have occurred in Great Britain, the location of the BSE epidemic
- BSE injected into monkeys produces a disease very similar to vCJD
- BSE and vCJD produce the same brain lesions after the same incubation period when injected into laboratory mice
- brain proteins isolated from vCJD victims, but not from the other forms of CJD, share similar molecular characteristics with brain proteins of animals that died from BSE

Researchers now treat the BSE-vCJD connection as solidly established.

Assuming that BSE is the source, the question that has loomed from the beginning has been how many people will eventually be affected. Epidemiological models once placed estimates at tens of thousands, but in 2003, scientists predicted a quicker end to the epidemic and have substantially lowered the numbers expected to contract the disease. The exact incubation period of vCJD in humans is about 10 to 20 years or longer, so it is more difficult to predict the number of cases. Researchers know that some people are more susceptible to vCJD, including young people age 10 to 20 years old.

Causes and symptoms

Causes

It is clear that Creutzfeldt-Jakob disease is caused by an infectious agent, but it is not yet clear what type of agent that is. Originally assumed to be a virus, evidence is accumulating that, instead, CJD is caused by a protein called a prion (PREE-on, for "proteinaceous infectious particle") transmitted from victim to victim. The other spongiform encephalopathies also are hypothesized to be due to prion infection.

If this hypothesis is proven true, it would represent one of the most radical new ideas in biology since the discovery of deoxyribonucleic acid (DNA). All infectious diseases, in fact all life, use nucleic acids—DNA or ribonucleic acid (RNA)—to code the instructions needed for reproduction. Inactivation of the nucleic acids destroys the capacity to reproduce. However, when these same measures are applied to infected tissue from spongiform encephalopathy victims, infectivity is not destroyed. Furthermore, purification of infected tissue to concentrate the infectious fraction yields protein, not nucleic acid. While it remains possible that some highly stable nucleic acid remains hidden within the purified protein, this is seemingly less and less likely as further experiments are done. The "prion hypothesis," as it is called, is now widely accepted, at least provisionally, by most researchers in the field. The most vocal proponent of the hypothesis, Stanley Prusiner, was awarded the Nobel Prize in 1997 for his work in the prion diseases.

A prion is an altered form of a normal brain protein. The normal protein has a helical shape along part of its length. In the prion form, a sheet structure replaces the helix. According to the hypothesis, when the normal form interacts with the prion form, some of its helical part is converted to a sheet, thus creating a new prion capable of transforming other normal forms. In this way, the disease process resembles crystallization more than typical viral infection, in which the virus commands the host's cellular machinery to reproduce more of the virus. Build-up of the sheet form causes accumulation of abnormal protein clumps and degeneration of brain cells, which is thought to cause the disease.

The brain protein affected by the prion, called PrP, is part of the membrane of brain cells, but its exact function is unknown. Exposure to the infectious agent is, of course, still required for disease development. Prion diseases are not contagious in the usual sense, and transmission from an infected person to another person requires direct inoculation of infectious material.

Familial CJD, on the other hand, does not require exposure, but develops through the inheritance of other, more disruptive mutations in the gene for the normal PrP protein. The other two inherited human prion diseases, Gerstmann-Straussler-Scheinker disease and fatal familial insomnia, involve different mutations in the same gene.

The large majority of CJD cases are sporadic, meaning they have no known route of infection or genetic link. Causes of sporadic CJD are likely to be diverse and may include spontaneous genetic mutation, spontaneous protein changes, or unrecognized exposure to infectious agents. It is highly likely that future research will identify more risk factors associated with sporadic CJD.

Symptoms

About one in four people with CJD begin their illness with weakness, changes in sleep patterns, weight loss, or loss of appetite or sexual drive. A person with CJD may first complain of visual disturbances, including double vision, blurry vision, or partial loss of vision. Some visual symptoms are secondary to cortical blindness related to death of nerve cells in the occipital lobe of the brain responsible for vision. This form of visual loss is unusual in that patients may be unaware that they are unable to see. These symptoms may appear weeks to months before the onset of dementia.

The most characteristic symptom of CJD is rapidly progressing dementia, or loss of mental function. Dementia is marked by:

- memory loss
- impaired abstraction and planning
- language and comprehension disturbances
- poor judgment
- disorientation
- decreased attention and increased restlessness
- personality changes and psychosis
- hallucinations

Muscle spasms and jerking movements, called myoclonus, are also a prominent symptom of CJD. Balance and coordination disturbance (ataxia), is common in CJD, and is more pronounced in nvCJD. Stiffness, difficulty moving, and other features representing Parkinson's disease are seen and can progress to akinetic **mutism**, which is a state of being unable to speak or move.

Diagnosis

CJD is diagnosed by a clinical **neurological exam** and **electroencephalography** (EEG), which shows characteristic spikes called triphasic sharp waves. **Magnetic resonance imaging** (MRI) or **computed tomography scans** (CT) should be done to exclude other forms of dementia, and in CJD typically shows atrophy or loss of brain tissue. **Lumbar puncture**, or spinal tap, may be done to rule out other causes of

KEY TERMS

Autosomal dominant inheritance—A pattern of inheritance in which a trait will be expressed if the gene is inherited from either parent.

Encephalopathy—Brain disorder characterized by memory impairment and other symptoms.

Iatrogenic—Caused by a medical procedure.

Nucleic acids—The cellular molecules DNA and RNA that act as coded instructions for the production of proteins and are copied for transmission of inherited traits.

dementia (as cell count, chemical analysis, and other routine tests are normal in CJD) and to identify elevated levels of marker proteins known as 14-3-3. Another marker, neuron-specific enolase, may also be increased in CJD. CJD is conclusively diagnosed after death by brain **autopsy**. Scientists are investigating whether testing lymphatic tissue such as the tonsil may be an early tool in vCJD diagnosis. Additionally, recent studies have suggested that other blood tests may be useful as well.

Treatment

There is no cure for CJD, and no treatment that slows the progression of the disease. Drug therapy and nursing care are aimed at minimizing psychiatric symptoms and increasing patient comfort. However, the rapid progression of CJD frustrates most attempts at treatment, since decreasing cognitive function and more prominent behavioral symptoms develop so quickly. Despite the generally grim prognosis, a few CJD patients progress more slowly and live longer than the average; for these patients, treatment will be more satisfactory. Scientists are investigating whether some medicines that can "break" the abnormal protein form may be useful and whether a vaccine could help.

Prognosis

Creutzfeldt-Jakob disease has proven invariably fatal, with death following symptom onset by an average of eight months. About 5% of patients live longer than two years. Death from vCJD has averaged approximately 12 months after onset. However, in 2003, clinicians reported improvement in a patient with vCJD who received a new experimental drug called Pentosan.

Prevention

There is no known way to prevent sporadic CJD, by far the most common type. Not everyone who inherits the gene mutation for familial CJD will develop the disease, but at present, there is no known way to predict who will and who will not succumb. The incidence of iatrogenic CJD has fallen with recognition of its sources, the development of better screening techniques for infected tissue, and the use of sterilization techniques for surgical instruments that inactivate prion proteins. Fortunately, scientists are making progress. In 2003, researchers announced that they had uncovered the basis for diagnosing, treating and possibly preventing prion diseases such as vCJD. Their research possibly could lead to a vaccine and immunotherapy drugs.

Strategies for prevention of vCJD are a controversial matter, as they involve a significant sector of the agricultural industry and a central feature of the diet in many countries. The infectious potential of contaminated meat is unknown, because the ability to detect prions within meat is limited. Surveillance of North American herds strongly suggests there is no BSE here, and strict regulations on imports of European livestock make future outbreaks highly unlikely. Therefore, avoidance of all meat originating in North America, simply on grounds of BSE risk, is a personal choice unsupported by current data.

Resources

PERIODICALS

Brown, Paul, et al. "Ultra-high Pressure Inactivation of Prion Infectivity in Processed Meat: A Practical Method to Prevent Human Infection." *Proceedings of the National Academy of Sciences of the United States* May 13, 2003: 6093–6095.

"GP Sees Patient with vCJD Improve." *Pulse* June 23, 2003: 12.

Kaye, Donald. "FDA Launches New Mad Cow Rules to Protect U.S. Food, Feed." *Clinical Infectious Diseases* March 15, 2004: 3–5.

"Large Human Mad Cow Epidemic Unlikely— Scientists." *Clinical Infectious Diseases* April 15, 2003: i.

"Report Appears to Confirm Blood-borne Transmission of Creutzfeldt-Jakob Disease." *Blood Weekly* January 8, 2004: 28.

"Researchers Discover Possible Diagnosis, Treatment, Vaccine." *Immunotherapy Weekly* June 25, 2003: 2.

"Scientists Predict Swift End to vCJD Epidemic." *British Medical Journal* May 24, 2003: 1104 –1111.

"U.S. Lawmakers Want Increase in Mad Cow Testing." *Healthcare Purchasing News* March 2004: 85.

Larry I. Lutwick, MD
Teresa G. Odle

Cri du chat syndrome

Definition

Cri du chat syndrome occurs when a piece of chromosomal material is missing from a particular region on chromosome 5. The disorder is also called cat cry syndrome or chromosome deletion 5p syndrome. Individuals with this syndrome have unusual facial features, poor muscle tone (hypotonia), small head size (microcephaly), and **mental retardation**. A classic feature of the syndrome is the cat-like cry made by infants with this disorder.

Description

Dr. Jerome Lejeune first described cri du chat syndrome in 1963. The syndrome is named for the cat-like cry made by infants with this genetic disorder. *Cri du chat* means "cat's cry" in French. This unusual cry is caused by abnormal development of the larynx (organ in the throat responsible for voice production). Cri du chat syndrome is also called 5p deletion syndrome because it is caused by a deletion, or removal, of genetic material from chromosome 5. The deletion that causes cri du chat syndrome occurs on the short or "p" arm of chromosome 5. This deleted genetic material is vital for normal development. Absence of this material results in the features associated with cri du chat syndrome.

A high-pitched mewing cry during infancy is a classic feature of cri du chat. Infants with cri du chat also typically have low birth weight, slow growth, a small head (microcephaly) and poor muscle tone (hypotonia). Infants with cri du chat may have congenital heart defects. Individuals with cri du chat syndrome have language difficulties, delayed motor skill development, and mental retardation. Behavioral problems may also develop as the child matures.

It has been estimated that cri du chat syndrome occurs in one of every 50,000 live births. It accounts for 1 in every 500 cases of mental retardation. According to the 5p minus Society, approximately 50–60 children are born with cri du chat syndrome in the United States each year. It can occur in all races and in both sexes, although there is a slight female predominance. The male:female ratio is 3:4.

Causes and symptoms

Cri du chat is the result of a chromosome abnormality—a deleted piece of chromosomal material on chromosome 5. In about 80% of patients, the defective chromosome comes from the father. In 90% of patients with cri du chat syndrome, the deletion is sporadic. This means that it happens randomly and is not hereditary. If a child has cri du chat due to a sporadic deletion, the chance the parents could have another child with cri du chat is 1%. In approximately 10% of patients with cri du chat, there is a hereditary chromosomal rearrangement that causes the deletion. If a parent has this rearrangement, the risk for them to have a child with cri du chat is greater than 1%.

The severity of mental retardation in cri du chat syndrome is correlated with the extent of deletion of delta-catenin, a protein with an important role in brain functioning. The more extensive the deletion, the more profound the mental dysfunction.

An abnormal larynx causes the unusual cat-like cry made by infants that is a hallmark of the syndrome. As children with cri du chat get older, the cat-like cry becomes less noticeable. This feature can make the diagnosis more difficult in older patients. In addition to the cat-like cry, individuals with cri du chat also have unusual facial features. These facial differences can be very subtle or more obvious. Microcephaly (small head size) is common. During infancy many patients with cri du chat do not gain weight or grow normally. Approximately 30% of infants with cri du chat have a congenital heart defect. Hypotonia (poor muscle tone) is also common, leading to problems with eating and slow, but normal development. Mental retardation is present in all patients with cri du chat, but the degree of mental retardation varies among patients.

Diagnosis

During infancy, the diagnosis of cri du chat syndrome is strongly suspected if the characteristic cat-like cry is heard. If a child has this unusual cry or other features seen in cri du chat syndrome, chromosome testing should be performed. Chromosome analysis provides the definitive diagnosis of cri du chat syndrome and can be performed from a blood test. Chromosome analysis, also called karyotyping, involves staining the chromosomes and examining them under a microscope. In some cases the deletion of material from chromosome 5 can be easily seen. In other cases, further testing must be performed. FISH (fluorescence in-situ hybridization) is a special technique that detects very small deletions. The majority of the deletions that cause cri du chat syndrome can be identified using the FISH technique.

Cri du chat syndrome can be detected before birth if the mother undergoes **amniocentesis** testing or **chorionic villus sampling** (CVS). This testing would only

Amniocentesis—A procedure performed at 16–18 weeks of pregnancy in which a needle is inserted through a woman's abdomen into her uterus to draw out a small sample of the amniotic fluid from around the baby. Either the fluid itself or cells from the fluid can be used for a variety of tests to obtain information about genetic disorders and other medical conditions in the fetus.

Centromere—The centromere is the constricted region of a chromosome. It performs certain functions during cell division.

Chorionic villus sampling (CVS)—A procedure used for prenatal diagnosis at 10–12 weeks gestation. Under ultrasound guidance a needle is inserted either through the mother's vagina or abdominal wall and a sample of cells is collected from around the early embryo. These cells are then tested for chromosome abnormalities or other genetic diseases.

Chromosome—A microscopic thread-like structure found within each cell of the body and consists of a complex of proteins and DNA. Humans have 46 chromosomes arranged into 23 pairs. Changes in either the total number of chromosomes or their shape and size (structure) may lead to physical or mental abnormalities.

Congenital—Refers to a disorder that is present at birth.

Deletion—The absence of genetic material that is normally found in a chromosome. Often, the genetic material is missing due to an error in replication of an egg or sperm cell.

Hypotonia—Reduced or diminished muscle tone.

Karyotyping—A laboratory procedure in which chromosomes are separated from cells, stained and arranged so that their structure can be studied under the microscope.

Microcephaly—An abnormally small head.

be recommended if the mother or father is known to have a chromosome rearrangement, or if they already have a child with cri du chat syndrome.

Treatment

There is no cure for cri du chat syndrome. Treatment consists of supportive care and developmental therapy. Behavioral modification therapy has been found to be useful to control head-banging, hyperactivity, and other behavioral problems that emerge during later childhood.

Prognosis

Individuals with cri du chat have a 10% mortality during infancy due to complications associated with congenital heart defects, hypotonia, and feeding difficulties. Once these problems are controlled, most individuals with cri du chat syndrome have a normal lifespan. The degree of mental retardation can be severe. However, a recent study suggested that the severity is somewhat affected by the amount of therapy received.

Resources

BOOKS

Beers, Mark H., Robert S. Porter, and Thomas V. Jones, eds. *The Merck Manual of Diagnosis and Therapy.* 18th ed. Whitehouse Station, NJ: Merck Research Laboratories, 2006.

Parker, Philip M. *Cri–Du–Chat Syndrome – A Bibliography and Dictionary for Physicians, Patients, and Genome Researchers.* San Diego: ICON Group International, 2007.

PERIODICALS

Israely, I., R. M. Costa, C. W. Xie, et al. "Deletion of the Neuron-Specific Protein Delta-Catenin Leads to Severe Cognitive and Synaptic Dysfunction." *Current Biology* 14 (September 21, 2004): 1657–1663.

OTHER

OMIM—Online Mendelian Inheritance in Man. http://www.ncbi.nlm.nih.gov/Omim/.

ORGANIZATIONS

5p-Society, 7108 Katella Ave. no. 502, Stanton, CA, 96080, (562) 804-4506, (562) 920-5240, (888) 970-0777, director@ fivepminus.org, http://www.fivepminus.org/.

Cri du Chat Syndrome Support Group, PO Box 3408, Norwich, England, NR3 3WE, 440845 094-2725, admin@criduchat.org.uk, http://www.criduchat.org.uk.

Genetic Alliance, Inc., 4301 Connecticut Ave., NW, Suite 404, Washington, DC, 20008-2369, (202) 966-5557, (202) 966-8553, info@geneticalliance.org, http://www.geneticalliance.org.

National Organization for Rare Disorders, P.O. Box 8923, New Fairfield, CT, 06812-8923, (800) 999-6673, http://www.rarediseases.org.

Holly Ann Ishmael, M.S.
Rebecca J. Frey, PhD

Crib death *see* **Sudden infant death syndrome**

Crohn's disease

Definition

Crohn's disease is a chronic inflammatory disorder that affects the digestive tract, characterized by cramping **pain**, **diarrhea**, and sometimes **nausea** or **vomiting**.

Demographics

It is estimated that there are about 500,000 persons with Crohn's disease in the United States, with another 500,000 suffering from ulcerative **colitis**. Another statistic that is given by some doctors is 7 cases per 100,000 in the general population in Canada and the United States. Crohn's is primarily a disorder of adults, most often beginning in late adolescence or

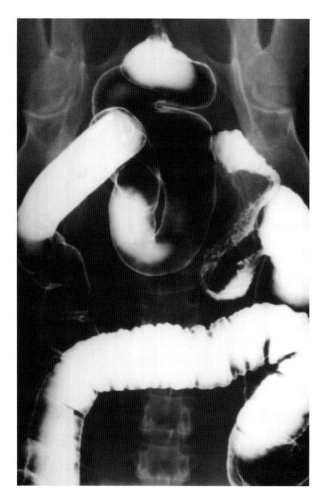

A barium x-ray showing the colon of a patient with Crohn's disease where the large and small intestines join (bottom left). *(Custom Medical Stock Photo, Inc. Reproduced by permission.)*

the early adult years. The most common age at onset is between 15 and 30 years, although the disorder may begin at any age.

The rate of Crohn's disease in North America has been increasing since the 1960s, although the reasons for the increase are not known as of 2009. Southern Europe, South America, Africa, and Asia have considerably lower rates of the disease —as low as 0.5–0.08 cases per 100,000 people. Around the world, however, the rates of Crohn's disease are higher in cities than in rural areas, and higher among people with higher incomes than among lower-income groups.

One argument for the presence of a genetic factor in Crohn's disease is that it runs in some families; people who have a sibling with the disease are 30 times more likely to develop it than the normal population. Crohn's disease is also relatively common among certain ethnic groups, particularly Jews of Eastern European origin. A two- to four-fold increase in the frequency of Crohn's disease has been found among the Jewish population in the United States, Europe, and South Africa compared to other ethnic groups.

In terms of other ethnic groups in the United States, Crohn's disease appears to be slightly more common in non-Jewish Caucasians than in African or Asian Americans. The disease is more common in men than in women; the male/female ratio is 1.8:1.

Description

Crohn's disease is named for Dr. Burrill Bernard Crohn (1884–1983) who, with his colleagues, first described the disease in 1932. Crohn's disease can affect any part of the digestive system, however, it develops most often in the section of the small intestine just before the large intestine begins. This region is called the ileum, and Crohn's disease that develops there is sometimes called ileitus. The other common site for Crohn's disease is in the colon or large intestine.

Crohn's disease is one of several inflammatory bowel diseases. It can be mistaken for ulcerative colitis. Both these diseases cause watery diarrhea or bloody diarrhea and abdominal cramps or pain. Ulcerative colitis, however, affects only the layer of cells that line the intestine forming sores or ulcers on this surface. Crohn's disease begins in these same surface cells, but eats its way inward, damaging all four layers of the intestine and sometimes creating a hole (**fistula**) through the intestine and into other tissue. Another major difference between Crohn's disease and ulcerative colitis is that Crohn's disease can develop simultaneously in several spots in the digestive tract, resulting in areas of damaged with patches with healthy tissue in between. Ulcerative colitis, on the other hand, spreads uniformly across an area. Crohn's disease is somewhat treatable but not curable, and can cause many complications beyond the digestive system. Eventually the walls of the intestine thicken and blockages may occur that can only be corrected by surgery.

In some cases of Crohn's disease, the underlying layers of intestinal tissue are damaged also, leading to complete perforation (puncturing) of the wall of the intestine. This form of the disease is sometimes called penetrating Crohn's disease. Penetrating disease may cause a serious infection in the abdomen or the formation of fistulas. In Crohn's disease, fistulas are most likely to form in the area around the anus, leading to the formation of abscesses (pus-filled sores). About 30 percent of patients with Crohn's disease develop fistulas.

Another subtype of Crohn's disease is called stricturing disease. Stricture is the medical term for an abnormal narrowing of a hollow organ such as the bowel. In stricturing disease, the inflammation and swelling of tissue inside the bowel leads to changes in the size of the patient's stools and eventual blockage of the intestinal passages. Severe abdominal cramping is often an indication of stricturing disease, as are **nausea and vomiting**.

Risk factors

Risk factors for Crohn's disease include a family history of the disorder; a history of heavy **smoking**; and Eastern European Jewish ethnicity.

Causes and symptoms

Causes

At one time, researchers thought that **stress** and diet caused Crohn's disease, particularly by eating sweet or high-fat foods. It is also known that smoking is a risk factor for developing Crohn's. Now researchers know that these are not causes in the strict sense, although both stress and diet can worsen symptoms in people who already have the disease. What researchers do know is that Crohn's disease is caused by an inappropriate immune system reaction that affects cells in the digestive tract. Beyond that, the reasons why some people develop the disease are not clear as of 2009.

There is almost certainly an inherited component that predisposes some people to the disease. Individuals who are blood relatives of a parent, sibling, or child with Crohn's disease are 30 times more likely to develop the disease than the general population. Scientists believe multiple genes are involved in development of the disease. However, more than genetics determines who gets Crohn's disease, because only about 44% of identical twins both develop the disease. Researchers have found mutated (altered) genes in many, but not all, people who have Crohn's disease but do not yet have a clear understanding of what these genes do. As of early 2009, about 30 different genes have been identified that are thought to play a role in the development of Crohn's disease.

Current thinking is that interactions among genes, the environment, the individual's health, and body chemistry affect a person's risk of developing Crohn's disease. When foreign materials (antigens) enter the body, the immune system produces antibodies, which are proteins that neutralize the foreign invader. One theory about Crohn's disease is that some foreign organism or material stimulates an immune system response in the digestive system, and then through an error in genetic control, the response cannot be "turned off." A second theory suggests that the cells of the immune system mistake good bacteria, food, or some other substance that is normally present in the digestive tract and make antibodies against this material as if it were a foreign substance. Either way, an inappropriate immune system response occurs that appears to be the root cause of the symptoms people with Crohn's disease experience.

Symptoms

Symptoms of Crohn's disease vary, depending on the location of the damaged cells and the length of time the individual has had the disease. Symptoms can be mild or severe. They can develop suddenly or gradually, and they may improve or even disappear, and then worsen many times throughout an individual's life. Some people may have only occasional episodes of diarrhea, for example, while others may have 20–30 bowel movements in a single day that interfere with sleep, work, school, or other activities. In general, symptoms can be divided into those that affect the digestive tract and those that affect the rest of the body.

The most common symptoms that affect the digestive tract are:

- chronic diarrhea, the most common symptom
- abdominal pain or cramps, often in the lower right portion of the abdomen
- rectal bleeding
- blood in the stool or black tarry stools

Abscess—A pus-filled sore surrounded by inflamed tissue.

Endoscope—A medical instrument that can be passed into an area of the body (e.g., the bladder or intestine) to allow examination of that area. The endoscope usually has a fiber-optic camera, which allows a greatly magnified image to be shown on a television screen viewed by the operator. Many endoscopes also allow the operator to retrieve a small sample (biopsy) of the area being examined.

Fistula—An abnormal tunnel or passage that forms between one part of the intestine and another or between the intestine and the body surface.

Gastroenterologist—A doctor who specializes in diagnosing and treating diseases of the digestive system.

Remission—A period in the course of a disease when symptoms disappear for a time.

Stoma—An opening made in the abdomen following surgery for colon cancer that allows wastes to pass from the body.

Stricture—The medical term for the abnormal narrowing of a hollow organ such as the bowel.

Ulceration—A pitted area or break in the continuity of a surface, such as the skin or mucous membrane.

- ulcers in the digestive tract, usually in the intestine
- fistulas, or holes in the intestine that connect the intestine to such other parts of the body as the bladder, stomach, vagina, or another section of bowel
- nausea and vomiting , usually from Crohn's disease in the stomach
- abscesses, fistulas, and ulcers around the anus, usually from Crohn's disease in the colon. These occur in about 45% of patients
- constipation, usually after many years when the bowel has thickened and the diameter of the intestine has narrowed

Symptoms of Crohn's disease also appear in other systems in the body. Some are the result of infection when fistulas develop. Others come from poor absorption of nutrients in the intestine over a long period. Some symptoms that occur outside the digestive tract include:

- persistent low-grade fever
- loss of appetite and weight loss
- fatigue
- anemia from blood loss and/or poor iron absorption
- skin infections
- eye infections
- arthritis and sore joints, usually in the large joints such as the knees or hips
- osteoporosis from poor calcium and vitamin D absorption
- poor blood clotting from inadequate vitamin K absorption
- stunted growth in children
- delayed puberty

Diagnosis

Examination

The most important aspect of diagnosing Crohn's disease is to distinguish it from other digestive disorders, including ulcerative colitis, intestinal parasites, and an intestinal obstruction. Normally the physician will begin the examination of a patient who might have Crohn's disease by taking a through medical and family history and standard blood and stool tests. Blood tests may reveal an increase in certain types of white blood cells, an indication that some type of inflammation or infection is occurring in the body. Blood tests may also reveal anemia and other signs of **malnutrition** due to malabsorption. Stool samples may be examined to make sure that no infectious agent is causing the diarrhea, and to see whether the waste products contain blood.

Special blood tests are available that can help differentiate between Crohn's disease and ulcerative colitis. These tests may be done if the results of other tests are questionable. According to the Crohn's & Colitis Foundation of America, it is quite difficult to tell these two diseases apart in about 10% of patients.

Tests

There is no single laboratory or imaging test that can be used to diagnose Crohn's disease. In addition to blood and stool tests, the four tests most commonly used to diagnose Crohn's are barium studies, computed tomography (CT) scans, sigmoidoscopies, and colonoscopies. In a barium study, the patient is given barium in enema form to coat the lining of the colon and rectum. Air is then blown into the colon in order to fill it. The resultant x-ray can be used to detect abnormalities in the lining of the intestine. CT scans are useful in detecting fistulas and abscesses.

Procedures

Sigmoidoscopies and colonoscopies are procedures that require special equipment inserted into the patient's body. A sigmoidoscope is a flexible lighted tube that can be inserted into the rectum and used to examine the last two feet of the colon. This procedure can be done in a doctor's office but does not provide a view of the entire colon. A colonoscope is a long flexible tube attached to a video camera and monitor that allows the doctor to examine the entire length of the patient's colon and rectum. The patient must take a laxative the night before to cleanse the bowel and may be given a sedative in the doctor's office to make them more comfortable. The doctor can also take tissue samples from the lining of the bowel for analysis.

Treatment

Traditional

As of 2009, there is no medical or surgical cure for Crohn's disease. Treatment consists of managing the patient's symptoms, getting the disease into remission, and preventing relapses. Patients with Crohn's disease are usually started on one or more different types of medications to relieve pain and discomfort. These medications may include cortisone and other drugs that reduce inflammation; drugs that block or lower the body's immune response; **antidiarrheal drugs** and fluid replacements; **antibiotics**; and **nutritional supplements**. Special high-calorie liquid formulas may be prescribed for patients whose intestines may need a rest.

Drugs

Individuals with mild to moderate Crohn's disease are usually treated first with such anti-inflammatory drugs as sulfasalazine (Azulfidine) or mesalamine (Asacol, Rowasa, Canasa). Individuals with moderate to severe Crohn's disease often are prescribed corticosteroid drugs. Prednisone (Deltasone, Orasone, Meticorten) is often the corticosteroid of choice. These drugs have significant side effects and cannot be used for long-term suppression of symptoms. Antibiotics are used to treat infection that may develop from fistula formation.

Biologic therapies use antibodies produced in the laboratory to treat disease. Infliximab (Remicade) is a laboratory-made antibody that blocks the production of an immune system factor that causes inflammation. This treatment is relatively new but appears to have a good success rate for relieving symptoms. Additional biologic therapies for Crohn's disease are under development. Individuals interested in participating in a clinical trial of a new drug or therapy for Crohn's disease at no cost can find a list of trials currently enrolling volunteers at http://www.clinicaltrials.gov.

Surgery

Patients who are not helped by medications or who have the stricturing form of the disease are usually treated by surgery. In most cases the surgeon removes the diseased part of the intestine and reconnects the healthy portions. This procedure may have to be repeated, however, as inflammation may develop in the area of the intestine next to where a diseased portion was removed. In cases in which the disease is located in the large intestine (colon), the surgeon may have to remove the entire colon in a procedure called a **colostomy**. In this procedure, an opening called a stoma is made in the wall of the abdomen and a portion of the remaining colon is attached to the stoma. The person's body wastes pass through the stoma and are collected in a special bag attached to the outside of the body.

Alternative

Acupuncture and **guided imagery** may be useful tools in treating pain associated with Crohn's disease. Acupuncture involves the placement of thin needles into the skin at targeted locations on the body known as acupoints in order to harmonize the energy flow within the human body. To treat chronic pain, such as that involved with Crohn's disease, an acupuncturist frequently places the acupuncture needles along what is known as the large intestine meridian.

Guided imagery involves creating a visual mental image of one's pain in one's mind. Once the pain can be visualized, the patient can adjust the image to make it more pleasing and, thus, more manageable. Other related alternative therapies include relaxation exercises, **yoga**, and **biofeedback**.

Several herbal remedies are also available to lessen pain symptoms and promote relaxation and healing. These include peppermint oil, slippery elm (*Ulmus rubra*), marsh mallow (*Althaea oficinalis*), and Chinese herbs. However, Crohn's patients should consult with their healthcare professional before taking them. Depending on the preparation and the type of herb, these remedies may aggravate the digestive tract or interact with prescription drugs that are being taken to control the inflammation of Crohn's disease.

Home remedies

Home treatment of Crohn's disease involves considerable adjustment of the patient's diet. Dietary changes are usually necessary to minimize pain, diarrhea, and other symptoms. In addition, regular physical **exercise** appears to be effective in lowering stress levels and regularizing bowel function.

Prognosis

Most people with Crohn's disease have periods of remission and are able to hold jobs and lead normal lives for the most part. Medical treatment of Crohn's disease, however, becomes less effective over time; about 80 percent of patients require surgery eventually. In addition, the disease can recur after surgery. The chance of a shortened life span or serious complications increases with the duration of the illness; patients with Crohn's disease also have an increased risk of colorectal **cancer**. The disease itself, however, is rarely fatal.

Prevention

There is no known way to prevent Crohn's disease as of 2009 because its causes are not yet understood.

Diet and nutrition

People with Crohn's disease tend to have vitamin and mineral deficiencies because damage to the lining of the intestine interferes with the absorption of nutrients, and chronic diarrhea hastens the loss of other nutrients. These deficiencies can cause specific disorders in other parts of the body. In addition, children with Crohn's disease also may need special high-calorie, high-nutrient liquid supplements to maintain normal growth. A nutritionist consulting with the patient's gastroenterologist can help determine the best diet and supplements to prevent nutritional deficiencies.

Although eating certain foods does not cause Crohn's disease, specific foods can worsen symptoms. Many people with Crohn's disease become lactose intolerant and must limit or eliminate dairy products from their diet. Alcohol, high fiber foods such as popcorn, and spicy foods can worsen diarrhea and abdominal cramping. Individuals must be alert to the effect of food on their symptoms until they figure out which foods to avoid.

Health care team roles

Crohn's disease is often diagnosed by primary care practitioners or gastroenterologists. In many instances, patients require surgical intervention. Imaging studies to assist in diagnosis are performed by x-ray technologists, and laboratory technologists may be involved in obtaining blood and stool samples for analysis.

Nurses, dieticians, and nutritional counselors have important roles in teaching patients about dietary changes to manage symptoms. Nurses, social workers, and **ostomy** specialists may also be involved in educating patients pre- and postoperatively about ostomy care.

Resources

BOOKS

Dahlman, David. *Why Doesn't My Doctor Know This? Conquering Irritable Bowel Syndrome, Inflammatory Bowel Disease, Crohn's Disease, and Colitis.* Garden City, NY: Morgan James, 2008.

Giddens, Sandra, and Owen Giddens. *Everything You Need to Know about Crohn's Disease and Ulcerative Colitis.* New York: Rosen Publishing Group, 2004.

Sklar, Jill. *Crohn's Disease and Ulcerative Colitis: An Essential Guide for the Newly Diagnosed*, rev. ed. New York: Marlowe and Co., 2007.

Warner, Andrew S., and Amy E. Barto. *100 Questions and Answers about Crohn's Disease and Ulcerative Colitis: A Lahey Clinic Guide.* Sudbury, MA: Jones and Bartlett Publishers, 2007.

Zonderman, Jon and Ronald Vender. *Understanding Crohn Disease and Ulcerative Colitis.* Jackson, MS: University Press of Mississippi, 2006.

PERIODICALS

American Academy of Family Practice (AAFP). "Patient Information: Crohn's Disease." *American Family Physician*, August 15, 2003. Available online at http://www.aafp.org/afp/20030815/717ph.html.

Bakalar, Nicholas. "Crohn's Disease and Colitis Are Linked to Mutant Gene." *New York Times*, November 7, 2006.

Bernard, André. "A Systematic Review of Patient Inflammatory Bowel Disease Information Resources on the World Wide Web." *American Journal of Gastroenterology* (September 2007): 2070–2077.

Clark, M., et al. "American Gastroenterological Association Consensus Development Conference on the Use of Biologics in the Treatment of Inflammatory Bowel Disease." *Gastroenterology* (July 2007): 312–339.

Feagan, Brian G., et al. "Health-Related Quality of Life During Natalizumab Maintenance Therapy for Crohn's Disease." *American Journal of Gastroenterology* (December 2007): 2737–2746.

Lucendo, A. J., and L. C. De Rezende. "Importance of Nutrition in Inflammatory Bowel Disease." *World Journal of Gastroenterology* 15 (May 7, 2009): 2081–8.

Noomen, C. G., D. W. Hommes, and H. H. Fidder. "Update on Genetics in Inflammatory Disease." *Best Practice and Research. Clinical Gastroenterology* 23 (2009): 233–43.

Van Limbergen, Johan, et al. "The Genetics of Inflammatory Bowel Disease." *American Journal of Gastroenterology* (December 2007): 2820–2831.

OTHER

Crohn's and Colitis Foundation of America (CCFA). *About Crohn's Disease.* http://www.ccfa.org/info/about/crohns

Mayo Clinic. *Crohn's Disease.* http://www.mayoclinic.com/health/crohns-disease/DS00104

National Institute of Diabetes and Digestive and Kidney Diseases (NIDDK). *Crohn's Disease.* http://digestive.niddk.nih.gov/ddiseases/pubs/crohns/index.htm

ORGANIZATIONS

American College of Gastroenterology, P.O. Box 342260, Bethesda, MD, 20827-2260, 301-263-9000, http://www.acg.gi.org/.

Crohn's & Colitis Foundation of America., 386 Park Ave. S., 17th Floor, New York, NY, 10016-8804, 800-932-2423, info@ccfa.org, http://www.ccfa.org/.

National Institute of Diabetes and Digestive and Kidney Diseases (NIDDK), Building 31. Rm 9A06, 31 Center Drive, MSC 2560, Bethesda, MD, 20892-2560, 301-496-3583, http://www2.niddk.nih.gov/Footer/Contact NIDDK.htm, http://www2.niddk.nih.gov/.

Tish Davidson, AM
David Edward Newton, EdD
Rebecca J. Frey, PhD

Cromolyn *see* **Antiasthmatic drugs**

Cross-eye *see* **Strabismus**

Cross-gender identification *see* **Gender identity disorder**

▌ Croup

Definition

Croup is a common childhood ailment. Typically, it arises from a viral infection of the larynx (voice box) and is associated with mild upper respiratory symptoms such as a runny nose and **cough**. The key symptom is a harsh barking cough. Croup usually is not serious, and most children recover within a few days. In a small percentage of cases, a child develops breathing difficulties and may need medical attention.

Demographics

Croup is most common in children between ages one and two years, with an incidence of 5–6 cases per 100 population. It accounts for about 15% of children's doctor and emergency room visits in the United States. The number of cases peaks in late fall and early winter.

Description

At one time, the term croup was primarily associated with **diphtheria**, a life-threatening respiratory infection. Owing to widespread immunization, diphtheria has become rare in the United States and other parts of the developed world, and croup currently refers to a mild viral infection of the larynx. Croup is also known as laryngotracheitis, a medical term that describes the inflammation of the trachea (windpipe) and larynx.

Parainfluenza viruses are the typical root cause of the infection, but influenza (flu) and cold viruses may sometimes be responsible. All of these viruses are highly contagious and easily transmitted between individuals via sneezing and coughing. Children between the ages of three months and six years are usually affected, with the greatest incidence at one to two years of age. The characteristic harsh barking of a croupy cough can be very distressing, but it rarely indicates a serious problem. Most children with croup can be treated very effectively at home; however, 1–5% may require medical treatment.

Croup may sometimes be confused with more serious conditions, such as **epiglottitis** or bacterial tracheitis. These ailments arise from bacterial infection and must receive medical treatment.

Causes and symptoms

The larynx and trachea may become inflamed or swollen from an upper respiratory viral infection. The hallmark sign of croup is a harsh, barking cough. This cough may be preceded by one to three days of symptoms that resemble a slight cold. A croupy cough is often accompanied by a runny nose, hoarseness, and a low **fever**. When the child inhales, there may be a raspy or high-pitched noise called **stridor**, owing to the narrowed airway and accumulated mucus. In the presence of stridor, medical attention is required.

Corticosteroid drug—A medication that acts like a type of hormone (cortisol) produced by the adrenal gland of the body. Corticosteroids produced by the body stimulate specific types of functional activity. As a drug, a corticosteroid (sometimes just called steroid) helps treat inflammation, infection, or trauma to the body.

Diphtheria—A serious, often fatal, bacterial infection that produces a toxin (poison) and an inflammation in the membrane lining of the throat, nose, trachea, and other tissues.

Epiglottitis—A bacterial infection that affects the epiglottis. The epiglottis is a flap of tissue that prevents food and fluid from entering the trachea. The infection causes it to become swollen, potentially blocking the airway. Other symptoms include a high fever, muffled voice, and an inability to swallow properly (possibly indicated by drooling).

Larynx—Also known as the voice box, the larynx is the part of the airway that lies between the pharynx and the trachea. It is composed of cartilage that contains the apparatus for voice production—the vocal cords and the muscles and ligaments that move the cords.

Reye's syndrome—A rare but often fatal disease that involves the brain, liver, and kidneys. It may brought on by giving salicylates (aspirin compounds) to children (but not adults) who have a viral infection.

Stridor—The high-pitched or rasping noise made when air is inhaled through narrowed airways.

Trachea—Commonly called the windpipe, it is the air pathway that connects the nose and mouth to the lungs.

However, the airway rarely narrows so much that breathing is impeded. Symptoms usually go away completely within a few days. Medical treatment may be sought if the child's symptoms do not respond to home treatment.

Emergency medical treatment is required immediately if the child has difficulty breathing, swallowing, or talking; develops a high fever (103°F [39.4°C] or more); seems unalert or confused; or has pale or blue-tinged skin.

Diagnosis

Croup is diagnosed based on the symptoms. If symptoms are particularly severe, or do not respond to treatment, an x ray of the throat area may be done to assess the possibility of epiglottitis or other blockage of the airway.

Treatment

Home remedies

Home treatment is the usual method of managing croup symptoms. It is important that the child is kept comfortable and calm to the best degree possible, because crying can make symptoms seem worse. Humid air can help a child with croup feel more comfortable. Recommended methods include sitting in a steamy bathroom with the hot water running or using a cool-water vaporizer or humidifier. However, although cool-mist therapy at home or in the hospital may add to the child's comfort, it does little to treat the actual condition. The child should drink frequently in order to stay well hydrated. To treat any fever, the child may be given an appropriate dose of **acetaminophen** (like Tylenol). Children should not be given **aspirin**, as it may cause **Reye's syndrome**, a life-threatening disease of the brain. **Antihistamines** and **decongestants** are ineffective in treating croup.

Medical treatment

If the child does not respond to home treatment, medical treatment at a doctor's office or an emergency room could be necessary. Based on the severity of symptoms and the response to treatment, the child may need to be admitted to a hospital.

For immediate symptom relief, epinephrine may be administered as an inhaled aerosol. Effects last for up to two hours, but there is a possibility that symptoms may return. For that reason, the child is kept under supervision for three or more hours. **Steroids (corticosteroids)** such as prednisone may be used to treat croup, particularly if the child has stridor when resting.

Of the 1–5% of children requiring medical treatment, approximately 1% need respiratory support. Such support involves intubation (inserting a tube into the trachea) and oxygen administration.

Alternative treatment

Botanical/herbal medicines can be helpful in healing the cough that is commonly associated with croup.

Several herbs to consider for cough treatment include aniseed (*Pimpinella anisum*), sundew (*Drosera rotundifolia*), thyme (*Thymus vulgaris*), and wild cherry bark (*Prunus serotina*). **Homeopathic medicine** can be very effective in treating cases of croup. Choosing the correct remedy (a common choice is aconite or monkshood, *Aconitum napellus*) is always the key to the success of this type of treatment.

Prognosis

Croup is a temporary condition and children typically recover completely within three to six days. Children can experience one or more episodes of croup during early childhood; however, croup is rarely a dangerous condition.

Prevention

Croup is caused by highly transmissible viruses and is often difficult to impossible to prevent.

Resources

OTHER

American Academy of Pediatrics. "Croup." HealthyChildren.org. August 12, 2010. http://www.healthychildren.org/English/health-issues/conditions/chest-lungs/pages/Croup.aspx (accessed December 22, 2010).

Mayo Foundation for Medical Education and Research. "Croup." MayoClinic.com. August 5, 2010. http://www.mayoclinic.com/health/croup/DS00312 (accessed December 22, 2010).

ORGANIZATIONS

American Academy of Family Physicians, P. O. Box 11210, Shawnee Mission, KS, 66207, (913) 906-6000, (800) 274-2237, (913) 906-6075, http://familydoctor.org.

American Academy of Pediatrics, 141 Northwest Point Boulevard, Elk Grove Village, IL, 60007-1098, (847) 434-4000, (847) 434-8000, http://www.aap.org.

Julia Barrett
Tish Davidson, A.M.

Cryoglobulin test

Definition

Cryoglobulin is an abnormal blood protein associated with several diseases. Testing for cryoglobulin is done when a person has symptoms of this protein or is being evaluated for one of the associated diseases.

Purpose

Cryoglobulin clumps in cold temperatures. This physical characteristic causes people with cryoglobulin to have symptoms during cold weather: blanching, **numbness**, and **pain** in their fingers or toes (Raynaud's phenomenon); bleeding into the skin (purpura); and pain in joints (arthralgia). People with these symptoms or any other symptoms that appear in cold weather should be tested for cryoglobulin.

Diseases that cause the body to make extra or abnormal proteins are often associated with cryoglobulin. These diseases include cancers involving white blood cells, infections, **autoimmune disorders**, and rheumatoid diseases.

This test provides information about the cause of symptoms in a person who already has a disease process. It does not diagnose a specific disease or monitor the course of a disease.

Precautions

This test is not a screening test for disease in a person without symptoms.

Description

Laboratory testing for cryoglobulin is based on the fact that cryoglobulin clumps when cooled and dissolves when warmed. The test is done on a person's serum (the yellow liquid part of blood that separates from the cells after the **blood clots**). The serum is kept warm from the time drawn until the cells and the serum are separated in the laboratory. The serum is placed at 33.8°F (1°C) for one to seven days. If there is clumping, cryoglobulins are present. The amount of cryoglobulins is determined by measuring the amount of clumping. Negative tests are checked through seven days.

Additional testing is done to find out what kind of cryoglobulin protein is present. There are three kinds of cryoglobulin, each associated with different diseases.

The test, also called the cold sensitivity antibodies test, is covered by insurance when medically necessary. Results are usually available the following day.

Preparation

This test requires 15–20 mL of blood. A healthcare worker ties a tourniquet on the person's upper arm, locates a vein in the inner elbow region, and inserts a needle into that vein. Vacuum action draws the blood through the needle into an attached tube. Collection of the sample takes only a few minutes. The blood must be kept warm, at body temperature, until the laboratory can separate the cells from the serum.

Aftercare

Discomfort or bruising may occur at the puncture site or the person may feel dizzy or faint. Pressure to the puncture site until the bleeding stops reduces bruising. Warm packs to the puncture site relieve discomfort.

Results

A normal result will be negative or absent.

If the person has cryoglobulin, the amount is reported. Larger amounts of cryoglobulin are associated with cancers or abnormalities involving white blood cells, moderate amounts are associated with autoimmune disorders and rheumatoid diseases, and smaller amounts are associated with infections.

The type of cryoglobulin is also reported. Type I cryoglobulin, also called monoclonal cryoglobulinemia, is found in cancers or abnormalities of white blood cells. Type II, also called mixed cryoglobulinemia, is associated with autoimmune disorders, rheumatoid diseases, and infections, particularly chronic **hepatitis B**.

The physician must interpret the cryoglobulin result along with other test results and the patient's clinical condition and medical history.

Resources

BOOKS

Pagana, Kathleen Deska, and Timothy J. Pagana. *Mosby's Manual of Diagnostic and Laboratory Tests.* 4th ed. St. Louis: Mosby, 2009.

Nancy J. Nordenson

Cryosurgery *see* **Cryotherapy**

Cryotherapy

Definition

Cryotherapy is a technique that uses an extremely cold liquid or instrument to freeze and destroy abnormal skin cells that require removal. The technique has been in use since the turn of the century, but modern techniques have made it widely available to dermatologists and primary care doctors. The technique is also called cryosurgery.

Purpose

Cryotherapy can be employed to destroy a variety of benign skin growths, such as **warts**, pre-cancerous lesions (such as actinic keratoses), and malignant lesions (such as basal cell and squamous cell cancers). The goal of cryotherapy is to freeze and destroy targeted skin growths while preserving the surrounding skin from injury.

Precautions

Cryotherapy is not recommended for certain areas of the body because of the danger of destruction of tissue or unacceptable scarring. These areas include: skin that overlies nerves, the corners of the eyes, the fold of skin between the nose and lip, the skin surrounding the nostrils, and the border between the lips and the rest of the face. Lesions that are suspected or known to be **malignant melanoma** should not be treated with cryotherapy, but should instead be removed surgically. Similarly, basal cell or squamous cell carcinomas that have reappeared at the site of a previously treated tumor should also be removed surgically. If it remains unclear whether a growth is benign or malignant, a sample of tissue should be removed for analysis (biopsy) by a pathologist before any attempts to destroy the lesion with cryotherapy. Care should be taken in people with diabetes or certain circulation problems when cryotherapy is considered for growths located on their lower legs, ankles, and feet. In these patients, healing can be poor and the risk of infection can be higher than for other patients.

Description

There are three main techniques to performing cryotherapy. In the simplest technique, usually reserved for warts and other benign skin growths, the physician will dip a cotton swab or other applicator into a cup containing a "cryogen," such as liquid nitrogen, and apply it directly to the skin growth to freeze it. At a temperature of $-320°F$ ($-196°C$), liquid nitrogen is the coldest cryogen available. The goal is to freeze the skin growth as quickly as possible, and then let it thaw slowly to cause maximum destruction of the skin cells. A second application may be necessary depending on the size of the growth. In another cryotherapy technique, a device is used to direct a small spray of liquid nitrogen or other cryogen directly onto the skin growth. Freezing may last from five to 20 seconds, depending on the size of the lesion. A second freeze-thaw cycle may be required. Sometimes, the physician will insert a small needle connected to a thermometer into the lesion to make certain the lesion is cooled to a low enough temperature to guarantee maximum destruction. In a third option, liquid nitrogen or another cryogen is circulated through a probe to cool it to low temperatures. The probe is then brought into direct contact with the skin lesion to freeze it. The freeze time can take two to three times longer than with the spray technique.

Preparation

Extensive preparation prior to cryotherapy is not required. The area to be treated should be clean and dry, but sterile preparation is not necessary. Patients should know that they will experience some **pain** at the time of the freezing, but **local anesthesia** is usually not required. The physician may want to reduce the size of certain growths, such as warts, prior to the cryotherapy procedure, and may have patients apply salicylic acid preparations to the growth over several weeks. Sometimes, the physician will pare away some of the tissue using a device called a curette or a scalpel.

Aftercare

Redness, swelling, and the formation of a blister at the site of cryotherapy are all expected results of the treatment. A gauze dressing is applied and patients should wash the site three or four times daily while fluid continues to ooze from the wound, usually for five to 14 days. A dry crust then forms that falls off by itself. **Wounds** on the head and neck may take four to six weeks to heal, but those on the body, arms, and legs can take longer. Some patients experience pain at the site following the treatment. This can usually be eased with **acetaminophen** (Tylenol), though in some cases a stronger pain reliever may be required.

Risks

Cryotherapy poses little risk and can be well-tolerated by elderly and other patients who are not good candidates for other surgical procedures. As with other surgical procedures, there is some risk of

scarring, infection, and damage to underlying skin and tissue. These risks are generally minimal in the hands of experienced users of cryotherapy.

Results

Some redness, swelling, blistering and oozing of fluid are all common results of cryotherapy. Healing time can vary by the site treated and the cryotherapy technique used. When cryogen is applied directly to the growth, healing may occur in three weeks. Growths treated on the head and neck with the spray technique may take four to six weeks to heal; growths treated on other areas of the body may take considerably longer. Cryotherapy boasts high success rates in permanently removing skin growths; even for malignant lesions such as squamous cell and basal cell cancers, studies have shown a cure rate of up to 98%. For certain types of growths, such as some forms of warts, repeat treatments over several weeks are necessary to prevent the growth's return.

Abnormal results

Although cryotherapy is a relatively low risk procedure, some side effects may occur as a result of the treatment. They include:

- Infection. Though uncommon, infection is more likely on the lower legs where healing can take several months.
- Pigmentary changes. Both hypopigmentation (lightening of the skin) and hyperpigmentation (darkening

of the skin) are possible after cryotherapy. Both generally last a few months, but can be longer lasting.

- Nerve damage. Though rare, damage to nerves is possible, particularly in areas where they lie closer to the surface of the skin, such as the fingers, the wrist, and the area behind the ear. Reports suggest this will disappear within several months.

ORGANIZATIONS

American Academy of Dermatology, PO Box 4014, Schaumburg, IL, 60168-4014, (847) 240-1859, (866) 503-SKIN (7546), http://www.aad.org.

American Society for Dermatologic Surgery, 5550 Meadowbrook Dr., Suite 120, Rolling Meadows, IL, 60008, (847) 956-0900, (847) 956-0999, http://www.asds.net/.

Richard H. Camer

Cryptococcosis

Definition

Cryptococcosis is an infection caused by inhaling the fungus *Cryptococcus neoformans*. It is one of the diseases most often affecting **AIDS** patients. Cryptococcosis may be limited to the lungs, but frequently spreads throughout the body. Although almost any organ can be infected, the fungus is often fatal if it infects the nervous system where it causes an inflammation of the membranes covering the brain and spinal cord (**meningitis**).

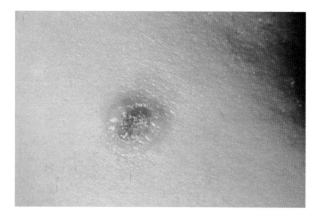

This lesion appearing on this person's body is due to exposure of the *C. neoformans* fungus. *(Photo Researchers, Inc.)*

Description

The fungus causing cryptococcis, *C. neoformans*, is found worldwide in soil contaminated with pigeon or other bird droppings. It has also been found on unwashed raw fruit. Cryptococcosis is a rare disease in healthy individuals, but is the most common fungal infection affecting people with AIDS.

People with Hodgkin's disease or who are taking large doses of drugs that suppress the functioning of the immune system (**corticosteroids, chemotherapy** drugs) are also more susceptible to cryptococcal infection. Cryptococcosis is also called cryptococcal meningitis (when the brain is infected), Busse-Buschke disease, European **blastomycosis**, torular meningitis, or torulosis.

Causes and symptoms

Once the cryptococcal fungus reaches the lungs, three things can happen. The immune system can heal the body without medical intervention, the disease can stay localized in the lungs, or it can spread throughout the body. In healthy people with normally functioning immune systems, the body usually heals itself, and the infected person notices no symptoms and has no complications (asymptomatic). The disease does not spread from one person to another.

Cryptococcosis is an opportunistic infection that puts people with immune system diseases at higher risk of developing more serious forms of the disease. In the United States, 6–10% of all patients with AIDS get cryptococcosis.

If the body does not heal itself, the fungus begins to grow in the lungs and form nodules that can be seen on chest x rays. In the early stages of infection, an individual usually only exhibits symptoms of a respiratory infection, such as a dry **cough**, so the disease is rarely diagnosed.

The fungus can remain dormant in the lungs and produce an active infection later if the immune system is weakened. If the disease becomes active, it can cause cryptococcal **pneumonia** in the lungs. Unfortunately, however, cryptococcal pneumonia has symptoms similar to other pneumonias (cough, chest **pain**, difficulty breathing), making it difficult to accurately diagnose. The infection can spread to other parts of the body, particularly the brain and central nervous system.

Most patients are not diagnosed as having cryptococcosis until they show signs of cryptococcal meningitis, or infection of the membranes surrounding the brain and spinal cord. Symptoms appear gradually

KEY TERMS

Adrenal gland—A pair of organs located above the kidneys. The outer tissue of the gland produces the hormones epinephrine (adrenaline) and norepinephrine, while the inner tissue produces several steroid hormones.

Amphotericin B (Fengizone)—An antifungal medication, prescribed for topical or systemic use in treating fungal infections.

Antibody—A specific protein produced by the immune system in response to a specific foreign protein or particle called an antigen.

Antigen—A foreign protein or particle capable of eliciting an immune response.

Asymptomatic—Persons who carry a disease but who do not exhibit symptoms of the disease are said to be asymptomatic.

Biopsy—The removal of a tissue sample for diagnostic purposes.

Cerebrospinal fluid (CSF)—The clear fluid that surrounds the spinal cord and brain and acts as a shock absorber.

Corticosteroids—A group of hormones produced naturally by the adrenal gland or manufactured synthetically. They are often used to treat inflammation. Examples include cortisone and prednisone.

Encephalitis—Inflammation of the brain.

Hodgkin's disease—A disease that causes chronic inflammation of the lymph nodes, spleen, liver and kidneys. It is also called malignant lymphoma.

Hydrocephalus—Build-up of fluid around the brain.

Immunocompromised—A state in which the immune system is suppressed or not functioning properly.

India ink test—A diagnostic test used to detect the cryptococcal organism *C. neoformans*. A dye, called India ink, is added to a sample of CSF fluid, and if the fungi is present, they will become visible as the dye binds to the capsule surrounding the fungus.

Lumbar puncture—Also called a spinal tap, a procedure in which a thin needle is used to withdraw a sample of cerebrospinal fluid for diagnostic purposes from the area surrounding the spine.

Meningitis—Inflammation of the membranes covering the brain and spinal cord called the meninges.

Molluscum contagiosum—A disease of the skin and mucuous membranes, caused by a poxvirus and found all over the world.

Opportunistic infection—An infection that is normally mild in a healthy individual, but which takes advantage of an ill person's weakened immune system to move into the body, grow, spread, and cause serious illness.

Pneumonia—Inflammation of the lungs, typically caused by a virus, bacteria, or other organism.

over a period of two to four weeks. **Fever** and **headache** are the most common symptoms, occurring in about 85% of patients. **Nausea**, **vomiting**, unwanted weight loss, and **fatigue** are also common. Other symptoms seen in 25–30% of patients are blurred vision, stiff neck, aversion to light, and seizures. Since the symptoms of classic meningitis, such as stiff neck and aversion to light, do not occur in many patients, diagnosis is often delayed. In addition to meningitis, inflammation of the brain (**encephalitis**) and brain lesions called cryptococcomas or tortulomas can also develop.

In addition to the brain, the cryptococcal infection can spread to the kidneys, bone marrow, heart, adrenal glands, lymph nodes, urinary tract, blood, and skin. Often times preceding the development of cryptococcal meningitis, painless **rashes** and lesions that mimic other skin diseases, such as *molluscum*

contagiosum, may develop. A small percentage of patients with brain infections show infections in other organs as well.

Diagnosis

Physicians who regularly work with AIDS patients have the most experience in diagnosing cryptococcosis. The preferred methods of diagnosis use simple and very accurate blood and cerebrospinal fluid (CSF) tests that detect the presence of an antigen produced by the fungus. The cerebrospinal fluid test is generally more sensitive to detecting the meningitis form of the infection. CSF is collected during a procedure called a **lumbar puncture**, during which an anesthetic is applied to a small area of the back near the spine and a needle is used to withdraw a sample of cerebrospinal fluid from the space between the vertebrae and the spinal cord. Once obtained, a small amount of ink (called India ink) is added to a sample of CSF or a sample prepared from **skin lesions**. If the fungus is present, it will become visible when the ink binds to the capsule or covering that surrounds the fungus. Faster results are obtained with the India ink test, but it is less accurate than the blood test (75–85% accuracy compared to 99% accuracy with the blood test) because some strains are not visible using this method. Antigen tests are routinely recommended for non-symptomatic patients with advanced AIDS.

Another way to diagnose cryptococcosis is to culture a sample of sputum, tissue from a **lung biopsy**, or CSF in the laboratory to isolate the fungus. Cultures are also done to assess the effectiveness of treatment.

Chest x rays are useful in assessing lung damage and may reveal a single mass or multiple distinct nodules, but the x ray alone does not lead to a definitive diagnosis of cryptococcosis.

Treatment

Once cryptococcosis is diagnosed, treatment begins with amphotericin B (Fungizone), sometimes in combination with 5-flucytosine (Ancobon). Amphotericin B is a powerful fungistatic drug with potentially toxic side effects, such as kidney toxicity and lower concentrations of an important blood component called hemoglobin. This medication can also cause fever, chills, **nausea and vomiting**, **diarrhea**, headache, and muscle aches. Treatment is generally given intravenously during a hospital stay and continues until the patient is stable or improving (no more than two to three weeks). 5-flucytosine is given orally. Patients may also receive other medication to minimize the side effects from these drugs.

Amphotericin B, with or without 5-flucytosine, is given for several weeks until the patient is stable, after which the patient receives oral fluconazole (Diflucan). Fluconazole is a broad-spectrum antifungal drug with few serious side effects. Patients with AIDS must continue taking fluconazole for the rest of their lives to prevent a relapse of cryptococcosis. Sometimes fluconazole is given to patients with advanced AIDS as a preventative (prophylactic) measure.

Because of the high cost of fluconazole, the manufacturer of the drug, Pfizer, has established a financial assistance plan to make the drug available at lower cost to those who meet certain criteria. Patients needing this drug should ask their doctors about this program.

Prognosis

Untreated cryptococcosis is always fatal. The acute mortality rate for patients with AIDS is 10–25%. Most deaths are attributable to cryptococcal meningitis and occur within two weeks after diagnosis. For AIDS patients who do not receive continued suppressive therapy (fluconazole), the relapse rate is 50–60% within six months and a shortened life expectancy. Once the cryptococcosis infection has been successfully treated, individuals may be left with a variety of neurologic symptoms, such as weakness, headache, and hearing or visual loss. In addition, fluid may accumulate around the brain (**hydrocephalus**).

Prevention

The best way to prevent cryptococcosis is to stay free of HIV infection. People with suppressed immune systems should try to stay away from areas contaminated with pigeon or other bird droppings, such as the attics of old buildings, barns, and areas under bridges where pigeons roost.

ORGANIZATIONS

Centers for Disease Control and Prevention (CDC), 1600 Clifton Road, Atlanta, GA, 30333, (800) 232-4636, cdcinfo@cdc.gov, http://www.cdc.gov.

National AIDS Hotline, CDC, 1600 Clifton Road, Atlanta, GA, 30333, (800) 232-4636, cdcinfo@cdc.gov, http://www.cdc.gov/hiv.

National Prevention Information Network, P.O. Box 6003, Rockville, MD, 20849-6003, (888) 282-7681, (800) 458-5231, info@cdcnpin.org, http://www.cdcnpin.org.

Project Inform, 1375 Mission Street, San Francisco, CA, 94103-2621, (415) 558-8669, (415) 558-0684, http://www.projinf.org.

Tish Davidson, A.M.

Cryptococcus neoformans infection *see* **Cryptococcosis**

Cryptorchidism *see* **Undescended testes**

Cryptosporidiosis

Definition

Cryptosporidiosis refers to infection by the spore-forming protozoan known as *Cryptosporidia*. Protozoa are a group of parasites that infect the human intestine, and include the better known *Giardia*. *Cryptosporidia*

KEY TERMS

Anti-motility medications—Medications such as loperamide (sold as Imodium), dephenoxylate (sold as Lomotil), or medications containing codeine or narcotics that decrease the ability of the intestine to contract. This can worsen the condition of a patient with dysentery or colitis.

Cyst—A protective sac that includes either fluid or the cell of an organism. The cyst enables many organisms to survive in the environment for long periods of time without need for food or water.

Immunocompromised—A change or alteration of the immune system that normally serves to fight off infections and other illnesses. This can involve changes in antibodies that the body produces (hygogammaglobulinemia), or defect in the cells that partake in the immune response. Diseases such as AIDS and cancer exhibit changes in the body's natural immunity.

Oral Rehydration Solution (ORS)—A liquid preparation developed by the World Health Organization that can decrease fluid loss in persons with diarrhea. Originally developed to be prepared with materials available in the home, commercial preparations have recently come into use.

Parasite—An organism that lives on or in another and takes nourishment (food and fluids) from that organism.

Protozoa—Group of extremely small single cell (unicellular) or acellular organisms that are found in moist soil or water. They tend to exist as parasites, living off other life forms.

Spore—A resistant form of certain species of bacteria, protozoa, and other organisms.

was first identified in 1976 as a cause of disease in humans.

Description

Cryptosporidia are normally passed in the feces of infected persons and animals in the form of cysts. The cysts can remain in the ground and water for months, and when ingested produce symptoms after maturing in the intestine and the bile ducts. When viewed under the microscope, they appear as small bluish-staining round bodies. Most common sources of infection are other humans, water supplies, or reservoirs. These are contaminated by animals that defecate in these areas. An outbreak in Milwaukee in 1993 in which over 400,000 persons were affected was traced to the city's water supply. Cysts of *Cryptosporidia* are extremely resistant to the disinfectants that are commonly used in most water treatment plants and are incompletely removed by filtration.

Most persons who experience significant symptoms have an altered immune system, and suffer from diseases such as **AIDS** and **cancer**. However, as shown in the Milwaukee outbreak, even those with normal immunity can experience symptoms.

Causes and symptoms

Cysts of *Cryptosporidia* mature in the intestine and bile ducts within three to five days of ingestion. As noted, large-scale infections from contaminated water supplies has been documented. However, human to human transmission (such as occurs in day care centers or through sexual behavior) is also an important cause.

Many individuals can be infected without any illness, but the major symptom is **diarrhea**, which is often watery and incapacitating. **Dehydration**, low-grade **fever**, **nausea**, and abdominal cramps are frequent.

In those with a normal immune system, the disease usually lasts about 10 days. For patients with altered immunity (immunocompromised), the story is quite different, with diarrhea becoming chronic, debilitating, and even fatal.

Complications

Dehydration and **malnutrition** are the most common effects of infection. In about 20% of AIDS patients, bile duct infection also occurs and causes symptoms similar to gallbladder attacks. Eighty percent or more of those with infection of the bile ducts die from the disease. The lungs and pancreas are also sometimes involved. *Cryptosporidia* are just one cause of the diarrhea wasting syndrome in AIDS, which results in severe weight loss and malnutrition.

Diagnosis

This is based on either finding the characteristic cysts in stool specimens, or on biopsy of an infected organ, such as the intestine.

Treatment

The first aim of treatment is to avoid dehydration. Oral Rehydration Solution (ORS) or intravenous fluids may be needed. Medications used to treat diarrhea by decreasing intestinal motility (Anti-Motility Agents), such as loperamide or diphenoxylate, are also useful, but should only be used with the advice of a physician.

Treatment aimed directly at *Cryptosporidia* is only partially effective, and rarely eliminates the organism. The medication most commonly used is paromomycin (Humatin), but others are presently under evaluation.

Prognosis

Cryptosporidia rarely cause a serious disease in persons with normal immune systems. Replacement of fluids is all that is usually needed. On the other hand, those with altered immune systems often suffer for months to years. Paramomycin and other drugs have been able to improve symptoms in over half of those treated. Unfortunately, many organisms are resistant, and recurrence is frequent.

Prevention

The best way to prevent cryptosporidiosis is to minimize exposure to cysts from infected humans and animals. Proper hand washing technique, especially in day care centers, is recommended.

Resources

OTHER

"Cryptosporidiosis." *Centers for Disease Control*. http://www.cdc.gov/ncidod/diseases/crypto/crypto.htm.

Vakil, Nimish B., et al. "Biliary Cryptosporidiosis in HIV-Infected People after the Waterborne Outbreak of Cryptosporidiosis in Milwaukee." *New England Journal of Medicine Online*. http://content.nejm.org.

ORGANIZATIONS

Centers for Disease Control and Prevention (CDC), 1600 Clifton Road, Atlanta, GA, 30333, (800) 232-4636, cdcinfo@cdc.gov, http://www.cdc.gov.

David Kaminstein, MD

CSF analysis *see* **Cerebrospinal fluid (CSF) analysis**

CT-guided biopsy

Definition

Computed tomography (CT) is a process that images anatomic information from a cross-sectional plane of the body. Biopsy is the process of taking a sample of tissue from the body for analysis. CT is commonly used in biopsies to provide images that help guide the tools or equipment necessary to perform the biopsy to the appropriate area of the body.

Purpose

CT is used in the process of performing a biopsy, such as a needle biopsy, in order to guide the needle to the site of the biopsy and to provide rapid and precise localization of the needle. CT enables imaging of areas that are normally beyond visible boundaries. This enables the physician to see the target area clearly and help to ensure that the tissue being removed is from the target lesion.

Precautions

The patient that suffers from claustrophobia will want to discuss this with their physician. This procedure involves the patient being placed into the CT scanner, typically a small, enclosed area. Depending on the specific type of biopsies being performed, certain anesthetics will be used, so discuss drug **allergies** with your physician.

Description

CT can assist in providing more enhanced images of a suspicious lesion. It helps to determine whether a tumor is truly solitary or not. CT can characterize the tumor and aid in the estimation of malignancy.

Preparation

Since there are many different types of biopsies, you should follow the instructions from your physician to prepare for your CT-guided biopsy. Patients who suffer from claustrophobia should discuss their concerns with the physician. In some cases, medicine can be given that will relax the patient during the procedure.

Risks

CT-guided biopsy does not increase the risk of the biopsy any more than any other radiologic imaging such as x ray.

Results

Because the area being biopsied, as well as the specific type of biopsy procedure can vary, results will vary. Before undergoing the procedure, notification procedure should be clearly defined.

Resources

BOOKS

McPhee, Stephen, and Maxine Papadakis. *Current Medical Diagnosis and Treatment, 2010*, 49th ed. New York: McGraw–Hill Medical, 2009.

Stedman, Thomas Lathrop. *Stedman's Medical Dictionary*. 28th ed. Philadelphia: Lippincott Williams & Wilkins, 2006.

PERIODICALS

Garpestad, E., et. al. "CT Fluoroscopy Guidance for Transbronchial Needle Aspiration." *Chest* 119 (February 2001).

Kim A. Sharp, M.Ln.

CT-myelogram *see* **Myelography**
CT scan *see* **Computed tomography scans**

Culture-fair test

Definition

A culture-fair test is test designed to be free of cultural bias, as far as possible, so that no one culture has an advantage over another. The test is designed to not be influenced by verbal ability, cultural climate, or educational level.

Purpose

The purpose of a culture-fair test is to eliminate any social or cultural advantages, or disadvantages, that a person may have due to their upbringing. The test can be administered to anyone, from any nation, speaking any language. A culture-fair test may help identify learning or emotional problems. The duration of the test varies for the individual types of tests available, but the time is approximately between 12–18 minutes per section (a test usually has two to four sections).

A culture-fair test is often administered by employers in order to determine the best location for new employees in a large company. The wide variety of culture-fair tests available allows the administrator to select which area is most vital, whether it be general intelligence, knowledge of a specific area, or emotional stability.

Precautions

There is doubt as to whether any test can truly be culturally unbiased or can ever be made completely fair to all persons independent of culture. There are no other precautions.

Description

A culture-fair test is a non-verbal paper-pencil test that can be administered to patients as young as four years old. The patient only needs the ability to recognize shapes and figures and perceive their respective relationships. Some examples of tasks in the test may include:

- completing series
- classifying
- solving matrices
- evaluating conditions

The culture-fair test is also often referred to as a culture-free test or unbiased test. There are many variations of the test including class, economic, and intelligence tests. The threading theme among the various tests is their design to be culturally unbiased.

Preparation

The only preparation necessary to administer the test is pre-ordered materials and a quiet and secluded location for the duration of the test.

Aftercare

Post-test treatment depends on the results of the test and the specifics of the individual patient. Any further treatment is best prescribed by the doctor.

Risks

There are no risks associated with the culture-fair test.

Results

The results can be compared to the key that comes with the purchase of a culture-fair test. All results should be compared to the included key.

Resources

BOOKS

Maddox, Taddy. *Tests*. 6th ed. Austin, Texas: Pro–Ed, 2008.

Michael Sherwin Walston
Ronald Watson, PhD

Cultures for sexually transmitted diseases *see*
Sexually transmitted diseases cultures

Cushing's syndrome

Definition

Cushing's syndrome is a relatively rare endocrine (hormonal) disorder resulting from excessive exposure to the hormone cortisol. The disorder, which leads to a variety of symptoms and physical abnormalities, is most commonly caused by taking medications containing the hormone over a long period of time. A more rare form of the disorder occurs when the body itself produces an excessive amount of cortisol.

Description

The adrenals are two glands, each of which is perched on the upper part of the two kidneys. The outer part of the gland is known as the cortex; the inner part is known as the medulla. Each of these parts of the adrenal gland is responsible for producing different types of hormones. Regulation of hormone production and release from the adrenal cortex involves the pituitary gland, a small gland located at the base of the brain. After the hypothalamus (the part of the brain containing secretions important to metabolic activities) sends "releasing hormones" to the pituitary gland, the pituitary secretes a hormone called adrenocorticotropic hormone (ACTH). The ACTH then travels through the bloodstream to the adrenal cortex, where it encourages the production and release of cortisol (sometimes called the "stress" hormone) and other adrenocortical hormones.

Cortisol, a very potent glucocorticoid—a group of adrenocortical hormones that protects the body from **stress** and affect protein and carbohydrate metabolism—is involved in regulating the functioning

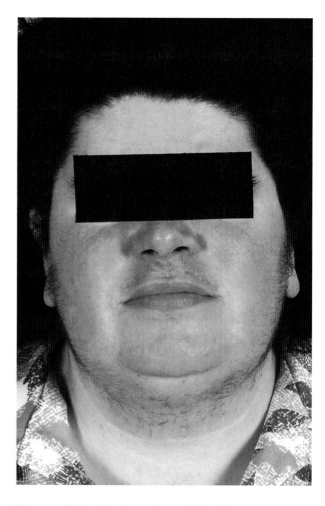

Woman with Cushing's syndrome. *(Photo Researchers, Inc.)*

of nearly every type of organ and tissue in the body, and is considered to be one of the few hormones absolutely necessary for life. Cortisol is involved in:

- complex processing and utilization of many nutrients, including sugars (carbohydrates), fats, and proteins
- normal functioning of the circulatory system and the heart
- functioning of muscles
- normal kidney function
- production of blood cells
- normal processes involved in maintaining the skeletal system
- proper functioning of the brain and nerves
- normal responses of the immune system

Cushing's syndrome, also called hypercortisolism, has an adverse effect on all of the processes described above. The syndrome occurs in approximately 10 to 15 out of every one million people per year, usually striking adults between the ages of 20 and 50.

Causes and symptoms

The most common cause of Cushing's syndrome is the long-term use of glucocorticoid hormones in medications. Medications such as prednisone are used in a number of inflammatory conditions. Such conditions include **rheumatoid arthritis**, **asthma**, **vasculitis**, lupus, and a variety of other **autoimmune disorders** in which the body's immune cells accidentally attack some part of the body itself. In these disorders, the glucocorticoids are used to dampen the immune response, thereby decreasing damage to the body.

Cushing's syndrome can also be caused by three different categories of disease:

- a pituitary tumor producing abnormally large quantities of ACTH
- the abnormal production of ACTH by some source other than the pituitary
- a tumor within the adrenal gland overproducing cortisol

Although it is rare, about two-thirds of endogenous (occurring within the body rather than from a source outside the body, like a medication) Cushing's syndrome which is caused by excessive secretion of ACTH by a pituitary tumor, usually an adenoma (noncancerous tumor). The pituitary tumor causes increased growth of the adrenal cortex (hyperplasia) and increased cortisol production. Cushing's disease affects women more often than men.

Tumors in locations other than the pituitary can also produce ACTH. This is called ectopic ACTH syndrome ("ectopic" refers to something existing out of its normal place). Tumors in the lung account for more than half of all cases of ectopic ACTH syndrome. Other types of tumors that may produce ACTH include tumors of the thymus, the pancreas, the thyroid, and the adrenal gland. Nearly all adrenal gland tumors are benign (noncancerous), although in rare instances a tumor may actually be cancerous.

Symptoms of cortisol excess (resulting from medication or from the body's excess production of the hormone) include:

- weight gain
- an abnormal accumulation of fatty pads in the face (creating the distinctive "moon face" of Cushing's syndrome); in the trunk (termed "truncal obesity");

and over the upper back and the back of the neck (giving the individual what has been called a "buffalo hump")

- purple and pink stretch marks across the abdomen and flanks
- high blood pressure
- weak, thinning bones (osteoporosis)
- weak muscles
- low energy
- thin, fragile skin, with a tendency toward both bruising and slow healing
- abnormalities in the processing of sugars (glucose), with occasional development of actual diabetes
- kidney stones
- increased risk of infections
- emotional disturbances, including mood swings, depression, irritability, confusion, or even a complete break with reality (psychosis)
- irregular menstrual periods in women
- decreased sex drive in men and difficulty maintaining an erection
- abormal hair growth in women (in a male pattern, such as in the beard and mustache area), as well as loss of hair from the head (receding hair line)

Diagnosis

Diagnosing Cushing's syndrome can be complex. Diagnosis must not only identify the cortisol excess, but also locate its source. Many of the symptoms listed above can be attributed to numerous other diseases. Although a number of these symptoms seen together would certainly suggest Cushing's syndrome, the symptoms are still not specific to Cushing's syndrome. Following a review of the patient's medical history, **physical examination**, and routine blood tests, a series of more sophisticated tests is available to achieve a diagnosis.

24-hour free cortisol test

This is the most specific diagnostic test for identifying Cushing's syndrome. It involves measuring the amount of cortisol present in the urine over a 24-hour period. When excess cortisol is present in the bloodstream, it is processed by the kidneys and removed as waste in the urine. This 24-hour free cortisol test requires that an individual collect exactly 24-hours' worth of urine in a single container. The urine is then analyzed in a laboratory to determine the quantity of cortisol present. This technique can also be paired with the administration of dexamethasone, which in a

KEY TERMS

Adenoma—A type of noncancerous (benign) tumor that often involves the overgrowth of certain cells of the type normally found within glands.

Adrenocorticotropic hormone (ACTH)—A pituitary hormone that stimulates the cortex of the adrenal glands to produce adrenal cortical hormones.

Cortisol—A hormone secreted by the cortex of the adrenal gland. Cortisol regulates the function of nearly every organ and tissue in the body.

Ectopic—In an abnormal position.

Endocrine—Pertaining to a gland that secretes directly into the bloodstream.

Gland—A collection of cells whose function is to release certain chemicals (hormones) that are

important to the functioning of other, sometimes distantly located, organs or body systems.

Glucocorticoids—General class of adrenal cortical hormones that are mainly active in protecting against stress and in protein and carbohydrate metabolism.

Hormone—A chemical produced in one part of the body that travels to another part of the body in order to exert its effect.

Hypothalamus—the part of the brain containing secretions important to metabolic activities.

Pituitary—A gland located at the base of the brain, the pituitary produces a number of hormones, including hormones that regulate growth and reproductive function.

normal individual would cause urine cortisol to be very low. Once a diagnosis has been made using the 24-hour free cortisol test, other tests are used to find the exact location of the abnormality causing excess cortisol production.

Dexamethasone suppression test

This test is useful in distinguishing individuals with excess ACTH production due to a pituitary adenoma from those with ectopic ACTH-producing tumors. Patients are given dexamethasone (a synthetic glucocorticoid) orally every six hours for four days. Low doses of dexamethasone are given during the first two days; for the last two days, higher doses are administered. Before dexamethasone is administered, as well as on each day of the test, 24-hour urine collections are obtained.

Because cortisol and other glucocorticoids signal the pituitary to decrease ACTH, the normal response after taking dexamethasone is a drop in blood and urine cortisol levels. Thus, the cortisol response to dexamethasone differs depending on whether the cause of Cushing's syndrome is a pituitary adenoma or an ectopic ACTH-producing tumor.

However, the dexamethasone suppression test may produce false-positive results in patients with conditions such as depression, alcohol **abuse**, high estrogen levels, acute illness, and stress. On the other hand, drugs such as phenytoin and phenobarbital may produce false-negative results. Thus, patients are

usually advised to stop taking these drugs at least one week prior to the test.

Corticotropin-releasing hormone (CRH) stimulation test

The CRH stimulation test is given to help distinguish between patients with pituitary adenomas and those with either ectopic ACTH syndrome or cortisol-secreting adrenal tumors. In this test, patients are given an injection of CRH, the corticotropin-releasing hormone that causes the pituitary to secrete ACTH. In patients with pituitary adenomas, blood levels of ACTH and cortisol usually rise. However, in patients with ectopic ACTH syndrome, this rise is rarely seen. In patients with cortisol-secreting adrenal tumors, this rise almost never occurs.

Petrosal sinus sampling

Although this test is not always necessary, it may be used to distinguish between a pituitary adenoma and an ectopic source of ACTH. Petrosal sinus sampling involves drawing blood directly from veins that drain the pituitary. This test, which is usually performed with **local anesthesia** and mild **sedation**, requires inserting tiny, flexible tubes (catheters) through a vein in the upper thigh or groin area. The catheters are then threaded up slowly until they reach veins in an area of the skull known as the petrosal sinuses. X rays are typically used to confirm the correct position of the catheters. Often CRH is also given during the test to increase the accuracy of results.

When blood tested from the petrosal sinuses reveals a higher ACTH level than blood drawn from a vein in the forearm, the likely diagnosis is a pituitary adenoma. When the two samples show similar levels of ACTH, the diagnosis indicates ectopic ACTH syndrome.

Radiologic imaging tests

Imaging tests such as **computed tomography scans** (CT) and **magnetic resonance imaging** (MRI) are only used to look at the pituitary and adrenal glands after a firm diagnosis has already been made. The presence of a pituitary or adrenal tumor does not necessarily guarantee that it is the source of increased ACTH production. Many healthy people with no symptoms or disease whatsoever have noncancerous tumors in the pituitary and adrenal glands. Thus, CT and MRI is often used to image the pituitary and adrenal glands in preparation for surgery.

Treatment

The choice of a specific treatment depends on the type of problem causing the cortisol excess. Pituitary and adrenal adenomas are usually removed surgically. Malignant adrenal tumors always require surgical removal.

Treatment of ectopic ACTH syndrome also involves removing all of the cancerous cells that are producing ACTH. This may be done through surgery, **chemotherapy** (using combinations of cancer-killing drugs), or **radiation therapy** (using x rays to kill **cancer** cells), depending on the type of cancer and how far it has spread. Radiation therapy may also be used on the pituitary (with or without surgery) for patients who cannot undergo surgery, or for patients whose surgery did not successfully decrease pituitary release of ACTH.

There are a number of drugs that are effective in decreasing adrenal production of cortisol. These medications include mitotane, ketoconazole, metyrapone, trilostane, aminoglutethimide, and **mifepristone**. These drugs are sometimes given prior to surgery in an effort to reverse the problems brought on by cortisol excess. However, the drugs may also need to be administered after surgery (sometimes along with radiation treatments) in patients who continue to have excess pituitary production of ACTH.

Because pituitary surgery can cause ACTH levels to drop too low, some patients require short-term treatment with a cortisol-like medication after surgery. Patients who need adrenal surgery may also require glucocorticoid replacement. If the entire adrenal gland has been removed, the patient must take oral glucocorticoids for the rest of his or her life.

Prognosis

Prognosis depends on the source of the problem. When pituitary adenomas are identified as the source of increased ACTH leading to cortisol excess, about 80% of patients are cured by surgery. When cortisol excess is due to some other form of cancer, the prognosis depends on the type of cancer and the extent of its spread.

Resources

BOOKS

Fauci, Anthony S., et al., eds.*Harrison's Principles of Internal Medicine*. 17th ed. New York: McGraw–Hill Professional, 2008.

PERIODICALS

Boscaro, Marco, Luisa Barzon, Francesco Fallo, and Nicoletta Sonino. "Cushing's Syndrome." *Lancet* 357 (2001): 783–91.

Kirk, Lawrence F., Robert B. Hash, Harold P. Katner, and Tom Jones. "Cushing's Disease: Clinical Manifestations and Diagnostic Evaluation."*American Family Physician* 62, no. 5 (September 1, 2001): 1119–27.

Rosalyn Carson-DeWitt, MD

Cutaneous larva migrans

Definition

Cutaneous larvae migrans is a parasitic skin disease caused by a hookworm larvae that usually infests dogs, cats, and other animals. Humans can pick up the infection by walking barefoot on soil or beaches contaminated with animal feces.

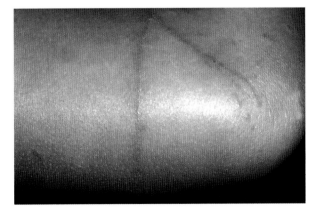

Linear red rashes around a patient's knee caused by burrowing larvae of the dog hookworm *Ancylostoma braziliensis*. (*Custom Medical Stock Photo, Inc. Reproduced by permission.*)

Description

Cutaneous larvae migrans (also called "creeping eruption" or "ground itch") is found in southeastern and Gulf states, and in tropical developing countries.

The hookworms that cause the condition are small, round blood-sucking worms that infest about 700 million people around the world. Cutaneous larvae migrans occurs most often among children, those who crawl beneath raised buildings, and sunbathers who lie down on wet sand contaminated with hookworm larvae.

Causes and symptoms

After an animal passes feces that are infested with hookworm eggs, the eggs hatch into infective larvae that are able to penetrate human skin (even through solid material, such as a beach towel). The larvae are commonly found in shaded, moist, or sandy areas (such as beaches, a child's sandbox, or areas underneath a house), where they are easily picked up by bare feet or buttocks.

In minor infestations, there may be no symptoms at all. In more severe cases, a red elevation of the skin (papule) appears within a few hours after the larvae have penetrated the skin. This usually arises first in areas that are in contact with the soil, such as the feet, hands, and buttocks.

Between a few days and a few months after infection, the larvae begin to migrate beneath the skin, leaving extremely itchy red lines that may be accompanied by blisters. These red lines usually appear at the top of the sole of the foot or on the buttocks.

Tyically, the larvae travel through the bloodstream, to the lungs, and then migrate into the mouth where they are swallowed and attach to the small intestine lining. There they mature into adult worms. In cases where the larvae migrate through the lungs, they can produce anemia, **cough**, and **pneumonia**, in addition to the itchy rash.

Diagnosis

The condition can be diagnosed by microscopic inspection of feces which can reveal hookworm eggs. In addition visual inspection of the skin would reveal telltale itchy red lines and blisters.

Treatment

People without intestinal symptoms do not need treatment, since the worms will eventually die or be excreted. Thiabendazole or albendazole are used to treat the infestation. Mild infections can be treated by applying one of the drugs to the skin along the

tracks and the normal skin surrounding the area. Thiabendazole also can be given internally, but taken this way it can cause side effects including **dizziness**, **nausea**, and **vomiting**

Prognosis

No matter how severe an infestation, with adequate treatment patients recover completely. However, if the patient scratches the lesions open, the areas can become vulnerable to bacterial infection.

Prevention

In the United States, the prevalence of dogs and cats with hookworms is the reason why the infective larvae are found so commonly in soil and sand. The play habits of children, together with their attraction to pets, puts them at high risk for hookworm infection and cutaneous larvae migrans.

Human hookworm infestation can be prevented by practicing good personal hygiene, deworming pets, and not allowing children to play in potentially contaminated environments.

Resources

BOOKS

Ferri, Fred F., James S Studdiford, and Amber Tully.*Ferri's Fast Facts in Dermatology: A Practical Guide to Skin Diseases and Disorders.* Philadelphia: Saunders/Elsevier, 2011.

Carol A. Turkington

Cutaneous T-cell lymphoma

Definition

Cutaneous T-cell lymphoma (CTCL) is a malignancy of the T-helper (CD4 +) cells of the immune system.

Description

CTCL, also known as mycosis fungoides, is a **cancer** of the white blood cells that primarily affects the skin and only secondarily affects other sites. This disease involves the uncontrollable proliferation of T-lymphocytes known as T-helper cells, so named because of their role in the immune response. T-helper cells are characterized by the presence of a protein receptor on their surface called CD4. Accordingly, T-helper cells are said to be CD4 + .

The proliferation of T-helper cells results in the penetration, or infiltration, of these abnormal cells into the epidermal layer of the skin. The skin reacts with slightly scaling lesions that itch, although the sites of greatest infiltration do not necessarily correspond to the sites of the lesions. The lesions are most often located on the trunk, but can be present on any part of the body. In the most common course of the disease, the patchy lesions progress to palpable plaques that are deeper red and have more defined edges. As the disease worsens, skin tumors develop that are often mushroom-shaped, hence the name mycosis fungoides. Finally, the cancer progresses to extracutanous involvement, often in the lymph nodes or the viscera.

CTCL is a rare disease, with an annual incidence of about 0.29 cases per 100,000 persons in the United States. It is about half as common in Eastern Europe. However, this discrepancy may be attributed to a differing physician awareness of the disease rather than a true difference in occurrence. In the United States, there are about 500–600 new cases a year and about 100–200 deaths. CTCL is usually seen in older adults; the median age at diagnosis is 55–60 years. It strikes twice as many men as women. The average life expectancy at diagnosis is 7–10 years, even without treatment.

Causes and symptoms

The cause of CTCL is unknown. Exposure to chemicals or pesticides has been suggested; however, the most recent study on the subject failed to show a connection between exposure and development of the disease. The ability to isolate various viruses from cell lines grown from cells of CTCL patients raises the question of a viral cause, but studies have been unable to confirm these suspicions.

The symptoms of CTCL are seen primarily in the skin, with itchy red patches or plaques and, usually over time, mushroom-shaped skin tumors. Any part of the skin can be involved and the extent and distribution of the rash or tumors vary greatly from patient to patient. The only really universal symptom of the disease is the itch and this symptom is usually what brings the patient to the doctor for treatment. If the disease spreads outside of the skin, the symptoms include swelling of the lymph nodes, usually most severe in those draining the areas with skin involvement. Spread to the viscera is most often manifested as disorders of

the lungs, upper digestive tract, central nervous system, or liver but virtually any organ can be shown to be involved at **autopsy**.

Some patients with CTCL develop a leukemic phase of the disorder known as Sézary syndrome, which is characterized by the appearance of malignant T cells in the bloodstream. It is named for the French dermatologist who first identified the abnormal T cells.

Diagnosis

Diagnosis of CTCL is often difficult in the early stages because of its slow progression and ability to mimic many other benign skin conditions. The early patches of CTCL resemble **eczema**, **psoriasis**, and **contact dermatitis**. In a further complication, the early manifestations of the disease can respond favorably to the topical corticosteroid treatments prescribed for these skin disorders. This has the unfortunate result of the disease being missed and the patient remaining untreated for years. CTCL is most likely discovered when a physician maintains a suspicion about the disease, performs multiple skin biopsies, and provides close follow-up after the initial presentation.

Skin biopsies showing penetration of abnormal cells into the epidermal tissue are necessary to make a firm diagnosis of CTCL. Several molecular studies can also help support the diagnosis. The first looks at the cellular proteins seen on the surface of the abnormal cells. Many cases of CTCL show the retention of the CD4 + protein, but the loss of other proteins usually seen on the surface of mature CD4 + cells, such as Leu-8 or Leu-9. The abnormal cells also show unusual rearrangements at the genetic level for the gene that encodes the T-cell receptors. These rearrangements can be identified using Southern blot analysis. The information from the molecular tests, combined with the presence of abnormal cells in the epidermis, strongly supports the CTCL diagnosis.

Treatment

Treatment of CTCL depends on the stage of the disease. The current staging of this disease was first presented at the International Consensus Conference on CTCL in 1997. The staging attempts to show the complex interaction between the various outward symptoms of the disease and prognosis. The system has seven clinical stages based on skin involvement (tumor = T), lymph node involvement (LN), and presence of visceral metastases (M).

The first stage, IA, is characterized by plaques covering less than 10% of the body (T1) and no visceral involvement (M0). Lymph node condition at this stage can be uninvolved, reactive to the skin disease, or dermatopathic (biopsies showing CTCL involvement) but not enlarged (LN0-2). The shorthand expression of this stage is therefore T1, LN0-2, M0. The next stage, IB, differs from IA in that greater than 10% of the body is covered by plaques (T2, LN0-2, M0). Stage IIA occurs with any amount of plaques in addition to the ability to palpate the lymph node and the lymph uninvolved, reactive, or dermatopathic (T1-2, LN0-2, M0).

Treatments applied to the skin are preferred for patients having these preliminary stages of the disease, commonly topical **chemotherapy** with mechlorethamine hydrochloride (nitrogen mustard) or **phototherapy** of psoralen plus ultraviolet A (PUVA). Topical chemotherapy involves application to the skin of nitrogen mustard, an alkylating agent, in a concentration of 10–20 mg/dL in an aqueous or ointment base. Treatment of affected skin is suggested at a minimum and application over the entire skin surface is often recommended. Care needs to be taken that coverage of involved skin is adequate, as patients who self-apply the drug often cannot reach all affected areas. The most common side effect is skin hypersensitivity to the drug. Nearly all patients respond favorably to this treatment, with a 32–61% complete response rate, based on amount of skin involvement. Unfortunately, only 10–15% of patients maintain a complete response rate after discontinuing the treatment.

Phototherapy involves treatment with an orally administered drug, 8-methyloxypsoralen, that renders the skin sensitive to long-wave ultraviolet light (UVA), followed by controlled exposure to the radiation. During the initial treatment period, which may last as long as six months, patients are treated two to three times weekly. This is reduced to about once monthly after initial clearing of the lesions. Redness of the skin and blistering are the most common side effects of the treatment and are much more common in patients presenting with overall skin redness, or erythroderma, so lower intensities of light are usually used in this case. About 50% of all patients experience complete clearance with this treatment. Some patients with very fair skin and limited skin involvement can successfully treat themselves at home with special lamps and no psoralen.

The next stage, IIB, involves one or more cutaneous tumors, in combination with absent or present palpable lymph nodes, lymph uninvolved, reactive, or dermatopathic, and no visceral involvement (T3, LN0-2, M0). Stage III is characterized by erythroderma, an abnormal redness over widespread areas of the skin (T4, LN0-2, M0).

For more extensive disease, **radiation therapy** is an effective treatment option. It is generally used after the topical treatments have proven ineffective. Individual plaques or tumors can be treated using electrons, orthovoltage x rays, or megavoltage photons with exposure in the range of 15 to 25 Gy. Photon therapy has proven particularly useful once the lymph nodes are involved. Another possibility is total-skin electron beam therapy (TSEB), although the availability of this treatment method is limited. It involves irradiation of the entire body with energized electrons. Side effects of this treatment include loss of finger and toe nails, acute redness of the skin, and inability to sweat for about six to 12 months after therapy. Almost all patients respond favorably to radiation treatment and any reoccurrence is usually much less severe.

Combination of different types of treatments is a very common approach to the management of CTCL. Topical nitrogen mustard or PUVA is often used after completion of radiation treatment to prolong the effects. The addition of genetically engineered interferon to PUVA therapy significantly increases the percentage of patients showing a complete response. Furthermore, although treatments using chemotherapy drugs alone, such as deoxycofomycin or etretinate, have been disappointing for CTCL, combining these drugs with interferon has shown promising results. Interferon has also been combined with retinoid treatments, although the mechanism of action of retinoids (Vitamin A analogues) against CTCL is unknown.

The final two stages of the disease are IVA and IVB. IVA presents as any amount of skin involvement, absent or present palpable lymph nodes, no visceral involvement, and lymph that contains large clusters of convoluted cells or obliterated nodes (T1-4, LN3-4). IVB differs in the addition of palpable lymph nodes and visceral involvement (T1-4, LN3-4, M1). All of the treatment methods described above are appropriate for the final two stages of the disease.

A newer drug that has been used to treat CTCL is bexarotene, a topical gel that is a synthetic retinoid analog. Bexarotene has been shown to be effective in clinical trials for stage IA or IB CTCL, and has fewer side effects than topical nitrogen mustard or electron beam radiotherapy. Another team of researchers at the University of Pennsylvania reported in 2003 that bexarotene combined with psoralen and UVA therapy

Alkylating agent—A chemical that alters the composition of the genetic material of rapidly dividing cells, such as cancer cells, causing selective cell death; used as a topical chemotherapeutic agent to treat CTCL.

Cutaneous—Pertaining to the skin.

Erythroderma—An abnormal reddening of the entire skin surface.

Monoclonal antibody—An antibody produced by the identical offspring of a single cloned antibody-producing cell.

Mycosis fungoides—Another name for cutaneous T-cell lymphoma.

Sézary syndrome—A leukemic phase of CTCL that develops in some patients, characterized by the appearance of malignant T cells in the peripheral blood and sometimes in the lymph nodes. The syndrome is named for Alfred Sézary (1880-1956), a French dermatologist.

T-helper cells—A cellular component of the immune system that plays a major role in ridding the body of bacteria and viruses, characterized by the presence of the CD4 protein on its surface; the type of cell that divides uncontrollable with CTCL.

Total-skin electron beam therapy—A method of radiation therapy used to treat CTCL that involves bombarding the entire body surface with high-energy electrons.

is also effective in treating patients with advanced CTCL.

A treatment for advanced CTCL that is considered experimental as of mid-2003 is **alemtuzumab**, a monoclonal antibody. A Swedish study of 22 patients with advanced CTCL and Sézary syndrome found that alemtuzumab relieved symptoms in 55% of patients, with 32% in complete remission and 23% in partial remission.

Alternative treatment

Itching of the skin is one of the most troublesome symptoms of CTCL. One alternative treatment for itchiness is the application of a brewed solution of chickweed that is applied to the skin using cloth compresses. Another suggested topical application is a mixture of vitamin E, vitamin A, unflavored yogurt, honey, and zinc oxide. Evening primrose oil applied topically is also claimed to reduce itch and promote healing.

Prognosis

The prognosis for CTCL is dependent on the stage of the disease. Prognosis is very good if the disease has only progressed to Stage IA, with a mean survival of 20 or more years. At this point, the disease is a very low mortality risk to the patient, with most deaths occurring to persons in this group unrelated to CTCL. For patients diagnosed at stages IB and IIA, the median survival is about 12 years. The disease in both of these stages involves intermediate risk to the patient. Patients in stage III and IVA have a mean life expectancy of about five years. At these later stages, the disease is high risk, with most deaths occurring by infection due to the depleted immune system of the later-stage patient. Once a patient has reached stage IVB, the mean life expectancy is one year.

Prevention

Studies have been unable to link CTCL to any environmental or genetic factors, so prevention at this time is not possible.

Resources

BOOKS

Beers, Mark H., Robert S. Porter, and Thomas V. Jones, eds. *The Merck Manual of Diagnosis and Therapy.* 18th ed. Whitehouse Station, NJ: Merck Research Laboratories, 2006.

Canellos, George Peter, Thomas Andrew Lister, and Bryan D Young. *The Lymphomas.* 2nd ed. Philadelphia: Saunders, 2006.

DeVita, Vincent T., Samuel Hellman, and Steven A Rosenberg. *Cancer: Principles and Practice of Oncology.* 7th ed. Philadelphia: Lippincott, Williams & Wilkins, 2005.

PERIODICALS

Dawe, R. S. "Ultraviolet A1 Phototherapy." *British Journal of Dermatology* 148 (April 2003): 626–637.

Kari, L., A. Loboda, M. Nebozhyn, et al. "Classification and Prediction of Survival in Patients with the Leukemic Phase of Cutaneous T Cell Lymphoma."

Journal of Experimental Medicine 197 (June 2, 2003): 1477–1488.

Lundin, J., H. Hagberg, R. Repp, et al. "Phase 2 Study of Alemtuzumab (Anti-CD52 Monoclonal Antibody) in Patients with Advanced Mycosis Fungoides/Sézary Syndrome." *Blood* 101 (June 1, 2003): 4267–4272.

Martin, A. G. "Bexarotene Gel: A New Skin-Directed Treatment Option for Cutaneous T-Cell Lymphomas." *Journal of Drugs in Dermatology* 2 (April 2003): 155–167.

McGinnis, K. S., M. Shapiro, C. C. Vittorio, et al. "Psoralen plus Long-Wave UV-A (PUVA) and Bexarotene Therapy: An Effective and Synergistic Combined Adjunct to Therapy for Patients with Advanced Cutaneous T-Cell Lymphoma." *Archives of Dermatology* 139 (June 2003): 771–775.

ORGANIZATIONS

American Academy of Dermatology, PO Box 4014, Schaumburg, IL, 60168-4014, (847) 240-1859, (866) 503-SKIN (7546), http://www.aad.org.

American Cancer Society, 1599 Clifton Rd. NE, Atlanta, GA, 30329, (800) 227-2345, http://www.cancer.org.

National Cancer Institute (National Institutes of Health), NCI Office of Communications and Education, 6116 Executive Blvd. Suite 300, Bethesda, MD, 20892-8322, (800) 4-CANCER (422-6237), cancergovstaff@mail.nih.gov, http://www.cancer.gov/.

Michelle Johnson, M.S., J.D.
Rebecca J. Frey, PhD

Cutis laxa

Definition

Cutis laxa (Latin for loose or lax skin) is a connective tissue disorder in which the skin lacks elasticity and hangs in loose folds.

Description

Cutis laxa is extremely rare; less than a few hundred cases worldwide have been described.

The several forms of cutis laxa are divided into primary cutis laxa, which is present from birth and is hereditary, secondary cutis laxa, which arises later in life and may be hereditary, and acquired cutis laxa, which arises later in life and is not hereditary. Loose skin, the primary and most obvious symptom of these diseases, is caused by underlying defects in connective tissue structure, which also cause more serious internal problems in vocal cords, bones, cartilage, blood vessels, bladder, kidney, digestive system, and lungs. The loose skin is particularly obvious on the face, and children with the disorder look sad or mournful.

There are four genetic forms of the disease: sex-linked, autosomal dominant, and two types of autosomal recessive inheritance. The recessive forms are the most common and are usually more severe than the other forms.

Causes and Symptoms

Sex-linked cutis laxa is caused by a defective gene on the X chromosome. In addition to loose skin, its symptoms are mild **mental retardation**, loose joints, bone abnormalities (like hooked nose, pigeon breast, and funnel breast), frequent loose stools, urinary tract blockages, and deficiencies in lysyl oxidase, an enzyme required for the formation of properly functioning connective tissue. (But the defective gene does not code for lysyl oxidase.)

Autosomal dominant cutis laxa is caused by a defective gene carried on an autosomal (not sex-linked) chromosome. Its symptoms are loose, hanging skin, missing elastic fibers, premature **aging**, and pulmonary **emphysema**. Only a few families are known with cutis laxa inherited as a dominant trait.

Autosomal recessive cutis laxa type 1 is caused by a defective gene on chromosome 5. Symptoms include emphysema; diverticula in the esophagus, duodenum, and bladder; lax and dislocated joints; tortuous arteries; hernias; lysyl oxidase deficiencies; and retarded growth.

Autosomal recessive cutis laxa type 2 is also inherited as a recessive trait. In addition to the loose skin, this form of the disease is characterized by bone abnormalities, the delayed joining of the cranial (skull) bones, hip dislocation, curvature of the spine, flat feet, and excessive **tooth decay**.

Acquired cutis laxa tends to follow (and may be caused by) severe illness characterized by **fever**, inflammation, and a severe skin rash (**erythema multiforme**); an injury to the nerves that control blood vessel dilation and contraction; or an autoimmune condition.

Diagnosis

The signs of cutis laxa are very obvious, and it is usually easy to diagnose by examining the skin. The determination of which form of cutis laxa is present is aided by information about the associated symptoms and by family histories.

Treatment

There is no effective cure for any of these disorders. Complications are treated by appropriate specialists,

KEY TERMS

Autosomal—Refers to the 22 pairs (in humans) of chromosomes not involved with sex determination.

Connective tissue—Tissue that supports and binds other tissue; much of it occurs outside of cells (extra-cellular) and consists of fibrous webs of the polymers, elastin and collagen. Cutis laxa is associated with defects in these fibers.

Diverticula—Pouches in the walls of organs.

Dominant trait—A genetic trait where one copy of the gene is sufficient to yield an outward display of the trait; dominant genes mask the presence of recessive genes; dominant traits can be inherited from only one parent.

Duodenum—The uppermost part of the small intestine, about 10 in (25 cm) long.

Esophagus— The tube connecting the throat to the stomach, about 10 in (25 cm) long.

Funnel breast (also known as pectus excavatum)— A condition where there is a hollow depression in the lower part of the chest.

Gene—A portion of a DNA molecule that either codes for a protein or RNA molecule or has a regulatory function.

Lysyl oxidase—An enzyme required for the cross-linking of elastin and collagen molecules to form properly functioning connective tissue; present in relatively low levels in at least some forms of cutis laxa.

Pigeon breast (also known as pectus carinatum)— A chest shape with a central projection resembling the keel of a boat.

Recessive trait—An inherited trait that is outwardly obvious only when two copies of the gene for that trait are present; an individual displaying a recessive trait must have inherited one copy of the defective gene from each parent.

Sex-linked—Refers to genes or traits carried on one of the sex chromosomes, usually the X.

Tortuous arteries—Arteries with many bends and twists.

X chromosome—One of the two types of sex chromosomes; females have two X chromosomes, while males have one X chromosome and one Y chromosome.

for example, cardiologists, gastroenterologists, rheumatologists, and dermatologists. **Plastic surgery** can be helpful for cosmetic purposes, but the skin may become loose again.

Prognosis

The prognosis for cutis laxa varies with the form of the disorder. The effects may be relatively mild with individuals living a fairly normal, full life, or the disease may be fatal.

Prevention

The inherited forms of cutis laxa are genetically determined and are not currently preventable. **Genetic counseling** can be helpful for anyone with a family history of cutis laxa. The cause of acquired cutis laxa is not known, so no preventive measures can be taken.

Resources

OTHER

OMIM Homepage, Online Mendelian Inheritance in Man. http://www.ncbi.nlm.nih.gov/Omim.

ORGANIZATIONS

Coalitiion for Hertiable Disorders of Connective Tissue, 4301 Connecticut Avenue, NW, Suite 404, Washington, DC, 20008, (202) 362-9599, (202) 966-8553, chdct@pxe.org, http://www.chdct.org.

Lorraine Lica, PhD

Cuts *see* **Wounds**

CVA *see* **Stroke**

CVS *see* **Chorionic villus sampling; Cyclic vomiting syndrome**

Cyanosis

Definition

Cyanosis is a physical sign causing bluish discoloration of the skin and mucous membranes. Cyanosis is caused by a lack of oxygen in the blood. Cyanosis is associated with cold temperatures, **heart failure**, lung diseases, and smothering. It is seen in infants at birth

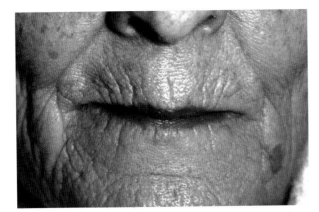

This elderly woman's lips turned purple due to central cyanosis, a condition most commonly due to slow blood circulation, leading to a bluish skin coloration. *(Photo Researchers, Inc.)*

as a result of heart defects, **respiratory distress syndrome**, or lung and breathing problems.

Description

Blood contains a red pigment (hemoglobin) in its red blood cells. Hemoglobin picks up oxygen from the lungs, then circulates it through arteries and releases it to cells through tiny capillaries. After giving up its oxygen, blood circulates back to the lungs through capillaries and veins. Hemoglobin, as well as blood, is bright red when it contains oxygen, but appears dark or "bluish" after it gives up oxygen.

The blue discoloration of cyanosis is seen most readily in the beds of the fingernails and toenails, and on the lips and tongue. It often appears transiently as a result of slowed blood flow through the skin due to the cold. As such, it is not a serious symptom. However, in other cases cyanosis is a serious symptom of underlying disease.

Causes and symptoms

The blue color of the skin and mucous membranes is caused by a lack of oxygen in the blood. Low blood oxygen may be caused by poor blood circulation, or heart or breathing problems. It can also be caused by being in a low-oxygen environment or by **carbon monoxide poisoning**. More rarely, cyanosis can be present at birth as a sign of **congenital heart disease**, in which some of the blood is not pumped to the lungs where oxygen would make the blood a bright red color. Instead, the blood goes to the rest of the body and remains unoxygenated. Cyanosis also may be caused by poisoning from chemicals, drugs, or contaminated food and water.

Other signs of low blood oxygen may accompany cyanosis, including feeling lightheaded or fainting.

Treatment

Treatment of the underlying disease can restore proper color to the skin.

Prognosis

If the underlying condition (such as heart or lung disease) can be properly treated, the skin will return to its normal shade.

Resources

BOOKS

Carlson, Karen J., Stephanie A. Eisenstat, and Terra Ziporyn. *The New Harvard Guide to Women's Health.* Cambridge, MA: Harvard University Press, 2004.

Carol A. Turkington

Cyclic vomiting syndrome

Definition

Cyclic **vomiting** syndrome (CVS) is a rare idiopathic disorder characterized by recurring periods of **vomiting** in an otherwise normal child or adult. It was first described in 1882 by an English physician, Samuel Jones Gee. CVS is sometimes called abdominal migraine because it may be caused by some of the same mechanisms in the central nervous system that cause migraine headaches.

Description

Children in the pre–school or early school years are most susceptible to CVS, although the disorder

KEY TERMS

Abdominal migraine—Another term that is sometimes used for CVS.

Idiopathic—Of unknown cause or spontaneous origin. CVS is sometimes called an idiopathic disorder because its cause(s) are still not known.

Prodrome—A symptom or group of symptoms that appears shortly before an acute attack of illness. The term comes from a Greek word that means "running ahead of."

can appear at any time from infancy to adulthood. One doctor reports that 43 of the 233 patients with CVS that he has treated were adults when their symptoms began. The average age of patients at onset is 5.2 years, but CVS has been diagnosed in patients as old as 73. This disorder was identified over a century ago, but its cause is still unknown. Episodes can be triggered by emotional **stress** or infections (particularly **sinusitis**), can last hours or days, and can return at any time. Abdominal **pain** is a frequent feature.

CVS appears to affect all races equally. The female:male ratio has been reported as 11:9.

Causes and symptoms

The cause of CVS is still unknown. Similarities to migraine suggest a common cause, but as yet no firm evidence has surfaced. It is known, however, that 82% of patients with CVS have a family history of migraine compared to 14% of control subjects. Patients can usually identify some factor that precedes an attack. Vomiting can be protracted and lead to such complications as **dehydration**; chemical imbalances; and tearing, burning, and bleeding of the esophagus (swallowing tube). Between attacks, there is no sign of any illness.

CVS has four distinct stages or phases:

- Prodrome. A prodrome is a warning symptom (or group of symptoms) that appears just before an acute attack of an illness. Patients with CVS often feel pain in the abdomen a few minutes or hours before the vomiting starts. Adults with CVS often have anxiety or panic attacks as a prodrome.
- Episode phase. During this phase, the patient is actively nauseated and vomiting. He or she may also feel drowsy or exhausted.

- Recovery phase.
- Symptom–free interval.

Diagnosis

The most important and difficult aspect of CVS is to be sure there is not an acute and life–threatening event in progress. So many different diseases can cause vomiting—from bowel obstruction to epilepsy—that an accurate and timely diagnosis is critical. Because there is no way to confirm a diagnosis of CVS, the physician must instead disprove every other diagnosis. This process, which is known as a diagnosis of exclusion, can be tedious, expensive, exhausting, and involving almost every system in the body. The first episode may be diagnosed as a stomach flu when nothing more serious turns up. Only after several episodes and several fruitless searches for a cause will a physician normally consider a diagnosis of CVS.

A careful history–taking is critical to making the correct diagnosis of CVS. A family history of migraine, particularly on the mother's side of the family, should alert the doctor to the possibility that the patient may have CVS.

In some cases, the doctor may refer the patient to a psychiatrist for evaluation in order to rule out **anxiety disorders** or an eating disorder.

Treatment

Several different medications have given good results in small trials. The antimigraine drugs amitriptyline and cyproheptadine performed well for one study group. Propranolol is sometimes effective, and erythromycin helped several patients in one study, not because it is an antibiotic but because it irritates the stomach and encourages it to move its contents forward instead of in reverse.

Another medication that has been reported to be successful in treating children with CVS is dexmedetomidine (Precedex), a drug originally developed to sedate patients on respirators in intensive care settings. Researchers found that dexmedetomidine relieved the **anxiety** as well as the **nausea** associated with CVS.

Antiemetic medication such as ondansetron (Zofran), antianxiety medication such as lorazepam (Ativan) and medication for stomach acid irritation such as ranitidine (Zantac) may be helpful during the prodrome phase.

Acupuncture treatments have also been found to be helpful to some children with CVS.

Patients are urged to drink plenty of water and electrolyte fluids to stay healthy during the recovery phase, moving slowly to solid food as tolerated.

Prognosis

The disease may go on for many years without a change in pattern. If the acute complications of prolonged vomiting can be successfully prevented or managed, most patients can lead normal lives between episodes. Medications may ease the symptoms during attacks.

Resources

BOOKS

Bean, Dianne. *Nutrition Ambition: Reaching Your Wellness Goals, Ages 8 - 12,* 2nd ed. Winter Park, FL: Baux Publishing LLC, 2009.

DiMario, Francis J., Jr. *Non–Epileptic Childhood Paroxysmal Disorders.* New York, NY: Oxford University Press, 2009.

Larson Duyff, R. *ADA Complete Food and Nutrition Guide,* 3rd ed. Chicago, IL: American Dietetic Association, 2006.

Pelletier, Kenneth R. *The Best Alternative Medicine*, Part II, "CAM Therapies for Specific Conditions: Anxiety." New York: Simon & Schuster, 2007.

Robertson, Cathie. *Safety, Nutrition and Health in Early Education*, 4th ed. Florence, KY: Wadsworth Publishing, 2009.

PERIODICALS

Fleisher, David R. "Cyclic Vomiting Syndrome in Adults." *Code "V": The Official Newsletter of the CVSA—USA/Canada* 11 (Spring 2003): 1– 3.

Khasawinah, T. A., A. Ramirez, J. W. Berkenbosch, and J. D. Tobias. "Preliminary Experience with Dexmedetomidine in the Treatment of Cyclic Vomiting Syndrome." *American Journal of Therapeutics* 10 (July–August 2003): 303–307.

Li, B. U., and L. Misiewicz. "Cyclic Vomiting Syndrome: A Brain-Gut Disorder." *Gastroenterology Clinics of North America* 32 (September 2003): 997–1019.

Lin, Yuan–Chi, and Brenda Golianu. "Acupuncture as Complementary Treatment for Cyclic Vomiting Syndrome." *Medical Acupuncture* 13 (March 1999): 1–4.

OTHER

Sundaram, Shikha, and B. Uk Li. "Cyclic Vomiting Syndrome." eMedicine August 10, 2002. http://www.emedicine.com/ped/topic2910.htm (accessed September 10, 2010).

ORGANIZATIONS

American Academy of Child and Adolescent Psychiatry, 3615 Wisconsin Ave., NW, Washington, DC, 20016–3007, (202) 966–7300, (202) 966–2891, http://www.aacap.org.

American Academy of Family Physicians, PO Box 11210, Shawnee Mission, KS, 66207 (913) 906–6000, (800) 274–2237, (913) 906–6075, http://www.aafp.org.

American Academy of Pediatrics, 141 Northwest Point Blvd., Elk Grove Village, IL, 60007–1098 (847) 434–4000, http://www.aap.org.

American Dietetic Association, 20 South Riverside Plaza, Suite 2000, Chicago, IL, 60605, (800) 877–1600, http://www.eatright.org.

Cyclic Vomiting Syndrome Association in the United States and Canada (CVSA—USA/Canada), 3585 Cedar Hill Road, NW, Canal Winchester, OH, 43110, (614) 837–2586, http://www.cvsaonline.or.

National Eating Disorders Association, 603 Stewart St., No. 803, Seattle, WA, 98101, (206) 382–3587, http://www.nationaleatingdisorders.org.

National Institute of Child Health and Human Development (NICHD), PO Box 3006, Rockville, MD, 30847, (800) 370–2943 TTY: (800) 320–6942, (866) 760–5947, NICHDInformationResourceCenter@mail.nih. gov, http://www.nichd.nih.gov.

National Organization for Rare Disorders, Inc. (NORD), 55 Kenosia Ave., PO Box 1968, Danbury, CT, 06813, (203) 744–0100, (800) 999–6673, http://www.rarediseases.org.

Nutrition.gov. USDA National Agricultural Library, Food and Nutrition Information Center, Nutrition.gov Staff, 10301 Baltimore Ave., Beltsville, MD, 20705–2351, http://www.nutrition.gov.

Rebecca J. Frey, Ph.D.
J. Ricker Polsdorfer, MD
Laura Jean Cataldo, RN, Ed.D.

Cyclobenzaprine *see* **Muscle relaxants**
Cyclophospha *see* **Anticancer drugs**
Cyclospora infection *see* **Cyclosporiasis**

Cyclosporiasis

Definition

Cyclosporiasis refers to infection by the spore-forming protozoan known as *Cyclospora*. Protozoa are a group of parasites that infect the human intestine. Parasites are organisms that live in another body, called the host, and get food and liquids from that host. This parasite is a member of the group of protozoa known

KEY TERMS

Anti-motility medications—Medications such as loperamide (sold as Imodium), dephenoxylate (sold as Lomotil), or medications containing codeine or narcotics that decrease the ability of the intestine to contract. This can worsen the condition of a patient with dysentery or colitis.

Cyst—A protective sac that includes either fluid or the cell of an organism. The cyst enables many organisms to survive in the environment for long periods of time without need for food or water.

Immunocompromised—A change or alteration of the immune system that normally serves to fight off infections other illnesses. This can involve changes in antibodies that the body produces (hygogammaglobulinemia), or a defect in the cells that partake in the immune response.

Diseases such as AIDS and cancer exhibit changes in the body's natural immunity.

Oral Rehydration Solution (ORS)—A liquid preparation developed by the World Health Organization that can decrease fluid loss in persons with diarrhea. Originally developed to be prepared with materials available in the home, commercial preparations have recently come into use.

Parasite—An organism that lives on or in another and takes nourishment (food and fluids) from that organism.

Protozoa—Group of extremely small single cell (unicellular) or acellular organisms that are found in moist soil or water. They tend to exist as parasites, living off other life forms.

Spore—A resistant form of certain species of bacteria, protozoa, and other organisms.

---

as coccidia, to which *Cryptosporidia* also belongs. This group of parasites infects the human intestine, and causes chronic recurrent infections in those with altered immunity or **AIDS**. Even in people with normal immune function, *Cyclopsora* can cause prolonged bouts of **diarrhea** and other gastrointestinal symptoms.

Description

Until recently, *Cyclospora* was considered to be a form of algae. The parasite causes a common form of waterborne infectious diarrhea throughout the world. Just how the parasite gets into water sources is not yet clear. It is known that ingestion of small cysts in contaminated water leads to disease.

Causes and symptoms

Symptoms begin after an incubation period of about a day or so following ingestion of cysts. A brief period of flu-like illness characterized by weakness and low-grade **fever** is followed by watery diarrhea, **nausea**, loss of appetite, and muscle aches. In some patients, symptoms may wax and wane for weeks, and there are those in whom nausea and burping may predominate. It is also believed that infection can occur without any symptoms at all.

In patients with abnormal immunity (immunocompromised patients), such as those with AIDS and **cancer**, prolonged diarrhea and severe weight loss

often become a major problem. The bile ducts are also susceptible to infection in AIDS patients.

Diagnosis

The disease should be suspected in anyone with a history of prolonged or recurrent diarrhea. The parasite is identified either by staining stool specimens or by applying certain fluorescent ultraviolet techniques to find the characteristic cysts. Biopsy of an infected organ such as the intestine through an endoscope is another way to make the diagnosis.

Treatment

The first aim of treatment as with any severe diarrheal illness is to avoid **dehydration** and **malnutrition**. Oral Rehydration Solution (ORS) or intravenous fluids are sometimes needed. Medications used to treat diarrhea by decreasing intestinal motility, such as loperamide or diphenoxylate are also useful, but should only be used with the advice of a physician.

The use of the medication, trimethoprim-sulfamethoxazole (Bactrim) for one week can be successful in treating intestinal infections and prevents relapse in those with a normal immune system. The same medicine can be prescribed to treat infections of both the intestine or bile ducts in immunocompromised individuals, but maintenance or continuous treatment is often needed.

Prognosis

The outlook is quite good for individuals in whom a diagnosis is made. Even without treatment, symptoms usually do not last much more than a month except in cases with altered immunity. Fortunately, treatment is usually successful even in those patients.

Prevention

Aside from a waterborne source as the origin of infection, little else is known about how the parasite is transmitted. Therefore, little can be done regarding prevention, except to maintain proper hand washing techniques and hygiene.

Resources

OTHER

"Cyclospora." *Centers for Disease Control.* http://www.cdc.gov/ncidod/diseases/cyclospo/cyclohp.htm.

ORGANIZATIONS

Centers for Disease Control and Prevention (CDC), 1600 Clifton Road, Atlanta, GA, 30333, (800) 232-4636, cdcinfo@cdc.gov, http://www.cdc.gov.

David Kaminstein, MD

Cyclosporine *see* **Immunosuppressant drugs**

Cystectomy

Definition

Cystectomy is a surgical procedure to remove the bladder.

Purpose

Cystectomy is performed to treat **cancer** of the bladder. Radiation and **chemotherapy** are also used to treat **bladder cancer**. Surgery is used to remove cancer when it is in the muscle of the bladder.

Precautions

Cystectomy is an aggressive treatment that may not be appropriate for patients with superficial tumors that respond to more conservative treatment.

Description

Cystectomy is a major surgical operation. The patient is placed under **general anesthesia**. An incision is made across the lower abdomen. The ureters are located, tied and cut. The ureters connect the kidneys to the bladder. Cutting them frees the bladder for removal. The bladder and associated organs are removed. In men the prostate is removed with the bladder. In women, the uterus, fallopian tubes, ovaries, and part of the vagina are removed with the bladder. The bladder collects urine from the kidneys for excretion at a later time. Since the bladder is removed, a new method must be created to remove the urine. A small piece of the small intestine is removed, cleaned, and tied at one end to form a tube. The other end is used to form a stoma, an opening through the abdominal wall to the outside. The ureters are then connected to the tube. Urine produced by the kidneys now flows down the ureters, into the tube, and through the stoma. The patient wears a bag to collect the urine.

Preparation

The medical team will discuss the procedure and tell the patient where the stoma will appear and what it will look like. The patient receives instruction on caring for a stoma and bag. Counseling may be initiated. A period of **fasting** and an enema may be required.

Aftercare

After the operation, the patient is given fluid-based **nutrition** until the intestines being to function normally again. **Antibiotics** are given to prevent infection of the incision sites. The nature of the organs removed mean that there will be major lifestyle changes for the person undergoing the operation. Men will become impotent because nerves controlling penile erection are cut during removal of the bladder. In women, **infertility** is a consequence because the ovaries and uterus are removed. However, most women who undergo cystectomy are postmenopausal and past their childbearing years.

Both men and women are fitted with an external bag that connects to the stoma and collects the urine. The bag is generally worn around the waist under the clothing. It takes a period of adjustment to get used to wearing the bag. Because there is no bladder, urine is excreted as it is produced, essentially continuously. The stoma must be treated properly to ensure that it does not become infected or blocked. Patients must be trained to care for their stoma. Often there is a period of psychological adjustment to the major change in life style created by the stoma and bag. Patients should be prepared for this by discussion with their physician.

Risks

As with any major surgery, there is a risk of infection; in this case infection of the intestine is especially dangerous as it can lead to **peritonitis** (inflammation of the membrane lining the abdomen).

Results

Normal results

The bladder is successfully removed and a stoma created. Intestinal function returns to normal and the patient learns proper care of the stoma and bag. He or she adjusts to lifestyle changes and returns to a normal routine of work and recreation, some sports excluded.

Abnormal results

The patient develops an infection at the incision site. The patient does not make a successful psychological adjustment to the long term consequences of **impotence** and urinary diversion. In some women, the vagina is constricted, which may require a secondary procedure.

Resources

BOOKS

Beers, Mark H., Robert S. Porter, and Thomas V. Jones, eds. *The Merck Manual of Diagnosis and Therapy*. 18th ed. Whitehouse Station, NJ: Merck Research Laboratories, 2006.

John T. Lohr, PhD

Cystic fibrosis

Definition

Cystic fibrosis (CF) is an inherited disease that affects the lungs, digestive system, sweat glands, and male fertility. Its name derives from the fibrous scar tissue that develops in the pancreas, one of the principal organs affected by the disease.

Demographics

According to the Cystic Fibrosis Foundation, about 30,000 people in the United States and 70,000 worldwide have cystic fibrosis. It is one of the most common inherited diseases among Caucasians. About 1,000 new cases are diagnosed each year. About 12 million Americans are carriers of a faulty CF gene and many do not know that they are CF carriers.

Description

Cystic fibrosis (CF) is a disease of the mucus glands that affects many body systems. CF affects the body's ability to move salt and water in and out of cells, resulting in progressive damage to the respiratory system and chronic digestive system problems. It causes the lungs and pancreas to secrete thick mucus, blocking passageways and preventing proper function.

Many of the symptoms of CF can be treated with drugs or **nutritional supplements**. Close attention to and prompt treatment of respiratory and digestive complications have dramatically increased the expected life span of a person with CF. Several decades ago most children with CF died by age two years; today, about half of all people with CF live past age 31. That median age is expected to grow as new treatments are developed, and it is estimated that a person born in 1998 with CF has a median expected life span of 40 years.

Risk factors

Cystic fibrosis affects males and females equally and people from all racial and ethnic groups. However, the disease is most common among Caucasians of Northern European descent. It also occurs among Latinos and Native Americans, especially the Pueblo and Zuni. Cystic fibrosis is much less common among African Americans and Asian Americans.

Causes and symptoms

Cystic fibrosis is a genetic disease, meaning it is caused by a defect in the person's genes. Genes, found in the nucleus of all the body's cells, control cell function by serving as the blueprint for the production of proteins. Proteins carry out a wide variety of functions within cells. The gene that, when defective, causes CF is called the CFTR gene, which stands for cystic fibrosis transmembrane conductance regulator. A simple change in this gene leads to all the consequences of CF. There are over 1000 known defects in the CFTR gene that can cause CF. However, 70% of all people with an abnormal CFTR gene have the same defect, known as delta–F508.

DOROTHY ANDERSEN (1901–1963)

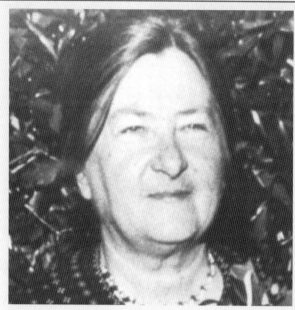

(The Library of Congress.)

Dorothy Andersen was born on May 15, 1901, in Asheville, North Carolina. She was the only child of Hans Peter Andersen and the former Mary Louise Mason. Orphaned as a young adult, Andersen put herself through Saint Johnsbury Academy and Mount Holyoke College before enrolling in the Johns Hopkins School of Medicine, from which she received her M.D. in 1926.

Andersen turned instead to medical research as a pathologist at Babies Hospital of the Columbia-Presbyterian Medical Center in New York City, where she stayed for more than 20 years, eventually becoming chief of pathology in 1952. Andersen is probably best known for her discovery of cystic fibrosis in 1935. That discovery came about during the postmortem examination of a child who had supposedly died of celiac disease, a nutritional disorder. She searched for similar cases in the autopsy files and in medical literature, eventually realizing that she had found a disease that had never been described and to which she gave the name cystic fibrosis.

Genes can be thought of as long strings of chemical words, each made of chemical letters, called nucleotides. Just as a sentence can be changed by rearranging its letters, genes can be mutated, or changed, by changes in the sequence of their nucleotide letters. The gene changes in CF are called point mutations, meaning that the gene is mutated only at one small spot along its length. In other words, the delta–F508 mutation is a loss of one "letter" out of thousands within the CFTR gene. As a result, the CFTR protein made from its blueprint is made incorrectly, and cannot perform its function properly.

The CFTR protein helps to produce mucus. Mucus is a complex mixture of salts, water, sugars, and proteins that cleanses, lubricates, and protects many passageways in the body, including those in the lungs and pancreas. The role of the CFTR protein is to allow chloride ions to exit the mucus–producing cells. When the chloride ions leave these cells, water follows, thinning the mucus. In this way, the CFTR protein helps to keep mucus from becoming thick and sluggish, thus allowing the mucus to be moved steadily along the passageways to aid in cleansing.

In CF, the CFTR protein does not allow chloride ions out of the mucus–producing cells. With less chloride leaving, less water leaves, and the mucus becomes thick and sticky. It can no longer move freely through the passageways, so they become clogged. In the pancreas, clogged passageways prevent secretion of digestive enzymes into the intestine, causing serious impairment of digestion—especially of fat—which may lead to **malnutrition**. Mucus in the lungs may plug the airways, preventing good air exchange and, ultimately, leading to **emphysema**. The mucus is also a rich source of nutrients for bacteria, leading to frequent infections.

To understand the inheritance pattern of CF, it is important to realize that genes actually have two functions. First, as noted above, they serve as the blueprint for the production of proteins. Second, they are the material of inheritance: parents pass on characteristics to their children by combining the genes in egg and sperm to make a new individual.

Each person actually has two copies of each gene, including the CFTR gene, in each of his or her body cells. During sperm and egg production, however, these two copies separate, so that each sperm or egg contains only one copy of each gene. When sperm and egg unite, the newly created cell once again has two copies of each gene.

The two gene copies may be the same or they may be slightly different. For the CFTR gene, for instance, a person may have two normal copies, or one normal and one mutated copy, or two mutated copies. A person with two mutated copies will develop cystic fibrosis. A person with one mutated copy is said to be a carrier. A carrier will not have symptoms of CF, but can pass on the mutated CFTR gene to his or her children.

When two carriers have children, they have a one in four chance of having a child with CF each time they conceive. They have a two in four chance of having a child who is a carrier, and a one in four chance of having a child with two normal CFTR genes.

Approximately one in every 25 Americans of northern European descent is a carrier of the mutated CF gene, while only one in 17,000 African Americans and one in 30,000 Asian Americans are carriers. Since carriers are symptom–free, very few people will know whether or not they are carriers, unless there is a family history of the disease. Two white Americans with no family history of CF have a one in 2,500 chance of having a child with CF.

It may seem puzzling that a mutated gene with such harmful consequences would remain so common; one might guess that the high mortality of CF would quickly lead to loss of the mutated gene from the population. Some researchers now believe the reason for the persistence of the CF gene is that carriers, those with only one copy of the gene, are protected from the full effects of **cholera**, a microorganism that infects the intestine, causing intense **diarrhea** and eventual **death** by **dehydration**. It is believed that having one copy of the CF gene is enough to prevent the full effects of cholera infection, while not enough to cause the symptoms of CF. This so–called "heterozygote advantage" is seen in some other genetic disorders, including sickle–cell anemia.

The most severe effects of cystic fibrosis are seen in two body systems: the gastrointestinal (digestive) system and the respiratory tract, from the nose to the lungs. CF also affects the sweat glands and male fertility. Symptoms develop gradually, with gastrointestinal symptoms often the first to appear.

Gastrointestinal system

Ten to fifteen percent of babies who inherit CF have meconium **ileus** at birth. Meconium is the first dark stool that a baby passes after birth; ileus is an obstruction of the digestive tract. The meconium of a newborn with meconium ileus is thickened and sticky, due to the presence of thickened mucus from the intestinal glands. Meconium ileus causes abdominal swelling and **vomiting**, and often requires surgery immediately after birth. Presence of meconium ileus is considered highly indicative of CF. Borderline cases may be misdiagnosed, however, and attributed instead to a "milk allergy."

Other abdominal symptoms are caused by the inability of the pancreas to supply digestive enzymes to the intestine. During normal digestion, as food passes from the stomach into the small intestine, it is mixed with pancreatic secretions, which help to break down the nutrients for absorption. While the intestines themselves also provide some digestive enzymes, the pancreas is the major source of enzymes for the digestion of all types of foods, especially fats and proteins.

In CF, thick mucus blocks the pancreatic duct, which is eventually closed off completely by scar tissue formation, leading to a condition known as pancreatic insufficiency. Without pancreatic enzymes, large amounts of undigested food pass into the large intestine. Bacterial action on this rich food source can cause gas and abdominal swelling. The large amount of fat remaining in the feces makes it bulky, oily, and foul–smelling.

Because nutrients are only poorly digested and absorbed, the person with CF is often ravenously hungry, underweight, and shorter than expected for his age. When CF is not treated for a longer period, a child may develop symptoms of malnutrition, including anemia, bloating, and, paradoxically, appetite loss.

Diabetes becomes increasingly likely as a person with CF ages. Scarring of the pancreas slowly destroys those pancreatic cells which produce insulin, producing type I, or insulin–dependent, diabetes.

Gallstones affect approximately 10% of adults with CF. Liver problems are less common, but can be caused by the build–up of fat within the liver. Complications of liver enlargement may include internal hemorrhaging, abdominal fluid (**ascites**), spleen enlargement, and liver failure.

Other gastrointestinal symptoms can include a prolapsed rectum, in which part of the rectal lining protrudes through the anus; intestinal obstruction; and rarely, **intussusception**, in which part of the intestinal tube slips over an adjoining part, cutting off blood supply.

Somewhat fewer than 10% of people with CF do not have gastrointestinal symptoms. Most of these people do not have the delta–F508 mutation, but rather a different one, which presumably allows at least some of their CFTR proteins to function normally in the pancreas.

Respiratory tract

The respiratory tract includes the nose, the throat, the trachea (or windpipe), the bronchi (which branch off from the trachea within each lung), the smaller bronchioles, and the blind sacs called alveoli, in which gas exchange takes place between air and blood.

Swelling of the sinuses within the nose is common in people with CF. This usually shows up on x ray, and may aid the diagnosis of CF. However, this swelling, called pansinusitis, rarely causes problems, and does not usually require treatment.

Nasal polyps, or growths, affect about one in five people with CF. These growths are not cancerous, and do not require removal unless they become annoying. While nasal polyps appear in older people without CF, especially those with **allergies**, they are rare in children without CF.

The lungs are the site of the most life–threatening effects of CF. The production of a thick, sticky mucus increases the likelihood of infection, decreases the ability to protect against infection, causes inflammation and swelling, decreases the functional capacity of the lungs, and may lead to emphysema. People with CF will live with chronic populations of bacteria in their lungs, and lung infection is the major cause of death for those with CF.

The bronchioles and bronchi normally produce a thin, clear mucus, which traps foreign particles including bacteria and viruses. Tiny hair-like projections called cilia on the surface of these passageways slowly sweep the mucus along, out of the lungs and up the trachea to the back of the throat, where it may be swallowed or coughed up. This "mucociliary escalator" is one of the principal defenses against lung infection.

The thickened mucus of CF prevents easy movement out of the lungs, and increases the irritation and inflammation of lung tissue. This inflammation swells the passageways, partially closing them down, further hampering the movement of mucus. A person with CF is likely to **cough** more frequently and more vigorously as the lungs attempt to clean themselves out.

At the same time, infection becomes more likely since the mucus is a rich source of nutrients. **Bronchitis**, **bronchiolitis**, and **pneumonia** are frequent in CF. The most common infecting organisms are the bacteria *Staphylococcus aureus*, *Haemophilus influenzae*, and *Pseudomonas aeruginosa*. A small percentage of people with CF have infections caused by *Burkholderia cepacia*, a bacterium which is resistant to most current **antibiotics** (*Burkholderia cepacia* was formerly known as *Pseudomonas cepacia*). The fungus *Aspergillus fumigatus* may infect older children and adults.

The body's response to infection is to increase mucus production; white blood cells fighting the infection thicken the mucus even further as they break down and release their cell contents. These white blood cells also provoke more inflammation, continuing the downward spiral that marks untreated CF.

As mucus accumulates, it can plug up the smaller passageways in the lungs, decreasing functional lung volume. Getting enough air can become difficult; tiredness, **shortness of breath**, and intolerance of **exercise** become more common. Because air passes obstructions more easily during inhalation than during exhalation, over time, air becomes trapped in the smallest chambers of the lungs, the alveoli. As millions of alveoli gradually expand, the chest takes on the enlarged, barrel-shaped appearance typical of emphysema.

For unknown reasons, recurrent respiratory infections lead to "digital clubbing," in which the last joint of the fingers and toes becomes slightly enlarged.

Sweat glands

The CFTR protein helps to regulate the amount of salt in sweat. People with CF have sweat that is much saltier than normal, and measuring the saltiness of a person's sweat is the most important diagnostic test for CF. Parents may notice that their infants taste salty when they kiss them. Excess salt loss is not usually a problem except during prolonged exercise or heat. While most older children and adults with CF compensate for this extra salt loss by eating more salty foods, infants and young children are in danger of suffering its effects (such as heat prostration), especially during summer. Heat prostration is marked by lethargy, weakness, and loss of appetite, and should be treated as an emergency condition.

Fertility

Ninety-eight percent of men with CF are sterile, due to complete obstruction or absence of the vas deferens, the tube carrying sperm out of the testes. While boys and men with CF form normal sperm and have normal levels of sex hormones, sperm are unable to leave the testes, and fertilization is not possible. Most women with CF are fertile, though they often have more trouble getting pregnant than women without CF. In both boys and girls, **puberty** is often delayed, most likely due to the effects of poor **nutrition** or chronic lung infection. Women with good lung health usually have no problems with **pregnancy**, while those with ongoing lung infection often do poorly.

Diagnosis

The decision to test a child for cystic fibrosis may be triggered by concerns about recurring gastrointestinal

KEY TERMS

Carrier—A person who possesses a gene for an abnormal trait without showing signs of the disorder. The person may pass the abnormal gene on to offspring.

CFTR—Cystic fibrosis transmembrane conductance regulator. The protein responsible for regulating chloride movement across cells in some tissues. When a person has two defective copies of the CFTR gene, cystic fibrosis is the result.

Emphysema—A chronic lung disease that begins with breathlessness during exertion and progresses to shortness of breath at all times, caused by destructive changes in the lungs.

Mucociliary escalator—The coordinated action of tiny projections on the surfaces of cells lining the respiratory tract, which moves mucus up and out of the lungs.

Mucolytic—An agent that dissolves or destroys mucin, the chief component of mucus.

Pancreatic insufficiency—Reduction or absence of pancreatic secretions into the digestive system due to scarring and blockage of the pancreatic duct.

---

or respiratory symptoms, or salty sweat. A child born with meconium ileus will be tested before leaving the hospital. Families with a history of CF may wish to have all children tested, especially if there is a child who already has the disease. Some hospitals now require routine screening of newborns for CF.

Sweat test

The sweat test is both the easiest and most accurate test for CF. In this test, a small amount of the drug pilocarpine is placed on the skin. A very small electrical current is then applied to the area, which drives the pilocarpine into the skin. The drug stimulates sweating in the treated area. The sweat is absorbed onto a piece of filter paper, and is then analyzed for its salt content. A person with CF will have salt concentrations that are one-and-one-half to two times greater than normal. The test can be done on persons of any age, including newborns, and its results can be determined within an hour. Virtually every person who has CF will test positively on it, and virtually everyone who does not will test negatively.

Genetic testing

The discovery of the CFTR gene in 1989 allowed the development of an accurate genetic test for CF. Genes from a small blood or tissue sample are analyzed for specific mutations; presence of two copies of the mutated gene confirms the diagnosis of CF in all but a very few cases. However, since there are so many different possible mutations, and since testing for all of them would be too expensive and time–consuming, a negative gene test cannot rule out the possibility of CF.

Couples planning a family may decide to have themselves tested if one or both have a family history of CF. Prenatal **genetic testing** is possible through **amniocentesis**. Many couples who already have one child with CF decide to undergo prenatal screening in subsequent pregnancies. Siblings in these families are also usually tested, both to determine if they will develop CF, and to determine if they are carriers, to aid in their own family planning. If the sibling has no symptoms, determining his or her carrier status is often delayed until the teen years or later, when he or she is closer to needing the information to make decisions.

Newborn screening

Some states now require screening of newborns for CF, using a test known as the IRT test. This is a blood test which measures the level of immunoreactive trypsinogen, which is generally higher in babies with CF than those without it. This test gives many false positive results immediately after birth, and so requires a second test several weeks later. A second positive result is usually followed by a sweat test.

Treatment

Traditional

There is no cure for cystic fibrosis. Treatment has advanced considerably in the past several decades, increasing both the life span and the quality of life for most people affected by CF. Early diagnosis is important to prevent malnutrition and infection from weakening the young child. With proper management, many people with CF engage in the full range of school and sports activities.

People with CF usually require high-calorie **diets** and vitamin supplements. Height, weight, and growth of a person with CF are monitored regularly. Most people with CF need to take pancreatic enzymes to supplement or replace the inadequate secretions of the pancreas. Tablets containing pancreatic enzymes are taken with every meal; depending on the size of the tablet and the meal, as many as 20 tablets may be needed. Because of incomplete absorption even with pancreatic enzymes, a person with CF needs to take in about 30% more food than a person without CF. Low–fat diets are *not* recommended except in special circumstances, since fat is a source of both essential fatty acids and abundant calories.

Some people with CF cannot absorb enough nutrients from the foods they eat, even with specialized diets and enzymes. For these people, tube feeding is an option. Nutrients can be introduced directly into the stomach through a tube inserted either through the nose (a nasogastric tube) or through the abdominal wall (a **gastrostomy** tube). A jejunostomy tube, inserted into the small intestine, is also an option. Tube feeding can provide nutrition at any time, including at night while the person is sleeping, allowing constant intake of high–quality nutrients. The feeding tube may be removed during the day, allowing normal meals to be taken.

The key to maintaining respiratory health in a person with CF is regular monitoring and early treatment. Lung function tests are done frequently to track changes in functional lung volume and respiratory effort. Sputum samples are analyzed to determine the types of bacteria present in the lungs. Chest x rays are usually taken at least once a year. Lung scans, using a radioactive gas, can show closed off areas not seen on the x ray. Circulation in the lungs may be monitored by injection of a radioactive substance into the bloodstream.

People with CF live with chronic bacterial colonization; that is, their lungs are constantly host to several species of bacteria. Good general health, especially good nutrition, can keep the immune system healthy, which decreases the frequency with which these colonies begin an infection, or attack on the lung tissue. Exercise is another important way to maintain health, and people with CF are encouraged to maintain a program of regular exercise.

In addition, clearing mucus from the lungs helps to prevent infection, and mucus control is an important aspect of CF management. Bronchial drainage is used to allow gravity to aid the mucociliary escalator.

For this technique, the person with CF lies on a tilted surface with head downward, alternately on the stomach, back, or side, depending on the section of lung to be drained. An assistant thumps the rib cage to help loosen the secretions. A device called a "flutter" offers another way to loosen secretions: it consists of a stainless steel ball in a tube. When a person exhales through it, the ball vibrates, sending vibrations back through the air in the lungs. Some special breathing techniques may also help clear the lungs.

Supplemental oxygen may be needed as lung disease progresses. **Respiratory failure** may develop, requiring temporary use of a ventilator to perform the work of breathing.

Drugs

Several drugs are available to prevent the airways from becoming clogged with mucus. **Bronchodilators** can help open up the airways; **steroids** reduce inflammation; and mucolytics loosen secretions. Acetylcysteine (Mucomyst) has been used as a mucolytic for many years but is not prescribed frequently now, while DNase (Pulmozyme) is a newer product gaining in popularity. DNase breaks down the DNA from dead white blood cells and bacteria found in thick mucus.

People with CF may pick up bacteria from other CF patients. This is especially true of *Burkholderia cepacia*, which is not usually found in people without CF. While the ideal recommendation from a health standpoint might be to avoid contact with others who have CF, this is not usually practical (since CF clinics are a major site of care), nor does it meet the psychological and social needs of many people with CF. At a minimum, CF centers recommend avoiding prolonged close contact between people with CF, and scrupulous hygiene, including frequent hand washing. Some CF clinics schedule appointments on different days for those with and without *B. cepacia* colonies.

Some doctors choose to prescribe antibiotics only during infection, while others prefer long–term antibiotic treatment against *S. aureus*. The choice of antibiotic depends on the particular organism or organisms found. Some antibiotics are given as aerosols directly into the lungs. Antibiotic treatment may be prolonged and aggressive.

Long-term use of ibuprofen has been shown to help some people with CF; presumably by reducing inflammation in the lungs. Close medical supervision is necessary, however, since the effective dose is high and not everyone benefits. Ibuprofen at the required doses interferes with kidney function, and together with aminoglycoside antibiotics, may cause kidney failure.

Alternative

Lung transplantation is another option for people with CF, although the number of people who receive them is still much lower than those who want them. Transplantation is not a cure, however, and has been likened to trading one disease for another. Long–term immunosuppression is required, increasing the likelihood of other types of infection. About 50% of adults and more than 80% of children who receive lung transplants live longer than two years. Some CF patients whose livers have been damaged by fibrosis also undergo liver transplants.

A number of experimental treatments are currently the subject of much research. Some evidence indicates that aminoglycoside antibiotics may help overcome the genetic defect in some CF mutations, allowing the protein to be made normally. While promising, these results would apply to only about 5% of those with CF.

Gene therapy is currently the most ambitious approach to curing CF. In this set of techniques, non–defective copies of the CFTR gene are delivered to affected cells, where they are taken up and used to create the CFTR protein. While elegant and simple in theory, gene therapy has met with a large number of difficulties in trials so far, including immune resistance, very short duration of the introduced gene, and inadequately widespread delivery.

In **homeopathic medicine**, the symptoms of the disease would be addressed to enhance the quality of life for the person with cystic fibrosis. Treating the cause of CF, because of the genetic basis for the disease, is not possible. Homeopathic medicine seeks to treat the whole person, however, and in cystic fibrosis, this approach might include:

- Mucolytics to help thin mucous.
- Supplementation of pancreatic enzymes to assist in digestion.
- Respiratory symptoms can be addressed to open lung passages.
- Hydrotherapy techniques to help ease the respiratory symptoms and help the body eliminate mucus.
- Immune enhancements can help prevent the development of secondary infections.
- Dietary enhancements and adjustments to treat digestive and nutritional problems.

Prognosis

People with CF may lead relatively normal lives. The possible effect of pregnancy on the health of a woman with CF requires careful consideration before beginning a family, as do issues of longevity, and their children's status as carriers. Although most men with CF are functionally sterile, new procedures for removing sperm from the testes are being tried, and may offer more men the chance to become fathers.

Approximately half of people with CF live past the age of 30. Because of better and earlier treatment, a person born today with CF is expected, on average, to live to age 40.

Prevention

CF is a genetic disorder that cannot be prevented. Screening people with a family history of CF may detect the cystic fibrosis gene in 60 to 90% of carriers, depending on the test used.

Resources

BOOKS

Davis, Lisa, et al. *A Way of Life: Cystic Fibrosis Nutrition Handbook and Cookbook*, 3rd ed., Madison, WI: University of Wisconsin Hospital, 2009.

Giddings, Sharon. *Cystic Fibrosis (Genes and Disease).* New York, NY: Chelsea House Publications, 2009.

Harris, Ann, and Anne Thomson. *Cystic Fibrosis.* New York, NY: Oxford University Press, 2008.

Langwith, Jacqueline, editor. *Cystic Fibrosis (Perspectives on Diseases and Disorders)*. Florence, KY: Greenhaven Press (Gale), 2008.

Sasso, Emilie. *Cystic Fibrosis and You.* Frederick, MD: PublishAmerica, 2008.

Stainback, Melissa Anne. *Living with Cystic Fibrosis.* Frederick, MD: PublishAmerica, 2008.

PERIODICALS

Jacquemin, E., et al. "Bioavailability of oral vitamin E formulations in adult volunteers and children with chronic cholestasis or cystic fibrosis." *Journal of Clinical Pharmacy and Therapeutics* 34, no. 5 (October 2009): 515–512.

Olveira, G., et al. "Markers for the validation of reported dietary intake in adults with cystic fibrosis." *Journal of the American Dietetic Association* 109, no. 10 (October 2009): 1704–1711.

O'Sullivan, B. P., and S. D. Freedman. "Cystic fibrosis." *Lancet* 373, no. 9678 (May 2009): 1891–1904.

Proesmans, M., et al. "What's new in cystic fibrosis? From treating symptoms to correction of the basic defect." *European Journal of Pediatrics* 167, no. 8 (August 2008): 839–849.

Ratjen, F. A. "Cystic fibrosis: pathogenesis and future treatment strategies." *Respiratory Care* 54, no. 5 (May 2009): 595–605.

Southern, K. W., et al. "Newborn screening for cystic fibrosis." *Cochrane Database of Systematic Reviews* 1
(January 2009): CD0011402.

Stark, L. J., et al. "Randomized clinical trial of behavioral
intervention and nutrition education to improve caloric
intake and weight in children with cystic fibrosis."
Archives of Pediatrics & Adolescent Medicine 163, no. 10
(October 2009): 915–921.

Torpy, J. M., et al. "JAMA patient page. Cystic fibrosis."
JAMA 302, no. 10 (September 2009): 1130.

Ward, C., et al. "Problem behaviours and parenting in preschool children with cystic fibrosis." *Archives of Disease
in Childhood* 94, no. 5 (May 2009): 341–347.

OTHER

"Cystic Fibrosis." *Medline Plus*. Health Topics. http://www.
nlm.nih.gov/medlineplus/cysticfibrosis.html (accessed
November 15, 2009)

"Cystic Fibrosis." *NIDDK*. Information Page. http://www2.
niddk.nih.gov/Research/ScientificAreas/GeneticGene-
Therapy/CFXX.htm (accessed November 15, 2009)

"Cystic Fibrosis." *Genetics Home Reference*. Information
Page. http://ghr.nlm.nih.gov/condition = cysticfibrosis
(accessed November 15, 2009)

"What Is Cystic Fibrosis?" *NHLBI*. Information Page.
http://www.nhlbi.nih.gov/health/dci/Diseases/cf/cf_
what.html (accessed November 15, 2009)

"What Is Cystic Fibrosis?" *Cystic Fibrosis Foundation*.
Information Page. http://www.cff.org/AboutCF
(accessed November 15, 2009)

ORGANIZATIONS

Cystic Fibrosis Foundation, 6931 Arlington Road,
Bethesda, MD, 20814, (301) 951-4422, (800) 344-4823,
(301) 951-6378, http://www.cff.org.

National Heart, Lung, and Blood Institute (NHLBI), Building
31, Room 5A52, 31 Center Drive MSC 2486, Bethesda,
MD, 20892, (301) 592-8573, (240) 629-3246, nhlbiin-
fo@nhlbi.nih.gov, http://www.nhlbi. nih.gov.

National Institute of Diabetes and Digestive and Kidney
Diseases (NIDDK), Building 31, Room 9A06, 31 Center Drive, MSC 2560, Bethesda, MD, 20892-2560, (301)
496-3583, http://www2.niddk.nih.gov.

Edward Rosick, DO, MPH, MS

Monique Laberge, PhD

Cystinuria

Definition

Cystinuria is an inborn error of amino acid transport that results in the defective absorption by the
kidneys of the amino acid called cystine. The name
means "cystine in the urine."

Description

Cystine is an amino acid. Amino acids are organic
compounds needed by the body to make proteins and
for many normal functions. When the kidneys do not
absorb cystine, this compound builds up in the urine.
When the amount of cystine in the urine exceeds its
solubility (the greatest amount that can be dissolved),
crystals form. As the amount of cystine continues to
increase in the urine, the number of crystals also
increases. When very large numbers of cystine crystals
form, they clump together into what is called a stone.

Causes and symptoms

Cystinuria is a rare disease that occurs when people inherit an abnormal gene from their parents. This
disease occurs in differing degrees of severity in people
who have inherited either one or two abnormal genes.
Humans have two copies of each gene. When both are
abnormal, the condition is called homozygous for the
disease. When one copy is normal and the other is
abnormal, the condition is called heterozygous for
the disease. Persons with one abnormal gene can
have a milder form of cystinuria that rarely results in
the formation of stones.

Severe cystinuria occurs when people are homozygous for the disease. For these individuals, the kidneys may excrete as much as 30 times the normal
amount of cystine. Research has shown that this condition is caused by mutations on chromosome number
two (humans have 23 pairs of chromosomes).

A person who has inherited cystinuria may have
other abnormal bodily functions. In addition to excess
levels of the amino acid cystine, high amounts of the
amino acids lysine, arginine, and ornithine are found in
the urine. This condition indicates that these amino
acids are not being reabsorbed by the body.

When excess cystine crystals clump together to
form a stone, the stone can block portions of the interior of the kidney or the tube (the ureter) that connects
the kidney to the urinary bladder. These cystine stones
can be painful, and depending upon where the stone
becomes trapped, the **pain** can be felt in the lower back
or the abdomen. **Nausea and vomiting** can also occur,
and patients may sometimes feel the need to urinate
often. Cystine stones can also cause blood in the urine.
When the urinary tract is blocked by a stone, urinary
tract infections or kidney failure may result.

Diagnosis

Small stones (called "silent") often do not cause
any symptoms, although they can be detected by an

KEY TERMS

Alkaline—A solution is considered alkaline if it contains fewer hydrogen atoms than pure water.

Amino acid—An organic compound made of an amino group (containing nitrogen and hydrogen) and a carbolic acid group. Amino acids are an essential part of protein molecules.

Nephroscope—An instrument made of a light source in a tube. The tube is inserted into the kidney through an incision in the back and used to locate

kidney stones. The stones are broken up with high frequency sound waves and removed by suction through the scope.

Nitroprusside—A compound that is used in laboratory tests to identify large amounts of cystine in urine samples.

Uretoscope—A tube-shaped device inserted into the body through the urinary system that allows objects to be both seen and grasped for removal.

---

x ray. Large stones are often painful and easily noticed by the patient. Blood in the urine can also mean that a stone has formed.

When the urine contains extremely high amounts of cystine, yellow-brown hexagonal crystals are visible when a sample is examined under the microscope. Urine samples can also be mixed with chemicals that change color when high levels of cystine are present. When the compound nitroprusside is added to urine that has been made alkaline by the addition of ammonia, the urine specimen turns red if it contains excess cystine.

Treatment

No treatment can decrease cystine excretion. The best treatment for cystinuria is to prevent stones from forming. Stones can be prevented by drinking enough liquid each day (about 5–7 qts) to produce at least 8 pts of urine, thus keeping the concentration of cystine in the urine low. Because a person does not drink throughout the night, less urine is produced, and the likelihood of stone formation increases. This risk can be minimized by drinking water or other liquids just before going to bed.

Drug treatments

In addition to drinking large amounts of fluids, it is helpful to make the urine more alkaline. Cystine dissolves more easily in alkaline urine. To increase urine alkalinity, a person may take **sodium** bicarbonate and acetazolamide. Penicillamine, a drug that increases the solubility of cystine, may be prescribed for patients who do not respond well to other therapies. This drug must be used with caution, however, because it can cause serious side effects or allergic reactions. For those unable to take penicillamine, another drug, alpha-mercaptopropionylglycine (Thiola), may be prescribed.

Surgical treatments

Most stones can be removed from the body by normal urination, helped by drinking large amounts of water. Large stones that cannot be passed this way must be removed by surgical procedures.

Large stones can be surgically removed by having a device called a uretoscope placed into the urethra, up through the bladder and into the ureter, where the trapped stone can be seen and removed. Another method involves using sound-wave energy aimed from outside the body to break the large stone into small pieces that can be passed by urination. This external technique is called extracorporeal shock-wave **lithotripsy** (ESWL).

For large stones in the kidney, a procedure called percutaneous nephrolithomy may be used. In this procedure, the surgeon makes a small incision in the back over the kidney. An instrument called a nephroscope is inserted through the incision into the kidney. The surgeon uses the nephroscope to locate and remove the stone. If the stone is very large, it may be broken up into smaller pieces by an ultrasonic or other kind of probe before removal.

Prognosis

As many as 50% of patients who have had surgical treatment for a kidney stone will have another stone within five years if no medicines are used to treat this condition.

Prevention

Cystinuria is a genetic disorder that currently cannot be prevented.

ORGANIZATIONS

Cystinuria Support Network, 21001 NE 36th St., Redmond, WA, 98053, (425) 868-2996, sue@cystinuria.com, http://www.cystinuria.com.

National Kidney Foundation, Inc. 30 East 33rd Street, New York, NY, 10016, (212) 889-2210, (212) 689-9261, (800) 622-9010, http://www.kidney.org/.

Dominic De Bellis, PhD

Cystitis

Definition

Cystitis is defined as inflammation of the urinary bladder. **Urethritis** is an inflammation of the urethra, which is the passageway that connects the bladder with the exterior of the body. Sometimes cystitis and urethritis are referred to collectively as a lower **urinary tract infection**, or UTI. Infection of the upper urinary tract involves the spread of bacteria to the kidney and is called **pyelonephritis**.

Description

The frequency of bladder infections in humans varies significantly according to age and sex. The male/female ratio of UTIs in children younger than 12 months is 4:1 because of the high rate of **birth defects** in the urinary tract of male infants. In adult life, the male/female ratio of UTIs is 1:50. After age 50, however, the incidence among males increases due to prostate disorders.

Cystitis in women

Cystitis is a common female problem. It is estimated that 50% of adult women experience at least one episode of dysuria (painful urination); half of these patients have a bacterial UTI. Between 2–5% of women's visits to primary care doctors are for UTI symptoms. About 90% of UTIs in women are uncomplicated but recurrent.

Cystitis in men

UTIs are uncommon in younger and middle-aged men, but may occur as complications of bacterial infections of the kidney or prostate gland.

Cystitis in children

In children, cystitis often is caused by congenital abnormalities (present at birth) of the urinary tract. **Vesicoureteral reflux** is a condition in which the child cannot completely empty the bladder. It allows urine to remain in or flow backward (reflux) into the partially empty bladder.

Causes and symptoms

The causes of cystitis vary according to sex because of the differences in anatomical structure of the urinary tract.

Females

Most bladder infections in women are so-called ascending infections, which means they are caused by disease agents traveling upward through the urethra to the bladder. The relative shortness of the female urethra (1.2–2 in. [3–5 cm] in length) makes it easy for bacteria to gain entry to the bladder and multiply. The most common bacteria associated with UTIs in women include **Escherichia coli** (about 80% of cases), *Staphylococcus saprophyticus*, *Klebsiella*, *Enterobacter*, and *Proteus* species. Risk factors for UTIs in women include:

- Sexual intercourse. The risk of infection increases if the woman has multiple partners.
- Use of a diaphragm for contraception
- An abnormally short urethra
- Diabetes or chronic dehydration
- The absence of a specific enzyme (fucosyltransferase) in vaginal secretions. The lack of this enzyme makes it easier for the vagina to harbor bacteria that cause UTIs.
- Inadequate personal hygiene. Bacteria from fecal matter or vaginal discharges can enter the female urethra because its opening is very close to the vagina and anus.
- History of previous UTIs. About 80% of women with cystitis develop recurrences within two years.

The early symptoms of cystitis in women are dysuria, or **pain** on urination; urgency, or a sudden strong desire to urinate; and increased frequency of urination. About 50% of female patients experience **fever**, pain in the lower back or flanks, **nausea and vomiting**, or shaking chills. These symptoms indicate pyelonephritis, or spread of the infection to the upper urinary tract.

Males

Most UTIs in adult males are complications of kidney or prostate infections. They usually are associated with a tumor or **kidney stones** that block the flow of urine and often are persistent infections caused by drug-resistant organisms. UTIs in men are most likely to be caused by *E. coli* or another gram-negative bacterium. *S. saprophyticus*, which is the second most common cause of UTIs in women, rarely causes infections in men. Risk factors for UTIs in men include:

- Lack of circumcision. The foreskin can harbor bacteria that cause UTIs.
- Urinary catheterization. The longer the period of catheterization, the higher the risk of UTIs.

The symptoms of cystitis and pyelonephritis in men are the same as in women.

Hemorrhagic cystitis

Hemorrhagic cystitis, which is marked by large quantities of blood in the urine, is caused by an acute bacterial infection of the bladder. In some cases, hemorrhagic cystitis is a side effect of **radiation therapy** or treatment with cyclophosphamide. Hemorrhagic cystitis in children is associated with adenovirus type 11.

Diagnosis

When cystitis is suspected, the doctor will first examine the patient's abdomen and lower back, to evaluate unusual enlargements of the kidneys or swelling of the bladder. In small children, the doctor will check for fever, abdominal masses, and a swollen bladder.

The next step in diagnosis is collection of a urine sample. The procedure differs somewhat for women and men. Laboratory testing of urine samples now can be performed with dipsticks that indicate immune system responses to infection, as well as with microscopic analysis of samples. Normal human urine is sterile. The presence of bacteria or pus in the urine usually indicates infection. The presence of hematuria, or blood in the urine, may indicate acute UTIs, **kidney disease**, kidney stones, inflammation of the prostate (in men), **endometriosis** (in women), or **cancer** of the urinary tract. In some cases, blood in the urine results from athletic training, particularly in runners.

Females

Female patients often require a pelvic examination as part of the diagnostic workup for bladder infections. Normally, however, a midstream urine sample of 200 mL is collected to test for infection.

A count of more than 104 bacteria CFU/mL (colony forming units per milliliter) in the midstream sample indicates a bladder or kidney infection. A colony is a large number of microorganisms that grow from a single cell within a substance called a culture. A bacterial count can be given in CFU or (colony forming units).

In recent years, many health providers and insurance companies have adopted telephone treatment of women with presumed cystitis. Trained nurses diagnose uncomplicated bladder infections over the telephone based on the patient's symptoms and a series of questions prepared by physicians. The practice has been found safe and cost-effective.

Males

In male patients, the doctor will cleanse the opening to the urethra with an antiseptic before collecting the urine sample. The first 10 mL of specimen are collected separately. The patient then voids a midstream sample of 200 mL. Following the second sample, the doctor will massage the patient's prostate and collect several drops of prostatic fluid. The patient then voids a third urine specimen for prostatic culture.

A high bacterial count in the first urine specimen or the prostatic specimens indicates urethritis or prostate infections respectively. A bacterial count greater than 100,000 bacteria CFU/mL in the midstream sample suggests a bladder or kidney infection.

Other tests

Women with recurrent UTIs can be given ultrasound exams of the kidneys and bladder together with a voiding cystourethrogram to test for structural abnormalities. (A cystourethrogram is an x-ray test in which an iodine dye is used to better view the urinary bladder and urethra.) Voiding cystourethrograms are also used to evaluate children with UTIs. In some cases, **computed tomography scans** (CT scans) can be used to evaluate patients for possible cancers in the urinary tract.

Treatment

Medications

Uncomplicated cystitis is treated with **antibiotics**. These include penicillin, ampicillin, and amoxicillin; sulfisoxazole or sulfamethoxazole; trimethoprim; nitrofurantoin; **cephalosporins**; or **fluoroquinolones**. (Flouroquinolones generally are not used in children under 18 years of age.) A 2003 study showed that fluoroquinolone was preferred over amoxicillin, however, for uncomplicated cystitis in young women. Treatment for women is short-term; most patients respond within three days. Men do not respond as well to short-term treatment and require seven to 10 days of oral antibiotics for uncomplicated UTIs.

Patients of either sex may be given phenazopyridine or flavoxate to relieve painful urination.

Trimethoprim and nitrofurantoin are preferred for treating recurrent UTIs in women.

Over 50% of older men with UTIs also suffer from infection of the prostate gland. Some antibiotics, including amoxicillin and the cephalosporins, do not affect the prostate gland. Fluoroquinolone antibiotics or trimethoprim are the drugs of choice for these patients.

Patients with pyelonephritis can be treated with oral antibiotics or intramuscular doses of cephalosporins. Medications are given for 10–14 days, and sometimes longer. If the patient requires hospitalization because of high fever and **dehydration** caused by **vomiting**, antibiotics can be given intravenously.

Surgery

A minority of women with complicated UTIs may require surgical treatment to prevent recurrent infections. Surgery also is used to treat reflux problems (movement of the urine backward) or other structural abnormalities in children and anatomical abnormalities in adult males.

Alternative treatment

Alternative treatment for cystitis may emphasize eliminating all sugar from the diet and drinking lots of water. Drinking unsweetened cranberry juice not only adds fluid, but also is thought to help prevent cystitis by making it more difficult for bacteria to cling to the bladder wall. A variety of herbal therapies also are recommended. Generally, the recommended herbs are antimicrobials, such as garlic (*Allium sativum*), goldenseal (*Hydrastis canadensis*), and bearberry (*Arctostaphylos uva-ursi*), and/or demulcents that soothe and coat the urinary tract, including corn silk and marsh mallow (*Althaea officinalis*).

Homeopathic medicine also can be effective in treating cystitis. Choosing the correct remedy based on the individual's symptoms is always key to the success of this type of treatment. **Acupuncture** and Chinese traditional herbal medicine can also be helpful in treating acute and chronic cases of cystitis.

Prognosis

Females

The prognosis for recovery from uncomplicated cystitis is excellent.

Males

The prognosis for recovery from uncomplicated UTIs is excellent; however, complicated UTIs in males are difficult to treat because they often involve bacteria that are resistant to commonly used antibiotics.

KEY TERMS

Bacteriuria—The presence of bacteria in the urine.

Dysuria—Painful or difficult urination.

Hematuria—The presence of blood in the urine.

Pyelonephritis—Bacterial inflammation of the upper urinary tract.

Urethritis—Inflammation of the urethra, which is the passage through which the urine moves from the bladder to the outside of the body.

Prevention

Females

Women with two or more UTIs within a six-month period sometimes are given prophylactic treatment, usually nitrofurantoin or trimethoprim for three to six months. In some cases the patient is advised to take an antibiotic tablet following sexual intercourse.

Other preventive measures for women include:

- drinking large amounts of fluid
- voiding frequently, particularly after intercourse
- proper cleansing of the area around the urethra

In recent clinical trials in humans, a possible vaccine for recurrent urinary tract infections was being tested. The vaccine was administered via a vaginal suppository.

Males

The primary preventive measure for males is prompt treatment of prostate infections. Chronic **prostatitis** may go unnoticed, but can trigger recurrent UTIs. In addition, males who require temporary catheterization following surgery can be given antibiotics to lower the risk of UTIs.

Resources

PERIODICALS

Harrar, Sari. "Bladder Infection Protection." *Prevention* November 2003: 174.

Jancin, Bruce. "Presumed Cystitis Well Managed Via Telephone: Large Kaiser Experience." *Family Practice News* November 1, 2003: 41.

Prescott, Lawrence M. "Presumed Quinolone Gets the Nod for Uncomplicated Cystitis." *Urology Times* November 2003: 11.

Rebecca J. Frey, PhD
Teresa G. Odle

Cystometry

Definition

Cystometry is a test of bladder function in which pressure and volume of fluid in the bladder is measured during filling, storage, and voiding.

Purpose

The urinary bladder stores urine produced by the kidneys. The main muscle of the bladder wall, the detrusor, relaxes to allow expansion of the bladder during filling. The urethra, the tube through which urine exits, is held closed by a ring of muscle, known as the urethral sphincter. As volume increases, stretching of the detrusor and pressure on the sphincter sends signals to the brain, indicating the need for urination, or voiding. Voluntary relaxation of the sphincter and automatic contractions of the detrusor allow successful and virtually complete voiding.

A cystometry study is performed to diagnose problems with urination, including incontinence, urinary retention, and recurrent urinary tract infections. Urinary difficulties may occur because of weak or hyperactive sphincter or detrusor, or incoordination of their two activities. Infection of the bladder or urethra may cause incontinence, as can obstruction of the urethra from scar tissue, prostate enlargement, or other benign or cancerous growths. Loss of sensation due to nerve damage can lead to chronic overfilling.

Precautions

The mild irritation of the urinary tract necessary for insertion of the catheter may occasionally cause flushing, sweating, and **nausea**.

Description

The patient begins by emptying the bladder as much as possible. A thin plastic catheter is then slowly inserted into the urethra until it reaches the bladder. Measurements are taken of the residual urine volume and bladder pressure. Pressure measurements may require a rectal probe to account for the contribution of the abdominal muscles to the pressure recording.

The bladder is then gradually filled with either warm water, room temperature water, saline solution, carbon dioxide gas, or a contrast solution for x-ray analysis, depending on the type of study being done. The patient is asked to describe sensations during filling, including temperature sensations and when the

---

first feeling of bladder fullness occurs. Once the bladder is completely full, the patient is asked to begin voiding, and measurements are again made of pressure and volume, as well as flow rate and pressure.

Preparation

There is no special preparation needed for this test. The patient may be asked to stop taking certain medications in advance of the test, including sedatives, cholinergics, and anticholinergics.

Aftercare

Cystometry can be somewhat uncomfortable. The patient may wish to reserve an hour or so afterward to recover. Urinary frequency or urgency, and some reddening of the urine, may last for a day. Increasing fluid intake helps to flush out the bladder, but caffeinated, carbonated, or alcoholic beverages are discouraged, because they may irritate the bladder lining. Signs of infection, such as **fever**, chills, **low back pain**, or persistent blood in the urine, should be reported to the examining physician.

Risks

There is a slight risk of infection due to tearing of the urethral lining.

Results

The normal bladder should not begin contractions during filling and should initially expand without resistance. A feeling of fullness occurs with a volume of 100–200 mL. The adult bladder capacity is 300–500 mL. The sphincter should relax and open when the patient wills it, accompanied by detrusor contractions. During voiding, detrusor contraction should be smooth and lead to a steady urine stream.

Abnormal results

Inability of the bladder to relax during filling, or low bladder volume, may indicate interstitial **cystitis**, prostate enlargement, or **bladder cancer**. Contraction of the bladder during filling may be due to irritation from infection or cysts, obstruction of the bladder outlet, or neurological disease such as **stroke**, **multiple sclerosis**, or **spinal cord injury**. Diminished sensation may occur with nerve lesions, **peripheral neuropathy**, or chronic overfilling.

Resources

OTHER

"Cystometrogram, Simple and Complex." *HealthGatePage*. www.healthgate.com/HealthGate/free/dph/static/dph. 0085.shtml.

Richard Robinson

Cystoscopy

Definition

Cystoscopy (cystourethroscopy) is a diagnostic procedure that uses a cystoscope, which is an endoscope especially designed for urological use to examine the bladder, lower urinary tract, and prostate gland. It can also be used to collect urine samples, perform biopsies, and remove small stones.

Purpose

Cystoscopy is performed by urologists to examine the entire bladder lining and take biopsies of any questionable areas. Cystoscopy may be prescribed for patients who display the following conditions:

- blood in the urine (hematuria)
- inability to control urination (incontinence)
- urinary tract infection (UTI)
- signs of congenital abnormalities in the urinary tract
- suspected tumors in the bladder
- bladder or kidney stones
- signs or symptoms of an enlarged prostate
- pain or difficulty urinating (dysuria)
- disorders of or injuries to the urinary tract
- symptoms of interstitial cystitis

Blood and urine studies, in addition to x rays of the kidneys, ureters, and bladder, may be performed before a cystoscopy to obtain as much diagnostic information as possible. During the cystoscopy, a retrograde pyelogram may also be performed to examine the kidneys and ureters.

Description

There are two types of cystoscopes used to carry out the procedure, a rigid type and a flexible type. Both types are used for the same purposes and differ only in their method of insertion. The rigid type requires that the patient adopt the lithotomy position, meaning that the patient lies on his or her back with knees up and apart. The flexible cystoscope does not require the lithotomy position.

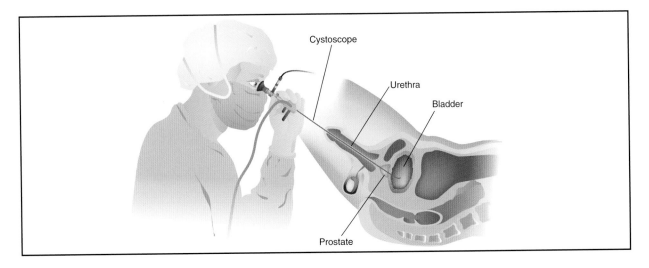

Cystoscope

Urethra

Bladder

Prostate

A cystoscope helps the doctor examine the urethra, bladder, and prostate. *(Illustration by Argosy, Inc. Reproduced by permission of Gale, a part of Cengage Learning.)*

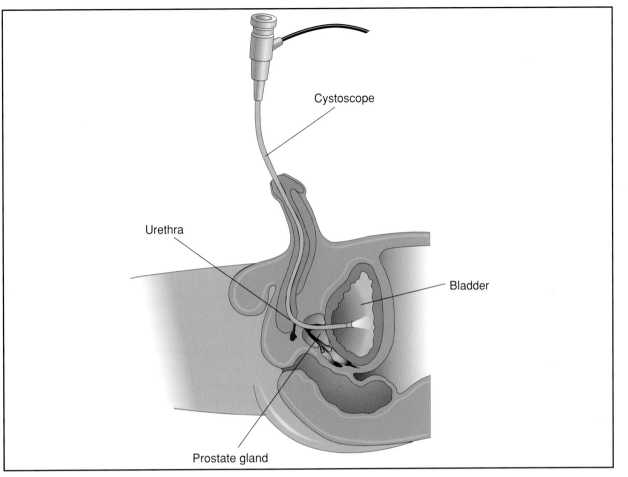

Cystoscope

Urethra

Bladder

Prostate gland

Cystoscopy is a diagnostic procedure which is used to view the bladder, collect urine samples, and examine the prostate gland. This procedure also enables biopsies to be taken. The primary instrument used in cystoscopy is the cystoscope, a tube which is inserted through the penis into the urethra, and ultimately into the bladder. *(Illustration by Electronic Illustrators Group. Reproduced by permission of Gale, a part of Cengage Learning.)*

A cystoscopy typically lasts from 10 to 40 minutes. The patient is asked to urinate before surgery and advised that relaxing pelvic muscles will help make this part of the procedure easier. A well-lubricated flexible or rigid cystoscope (urethroscope) is passed through the urethra into the bladder where a urine sample is taken. There may be some discomfort as the instrument is inserted. Fluid is then injected to inflate the bladder and allow the urologist to examine the entire bladder wall. The cystoscope uses a lighted tip for guidance and enables biopsies to be taken or small stones to be removed through a hollow channel in the cystoscope.

During a cystoscopy, the urologist may remove **bladder stones** or **kidney stones**, gather tissue samples, and perform x-ray studies. To remove stones, an instrument that looks like a tiny basket or grasper is inserted through the cystoscope so that small stones can be extracted through the scope's channel. For a biopsy, special forceps are inserted through the cystoscope to pinch off a tissue sample. Alternatively, a small brush-like instrument may be inserted to scrape off some tissue. To perform x-ray studies such as a retrograde pyelogram, a dye is injected into the ureter by way of a catheter passed through the cystoscope. After completion of all required tests, the cystoscope is removed.

Preparation

Before cytoscopy, patients may be asked to give a urine sample to check for infection and to avoid urinating for an hour before the procedure. A sedative may be given about one hour prior to the operation to help the patient relax. The region of the urethra is cleansed and a local anesthetic is applied. Spinal or **general anesthesia** may also be used for the procedure.

KEY TERMS

Anesthetic—A drug that causes loss of sensation. It is used to lessen the pain of surgery and other medical procedures.

Bladder—The bladder is located in the lower part of the abdomen; it is a structure like a small balloon that collects urine for temporary storage and is emptied from time to time by urinating.

Catheter—A tubular, flexible surgical instrument for withdrawing fluids from (or introducing fluids into) a body cavity, especially one for introduction into the bladder through the urethra for the withdrawal of urine.

Cystoscope—Endoscope especially designed for urological use to examine the bladder, lower urinary tract, and prostate gland.

Diverticula—A pouch or sac occurring normally or from a herniation or defect in a membrane.

Endoscope—A highly flexible, thin viewing instrument used to see inside body cavities.

Endoscopy—A minimally invasive procedure that involves examination of body organs or cavities using an endoscope.

Interstitial cystitis—A chronic inflammatory condition of the bladder involving symptoms of bladder pain, frequent urination, and burning during urination.

Retrograde pyelogram—A pyelography or x-ray technique in which a dye is injected into the kidneys through the ureters.

Ureter—The tube that carries urine from each kidney to the bladder.

Urethra—The tube that carries urine from the bladder to outside the body. In females, the urethral opening is between the vagina and clitoris; in males, the urethra travels through the penis, opening at the tip.

Urogynecologist—A physician that specializes in female medical conditions concerning the urinary and reproductive systems.

Uroradiologist—A radiologist that specializes in diagnostic imaging of the urinary tract and kidneys.

Distension of the bladder with fluid is particularly painful, and if it needs to be done, as in the case of evaluating interstitial **cystitis**, general anesthesia is required. A signed consent form is necessary for this procedure.

Aftercare

After removal of the cystoscope, the urethra is usually sore, and patients should expect to feel a burning sensation while urinating for one or two days following the procedure. To alleviate discomfort or **pain**, patients may be prescribed pain medication, and **antibiotics** may also be required to prevent infection. Minor pain may also be treated with over-the-counter, nonprescription drugs such as **acetaminophen**. To relieve discomfort, patients may be advised to drink two 8-oz glasses of water each hour for two hours and to take a warm bath to relieve the burning feeling. If not able to bathe, they may be advised to hold a warm, damp washcloth over the urethral opening.

Patients who have undergone a cystoscopy are instructed to:

- take warm baths to relieve pain
- rest and refrain from driving for several days, especially if general anesthesia was used
- expect any blood in the urine to clear up in one to two days
- avoid strenuous exercise during recovery
- postpone sexual relations until the urologist determines that healing is complete

Risks

As with any surgical procedure, there are some risks involved with a cystoscopy. Complications may include profuse bleeding, a damaged urethra, a perforated bladder, a **urinary tract infection**, or an injured penis.

Patients should contact their physician if they experience any of the following symptoms after the procedure, including pain, redness, swelling, drainage, or bleeding from the surgical site; signs of generalized infection, which may include **headache**, muscle aches, **dizziness**, or an overall ill feeling and **fever**; **nausea** or **vomiting**; or difficult or painful urination.

Cystoscopy is a commonly performed procedure, but it is an invasive technique that involves small yet significant risk. If anesthesia is required, there is additional risk, particularly for people who are obese, smoke, or are in poor health. Those undergoing anesthesia must inform the doctor of any medications they are taking.

Results

A successful cystoscopy includes a thorough examination of the bladder and collection of urine samples for cultures. If no abnormalities are seen, the results are indicated as normal. In this case, the bladder wall appears smooth and the bladder is seen to be of normal size, shape, and position, without obstructions, growths, or stones.

The treating physician can tell the patient what was seen inside the bladder right after the procedure. If a biopsy sample was taken, this will take several days to be examined and tested.

Cystoscopy allows the urologist to detect inflammation of the bladder lining, prostatic enlargement, or tumors. If these are seen, further evaluation or biopsies may be needed. Cystoscopy with bladder distention can also evaluate interstitial cystitis. Bladder stones, urethral strictures, diverticula, or congenital abnormalities can also be detected.

Alternatives

There are procedures that can provide some information about the lining of the bladder, for example, x rays; however, none of these provide as much information to the doctor as a cystoscopy.

Resources

BOOKS

Khatri, V. P., and J. A. Asensio. *Operative Surgery Manual*, 1st ed. Philadelphia: Saunders, 2003.

Townsend, C. M., et al. *Sabiston Textbook of Surgery*, 18th ed. Philadelphia: Saunders, 2007.

Wein, A. J., et al. *Campbell-Walsh Urology*, 9th ed. Philadelphia: Saunders, 2007.

OTHER

"Cystoscopy." *Harvard Medical School.* http://www.health. harvard.edu/fhg/diagnostics/cysto/cystoWhat.shtml (accessed March 11, 2008).

"Cystoscopy." *Medline Plus.* http://www.nlm.nih.gov/medlineplus/ency/article/003903.htm (accessed March 11, 2008).

"What Is IC? Interstitial Cystitis Fact Sheet." *Interstitial Cystitis Association.* http://www.ichelp.org/whatisic/ICFActSheet.html (accessed March 11, 2008).

ORGANIZATIONS

American Urologic Association Foundation, 1000 Corporate Boulevard, Linthicum, MD, 21090, (410) 689-3700, (800) 828-7866, (410) 689-3800, auafoundation@auafoundation.org, http://www.urologyhealth.org.

American Urological Association, 1000 Corporate Boulevard, Baltimore, MD, 21090, (410) 689-3700, (866) 746-4282, (410) 689-3800, aua@AUAnet.org, http://www.auanet.org.

Interstitial Cystitis Association, 100 Park Avenue, Suite 108-A, Rockville, MD, 20850, (800) 435-7422, (301) 610-5308, ICAmail@ichelp.org, http://www.ichelp.org.

Society of Urologic Nurses and Associates, P.O. Box 56, East Holly Avenue, Pitman, NJ, 08071-0056, (856) 256-2335, (888) 827-7862, suna@ajj.com, http://www.suna.org.

Monique Laberge, PhD
Rosalyn Carson-DeWitt, MD
Brenda W. Lerner

Cystourethroscopy *see* **Cystoscopy**

Cytomegalic inclusion disease *see* **Cytomegalovirus infection**

Cytomegalovirus antibody screening test

Definition

Cytomegalovirus (CMV) is a common human herpes virus. Detected by a blood test, antibodies to CMV are evidence of a current or past infection.

Purpose

Transmission of the virus can occur by coming into direct contact with oral, respiratory, or genital secretions of a person infected with the virus. Consequences of a CMV infection can be devastating in a pregnant woman; a patient who has recently undergone an organ, bone marrow, or stem cell transplant; or a person with human **immunodeficiency** virus (HIV). Blood products that are to be transfused to persons in these high risk groups should be screened for CMV antibodies. Antibody screening helps control the infection risk for these groups.

In a healthy, nonpregnant person, CMV infection is almost never serious. Symptoms, if present, are mild, often resembling **infectious mononucleosis** due to **Epstein-Barr virus**. Antibody screening distinguishes between these two infections.

Description

When first exposed to CMV, a person's immune system is triggered and quickly makes antibodies to fight the virus. Antibodies are special proteins designed to attack and destroy foreign material, in this case, the cytomegalovirus.

The test combines a person's serum with a substance to which CMV antibodies attach. This antibody-antigen complex is measured and the amount of original antibody determined. If positive for antibodies, the serum is diluted, or titered, and the test repeated until the serum is so dilute it no longer gives a positive result. The last dilution that gives a positive result is the titer reported.

A test positive for CMV antibodies means the person has been infected with the virus, either currently or in the past; it does not mean the person has lifetime immunity. After an infection, this virus, like all members of the herpes virus group, can stay hidden inside a person and cause infection if the person's immune system later weakens and antibody protection decreases. In fact, reactivation of such hidden (or latent) infection is not at all uncommon and usually occurs without symptoms.

Transplant patients and people with weakened immune systems, including those with HIV, are vulnerable to infection from several routes, including from another person, from a donated organ or transfused blood, or from reactivation of a past infection. Before transplant, both the recipient and donor are usually tested for antibodies. A recipient who has never had CMV (negative for antibodies), should not receive an organ from a donor who has had CMV (positive for antibodies). CVM infection can be associated with organ rejection, or can cause illness such as **pneumonia**, hepatitis, or **death**. Similarly, blood is usually screened for CMV antibodies before being transfused into a person with a weakened immune system.

CMV infection is the most common congenital infection (existing at birth). The infection, passed from mother to baby, can cause permanent mental or physical damage, or death. The antibody screening test tells a woman whether or not she has antibody protection against the virus in case she is exposed during **pregnancy**. Pregnant women 25 years and older who are immune to CMV are much less likely to pass the virus to their babies than younger women who have never been exposed to CMV.

Tests that measure a specific type of antibody help tell the difference between a current and a past infection. Immunoglobulin M (IgM) antibodies appear at the beginning of an infection and last only weeks. Immunoglobulin G (IgG) antibodies appear 10–14 days later and can last a lifetime. A person suspected of having a current infection should be tested at the beginning of the infection and again 10–14 days later.

KEY TERMS

Antibody—A special protein built by the body as a defense against foreign material entering the body.

Cytomegalovirus (CMV)—A common human virus causing mild or no symptoms in healthy people, but permanent damage or death to an infected fetus, a transplant patient, or a person with HIV.

Titer—A dilution of a substance with an exact known amount of fluid. For example, one part of serum diluted with four parts of saline is a titer of 1:4.

The CMV antibody screening test is also called the transplant reaction screening test. Results are usually available the following day.

A newer test, the anti-CMV immediate early antigen monoclonal test, can detect CMV infection as early as three hours after infection.

It may be possible to test fetal blood for certain antibodies to CMV virus by drawing a blood sample from the umbilical cord. This may be an important test to add to prenatal care, since newborn babies with CMV often show no symptoms.

Preparation

The adult CMV antibody screening test requires 1 mL of blood. Collection of the sample takes only a few minutes.

Aftercare

Discomfort or bruising may occur at the puncture site or the person may feel dizzy or faint. Pressure to the puncture site until the bleeding stops reduces bruising. Warm packs to the puncture site relieve discomfort.

Risks

There are no major risks involved with this testing.

Results

Normal results

A person without previous exposure to CMV will test negative.

Abnormal results

The presence of antibodies means the person has been infected with CMV, either now or in the past. An antibody titer at least four times higher at the end of the illness than at the beginning, or the presence of IgM antibodies, indicates a recent or current first time infection.

People with weak immune systems may not generate antibodies against CMV. A current infection in a transplant patient or a person with HIV is confirmed with other tests, such as viral culture.

Resources

PERIODICALS

Anderson, B., et al. "Knowledge and Practices of Obstetricians and Gynecologists Regarding Cytomegalovirus Infection During Pregnancy—2007." *Morbidity and Mortality Weekly Report* 57, no. 3 (2008): 65–68

Stratta, R.J., C. Pietrangeli, and M. Baillie. "Defining the Risks for Cytomegalovirus Infection and Disease after Solid Organ Transplantation." *Pharmacotherapy* 30, no. 2 (2010): 144–57.

Nancy J. Nordenson
Teresa G. Odle
Melinda Granger Oberleitner
RN, DNS, APRN, CNS

Cytomegalovirus infection

Definition

Cytomegalovirus (CMV) is a virus related to the group of herpes viruses. Infection with CMV can cause no symptoms, or can be the source of serious illness in people with weakened immune systems. CMV infection is also an important cause of **birth defects**.

Demographics

CMV is an extremely common organism worldwide. It is believed that about 60% of people in the United States have been infected by CMV at some point in their lives. Up to 90% of high risk groups, such as male homosexuals, are thought to be infected with CMV. CMV prevalence increases with age.

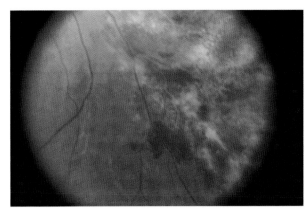

An infected retina of an AIDS patient. Cytomegaloviruses are herpes viruses that can, among other problems, act as opportunistic infectious agents in suppressed immune systems, a common problem with AIDS sufferers. *(Custom Medical Stock Photo, Inc. Reproduced by permission.)*

Description

CMV is found in almost all of the body's organs. It is also found in body fluids, including semen, saliva, urine, feces, breast milk, blood, and secretions of the cervix (the narrow, lower section of the uterus).

CMV is able to cross the placenta (the organ that provides oxygen and nutrients to the unborn baby in the uterus). Because of this, initial infection in a pregnant woman can lead to infection of the developing baby.

Risk factors

Individuals at high risk for infection with CMV include:

- children who attend day care at day care centers
- individuals who work in day care centers
- patients who receive blood transfusions
- organ transplant or bone marrow transplant patients who receive CMV mismatched organs or bone marrow from donors
- individuals with multiple sexual partners

Causes and symptoms

CMV is passed between people through contact with body fluids. CMV also can be passed through sexual contact. Babies can be born infected with CMV, either becoming infected in the uterus (congenital infection) or during birth (from infected cervical secretions). Congenital infection of CMV causes significant neurological problems and deafness in about 8,000 American newborns every year. The virus can also be spread through blood transfusions and during organ transplants.

Like other herpes viruses, CMV remains inactive (dormant) within the body for life after the initial infection. Some of the more serious types of CMV infections occur in people who have been harboring the dormant virus, only to have it reactivate when their immune system is stressed. Immune systems may be weakened because of treatment with **cancerchemotherapy**, medications given after organ transplantation, or diseases that significantly lower immune resistance like acquired **immunodeficiency** syndrome (**AIDS**).

In a healthy person, initial CMV infection often occurs without symptoms and is rarely noticed. If symptoms do occur, they typically occur 9–60 days after the first infection. Occasionally, a first-time infection with CMV may cause a mild illness called mononucleosis. Symptoms include **swollen glands**, liver, and spleen; **fever**; increased white blood cells; **headache**; **fatigue**; and **sore throat**. About 8% of all mononucleosis cases are due to CMV infection. A similar infection, though slightly more serious, may occur two to four weeks after receiving a blood **transfusion** containing CMV.

In people with weakened immune systems, CMV infection can cause more serious and potentially life-threatening illnesses. These illnesses include **pneumonia**, and inflammations of the liver (hepatitis), brain (**encephalitis**), esophagus (esophagitis), large intestine (**colitis**), and retina of the eye (retinitis).

Babies who contract CMV from their mothers during birth rarely develop any illness from these infections. Infants born prematurely who become CMV infected during birth have a greater chance of complications, including pneumonia, hepatitis, decreased blood platelets.

An unborn baby is at greatest risk for serious problems when the mother becomes infected with CMV for the first time while pregnant. About 10% of these babies will be born with obvious problems, including **prematurity**, lung problems, an enlarged liver and spleen, **jaundice**, anemia, low birth weight, small head size, and inflammation of the retina. About 90% of these babies may appear normal at birth. About 20% will later develop severe hearing impairments and **mental retardation**. Pregnant women 25 years and older who are immune to CMV are much less likely to pass the virus to their babies than younger women who have never been exposed to CMV.

KEY TERMS

Cervix—The narrowed, lowest part of the uterus through which a baby must pass in order to enter the birth canal.

Congenital—A condition that exists before birth and at birth.

Placenta—The organ that provides oxygen and nutrition from the mother to the unborn baby during pregnancy. The placenta is attached to the wall of the uterus and leads to the unborn baby via the umbilical cord.

Diagnosis

Tests

CMV can be detected using fluid or tissue cultures, blood testing, antigen assays, qualitative polymerase chain reaction (PCR) testing of blood and tissue samples, and by cytopathology.

Body fluids or tissues can be tested to reveal CMV infection. However, this information is not always particularly helpful because CMV stays dormant in the cells for life. Tests to look for special immune cells (antibodies) directed specifically against CMV are useful in proving that a person has been infected with CMV. These tests do not give any information regarding when the CMV infection first occurred.

A newer test, the anti-CMV immediate early antigen monoclonal antibody test, can detect CMV infection as early as three hours after infection with CMV.

Treatment

Drugs

Ganciclovir (Cytovene) and valganciclovir (Valcyte) are antiviral medications that have been used to prevent CMV in high-risk patients (such as solid organ transplant patients) or to treat patients infected with CMV. Treatment with intravenous ganciclovir is the preferred treatment for CMV. Valganciclovir, which is given orally once per day, may be used to treat some cases of existing CMV and has proved to be very effective when used for CMV **prophylaxis** in high-risk patients. It should not be used in patients with pre-existing **kidney disease**. Another antiviral medication, foscarnet (Foscavir), may be used to treat patients whose CMV infection has not responded to treatment with ganciclovir.

Antiviral drugs are not used to treat CMV infection in otherwise healthy patients because the drugs have significant side effects that outweigh their benefits.

Prognosis

Prognosis in healthy people with CMV infection is excellent.

About 0.1% of all newborn babies will have serious damage from CMV infection occurring while they were developing in the uterus.

Despite lengthy treatment courses with valganciclovir, relapse of CMV disease remains common among organ transplant recipients.

Prevention

Prevention of CMV infection in the normal, healthy person involves good handwashing. Blood products can be screened or treated to insure that they do not contain CMV.

Individuals who engage in high-risk behaviors, such as engaging in sexual activities with multiple sexual partners, should be educated as to their risk for infection with CMV.

Resources

PERIODICALS

Drew, W.L. "Cytomegalovirus Resistance Testing: Pitfalls and Problems for the Clinician." *Clinical Infectious Diseases* 50, no. 5 (March 1, 2010): 733–6.

Eid, A.J., et al. "Clinical Predictors of Relapse After Treatment of Primary Gastrointestinal Cytomegalovirus Disease in Solid Organ Transplant Recipients." *American Journal of Transplantation* 10, no. 1 (January 2010): 157–61.

Fishman, J.A., et al. "Cytomegalovirus in Transplantation—Challenging the Status Quo." *Clinical Transplantation* 21, no. 2 (March-April 2007): 149–58.

OTHER

Akhter, Kauser, and Todd S. Willis. "Cytomegalovirus." *eMedicine*. May 12, 2010. http://emedicine.medscape.com/article/215702-overview (accessed October 3, 2010).

Rosalyn Carson-DeWitt, MD
Teresa G. Odle
Melinda Granger Oberleitner
RN, DNS, APRN, CNS

D

D & C *see* **Dilatation and curettage**

Dacryocystitis

Definition

Dacryocystitis is an inflammation of the tear sac (lacrimal sac) at the inner corner of the eye.

Description

Tears drain into little openings (puncta) in the inner corners of the eyelids. From there, the tears travel through little tube-like structures (canaliculi) to the lacrimal sac. The nasolacrimal ducts then take the tears from the lacrimal sac to the nose. That's why people need to blow their nose when they cry a lot.

Dacryocystitis is usually caused by a blockage of the nasolacrimal duct, which allows fluid to drain into the nasal passages. When the lacrimal sac does not drain, bacteria can grow in the trapped fluid. This condition is most common in infants and people over 40 years old.

Causes and symptoms

In newborn infants, the nasolacrimal duct may fail to form an opening–a condition called dacryostenosis. The cause of dacryocystitis in adults is usually associated with inflammation and infection in the nasal region. Dacryocystitis can be acute, having a sudden onset, or it can be chronic, with symptoms occurring over the course of weeks or months. Symptoms of acute dacryocystitis can include **pain**, redness, tearing, and swelling at the inner corner of the eye by the nose. In chronic dacryocystitis, the eye area may be swollen, watery or teary, and, when pressure is applied to the area, there may be a discharge of pus or mucus through the punctum.

Diagnosis

Dacryocystitis usually occurs in only one eye. As mentioned, the symptoms can range from watery eyes, pain, swelling, and redness to a discharge of pus when pressure is applied to the area between the bridge of the nose and the inner eyelids. A sample of the pus may be collected on a swab or in a tube for laboratory analysis. The type of antibiotic and treatment may depend on which bacteria is present. In the acute form, a blood test may reveal an elevated white blood cell (WBC) count; with a chronic infection, the WBC count is usually normal. To identify the exact location of the blockage,

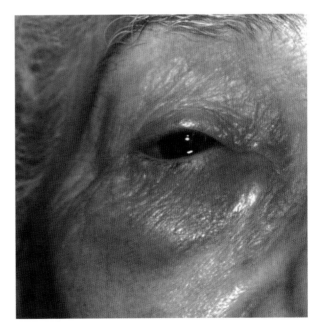

Dacryocystitis of the right eye. The inner corner of the lower lid is bulging from an inflamed tear sac. Blockage of the tear duct causes fluid to be trapped in the tear sac, which becomes infected. *(Custom Medical Stock Photo, Inc. Reproduced by permission.)*

an x ray can be taken after a dye is injected into the duct in a procedure called dacryocystography.

Treatment

A warm compress applied to the area can help relieve pain and promote drainage. Topical and oral **antibiotics** may be prescribed if an infection is present. Intravenous antibiotics may be needed if the infection is severe. In some cases, a tiny tube (cannula) is inserted into the tear duct which is then flushed with a sterile salt water solution (sterile saline). If other treatments fail to clear up the symptoms, surgery (dacryocystorhinostomy) to drain the lacrimal sac into the nasal cavity can be performed. In extreme cases, the lacrimal sac will be removed completely.

In infants, gentle massage of the lacrimal sac four times daily for up to nine months can drain the sac and sometimes clear a blockage. As the infant grows, the duct may open by itself. If the duct does not open, it may need to be dilated with a minor surgical procedure.

Prognosis

Treatment of dacryocystitis with antibiotics is usually successful in clearing the infection that is present. If there is a permanent blockage that prevents drainage, infection may recur and surgery may be required to

open the duct. If left untreated, the infected sac can rupture, forming an open, draining sore.

Prevention

There are no specific recommendations for the prevention of dacryocystitis, however, good hygiene may decrease the chances of infection.

Resources

BOOKS

Gorbach, Sherwood F., John S. Bartlett, and Neil R. Blacklow, eds. *Infectious Diseases*, 3rd ed. Philadelphia: W. B. Saunders Co., 2004.

Altha Roberts Edgren

Dandruff *see* **Seborrheic dermatitis**

Death

Definition

Death is defined as the cessation of all vital functions of the body including the heartbeat, brain activity (including the brain stem), and breathing.

Description

Death comes in many forms, whether it be expected after a diagnosis of terminal illness or an unexpected accident or medical condition.

Terminal illness

When a terminal illness is diagnosed, a person, family, friends, and physicians are all able to prepare for the impending death. A terminally ill individual goes through several levels of emotional acceptance while in the process of dying. First, there is denial and isolation. This is followed by anger and resentment. Thirdly, a person tries to escape the inevitable. With the realization that death is eminent, most people suffer from depression. Lastly, the reality of death is realized and accepted.

Causes and symptoms

The two leading causes of death for both men and women in the United States are heart disease and **cancer**. Accidental death was a distant third followed by such problems as **stroke**, chronic lung disorders, **pneumonia**, **suicide**, **cirrhosis**, **diabetes mellitus**, and murder. The order of these causes of death varies among persons of different age, ethnicity, and gender.

KEY TERMS

Angiography—X rays of blood vessels filled with a contrast agent.

Caloric testing—Flushing warm and cold water into the ear stimulates the labyrinth and causes vertigo and nystagmus if all the nerve pathways are intact.

Electroencephalogram—Recording of electrical activity in the brain.

Hospice—Systematized care of dying persons.

Living will—A legal document detailing a person's wishes during the end of life, to be carried out by designated decision makers.

Stroke—Interruption of blood flow to a part of the brain with consequent brain damage, also known as a cerebrovascular accident (CVA).

Diagnosis

In an age of organ transplantation, identifying the moment of death may now involve another life. It thereby takes on supreme legal importance. It is largely due to the need for transplant organs that death has been so precisely defined.

The official signs of death include the following:

- no pupil reaction to light
- no response of the eyes to caloric (warm or cold) stimulation
- no jaw reflex (the jaw will react like the knee if hit with a reflex hammer)
- no gag reflex (touching the back of the throat induces vomiting)
- no response to pain
- no breathing
- a body temperature above 86 °F (30 °C), which eliminates the possibility of resuscitation following cold-water drowning
- no other cause for the above, such as a head injury
- no drugs present in the body that could cause apparent death
- all of the above for 12 hours
- all of the above for six hours and a flat-line electroencephalogram (brain wave study)
- no blood circulating to the brain, as demonstrated by angiography

Current ability to resuscitate people who have "died" has produced some remarkable stories. Drowning in cold water (under 50 °F/10 °C) so effectively slows metabolism that some persons have been revived after a half hour under water.

Treatment

Only recently has there been concerted public effort to address the care of the dying in an effort to improve their comfort and lessen their alienation from those still living. Hospice care represents one of the greatest advances made in this direction. There has also been a liberalization of the use of **narcotics** and other drugs for symptomatic relief and improvement in the quality of life for the dying.

Living will

One of the most difficult issues surrounding death in the era of technology is that there is now a choice, not of the event itself, but of its timing. When to die, and more often, when to let a loved one die, is coming within people's power to determine. This is both a blessing and a dilemma. Insofar as the decision can be made ahead of time, a living will is an attempt to address this dilemma. By outlining the conditions under which one would rather be allowed to die, a person can contribute significantly to that final decision, even if not competent to do so at the time of actual death. The problem is that there are uncertainties surrounding every severely ill person. Each instance presents a greater or lesser chance of survival. The chance is often greater than zero. The best living will follows an intimate discussion with decision makers covering the many possible scenarios surrounding the end of life. This discussion is difficult, for few people like to contemplate their own demise. However, the benefits of a living will are substantial, both to physicians and to loved ones who are faced with making final decisions. Most states have passed living will laws, honoring instructions on artificial **life support** that were made while a person was still mentally competent.

Euthanasia

Another issue that has received much attention is assisted suicide (euthanasia). In 1997, the State of Oregon placed the issue on the ballot, amid much consternation and dispute. Perhaps the main reason euthanasia has become front page news is because Dr. Jack Kevorkian, a pathologist from Michigan, is one of its most vocal advocates. The issue highlights the many new problems generated by increasing ability to intervene effectively in the final moments of life and unnaturally

ELISABETH KÜBLER-ROSS
(1926–2004)

Kübler-Ross was a contemporary physician who was a world authority on the subject of death and after-death states. Born in Switzerland on July 8, 1926, she worked as a country doctor before moving to the United States. During World War II she spent weekends at the Kantonspital (Cantonai Hospital) in Zürich, where she volunteered to assist escaped refugees. After the war she visited Majdanek concentration camp, where the horrors of the death chambers stimulated in her a desire to help people facing death and to understand the human impulses of love and destruction. She extended her medical background by becoming a practicing psychiatrist. Her formal work with dying patients began in 1965 when she was a faculty member at the University of Chicago. She also conducted research on basic questions concerning life after death at the Manhattan State Hospital, New York. Her studies of death and dying involved accounts by patients who reported out-of-the-body travel. Her research tends to show that while dying can be painful, death itself is a peaceful condition. Her 1969 text, *On Death and Dying*, was hailed by her colleagues and also became a popular best-seller.

In 1978 Kübler-Ross helped to found Shanti Nilaya (Final Home of Peace), a healing and growth center in Escondido, California. This was an extension of her well-known "Life-Death and Transition" workshops conducted in various parts of the United States and Canada, involving physicians, nurses, social workers, laypeople, and terminally ill patients. Much of Kübler-Ross's later research was directed toward proving the existence of life after death. Her publication *To Live Until We Say Goodbye* (1979) was both praised as a "celebration of life" and criticized as "prettifying" the real situation. She also dealt with issues such as AIDS and "near death" experiences. In the mid-1980s, Shanti Nilaya moved from San Diego County, California, to Head Waters, Virginia, where it continues to offer courses and short- and long-term therapeutic sessions. Information on the foundation that bears her name and continues her work can be found at http://www.ekrfoundation.org/

prolong the process of dying. The public appearance of euthanasia has also stimulated discussion about more compassionate care of the dying.

Prevention

Autopsy after death is a way to precisely determine a cause of death. The word autopsy is derived from Greek meaning to see with one's own eyes. A pathologist extensively examines a body and submits a detailed report to an attending physician. Although an autopsy can do nothing for an individual after death, it can benefit the family and, in some cases, medical science. Hereditary disorders and disease may be found. This knowledge could be used to prevent illness in other family members. Information culled from an autopsy can be used to further medical research. The link between **smoking** and lung cancer was confirmed from data gathered through autopsy. Early information about **AIDS** was also compiled through autopsy reports.

Resources

BOOKS

Cecil, Russell L., Lee Goldman, and D. A. Audiello. *Cecil Medicine*. 23rd ed, Philadelphia: Saunders Elsevier, 2008.

Finkbeiner, Walter E., Philip C. Ursell, and Richard L. Davis. *Autopsy Pathology: A Manual and Atlas*. 2nd ed. Philadelphia: Saunders/Elsevier, 2009.

Keegan, Lynn, and Carole Ann Drick. *End of Life: Nursing Solutions for Death with Dignity*. New York: Springer, 2011.

Sheaff, Michael T., and Deborah J. Hopster. *Post Mortem Technique Handbook*. 2nd ed. New York: Springer, 2005.

PERIODICALS

Roger, V. L., et al. "Time Trends in the Prevalence of Atherosclerosis: A Population-based Autopsy Study." *American Journal of Medicine* 110, no. 4 (2001): 267–273.

Targonski, P., et al. "Referral to Autopsy: Effect of Atemortem Cardiovascular Disease. A Population-based Study in Olmsted County, Minnesota." *Annals of Epidemiology* 11, no. 4 (2001): 264–270.

OTHER

American Association of Retired Persons. http://www.aarp.org.

Association for Death Education and Counseling. http://www.adec.org.

Death and Dying Grief Support. http://www.death-dying.com.

National Center for Health Statistics. http://www.cdc.gov/nchs.

ORGANIZATIONS

American Academy of Family Physicians (AAFP), 11400 Tomahawk Creek Parkway, Leawood, KS, 66211-2680, (913) 906-6000, (913) 906-6075, (800) 271-2237, http://www. aafp.org/.

American Medical Association, 515 N. State St., Chicago, IL, 60654, (800) 621-8335, http://www.ama-assn.org/.

American Society for Clinical Pathologists, 33 West Monroe Street, Suite 1600, Chicago, IL, 60603, (312) 541-4999, (312) 541-4998, (800) 267-2727, option 2, info@ ascp.org, http://www.ascp.org/.

College of American Pathologists, 325 Waukegan Road, Northfield, IL, 60093-2750, (847) 832-7000, (847) 832-8000, (800) 323-4040, http://www.cap.org.

Hospice Foundation of America, 1710 Rhode Island Ave., NW, Suite 400, Washington, DC, 20036, (202) 457-5811, (202) 457-5815, (800) 854-3402, hfaoffice@hospice foundation. org, http://www.hospice foundation.org.

L. Fleming Fallon, Jr., MD, DrPH

Debridement

Definition

Debridement is the process of removing non-living tissue from pressure ulcers, **burns**, and other **wounds**.

Purpose

Debridement speeds the healing of pressure ulcers, burns, and other wounds. Wounds that contain non-living (necrotic) tissue take longer to heal. The necrotic tissue may become colonized with bacteria, producing an unpleasant odor. Though the wound is not necessarily infected, the bacteria can cause inflammation and strain the body's ability to fight infection. Necrotic tissue may also hide pockets of pus called abscesses. Abscesses can develop into a general infection that may lead to **amputation** or **death**.

Precautions

Not all wounds need debridement. Sometimes it is better to leave a hardened crust of dead tissue, called an eschar, than to remove it and create an open wound, particularly if the crust is stable and the wound is not inflamed. Before performing debridement, the physician will take a medical history with attention to factors that might complicate healing, such as medications being taken and **smoking**. The physician will also note the cause of the wound and the ways it has been treated. Some ulcers and other wounds occur in places where blood flow is impaired, for example, the foot ulcers that can accompany **diabetes mellitus**. In such cases, the physician or nurse may decide not to debride the wound because blood flow may be insufficient for proper healing.

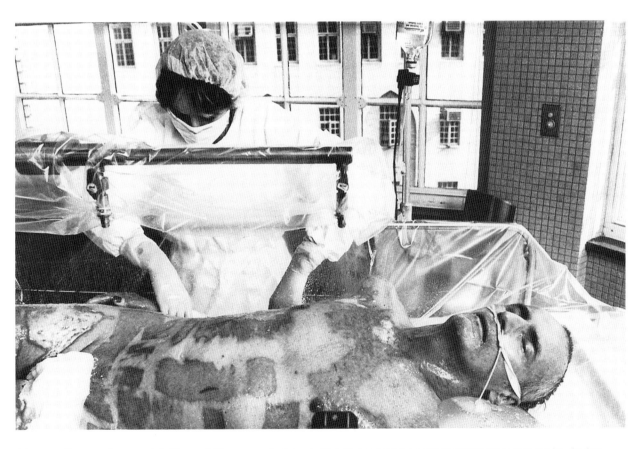

A burn sufferer undergoes debridement (the removal of dead skin). The patterns on his chest are from skin grafts. *(© Ann Chawatsky/Phototake. — All rights reserved.)*

Description

In debridement, dead tissue is removed so that the remaining living tissue can adequately heal. Dead tissue exposed to the air will form a hard black crust, called an eschar. Deeper tissue will remain moist and may appear white, or yellow and soft, or flimsy. The four major debridement techniques are surgical, mechanical, chemical, and autolytic.

Surgical debridement

Surgical debridement (also known as sharp debridement) uses a scalpel, scissors, or other instrument to cut dead tissue from a wound. It is the quickest and most efficient method of debridement. It is the preferred method if there is rapidly developing inflammation of the body's connective tissues (**cellulitis**) or a more generalized infection (**sepsis**) that has entered the bloodstream. The procedure can be performed at a patient's bedside. If the target tissue is deep or close to another organ, however, or if the patient is experiencing extreme **pain**, the procedure may be done in an operating room. Surgical debridement is generally performed by a physician, but in some areas of the country an advance practice nurse or physician assistant may perform the procedure.

The physician will begin by flushing the area with a saline (salt water) solution, and then will apply a topical anesthetic gel to the edges of the wound to minimize pain. Using a forceps to grip the dead tissue, the physician will cut it away bit by bit with a scalpel or scissors. Sometimes it is necessary to leave some dead tissue behind rather than disturb living tissue. The physician may repeat the process again at another session.

Mechanical debridement

In mechanical debridement, a saline-moistened dressing is allowed to dry overnight and adhere to the dead tissue. When the dressing is removed, the dead tissue is pulled away too. This process is one of the oldest methods of debridement. It can be very painful because the dressing can adhere to living as well as nonliving tissue. Because mechanical debridement cannot select between good and bad tissue, it is an unacceptable debridement method for clean wounds where a new layer of healing cells is already developing.

Chemical debridement

Chemical debridement makes use of certain enzymes and other compounds to dissolve necrotic tissue. It is more selective than mechanical debridement. In fact, the body makes its own enzyme, collagenase, to break down collagen, one of the major building blocks of skin. A pharmaceutical version of

collagenase is available and is highly effective as a debridement agent. As with other debridement techniques, the area first is flushed with saline. Any crust of dead tissue is etched in a cross-hatched pattern to allow the enzyme to penetrate. A topical antibiotic is also applied to prevent introducing infection into the bloodstream. A moist dressing is then placed over the wound.

Autolytic debridement

Autolytic debridement takes advantage of the body's own ability to dissolve dead tissue. The key to the technique is keeping the wound moist, which can be accomplished with a variety of **dressings**. These dressings help to trap wound fluid that contains growth factors, enzymes, and immune cells that promote wound healing. Autolytic debridement is more selective than any other debridement method, but it also takes the longest to work. It is inappropriate for wounds that have become infected.

Preparation

The physician or nurse will begin by assessing the need for debridement. The wound will be examined, frequently by inserting a gloved finger into the wound to estimate the depth of dead tissue and evaluate whether it lies close to other organs, bone, or important body features. The area may be flushed with a saline solution before debridement begins, and a topical anesthetic gel or injection may be applied if surgical or mechanical debridement is being performed.

Aftercare

After surgical debridement, the wound will be packed with a dry dressing for a day to control bleeding.

Afterward, moist dressings are applied to promote wound healing. Moist dressings are also used after mechanical, chemical, and autolytic debridement. Many factors contribute to wound healing, which frequently can take considerable time. Debridement may need to be repeated.

Risks

It is possible that underlying tendons, blood vessels or other structures will be damaged during the examination of the wound and during surgical debridement. Surface bacteria may also be introduced deeper into the body, causing infection.

Normal results

Removal of dead tissue from pressure ulcers and other wounds speeds healing. Although these procedures cause some pain, they are generally well tolerated by patients and can be managed more aggressively. It is not uncommon to debride a wound again in a subsequent session.

ORGANIZATIONS
American Academy of Wound Management, 1155 15th Street, NW, Suite 500, Washington, DC, 20005, (202) 457-8408, (202) 530-0659, http://www.aawm.org.
Wound Care Institute, 1100 N.E. 163rd Street, Suite #101, North Miami Beach, FL, 33162, FishmanTamara@ hotmail.com, http://www.woundcare.org.

Richard H. Camer

Decompression sickness

Definition

Decompression sickness (DCS) is a dangerous and occasionally lethal condition caused by nitrogen bubbles that form in the blood and other tissues of scuba divers who surface too quickly.

Description

According to the Divers Alert Network (DAN), a worldwide organization devoted to safe-diving research and promotion, less than 1% of divers fall victim to DCS or the rarer bubble problem called **gas embolism**, air **embolism**, or arterial gas embolism (AGE). A study of the United States military community in Okinawa, where tens of thousands of sport and military dives are made each year, identified 84 DCS and 10 AGE cases in 1989–95, including nine deaths. This translated into estimates of one case in every 7,400 dives and one **death** in every 76,900 dives. DCS symptoms can be quite mild, however, and many cases certainly go unnoticed by divers.

At times the terminology adopted by writers on DCS can be confusing. Some substitute the term decompression illness (DCI) for DCS. Others treat DCI as a label encompassing both DCS and AGE. An older term for DCS is caisson disease, coined in the nineteenth century when it was discovered that bridge construction crews working at the bottom of lakes and rivers in large pressurized enclosures (caissons) were experiencing joint **pain** (a typical DCS symptom) on returning to the surface.

Causes and symptoms

The air we breathe is mostly a mixture of two gases, nitrogen (78%) and oxygen (21%). Unlike oxygen, nitrogen is a biologically inert gas, meaning that it is not metabolized (converted into other substances) by the body. For this reason, most of the nitrogen we inhale is expelled when we exhale, but some is dissolved into the blood and other tissues. During a dive, however, the lungs take in more nitrogen than usual. This happens because the surrounding water pressure is greater than the air pressure at sea level (twice as great at 33 ft [10 m], for instance). As the water pressure increases, so does the pressure of the nitrogen in the compressed air inhaled by the diver. Because increased pressure causes an increase in gas density, the diver takes in more nitrogen with each breath than he or she would at sea level. Instead of being exhaled, however, the extra nitrogen safely dissolves into the tissues, where it remains until the diver begins his or her return to the surface (under some circumstances the extra nitrogen can cause **nitrogen narcosis**, but that condition is distinct from DCS). On the way up, decompression occurs (in other words, the water pressure drops), and with the change in pressure, the extra nitrogen gradually diffuses out of the tissues and is delivered by the bloodstream to the lungs, which expel it from the body. If the diver surfaces too quickly, however, potentially dangerous nitrogen bubbles can form in the tissues and cause DCS. These bubbles can compress nerves, obstruct arteries, veins, and lymphatic vessels, and trigger harmful chemical reactions in the blood. The precise reasons for bubble formation remain unclear.

How much extra nitrogen enters the tissues varies with the dive's depth and duration. Dive tables prepared by the U.S. Navy and other organizations specify how long most divers can safely remain at a particular depth. If the dive table limits are exceeded, the diver must pause on the way up to allow the nitrogen to diffuse into the

KEY TERMS

Gas embolism—The presence of a gas bubble in the bloodstream that obstructs circulation.

Hyperbaric chamber—A sealed compartment in which air pressure is gradually increased and then gradually decreased, allowing nitrogen bubbles to shrink and the nitrogen to safely diffuse out of body tissue.

Lymphatic vessels—Vessels that carry a fluid called lymph from the tissues to the bloodstream.

Nitrogen narcosis—Also called "rapture of the deep," the condition is caused by increased nitrogen pressure at depth and is characterized by symptoms similar to alcohol intoxication.

bloodstream without forming bubbles; these pauses are called decompression stops, and are carefully calibrated. DCS can occur, however, even when a diver obeys safe diving rules. In such cases, the predisposing factors include **fatigue**, **obesity**, **dehydration**, **hypothermia**, and recent alcohol use. People who fly or travel to high-altitude locations without letting 12–24 hours pass after their last dive are at risk for DCS as well because their bodies undergo further decompression. This is true even when flying in commercial aircraft. Many travelers are unaware that to save money on fuel the cabin pressure in commercial aircraft is set much lower than the pressure at sea level. At 30,000 ft (9,144 m), for instance, cabin pressure is usually equivalent to the pressure at 7,000–8,000 ft (2,133–2,438 m) above sea level, a safe setting for everyone but recent divers. Exactly how long a diver should wait before flying or traveling to a high-altitude location depends on how much diving he or she has done and other considerations. If there is uncertainty about the appropriate waiting period, the sensible course of action is to let the full 24 hours pass.

Because the nitrogen bubbles that cause DCS can affect any of the body's tissues, including the blood, bones, nerves, and muscles, many kinds of symptoms are possible. Symptoms can appear minutes after a diver surfaces, and in about 80% of cases do so within eight hours. Pain is often the only symptom; this is sometimes called the bends, although many people incorrectly use that term as a synonym for DCS itself. The pain, which ranges from mild to severe, is usually limited to the joints, but can be felt anywhere. Severe **itching** (pruritis), skin **rashes**, and skin mottling (cutis marmorata) are other possible symptoms. All of these are sometimes

classified as manifestations of type 1 or "mild" DCS. Type 2 or "serious" DCS can lead, among other things, to **paralysis**, brain damage, heart attacks, and death. Many DCS victims, however, experience both type 1 and type 2 symptoms.

Diagnosis

Diagnosis requires taking a medical history (questioning the patient about his or her health and recent activities) and conducting a **physical examination**.

Treatment

DCS is treated by giving the patient oxygen and placing him or her in a **hyperbaric chamber**, an enclosure in which the air pressure is first gradually increased and then gradually decreased. This shrinks the bubbles and allows the nitrogen to safely diffuse out of the tissues. Hyperbaric chamber facilities exist throughout the United States. No matter how mild one's symptoms may appear, immediate transportation to a facility is essential. Treatment is necessary even if the symptoms clear up before the facility is reached, because bubbles may still be in the bloodstream and pose a threat. DAN maintains a list of facilities and a 24-hour hotline that can provide advice on handling DCS and other diving emergencies.

Prognosis

DCS sufferers who undergo chamber treatment within a few hours of symptom onset usually enjoy a full recovery. If treatment is delayed the consequences are less predictable, although many people have been helped even after several days have passed. A 1992 DAN report on diving accidents indicated that full recovery following chamber treatment was immediate for about 50% of divers. Some people, however, suffer **numbness**, **tingling**, or other symptoms that last weeks, months, or even a lifetime. In the Okinawa study, six of the 94 patients experienced "long-lasting" symptoms even after repeated chamber treatments.

Prevention

The obvious way to minimize the risk of falling victim to DCS is to follow the rules on safe diving and air travel after a dive. People who are obese, suffer from lung or heart problems, or are otherwise in poor health should not dive. And because the effect of nitrogen diffusion on the fetus remains unknown, diving while pregnant is not recommended.

ORGANIZATIONS

American College of Hyperbaric Medicine, 9875 South Franklin Drive, Suite 300, Franklin, Wisconsin, 53132, (414) 385-2943, (414) 385-8721, http://www.achm.org.

Divers Alert Network, 6 West Colony Place, Durham, NC, 27705, (919) 684-2948, (919) 490-6630, (800) 446-2671, http://www.diversalertnetwork.org.

Undersea and Hyperbaric Medical Society, 21 West Colony Place, Suite 280, Durham, NC, 27705, (919) 490-5140, (919) 490-5149, (877) 533-UHMS (8467), uhms@uhms@org, http://www.uhms.org.

Howard Baker

Decongestants

Definition

Decongestants are medicines used to relieve nasal congestion (stuffy nose).

Purpose

A congested or stuffy nose is a common symptom of colds and **allergies**. This congestion results when membranes lining the nose become swollen. Decongestants relieve the swelling by narrowing the blood vessels that supply the nose. This reduces the blood supply to the swollen membranes, causing the membranes to shrink.

These medicines do not cure colds or reverse the effects of histamines—chemicals released as part of the allergic reaction. They will not relieve all of the symptoms associated with colds and allergies, only the stuffiness.

When considering whether to use a decongestant for cold symptoms, keep in mind that most colds go away with or without treatment and that taking medicine is not the only way to relieve a stuffy nose. Drinking hot tea or broth or eating chicken soup may help. There are also adhesive strips can be placed on the nose to help widen the nasal passages, making breathing through the nasal passages a bit easier when congestion is present.

Precautions

Decongestant nasal sprays and nose drops may cause a problem called rebound congestion if used repeatedly over several days. When this happens, the nose remains stuffy or gets worse with every dose. The only way to stop the cycle is to stop using the drug. The stuffiness should then go away within about a week. Anyone who shows signs of severe rebound congestion should also contact his or her physician.

Do not use decongestant nasal sprays for more than three days. Decongestants taken by mouth should not be used for more than seven days. If the congestion has not gone away in this time, or if the symptoms are accompanied by **fever**, call a physician.

Do not use a decongestant nasal spray after the product's expiration date. If the product has become cloudy or discolored, throw it away and do not use it. Do not share droppers or spray bottles with anyone else, as this could spread infection. Do not let droppers and bottle tips touch countertops or other surfaces.

Some decongestants cause drowsiness. People who takes these drugs should not drive, use machines or do anything else that might be dangerous until they have found out how the drugs affect them.

In general, older people may be more sensitive to the effects of decongestants and may need to take lower doses to avoid side effects. People in this age group should not take long-acting (extended release) forms of decongestants unless they have previously taken a short-acting form with no ill effects.

Children may also be more sensitive to the effects of decongestants. Before giving any decongestant to a child, check the package label carefully. Some of these medicines are too strong for use in children. Serious side effects are possible if they are given large amounts of these drugs or if they swallow nose drops, nasal spray or eye drops. If this happens, call a physician or poison center immediately.

Special conditions

People with certain medical conditions or who are taking certain other medicines can have problems if they take decongestants. Before taking these drugs, be sure to let the physician know about any of these conditions:

ALLERGIES. Anyone who has had unusual reactions to decongestants in the past should let his or her physician know before these drugs or any similar drugs are prescribed. The physician should also be told about any allergies to foods, dyes, preservatives, or other substances.

PREGNANCY. In studies of laboratory animals, some decongestants have had unwanted effects on fetuses. However, it is not known whether such effects also occur in people. Women who are pregnant or who plan to become pregnant should check with their physicians before taking decongestants.

BREASTFEEDING. Some decongestants pass into breast milk and may have unwanted effects on nursing babies whose mothers take the drugs. Women who are **breastfeeding** should check with their physicians before using decongestants. If they need to take the medicine, it may be necessary to bottle feed the baby with formula while taking it.

OTHER MEDICAL CONDITIONS. Anyone with heart or blood vessel disease, high blood pressure, diabetes, **enlarged prostate**, or overactive thyroid should not take decongestants unless under a physician's supervision. The medicine can increase blood sugar in people with diabetes. It can be especially dangerous in people with high blood pressure, as it may increase blood pressure.

Before using decongestants, people with any of these medical problems should make sure their physicians are aware of their conditions:

• glaucoma
• history of mental illness

Decongestants may have a variety of side effects, and may also interact with other medications the patient is taking.

Side effects

DECONGESTANT NASAL SPRAYS AND NOSE DROPS. The most common side effects from decongestant nasal sprays and nose drops are sneezing and temporary burning, stinging, or dryness. These effects are usually temporary and do not need medical attention. If any of the following side effects occur after using a decongestant nasal spray or nose drops, stop using the medicine immediately and call the physician:

• increased blood pressure
• headache
• fast, slow, or fluttery heartbeat
• nervousness
• dizziness
• nausea
• sleep problems

DECONGESTANTS TAKEN BY MOUTH. The most common side effects of decongestants taken by mouth are nervousness, restlessness, excitability, **dizziness**, drowsiness, **headache**, **nausea**, weakness, and sleep problems. Anyone who has these symptoms while taking decongestants should stop taking them immediately.

Patients who have these symptoms while taking decongestants should call the physician immediately:

• increased blood pressure
• fast, irregular, or fluttery heartbeat
• severe headache
• tightness or discomfort in the chest

• breathing problems
• fear or anxiety
• hallucinations
• trembling or shaking
• convulsions (seizures)
• pale skin
• painful or difficult urination

Other side effects may occur. Anyone who has unusual symptoms after taking a decongestant should get in touch with his or her physician.

Interactions with other medicines

Decongestants may interact with a variety of other medicines. When this happens, the effects of one or both of the drugs may change or the risk of side effects may be greater. Do not take decongestants at the same time as these drugs:

• Monoamine oxidase inhibitors (MAO inhibitors) such as phenzeline (Nardil) or tranylcypromine (Parnate), used to treat conditions including depression and **Parkinson's disease**. Do not take decongestants at the same time as a MAO inhibitor or within two weeks of stopping treatment with an MAO inhibitor unless a physician approves.
• Other products containing the same or other decongestants
• Caffeine.

In addition, anyone who takes decongestants should let the physician know all other medicines he or she is taking. Among the drugs that may interact with decongestants are:

• tricyclic antidepressants such as imipramine (Tofranil) or desipramine (Norpramin)
• the antidepressant maprotiline (Ludiomil)
• amantadine (Symmetrel)
• amphetamines
• medicine to relieve asthma or other breathing problems
• methylphenidate (Ritalin)
• appetite suppressants
• other medicine for colds, sinus problems, hay fever or other allergies
• beta-blockers such as atenolol (Tenormin) and propranolol (Inderal)
• digitalis glycosides, used to treat heart conditions

The list above does not include every drug that may interact with decongestants. Be sure to check with a physician or pharmacist before combining decongestants with any other prescription or nonprescription (over-the-counter) medicine.

Description

Decongestants are sold in many forms, including tablets, capsules, caplets, gelcaps, liqui-caps, liquids, nasal sprays, and nose drops. These drugs are sometimes combined with other medicines in cold and allergy products designed to relieve several symptoms. Some decongestant products require a physician's prescription, but there are also many nonprescription (over-the-counter) products. Ask a physician or pharmacist about choosing an appropriate decongestant.

Commonly used decongestants include oxymetazoline (Afrin and other brands) and pseudoephedrine (Sudafed, Actifed, and other brands). The decongestant oxymetazoline is also used in some eye drops to relieve redness and **itching**.

The recommended dosage depends on the drug. Check with the physician who prescribed the drug or the pharmacist who filled the prescription for the correct dosage, and always take the medicine exactly as directed. If using nonprescription (over-the-counter) types, follow the directions on the package label or ask a pharmacist for assistance. Never take larger or more frequent doses, and do not take the drug for longer than directed.

Risks

Anyone considering taking a decongestant should take a close look at the labels of any already in their medicine cabinet. In 2000, the Food and Drug Administration prohibited over-the-counter sales of medicines containing the decongestant phenylpropanolamine. The medicine is associated with an increased risk of **stroke** in people ages 18 to 49, especially women. Many cold remedies contained this medicine. Contact a pharmacist if there is any question about the ingredients in a medication. Over-the-counter remedies containing phenylpropanolamine should be discarded.

Normal results

The desired result when taking decongestants is the short-term relief of nasal congestion.

Resources

OTHER

Medline Plus Health Information. U.S.National Library of Medicine. http://www.nlm.nih.gov/medlineplus.

Deanna M. Swartout-Corbeil, R.N.

Decubitus ulcers *see* **Bedsores**

Deep vein thrombosis

Definition

Deep vein thrombosis (DVT) is a blood clot in a major vein that usually develops in the legs and/or pelvis.

Description

Deep vein thrombosis is a common but difficult to detect illness that can be fatal if not treated effectively. The disorder is estimated to affect 80 people per 100,000 population annually, but some experts feel this is an underestimate of the disorder because the condition often remains undetected and resolves on its on without complications. About 600,000 people are hospitalized in the United States for DVT each year. If left untreated, DVT can cause pulmonary emboli. This is a potentially fatal complication in which **blood clots** break off, travel through the circulatory system, and become lodged in and block an artery going to the lungs. Each year about 200,000 people die of pulmonary emboli caused by DVT. Deep vein thrombosis is also called venous thromboembolism, **thrombophlebitis** or phlebothrombosis.

Deep vein thrombosis is a major complication in patients who have had **orthopedic surgery** or pelvic, abdominal, or **thoracic surgery**. Patients with **cancer** and other chronic illnesses (including congestive **heart failure**), as well as those who have experienced a recent **heart attack** (myocardial infarction), are also at high risk for developing DVT. Deep vein thrombosis can be chronic, with recurrent episodes.

Causes and symptoms

Deep vein thrombosis is caused by blood clots in blood vessels that form in veins where blood flow is sluggish or has been disturbed, in pockets in the deep

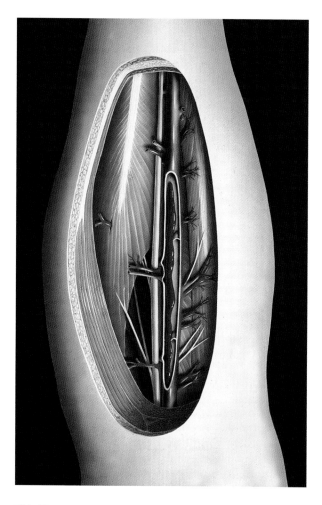

This illustration features a dissected human lower leg showing clot formation (thrombosis) along the length of a vein. *(Custom Medical Stock Photo, Inc. Reproduced by permission.)*

veins of the calf, or in veins that have been traumatized. Symptoms include swelling and tenderness, **pain** in the calf or thigh, and possibly warmth. Fewer than half of all people with the condition experience symptoms, and symptoms tend to be nonspecific (e.g., leg pain may be caused by many other conditions). Some individuals and families have underlying clotting tendencies that can be tested for.

Diagnosis

Deep vein thrombosis can be detected through **venography** and radionuclide venography, **Doppler ultrasonography**, and impedance plethysmography. Venography is the most accurate test, but it is not used much because it is often painful, expensive, exposes the patient to radiation, and can cause allergic reactions and complications. Venography identifies the location, extent, and degree of attachment of the blood clots and enables the condition of the deep leg veins to be assessed. A contrast solution is injected into a foot vein through a catheter. The physician observes the movement of the solution through the vein with a fluoroscope while a series of x rays are taken. Venography takes 30–45 minutes and can be done in a physician's office, a laboratory, or a hospital. Radionuclide venography, in which a radioactive isotope is injected, is occasionally used, especially if a patient has had an allergic reaction to contrast solutions.

Doppler ultrasonography usually is the preferred procedure for detecting deep vein thrombosis. This technique uses sound waves to measure blood flow through leg veins and arteries. A blood pressure cuff is wrapped around the patient's ankle and a transducer with gel on it is placed over pulse points of the foot and lower leg. High-frequency sound waves bounce off the soft tissue, and the echoes are converted into images on a monitor. This procedure is very accurate in detecting clots above the knee that can become pulmonary embolisms. Usually performed in a physician's office or hospital outpatient diagnostic center, Doppler ultrasound takes about 30–45 minutes.

Impedance plethysmography is a noninvasive way to record changes in blood volume and vessel resistance. A blood pressure cuff is wrapped around the leg above the knee, four electrodes are placed near the knee and the ankle, and the cuff is inflated to compress the veins and reduce blood flow. The efficiency with which the veins return to normal is then measured. Performed in a physician's office, impedance plethysmography takes about 15 minutes.

Treatment

Deep vein thrombosis can be treated with drug therapy, bed rest, and gradient elastic stockings. Medications include anticoagulants that "thin" blood to prevent further growth of blood clots, as well as clot-dissolving drugs. Heparin is a common injectable anticoagulant and is usually followed by warfarin (Coumadin) tablets for at least three months. Bed rest with the patient's legs elevated is necessary until the condition improves. Gradient elastic stockings should then be worn, and standing for long periods avoided. In some cases, a filter is surgically placed in the major vein (the inferior vena cava) to trap emboli or clots before they get to the heart and lungs. In another surgical procedure, a catheter is inserted into the vein. When the clot is reached, a balloon at the end of the catheter is inflated, and then withdrawn along with the clot. However, this procedure risks dislodging the clot.

Alternative treatment

Deep vein thrombosis can be life threatening and must be treated with conventional medical therapies. However, some alternative therapies may be used in conjunction with conventional treatments to dissolve the clot. These therapies may help support the body and prevent recurrence. A conventional physician as well as a trained alternative health care practitioner should be consulted due to the severity of this condition.

Prognosis

Complications from DVT can be life threatening or chronically debilitating. Pulmonary emboli develop in about 10% of people with DVT and account for about 10% of all hospital deaths. DVT also can cause inflammation of the blood vessels resulting in loss of contractility and chronically decreased function. On the other hand, about three-quarters of people with DVT remain free of symptoms, and in many cases, the condition resolves with minimal treatment.

Prevention

Deep vein thrombosis can be prevented through prophylactic **anticoagulant drugs** and venous stasis prevention with gradient elastic stockings and intermittent pneumatic compression of the legs. Individuals should avoid standing or sitting for long periods without moving; walking or exercising the legs on long airplane and car trips helps keep blood from pooling in the legs and helps to prevent DVT. High-risk individuals often need to remain on oral anticoagulants (e.g., Coumadin) indefinitely.

Resources

OTHER

"Deep Vein Thrombosis." *MedlinePlus*. February 17, 2009 [cited February 18, 2009]. http://www.nlm.nih.gov/medlineplus/deepveinthrombosis.html

"Deep Vein Thrombosis, Thrombophlebitis, and Phlebitis." *VascularWeb*. 2009 [cited February 18, 2009]. http://www.vascularweb.org/vascularhealth/Pages/Deep Veinthrombosis%28DVT%29.aspx
Wedro, Benjamin C. "Deep Vein Thrombosis." *MedicineNet.com*. April 30, 2008 [cited February 18, 2009]. http://www.medicinenet.com/deep_vein_thrombosis/article.htm

ORGANIZATIONS

American Heart Association National Center, 7272 Greenville Avenue, Dallas, TX, 75231, (800) 242-8721, Review.personal.info@heart.org.
National Heart Lung and Blood Institute Health Information Center, P.O. Box 30105, Bethesda, MD, 20824-0105, (301) 592-8573, (240) 629-3246, http://www.nhlbi.nih.gov.
Society for Vascular Surgery, 633 North Saint Clair Street, 22nd Floor, Chicago, IL, 60611, (312) 334-2300, (312) 334-2320, (800) 258-7188, vascular@vascularsociety.org, http://www.vascularweb.org.

Lori De Milto
Tish Davidson, A. M.

Deer-fly fever *see* **Tularemia**

Defibrillation

Definition

Defibrillation is a process in which an electronic device—which may be an external or an implantable device—sends an electric shock to the heart to stop an extremely rapid irregular heartbeat, and restore the normal heart rhythm.

Purpose

Defibrillation is performed to correct life-threatening fibrillations of the heart or such other **arrhythmias** as **ventricular tachycardia** that may result in cardiac arrest. It should be performed immediately after identifying that the patient is experiencing a cardiac emergency, has no pulse, and is unresponsive.

Precautions

Defibrillation should not be performed on a patient who has a pulse or is alert, as this could cause a lethal heart rhythm disturbance or cardiac arrest. The paddles used in the procedure should not be placed on a woman's breasts or over a pacemaker.

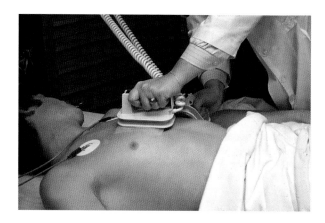

Defibrillation by paddles. *(Custom Medical Stock Photo, Inc. Reproduced by permission.)*

Description

Normal and abnormal heart rhythms

Normal heart rhythm is established by the sino-atrial node (SAN), a group of cells located in the wall of the right atrium (upper chamber) of the heart near the entry of the superior vena cava. The superior vena cava is a major vein that carries deoxygenated blood from the upper part of the body to the heart. The SAN, sometimes called the body's natural pacemaker, discharges electrical impulses at the rate of 60–100 per minute that trigger the contractions of the heart muscle (myocardium). It is the regular contractions of the myocardium that enable blood to pumped efficiently throughout the rest of the body.

The contractions of the heart muscle result from depolarization, which is the change in a cell's membrane potential, making its electrical charge either more positive or less negative. The electrical impulses discharged by the sinoatrial node produce a wave of depolarization that moves from the right atrium to the left atrium and causes these two upper chambers of the heart to contract. The impulses then travel to another node in the heart known as the atrioventricular node or AV node. The AV node functions as a timing device that delays the conduction of the electrical impulses to the ventricles (lower chambers), thus preventing the atria and the ventricles from contracting at the same time. At the end of the cycle, the ventricles of the heart repolarize in preparation for the next heartbeat.

Ventricular fibrillation is a medical emergency in which the muscle of the ventricles twitches randomly rather than contracting in a coordinated manner from the apex of the heart to the outflow of the ventricles. It thus causes the heart to stop pumping blood into the arteries and general body circulation, leading to brain

damage and/or cardiac arrest. The mechanisms leading to ventricular fibrillation are not completely understood as of 2010, and research into this type of cardiac emergency is ongoing. Most episodes of fibrillation occur in diseased or damaged hearts; however, others occur in so-called normal hearts. **Sudden cardiac death** accounts for approximately 300,000 deaths per year in the United States, of which 75–80% are due to ventricular fibrillation. Ventricular fibrillation is linked to more deaths each year in North America than lung **cancer**, **breast cancer**, or **AIDS**.

Emergency defibrillation

About 10% of the ability to restart the heart is lost with every minute that the heart stays in fibrillation. Irreversible brain damage leading to **death** can occur within 3–5 minutes unless the normal heart rhythm is restored through defibrillation. Because immediate defibrillation is crucial to the patient's survival, the American Heart Association (AHA) has called for the integration of defibrillation into an effective emergency cardiac care system. The system should include early access, early **cardiopulmonary resuscitation**, early defibrillation, and early advanced cardiac care.

The AHA has also drawn up guidelines for advanced cardiac **life support** (ACLS), a set of interventions for cardiac arrest and other heart-related medical emergencies. Only qualified health care providers can supply ACLS when needed, as the guidelines require the ability to manage the patient's airway, initiate intravenous treatment, read and interpret electrocardiograms (EKGs), and understand emergency drug administration. The present ACLS provider course requires about 14 hours of classroom work, including simulations, and the successful completion of a written examination.

How defibrillators work

Defibrillators deliver a brief electric shock to the heart, which enables the heart's natural pacemaker to regain control and establish a normal heart rhythm. The defibrillator is an electronic device with electrocardiogram leads and paddles. During defibrillation, the paddles are placed on the patient's chest, caregivers stand back, and the electric shock is delivered. The patient's pulse and heart rhythm are continually monitored. Medications to treat possible causes of the abnormal heart rhythm may be administered. Defibrillation continues until the patient's condition stabilizes or the procedure is ordered to be discontinued.

Some patients with a history of ventricular tachycardia or ventricular fibrillation may benefit from an **implantable cardioverter-defibrillator** or ICD. ICDs, in use since 1980, are small battery-powered devices

Arrhythmia—Any of a number of conditions in which there is abnormal electrical activity in the heart. Some arrhythmias are minor while others are potentially life-threatening. They are also called cardiac dysrhythmias.

Automated external defibrillator (AED)—A portable electronic device that automatically diagnoses potentially life-threatening cardiac arrhythmias (ventricular fibrillation and ventricular tachycardia) and is able to treat them through defibrillation.

Cardiac arrest—A condition in which the heart stops functioning. Fibrillation can lead to cardiac arrest if not corrected quickly.

Depolarization—A change in a cell's membrane potential, making its electrical charge more positive or less negative. Defibrillation essentially depolarizes a portion of the heart muscle, allowing the heart's natural pacemaker to reestablish normal heart rhythm.

Myocardium—The medical term for the specialized involuntary muscle tissue found in the walls of the heart.

Pacemaker—A surgically implanted electronic device that sends out electrical impulses to regulate a slow or erratic heartbeat.

Sinoatrial node (SAN)—The heart's natural pacemaker, a group of cells located in the wall of the right atrium (upper chamber) of the heart near the entry of the superior vena cava, a major vein that carries deoxygenated blood from the upper part of the body to the heart.

Ventricular fibrillation—Uncoordinated contraction of the muscle in the ventricles (lower chambers) of the heart.

Ventricular tachycardia—An abnormally rapid heartbeat originating in one of the lower chambers of the heart. It can lead to ventricular fibrillation.

similar to **pacemakers** implanted by the surgeon in the patient's heart. It is estimated that over a million of these devices have been implanted as of 2010. ICDs continuously monitor the patient's heart rhythm and deliver an electrical shock when the rate of electrical activity in the patient's heart exceeds a preset number. The newest ICDs are programmed to detect the differences among a normal fast heart rhythm, ventricular tachycardia, and ventricular fibrillation. They can correct ventricular tachycardia before it progresses to ventricular fibrillation. The very newest ICDs are implanted under the skin of the patient's rib cage near the heart. Known as subcutaneous ICDs, these devices can deliver enough electricity to correct an abnormal heart rhythm without the need for wires or electrodes placed in or on the heart itself, thus lowering the risk of infection.

Early defibrillators, about the size and weight of a car battery, were used primarily in ambulances and hospitals. The newer automated external defibrillators (AEDs) are smaller, lighter, less expensive, and easier to use than the early defibrillators. They are computerized to provide simple verbal instructions to the operator and to make it impossible to deliver a shock to a patient whose heart is not fibrillating. The placement of public-access AEDs, urged by the American Heart Association, has expanded to cover many public locations in Canada and the United States as of 2010, including corporate and government offices, shopping centers, airports, casinos, hotels, sports arenas, universities, community centers, fitness

centers, health clubs, and even some workplaces. Public-access AEDs often are brightly colored to increase their visibility, and mounted in protective cases near the entrances of buildings. The use of AEDs is now taught in **first aid**, first responder, and basic life support (BLS) level CPR classes as well as in military combat and front line hospitals.

Preparation

After help is called for, the emergency response team begins cardiopulmonary resuscitation (CPR) and continues until the defibrillator arrives. Electrocardiogram leads are attached to the patient's chest. Gel or paste is applied to the defibrillator paddles, or two gel pads are placed on the patient's chest. The caregivers verify lack of a pulse, and select a charge.

Preparation for the implantation of an ICD includes an electrocardiogram (EKG) and a series of other tests of the heart's function to determine what type of arrhythmia the patient is experiencing and whether he or she can benefit from an implanted device. As with most other procedures requiring **general anesthesia**, the patient will be asked not to eat or drink anything for a minimum of eight hours before the surgery.

Aftercare

After defibrillation, the patient's cardiac status, breathing, and vital signs are monitored until he or she is stable. Typically, this monitoring takes place after the patient has been removed to an intensive care or cardiac care unit in a hospital. An electrocardiogram and **chest x ray** are taken. The patient's skin is cleansed to remove gel or paste, and, if necessary, ointment is applied to **burns**. An intravenous line provides additional medication, as needed.

Patients who have received an ICD usually remain in the hospital for one or two days after the procedure so that doctors can test the device for proper functioning. They may need to use over-the-counter **pain** relievers for several days or weeks to relieve soreness after returning home. While patients with ICDs can lead relatively normal lives, they should avoid sports that involve vigorous movements of the shoulder, arm, or torso close to the implant site. They must also avoid equipment that uses large magnets or produces intense magnetic fields. Such equipment includes **magnetic resonance imaging** (MRI) devices.

Risks

Skin burns from the defibrillator paddles are the most common complication of defibrillation. Other risks include injury to the heart muscle, abnormal heart rhythms, and **blood clots**.

The risks of ICD placement include infection; swelling or bruising at the site of implantation; bleeding around the heart, a potentially life-threatening complication; and damage to the vein where the ICD leads are placed.

Resources

BOOKS

Hayes, David L., and Paul A. Friedman, eds. *Cardiac Pacing, Defibrillation and Resynchronization: A Clinical Approach*, 2nd ed. Hoboken, NJ: Wiley-Blackwell, 2008.

Jevon, Phil. *Advanced Cardiac Life Support: A Guide for Nurses*, 2nd ed. Ames, IA: Wiley-Blackwell, 2010.

Sankaranarayanan, Rajiv, Hanney Gonna, and Michael James. *Treatment of Ventricular Fibrillation*. Hauppauge, NY: Nova Science, 2009.

PERIODICALS

Adams, B.D., et al. "Cardiopulmonary Resuscitation in the Combat Hospital and Forward Operating Base: Use of Automated External Defibrillators." *Military Medicine* 174 (June 2009): 584–87.

Andresen, D., et al. "Public Access Resuscitation Program Including Defibrillator Training for Laypersons: A Randomized Trial to Evaluate the Impact of Training Course Duration." *Resuscitation* 76 (March 2008): 419–24.

Hoadley, T.A. "Learning Advanced Cardiac Life Support: A Comparison Study of the Effects of Low- and High-fidelity Simulation." *Nursing Education Perspectives* 30 (March-April 2009): 91–95.

Moss, A.J., et al. "Cardiac-Resynchronization Therapy for the Prevention of Heart-Failure Events." *New England Journal of Medicine* 361 (October 1, 2009): 1329–38.

Stewart, G.C., et al. "Patient Expectations from Implantable Defibrillators to Prevent Death in Heart Failure." *Journal of Cardiac Failure* 16 (February 2010): 106–113.

OTHER

American Heart Association (AHA). *ACLS Provider Course*. http://www.americanheart.org/presenter.jhtml?identifier=3011972

Mayo Clinic. *Implantable Cardioverter-Defibrillators (ICDs)*. http://www.mayoclinic.com/health/implantable-cardioverter-defibrillator/MY00336

Mayo Clinic. *Ventricular Fibrillation*. http://www.mayoclinic.com/health/ventricular-fibrillation/DS01158

Web MD. *Normal Sinus Rhythm Animation*. http://www.webmd.com/heart-disease/healthtool-heart-rhythm-disorders-illustrated-guide

Zevitz, Michael E. "Ventricular Fibrillation." *eMedicine*, January 12, 2009. http://emedicine.medscape.com/article/158712-overview

ORGANIZATIONS

American Heart Association, 7320 Greenvilee Ave., Dallas, TX, 75231, (214) 373-6300, http://www.american heart.org.

Lori De Milto
Rebecca J. Frey, Ph.D.
Brenda W. Lerner

Definitive cancer therapy *see* **Cancer therapy, definitive**

Degenerative arthritis *see* **Osteoarthritis**

Dehydration

Definition

Dehydration is a condition in which the body loses too much water usually as a result of excess sweating, **vomiting**, and/or **diarrhea**. Hydration describes a condition of fluid balance (water homeostasis) when adequate fluid levels are maintained. When fluid balance is not maintained, the individual is said to be dehydrated.

Demographics

The very young and the very old are most likely to become dehydrated. Young children are at greater risk because they are more likely to get diseases that cause **vomiting**, diarrhea, and **fever**. Worldwide, dehydration is the leading cause of **death** in children. In the United States, 400–500 children under the age of 5 die every year of dehydration. The elderly are at risk because they are less likely to drink when they become dehydrated. The thirst mechanism often becomes less sensitive as people age. Also, their kidneys lose the ability to make highly concentrated urine. Older individuals who are confined to wheelchairs or bed and cannot get water for themselves (e.g. nursing home and hospital patients) are at risk of developing chronic dehydration.

Description

Dehydration occurs when more fluid is lost from the body than is taken in. Water is essential to life. Transporting nutrients throughout the body, removing wastes, regulating body temperature, lubrication of joints and membranes, and chemical reactions that occur during cellular metabolism all require water.

Water is distributed throughout three compartments in the body: inside the cells (intracellular), in the tissue (interstitial), and in the bloodstream (intravascular). Each compartment contains differing amounts of electrolytes that must remain in balance in order for body organs and systems to function correctly. Dehydration upsets this delicate balance. Total body water also varies in relation to age, gender, and amount of body fat. Adult males have approximately 60% water content, adult females have 50%, infants have an estimated 77%, and the elderly have 46% to 52%. An increase in body fat causes a decrease in the percent fluid content because fat does not contain significant amounts of water.

The amount of water a person needs to prevent dehydration varies widely depending on the individual's age, weight, level of physical activity, and the environmental temperature. The individual's health and the medications they take may also affect the amount of water a person needs. Most dehydration results from an acute, or sudden, loss of fluid. Slow-developing chronic dehydration can occur, however, most often in the frail elderly and infants and young children who must rely on others to supply them with liquids. Infants are also more likely to develop dehydration than adults because they have a higher metabolic rate and their immature kidneys have difficulty concentrating urine. Children who do not wet their diapers for three hours or more are dehydrated.

Healthy people lose water through urination, elimination of solid wastes, sweating, and breathing out water vapor. This water must be replaced through the diet. The United States Institute of Medicine (IOM) recommended in 2004 that relatively inactive adult men take in about 3.7 L (about 15 cups) of fluids daily and that women take in about of 2.7 liters (about 10 cups) to replace lost water. These recommendations are for total fluid intake from both beverages and food. Highly active adults and those living in very warm climates need more fluid.

About 80% of the water the average person needs is replaced by drinking liquids. The other 20% is found in food. Below are listed some foods and the percentage of water that they contain:

- iceberg lettuce 96%
- squash, cooked 90%
- cantaloupe, raw, 90%
- 2% milk 89%
- apple, raw 86%
- cottage cheese 76%
- potato, baked 75%
- macaroni, cooked 66%
- turkey, roasted 62%
- steak, cooked 50%
- cheese, cheddar 37%
- bread, white 36%
- peanuts, dry roasted 2%

Dehydration involves more than just water deficiency. Electrolytes are ions that form when salts dissolve in water or body fluids. In order for cells to function adequately, the various electrolytes, such as **sodium** (Na+) and potassium (K+), must remain within a very narrow range of concentrations. Often electrolytes are lost along with water. For example, sodium is lost in sweat. To prevent the effects of dehydration, both water and electrolytes must be replaced in the correct proportions.

Risk factors

Risk factors for dehydration in the general population include:

- Geographical location. People lose more water from the body in dry climates and at high altitudes.
- Environmental conditions. Heat waves and natural disasters affecting sanitation can lead to dehydration.
- Occupations requiring outdoor work in warm weather.
- Diseases and disorders that affect the body's water balance. These include diabetes, kidney disease, diseases of the adrenal gland, eating disorders, intestinal parasites, and alcoholism.
- Travel to countries where cholera, dengue, and other diarrheal diseases are endemic.
- Methamphetamine abuse.
- Malnutrition.

Risk factors for dehydration in seniors include:

- Age over age 85
- Living alone and not drinking enough or having access to fluids
- Heavy alcohol consumption
- Taking such medications as diuretics, laxatives, and sedatives
- Having acute or chronic illnesses that affect normal eating and drinking habits
- Are confused or have mental problems or communication problems
- Having difficulty swallowing

Causes and symptoms

There are three basic types of dehydration, defined by the sodium/water balance in body fluids. Doctors who are treating patients with dehydration must determine the type of water loss to ensure appropriate treatment. In addition, water and sodium levels in the body are closely related; if one is abnormal, the other often is too.

Isotonic dehydration is an equal loss of water and sodium. Isotonic means that the number of particles contained on one side of a permeable membrane is the same as on the other side, thus there is no fluid shift in either direction. The amount of intracellular and extracellular water remains in balance. Isotonic dehydration can be caused by a complete fast, vomiting, and diarrhea.

Hypertonic dehydration occurs when water loss is greater than sodium loss. Blood sodium levels may be 145 mmol/l (normal range = 135 to 145 mmol/l). Higher blood sodium levels combined with decreased water in the intravascular space increases the osmotic pressure in the bloodstream, which, in turn, pulls more fluid out of the cells. This type of dehydration is usually caused by extended fever with limited oral rehydration. Mortality is more likely to occur from hypertonic than from isotonic dehydration.

Hypotonic dehydration occurs when sodium loss is greater than water loss. Blood sodium levels may be less than 135 mmol/l; and the osmotic pressure is greater inside the cells, which pulls more fluid out of the intravascular space into the intracellular space. This type of dehydration occurs with overuse of **diuretics**, which causes excessive sodium and potassium loss. Potassium depletion affects respiration, increases **nausea**, and, if severe enough, may cause respiratory arrest or central nervous system (CNS) seizures. Potassium depletion may also cause **arrhythmias** (irregular heartbeat). As a result, patients are told to take diuretics with orange juice or to eat a banana, both of which are high in potassium.

Causes

Diarrhea, often accompanied by vomiting, is the leading cause of dehydration. Both water and electrolytes are lost in large quantities. Diarrhea is often caused by bacteria, viruses, or parasites. Fever that often accompanies disease accelerates the amount of water that is lost through the skin. The smaller the child, the greater the risk of dehydration. Worldwide, acute diarrhea accounts for the death of about 4 million children each year. In the United States, about 220,000 children are hospitalized for dehydration caused by diarrhea annually.

Heavy sweating also causes dehydration and loss of electrolytes. Athletes, especially endurance athletes and individuals with active outdoor professions as roofers and road crew workers are at high risk of becoming dehydrated. Children who play sports outdoors can also be vulnerable to dehydration.

Certain chronic illnesses that disrupt fluid balance can cause dehydration. **Kidney disease** and hormonal disorders, such as diabetes, adrenal gland, or pituitary gland disorders, can cause fluid and electrolyte loss through excessive urination. Such disorders as **cystic fibrosis** or other genetic disorders resulting in inadequate absorption of nutrients from the intestines can cause chronic diarrhea that leads to dehydration. Individuals with **eating disorders** who abuse **laxatives**, diuretics, and **enemas**, or regularly cause themselves to vomit are vulnerable to severe electrolyte imbalances and dehydration. The same is true of people with **alcoholism**. People who have severe **burns** over a large part of their body also are likely to become dehydrated because they no longer have unbroken skin to act as a barrier to evaporation.

Symptoms

Dehydration can be mild, moderate or severe. Mild dehydration occurs when fluid losses equal 3–5%. At this point, the thirst sensation is felt, and is often accompanied by **dry mouth** and thick saliva.

Moderate dehydration occurs when fluid losses equal 6–9% of their body weight. This condition can occur rapidly in young children who are vomiting and/or have diarrhea. In an infant, a loss of as little as 2–3 cups of liquids can result in moderate dehydration. Signs of moderate dehydration include intense thirst, severely reduced urine production, sunken eyes, **headache**, **dizziness**, irritability, and decreased activity.

Severe dehydration occurs when fluid losses are 10% or more of their body weight. Severe dehydration is a medical emergency for individuals of any age. A loss of fluids equaling 15–20% of a person's body weight is fatal. Signs of severe dehydration include all those of

KEY TERMS

Antiemetic—A type of drug given to stop vomiting.

Diuretic—A drug designed to encourage excretion of urine in people who accumulate excess fluid such as individuals with high blood pressure or heart conditions.

Electrolytes—Substances in the body that are able to conduct electricity. Electrolytes are essential in the normal functioning of body cells and organs.

Endemic—Referring to a disease that is prevalent in a particular location.

Hydration—Taking in water or fluid to replace loss of fluid.

Incontinence—Loss of ability to control urination or to control bowel movements (fecal incontinence).

Postural hypotension (orthostatic hypotension)—A sudden drop in blood pressure when rising from a sitting or lying down position.

Rupture—A tear or break in body tissue of an organ.

Water homeostasis—A condition of adequate fluid level in the body in which fluid loss and fluid intake are equally matched and sodium levels are within normal range.

moderate dehydration as well as lack of sweating, little or no urine production, dry skin that has little elasticity, low blood pressure, rapid heartbeat, fever, **delirium**, or **coma**.

Diagnosis

Mild dehydration can often be treated at home. However, a doctor should be consulted whenever:

- A child less than three months old develops a fever higher than 100 °F (37.8 °C)
- A child more than three months old develops a fever higher than 102 °F (38.9 °C)
- Symptoms of dehydration in an older child or adult worsen
- An individual urinates very sparingly, passes dark-colored urine, or does not urinate at all during a six-hour period
- Dizziness, listlessness, or excessive thirst occur
- A person who is dieting and using diuretics loses more than 3 lb (1.3 kg) in a day or more than 5 lb (2.3 kg) a week

A doctor's diagnosis of dehydration includes taking a recent health history, especially checking for the presence of specific illnesses, vomiting, diarrhea, **constipation**, fever, or such other noticeable symptoms as less frequent urination or lack of thirst. The doctor will also want to know about chronic illnesses and current medications.

Examination

In addition to taking the patient's history, dehydration is diagnosed by a **physical examination**. A healthcare professional or observant adult can usually tell by looking at someone that they are moderately or severely dehydrated. Visual signs are often enough to begin treatment.

Tests

Laboratory tests are important indicators of dehydration; blood tests include **complete blood count** (CBC), blood chemistries such as electrolytes (i.e., sodium, potassium, chloride), blood urea nitrogen (BUN), and creatinine, among others. Examination of urine and measurement of a 24-hour urine sample may be done to determine if output is normal or decreased. Heart rate and blood pressure will be measured and an electrocardiogram may be taken to see if heart rhythm is altered. In hospitalized patients with possible dehydration, fluid intake and output may be measured to determine if kidney function is impaired.

Other laboratory tests may be ordered to determine if an underlying condition (e.g., diabetes or an adrenal gland disorder) is the cause of the dehydration.

Treatment

Traditional

The goal of treatment is to restore fluid and electrolyte balance. For individuals with mild dehydration, this can be done in infants and children by giving them oral rehydration solutions such as Pedialyte, Infalyte, Naturalyte, Oralyte, or Rehydralyte. These are available in supermarkets and pharmacies without a prescription. These solutions have the proper balance of salts and sugars to restore the electrolyte balance. Water, apple juice, chicken broth, sodas, and similar fluids are effective in treating mild dehydration. Oral rehydration fluids can be given young children in small sips as soon as vomiting and diarrhea start. They may continue to vomit and have diarrhea, but some of the fluid will be absorbed.

A child who is vomiting should sip one or two teaspoons of liquid every 10 minutes. A child who is less than a year old and who is not vomiting should be given one tablespoon of liquid every 20 minutes. A child who is more than one year old and who is not vomiting should take two tablespoons of liquid every 30 minutes. A baby who is being breastfed should be given clear liquids for two consecutive feedings before **breastfeeding** is resumed. A bottle-fed baby should be given formula diluted with water to half the formula strength for the first 24 hours after symptoms of dehydration are identified.

To calculate fluid loss accurately, weight changes should be charted every day and a record kept of how many times a patient vomits or has diarrhea. A record of fluid output (including sputum or vomit) and of fluid intake or replacement should be kept for at least 24 to 48 hours to see if balance is being accomplished. Parents should note how many times a baby's diaper must be changed. If dehydration continues, emergency department treatment or hospitalization to receive intravenous fluids and electrolytes may be necessary.

Older children who are dehydrated can be given oral rehydration solutions or sports drinks such as Gatorade for moderate and severe dehydration, otherwise general fluids are fine. Athletes who are dehydrated should be given sports drinks. According to the American College of Sports Medicine, sports drinks are effective in supplying energy for muscles, maintaining blood sugar levels, preventing dehydration, and replacing electrolytes lost in sweat. Adults who are mildly or moderately dehydrated usually improve by drinking water and avoiding coffee, tea, and soft drinks that do not contain **caffeine**.

Individuals of all ages who are seriously dehydrated need to be treated by a medical professional. In the case of severe dehydration, the individual may be hospitalized and fluids given intravenously (IV; directly into the vein). Hospital care will include not only immediate replacement of fluids but may also involve treating an underlying chronic illness such as diabetes, kidney disease, or heart disease, which has resulted in fluid loss and dehydration.

Drugs

Treatment of dehydration may involve changing medications that have caused excessive fluid loss. In some cases patients may be given antiemetics or **antidiarrheal drugs** to stop the vomiting or diarrhea that may be causing the dehydration.

Home remedies

People can keep rehydration products in the home in case they are needed. Fluid replacement products that contain essential body chemicals and nutrients are available at pharmacies and some supermarkets; pharmacists can offer advice about the best ones to help correct or prevent dehydration and to restore electrolyte balance.

The World Health Organization (WHO) recommends a homemade solution to help the dehydrated person correct fluid levels and also receive needed sugars and nourishment. To rehydrate the body, the following ingredients can be combined and sipped frequently over several hours:

- 1 quart of water
- three-fourths teaspoon of table salt
- 1 teaspoon of baking powder
- 4 tablespoons of sugar
- 1 cup of orange juice

Prognosis

Mild dehydration rarely results in complications. It can usually be reversed by correcting fluid levels through drinking or receiving fluids intravenously. If the cause is eliminated and lost fluid is replaced, mild dehydration can usually be resolved in 24 to 48 hours.

On the other hand, vomiting and diarrhea that continue for several days without adequate fluid replacement can be fatal since more is lost than water and sodium. Severe potassium loss may lead to cardiac arrhythmias, respiratory distress or arrest, or convulsions (seizures). The risk of life-threatening complications is greater for young children and the elderly. Imbalances in the electrolyte sodium can cause too much water to be absorbed by brain cells, causing them to swell and rupture—a serious complication of dehydration. Underlying chronic diseases can complicate the correction of dehydration, resulting in organ system dysfunction. Severe dehydration can lead to **shock** and kidney failure, which can be life-threatening.

Prevention

Preventing dehydration is easier than treating it once it occurs. Drinking at least eight glasses of water a day prevents dehydration. More may be needed in hot weather. Beginning each day with a glass of water containing a small amount of lemon or other citrus juice helps restore fluid and blood sugar (glucose) levels that have diminished overnight. Water and other clear liquids (tea, juices, and clear soups) can be consumed slowly throughout the day rather than drinking too much at mealtimes, which will dilute digestive juices. Alcoholic beverages and excessive amounts of caffeine–containing drinks, which dehydrate the body, should be avoided.

Another way to prevent dehydration is to be alert to situations in which it could occur, such as exercising in hot weather or vomiting and diarrhea in infants and young children. Athletes and people who work in hot conditions should drink regularly whether or not they feel thirsty. Rehydration of young children should begin at the first sign of fluid loss. A healthcare provider should be consulted before the situation becomes serious. Caregivers of the mobility-impaired elderly and infants and young children who cannot get water for themselves should be offered fluids on a regular basis.

Nutrition/Dietetic concerns

Besides drinking to restore fluid balance, normal consumption of food is necessary when someone is dehydrated. Because intestinal upsets with either diarrhea or vomiting can result in loss of interest in eating or the temporary inability to keep food down or digest it, foods should be kept simple and as soft or liquid as possible, including weak tea, broth, bouillon, plain soups, and lightly cooked vegetables. Large amounts of fluids should not be consumed all at once as this delays gastric emptying and encourages urination. It is recommended that dehydrated individuals sip fluids in small amounts at frequent intervals (e.g. 100–200 mL every 20 minutes) to achieve effective rehydration. Flavored gelatin is often a good fluid replacement and is easy to digest. Such high-fiber foods as whole fruit, bread, grains, and meat should be avoided until the intestinal tract has had a rest. Milk is not a clear liquid and may not be tolerated; milk is not ideal for fluid replacement. Caffeine–containing drinks and alcohol encourage excess urination and should be avoided.

Caregiver concerns for the elderly

Any older individual who has an illness that causes fever, diarrhea, or vomiting may become dehydrated if fluid is not replaced through drinking water and other clear fluids. In these situations, caretakers must always watch for early signs of dehydration such as dry mouth, dark urine, and **fatigue** or irritability. Older individuals may not drink enough for various reasons: They may not feel thirsty; it may be difficult to hold a glass containing liquid; or they may have difficulty getting up from a chair or bed and want to avoid trips to the bathroom. Some elderly people take diuretic medications and have a time during the day, usually morning, when they urinate frequently. Some will not drink because they are incontinent and want

to reduce the possibility of having accidents. Caregivers must always encourage drinking to replace what is excreted or replace fluid loss during certain illnesses through diarrhea, vomiting, or fever. Caregivers should also understand the symptoms of severe dehydration described above and know when to call the doctor or an ambulance.

Resources

BOOKS

"Dehydration." *The Merck Manual of Diagnosis and Therapy,* Section 6, edited by R. S. Porter. White House Station, NJ: Merck Research Laboratories, 2007.

Isaac, Jeff. *Outward Bound Wilderness First-Aid Handbook,* revised and updated. Guilford, CT: Falcon Guides, 2008.

Knoop, Kevin J. et al., eds. *Atlas of Emergency Medicine,* 3rd ed. New York: McGraw-Hill Professional, 2009.

Maughn, Ronald J., and Louise M. Burke, eds. *Sports Nutrition.* Malden, MA: Blackwell Science, 2002.

Panel on Dietary Reference Intakes for Electrolytes and Water, Standing Committee on the Scientific Evaluation of Dietary Reference Intakes, Food and Nutrition Board. *DRI, Dietary Reference Intakes for Water, Potassium, Sodium, Chloride, and Sulfate.* Washington, DC: National Academies Press, 2005.

Rich, Brent E., and Mitchell K. Pratte. *Tarascon Sports Medicine Pocketbook.* Sudbury, MA: Jones and Bartlett Publishers, 2010.

PERIODICALS

Gregorio, G. V., et al. "Polymer-based Oral Rehydration Solution for Treating Acute Watery Diarrhoea." *Cochrane Database of Systematic Reviews,* April 15, 2009: CD006519.

Levine, D. A. "Antiemetics for Acute Gastroenteritis in Children." *Current Opinion in Pediatrics* 21 (June 2009): 294–8.

Scherb, C. A., et al. "Outcomes Related to Dehydration in the Pediatric Population." *Journal of Pediatric Nursing* 22 (October 2007): 376–382.

Wakefield, B. J., et al. "Risk Factors and Outcomes Associated with Hospital Admission for Dehydration." *Rehabilitation Nursing* 33 (November-December 2008): 233–241.

Wotton, K., et al. "Prevalence, Risk Factors, and Strategies to Prevent Dehydration in Older Adults." *Contemporary Nurse* 31 (December 2008): 44–56.

OTHER

Centers for Disease Control and Prevention (CDC). *Guidelines for the Management of Acute Diarrhea.* http://emergency.cdc.gov/disasters/hurricanes/pdf/dguidelines.pdf

Lozner, Alison Wiley. "Pediatrics, Dehydration." *eMedicine,* February 5, 2009. http://emedicine.medscape.com/article/801012-overview

Mayo Clinic. *Dehydration.* http://www.mayoclinic.com/health/dehydration/DS00561

Medline Plus. *Dehydration.* http://www.nlm.nih.gov/medlineplus/ency/article/000982.htm#visualContent

Prakash, Chandra. *Patient Information: Nausea and Vomiting.* http://www.acg.gi.org/patients/gihealth/nausea.asp

Water UK. *Water Requirements in Adults.* http://www.water.org.uk/home/water-for-health/medical-facts/adults

ORGANIZATIONS

American College of Gastroenterology, P.O. Box 342260, Bethesda, MD, 20827-2260, 301-263-9000, http://www.acg.gi.org/.

American College of Sports Medicine (ACSM), P.O. Box 1440, Indianapolis, IN, 46206-1440, 317-637-9200, 317-634-7817, http://www.acsm.org//AM/Template.cfm?Section = Home_Page.

Centers for Disease Control and Prevention (CDC), 1600 Clifton Road, Atlanta, GA, 30333, 800-232-4636, cdcinfo@cdc.gov, http://www.cdc.gov.

International Society of Travel Medicine (ISTM), 2386 Clower Street, Suite A-102, Snellvile, GA, United States, 30078, + 1 770 736 060, +1-770 736 0313, istm @istm.org, https://www.istm.org/.

World Health Organization (WHO), Avenue Appia 20, 1211 Geneva 27, Switzerland, + 41 22 791 21 11, + 41 22 791 31 11, info@who.int, http://www.who.int/en/.

Tish Davidson, A.M.
L. Lee Culvert
Rebecca J. Frey, PhD

Delavirdine *see* **Non-nucleoside reverse transcriptase inhibitors**

Delayed hypersensitivity skin test

Definition

A delayed hypersensitivity test (DHT) is an immune function test measuring the presence of activated T cells that recognize a certain substance.

Purpose

The immune system protects against infection by viruses, bacteria, fungi, and parasites. After initial exposure to a foreign substance, or antigen, the immune system creates both antibodies and sensitized T cells. Both these immune agents respond when the body is reexposed to the antigen. Antibodies, which are circulating proteins, respond within minutes, to give what, is termed an immediate hypersensitivity reaction. T cells responses occur over several days, and are thus called delayed hypersensitivity reactions. The cascade of events initiated by the T cells leads to hardening (induration) and redness (erythema) at the injection site.

A DHT is performed for one of three reasons:

- To test for exposure to specific diseases, such as tuberculosis (TB). Tuberculosis testing is done by injecting into the skin a small volume of TB antigen, which contains no organisms (live or dead) but can still provoke an immune response.

- To test for allergic sensitivity to potential skin irritants, such as poison ivy. Skin allergy testing is usually done by placing a series of adhesive patches on the skin containing potential allergens, or allergy-causing substances.

- To assess the vitality of the T cell response as part of the evaluation of immune system health in infection, cancer, immune disorders, pre-transplantation screening, aging, and malnutrition. DHT can help predict survival in immunocompromised patients, and evaluate the success of restorative therapy. Antigens used for these tests must be ones the patient has been exposed to before, and, therefore, include inactivated antigens from common infectious agents to which the patient might have been exposed, such as mumps, *Candida albicans*, tetanus toxoid, and trichophyton (a skin fungus).

Precautions

No special precautions are necessary for most patients. Those with known hypersensitivity to certain skin irritants should alert the clinician performing the test. Some commercial preparations of fungal antigens contain mercury, a source of irritation to some patients.

Description

The most accurate TB test is the Mantoux test, in which a small amount of TB antigen is injected into the skin. The area is examined 48–72 hours after the injection.

In the patch test, 20–30 adhesive patches are usually placed on the upper back. The patches are kept in place and the area is kept dry for 48 hours. The patches are then removed, and the skin is examined 24 hours afterward, and possibly again a day or more following that. Patch testing is usually performed following a patient complaint of skin irritation from an unknown substance. Testing may suggest several candidates; identifying the right one requires careful review of the patient's possible exposure.

The test of overall T cell responsiveness is performed with several injections. Each area injected is circled and marked. Results are read 48 hours after the injection.

KEY TERMS

Allergen—A foreign substance that provokes an immune reaction in some sensitive people but not in most others.

Anaphylaxis—An exaggerated, life-threatening hypersensitivity reaction to a previously encountered antigen.

Antibody—An immune system protein made to fight infection.

Antigen—A foreign substance detected that provokes an immune reaction.

Preparation

No special preparation is necessary.

Aftercare

Patches should be kept dry. Injection sites may be washed, but excessive rubbing should be avoided. Patches and injection sites may become reddened or irritated. If a patch causes severe **itching** or discomfort, the patient should remove it immediately.

Risks

DHT is quite safe for virtually all people. There is no risk of infection from the agents injected, since they are purified antigens, not whole organisms. Life threatening, hypersensitive reactions (**anaphylaxis**) are a very small risk; patients should notify the administering physician immediately if signs of **wheezing**, swelling, or diffuse redness of the skin develops.

Normal results

Absence of exposure to TB is indicated by absent or very little skin reaction; redness or hardness smaller than 5 mm (about 0.25 in) is considered normal for a person not exposed or infected with TB.

Patch test sites should be normal or only slightly red.

T cell responsiveness tests should be positive; that is, the injected areas should be reddened and hard. Two affected areas of 2 mm or more is considered a positive result.

Abnormal results

TB exposure is indicated by a reaction of 10 mm or more. The degree of redness is not important. A 5–10

mm area could indicate exposure if there is an underlying risk to TB.

Patch test areas that become reddened and irritated indicate reaction to the substance in the patch.

Absence of any reaction to injected areas indicates lack of T cell responsiveness, a condition called anergy. T cell anergy is seen in immune deficiency diseases including **AIDS**, some cases of infectious diseases, malignancies, immunosuppressive therapy (including corticosteroid treatment), some autoimmune diseases, **malnutrition**, major surgery, and some viral immunizations.

Resources

BOOKS

Spickett, Gavin. *Oxford Handbook of Clinical Immunology and Allergy*. Oxford, UK; New York: Oxford University Press, 2006.

Richard Robinson

Delirium

Definition

Delirium is a state of mental confusion that develops quickly and usually fluctuates in intensity.

Description

Delirium is a syndrome, or group of symptoms, caused by a disturbance in the normal functioning of the brain. The delirious patient has a reduced awareness of and responsiveness to the environment, which may be manifested as disorientation, incoherence, and memory disturbance. Delirium is often marked by **hallucinations**, **delusions**, and a dream-like state.

Delirium affects at least one in ten hospitalized patients, and is a common part of many terminal illnesses. Delirium is more common in the elderly than in the general population. While it is not a specific disease itself, patients with delirium usually fare worse than those with the same illness who do not have delirium.

Causes and symptoms

Causes

There are a large number of possible causes of delirium. Metabolic disorders are the single most common cause, accounting for 20–40% of all cases. This type of delirium, termed "metabolic encephalopathy," may result from organ failure, including liver or kidney failure. Other metabolic causes include **diabetes mellitus**, **hyperthyroidism** and **hypothyroidism**, vitamin deficiencies, and imbalances of fluids and electrolytes in the blood. Severe **dehydration** can also cause delirium.

Drug intoxication (intoxication confusional state) is responsible for up to 20% of delirium cases, either from side effects, overdose, or deliberate ingestion of a mind-altering substance. Medicinal drugs with delirium as a possible side effect or result of overdose include:

- anticholinergics, including atropine, scopolamine, chlorpromazine (an antipsychotic), and diphenhydramine (an antihistamine)
- sedatives, including barbiturates, benzodiazepines, and ethanol (drinking alcohol)
- antidepressant drugs
- anticonvulsant drugs
- nonsteroidal anti-inflammatory drugs (NSAIDs), including ibuprofen and acetaminophen
- corticosteroids, including prednisone
- anticancer drugs, including methotrexate and procarbazine
- lithium
- cimetidine
- antibiotics
- L-dopa

Delirium may result from ingestion of legal or illegal psychoactive drugs, such as:

- ethanol (drinking alcohol)
- marijuana
- LSD (lysergic acid diethylamide) and other hallucinogens
- amphetamines
- cocaine
- opiates, including heroin and morphine
- PCP (phencyclidine)
- inhalants

Drug withdrawal may cause delirium. Delirium tremens, or "DTs," may occur during alcohol withdrawal after prolonged or intense consumption. Withdrawal symptoms are possible from many of the psychoactive prescription drugs as well.

Poisons may cause delirium (toxic encephalopathy), including:

- solvents, such as gasoline, kerosene, turpentine, benzene, and alcohols
- carbon monoxide

- refrigerants (Freon)
- heavy metals, such as lead, mercury, and arsenic
- insecticides, such as Parathion and Sevin
- mushrooms, such as *Amanita* species
- plants such as jimsonweed (*Datura stramonium*) and morning glory (*Ipomoea* spp.)
- animal venoms

Other causes of delirium include:

- infection
- fever
- head trauma
- epilepsy
- brain hemorrhage or infarction
- brain tumor
- low blood oxygen (hypoxemia)
- high blood carbon dioxide (hypercapnia)
- post-surgical complication

Symptoms

The symptoms of delirium come on quickly, in hours or days, in contrast to those of **dementia**, which develop much more slowly. Delirium symptoms typically fluctuate through the day, with periods of relative calm and lucidity alternating with periods of florid delirium. The hallmark of delirium is a fluctuating level of consciousness. Symptoms may include:

- decreased awareness of the environment
- confusion or disorientation, especially of time
- memory impairment, especially of recent events
- hallucinations
- illusions and misinterpreted stimuli
- increased or decreased activity level
- mood disturbance, possibly including anxiety, euphoria or depression
- language or speech impairment

Diagnosis

Delirium is diagnosed through the medical history and recognition of symptoms during **mental status examination**. The most important part of diagnosis is determining the cause of the delirium.

Tests

Tests may include blood and urine analysis for levels of drugs, fluids, electrolytes, and blood gases, and to test for infection; **lumbar puncture** (spinal tap) to test for central nervous system infection; x ray, **computed tomography scans** (CT), or **magnetic**

KEY TERMS

Dementia—A loss of mental ability severe enough to interfere with functioning. While dementia and delirium have some of the same symptoms, dementia has a much slower onset.

Electroencephalogram (EEG)—A chart of the brain wave patterns picked up by electrodes placed on the scalp. This is useful for diagnosing central nervous system disorders.

Encephalopathy—A brain dysfunction or disorder.

resonance imaging (MRI) scans to look for tumors, hemorrhage, or other brain abnormality; thyroid tests; **electroencephalography** (EEG); **electrocardiography** (ECG); and possibly others as dictated by the likely cause.

Treatment

Treatment of delirium begins with recognizing and treating the underlying cause. Delirium itself is managed by reducing disturbing stimuli, or providing soothing ones; use of simple, clear language in communication; and reassurance, especially from family members. Physical restraints may be needed if the patient is a danger to himself or others, or if he insists on removing necessary medical equipment such as intravenous lines or monitors. Sedatives or **antipsychotic drugs** may be used to reduce **anxiety**, hallucinations, and delusions.

Prognosis

Persons with delirium usually have a worse prognosis for the underlying disease than the person without delirium. Nonetheless, those without terminal illness usually recover from delirium. They may not regain all their original cognitive abilities, and may be left with some permanent impairments, including **fatigue**, irritability, difficulty concentrating, or mood changes.

Prevention

Prevention of delirium is focused on treating or avoiding its underlying causes. The most preventable forms are those induced by drugs. Strategies for reducing delirium include following prescriptions, consulting the prescribing physician immediately if symptoms

occur, and consulting the physician before discontinuing the drug, even if it has been ineffective; avoiding intoxication with legal or illegal drugs, and seeking professional assistance before suddenly discontinuing an addictive drug such as alcohol or heroin. Maintaining good **nutrition**, which promotes general health, can minimize the likelihood of delirium from alcohol intoxication and withdrawal. Avoidance of exposure to solvents, insecticides, heavy metals, or biological poisons in the home or workplace is also important.

Resources

BOOKS

First, Michael B., and Allan Tasman. *Clinical Guide to the Diagnosis and Treatment of Mental Disorders.* 2nd ed. Hoboken, NJ: Wiley, 2010.

Miller, Bruce L., and Bradley F. Boeve, eds. *The Behavioral Neurology of Dementia.* New York: Cambridge University Press, 2009.

Richard Robinson
Laura Jean Cataldo, RN, EdD

Delta virus hepatitis *see* **Hepatitis D**

Delusions

Definition

A delusion is an unshakable belief in something untrue. These irrational beliefs defy normal reasoning, and remain firm even when overwhelming proof is presented to dispute them. Delusions are often accompanied by **hallucinations** and/or feelings of **paranoia**, which act to strengthen confidence in the delusion. They are distinct from culturally or religiously based beliefs that may be seen as untrue by outsiders.

Description

Delusions are a common symptom of several mood and personality-related mental illnesses, including **schizoaffective disorder**, **schizophrenia**, shared psychotic disorder, major depressive disorder, and **bipolar disorder**. They are also the major feature of delusional disorder. Individuals with delusional disorder have long-term, complex delusions that fall into one of six categories: persecutory, grandiose, jealousy, erotomanic, somatic, or mixed. There are also delusional disorders such as **dementia** that clearly have organic or physical causes.

Persecutory

Individuals with persecutory delusional disorder are plagued by feelings of paranoia and an irrational, unshakable belief that someone is plotting against them, or out to harm them.

Grandiose

Individuals with grandiose delusional disorder have an inflated sense of self-worth. Their delusions center on their own importance, such as believing that they have done or created something of extreme value or have a "special mission."

Jealousy

Jealous delusions are unjustified and irrational beliefs that an individual's spouse or significant other has been unfaithful.

Erotomanic

Individuals with erotomanic delusional disorder believe that another person, often a stranger, is in love with them. The object of their affection is typically of a higher social status, sometimes a celebrity. This type of delusional disorder may lead to stalking or other potentially dangerous behavior.

Somatic

Somatic delusions involve the belief that something is physically wrong with the individual. The delusion may involve a medical condition or illness or a perceived deformity. This condition differs from **hypochondriasis** in that the deformity is perceived as a fixed condition not a temporary illness.

Mixed

Mixed delusions are characterized by two or more of persecutory, grandiose, jealousy, erotomanic, or somatic themes.

Causes and symptoms

Some studies have indicated that delusions may be generated by abnormalities in the limbic system, the portion of the brain on the inner edge of the cerebral cortex that is believed to regulate emotions. The exact source of delusions has not been conclusively found, but potential causes include genetics, neurological abnormalities, and changes in brain chemistry. Delusions are a known possible side effect of drug use and **abuse** (e.g., amphetamines, **cocaine**, PCP).

Diagnosis

Patients with delusional symptoms should undergo a thorough **physical examination** and patient history to rule out possible organic causes (such as dementia). If a psychological cause is suspected, a mental health professional will typically conduct an interview with the patient and administer one of several clinical inventories, or tests, to evaluate mental status.

Treatment

Delusions that are symptomatic of delusional disorder should be treated by a psychologist and/or psychiatrist. Though **antipsychotic drugs** are often not effective, antipsychotic medication such as thioridazine (Mellaril), haloperidol (Haldol), chlorpromazine (Thorazine), clozapine (Clozaril), or risperidone (Risperdal) may be prescribed, and cognitive therapy or **psychotherapy** may be attempted.

If an underlying condition such as schizophrenia, depression, or drug abuse is found to be triggering the delusions, an appropriate course of medication and/or psychosocial therapy is employed to treat the primary disorder. The medication typically includes an antipsychotic agent.

Prognosis

Delusional disorder is typically a chronic condition, but with appropriate treatment, a remission of delusional symptoms occurs in up to 50% of patients. However, because of their strong belief in the reality of their delusions and a lack of insight into their condition, individuals with this disorder may never seek treatment, or may be resistant to exploring their condition in psychotherapy.

Resources

BOOKS

DeLisi Lynn E. *100 Questions & Answers About Schizophrenia: Painful Minds.* 2nd ed. Sudbury, MA: Jones & Bartlett, 2009.

Graham, George. *The Disordered Mind: An Introduction to Philosophy of Mind and Mental Illness.* New York: Routledge, 2010.

Wootton, Tom, et al. *Bipolar In Order: Looking At Depression, Mania, Hallucination, and Delusion From The Other Side.* Tiburon, CA: Bipolar Advantage, 2010.

ORGANIZATIONS

American Psychiatric Association, 1000 Wilson Boulevard, Suite 1825, Arlington, VA, 22209, (703) 907-7300, apa@psych.org, http://www.psych.org.

National Alliance on Mental Illness (NAMI), Colonial Place Three, 2107 Wilson Blvd., Suite 300, Arlington, VA, 22201, (703) 524-7600, (800) 950-NAMI (6264), (703) 524-9094, http://www.nami.org.

National Institute of Mental Health (NIMH), 6001 Executive Boulevard, Room 8184, MSC 9663, Bethesda, MD, 20892, (301) 443-4513, (866) 615-6464, (301) 443-4279, nimhinfo@nih.gov, http://www.nimh.nih.gov.

National Mental Health Association (NMHA), 2000 N. Beauregard Street, 6th Floor, Alexandria, VA, 22311, (703) 684-7722, (800) 969-NMHA, (703) 684-5968, http://www1.nmha.org.

Paula Anne Ford-Martin
Laura Jean Cataldo, RN, EdD

Dementia

Definition

Dementia is a condition characterized by a progressive, irreversible decline in mental ability, accompanied by changes in behavior, personality, and in the late stage, motor functions. There is commonly a loss of memory and skills required to carry out activities of daily living. These declining changes are severe enough to impair the ability of a person to perform a function or to interact socially. This operating definition encompasses 70–80 different types of dementia. They include changes due to diseases (e.g., **Alzheimer** and **Creutzfeldt-Jakob** diseases), changes due to **stroke** or repeated blows to the head (as suffered by boxers), and damage due to long-term alcohol **abuse**.

Demographics

The prevalence of dementia increases rapidly with age. It affects about 1% of people age 60–64 and approximately doubles every five years after age 60. By age 85, dementia affects between 30% and 50% of the population, or about five million individuals in the United States. The condition is somewhat more common among women than men. Some studies suggest that the risk for dementia is higher among African Americans and Hispanic Americans than it is for Caucasians. More than half of all nursing home admissions occur because of dementia. Surveys have found that dementia is the condition most feared by older adults in the United States.

The demographic distribution of dementia varies somewhat according to its cause. Moreover, recent research indicates that dementia in many individuals has overlapping causes, so that it is not always easy to assess the true rates of occurrence of the different types. For example, Alzheimer disease (AD) and multi-infarct dementia (MID) are found together in about 15–20% of cases.

Alzheimer disease

AD is by far the most common cause of dementia in the elderly, accounting for 60–80% of cases. It is estimated that about 5 million adults in the United States suffer from AD. The disease strikes women more often than men, but researchers do not know yet whether the sex ratio simply reflects the fact that women tend to live longer than men or whether female sex is itself a risk factor for AD.

Multi-infarct dementia

MID is responsible for between 15% and 20% of cases of dementia (not counting cases in which it coexists with AD). Unlike AD, MID is more common in men than in women. Diabetes, high blood pressure, a history of **smoking**, and heart disease are all risk factors for MID. Researchers in Sweden have suggested that MID is underdiagnosed, and may coexist with other dementias more frequently than is presently recognized.

Dementia with Lewy bodies

Dementia with Lewy bodies is now thought to be the second most common form of dementia after Alzheimer disease, but because researchers do not completely understand the relationship between Lewy bodies, AD, and **Parkinson's disease**, the demographic distribution of this type of dementia is also unclear.

Other dementias

FLD, Pick disease, **Huntington disease**, Parkinson's disease, HIV infection, **alcoholism**, head trauma, and other causes of dementia account for about 10% of all cases. In FLD and Pick dementia, women appear to be affected slightly more often than men.

Description

The definition of dementia has become more inclusive over the past several decades. Whereas earlier descriptions of dementia emphasized **memory loss**, the current *Diagnostic and Statistical Manual of Mental Disorders, Text Revision (DSM-IV-TR)* of the American Psychiatric Association defines dementia as an overall decline in intellectual function, including difficulties with language, simple calculations, planning and judgment, and abstract reasoning, as well as loss of memory. Dementia is not caused simply by **aging**, although it is quite common in older people. Many researchers regard it as resulting from injuries, infections, brain diseases, tumors, biochemical changes within the brain, or other disorders.

One of the challenges for health care professionals is to differentiate the early-stage cognitive deficits of dementia from normal age-related memory impairment. Individuals with age-related memory impairment may tend to learn new information more slowly, given additional time, their cognitive performance usually is adequate. Other problems that may be mistakenly labeled dementia include **delirium, psychosis**, depression, and the side effects of various medications

Dementia can be caused by as many as eighty different diseases and conditions, ranging from dietary deficiencies and metabolic disorders to head injuries and inherited diseases. The possible causes of dementia can be categorized as follows:

- Primary dementia. These dementias are characterized by damage to or wasting away of the brain tissue itself. They include Alzheimer disease (AD), Pick disease, and frontal lobe dementia (FLD).
- Multi-infarct dementia (MID). Sometimes called vascular dementia, this type is caused by blood clots in the small blood vessels of the brain. When the clots cut off the blood supply to the brain tissue, the brain cells are damaged and may die.
- Lewy body dementia. Lewy bodies are areas of injury found on damaged nerve cells in certain parts of the brain. They are associated with AD and Parkinson's disease, but researchers do not yet know whether dementia with Lewy bodies is a distinct type of dementia or a variation of AD or Parkinson's disease.
- Dementia related to alcoholism or exposure to heavy metals (e.g., arsenic, antimony, bismuth, mercury).
- Dementia related to infectious diseases. These infections may be caused by viruses (e.g., HIV, viral

encephalitis); spirochetes (e.g., Lyme disease, syphilis); or prions (e.g., Creutzfeldt-Jakob disease).
- Dementia related to abnormalities in the structure of the brain. These may include a buildup of spinal fluid in the brain (hydrocephalus), tumors, or blood collecting beneath the membrane that covers the brain (subdural hematoma).

Dementia may also be associated with depression, low levels of thyroid hormone, niacin, or vitamin (B_{12}) deficiency. Dementia related to these conditions is often reversible.

Risk factors

Genetic factors play a role in several types of dementia, but the importance of these factors in the development of the dementia varies considerably. Alzheimer disease (AD) is known, for example, to have an autosomal (non-sex-related) dominant pattern in most early-onset cases as well as in some late-onset cases, and to show different degrees of penetrance (frequency of expression) in late-life cases. Researchers have not yet discovered how the genes associated with dementia interact with other risk factors to produce or trigger the dementia. One non-genetic risk factor presently being investigated is toxic substances in the environment.

Causes and symptoms

As indicated above, there are many different causes of dementia. What they all have in common is damage to or degeneration of nerve cells in the brain.

Dementia is marked by a gradual impoverishment of thought and other mental activities. Losses eventually affect virtually every aspect of mental functioning. The slow progression of dementia is in contrast with delirium, which involves some of the same symptoms, but has a very rapid onset and fluctuating course with alteration in the level of consciousness. However, delirium may occur with dementia, especially since the person with dementia is more susceptible to the delirium-inducing effects of many types of drugs.

Early-onset Alzheimer disease

In early-onset AD, which accounts for 2–7% of cases of AD, the symptoms develop before age 60. Early-onset AD usually is caused by an inherited genetic mutation. Early-onset AD is also associated with **Down syndrome**, in that persons with trisomy 21 (three forms of human chromosome 21 instead of a pair) often develop early-onset AD.

Late-onset Alzheimer disease

Research indicates that late-onset Alzheimer disease is a polygenic disorder; that is, its development is influenced by more than one gene. It has been known since 1993 that a specific form of a gene for apolipoprotein E (APOE) on human chromosome 19 is a genetic risk factor for late-onset AD. In 1998 researchers at the University of Pittsburgh reported on another gene that controls the production of bleomycin hydrolase (BH) as a second genetic risk factor that acts independently of the APOE gene. In December 2000, three separate research studies reported that a gene on chromosome 10 that may affect the processing of amyloid-beta protein is also involved in the development of late-onset AD. Research in the genetic factors affecting AD is ongoing.

Multi-infarct dementia (MID)

While the chief risk factors for MID are high blood pressure, advanced age, and male sex, there is an inherited form of MID called CADASIL, which stands for cerebral autosomal dominant arteriopathy with subcortical infarcts and leukoencephalopathy. CADASIL can cause psychiatric disturbances and severe headaches as well as dementia.

Several studies have documented a link between elevated levels of an amino acid called **homocysteine** in the blood and the risk of developing dementia, likely vascular dementia. As homocysteine concentration can be modified by diet, the finding holds the potential that one risk factor for dementia may be controllable.

Frontal lobe dementias

Researchers think that between 25% and 50% of cases of frontal lobe dementia involve genetic factors. Pick dementia appears to have a much smaller genetic component than FLD. It is not yet known what other risk factors combine with inherited traits to influence the development of frontal lobe dementias.

Familial British dementia (FBD)

FBD is a rare autosomal dominant disorder that was first reported in the 1940s in a large British family extending over nine generations. FBD resembles Alzheimer in that the individual develops a progressive dementia related to amyloid deposits in the brain. In 1999 a mutated gene that produces the amyloid responsible for FBD was discovered on human chromosome 13. Studies of this mutation may yield further clues to the development of Alzheimer disease as well as FBD itself.

Creutzfeldt-Jakob disease

Although Creutzfeldt-Jakob disease is caused by a prion, researchers think that 5–15% of cases may have a genetic component.

Symptoms

The *DSM-IV-TR* specifies that certain criteria must be met for a individual to be diagnosed with dementia. One criterion is significant weakening of the individual's memory with regard to learning new information as well as recalling previously learned information. In addition, the individual must be found to have one or more of the following disturbances:

- Aphasia. Aphasia refers to loss of language function. People with dementia may use vague words like "it" or "thing" often because they cannot recall the exact name of an object. They also may echo what other people say, or repeat a word or phrase over and over. People in the later stages of dementia may totally stop speaking.

- Apraxia. Apraxia refers to loss of the ability to perform intentional movements even though the person is not paralyzed, has not lost their sense of touch, and knows what they are trying to do. For example, a individual with apraxia may stop brushing their teeth, or have trouble tying their shoelaces.

- Agnosia. Agnosia refers to loss of the ability to recognize objects even though the person's sight and sense of touch are normal. People with severe agnosia may fail to recognize family members or their own face reflected in a mirror.

- Problems with abstract thinking and complex behavior. This criterion refers to the loss of the ability to make plans, carry out the steps of a task in the proper order, make appropriate decisions, evaluate situations, show good judgment, etc. For example, a person with dementia might light a stove burner under a saucepan before putting food or water in the pan or be unable to record checks and balance his or her checkbook.

The *DSM-IV-TR* also specifies that these disturbances must be severe enough to cause problems in the person's daily life, and these disturbances they must represent a decline from a previously higher level of functioning.

The following sections will focus on the signs and symptoms that are used to differentiate among the various types of dementia during a diagnostic evaluation.

ALZHEIMER DISEASE. Dementia related to AD often progresses slowly; it may be accompanied by irritability, wide mood swings, and personality changes in the early stage. In second-stage AD, the individual typically gets

KEY TERMS

Agnosia—Loss of the ability to recognize objects by use of the physical senses.

Amyloid—A waxy translucent substance composed mostly of protein, that forms plaques (abnormal deposits) in the brain.

Aphasia—Loss of previously acquired ability to speak, or to understand written or spoken language.

Apraxia—Impairment of the ability to make purposeful movements, but not paralysis or loss of sensation.

Creutzfeldt-Jakob disease—A degenerative disease of the central nervous system caused by a prion, or "slow virus."

Delirium—A disturbance of consciousness marked by confusion, difficulty paying attention, delusions, hallucinations, or restlessness. It can be distinguished from dementia by its relatively sudden onset and variation in the severity of the symptoms.

Hematoma—An accumulation of blood, often clotted, in a body tissue or organ, usually caused by a break or tear in a blood vessel.

Huntington disease—A midlife-onset inherited disorder characterized by progressive dementia and loss of control over voluntary movements. It is sometimes called Huntington's chorea.

Hydrocephalus—The excess accumulation of cerebrospinal fluid around the brain, often causing enlargement of the head.

Lewy bodies—Areas of injury found on damaged nerve cells in certain parts of the brain associated with dementia.

Multi-infarct dementia—Dementia caused by damage to brain tissue resulting from a series of blood clots or clogs in the blood vessels. It is also called vascular dementia.

Parkinson's disease—A disease of the nervous system most common in people over 60, characterized by a shuffling gait, trembling of the fingers and hands, and muscle stiffness. It may be related in some way to Lewy body dementia.

Pick's disease—A rare type of primary dementia that affects the frontal lobes of the brain. It is characterized by a progressive loss of social skills, language, and memory, leading to personality changes and sometimes loss of moral judgment.

Pseudodementia—A term for a depression with symptoms resembling those of dementia. The term dementia of depression is now preferred.

lost easily, is completely disoriented with regard to time and space, and may become angry, uncooperative, or aggressive. In final-stage AD, the individual is completely bedridden, has lost control over bowel and bladder functions, and may be unable to swallow or eat. The risk of seizures increases as the individual progresses from early to end-stage AD. **Death** usually results from an infection or **malnutrition**.

Multi-infarct dementia

In MID, symptoms are more likely to occur after age 70. In the early stages, the individual retains his or her personality more fully than a individual with AD. Another distinctive feature of this type of dementia is that it often progresses in a stepwise fashion; that is, the individual shows rapid changes in functioning, then remains at a plateau for awhile rather than showing a continuous decline. The symptoms of MID may also have a "patchy" quality; that is, some of the individual's mental functions may be severely affected while others are relatively undamaged. Other symptoms of MID include exaggerated reflexes, an abnormal gait (manner of walking), loss of bladder or bowel control, and inappropriate laughing or crying.

Dementia with Lewy bodies

This type of dementia may combine some features of AD, such as severe memory loss and confusion, with certain symptoms associated with Parkinson's disease including stiff muscles, a shuffling gait, and trembling or shaking of the hands. Visual **hallucinations** may be one of the first symptoms of dementia with Lewy bodies.

Frontal lobe dementias

The frontal lobe dementias are gradual in onset. Pick dementia is most likely to develop in persons between ages 40 and 60, while FLD typically begins before age 65. The first symptoms of the frontal lobe dementias often include socially inappropriate behavior (e.g., rude remarks, sexual acting-out, lack of personal hygiene). Individuals often are obsessed with eating and may put non-food items in their mouths as well as making frequent sucking or smacking noises. In the later stages of frontal lobe dementia or Pick's disease, the individual may develop muscle weakness, twitching, and **delusions** or hallucinations.

Creutzfeldt-Jakob disease

The dementia associated with Creutzfeldt-Jakob disease occurs most often in persons between ages 40 and 60. It is typically preceded by a period of several weeks in which the individual complains of unusual tiredness, **anxiety**, loss of appetite, or difficulty concentrating. This type of dementia also usually progresses much more rapidly than other dementias, usually over a span of a few months.

In some cases, a patient's primary physician may be able to diagnose the dementia; in many instances, however, the patient will be referred to a neurologist or a specialist in geriatric medicine. The differential diagnosis of dementia is complicated because of the number of possible causes, because more than one cause may be present, and because dementia can coexist with other conditions such as depression and delirium. Delirium is a temporary disturbance of consciousness marked by confusion, restlessness, inability to focus one's attention, hallucinations, or delusions. In elderly people, delirium is frequently a side effect of surgery, medications, infectious illnesses, or **dehydration**. Delirium can be distinguished from dementia by the fact that delirium usually comes on suddenly (in a few hours or days) and may vary in severity—it is often worse at night. Dementia develops much more slowly, over a period of months or years, and the patient's symptoms are relatively stable. It is possible for a person to have delirium and dementia at the same time.

Another significant diagnostic distinction in elderly patients is the distinction between dementia and age-associated memory impairment (AAMI). Older people with AAMI have a mild degree of memory loss; they do not learn new information as quickly as younger people, and they may take longer to recall a certain fact or to balance their checkbook, but they do not suffer the degree of memory impairment that characterizes dementia, and they do not get progressively worse.

Patient history

The doctor will begin by taking a full history, including the patient's occupation and educational level as well as medical history. The occupational and educational history allows the examiner to make a more accurate assessment of the extent of the patient's memory loss and other evidence of intellectual decline. In some cases the occupational history may indicate exposure to heavy metals or other toxins. A complete medical history allows the doctor to assess possibilities such as delirium, depression, alcohol-related dementia, dementia related to **head injury**, or dementia caused by infection. It is particularly important for the doctor to have a list of all the patient's medications, including over-the-counter preparations, because of the possibility that the patient's symptoms are related to side effects.

Mental status examination

A **mental status examination** (MSE) evaluates the patient's ability to communicate, follow instructions, recall information, perform simple tasks involving movement and coordination, as well as his or her emotional state and general sense of space and time. The MSE includes the doctor's informal evaluation of the patient's appearance, vocal tone, facial expressions, posture, and gait as well as formal questions or instructions. A common form that has been used since 1975 is the so-called Folstein Mini-Mental Status Examination, or MMSE. Questions that are relevant to diagnosing dementia include asking the patient to count backward from 100 by 7s, to make change, to name the current President, to repeat a short phrase after the examiner (e.g., "no ifs, ands, or buts") to draw a clock face or geometric figure, and to follow a set of instructions involving movement (e.g., "Show me how to throw a ball" or "Fold this piece of paper and place it under the lamp on the bookshelf"). The examiner may test the patient's abstract reasoning ability by asking him or her to explain a familiar proverb (e.g. "People who live in glass houses shouldn't throw stones") or test the patient's judgment by asking about a problem with a common-sense solution, such as what one does when a prescription runs out.

Neurological examination

A neurological examination includes an evaluation of the patient's cranial nerves and reflexes. The cranial nerves govern the ability to speak as well as sight, hearing, taste, and smell. The patient will be asked to stick out the tongue, follow the examiner's finger with the eyes, raise the eyebrows, etc. The patient is also asked to perform certain actions (e.g., touching the nose with the eyes closed) that test coordination and spatial orientation. The doctor will usually touch or tap certain areas of the body, such as the knee or the sole of the foot, to test the patient's reflexes. Failure to respond to the touch or tap may indicate damage to certain parts of the brain.

Tests

Laboratory tests

Blood and urine samples are collected in order to rule out such conditions as thyroid deficiency, niacin (vitamin B$_{12}$) deficiency, **heavy metal poisoning**, **liver disease**, HIV infection, **syphilis**, anemia, medication reactions, or kidney failure. A **lumbar puncture** (spinal tap) may be done to rule out neurosyphilis.

Diagnostic imaging

The patient may be given a CT (computed tomography) scan or MRI (**magnetic resonance imaging**) to detect evidence of strokes, disintegration of the brain tissue in certain areas, **blood clots** or tumors, a buildup of spinal fluid, or bleeding into the brain tissue. **PET** (positron-emission tomography) or SPECT (single-emission computed tomography) imaging is not used routinely to diagnose dementia, but may be used to rule out Alzheimer disease or frontal lobe degeneration if a patient's CT scan or MRI is unrevealing.

Treatment and management

Reversible and responsive dementias

Some types of dementia are reversible, and a few types respond to specific treatments related to their causes. Dementia related to dietary deficiencies or metabolic disorders is treated with the appropriate **vitamins** or thyroid medication. Dementia related to HIV infection often responds well to zidovudine (Retrovir), a drug given to prevent the **AIDS** virus from replicating. Multi-infarct dementia is usually treated by controlling the patient's blood pressure and/or diabetes; while treatments for these disorders cannot undo damage already caused to brain tissue, they can slow the progress of the dementia. Patients with alcohol-related dementia often improve over the long term if they are able to stop drinking. Dementias related to head injuries, **hydrocephalus**, and tumors are treated by surgery.

It is important to evaluate and treat elderly patients for depression, because the symptoms of depression in older people often mimic dementia. This condition is sometimes called pseudodementia. In addition, patients who suffer from both depression and dementia often show some improvement in intellectual functioning when the depression is treated.

Irreversible dementias

As of 2009, there were no medications or surgical techniques that can cure Alzheimer disease, the frontal lobe dementias, MID, or dementia with Lewy bodies.

There are also no "magic bullets" that can reverse or stop the progression of these dementias.

Early intervention may allow the patient to compensate for the alterations in functioning, help to minimize complications, and have an improved quality of life. It may also allow the patient and family to plan for the future and to identify resources.

Drugs

Periodically, new drugs are studied for the treatment of dementia. The only drugs approved as of 2009 for the symptomatic treatment of AD were tacrine (Cognex), donepazil (Aricept), rivastigmine (Exelon) and galantamine (Razadyne). These drugs may provide temporary improvement in cognitive functioning for about 40% of patients with mild-to-moderate AD. However, drug therapy can be complicated by forgetfulness, especially if the drug must be taken several times a day.

Psychotic symptoms, including **paranoia**, delusions, and hallucinations, may be treated with **antipsychotic drugs** such as haloperidol, chlorpromazine, risperidone, and clozapine. Side effects of these drugs can be significant. **Antianxiety drugs** such as diazepam (Valium) may improve behavioral symptoms, especially agitation and anxiety although buspirone (BuSpar) has fewer side effects. The anticonvulsant carbamazepine (Tegretol) is also sometimes prescribed for agitation. Depression is treated with antidepressants, usually beginning with **selective serotonin reuptake inhibitors** (SSRIs) such as fluoxetine (Prozac) or paroxetine (Paxil).

In general, medications are administered cautiously in the lowest possible effective doses to individuals with dementia in order to minimize side effects. Supervision of taking medications is generally required.

The primary goals of treatment for progressive dementias are to preserve as much functioning and independence as possible and to maintain quality of life as long as possible. Caring for a person with dementia can be difficult and complex. The patient must cope with functional and cognitive limitations, while family members or other caregivers must assume increasing responsibility for the person's physical needs. The patient and family should be educated early on in the disease progression to help them anticipate and plan for inevitable changes.

Behavioral treatment

Behavioral approaches may be used to reduce the frequency or severity of problem behaviors such as aggression or socially inappropriate conduct. Problem behavior may be a reaction to frustration or over-stimulation. Understanding and modifying the situations that trigger it can be effective; strategies may include breaking down complex tasks such as dressing or feeding into simpler steps, or reducing the amount of activity in the environment to avoid confusion and agitation. Pleasurable activities such as crafts, games, and music can provide therapeutic stimulation and improve mood.

Home modification

Modifying the environment can increase safety and comfort while decreasing agitation. Home modifications for safety include removal or lock-up of hazards such as sharp knives, dangerous chemicals, and tools. Childproof latches may be used to limit access as well. Bed rails and bathroom safety rails can be important safety measures. Confusion may be reduced with the use of simpler decorative schemes and the presence of familiar objects. Covering or disguising doors may reduce the tendency to wander. Positioning the bed in view of the bathroom can decrease incontinence.

Long-term institutional care may be required for the person with dementia, as profound cognitive losses often precede death by a number of years. Early planning for the financial burden of nursing home care is critical. Useful information about financial planning for long-term care is available through the Alzheimer's Association.

Family members or others caring for a person with dementia are often subject to extreme **stress**, and may develop feelings of anger, resentment, guilt, and hopelessness, in addition to the sorrow they feel for their loved one and for themselves. Depression is an extremely common consequence of being a full-time caregiver for a person with dementia. Support groups can be an important way to deal with the stress of caregiving. Contact numbers are available from the Alzheimer's Association; they may also be available through a local social service agency.

Alternative therapies

No alternative therapies have been found to conclusively prevent, reverse, or slow dementias except for those caused by nutrient deficiencies. However, alternative practitioners find some of the following helpful to individual patients.

NUTRITIONAL SUPPLEMENTS. Some **nutritional supplements** may be helpful, especially if dementia is caused by deficiency of these essential nutrients:

- Acetyl-L-carnitine may improve brain function and increases attention span, enhances ability to concentrate and increases energy in individuals with Alzheimer's disease.
- Antioxidants (vitamin E, vitamin C, beta-carotene, or selenium): may reduce the risk of contracting dementia by reducing the damaging effects of free radicals.

- B-complex vitamins and vitamin B_{12} may significantly improve mental function in individuals who have low levels of these essential nutrients.
- Coenzyme Q10 may help deliver more oxygen to the brain.
- DHEA may increase brain function in the elderly.
- Magnesium may be helpful if the dementia is caused by magnesium deficiency and/or accumulation of aluminum in the brain.
- Phosphotidylserine deficiency may decrease mental function and cause depression.
- Zinc may boost short-term memory and increase attention span.

Herbal treatment

Herbal remedies that may be helpful in treating dementia include Chinese or Korean **ginseng**, Siberian ginseng, gotu kola, and *Ginkgo biloba*. Of these, **ginkgo biloba** is the most well known and widely accepted by Western medicine.

Homeopathy

A homeopathic physician may prescribe patient-specific homeopathic remedies to alleviate symptoms of dementia.

Acupressure

This form of therapy uses hands to apply pressure on specific acupressure points to improve blood circulation and calm the nervous system.

Aromatherapy

Aromatherapists use essential oils as inhalants or in baths to improve mental performances and to calm the nerves.

Prognosis

The prognosis for reversible dementia related to nutritional or thyroid problems are usually good once the cause has been identified and treated. The prognoses for dementias related to alcoholism or HIV infection depend on the patient's age and the severity of the underlying disorder.

For those with irreversible progressive dementia, the outlook often includes slow deterioration in mental and physical capacities ending in death. Eventually, help is often required when swallowing, walking, and even sitting become difficult. Aid can consist of preparing special **diets** that can be more easily consumed and making surroundings safe in case of falls. Lift assists in areas such as the bathroom can also be useful. On average, people with Alzheimer disease live eight years past their diagnosis, with a range from one to 20 years. Patients with frontal lobe dementia or Pick disease live on average between 5 and 10 years after diagnosis. The course of Creutzfeldt-Jakob disease is much more rapid, with patients living between 5 and 12 months after diagnosis. Vascular dementia is usually progressive, with death resulting from stroke, infection, or heart disease.

Prevention

Dementia caused by repeated blows to the head can be prevented by avoiding sports where head trauma is common. Alcohol-abuse related dementia can be prevented by avoiding alcohol or minimized by receiving early treatment for alcoholism. Good **nutrition** can prevent nutrient-deficiency dementia. Unfortunately, most forms of dementia cannot be prevented.

Resources

BOOKS

Glenner, Joy A. et al. *When Your Loved One Has Dementia: A Simple Guide for Caregivers* Baltimore MD: Johns Hopkins Press, 2005.

OTHER

"Dementia." Mayo Foundation for Education and Research. April 17. 2009 [August 27, 2009]. http://www.mayoclinic.com/health/dementia/DS01131

"Dementia." MedlinePlus. August 17, 2009 [August 27, 2009]. http://www.nlm.nih.gov/medlineplus/dementia.html

Hale, Kathryn and Julia Frank. "Dementia." Emedicine-Health October 27, 2005 [August 27, 2009]. http://www.emedicinehealth.com/dementia_overview/article_em.htm

ORGANIZATIONS

American Geriatrics Society (AGS), Empire State Building, 350 Fifth Avenue, Suite 801, New York, NY, 10118, (212) 308-1414, (212) 832-8646, info@americangeriatrics.org, http://www.americangeriatrics.org.

National Institute of Neurological Disorders and Stroke (NINDS), P.O. Box 5801, Bethesda, MD, 20828, (301) 496-5751. TTY: (301) 468-5981, (800) 352-9424, http://www.ninds.nih.gov.

National Institute on Aging, Building 31, Room 5C27, 31 Center Drive, MSC 2292, Bethesda, MD, 20892, (301) 496-1752, TTY: (800) 222-4225, (301) 496-1072, http://www.nia.nih.gov.

Deanna M. Swartout-Corbeil, R. N.
Tish Davidson, A.M.

Demyelinating disease *see* **Multiple sclerosis**

Dengue fever

Definition

Dengue **fever** is a disease caused by one of a number of viruses that are carried by mosquitoes. These mosquitoes then transmit the virus to humans.

Description

The virus that causes dengue fever is called an arbovirus, which stands for arthropod-borne virus. Mosquitoes are a type of arthropod. In a number of regions, mosquitoes carry this virus and are responsible for passing it along to humans. These regions include the Middle East, the far East, Africa, and the Caribbean Islands. In these locations, the dengue fever arbovirus is endemic, meaning that the virus naturally and consistently lives in that location. The disease only shows up in the United States sporadically.

In order to understand how dengue fever is transmitted, several terms need to be defined. The word "host" means an animal (including a human) that can be infected with a particular disease. The word "vector" means an organism that can carry a particular disease-causing agent (like a virus or bacteria) without actually developing the disease. The vector can then pass the virus or bacteria on to a new host.

Many of the common illnesses in the United States (including the **common cold**, many viral causes of **diarrhea**, and **influenza** or "flu") are spread because the viruses that cause these illness can be passed directly from person to person. However, dengue fever cannot be passed directly from one infected person to another. Instead, the virus responsible for dengue fever requires an intermediate vector, a mosquito, that carries the virus from one host to another. The mosquito that carries the arbovirus responsible for dengue fever is the same type of mosquito that can transmit other diseases, including **yellow fever**. This mosquito is called *Aedes egypti*. The most common victims are children younger than 10 years of age.

Causes and symptoms

Dengue fever can occur when a mosquito carrying the arbovirus **bites** a human, passing the virus on to the new host. Once in the body, the virus travels to various glands where it multiplies. The virus can then enter the bloodstream. The presence of the virus within the blood vessels, especially those feeding the skin, causes changes to these blood vessels. The vessels swell and leak. The spleen and lymph nodes become enlarged, and patches of liver tissue die. A process called disseminated intravascular coagulation (DIC) occurs, where chemicals responsible for clotting are used up and lead to a risk of severe bleeding (hemorrhage).

After the virus has been transmitted to the human host, a period of incubation occurs. During this time (lasting about five to eight days) the virus multiplies. Symptoms of the disease appear suddenly and include high fever, chills, **headache**, eye **pain**, red eyes, enlarged lymph nodes, a red flush to the face, lower back pain, extreme weakness, and severe aches in the legs and joints.

This initial period of illness lasts about two or three days. After this time, the fever drops rapidly and the patient sweats heavily. After about a day of feeling relatively well, the patient's temperature increases again, although not as much as the first time. A rash of small red bumps begins on the arms and legs, spreading to the chest, abdomen, and back. It rarely affects the face. The palms of the hands and the soles of the feet become swollen and turn bright red. The characteristic combination of fever, rash, and headache are called the "dengue triad." Most people recover fully from dengue fever, although weakness and **fatigue** may last for several weeks. Once a person has been infected with dengue fever, his or her immune system keeps producing cells that prevent reinfection for about a year.

More severe illness may occur in some people. These people may be experiencing dengue fever for the first time. However, in some cases a person may have already had dengue fever at one time, recovered, and then is reinfected with the virus. In these cases, the first infection teaches the immune system to recognize the presence of the arbovirus. When the immune cells encounter the virus during later infections, the immune system over-reacts. These types of illnesses, called dengue hemorrhagic fever (DHF) or dengue shock syndrome (DSS), involve more severe symptoms. Fever and headache are the first symptoms, but the other initial symptoms of dengue fever are absent. The patient develops a **cough**, followed by the appearance of small purplish spots (petechiae) on the skin. These petechiae are areas where blood is leaking out of the vessels. Large bruised areas appear as the bleeding worsens and abdominal pain may be severe. The patient may begin to vomit a substance that looks like coffee grounds. This is actually a sign of bleeding into the stomach. As the blood vessels become more damaged, they leak more and continue to increase in diameter (dilate), causing a decrease in blood flow to all tissues of the body. This state of low blood flow is called shock. Shock can result in damage to the body's organs (especially the heart and kidneys) because low blood flow deprives them of oxygen.

KEY TERMS

Endemic—Naturally and consistently present in a certain geographical region.

Host—The organism (such as a monkey or human) in which another organism (such as a virus or bacteria) is living.

Vector—A carrier organism (such as a fly or mosquito) that delivers a virus (or other agent of infection) to a host.

Diagnosis

Diagnosis should be suspected in endemic areas whenever a high fever goes on for two to seven days, especially if accompanied by a bleeding tendency. Symptoms of shock should suggest the progression of the disease to DSS.

The arbovirus causing dengue fever is one of the few types of arbovirus that can be isolated from the serum of the blood. The serum is the fluid in which blood cells are suspended. Serum can be tested because the phase in which the virus travels throughout the bloodstream is longer in dengue fever than in other arboviral infections. A number of tests are used to look for reactions between the patient's serum and laboratory-produced antibodies. Antibodies are special cells that recognize the markers (or antigens) present on invading organisms. During these tests, antibodies are added to a sample of the patient's serum. Healthcare workers then look for reactions that would only occur if viral antigens were present in that serum.

Treatment

There is no treatment available to shorten the course of dengue fever, DHF, or DSS. Medications can be given to lower the fever and to decrease the pain of muscle aches and headaches. Fluids are given through a needle in a vein to prevent **dehydration**. Blood transfusions may be necessary if severe hemorrhaging occurs. Oxygen should be administered to patients in shock.

Prognosis

The prognosis for uncomplicated dengue fever is very good, and almost 100% of patients fully recover. However, as many as 6–30% of all patients die when DHF occurs. The **death** rate is especially high among the youngest patients (under one year old). In places where excellent medical care is available, very close monitoring and immediate treatment of complications lowers the death rate among DHF and DSS patients to about 1%.

Prevention

Prevention of dengue fever means decreasing the mosquito population. Any sources of standing water (buckets, vases, etc.) where the mosquitoes can breed must be eliminated. Mosquito repellant is recommended for those areas where dengue fever is endemic. To help break the cycle of transmission, sick patients should be placed in bed nets so that mosquitoes cannot bite them and become arboviral vectors.

ORGANIZATIONS

Centers for Disease Control and Prevention (CDC), 1600 Clifton Road, Atlanta, GA, 30333, (800) 232-4636, cdcinfo@cdc.gov, http://www.cdc.gov.

Rosalyn Carson-DeWitt, MD

Dental caries *see* **Tooth decay**
Dental cavity *see* **Tooth decay**

Dental fillings

Definition

Dental fillings are metal amalgams or composite resins used to fill a cavity.

Purpose

Dentists use dental fillings to restore teeth damaged by dental caries (**tooth decay**). Dental caries are caused by microorganisms that convert sugars in food to acids that erode the enamel of a tooth, creating a hole or cavity. The dentist cleans out the decayed part of the tooth and fills the opening with an artificial material (a filling) to protect the tooth's structure and restore the appearance and utility of the tooth.

Precautions

As in any dental procedure, the dentist and dental assistant will need to use sterile techniques. Gloves and masks are essential as well as the sterilization of equipment and tools. This not only helps prevent the spread of infectious diseases like **AIDS** and hepatitis, but also the **common cold**.

The patient's reaction to anesthesia is the other main concern of the dentist and dental assistant when performing dental fillings. Nitrous oxide should be avoided with pregnant patients, and local anesthetics should be used with caution, though they are considered safe. Local anesthetics like Novocain and lidocaine have been in practical use for decades with few side effects reported. Some patients, however, are allergic to these drugs.

Description

Though dentists are encountering fewer and smaller cavities in their patients, there is still a need for dentists to fill cavities. Old fillings wear out over time and need to be replaced. Recently, patients have begun to request more restorative work on their teeth, sometimes opting for full mouth restorations that involve installing crowns, bleaching teeth or applying veneers, and replacing dark metal fillings with tooth-colored ones that create a monochromatic view in a patient's mouth.

The dentist begins by removing the decayed area of the tooth and preparing the tooth to receive the filling. The dentist has a wide choice of dental filling materials to choose from.

Amalgam fillings

The most common and strongest filling material is amalgam. It is a silver filling that is usually placed on the rear molars, which endure more stress during chewing. Amalgam fillings—used for large, deep cavities—are strong and very resistant to wear. Amalgam has been in use since 1833.

Amalgam is a mixture (which is what the word means) of several metals, including liquid mercury (35% silver, 15% tin or tin and copper, a trace of zinc, and 50% mercury). When it is prepared, it has a malleable consistency that can easily be shaped to fit the prepared tooth. It hardens to a durable metal.

Despite its durability, many dentists and patients avoid amalgam fillings. Dentists have found that amalgam has a tendency to expand with time. As a result, teeth become fractured from the inside, often splitting the tooth. Patients often avoid amalgam for strictly aesthetic reasons. Amalgam fillings darken over time and make teeth look as if they are decayed.

The biggest reason amalgam has lost favor is a health concern due to its 50% mercury content. Although the American Dental Association (ADA) has pronounced amalgam safe in the quantity and composition of amalgam, some patients and dentists are disturbed by various

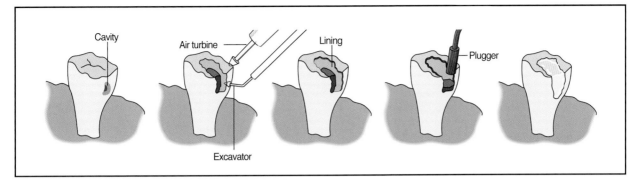

Cavity

Air turbine

Lining

Plugger

Excavator

The process of filling a cavity. *(Illustration by Hans & Cassady, Inc. Reproduced by permission of Gale, a part of Cengage Learning.)*

reports of illness in relation to the mercury in amalgam fillings. Mercury is a toxic material. Some states are required to dispose of mercury waste as if it were a hazardous product. There is also an added risk of inhaling mercury particles when old fillings are removed.

Gold fillings

Gold fillings or inlays are created outside of the mouth by a dental technician and then cemented into place. They are also used to fill the back molars. Gold fillings are very durable. Like amalgam, however, they are not as aesthetically pleasing as tooth-colored fillings.

Composite fillings

Composite fillings, often called white fillings, are made of a plastic resin and finely ground glass. They must be applied to the tooth surface in thin layers. Dentists try to match the color of composites with neighboring teeth for a more natural look, making the filling appear invisible. Composite resin fillings often are made smaller than amalgam fillings and require less tooth preparation, thereby saving more natural tooth surface.

Composite fillings are bonded to the tooth so that the tooth becomes stronger than it was before. They are also less sensitive to temperature changes in the mouth that can damage the tooth; therefore there is less chance that the tooth will shatter because of the filling.

These fillings may not be suitable for large cavities in molars. Though composite durability increased in the 1990s, a porcelain inlay or crown may be the best choice for a durable, natural-looking restoration of a molar.

The major drawback of composite resin fillings is cost. They average one-and-a-half to two times more than the price of amalgam fillings. They also can be stained from drinking coffee and tea. Large composite fillings tend to wear out sooner than amalgam fillings.

Composite fillings can last seven to 10 years, which is similar to the lifespan of amalgam fillings.

Resin ionomer

Resin ionomers are new, tooth-colored filling materials that contain a resin and fluoride. They are very suitable for children and for older adults who suffer from root decay that is more likely to occur as a person ages. These fillings seal the tooth and also protect it from future decay because of the fluoride that they release.

Preparation

During a routine checkup, the dentist may find a cavity in a tooth with a metal tooth probe. A new diagnostic tool, the DIAGNOdent, can detect evidence of cavities and pre-cavity conditions on the tooth's surface. A low-powered laser, the DIAGNOdent is able to detect decay so early that a dental cavity can be avoided. These pre-cavity areas can be protected with a sealant, thereby preventing further decay.

If the cavities found are relatively small and not very deep, there may be no need to anesthetize the area where the dental work will be done. High-speed drills often are able to clean out the decay quickly and with little discomfort. If the cavity is not very deep, the drill may not reach the sensitive nerves in the teeth, which usually cause **pain**. Children and some adults may need anesthesia in any case. The dentist and the dental assistant need to be aware of the patient's history and if the patient reacts adversely to **local anesthesia**.

There are some dentists who use electronic dental anesthesia (EDA), a device that sends electrical charges to the gum through electrodes. Sometimes this is enough anesthesia for the procedure. At other times, EDA numbs the area where the anesthesia is administered, so that the patient does not feel the needle as it goes into the gum. Some dentists also provide soothing

KEY TERMS

Amalgam—A mixture of metals, primarily mercury used to make large, durable fillings. Also called silver fillings.

Anesthesia—A condition created by drugs that produces a numb feeling. General anesthesia produces unconsciousness whereas a local anesthesia produces numbness around the site where the drug was introduced.

Composite filling—A resin material that is tooth colored and is used to fill a tooth once decay has been removed. It is used most often in front teeth, but may be used in any tooth for aesthetic reasons.

Crown—An artificial covering prepared by a lab technician to fit over a damaged tooth or one weakened by decay.

Dental caries—Tooth decay caused by microorganisms that convert sugars in food to acids which erode the enamel of a tooth.

Dental laser—A device that generates a low-powered beam of light that is used in place of a dentist's drill to cut away decay from a tooth or remove gum tissue.

Enamel—The hard outer surface of a tooth.

music to calm patients during the procedure. Other dentists will use local anesthesia in combination with nitrous oxide-oxygen analgesia to minimize discomfort through the drilling phase of a filling.

Dental lasers that generate a low-powered beam of light are being used to cut away decay, but without the whine of the drill and without using anesthesia. Though a bit slower than the conventional drill, lasers are very efficient at preparing a tooth to receive a filling. Unfortunately, lasers cannot yet remove old fillings or prepare a tooth surface to receive a crown.

Air abrasion is another way to remove decay without using anesthesia. Air abrasion machines produce a spray of air and powder. There is no vibration or heat. Because it has no vibration, it avoids microfractures in the tooth that sometimes occur with drills. Air abrasion removes only a small amount of the tooth's structure. Therefore, it is suitable for small cavities and the repair and replacement of old fillings. It also can repair chipped teeth and clean discolored or stained teeth.

After the cavity is cleaned of decay, the walls of the tooth are shaped and are ready to receive a filling material. If a composite resin filling is used, the tooth next needs to be etched so that the resin will adhere to the tooth. The tooth then is filled, shaped, and polished. The composite filling then must be hardened by shining a special light on it.

Aftercare

The dentist and dental assistant should advise the patient that the teeth, lips, and tongue may be numb for several hours after the procedure, if a local anesthetic was used. Some patients experience sore gums or a sensitivity to hot and cold in the tooth that has just been filled. Normally, patients are advised to avoid chewing hard foods directly on new amalgam fillings for 24 hours. Composite fillings require no special caution since they set immediately. If patients experience continued pain or an uncomfortable bite, they should call their dentist.

Complications

Some patient's have allergic reactions to local anesthesia. The tooth that received a filling may be sensitive to changes in temperature or may be sore for a short time after the procedure.

Results

Fillings restore a tooth's function and appearance. They permit the patient to continue to eat and chew properly and last for several years. Normal fillings will need to be replaced over a patient's lifetime. Since fewer dental caries had been observed since the last decade of the twentieth century, dentists are initially filling fewer teeth, but are replacing fillings as they fail and sometimes systematically, especially if the patient decides to cosmetically enhance his or her teeth. Since many of the initial cavities are quite small, patients are opting for more aesthetically pleasing filling materials even if they are not as durable.

Health care team roles

When the dentist discovers a cavity, filling options are discussed with the patient. The dental assistant prepares the dentist's workstation and lays out the specific instruments that are needed. The dental assistant prepares the filling material according to the manufacturer's directions and assists the dentist in preparing the tooth for filling and in the filling procedure itself. The dental assistant cleans the patient's mouth and returns the procedure room to order. All of the instruments that have been used are sterilized by the dental assistant.

Resources

BOOKS

Landau, Elaine. *Cavities and Toothaches.* New York: Marshall Cavendish Benchmark, 2008.

Pitts, Nigel, ed. *Detection, Assessment, Diagnosis and Monitoring of Caries.* New York: Krager, 2009.

Sroda, Rebecca. *Nutrition for a Healthy Mouth,* 2nd ed. Philadelphia: Wolters Kluwer Health/Lippincott Williams and Wilkins, 2010.

PERIODICALS

"Improving Patient Awareness: Methods For Optimal Caries Detection." *Practical Procedures and Aesthetic Dentistry.* (September 2008) 20(8):282–284.

Kolahi, Jafar, Fazilati, Mohamad, and Kadivar, Mahdi. "Towards Tooth Friendly Soft Drinks." *Medical Hypotheses* (October 2009) 73(4):524–525.

ORGANIZATIONS

American Dental Association, 211 East Chicago Avenue, Chicago, IL, 60611-2678, (312) 440-2500, www.ada.org.

American Dental Education Association, 1400 K Street, Suite 1100, Washington, DC, 20005, (202) 289-7201, (202) 289-7204, www.adea.org.

American Dental Hygienists' Association, 444 North Michigan Avenue, Suite 3400, Chicago, IL, 60611, (312) 440-8900, mail@adha.net, www.adha.org.

Janie F. Franz
Tish Davidson, AM

Dental hygiene *see* **Oral hygiene**

Dental implants

Definition

Dental implants are surgically fixed substitutes for roots of missing teeth. Embedded in the jawbone, they act as anchors for a replacement tooth, also known as a crown, or a full set of replacement teeth.

Purpose

The purpose of dental implant surgery is to position metallic anchors in the jawbone so that they can receive the replacement teeth and hold them in place. Dental implants should be considered as an option for replacing failing or missing teeth, and often

provide more predictable results than bridgework, resin bonded bridges, or endodontic treatment.

Demographics

In 2000, the estimated number of dental implants placed in the United States was 910,000, and this number is expected to increase at a rate of about 18% per year through 2010. Dental implants are equally popular in Europe, especially in Germany where the procedure is reimbursed by the national healthcare system.

Description

By replacing a lost tooth with a dental implant, the overall health and function of the surrounding teeth is maintained. The implant can prevent tooth migration and loss of structure and will help avoid loss of bone from the jaw in that area. Further, implants reduce the impact of the lost tooth on surrounding teeth, as traditional bridge structures often require reduction (filing down) of the two flanking teeth to hold the bridge in place with a crown. Implanting avoids such alterations to the surrounding teeth when replacing a lost tooth.

When replacing dentures, implants can provide even more benefits. Implants do not slip nor do they have the potential of limiting the diet to easily chewed

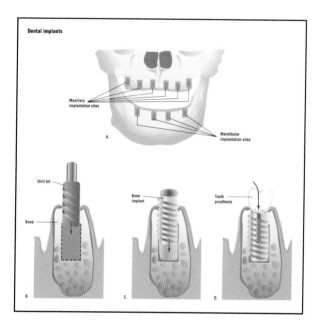

A dental drill is used to make a hole for the implant in the jawbone (B). The bone implant is secured into the drilled hole (C), and the tooth prosthesis is built onto the implant (D). (*Illustration by PreMediaGlobal. Reproduced by permission of Gale, a part of Cengage Learning.*)

KEY TERMS

Computed tomography (CT) scan—A method of imaging both hard and soft tissue of the body used in placement of dental implants that are not within the bone.

Crown—An artificial replacement tooth.

Endosteal implants—Dental implants that are placed within the bone.

Prosthetic tooth—The final tooth that is held in place by the dental implant anchor.

Resorbed—Absorbed by the body because of lack of function. This happens to the jawbone after tooth loss.

foods as can happen with poorly fitting dentures. If appropriate, implants are the method most able to surgically restore one or more missing teeth to their original conditions.

Under **local anesthesia**, the first step for most implant procedures is the exposure of the bone where the implant is to be made. This is followed by placement of the implant into the exposed jawbone. Implants that are placed in the bone are called endosteal implants and are made of titanium or a titanium alloy because this metal does not adversely interact with biological tissue. After placement of the implant, a cover screw is put in and the wound is closed with stitches and allowed to heal. In general, placements in the lower jaw need to heal about three months, while placements in the upper jaw need to heal about six months.

After healing, in a second surgical procedure, the implant is uncovered, the cover screw is removed, and a healing abutment or a temporary crown is placed in the implant. Temporary crowns are generally used for esthetic reasons, when the implant is in a place that is visible. Both healing abutments and temporary crowns allow the tissue around the implant to be trained to grow around the final prosthetic tooth.

After about two months, the soft tissue will be healed enough to receive the final prosthetic tooth. Impressions are used to make custom abutments that take into account the neck morphology of the implant. The prosthetic tooth is sometimes attached to a gold cylinder that can be screwed into the abutment or it can be directly cemented onto the abutment. This multi-stage process, where the two surgical procedures are separated by a lengthy healing time, has proven to provide excellent stability in the final implant. Single-step surgical implants are available, but some stability

of the final implant is often lost by eliminating the healing step.

Preparation/Diagnosis

At the first appointment, the dentist or oral surgeon performs a thorough examination to determine whether implants are appropriate to replace the missing teeth. Often, x rays are necessary to discover the state of the jawbone, particularly if the teeth have been lost for some time. This information is used to determine if implants are appropriate and, if so, what particular type of implant would be best for the clinical situation.

There are two solutions commonly used if the initial examination indicates that the bone in the area where the implant is to occur is too resorbed to support the implant. The first is **bone grafting**. This involves undergoing a procedure that moves bone from one place in the body to another to enlarge the bone structure at the implant site. Often, bone can be moved from one place in the mouth to another. Sometimes a graft from a donor, or an animal, or artificial bone can be used if bone from the patient is not available. Grafting usually is done four to eight months before the implant procedure to allow the graft a chance to heal before it is disturbed with the implant process.

A second solution is the use of subperiosteal implants that ride above the bone but beneath the gum. These types of implants are not placed in the bone. A computed tomography (CT) scan is commonly used to obtain a model of the bone structure and then the implant fixture is molded to precisely fit the bone model.

Risks

The greatest risk following the surgical procedures is that the implant will fail. For implants placed within the bone, most failures occur within the first year and then occur at a rate of less than 1% per year thereafter. Recent research has indicated that tobacco use by the patient and use of a single-stage implant procedure are two risk factors that increase failure rate.

Normal results

Overall, the success rate for all implants runs from 90–95%. Most failed implants can be replaced with a second attempt.

Resources

BOOKS

Babbush, Charles A. *As Good as New: A Consumer's Guide to Dental Implants.* Lyndhurst, OH: Dental Implant Center Press, 2004.

Misch, Carl E. *Contemporary Implant Dentistry*. St. Louis, MO: Mosby, 2007.

PERIODICALS

Bartlett, D. "Implants for Life? A Critical Review of Implant-supported Restorations." *Journal of Dentistry* 35 no.10 (2007): 768–7721.

ORGANIZATIONS

American Dental Association, 211 East Chicago Avenue, Chicago, IL, 60611-2678, (312) 440-2500, www.ada.org.

American Dental Education Association, 1400 K Street, Suite 1100, Washington, DC, 20005, (202) 289-7201, (202) 289-7204, www.adea.org.

American Dental Hygienists' Association, 444 North Michigan Avenue, Suite 3400, Chicago, IL, 60611, (312) 440-8900, mail@adha.net, www.adha.org.

Michelle Johnson, MS, JD
Tish Davidson, A M

Dental injuries *see* **Dental trauma**

Dental sealants

Definition

A dental sealant is a thin layer of plastic substance that is painted over teeth to discourage the formation of dental caries (cavities).

Demographics

Dental sealants normally are applied to the permanent back teeth (pre-molars and molars) of children soon after these teeth erupt through the gum, most often between the ages of six and 12 years. In a 2005 study, the United States Centers for Disease Control and Prevention (CDC) found that only 32% of children aged 6–19 years had received dental sealants. One of the goals of the United States Department of Health and Human Services Initiative Healthy People 2010 is to increase the percentage of children who receive dental sealants to 50%.

Purpose

The purpose of applying dental sealants is to protect the teeth by sealing out food particles and acids produced by bacteria so that they do not accumulate on the tooth surface and cause decay.

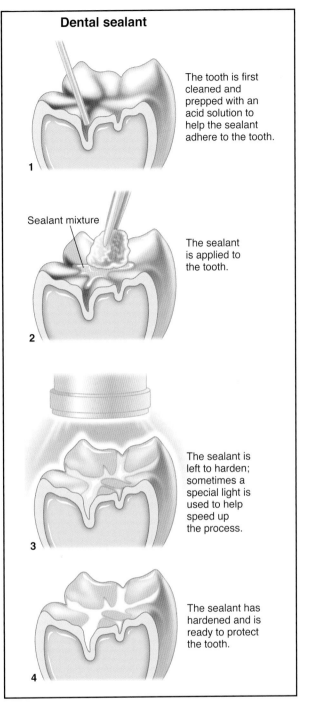

Dental sealant

1. The tooth is first cleaned and prepped with an acid solution to help the sealant adhere to the tooth.

Sealant mixture

2. The sealant is applied to the tooth.

3. The sealant is left to harden; sometimes a special light is used to help speed up the process.

4. The sealant has hardened and is ready to protect the tooth.

Illustration showing how a dental sealant is applied. *(Illustration by Electronic Illustrators Group. Reproduced by permission of Gale, a part of Cengage Learning.)*

Description

Dental sealants, sometimes called tooth sealants, are plastic material that first appeared in the 1960s. Sealants usually are applied to the chewing teeth—the pre-molars and molars. These are teeth that have what dentists call "pits and fissures" or rough surfaces with deep grooves that a toothbrush has trouble cleaning.

Teeth continuously develop a coating plaque that consists of bacteria and mucin. In order to prevent **tooth decay**, plaque must be removed daily through brushing and flossing. The structure of the pre-molars and molars makes it very difficult to reach all surfaces with a toothbrush. When dental sealant is applied to these teeth, it protects the tooth enamel from plaque. This helps prevent tooth decay and may ultimately save the individual money by eliminating the need for fillings, crowns, or other treatment for tooth decay. Some dental insurance will pay for sealants but may put restrictions on when or to which teeth they may be applied. Individuals should check with their insurance company.

Dental sealants can be applied quickly and painlessly. The procedure is as follows:

- The tooth is cleaned and dried.
- An acid solution is painted on the tooth in order to roughen the surface so that the dental sealant adheres to the tooth better.
- The tooth is rinsed and dried.
- A liquid sealant is applied to the tooth.
- The sealant quickly hardens

In March 2008, the American Dental Association (ADA) made the following recommendations based on critical evaluation of studies conducted on dental sealants (evidence based medicine):

- Sealants should be placed on pits and fissures of children's and adolescent's permanent teeth when these teeth are at risk for developing dental caries.
- Sealants should be placed on teeth early before cavities develop.
- Resin-based sealants are the preferred type of sealant.

The expert committee appointed by the ADA to investigate sealants suggested that sealants be placed on adult teeth in danger of developing dental caries, However, studies of sealants in adults have not been adequate to make this a firm, evidence-based recommendation. The use of sealants in primary (baby) teeth is left to the discretion of the dentist and the parent.

Benefits

There is clear evidence that sealant applied when secondary pre-molars or molars erupt from the gum will reduce the likelihood of developing dental caries

KEY TERMS

Cavity—A hole or weak spot in the tooth surface caused by decay.

Dental caries—The medical term for tooth decay.

Enamel—The hard, outermost surface of a tooth.

Evidence-based medicine—Recommendations that are based on an evaluation of randomized, controlled trials; non-randomized trials; other experiments; descriptive studies; and reports of expert committees. Each class of evidence is graded (A to D, with A being the most reliable) based on the type and size of study. Recommendations and clinical practice guides can then be made using these grades.

Fluoride—A chemical compound containing fluorine that is used to treat water or applied directly to teeth to prevent decay.

Mucin—A protein in saliva that combines with sugars in the mouth to form plaque.

Plaque—A thin, sticky, colorless film that forms on teeth. Plaque is composed of mucin, sugars from food, and bacteria that live in the plaque.

in these teeth. Adults may have sealants applied, but the benefit to adults has not been proven.

Precautions

The tooth must be free of decay before the sealant is applied. If tooth decay has already begun, there exists the possibility that they tooth will continue to decay under the sealant and that this will not be detected until much damage has already been done.

The sealant material may contain small amounts of bisphenol A (BPA), a material found in plastics that has been shown to cause **cancer** in animals. As of 2010, the ADA has stated that BPA is rarely used in dental sealants and that the small amount that may be present should not cause health concerns. Some European countries and Canada are considerably more concerned about the health risks of BPA than the United States. They are more likely to regulate the use of this material.

Preparation

The tooth is examined for any sign of decay. If no decay is found, the tooth is cleaned before the sealant is applied. If there is any sign of dental caries, the sealant should not be applied; instead, the decay should be removed and the tooth filled.

Aftercare

Sealants harden very quickly. No aftercare is needed. Sealants last on average five to ten years.

Risks

There are no known risks related to the application of dental sealants except for the concerns mentioned in the Precautions section.

Research and general acceptance

The American Dental Association and most other dental associations in developed countries endorse the use of dental sealants on secondary premolars and molars of children. Use of sealants in adults and on primary teeth of children is not specifically endorsed, but is left up to the discretion of the dentist and the patient.

Holistic dentists tend to be less enthusiastic about the use of dental sealants, citing concerns about trapping decay in the tooth and the presence of BPA in the sealant material.

Training and certification

Sealants are applied by a licensed dentist, often with the assistance of a certified dental hygienist.

Resources

BOOKS

Harris, Norman O., Garcia-Godoy, Franklin, and Nathe, Christine Nielsen. *Primary Preventive Dentistry,* 7th ed. Upper Saddle River, NJ: Pearson, 2009.

Hollins, Carole. *Basic Guide to Dental Procedures.* Oxford: Blackwell Publishing, 2008.

Runkle, Richard S. *Taking a Giant Bite Out of Dental Confusion: The Consumer's Guide to 21st Century Dentistry.* Moscow, ID: Luminary Media Group, 2008.

Taggart, Jose C., ed. *Handbook of Dental Care: Diagnostic, Preventive, and Restorative Services.* Hauppauge, NY: Nova Science Publishers, 2009.

PERIODICALS

Hyde, Susan, et al. "Developing an Acceptability Assessment of Preventive Dental Treatments." *Journal of Public Health Dentistry,* (2009) 69(1):18–23.

OTHER

Pit-and-Fissure Sealants. American Dental Association. Undated [accessed January 10, 2010]. http://www.ada.org/prof/resources/topics/sealants.asp

Things to Know About Tooth Sealants. Dental Health Directory Library. Undated [accessed January 10, 2010]. http://www.dental–health.com/tooth_sealants.html

Weil, Andrew. Are Dental Sealants Safe? October 12, 2009. http://www.drweil.com/drw/u/QAA400629/Are-Dental-Sealants-Safe.html

ORGANIZATIONS

American Dental Association, 211 East Chicago Avenue, Chicago, IL, 60611-2678, (312) 440-2500, http://www.ada.org.

American Dental Education Association, 1400 K Street, Suite 1100, Washington, DC, 20005, (202) 289-7201, (202) 289-7204, http://www.adea.org.

American Dental Hygienists' Association, 444 North Michigan Avenue, Suite 3400, Chicago, IL, 60611, (312) 440-8900, mail@adha.net, http://www.adha.org.

Tish Davidson, A.M.
Brenda Lerner

Dental trauma

Definition

Dental trauma is injury to the mouth, including teeth, lips, gums, tongue, and jawbones. The most common dental trauma is a broken or lost tooth.

Description

Dental trauma may be inflicted in a number of ways: contact sports, motor vehicle accidents, fights, falls, eating hard foods, drinking hot liquids, and other such mishaps. As oral tissues are highly sensitive, injuries to the mouth are typically very painful. Dental trauma should receive prompt treatment from a dentist.

Causes and symptoms

Soft tissue injuries, such as a "fat lip," a burned tongue, or a cut inside the cheek, are characterized by **pain**, redness, and swelling with or without bleeding. A broken tooth often has a sharp edge that may cut the tongue and cheek. Depending on the position of the fracture, the tooth may or may not cause **toothache** pain. When a tooth is knocked out (evulsed), the socket is swollen, painful, and bloody. A jawbone may be broken if the upper and lower teeth no longer fit together properly (**malocclusion**), or if the jaws have pain with limited ability to open and close (mobility), especially around the temporomandibular joint (TMJ).

Diagnosis

Dental trauma is readily apparent upon examination. **Dental x rays** may be taken to determine the extent of the damage to broken teeth. More comprehensive x rays are needed to diagnose a broken jaw.

Treatment

Soft tissue injuries may require only cold compresses to reduce swelling. Bleeding may be controlled with direct pressure applied with clean gauze. Deep lacerations and punctures may require stitches. Pain may be managed with **aspirin** or **acetaminophen** (Tylenol, Aspirin Free Excedrin) or ibuprofen (Motrin, Advil).

Treatment of a broken tooth will vary depending on the severity of the fracture. For immediate **first aid**, the injured tooth and surrounding area should be rinsed gently with warm water to remove dirt, then covered with a cold compress to reduce swelling and ease pain. A dentist should examine the injury as soon as possible. Any pieces from the broken tooth should be saved and brought along.

If a piece of the outer tooth has chipped off, but the inner core (pulp) is undisturbed, the dentist may simply smooth the rough edges or replace the missing section with a small composite filling. In some cases, a fragment of broken tooth may be bonded back into place. If enough tooth is missing to compromise the entire tooth structure, but the pulp is not permanently damaged, the tooth will require a protective coverage with a gold or porcelain crown. If the pulp has been seriously damaged, the tooth will require **root canal treatment** before it receives a crown. A tooth, that is vertically fractured or fractured below the gumline will require root canal treatment and protective restoration. A tooth that no longer has enough remaining structure to retain a crown may have to be extracted (surgically removed).

When a permanent tooth has been knocked out, it may be saved with prompt action. The tooth must be found immediately after it has been lost. It should be picked up by the natural crown (the top part covered by hard enamel). It must not be handled by the root. If the tooth is dirty, it may be gently rinsed under running water. It should never be scrubbed, and it should never be washed with soap, toothpaste, mouthwash, or other chemicals. The tooth should not be dried or wrapped in a tissue or cloth. It must be kept moist at all times.

The tooth may be placed in a clean container of milk, cool water with or without a pinch of salt, or in saliva. If possible, the patient and the tooth should be brought to the dentist within 30 minutes of the tooth

---

KEY TERMS

Crown—The natural part of the tooth covered by enamel. A restorative crown is a protective shell that fits over a tooth.

Eruption—The process of a tooth breaking through the gum tissue to grow into place in the mouth.

Evulsion—The forceful, and usually accidental, removal of a tooth from its socket in the bone.

Extraction—The surgical removal of a tooth from its socket in the bone.

Malocclusion—A problem in the way the upper and lower teeth fit together in biting or chewing.

Pulp—The soft innermost layer of a tooth containing blood vessels and nerves.

Root canal treatment—The process of removing diseased or damaged pulp from a tooth, then filling and sealing the pulp chamber and root canals.

Temporomandibular joint (TMJ)—The jaw joint formed by the mandible (lower jaw bone) moving against the temporal (temple and side) bone of the skull.

---

loss. Rapid action improves the chances of successful re-implantation; however, it is possible to save a tooth after 30 minutes, if the tooth has been kept moist and handled properly.

The body usually rejects re-implantation of a primary (baby) tooth. In this case, the empty socket is treated as a soft tissue injury and monitored until the permanent tooth erupts.

A broken jaw must be set back into its proper position and stabilized with wires while it heals. Healing may take six weeks or longer, depending on the patient's age and the severity of the fracture.

Alternative treatment

There is no substitute for treatment by a dentist or other medical professional. There are, however, homeopathic remedies and herbs that can be used simultaneously with dental care and throughout the healing process. Homeopathic arnica (*Arnica montana*) should be taken as soon as possible after the injury to help the body deal with the trauma. Repeating a dose several times daily for the duration of healing is also useful. Homeopathic hypericum (*Hypericum perforatum*) can be taken if nerve pain is involved, especially with a **tooth extraction** or root canal. Homeopathic comfrey (officinale) *Symphytum* may be helpful in treating pain due to broken jaw bones, but should only be used after the bones have been reset. Calendula (*Calendula officinalis*) and plantain (*Plantago major*) can be used as a mouth rinse to enhance tissue healing. These herbs should not be used with deep lacerations that need to heal from the inside first.

Prognosis

When dental trauma receives timely attention and proper treatment, the prognosis for healing is good. As with other types of trauma, infection may be a complication, but a course of **antibiotics** is generally effective.

Prevention

Most dental trauma is preventable. Car seat belts should always be worn, and young children should be secured in appropriate car seats. Homes should be monitored for potential tripping and slipping hazards. Child-proofing measures should be taken, especially for toddlers. In addition to placing gates across stairs and padding sharp table edges, electrical cords should be tucked away. Young children may receive severe oral **burns** from gnawing on live power cords.

Everyone who participates in contact sports should wear a mouthguard to avoid dental trauma. Athletes in football, ice hockey, wrestling, and boxing commonly wear mouthguards. The mandatory use of mouthguards in football prevents about 200,000 oral injuries annually. Mouthguards should also be worn along with helmets in noncontact sports such as skateboarding, in-line skating, and bicycling. An athlete who does not wear a mouthguard is 60 times more likely to sustain dental trauma than one who does. Any activity involving speed, an increased chance of falling, and potential contact with a hard piece of equipment has the likelihood of dental trauma that may be prevented or substantially reduced in severity with the use of mouthguards.

ORGANIZATIONS

American Academy of Pediatric Dentistry, 211 East Chicago Ave., Ste. 1700, Chicago, IL, 60611-2637, (312) 337-2169, (312) 337-6329, http://www.aapd.org.

American Association of Endodontists, 211 East Chicago Ave., Ste. 1100, Chicago, IL, 60611-2691, (312) 266-7255, (866) 451-9020, (800) 872-3636, info@aae.org, http://ww.aae.org.

American Association of Oral & Maxillofacial Surgeons, 9700 West Bryn Mawr Avenue, Rosemont, IL, 60018-5701, (847) 678-6200, (847) 678-6286, (800) 822-6637, http://www.aaoms.org.

American Dental Association, 211 E. Chicago Ave., Chicago, IL, 60611-2678, (312) 440-2500, http://www.ada.org.

Bethany Thivierge

Dental x rays

Definition

Dental x rays are pictures taken of the mouth area using high-energy photons with very short wavelengths. They show the teeth and surrounding bone.

Purpose

Dental x rays are effective in discovering **tooth decay**, broken fillings, fractured teeth, tumors, occlusal trauma, or impacted or ectopic teeth that would otherwise be unseen by the eye, in between the teeth and below the gum tissue.

Description

Dental x rays are part of the dental examination for aiding in the diagnostic process. X rays are vital in the diagnosis of **root canal treatment** on checking the apical of the tooth and the surrounding structures for abscesses or bone loss. Without the aid of dental x rays, 60% of dental decay would be missed. Diagnostic x rays are essential in providing accurate information. The most common x rays taken are:

- bitewing x rays (vertical and horizontal bitewings)
- panoramic x rays
- periapical x rays
- occlusal x rays

Each is used in its own respective degree of diagnosis, with the bitewing x ray being the most common. Bitewings are the most effective in discovering tooth decay in between the teeth and on adjacent teeth. A bitewing shows only the top crown portion of the tooth structure. It is called a bitewing due to the way the patient can bite down and hold the film securely in place. The bitewing is good in diagnosing and evaluating periodontal conditions and bone levels between the teeth. They are also good in detecting tartar buildup.

The panoramic (a type of film used), or Panorex (brand name) is also commonly taken on the initial visit to the dental office. This type of x ray makes a complete circle of the head from one ear to the other, to produce a complete two-dimensional representation of all the teeth. This x ray will also show bone structure beneath the teeth and the temporomandibular joint (TMJ). The panoramic is the most commonly used x ray in the aid of diagnostic decisions regarding third molar extractions (wisdom teeth) for people who are edentulous (the tooth is not there/has not erupted). This special x ray, however, has its advantages and disadvantages.

One advantage of the panoramic is that a broad area is imaged, showing many structures. Furthermore, the exposure level emits low radiation. The panoramic is excellent for evaluation of trauma, tooth development, and certain anomalies. In some cases dental x rays can even reveal non-dental medical conditions. One study at the University of Buffalo School of Dental Medicine demonstrated that calcifications in the carotid arteries, which were exposed on standard panoramic x rays, served as predictors of **death** from cardiovascular disease.

The main disadvantage of panoramic x rays is that the image shown does not provide the fine detail of a bitewing x ray. The procedure for taking a panoramic x ray is also somewhat confining to the patient, as the x-ray machine takes a minute or more to fully encircle the head for the complete picture. These films are not good in aiding the diagnosis of decay, bone level, and certain types of periapical problems.

A periapical x ray is similar to a bitewing. This type of x ray shows the entire tooth area, from crown to root, and the bone surrounding the root from a side view. This type of film will reveal any root anomalies, changes in the bone and surrounding tissue, cysts, bone tumors, and abscesses. The fine detail in the periapical film is necessary in diagnosis and treatment planning, and is commonly taken during root canal treatment and crown restoration procedures.

Occlusal films are least common. These films show the whole bite of the lower or upper jaw. Occlusal x rays, when taken, are mainly taken on children to show the eruption order of the permanent teeth.

X rays pass through hard and soft tissue in the mouth. The x-ray beam is blocked by denser structures, such as teeth, fillings, jaws, and bones. Teeth appear lighter because fewer x rays go through the teeth to reach the film. Cavities and gum disease appear darker (shown by a dark spot in the tooth or loss of bone structure around the tooth) because of more x-ray penetration. On the film, the white images are the dense structures.

Operation

William Roentgen, a German scientist, discovered the x ray in 1895. He found that x rays are energy in the form of waves, similar to visible light. The only difference between light and x rays is that light does not have the ability to penetrate the body as x ray energy does. Light makes pictures of the outside of objects, while x rays have the ability to make pictures of the inside of objects. The roentgen represents the amount of exposure given off by one single energy photon. The amount of absorbed x ray in the body is a unit called a rad. A unit called "rem" accounts for the difference in biological effectiveness of different types of radiation, such as secondary radiation, or cosmic radiation. One rem equals one rad. One rad equals one R and one thousand milliroentgens, more commonly known as mrad; it is equal to one roentgen (R).

Research conducted by the Idaho Radiation Network set a maximum permissible x ray dose for one year at 5R (roentgens). A full mouth set of dental x rays consists of 18 to 20 films (bitewings, periapicals, occlusals, and panoramic x rays). The amount of radiation for receiving the full-mouth set of x rays is 10 to 20 mrads (milliroentgens). The benefits derived from x rays greatly outweigh the radiation concerns. The amount of radiation an average person receives each year from background sources (e.g., outer space, materials in the earth, foods consumed, and naturally radioactive materials in the body) is about 360 mrads.

Secondary radiation consists of the radiation waves left over after the source of radiation is stopped. Most secondary waves can penetrate tissue and are the most damaging waves from radiation. Measures taken to prevent damaging rays are:

- setting radiation exposure to lower settings depending on the patient's age, height, build and structure
- using high-speed films to minimize exposure time
- using lead-filled aprons to shield sensitive body parts, such as thyroid glands and gonads
- x-ray badges worn by dental staff to monitor the amount of radiation exposure in the workplace

Maintenance

Dental x rays are essential in diagnosing and treating oral disease, abnormal tooth development, or trauma. At the initial dental examination, a full-mouth set of x rays may be taken (bitewings and panoramic). Thereafter, it is the dentist who should determine when and how often x rays will be required.

KEY TERMS

Apical—Rounded end of the root of a tooth that is embedded in hard tissue (bone); toward the apex of the root.

Crown—1. The upper part of the tooth, covered by enamel. 2. A dental restoration that is a protective shell fitting over a tooth.

Eruption—The process of a tooth breaking through the gum tissue to grow into place in the mouth.

Pulp—The soft, innermost part of a tooth containing blood and lymph vessels, and nerves.

Root canal treatment—The process of removing diseased or damaged pulp tissue from a tooth, then filling and sealing the pulp chamber and root canals.

Children are usually more cavity prone than adults; x rays may be taken with regard to degree of risk, or at the check-up examination every six months.

An adult presenting a **dental trauma** will need x rays to diagnose what the treatment should be. More x rays may be needed depending on the treatment plan and the extent of the injury.

The American Dental Association (ADA) recommends basic guidelines on taking dental x rays. On average, bitewing x rays should be taken approximately once a year. This is mainly to detect and treat any conditions early in their development. If the overall general health of the mouth is good, x rays can be taken every 18 to 24 months. The ADA also recommends that the type and frequency of dental x rays taken at an examination be based upon clinical judgment after the examination and consideration of the dental health and the general health of the patient.

Health care team roles

A registered dental assistant (RDA) or registered dental hygienist (RDH) commonly takes the x rays during a dental examination. They review the health and dental history, chart, and age of the patient to be x rayed. Adjustments are made to the x-ray unit depending on the size and age of the patient. The RDA then develops and mounts the x rays and presents them to the dentist. The dentist will interpret the x rays and complete the oral examination. A treatment plan will follow.

Training

An RDA and an RDH must have an x-ray certification in order to take and develop x rays. To become certified, full-mouth sets of x rays need to be taken. Knowledge of the x-ray machine unit is needed, as is the number of roentgens emitted from a variety of different x-ray machines. Furthermore, a working knowledge of angles and height of the x-ray unit is needed; this is necessary for taking fine-detailed images. Certification also requires knowledge of the principles of radiation safety.

Classes leading to certification as an RDA or RDH are available outside the work setting. Each state has different bylaws regarding x-ray licensing for technicians. The rules of the state in which one is interested in working should be consulted.

Resources

BOOKS

Hollins, Carole. *Basic Guide to Dental Procedures*. Oxford: Blackwell Publishing, 2008.

Bunkle, Richard S. *Taking a Giant Bite Out of Dental Confusion: The Consumer's Guide to 21st Century Dentistry*. Moscow, ID: Luminary Media Group, 2008.

Whaites, Eric. *Radiography and Radiology for Dental Nurses*, 2nd ed. New York: Saunders, 2009.

PERIODICALS

Barge, Katie. "Dental X Rays Accurately Predict Osteoporosis Risk." *Journal of Dental Hygiene* (2007) 81(2):42.

Robb-Nicholson, Celeste. "By The Way, Doctor. What Kind of Radiation Causes Thyroid Cancer? What About Microwave Ovens and Dental X Rays?" *Harvard Women's Health Watch* (February 2007) 14(6):8.

ORGANIZATIONS

American Dental Association, 211 East Chicago Avenue, Chicago, IL, 60611-2678, (312) 440-2500, www.ada.org.

American Dental Education Association, 1400 K Street, Suite 1100, Washington, DC, 20005, (202) 289-7201, (202) 289-7204, www.adea.org.

American Dental Hygienists' Association, 444 North Michigan Avenue, Suite 3400, Chicago, IL, 60611, (312) 440-8900, mail@adha.net, www.adha.org.

Cindy F. Ovard, RDA
Tish Davidson, AM
Brenda Lerner

Depersonalization disorder *see* **Dissociative disorders**

Depo-Provera/Norplant

Definition

Medroxyprogesterone is a long-acting progestin hormone that is inserted under the skin and prevents conception for up to five years. Depo-Provera is also a hormone, but is administered by intramuscular injection and provides protection against **pregnancy** for three months. Lunelle is another injectable contraceptive that is administered monthly (every 28 to 30 days); it was approved by the Food and Drug Administration (FDA) in October 2000. The hormone in Norplant and Depo-Provera is progestin, a synthetic hormone similar to one found naturally in a woman's body; Lunelle contains the hormones progestin and estrogen.

Purpose

The purpose of these hormones is to prevent pregnancy; they are about 99% effective in achieving this goal. No hormonal contraceptive methods provide protection from **AIDS** or other **sexually transmitted diseases**.

Depo-Provera and Lunelle are given as an injection and work in several ways to prevent conception. First, the egg (ovum) is prevented from maturing and being released. The mucus in the cervix (opening into the uterus or womb) becomes thicker, making it difficult for the sperm to enter. Depo-Provera and Lunelle also cause the lining of the uterus to become thinner, making implantation of a fertilized egg unlikely.

An injection of Depo-Provera or Lunelle must be given within the first five days of a normal period. Depo-Provera provides protection against pregnancy for three months, while Lunelle provides similar

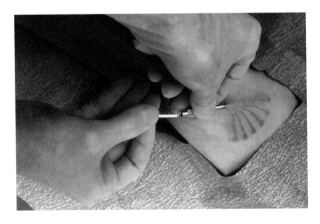

A physician inserts a contraceptive implant under the skin of a woman's arm. *(Photo Researchers, Inc.)*

protection for one month. Ovulation (release of a mature egg) typically occurs within 60 days of the last injection of Lunelle, about twice as fast after use of Depo-Provera. Also, because Lunelle is a combined hormone contraceptive as opposed to progestin-only Depo-Provera and Norplant, it is less likely to cause irregular or absent menstruation.

Norplant capsules contain a synthetic hormone that is slowly released over a period of up to five years. It functions like Depo-Provera in that it prevents the ovaries from producing ova (eggs) and also results in thicker mucus in the cervix, which prevents the sperm from passing through the cervix. Norplant can be inserted at any time.

Preparation

The woman being considered for Depo-Provera or Lunelle will have a pelvic and breast examination, a **Pap test** (a microscopic examination of cell samples taken from the cervix), blood pressure check, weight check, and a review of her medical history. Women who have **diabetes mellitus**, major depression, blood clotting problems, **liver disease**, or weight problems should use these methods only under strict medical supervision. Depo-Provera or Lunelle should not be used if the woman is pregnant, has unexplained vaginal bleeding, suffers from severe liver disease, has **breast cancer**, or has a history of **blood clots** or **stroke**.

Individuals who select Norplant will receive the same basic **physical examination**. If approved for this method, a site of implantation will be selected (usually the inside of the upper arm), and the area prepared for minor surgery. The skin will be washed with soap and water, and an antiseptic, such as iodine solution, will be applied. The physician will use a local anesthetic to numb the area, a small incision will be made, the six

Norplant capsules will be inserted, and the incision sewn up (sutured). Protection against pregnancy normally begins within 24 hours. If necessary, the implants can be removed in 15–20 minutes. Norplant should not be used by women who are pregnant, have blood clotting problems, or have unexplained vaginal bleeding. Advantages include light periods with less cramping and decreased anemia. This form of birth control may also be protective against **endometrial cancer**.

Because Depo-Provera and Norplant use only the hormone progestin, they may provide an alternative for women who can not use estrogen-containing birth control pills. One benefit of Lunelle, however, is that its effects wear off more quickly than Depo-Provera, an important factor in the event that a woman has serious side effects or wants to become pregnant.

Risks

The most common side effects associated with Depo-Provera and Lunelle are yellowing of the skin, **headache**, nervousness, **dizziness**, abdominal **pain**, hair loss, rash, increase in the number of migraine headaches, increased or decreased interest in sexual intercourse, the development of dark spots on the skin, depression, and weakness; more serious is, liver disease and breast **cancer**. Danger signs that need to reported immediately include weight gain, heavy vaginal bleeding, frequent urination, blurred vision, **fainting**, severe abdominal pain, and coughing up blood. Because the effects of Depo-Provera may last up to 12 weeks, it may take a longer time for women trying to conceive to become pregnant after discontinuing the injections.

The main reactions to Norplant include headache, weight gain, irregular periods or no period at all, breast tenderness, **acne**, gain or loss of facial hair, color changes of the skin over the area of insertion, and **ovarian cysts**. The doctor should be notified immediately of lumps in the breast, heavy vaginal bleeding, yellowing of the skin or eyes, or infection of the incision. Women who use Norplant are discouraged from **smoking**.

As of 2010, Depo-Provera comes with a special warning that links prolonged use of the drug with bone density loss. The Food and Drug Administration's strident warning informs women that the drug can cause significant loss of bone density. Losses are greater when the drug is used longer. In addition, bone density loss may not reverse completely when women stop using Depo-Provera. The FDA's decision to add such a warning followed analyses by the agency and Pfizer of data about the drug's long-term effect on bone density among teens and adult women. The women's study ran from 1994 to 2010 and enrolled 540 women aged 25 to 38.

Normal results

These hormone contraceptive methods normally result in a success rate of 99%.

Resources

BOOKS

Goldberg, A.B., et al. "Injectable contraceptives." In *Contraceptive Technology*, 19th ed., Hatcher, R.A., et al., 157. New York: Ardent Media Inc., 2007.

PERIODICALS

Jain, J. "Contraception: Subcutaneous Depot Medroxyprogesterone Acetate for Birth Control and Endometriosis Pain." *OBG Management* Vol. 17, No 8. (2005).

OTHER

Birth control. *The American College of Obstetricians and Gynecologists.* Accessed July 20, 2010. http://www.plannedparenthood.org/Library/birthcontrol/depoforyou.html.

James Waun, MD, RPh
Karl Finley

Depressive disorders

Definition

Depression or depressive disorders (unipolar depression) are mental illnesses characterized by a profound and persistent feeling of sadness or despair and/or a loss of interest in things that once were pleasurable. Disturbance in sleep, appetite, and mental processes are a common accompaniment.

Description

Everyone experiences feelings of unhappiness and sadness occasionally. But when these depressed feelings start to dominate everyday life and cause physical and mental deterioration, they become what are known as depressive disorders. There are two main categories of depressive disorders: major depressive disorder and dysthymic disorder. Major depressive disorder is a moderate to severe episode of depression lasting two or more weeks. Individuals experiencing this major depressive episode may have trouble sleeping, lose interest in activities they once took pleasure in, experience a change in weight, have difficulty concentrating, feel worthless and hopeless, or have a preoccupation with **death** or **suicide**. In children, major depression may be characterized by irritability.

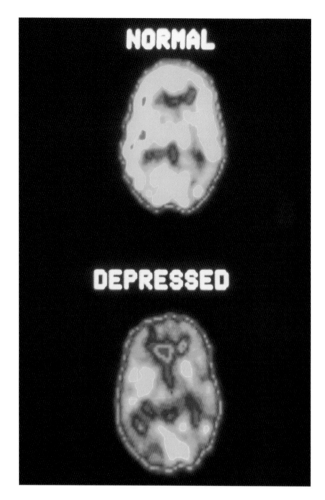

Positron emission tomography (PET) scans comparing a normal brain with that of someone with a depressed mental disorder. *(Photo Researchers, Inc.)*

In 2006 The National Institutes of Mental Health estimated that about 6.7% of Americans adults are affected by major depressive disorder, and about 1.5% are affected by dyrthmic disorder in a given year. Major depressive disorder has a median age of onset of 32 years, and affects women more frequently than men. Dyrthmic disorder has a median age of onset of 31 years. Both disorders may occur in any age group, from children to the elderly.

While major depressive episodes may be acute (intense but short-lived), dysthymic disorder is an ongoing, chronic depression that lasts two or more years (one or more years in children) and has an average duration of 16 years. The mild to moderate depression of dysthymic disorder may rise and fall in intensity, and those afflicted with the disorder may experience some periods of normal, non-depressed mood of up to two months in length. Its onset is gradual, and dysthymic

patients may not be able to pinpoint exactly when they started feeling depressed. Individuals with dysthymic disorder may experience a change in sleeping and eating patterns, low self-esteem, **fatigue**, trouble concentrating, and feelings of hopelessness.

Depression also can occur in **bipolar disorder**, an affective mental illness that causes radical emotional changes and mood swings, from manic highs to depressive lows. The majority of bipolar individuals experience alternating episodes of **mania** and depression.

Causes and symptoms

The causes behind depression are complex and not yet fully understood. While an imbalance of certain neurotransmitters—the chemicals in the brain that transmit messages between nerve cells—is believed to play a key role in depression, external factors such as upbringing and environment (more so in dysthymia than major depression) may be as important. For example, it is speculated that, if an individual is abused and neglected throughout childhood and adolescence, a pattern of low self-esteem and negative thinking may emerge. From that, a lifelong pattern of depression may follow. Many different factors have been linked to major depression, including chronic **pain**, severe **obesity**, and **smoking** (among teenagers).

Heredity seems to play a role in who develops depressive disorders. Individuals with major depression in their immediate family are up to three times more likely to have the disorder themselves. It would seem that biological and genetic factors may make certain individuals pre-disposed or prone to depressive disorders, but environmental circumstances often may trigger the disorder.

External stressors and significant life changes, such as chronic medical problems, death of a loved one, divorce or estrangement, **miscarriage**, or loss of a job, also can result in a form of depression known as adjustment disorder. Although periods of adjustment disorder usually resolve themselves, occasionally they may evolve into a major depressive disorder.

Major depressive episode

Individuals experiencing a major depressive episode have a depressed mood and/or a diminished interest or pleasure in activities. Children experiencing a major depressive episode may appear or feel irritable rather than depressed. In addition, five or more of the following symptoms will occur on an almost daily basis for a period of at least two weeks:

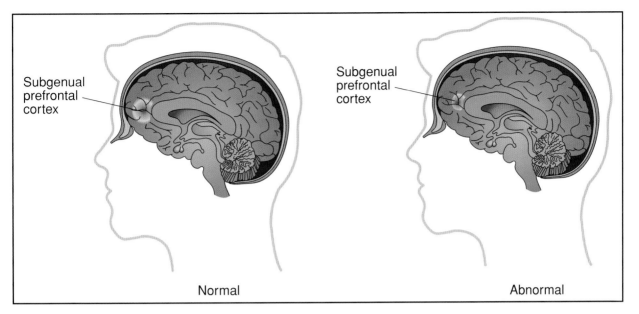

Subgenual prefrontal cortex

Subgenual prefrontal cortex

Normal

Abnormal

Recent scientific research has indicated that the size of the subgenual prefrontal cortex of the brain (located behind the bridge of the nose) may be a determining factor in hereditary depressive disorders. *(Illustration by Electronic Illustrators Group. Reproduced by permission of Gale, a part of Cengage Learning.)*

- Significant change in weight.
- Insomnia or hypersomnia (excessive sleep).
- Psychomotor agitation or retardation.
- Fatigue or loss of energy.
- Feelings of worthlessness or inappropriate guilt.
- Diminished ability to think or to concentrate, or indecisiveness.
- Recurrent thoughts of death or suicide and/or suicide attempts.

Dysthymic disorder

Dysthymia commonly occurs in tandem with other psychiatric and physical conditions. Up to 70% of dysthymic patients have both dysthymic disorder and major depressive disorder, known as double depression. **Substance abuse**, panic disorders, **personality disorders**, social **phobias**, and other psychiatric conditions also are found in many dysthymic patients. Dysthymia and medical conditions often co-occur. The connection between them is unclear, but it may be related to the way the medical condition and/or its pharmacological treatment affects neurotransmitters. Dysthymia is prevalent in patients with **multiple sclerosis, AIDS, hypothyroidism, chronic fatigue syndrome, Parkinson's disease,** diabetes, and post-cardiac transplantation. Dysthymic disorder can lengthen or complicate the recovery of patients with these and other medical conditions.

Along with an underlying feeling of depression, people with dysthymic disorder experience two or more of the following symptoms on an almost daily basis for a period for two or more years (many experience them for five or more years), or one year or more for children:

- under or overeating
- insomnia or hypersomnia
- low energy or fatigue
- low self-esteem
- poor concentration or trouble making decisions
- feelings of hopelessness

Diagnosis

In addition to an interview, several clinical inventories or scales may be used to assess a patient's mental status and determine the presence of depressive symptoms. Among these tests are: the Hamilton Depression Scale (HAM-D), Child Depression Inventory (CDI), Geriatric Depression Scale (GDS), Beck Depression Inventory (BDI), and the Zung Self-Rating Scale for Depression. These tests may be administered in an outpatient or hospital setting by a general practitioner, social worker, psychiatrist, or psychologist.

Treatment

Major depressive and dysthymic disorders are typically treated with a combination of antidepressants and psychosocial therapy. Psychosocial therapy focuses on the personal and interpersonal issues

Signs of depression

Lack of interest or pleasure in daily activities
Significant weight loss (without dieting) or weight gain
Difficulty sleeping or excessive sleeping
Loss of energy
Feelings of worthlessness or guilt
Difficulty in making decisions
Restlessness
Recurrent thoughts of death

(Table by PreMediaGlobal. Reproduced by permission of Gale, a part of Cengage Learning.)

behind depression, while antidepressant medication is prescribed to provide more immediate relief for the symptoms of the disorder. When used together correctly, therapy and antidepressants are a powerful treatment plan for the depressed patient.

Antidepressants

Selective serotonin reuptake inhibitors (SSRIs) such as fluoxetine (Prozac) and sertraline (Zoloft) reduce depression by increasing levels of serotonin, a neurotransmitter. Some clinicians prefer SSRIs for treatment of dysthymic disorder. **Anxiety**, **diarrhea**, drowsiness, **headache**, sweating, **nausea**, poor sexual functioning, and **insomnia** all are possible side effects of SSRIs. In early 2004, the U.S. Food and Drug Administration (FDA) issued warnings to physicians and parents about increased risk of suicide among children and adolescents taking SSRIs.

Tricyclic antidepressants (TCAs) are less expensive than SSRIs, but have more severe side-effects, which may include persistent **dry mouth, sedation, dizziness**, and cardiac **arrhythmias**. Because of these side effects, caution is taken when prescribing TCAs to elderly patients. TCAs include amitriptyline (Elavil), imipramine (Tofranil), and nortriptyline (Aventyl, Pamelor). A 10-day supply of TCAs can be lethal if ingested all at once, so these drugs may not be a preferred treatment option for patients at risk for suicide.

Monoamine oxidase inhibitors (MAOIs) such as tranylcypromine (Parnate) and phenelzine (Nardil) block the action of monoamine oxidase (MAO), an enzyme in the central nervous system. Patients taking MAOIs must cut foods high in tyramine (found in aged cheeses and meats) out of their diet to avoid potentially serious hypertensive side effects.

Heterocyclics include bupropion (Wellbutrin) and trazodone (Desyrel). Bupropion should not be prescribed to patients with a **seizure disorder**. Side effects of the drug may include agitation, anxiety, confusion, tremor, dry mouth, fast or irregular heartbeat, headache, low blood pressure, and insomnia. Because trazodone has a sedative effect, it is useful in treating depressed patients with insomnia. Other possible side effects of trazodone include dry mouth, gastrointestinal distress, dizziness, and headache.

Psychosocial therapy

Psychotherapy explores an individual's life to bring to light possible contributing causes of the present depression. During treatment, the therapist helps the patient to become self-aware of his or her thinking patterns and how they came to be. There are several different subtypes of psychotherapy, but all have the common goal of helping the patient develop healthy problem solving and coping skills.

Cognitive-behavioral therapy assumes that the patient's problematic thinking is causing the current depression and focuses on changing the depressed patient's thought patterns and perceptions. The therapist helps the patient identify negative or distorted thought patterns and the emotions and the behaviors that accompany them, and then retrains the depressed individual to recognize the thinking and react differently to it.

Electroconvulsant therapy

ECT, or **electroconvulsive therapy**, usually is employed after all psychosocial therapy and pharmaceutical treatment options have been explored. However, it is sometimes used early in treatment when severe depression is present and the patient refuses oral medication, or when the patient is becoming dehydrated, extremely suicidal, or psychotic.

The treatment consists of a series of electrical pulses that move into the brain through electrodes on the patient's head. ECT is given under **general anesthesia** and patients are administered a muscle relaxant to prevent convulsions. Although the exact mechanisms behind the success of ECT therapy are not known, it is believed that the electrical current modifies the electrochemical processes of the brain, consequently relieving depression. Headaches, muscle soreness, nausea, and confusion are possible side effects immediately following an ECT procedure. **Memory loss**, typically transient, also has been reported in ECT patients.

Alternative treatment

St. John's wort (*Hypericum perforatum*) is used throughout Europe to treat depressive symptoms.

KEY TERMS

Hypersomnia—The need to sleep excessively; a symptom of dysthymic and major depressive disorder.

Neurotransmitter—A chemical in the brain that transmits messages between neurons, or nerve cells. Changes in the levels of certain neurotransmitters, such as serotonin, norepinephrine, and dopamine, are thought to be related to depressive disorders.

Psychomotor agitation—Disturbed physical and mental processes (e.g., fidgeting, wringing of hands, racing thoughts); a symptom of major depressive disorder.

Psychomotor retardation—Slowed physical and mental processes (e.g., slowed thinking, walking, and talking); a symptom of major depressive disorder.

Unlike traditional prescription antidepressants, this herbal antidepressant has few reported side effects. Despite uncertainty concerning its effectiveness, it is accepted by many practitioners of alternative medicine. Although St. John's wort appears to be a safe alternative to conventional antidepressants, care should be taken, as the herb can interfere with the actions of some pharmaceuticals, and because herbal supplements are not regulated by the FDA in the same way as conventional medications.

Homeopathic treatment also can be therapeutic in treating depression. Good **nutrition**, proper sleep, **exercise**, and full engagement in life are very important to a healthy mental state.

In several small studies, S-adenosyl-methionine (SAM, SAMe) was shown to be more effective than placebo and equally effective as tricyclic antidepressants in treating depression. The usual dosage is 200 mg to 400 mg twice daily. It may however cause some side effects, and an individual should discuss the possible risks and benefits with a doctor.

Prognosis

Untreated or improperly treated depression is the number one cause of suicide in the United States. Proper treatment relieves symptoms in 80–90% of depressed patients. After each major depressive episode, the risk of recurrence climbs significantly—50% after one episode, 70% after two episodes, and 90% after three episodes. For this reason, patients need to be aware of the symptoms of recurring depression and may require long-term maintenance treatment of antidepressants and/or therapy.

Research has found that depression may lead to other problems as well. Increased risk of heart disease has been linked to depression, particularly in postmenopausal women. And while chronic pain may cause depression, some studies indicate that depression may also cause chronic pain.

Prevention

Patient education in the form of therapy or self-help groups is crucial for training patients with depressive disorders to recognize symptoms of depression and to take an active part in their treatment program. Extended maintenance treatment with antidepressants may be required in some patients to prevent relapse. Early intervention for children with depression is usually effective in arresting development of more severe problems.

Resources

BOOKS

Henri, Maurice J., ed. *Trends in Depression Research.* New York: Nova Science Publishers, 2007.

PERIODICALS

"Depression Can Lead to Back Pain." *Biotech Week*, March 24, 2004: 576.

"Depression May Be a Risk Factor for Heart Disease, Death in Older Women." *Women's Health Weekly*, March 4, 2004: 90.

"FDA Panel Urges Stronger Warnings of Child Suicide." *SCRIP World Pharmaceutical News*, February 6, 2004: 24.

"National Study Indicates Obesity Is Linked to Major Depression." *Drug Week*, February 13, 2004: 338.

"Researchers See Link Between Depression, Smoking." *Mental Health Weekly*, March 1, 2004: 8.

ORGANIZATIONS

American Psychiatric Association (APA), 1000 Wilson Boulevard, Suite 1825, Arlington, VA, 22209, (888) 357-7924, apa@psych.org, http://www.psych.org.

American Psychological Association (APA), 750 First St. NE, Washington, DC, 20002-4242, (202) 336-5500, (800) 374-2721, http://www.apa.org/.

Depression and Bipolar Support Alliance (DBSA), 730 N. Franklin Street, Suite 501, Chicago, IL, 60654-7225, (312) 642-7243, (800) 826-3632, http://www.dbsalliance.org.

National Alliance for the Mentally Ill (NAMI), 3803 N. Fairfax Dr., Ste. 100, Arlington, VA, 22203, (703) 524-7600, (703) 524-9094, (800) 950-6264, http://www.nami.org.

National Institute of Mental Health (NIMH), 6001 Executive Boulevard, Room 8184, MSC 9663, Bethesda, MD 20892-9663, (866) 615-6464, http://www.nimh.nih.gov.

Paula Anne Ford-Martin
Teresa G. Odle

Depression *see* **Depressive disorders; Postpartum depression**

Dermabrasion *see* **Skin resurfacing**

Dermatitis

Definition

Dermatitis is a general term used to describe inflammation of the skin.

Description

Most types of dermatitis are characterized by an itchy pink or red rash.

Contact dermatitis is an allergic reaction to something that irritates the skin and is manifested by one or more lines of red, swollen, blistered skin that may itch or seep. It usually appears within 48 hours after touching or brushing against a substance to which the skin is sensitive. The condition is more common in adults than in children.

Contact dermatitis can occur on any part of the body, but it usually affects the hands, feet, and groin. Contact dermatitis usually does not spread from one

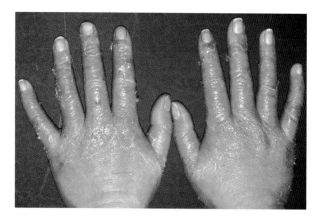

Dermatitis on hands and fingers. *(Custom Medical Stock Photo, Inc. Reproduced by permission.)*

person to another, nor does it spread beyond the area exposed to the irritant unless affected skin comes into contact with another part of the body. However, in the case of some irritants, such as **poison ivy**, contact dermatitis can be passed to another person or to another part of the body.

Stasis dermatitis is characterized by scaly, greasy looking skin on the lower legs and around the ankles. Stasis dermatitis is most apt to affect the inner side of the calf.

Nummular dermatitis, which is also called nummular eczematous dermatitis or nummular **eczema**, generally affects the hands, arms, legs, and buttocks of men and women older than 55 years of age. This stubborn inflamed rash forms circular, sometimes itchy, patches and is characterized by flares and periods of inactivity.

Atopic dermatitis is characterized by **itching**, scaling, swelling, and sometimes blistering. In early childhood it is called infantile eczema and is characterized by redness, oozing, and crusting. It is usually found on the face, inside the elbows, and behind the knees.

Seborrheic dermatitis may be dry or moist and is characterized by greasy scales and yellowish crusts on the scalp, eyelids, face, external surfaces of the ears, underarms, breasts, and groin. In infants it is called "cradle cap."

Causes and symptoms

Allergic reactions are genetically determined, and different substances cause contact dermatitis to develop in different people. A reaction to resin produced by poison ivy, **poison oak**, or poison sumac is the most common source of symptoms. It is, in fact, the most common allergy in this country, affecting one of every two people in the United States.

Flowers, herbs, and vegetables can also affect the skin of some people. **Burns** and **sunburn** increase the risk of dermatitis developing, and chemical irritants that can cause the condition include:

- chlorine
- cleansers
- detergents and soaps
- fabric softeners
- glues used on artificial nails
- perfumes
- topical medications

Contact dermatitis can develop when the first contact occurs or after years of use or exposure.

Stasis dermatitis, a consequence of poor circulation, occurs when leg veins can no longer return blood to the heart as efficiently as they once did. When that happens, fluid collects in the lower legs and causes them to swell. Stasis dermatitis can also result in a rash that can break down into sores known as stasis ulcers.

The cause of nummular dermatitis is not known, but it usually occurs in cold weather and is most common in people who have dry skin. Hot weather and **stress** can aggravate this condition, as can the following:

- allergies
- fabric softeners
- soaps and detergents
- wool clothing
- bathing more than once a day

Atopic dermatitis can be caused by **allergies**, **asthma**, or stress, and there seems to be a genetic predisposition for atopic conditions. It is sometimes caused by an allergy to nickel in jewelry.

Seborrheic dermatitis (for which there may also be a genetic predisposition) is usually caused by overproduction of the oil glands. In adults it can be associated with **diabetes mellitus** or gold allergy. In infants and adults it may be caused by a biotin deficiency.

Diagnosis

The diagnosis of dermatitis is made on the basis of how the rash looks and its location. The doctor may scrape off a small piece of affected skin for microscopic examination or direct the patient to discontinue use of any potential irritant that has recently come into contact with the affected area. Two weeks after the rash disappears, the patient may resume use of the substances, one at a time, until the condition recurs. Eliminating the substance most recently added should eliminate the irritation.

If the origin of the irritation has still not been identified, a dermatologist may perform one or more patch tests. This involves dabbing a small amount of a suspected irritant onto skin on the patient's back. If no irritation develops within a few days, another patch test is performed. The process continues until the patient experiences an allergic reaction at the spot where the irritant was applied.

Treatment

Treating contact dermatitis begins with eliminating or avoiding the source of irritation. Prescription or over-the-counter corticosteroid creams can lessen inflammation and relieve irritation. Creams, lotions, or ointments not specifically formulated for dermatitis can intensify the irritation. Oral **antihistamines** are sometimes recommended to alleviate itching, and **antibiotics** are prescribed if the rash becomes infected. Medications taken by mouth to relieve symptoms of dermatitis can make skin red and scaly and cause hair loss.

Patients who have a history of dermatitis should remove their rings before washing their hands. They should use bath oils or glycerine-based soaps and bathe in lukewarm saltwater.

Patting rather than rubbing the skin after bathing and thoroughly massaging lubricating lotion or non-prescription cortisone creams into still-damp skin can soothe red, irritated nummular dermatitis. Highly concentrated cortisone preparations should not be applied to the face, armpits, groin, or rectal area. Periodic medical monitoring is necessary to detect side effects in patients who use such preparations on **rashes** covering large areas of the body.

Coal-tar salves can help relieve symptoms of nummular dermatitis that have not responded to other treatments, but these ointments have an unpleasant odor and stain clothing.

Patients who have stasis dermatitis should elevate their legs as often as possible and sleep with a pillow between the lower legs.

Tar or zinc paste may also be used to treat stasis dermatitis. Because these compounds must remain in contact with the rash for as long as two weeks, the paste and **bandages** must be applied by a nurse or a doctor.

Coal-tar shampoos may be used for seborrheic dermatitis that occurs on the scalp. Sun exposure after the use of these shampoos should be avoided because the risk of sunburn of the scalp is increased.

Alternative treatment

Some herbal therapies can be useful for skin conditions. Among the herbs most often recommended are:

- Burdock root (*Arctium lappa*)
- Calendula (*Calendula officinalis*) ointment
- Chamomile (*Matricaria recutita*) ointment
- Cleavers (*Galium* ssp.)
- Evening primrose oil (*Oenothera biennis*)
- Nettles (*Urtica dioica*)

Contact dermatitis can be treated botanically and homeopathically. Grindelia (*Grindelia* spp.) and sassafras (*Sassafras albidum*) can help when applied topically. Determining the source of the problem and

KEY TERMS

Allergic reaction—An inappropriate or exaggerated genetically determined reaction to a chemical that occurs only on the second or subsequent exposures to the offending agent, after the first contact has sensitized the body.

Corticosteriod—A group of synthetic hormones that are used to prevent or reduce inflammation. Toxic effects may result from rapid withdrawal after prolonged use or from continued use of large doses.

Patch test—A skin test that is done to identify allergens. A suspected substance is applied to the skin.

After 24–48 hours, if the area is red and swollen, the test is positive for that substance. If no reaction occurs, another substance is applied. This is continued until the patient experiences an allergic reaction where the irritant was applied to the skin.

Rash—A spotted, pink or red skin eruption that may be accompanied by itching and is caused by disease, contact with an allergen, food ingestion, or drug reaction.

Ulcer—An open sore on the skin, resulting from tissue destruction, that is usually accompanied by redness, pain, or infection.

eliminating it is essential. Oatmeal baths are very helpful in relieving the itch. Bentonite clay packs or any mud pack draws the fluid out and helps dry up the lesions. Cortisone creams are not recommended.

Stasis dermatitis should be treated by a trained practitioner. This condition responds well to topical herbal therapies, however, the cause must also be addressed. Selenium-based shampoos, topical applications of flax oil and/or olive oil, and biotin supplementation are among the therapies recommended for seborrheic dermatitis.

Prognosis

Dermatitis is often chronic, but symptoms can generally be controlled.

Prevention

Contact dermatitis can be prevented by avoiding the source of irritation. If the irritant cannot be avoided completely, the patient should wear gloves and other protective clothing whenever exposure is likely to occur.

Immediately washing the exposed area with soap and water can stem allergic reactions to poison ivy, poison oak, or poison sumac, but because soaps can dry the skin, patients susceptible to dermatitis should use them only on the face, feet, genitals, and underarms.

Clothing should be loose fitting and 100% cotton. New clothing should be washed in dye-free, unscented detergent before being worn.

Injury to the lower leg can cause stasis dermatitis to ulcerate (form open sores). If stasis ulcers develop, a doctor should be notified immediately.

Yoga and other relaxation techniques may help prevent atopic dermatitis caused by stress.

Avoidance of sweating may aid in preventing seborrheic dermatitis.

A patient who has dermatitis should also notify a doctor if any of the following occurs:

• fever develops

• skin oozes or other signs of infection appear

• symptoms do not begin to subside after seven days' treatment

• he/she comes into contact with someone who has a wart, cold sore, or other viral skin infection

Resources

OTHER

"Allergic Contact Dermatitis." *The Skin Site*. April 10, 1998 (January 11, 2006). http://www.skinsite.com/info_allergic.htm.

Maureen Haggerty

Dermatomyositis

Definition

Dermatomyositis (DM) is a rare inflammatory muscle disease that leads to destruction of muscle tissue usually accompanied by **pain** and weakness.

Description

Dermatomyositis is one of a group of three related diseases called inflammatory **myopathies**. The other two are **polymyositis** and inclusion-body **myositis**. These diseases are rare; only about 20,000 people in the United States have dermatomyositis. Another estimates suggest that DM occurs in about 5.5 individuals out of every one million. The disease is of unknown origin and can develop in children and adults. Most often individuals either develop DM either between the ages of five and 14 or they do not develop it until they are over age 45. In all age groups, females are twice as likely to develop the disease than males. Although DM causes pain and weakness, it is not necessarily life threatening. However, adults, but not children, who develop DM have an increased risk of developing **cancer** and should be screened for malignancies regularly.

Causes and symptoms

The exact cause of dermatomyositis is unknown. It is an autoimmune disease. In a healthy body, cells of immune system attack only foreign or defective cells in the body to protect it from disease. In an autoimmune disease, the immune system attacks normal body cells. In the case of DM, immune system cells attack healthy cells of small blood vessels in the muscle and skin. Over time, this causes muscle fiber to shrink and sometimes cuts off blood supply to the muscle. DM tends to develop in muscles closest to the center of the body.

As yet, there is no clear explanation of what causes an individual to develop DM. It is thought that the disease may be triggered by a virus or exposure to certain drugs or vaccines. According to the **Muscular Dystrophy** Association, recent research suggests developing DM may be related to the mixing of blood cells that sometimes occurs between the mother and fetus during **pregnancy**. The disease is not directly inherited, although there may be some genetic sensitivity toward whatever triggers it.

Often the first sign of DM is the development of a patchy, scaly, violet to dark red skin rash on the face, neck, shoulders, upper chest, knees, or back. Often the rash appears before any signs of illness or muscle weakness. About 40% of children and teens develop hard, painful bumps under the skin that are deposits of **calcium**, a mineral used in bone formation. This condition, called calcinosis, is much less common in adults.

Muscle weakness, especially in the upper arms, hips, thighs, and neck, becomes apparent in activities such as climbing stairs or reaching up over the head. This weakness develops after the rash appears. Some people have difficulty swallowing and chewing when the muscles of the face and esophagus are affected.

Individuals may also feel tried, weak, have a low-grade **fever**, weight loss, and joint stiffness. Some individuals have the rash for years before they progress to these symptoms, while in others the onset of symptoms is rapid. In children the development of symptoms is almost always gradual, making diagnosis especially difficult.

Diagnosis

DM can be difficult to diagnose, and often the first doctor an individual sees is a dermatologist for treatment of the rash and then is referred to a rheumatologist, specialist in internal medicine or neurologist when DM is suspected. Many tests may be done to rule out other diseases before a firm diagnosis is made. A blood test is done to measure the level of creatine kinase. Creatine kinase is an enzyme found in muscle tissue. When muscle is damaged, this enzyme leaks out into the blood. An increased level of creatine kinase in the blood suggests DM as a possible diagnosis. Another blood test may be done to test for specific immune system antibodies. Antibodies are proteins made in response to material the body thinks is foreign.

An electromyogram (EMG) is a test that measures electrical activity in muscles as they contract. Individuals with inflammatory myopathies usually have distinct patterns of electrical activity in the affected muscles. However, up to 15% of people with DM have normal electromyogram readings, so this test is not definitive. The definitive test is a muscle biopsy. The doctor takes a small sample of muscle tissue and examines it under a microscope. From this sample, the doctor can differentiate DM from other inflammatory myopathies and other muscle wasting diseases.

Treatment

The goal of treatment is to improve muscle strength and allow the individual to participate in normal daily activities. Individuals are given steroid drugs (prednisone, **corticosteroids**) that suppress the immune system. Over time, these drugs often produce undesirable side effects, so treatment is usually begun with a large dose, then tapered to the minimum dose needed for maintenance. People who do not respond well to steroid treatment may be treated with other immunosuppressive drugs or intravenous immunoglobulin. Individuals with DM are advised to avoid exposure to the sun, as sunlight worsens the skin rash. **Physical therapy** is often helpful in keeping joints from stiffening and freezing. Moderate **exercise** is also recommended.

Alternative treatment

A healthy diet high is recommended for all individuals with supplemental protein for those with severe muscle damage.

Prognosis

The course of DM is highly variable. In about 20% of people, the disease spontaneously goes into remission and individuals are able to lead symptom-free lives for long periods. On the other hand, in about 5% of individuals the disease progresses to **death** because of heart and lung involvement. The majority of people continue to have some symptoms and require long-term treatment, but their degree of daily activity varies greatly.

Serious complications from DM include involvement of the muscles of the heart and lungs, difficulty eating and swallowing, and a tendency to develop cancer. This association is seen only in adults and not in children. Individuals over age 60 are more likely to have serious complications than younger individuals.

Prevention

There is no known way to prevent this disease.

Resources

PERIODICALS

Koler, Ric A. and Andrew Montemarano. "Dermatomyositis." *American Family Physician*, 24, no. 9 (1 November 2001) 1565–1574.

OTHER

Callen, Jeffrey P. *Dermatomyositis*, 5 December 2002 [cited 16 February 2005]. http://www.emedicine.com/derm/topic98.htm.

Hashmat, Aamir and Zaineb Daud. *Dermatomyositis/Polymyositis*, 16 January 2004 [cited 16 February 2005]. http://www.emedicine.com/neuro/topic85.htm.

ORGANIZATIONS

American Autoimmune Related Diseases Association, Inc., 22100 Gratiot Avenue, East Detroit, MI, 48021, (586) 776-3900, (586) 776-3903, http://www.aarda.org.

Muscular Dystrophy Association, 3300 East Sunrise Drive, Tucson, AZ, 85718, (800) 572-1717, http://www.mdausa.org.

National Organization for Rare Disorders, P.O. Box 8923, New Fairfield, CT, 06812-8923, (800) 999-6673, http://www.rarediseases.org.

The Myositis Association, 1737 King Street, Suite 600, Alexandria, VA, 22314, (800) 821-7356, TMA@myositis.org, http://www.myositis.org.

Tish Davidson, A.M.

Dermatophyte infections *see* **Ringworm**

DES exposure

Definition

DES (diethylstilbestrol) is a hormone that was prescribed for pregnant women in the 1950s and early 1960s. Many years later, doctors discovered that the daughters of the women who received DES were at high risk for a variety of problems, including **infertility**, **premature labor**, and **cancer** of the vagina and cervix. Sons of DES mothers were also affected.

Demographics

It is estimated that five to 10 million people in the United States were exposed to DES between 1938 and 1971. The United States has approximately 250,000 to one million DES daughters.

Description

In the 1950s and early 1960s, several drug companies claimed that DES (diethylstilbestrol) could prevent miscarriages. DES is a synthetic hormone, related to estrogen. At the time, up to 20% of all pregnancies ended in **miscarriage**, making this an important breakthrough and DES was prescribed for many women who had bleeding in early **pregnancy**. Ultimately, it was found to have no effect on miscarriages and the practice of prescribing DES was stopped in the 1960s. Almost 10 years later, the daughters of women who had taken DES during pregnancy began to develop unusual symptoms.

Doctors discovered that when these young women reached their teens, they were at higher risk for a variety of problems, including:

- clear cell adenocarcinoma of the vagina and cervix
- infertility
- premature labor and other problems in pregnancy

Sons of DES mothers were also affected, although fertility issues are not as common among DES sons as in DES daughters. Sons of DES mothers are more likely to be diagnosed with:

- increased rate of cryptorchidism (undescended testicles)
- increased incidence of epididymal cysts
- increased incidence of hypoplastic testes

Causes and symptoms

DES has affected a very specific group of women. These are women who were exposed to DES in utero before 18 weeks of pregnancy. In other words, their mothers must have taken DES within the first four-to-five months of pregnancy. It is now known that the female reproductive organs are formed during that time. DES appears to interfere with proper growth and development of the uterus, cervix, vagina, and fallopian tubes. In some studies, DES was also associated with a modestly increased risk of **breast cancer** for DES mothers.

In the early 1970s, there was an increase in a rare form of cancer, clear cell adenocarcinoma of the vagina and cervix. Up until that time, doctors had seen these cancers only in elderly women. Suddenly, young women who had the disease appeared.

Researchers studied these women to see if they had anything in common. After extensive questioning and examination, it was found that all of the young women had been exposed to DES in utero in the early weeks of pregnancy.

It was a shocking discovery. Doctors had only recently recognized that medications and exposure to chemicals during pregnancy could cause **birth defects**. This was a birth defect that had gone undetected for almost two decades.

Since then, doctors have studied DES daughters very carefully. Fortunately, the risk of clear cell adenocarcinoma is actually quite low. In fact, it appears that if a DES daughter has not developed this cancer by age 30, she will not develop it. Since all DES daughters are now over age 30, there should be no further cases related to DES exposure. However, there are a number

KEY TERMS

Cervix—The opening at the bottom of the uterus.

Colposcopy—A special examination of the cervix using a magnifying scope. This is a procedure that can be done in the doctor's office.

Fallopian tubes—The tubes that carry the ovum (egg) from the ovary to the uterus.

Pap smear—A screening test for precancerous and cancerous cells on the cervix. This simple test is done during a routine pelvic exam and involves scraping cells from the cervix.

of other symptoms and problems associated with DES exposure.

- Cervix and vagina. DES daughters often have distinctive changes of the cervix and vagina that can be seen during a pelvic exam. These changes include a cervical hood (a vaginal fold draped over the cervix), cockscomb cervix (an abnormally shaped cervix), and adenosis (glandular cells normally located within the cervix that appear on the outside of the cervix and in the vagina).

- Fallopian tubes. Some DES daughters have fallopian tube abnormalities that lead to infertility.

- Uterus. Many DES daughters have a uterus that is abnormal in size and shape. The classic sign is the T-shaped uterus. In the normal uterus, the cavity (hollow space inside) is rounded. In a T-shaped uterus, the cavity is reduced to a thin T. The abnormal shape of the inside of the uterus makes it harder for a woman to get pregnant and leads to a higher risk of premature labor and birth.

Diagnosis

Women who have been exposed to DES should have a **pelvic exam** at least once a year. In addition to the usual pelvic exam and Pap smear, DES daughters should have Pap smears of the vagina and, if possible, **colposcopy**. During colposcopy, the doctor looks at the cervix and vagina through a special magnifying scope. In this way, tiny areas of abnormal cells can be seen. This procedure is easily performed in the doctor's office.

When DES daughters get pregnant, they may be at high risk for premature labor and birth and should be monitored very carefully.

Not all women who were exposed to DES develop problems in pregnancy. However, if problems like infertility or miscarriage occur, the doctor may recommend a special x-ray test to check the woman's fallopian tubes and uterus. This special test is called a hysterosalpingogram.

Treatment

There is no treatment for the abnormalities of the fallopian tubes and uterus caused by DES exposure. Fortunately, there are treatments that can help with infertility and premature labor. Clear cell adenocarcinoma of the vagina or cervix must be treated with surgery and, possibly, **chemotherapy**.

Prevention

The practice of prescribing DES to prevent miscarriages has been banned in the United States for about five decades. Individuals, especially women, who were exposed to DES in utero, should notify their health care providers and should continue to be monitored.

The Centers for Disease Control and other agencies around the world continue to monitor the women who were prescribed DES and their offspring, including the third generation (grandchildren of the original mothers prescribed DES), to determine the effects, if any, of DES exposure on successive generations.

Resources

PERIODICALS

Kruse, Kelly, Diane Lauver, and Karen Hanson. "Clinical Implications of DES." *Nurse Practitioner* (July 2003): 26–29.

Newbold, R.R. "Pre-Natal Exposure to Diethylstilbesterol (DES)." *Fertility and Sterility* 2 supplement (February 2008): e55–6.

Rubin, M.M. "Antenatal Exposure to DES: Lessons Learned...Future Concerns." *Obstetrics and Gynecology Survey* 62, no. 8 (August 2007): 548–55.

OTHER

DES Update Home. Centers for Disease Control and Prevention. http://www.cdc.gov/DES (accessed October 3, 2010).

Amy B. Tuteur, MD
Teresa G. Odle
Melinda Granger Oberleitner
RN, DNS, APRN, CNS

Detached retina *see* **Retinal detachment**

Detoxification

Definition

Detoxification is one of the more widely used treatments and concepts in alternative medicine. It is based on the principle that illnesses can be caused by the accumulation of toxic substances (toxins) in the body. Eliminating existing toxins and avoiding new toxins are essential parts of the healing process. Detoxification utilizes a variety of tests and techniques.

Purpose

Detoxification is helpful for those patients suffering from many chronic diseases and conditions, including **allergies**, **anxiety**, arthritis, **asthma**, chronic infections, depression, diabetes, headaches, heart disease, high cholesterol, low blood sugar levels, digestive disorders, mental illness, and **obesity**. It is helpful for those with conditions that are influenced by environmental factors, such as **cancer**, as well as for those who have been exposed to high levels of toxic materials due to accident or occupation. Detoxification therapy is useful for those suffering from allergies or immune system problems that conventional medicine is unable to diagnose or treat, including **chronic fatigue syndrome**, environmental

Common herbs used for detoxification		
Antibiotics	**Anticatarrhals (help eliminate mucus)**	**Blood cleaners**
Clove	Boneset	Buckthorn
Echinacea	Echinacea	Burdock root
Eucalyptus	Garlic	Dandelion root
Garlic	Goldenseal root	Echinacea
Myrrh	Hyssop	Red clover blossoms
Prickly ash bark	Sage	Yellow dock root
Propolis	Yarrow	
Wormwood		
Diaphoretics/skin cleaners	**Diuretics**	**Laxatives**
Boneset	Cleavers	Buckthorn
Burdock root	Corn silk	Cascara sagrada
Cayenne pepper	Horsetail	Dandelion root
Elder flowers	Juniper berries	Licorice root
Ginger root	Parsley leaf	Rhubarb root
Goldenseal root	Uva ursi	Senna
Oregon grape root	Yarrow	Yellow dock
Peppermint		
Yellow dock		

(Table by PreMediaGlobal. Reproduced by permission of Gale, a part of Cengage Learning.)

illness/multiple chemical sensitivity, and fibromyalgia. Symptoms for those suffering these conditions may include unexplained **fatigue**, increased allergies, hypersensitivity to common materials, intolerance to certain foods and **indigestion**, aches and pains, low grade **fever**, headaches, **insomnia**, depression, sore throats, sudden weight loss or gain, lowered resistance to infection, general malaise, and disability. Detoxification can be used as a beneficial preventative measure and as a tool to increase overall health, vitality, and resistance to disease.

Description

Origins

Detoxification methods of healing have been used for thousands of years. **Fasting** is one of the oldest therapeutic practices in medicine. Hippocrates, the ancient Greek known as the "Father of Western medicine," recommended fasting as a means for improving health. **Ayurvedic medicine**, a traditional healing system that has developed over thousands of years, utilizes detoxification methods to treat many chronic conditions and to prevent illness.

Detoxification treatment has become one of the cornerstones of alternative medicine. Conventional medicine notes that environmental factors can play a significant role in many illnesses. Environmental medicine is a field that studies exactly how those environmental factors influence disease. Conditions such as asthma, cancer, chronic fatigue syndrome, **multiple chemical sensitivity**, and many others are strongly influenced by exposure to toxic or allergenic substances in the environment. The United States Centers for Disease Control estimate that over 80% of all illnesses have environmental and lifestyle causes.

Detoxification has also become a prominent treatment as people have become more aware of environmental pollution. It is estimated that one in every four Americans suffers from some level of **heavy metal poisoning**. Heavy metals, such as lead, mercury, cadmium, and arsenic, are by-products of industry. Synthetic agriculture chemicals, many of which are known to cause health problems, are also found in food, air, and water. American agriculture uses nearly 10lb (4.5 kg) of pesticides per person on the food supply each year. These toxins have become almost unavoidable. Pesticides that are used only on crops in the southern United States have been found in the tissue of animals in the far north of Canada. DDT, a cancer-causing insecticide that has been banned for decades, is still regularly found in the fatty tissue of animals, birds, and fish, even in extremely remote regions such as the North Pole.

The problem of toxins in the environment is compounded because humans are at the top of the food chain and are more likely to be exposed to an accumulation of toxic substances in the food supply. For instance, pesticides and herbicides are sprayed on grains that are then fed to farm animals. Toxic substances are stored in the fatty tissue of those animals. In addition, those animals are often injected with synthetic hormones, **antibiotics**, and other chemicals. When people eat meat products, they are exposed to the full range of chemicals and additives used along the entire agricultural chain. Detoxification specialists call this build up of toxins *bioaccumulation*. They assert that the bioaccumulation of toxic substances over time is responsible for many physical and mental disorders, especially ones that are increasing rapidly (like asthma, cancer, and mental illness). As a result, detoxification therapies are increasing in importance and popularity.

Toxins in the body include heavy metals and various chemicals such as pesticides, pollutants, and food additives. Drugs and alcohol have toxic effects in the body. Toxins are produced as normal by-products in the intestines by the bacteria that break down food. The digestion of protein also creates toxic by-products in the body.

The body has natural methods of detoxification. Individual cells get detoxified in the lymph and circulatory system. The liver is the principle organ of detoxification, assisted by the kidneys and intestines. Toxins can be excreted from the body by the kidneys, bowels, skin, and lungs. Detoxification treatments become necessary when the body's natural detoxification systems become overwhelmed. This can be caused by long-term effects of improper diet, **stress**, overeating, sedentary lifestyles, illness, and poor health habits in general. When a build up of toxic substances in the body creates illness, it's called toxemia. Some people's digestive tracts become unable to digest food properly, due to years of overeating and **diets** that are high in fat and processed foods and low in fiber (the average American diet). When this happens, food cannot pass through the digestive tract efficiently. Instead of being digested properly or eliminated from the bowel, food can literally rot inside the digestive tract and produce toxic by-products. This state is known as toxic colon syndrome or intestinal toxemia.

Detoxification therapies try to activate and assist the body's own detoxification processes. They also try to eliminate additional exposure to toxins and strengthen the body and immune system so that toxic imbalances won't occur in the future.

Testing for toxic substances

Detoxification specialists use a variety of tests to determine the causes contributing to toxic conditions. These causes include infections, allergies, addictions, toxic chemicals, and digestive and organ dysfunction. Blood, urine, stool, and hair analyses, as well as **allergy tests**, are used to measure a variety of bodily functions that may indicate problems. Detoxification therapists usually have access to laboratories that specialize in sophisticated diagnostic tests for toxic conditions.

People who have toxemia are often susceptible to infection because their immune systems are weakened. Infections can be caused by parasites, bacteria, viruses, and a common yeast. Therapists will screen patients for underlying infections that may be contributing to illness.

Liver function is studied closely with blood and urine tests because the liver is the principle organ in the body responsible for removing toxic compounds. When the liver detoxifies a substance from the body, it does so in two phases. Tests are performed that indicate where problems may be occurring in these phases, which may point to specific types of toxins. Blood and urine tests can also be completed that screen for toxic chemicals such as PCBs (environmental poisons), formaldehyde (a common preservative), pesticides, and heavy metals. Another useful blood test is a test for zinc deficiency, which may reveal heavy metal **poisoning**. Hair analysis is used to test for heavy metal levels in the body. Blood and urine tests check immune system activity, and hormone levels can also indicate specific toxic compounds. A 24-hour urine analysis, where samples are taken around the clock, allows therapists to determine the efficiency of the digestive tract and kidneys. Together with stool analysis, these tests may indicate toxic bowel syndrome and digestive system disorders. Certain blood and urine tests may point to nutritional deficiencies and proper recovery diets can be designed for patients as well.

Detoxification therapists may also perform extensive allergy and hypersensitivity tests. Intradermal (between layers of the skin) and sublingual (under the tongue) allergy tests are used to determine a patient's sensitivity to a variety of common substances, including formaldehyde, auto exhaust, perfume, tobacco, chlorine, jet fuel, and other chemicals.

Food allergies require additional tests because these allergies often cause reactions that are delayed for several days after the food is eaten. The RAST (radioallergosorbent test) is a blood test that determines the level of antibodies (immunoglobulins) in the blood after specific foods are eaten. The cytotoxic test is a blood test that determines if certain substances affect blood cells, including foods and chemicals. The ELISA-ACT (enzyme-linked immunoserological assay activated cell test) is considered to be one of the most accurate tests for allergies and hypersensitivity to foods, chemicals, and other agents. Other tests for food allergies are the elimination and rotation diets, in which foods are systematically evaluated to determine the ones that are causing problems.

Detoxification therapists usually interview and counsel patients closely to determine and correct lifestyle, occupational, psychological, and emotional factors that may also be contributing to illness.

Detoxification therapies

Detoxification therapists use a variety of healing techniques after a diagnosis is made. The first step is to eliminate a patient's exposure to all toxic or allergenic substances. These include heavy metals, chemicals, radiation (from x rays, power lines, cell phones, computer screens, and microwaves), smog, polluted water, foods, drugs, **caffeine**, alcohol, perfume, excess noise, and stress. If **mercury poisoning** has been determined, the patient will be advised to have mercury fillings from the teeth removed, preferably by a holistic dentist.

Specific treatments are used to stimulate and assist the body's detoxification process. Dietary change is immediately enacted, eliminating allergic and unhealthy foods, and emphasizing foods that assist detoxification and support healing. **Detoxification diets** are generally low in fat, high in fiber, and vegetarian with a raw food emphasis. Processed foods, alcohol, and caffeine are avoided. **Nutritional supplements** such as **vitamins**, **minerals**, **antioxidants**, amino acids, and essential fatty acids are often prescribed. Spirulina is a sea algae that is frequently given to assist in eliminating heavy metals. Lipotropic agents are certain vitamins and nutrients that promote the flow of bile and fat from the liver.

Many herbal supplements are used in detoxification therapies as well. Milk thistle extract, called silymarin, is one of the more potent herbs for detoxifying the liver. Naturopathy, Ayurvedic medicine, and **traditional Chinese medicine** (TCM) recommend numerous herbal formulas for detoxification and immune strengthening. If infections or parasites have been found, these are treated with herbal formulas and, in difficult cases, antibiotics.

For toxic bowel syndrome and digestive tract disorders, herbal **laxatives** and high fiber foods such as psyllium seeds may be given to cleanse the digestive

KEY TERMS

Allergen—A foreign substance, such as mites in house dust or animal dander, that when inhaled causes the airways to narrow and produces symptoms of asthma.

Antibody—A protein, also called immunoglobulin, produced by immune system cells to remove antigens (the foreign substances that trigger the immune response).

Fibromyalgia—A condition of debilitating pain, among other symptoms, in the muscles and the

myofascia (the thin connective tissue that surrounds muscles, bones, and organs).

Hypersensitivity—The state where even a tiny amount of allergen can cause severe allergic reactions.

Multiple chemical sensitivity—A condition characterized by severe and crippling allergic reactions to commonly used substances, particularly chemicals. Also called environmental illness.

---

tract and promote elimination. Colonics are used to cleanse the lower intestines. Digestive enzymes are prescribed to improve digestion, and acidophilus and other friendly bacteria are reintroduced into the system with nutritional supplements.

Fasting is another major therapy in detoxification. Fasting is one of the quickest ways to promote the elimination of stored toxins in the body and to prompt the healing process. People with severe toxic conditions are supervised closely during fasting because the number of toxins in the body temporarily increases as they are being released.

Chelation therapy is used by detoxification specialists to rid the body of heavy metals. Chelates are particular substances that bind to heavy metals and speed their elimination. Homeopathic remedies have also been shown to be effective for removing heavy metals.

Sweating therapies can also detoxify the body because the skin is a major organ of elimination. Sweating helps release those toxins that are stored in the subcutaneous (under the skin) fat cells. Saunas, **therapeutic baths**, and **exercise** are some of these treatments. Body therapies may also be prescribed, including **massage therapy**, **acupressure**, **shiatsu**, manual lymph drainage, and **polarity therapy**. These body therapies seek to improve circulatory and structural problems, reduce stress, and promote healing responses in the body. Mind/body therapies such as **psychotherapy**, counseling, and stress management techniques may be used to heal the psychological components of illness and to help patients overcome their negative patterns contributing to illness.

Practitioners and treatment costs

The costs of detoxification therapies can vary widely, depending on the number of tests and treatments required. Detoxification treatments can be

lengthy and involved since illnesses associated with toxic conditions usually develop over many years and may not clear up quickly. Detoxification treatments may be lengthy because they often strive for the holistic healing of the body, mind, and emotions.

Practitioners may be conventionally trained medical doctors with specialties in environmental medicine or interests in alternative treatment. The majority of detoxification therapists are alternative practitioners, such as naturopaths, homeopaths, ayurvedic doctors, or traditional Chinese doctors. Insurance coverage varies, depending on the practitioner and the treatment involved. Consumers should review their individual insurance policies regarding treatment coverage.

Preparations

Patients can assist diagnosis and treatment by keeping detailed diaries of their activities, symptoms, and contact with environmental factors that may be affecting their health. Reducing exposure to environmental toxins and making immediate dietary and lifestyle changes may speed the detoxification process.

Side effects

During the detoxification process, patients may experience side effects of fatigue, malaise, aches and pains, emotional duress, **acne**, headaches, allergies, and symptoms of colds and flu. Detoxification specialists claim that these negative side effects are part of the healing process. These reactions are sometimes called *healing crises*, which are caused by temporarily increased levels of toxins in the body due to elimination and cleansing.

Research and general acceptance

Although environmental medicine is gaining more respect within conventional medicine, detoxification treatment is scarcely mentioned by the medical establishment. The research that exists on detoxification is largely testimonial, consisting of individual personal accounts of healing without statistics or controlled scientific experiments. In the alternative medical community, detoxification is an essential and widely accepted treatment for many illnesses and chronic conditions.

Resources

OTHER

A Citizens Toxic Waste Manual. Greenpeace USA, 1436 U St. NW, Washington, DC 20009. (202) 462-1177.

ORGANIZATIONS

American Holistic Medical Association, 23366 Commerce Park, Suite 101B, Beachwood, OH, 44122, (216) 292-6644, (216) 292-6688, info@holisticmedicine.org, http://www.holisticmedicine.org.

Cancer Prevention Coalition, c/o University of Illinois at Chicago; School of Public Health, MC 922; 2121 West Taylor Street, Chicago, IL, 60612, (312) 996-2297, (312) 413-9898, http://www.preventcancer.com/.

Center for Occupational and Environmental Medicine, 7510 Northforest Dr, North Charleston, SC, 29420, (843) 572-1600, (843) 572-1795, allanl@coem.com, http://www. coem.com.

Douglas Dupler, MA

Detoxification diets

Definition

Detoxification diets, or detox diets for short, are a group of short-term diets intended to release accumulated toxins and waste products from the body. They are based on a theory of digestion and elimination usually associated with naturopathy, an alternative medical system that emphasizes the role of **nutrition** in restoring or improving the body's own self-healing properties. In general, detox diets emphasize the following:

- Minimal intake of chemicals on or in food by choosing organic or non-processed foods
- Increased intake of fruits, vegetables, and other foods thought to aid the process of detoxification
- Increased intake of foods and fluids that speed up the processes of urination and defecation

Detoxification diets can be categorized into several subgroups: raw food diets, which are based on the premise that uncooked foods prevent the accumulation of toxins in the digestive system; mono diets, in which the dieter consumes only one or two foods (sometimes in liquid form only) for a period of 10–14 days; juice **fasting**, in which the dieter consumes large quantities of fruit and vegetable juices along with water and herbal teas for one to three days; and vegetarian or semi-vegetarian detox diets, which allow the dieter some variety of cooked whole grains, steamed vegetables, fresh fruit, and small amounts of protein foods as well as several glasses of water and herbal teas each day.

Origins

Detoxification diets as a general practice can be traced back for over 5,500 years to an annual ritual of bodily and spiritual preparation known as *pancha karma*, which is part of the practice of **Ayurvedic medicine** in India. Ayurveda is a traditional system of health care that dates back to about 3500 BC; its name is Sanskrit for "science of long life." Pancha karma is undergone for disease prevention, which in Ayurvedic practice requires spiritual renewal and the breaking of negative emotional patterns as well as physical purification. It has three phases: a preparation phase, in which the person eliminates sweets, caffeinated drinks, and processed foods from the diet, as well as spending more time in **meditation** and taking walks in natural surroundings; the cleansing phase, which includes bloodletting, emesis (forced **vomiting**), nasal cleansing, and the use of **enemas** and **laxatives** as well as a very restricted diet of grains and vegetables; and a rejuvenation phase, in which solid foods are gradually reintroduced to the diet. Practitioners of Ayurveda in Canada and the United States generally omit **vomiting** and bloodletting in the second phase of pancha karma.

In Europe and North America the most important factor in the popularity of detoxification diets is naturopathy, an alternative approach to health care developed out of the natural healing movement in Germany and North America in the late nineteenth century. Naturopathy is closely connected with **vegetarianism**, particularly its raw-food offshoot. Naturopaths of the twenty-first century use a variety of techniques in treating patients, including **hydrotherapy**, spinal manipulation, and **physical therapy** as well as nutrition and dietary advice. There has been a revival of interest in naturopathy in the United States since the 1980s.

Naturopaths frequently recommend detoxification diets as a way of ridding the body of various toxins that they identify as coming from several sources:

- Heavy metals. These include such substances as cadmium, arsenic, nickel, aluminum, chromium, mercury, vanadium, strontium, antimony, cobalt, and lead, which are used in various manufacturing processes and some medical procedures as well as being present in batteries, electronic equipment, coins, cookware, food containers, and other common household items.

- Toxic chemicals taken directly into the digestive tract through alcoholic beverages, pesticide residues on supermarket produce, additives in processed foods, or drugs of abuse; or taken into the respiratory tract through breathing household solvents (nail polish remover, spot or stain removers containing benzene, etc.).

- Toxins in the digestive tract produced by yeast and other microorganisms. Ridding the body of this group of toxins is frequently cited as a reason for combining laxatives or enemas with detoxification diets. Mainstream physicians dispute the notion that normal digestion produces toxic substances in the colon that must be removed by a laxative or enema.

- Ammonia, urea, and other breakdown products of protein metabolism. Naturopaths often recommend a vegetarian lifestyle as well as periodic intensive detoxification practices in order to minimize the production of these byproducts of meat and dairy products consumption.

A third factor that has contributed to interest in detox diets in the 1990s and early 2000s is the environmental movement. Some people who are concerned about the impact on the environment of raising animals for food use detox diets as a transition into a long-term vegetarian or vegan lifestyle. In addition, growing awareness of the effects of exposure to industrial chemicals, pesticides, secondhand tobacco smoke, and other contaminants in the home environment as well as the workplace has led many people to consider detoxification diets as a preventive health practice to lower their risk of arthritis and other degenerative diseases.

Description

Practitioners of alternative medicine generally recommend the warmer months as the best time of year for a detox diet, although some dieters prefer January in order to counteract the effects of overindulgence in food and drink during the holidays. Many people suggest beginning a detox diet on the weekend or scheduling time off from work in order to allow time for extra rest if needed. Detox diets are usually used only once or twice a year.

Many detoxification diet books include a questionnaire or symptom checklist to help readers evaluate whether they need detoxification. The following list is typical; more than four "yes" answers indicates the individual could benefit from a detox diet:

- Do you have only one bowel movement per day, or only one every other day?
- Do you take prescription, recreational, or over-the-counter drugs?
- Do you eat meat more than twice a week?
- Do you eat fast foods or processed foods?
- Do you smoke, or are you exposed to secondhand smoke?
- Do you have any skin problems or digestive gas and bloating?
- Do you drink alcohol?
- Do you live in a major city?
- Do you drink tap water, coffee, or soda?
- Do you feel tired, sleep poorly, or have low energy?

Individuals considering a detox diet should prepare by cutting down gradually on caffeinated beverages a week to 10 days before the diet, as sudden elimination of these drinks often causes headaches. Dieters should also reduce their intake of sugary foods, chocolate, alcohol, dairy products, foods high in fat, foods containing wheat or yeast, and grains containing gluten (an elastic protein found in barley and rye). Recommended foods for detox diets (except the mono diets) include fresh organic fruits and vegetables; rice (both brown and basmati rice), rice cakes, and rice pasta; other grains such as millet, quinoa, and buckwheat; beans, lentils, and dried green or yellow peas; unsalted nuts; seeds; olive oil; and herbal teas. The dieter should plan to drink at least eight glasses of filtered or other non-tap water per day on a detox diet.

At the end of a detox diet, the dieter should return gradually to a full diet, perhaps vegetable soup or steamed vegetables the first day. They should not add fruits or vegetables until the second or third day.

Raw food diets

Raw food detox diets consist of foods that have not been heated above 92° to 118°F (33° to 48°C). These diets are based on the belief that raw foods have higher nutrient value and contain enzymes that assist digestion, allowing the other enzymes in the body to regulate other biological processes. Raw foodists also believe raw foods prevent **obesity** by lowering excessive food consumption, and their high fiber content helps detoxify the body by speeding up digestion and elimination.

Juice fasting

In a juice fast, the dieter is instructed to drink between 32 and 64 oz of fruit or vegetable juice per day, in addition to six glasses of warm filtered water.

Although some modified juice fasts allow a small quantity of steamed vegetables, most are short-term liquid diets. Some therapists recommend one or more cups of herbal tea each day in addition to the juice and water. The juice must be fresh, obtained from organic fruits and vegetables processed through a juicer or juice extractor. Prepackaged juices cannot be used for a juice fast because they have been pasteurized. In addition, fresh juice must be consumed within a half hour of extraction; it cannot be refrigerated.

Mono diets

Mono diets are detox diets in which the dieter consumes only one food, usually apples, grapes, or some other fruit or vegetable, or one liquid, for a period of 10 to 14 days. The oldest mono diet is the so-called Miracle Grape Cure, attributed to Johanna Brandt, a woman from South Africa who claimed that eating grapes cured her of **stomach cancer**. In a book she published in 1928, Brandt stated that she alternated 12 hours of drinking only natural (unchlorinated) water with 12 hours of eating only purple grapes or drinking grape juice made from purple grapes. Recent modifications of this diet recommend following Brandt's plan to the letter for five weeks, followed by one week of a raw-food vegetarian diet.

The best-known mono diet is variously known as the Master Cleanser, lemonade diet, or maple syrup diet. Stanley Burroughs is generally credited with inventing this diet in 1941, although he did not publish it in book form until 1976. His book, which is only about fifty pages long, is still in print even though Burroughs died in 1991. The Master Cleanser involves drinking a mixture of lemon juice, cayenne pepper, and grade B maple syrup for a period of 10 to 14 days. The lemon/maple syrup drink is then followed by drinking a "saltwater flush," which is supposed to purge toxins from the stomach and bowels. This diet was popularized in the early 2000s by a book by Peter Glickman titled *Lose Weight, Have More Energy and Be Happier in 10 Days*, which is a modernization of Burrough's regimen.

Vegetarian or semivegetarian diets

Less stringent detox diets that allow some protein foods have been published; a typical example is the following diet plan for a week-long detox regimen by Elson Haas. Haas begins with general guidelines for the dieter:

- Eat slowly and chew the food well.
- Relax for a few minutes before and after each meal.
- Eat in a comfortable sitting position.

- Drink only herbal teas (peppermint, chamomile, or pau d'arco) after dinner.

The daily diet plan:

- Morning: two glasses of filtered or spring water, one glass with half a lemon squeezed into it.
- Breakfast: One piece of fresh fruit at room temperature, followed 15 to 30 minutes later by a bowl of cooked whole grains (millet, buckwheat, quinoa, brown rice, or amaranth), flavored with 2 tbsp of fruit juice.
- Lunch: One or two medium bowls of steamed vegetables, using a variety of root vegetables, leafy vegetables, asparagus, cabbage, kale, or others. A maximum of 3 tsp daily of a mixture of butter and canola or olive oil can be used for seasoning.
- Dinner: Same as lunch.
- Midmorning and midafternoon: One or two cups of vegetable water saved from the steamed vegetables, with a little sea salt or kelp added.
- A small portion (3 or 4 oz) of a protein food (fish, organic chicken, lentils, black beans, or garbanzo beans) may be eaten midafternoon if the dieter feels weak or extremely hungry.

Supplemental recommendations

An important part of many detoxification diets is the use of laxatives or enemas to cleanse the lower digestive tract. The removal of wastes is considered essential to prevent toxins in the intestines from being reabsorbed into the bloodstream. Some alternative therapists recommend mixtures of slippery elm or other herbs to cleanse the colon; others prefer saltwater laxatives, enemas, or colonics for cleansing the bowel. A colonic is a procedure in which a large amount of water, sometimes as much as 20 gal (76 L), is infused into the colon through the rectum a few pints at a time. It differs from an enema in that much more fluid is used; and a colonic is infused into the colon, whereas an enema infuses water or a cleansing solution into the rectum only. Mainstream physicians do not recommend colonics on the grounds that they are unnecessary, based on a nineteenth-century misunderstanding of the process of digestion, and very often uncomfortable for the patient. In some cases they pose serious risks to health.

Some therapists recommend the use of such dietary supplements as multivitamins, vitamin C, choline and methionine, milk thistle, or a laxative tea known as Smooth Move during a detox diet. These supplements are supposed to aid liver function and decrease such side effects of detox diets as headaches and **nausea**.

Many advocates of detox diets suggest the use of meditation, affirmations, **yoga**, and other spiritual practices in order to improve the mental and emotional well-being. Others recommend undertaking the detox diet at a health spa, where such services as **massage therapy**, sauna baths, and whirlpool therapy or other forms of hydrotherapy are available.

Function

The primary function of detoxification diets is physical purification—removal of toxic substances from the body including the skin and respiratory system as well as the digestive tract—in order to raise energy levels; relieve such minor health complaints as poor skin, **bad breath**, or headaches; and improve the body's ability to heal from various diseases. These diets are not primarily intended as weight reduction regimens.

Spiritual or religious practice

Some people undertake detoxification diets as part of a general religious or spiritual retreat. The first stage of Ayurvedic pancha karma includes extra time given to meditation and nature walks as well as gradual exclusion of stimulants and solid foods from the diet. Many people also report relief from **insomnia** or other symptoms of emotional **stress** as a side benefit of detoxification diets.

Treatment of specific illnesses

Detoxification diets are sometimes recommended for the treatment of specific diseases and disorders, most commonly arthritis, **autoimmune disorders**, and depression, but they have also been claimed to be an effective treatment for severe infections (including **AIDS**) and **cancer**. However, there is insufficient evidence to support such claims.

Benefits

Claimed benefits of detox diets include higher energy levels, increased mental clarity and ability to concentrate, clearer skin, improved digestion, and more restful sleep. Many of these improvements may simply be due to better hydration as such diets encourage high fluid intake. Some people also lose weight on detox diets, but emphasize that weight reduction should never be the primary purpose of following one of these regimens.

Precautions

In general, anyone considering a detoxification diet should consult a health professional beforehand. Some serious diseases, including cancer, may have minor symptoms at onset, including headaches, **low back pain**, and **fatigue**. These symptoms can easily be misattributed to stress or poor eating habits. Some therapists recommend requesting blood, urine, stool, and **liver function tests** from a physician before undergoing a detoxification diet.

Individuals who should not undertake a detoxification diet are:

- Pregnant or lactating women.
- Children.
- People with diabetes, hypothyroidism, heart disease, anorexia or bulimia nervosa, kidney or liver disease, stomach ulcers, impaired immune function, epilepsy, cancer, terminal illness, active infections, or ulcerative colitis.
- People who are underweight.
- People with alcohol or drug addictions.
- People who have recently undergone surgery or treatment for severe burns.

Prescription medications should be taken as usual during a detoxification diet. The dieter should not discontinue medications or reduce dosages without consulting a physician.

Anyone on a detoxification diet who feels faint or dizzy, develops an abnormal heart rhythm, feels nauseated or vomits, or has signs of low blood pressure, should discontinue the fast and consult their doctor at once.

Detox diets may encourage yo-yo dieting, which is detrimental to health. They should not be undertaken more than three times a year without medical supervision.

Risks

The major risks to health from detoxification diets include metabolic crises in patients with undiagnosed diabetes; flare-ups or worsening of stomach ulcers; **dizziness** or **fainting** due to sudden lowering of blood pressure; **diarrhea** that may result in **dehydration** and an imbalance of electrolytes in the body; and protein or **calcium** deficiencies from unsupervised long-term juice fasts. Some people develop dental erosion from raw-food detoxification diets.

Other side effects reported include headaches (often caused by sudden withdrawal from **caffeine**), fatigue, **constipation** (from extra fiber combined with inadequate water intake), **acne**, irritability, **dysmenorrhea** (painful periods) in women, and intense hunger.

Raw-food detoxification diets increase the risk of contracting parasites or other foodborne illnesses caused by organisms normally destroyed in cooking or pasteurization. In addition, some raw vegetables, such as rhubarb leaves and stalks, buckwheat greens, kidney beans, kidney bean sprouts, and raw potatoes that have turned green are toxic, particularly if consumed in large quantities.

People on detoxification diets who undergo colonics are at risk of contracting an infection from improperly sterilized colonic equipment; of serious illness or **death** from electrolyte imbalances in the blood; or of serious illness or death resulting from perforation of the intestinal wall by improperly inserted equipment. Colonics can also worsen the symptoms of ulcerative **colitis**.

Research and general acceptance

Detoxification diets are generally dismissed as fads by such professional nutritionists' organizations as the American Dietetic Association (ADA) and other mainstream medical groups. Most physicians point out that the human body is a remarkably efficient organism that can rid itself of toxins through normal digestion, respiration, and excretion without elaborate diets or the assistance of enemas and laxatives. In addition, some fruits and vegetables may contain more toxins than meat, fish, and other protein-rich foods usually condemned by proponents of detoxification diets. Lastly, many physicians object to the naturopathic view of the digestive tract as a source of illness or toxicity.

Resources

BOOKS

Andrews, Sheila. *The No-Cooking Fruitarian Recipe Book*. Wellingborough, UK: Thorsons Publishers, 1975.

Brandt, Johanna. *The Grape Cure*. New York: The Order of Harmony, 1928.

Burroughs, Stanley. *The Master Cleanser with Special Needs and Problems*. N.p.: Burroughs Books, 1976.

Gittleman, Ann Louise. *The Fat Flush Cookbook*. New York: McGraw-Hill, 2003.

Jensen, Bernard. *Dr. Jensen's Guide to Diet and Detoxification*. Los Angeles: Keats Publishing, 2000.

Karas, Jim, and Carolyn Griesse. *The Raw Foods Diet: The Vital Gift of Enzymes*. Piscataway, NJ: New Century, 1981.

Kenton, Leslie. *Leslie Kenton's 10-day Clean-up Plan: Detoxify Your Body for Natural Health and Vitality*. London: Century, 1986.

Meyerowitz, Steve. *Juice Fasting and Detoxification: Use the Healing Power of Fresh Juice to Feel Young and Look Great*, 6th ed. Great Barrington, MA: Sproutman Publications, 1999.

Murray, Michael, ND, and Joseph Pizzorno, ND. *Encyclopedia of Natural Medicine*, 2nd ed. Rocklin, CA: Prima Publishing, 1998.

Pelletier, Kenneth R., MD. *The Best Alternative Medicine*, Chapter 7, "Naturopathic Medicine," and Chapter 10, "Ayurvedic Medicine and Yoga" New York: Fireside Books, 2002.

Vasey, Christopher, ND. *The Detox Mono Diet: The Miracle Grape Cure and Other Cleansing Diets*. Translated from the French by Jon E. Graham. Rochester, VT: Healing Arts Press, 2006.

Wigmore, Ann. *The Sprouting Book*. Wayne, NJ: Avery Publishing Group, 1986.

PERIODICALS

Alexander, Jane. "Demystifying Detox." *Experience Life* 6 (May 2004). [cited May 4, 2007]. http://www.lifetimefitness.com/.

Griffin, J. "Health and Fitness Series: Popular Dietary Fads: How Should Health Professionals Respond?" *Journal of Family Health Care* 13 (2003): 65–67.

Haas, Elson, MD. "The Purification Process: Healing for Modern Times." San Rafael, CA: Preventive Medical Center of Marin, 2002. [cited May 4, 2007]. http://www.elsonhaas.com/articles/article_20.html.

OTHER

Haas, Elson, MD. "Detoxification and the Detox Diet." 1999. http://www.elsonhaas.com/articles/article_01.html.

"Scientists Dismiss Detox Schemes." *BBC News*. January 3, 2006. [cited May 4, 2007]. http://news.bbc.co.uk/2/hi/health/4576574.stm.

ORGANIZATIONS

American Dietetic Association, 120 S. Riverside Plaza, Suite 2000, Chicago, IL, 60606-6995, (312) 899-0040, (800) 877-1600, http://www.eatright.org.

American Holistic Medical Association, 23366 Commerce Park, Suite 101B, Beachwood, OH, 44122, (216) 292-6644, (216) 292-6688, http://www.holisticmedicine.org.

Rebecca J. Frey, PhD

Deviated septum

Definition

The nasal septum is a thin structure, separating the two sides of the nose. If it is not in the middle of the nose, then it is deviated.

Description

The nasal septum is composed of two parts. Toward the back of the head the nasal septum is rigid bone, but further forward the bone becomes cartilage. With one finger in each nostril this cartilage

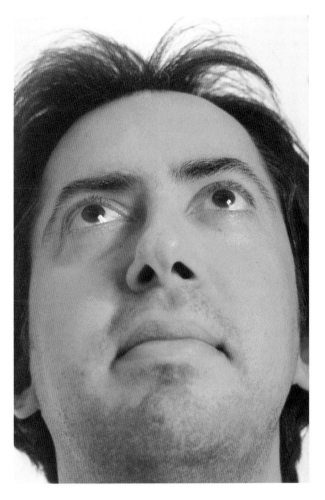

A close-up of person with a deviated septum. *(Custom Medical Stock Photo, Inc. Reproduced by permission.)*

can easily be bent back and forth. If the nasal septum is sufficiently displaced to one side, it will impede the flow of air and mucus through the nose. This condition, called a deviated septum, can cause symptoms and disease.

Causes and symptoms

A deviated septum can be a simple variation in normal structure or the result of a broken nose. Any narrowing of the nasal passageway that it causes will threaten the drainage of secretions from the sinuses, which must pass through the nose. It is a general rule of medicine that when flow is obstructed, whether it is mucus from the sinuses or bile from the gall bladder, infection results. People with **allergic rhinitis** (hay fever) are at greater risk of obstruction because their nasal passageways are already narrowed by the swollen membranes lining them. The result is **sinusitis**, which can be acute and severe or chronic and lingering.

Diagnosis

It is easy to see that a septum is deviated. It is more difficult to determine if that deviation needs correction. It is common for a patient to complain that he/she can breathe through only one nostril. Then the diagnosis is easy. A deviated septum may also contribute to **snoring**, **sleep apnea**, and other breathing disorders.

Treatment

The definitive treatment is surgical repositioning of the septum, accomplished by breaking it loose and fixing it in a proper place while it heals. **Decongestants** like pseudoephedrine or phenylpropanolamine will shrink the membranes and thereby enlarge the passages. **Antihistamines**, nasal cortisone spray, and other allergy treatments may also be temporarily beneficial.

Alternative treatment

As a palliative, saline drops and sprays are very helpful in loosening mucus in the obstructed side and preventing drying in the other side, where all the air blows. Hot peppers, such as jalapenos, can produce enough tears and discharge to flush out a stopped-up nose. An even more effective treatment is called a nasal lavage, often done using a small pot with a spout. Saline solution is poured into one nostril and allowed to flow out the other nostril. Then, the process is repeated in reverse. These therapies are all useful to take care of symptoms, but do not correct the problem. Nasospecific, a procedure where a deflated balloon is inserted in the nostril and inflated to a large enough degree to adjust the septal deviation, can be an alternative to surgery. A trained practitioner in the nasospecific procedure is necessary.

Prognosis

Surgical repair is curative and carries little risk. Chronic infection can be painful and lead to complications until it is resolved. If there is continued obstruction, the infection will very likely return.

Prevention

Avoidance of virus colds, airborne dusts, air pollution, and known allergens will minimize the irritation and swelling of the membranes lining the nasal passages.

KEY TERMS

Allergen—Any substance that irritates people sensitive (allergic) to it.

Allergic rhinitis—Swelling and inflammation of the nasal membranes caused by sensitivity to airborne matter like pollen or cat hair.

Saline—A salt solution in water. Normal saline has the same salt concentration as the body, 0.9%.

Sinuses—The nasal sinuses, air-filled cavities surrounding the eyes and nose, like the nose itself are lined with mucus-producing membranes. They provide cleansing to the nose, resonance to the voice, and structure to the face.

Sinusitis—Infection of the sinuses.

Sleep apnea—A condition in which breathing is temporarily interrupted during sleep. It leads to high blood pressure, sleepiness, and a variety of other problems.

Resources

BOOKS

Daniel, Rollin K.*Mastering Rhinoplasty*. 2nd ed. Berlin; Heidelberg: Springer, 2010.

J. Ricker Polsdorfer, MD

Dextromethorphan *see* **Cough suppressants**

Diabetes insipidus

Definition

Diabetes insipidus (DI) is a disorder that causes the patient to produce tremendous quantities of urine. The massively increased urine output is usually accompanied by intense thirst.

Description

The balance of fluid within the body is maintained through a number of mechanisms. One important chemical involved in fluid balance is called antidiuretic hormone (ADH). ADH is produced by the pituitary, a small gland located at the base of the brain. In a healthy person and under normal conditions, ADH is continuously released. ADH influences the amount of fluid that the kidneys reabsorb into the circulatory system and the amount of fluid that the kidneys pass out of the body in the form of urine.

Production of ADH is regulated by the osmolality of the circulating blood. Osmolality refers to the concentration of dissolved chemicals (such as **sodium**, potassium, and chloride; together called solute) circulating in the fluid base of the blood (plasma). When there is very little fluid compared to the concentration of solute, the pituitary will increase ADH production. This tells the kidneys to retain more water and to decrease the amount of urine produced. As fluid is retained, the concentration of solute will normalize. At other times, when the fluid content of the blood is high in comparison to the concentration of solute, ADH production will decrease. The kidneys are then free to pass an increased amount of fluid out of the body in the urine. Again, this will allow the plasma osmolality to return to normal.

Diabetes insipidus occurs when either the amount of ADH produced by the pituitary is below normal (central DI), or the kidneys' ability to respond to ADH is defective (nephrogenic DI). In either case, a person with DI will pass extraordinarily large quantities of urine, sometimes reaching 10 or more liters each day. At the same time, the patient's blood will be very highly concentrated, with low fluid volume and high concentrations of solute.

DI occurs on average when a person is about 24 years old, and occurs more frequently in males than in females.

Causes and symptoms

DI may run in families. The cause of this type of DI is unknown. Other times, central DI can be caused by:

- an injury to the head
- brain surgery
- cancers that have spread to the pituitary gland (most commonly occurring with breast cancer)
- sarcoidosis (or other related disorders), causing destruction of the pituitary gland
- any condition or illness that causes decreased oxygen delivery to the brain

- the use of certain medications that decrease ADH production (like the antiseizure drug phenytoin)
- the excessive use of alcohol

Central DI may also occur in women who are pregnant or have just given birth, and in patients with **AIDS** who have suffered certain types of brain infections. Nephrogenic DI sometimes occurs in patients who are taking the medication lithium, patients who have high levels of blood **calcium**, and patients who are pregnant.

DI is easily confused with an entirely unrelated disorder, psychogenic polydipsia. Polydipsia refers to drinking large amounts of water. Psychogenic polydipsia is a psychiatric problem that makes a person drink huge quantities of water uncontrollably.

Symptoms of DI include extreme thirst and the production of tremendous quantities of urine. Patients with DI typically drink huge amounts of water, and usually report a specific craving for cold water. When the amount of water passed in the urine exceeds the patient's ability to drink ample replacement water, the patient may begin to suffer from symptoms of **dehydration**. These symptoms include weakness, **fatigue**, **fever**, low blood pressure, increased heart rate, **dizziness**, and confusion. If left untreated, the patient could lapse into unconsciousness and die.

Diagnosis

Diagnosis should be suspected in any patient with sudden increased thirst and urination. Laboratory examination of urine will reveal very dilute urine, made up mostly of water with no solute. Examination of the blood will reveal very concentrated blood, high in solute and low in fluid volume.

A water deprivation test may be performed. This test requires a patient to stop all fluid intake. The patient is weighed just before the test begins, and urine is collected and examined hourly. The test is stopped when:

- the patient has lost more than 5% of his or her original body weight
- the patient has reached certain limits of low blood pressure and increased heart rate
- the urine is no longer changing significantly from one sample to the next in terms of solute concentration.

The next step of the test involves injecting a synthetic form of ADH, with one last urine sample examined 60 minutes later. Comparing plasma and urine osmolality allows the doctor to diagnose either central DI, nephrogenic DI, partial DI, or psychogenic polydipsia.

KEY TERMS

Concentration—Refers to the amount of solute present in a solution, compared to the total amount of solvent.

Dilute—A solution that has comparatively more fluid in it, relative to the quantity of solute.

Osmolality—A measure of the solute-to-solvent concentration of a solution.

Solute—Solid substances that are dissolved in liquid in order to make a solution.

Treatment

A number of medications can be given to decrease the quantity of fluid passed out into the urine. These include vasoprassin (Pitressin) injected and desmopressin acetate (DDAVP) inhaled through the nose, injected under the skin, or taken orally. Other medications that may be given include some antidiuretic drugs (chlorpropamide, clofibrate, carbamazepine). Patients with nephrogenic DI, however, will also require special **diets** that restrict the amount of solute taken in. These patients are also treated with a type of medication called a thiazide diuretic.

Prognosis

Uncomplicated diabetes insipidus is controllable with adequate intake of water and most patients can lead normal lives.

Resources

BOOKS

American Diabetes Association. *American Diabetes Association Complete Guide to Diabetes.* New York: Bantam, 2006.

Remedios, David M. *The Great Physician's Rx for Diabetes.* Nashville, TN: Thomas Nelson, 2006.

PERIODICALS

Hudson, Mary Jane. "Complications of Diabetes Insipidus: The Significance of Headache." *Pediatric Nursing* (January-February 2007): 58–59.

ORGANIZATIONS

American Diabetes Association, 1701 North Beauregard Street, Alexandria, VA, 22311, (800) 342-2383, AskADA@ diabetes.org, http://www.diabetes.org/.

Australian Diabetes Society, 145 Macquarie Street, Sydney, Australia, NSW 2000, 61(2) 9256 5462, 61(2) 9251-8174, suzie@diabetessociety.com.au, http://www. diabetes society.com.au.

Canadian Diabetes Association, 1400-522 University Ave., Toronto, CanadaOntario, M5G 2R5, (800) 226-8464, info@diabetes.ca, http://www.diabetes.ca.

Juvenile Diabetes Research Foundation International, 26 Broadway, 14th Floor, New York, NY, 10004, (212) 785-9595, (800) 533-2873, info@jdrf.org, http://www.jdf.org.

Rosalyn Carson-DeWitt, MD
Ken R. Wells

Diabetes mellitus

Definition

Diabetes mellitus is a condition in which the pancreas no longer produces enough insulin or cells stop responding to the insulin that is produced, so that glucose in the blood cannot be absorbed into the cells of the body. Symptoms include frequent urination, lethargy, weight loss, excessive thirst, and hunger. Treatment includes changes in diet, oral medications, and in some cases, daily injections of insulin or other hormone–like medications designed to boost insulin or lower blood sugar.

Demographics

Approximately 23 million Americans have diabetes, according to the American Diabetes Association. Unfortunately, as many as one-half are unaware they have it. The World Health Organization (WHO) estimates that as of 2010, 230 million people worldwide have diabetes, including 20 million in China, 31 million in India, 8.4 million in Indonesia, 33 million in Europe, 11 million in Africa, and two million in Mexico. WHO estimates that without large-scale, strategic intervention, the number of people with diabetes worldwide could double by 2030.

Description

Diabetes mellitus is a chronic disease that causes serious health complications including renal (kidney) failure, heart disease, **stroke**, limb **amputation**, and blindness. Every cell in the human body needs energy in order to function. The body's primary energy source is glucose, a simple sugar resulting from the digestion of foods containing carbohydrates (sugars and starches). Glucose from digested food circulates in the blood as a ready energy source for cells. Insulin is a hormone or chemical produced by cells in the pancreas, an organ located behind the stomach. Insulin bonds to a receptor site on the outside of cell and acts like a key to open a doorway into the cell, through which glucose can enter. Some of the glucose can be converted to concentrated energy sources like glycogen or fatty acids and saved for later use. When there is not enough insulin produced or when the doorway no longer recognizes the insulin key, glucose stays in the blood rather entering the cells.

The body will attempt to dilute the high level of glucose in the blood, a condition called hyperglycemia, by drawing water out of cells and into the bloodstream in an effort to dilute the sugar and excrete it in the urine. It is not unusual for people with undiagnosed diabetes to be constantly thirsty, drink large quantities of water, and to urinate frequently as their bodies try to get rid of the extra glucose. This creates high levels of glucose in the urine.

At the same time that the body is trying to get rid of glucose from the blood, cells are starving for glucose and sending signals to the body to eat more food, thus making patients extremely hungry. To provide energy for the starving cells, the body also tries to convert fats and proteins to glucose. The breakdown of fats and proteins for energy causes acid compounds called ketones to form in the blood. Ketones also will be excreted in the urine. As ketones build up in the blood, a condition called ketoacidosis can occur. This condition can be life–threatening if left untreated, leading to **coma** and **death**.

Types of diabetes mellitus

Type I diabetes, earlier called juvenile diabetes, begins most commonly in childhood, adolescence, or early adulthood. In this form of diabetes, the body produces little or no insulin. The disease is characterized

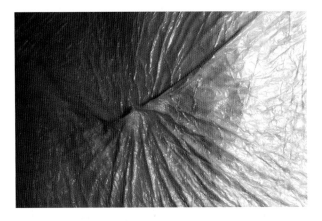

Wrinkled, dehydrated skin of a person in a diabetic coma. Untreated diabetes mellitus results in elevated blood glucose levels, causing a variety of symptoms that can culminate in a diabetic coma. (Dr. P. Marazzi/SPL/Photo Researchers, Inc.)

by a sudden onset and occurs more frequently in populations descended from Northern European countries (Finland, Scotland, Scandinavia) than in those from Southern European countries, the Middle East, or Asia. In the United States, approximately three people in 1,000 develop Type I diabetes. This form is also called insulin–dependent diabetes because people who develop this type require daily injections of insulin.

Brittle diabetics are a subgroup of Type I in which patients have frequent and rapid swings of blood sugar levels between hyperglycemia (a condition where there is too much glucose or sugar in the blood) and **hypoglycemia** (a condition where there are abnormally low levels of glucose or sugar in the blood). These diabetics require several injections of different types of insulin during the day to keep the blood sugar level within a fairly normal range.

The more common form of diabetes, Type II diabetes, occurs in approximately three to five percent of Americans under 50 years of age, and increases to 10–15% in those over 50. More than 90% of the diabetics in the United States are Type II diabetics. Sometimes called adult–onset diabetes, this form of diabetes occurs most often in people who are overweight and who do not **exercise** enough. It is also more common in people of Native American, Hispanic, and African American descent. People who have migrated to Western cultures from East India, Japan, and Australian Aboriginal cultures also are more likely to develop Type II diabetes than those who remain in their original countries.

Type II is considered a milder form of diabetes because of its slow onset (sometimes developing over the course of several years) and because it frequently can be controlled with diet and oral medication. The consequences of uncontrolled and untreated Type II diabetes, however, are the just as serious as those for Type I. This form is also called non–insulin–dependent diabetes, a term that is somewhat misleading. Many people with Type II diabetes can control the condition with diet and oral medications, however, insulin injections are sometimes necessary if treatment with diet and oral medication is inadequate to maintain normal blood glucose levels

Another form of diabetes called **gestational diabetes** can develop during **pregnancy** and generally resolves after the baby is delivered. This diabetic condition develops during the second or third trimester of pregnancy in about two percent of pregnancies. In 2004, the incidence of gestational diabetes was reported to have increased 35% in 10 years. Children of women with gestational diabetes are more likely to be born prematurely, have hypoglycemia, have an excess of

body fat, or have severe **jaundice** at birth. The condition usually is treated by diet; however, insulin injections may be required. Women who have diabetes during pregnancy are at higher risk for developing Type II diabetes within 5–10 years.

Diabetes also can develop as a result of pancreatic disease, **alcoholism**, **malnutrition**, or other severe illnesses that stress the body.

Causes and symptoms

Causes

The causes of diabetes mellitus are unclear, however, there seem to be both hereditary (genetic factors passed on in families) and environmental factors involved. Research has shown that some people who develop diabetes have common genetic markers. In Type I diabetes, the immune system, the body's defense system against infection, is assumed to be triggered by a virus or another microorganism that destroys cells in the pancreas that produce insulin. In Type II diabetes, age, **obesity**, and family history of diabetes play a role.

In Type II diabetes, the pancreas may produce enough insulin. However, cells have become resistant to the insulin produced and it may not work as effectively. Symptoms of Type II diabetes can begin so gradually that a person may not know that he or she has it. Early signs are lethargy, extreme thirst, and frequent urination. Other symptoms may include sudden weight loss, slow wound healing, urinary tract infections, gum disease, or blurred vision. It is not unusual for Type II diabetes to be detected while a patient is seeing a doctor about another health concern that is actually being caused by the yet undiagnosed diabetes.

Individuals who are at high risk of developing Type II diabetes mellitus include people who:

- are obese (more than 20% above their ideal body weight)
- have a relative with diabetes mellitus
- belong to a high–risk ethnic population (African American, Native American, Hispanic, or Native Hawaiian)
- have been diagnosed with gestational diabetes or have delivered a baby weighing more than nine lb (four kg)
- have high blood pressure (140/90 mmHg or above)
- have a high–density lipoprotein cholesterol level less than or equal to 35 mg/dL and/or a triglyceride level greater than or equal to 250 mg/dL
- have had impaired glucose tolerance or impaired fasting glucose on previous testing

Cataract—A condition in which the lens of the eye becomes cloudy.

Diabetic peripheral neuropathy—A condition in which the sensitivity of nerves to pain, temperature, and pressure is dulled, particularly in the legs and feet.

Diabetic retinopathy—A condition in which the tiny blood vessels to the retina, the tissues that sense light at the back of the eye, are damaged, leading to blurred vision, sudden blindness, or black spots, lines, or flashing lights in the field of vision.

Glaucoma—A condition in which pressure within the eye causes damage to the optic nerve, which sends visual images to the brain.

Hyperglycemia—A condition in which there is too much glucose or sugar in the blood.

Hypoglycemia—A condition in which there is too little glucose or sugar in the blood.

Insulin—A hormone or chemical produced by the pancreas that is needed by cells of the body in order to use glucose (sugar), the body's main source of energy.

Ketoacidosis—A condition due to starvation or uncontrolled Type I diabetes. Ketones are acid compounds that form in the blood when the body breaks down fats and proteins. Symptoms include abdominal pain, vomiting, rapid breathing, extreme tiredness, and drowsiness.

Kidney dialysis—A process during which blood is filtered through a dialysis machine to remove waste products that would normally be removed by the kidneys. The filtered blood is then circulated back into the patient. This process also is called renal dialysis.

Pancreas—A gland located behind the stomach that produces insulin.

Several common medications can impair the body's use of insulin, causing a condition known as secondary diabetes. These medications include treatments for high blood pressure (furosemide, clonidine, and thiazide **diuretics**), drugs with hormonal activity (**oral contraceptives**, thyroid hormone, progestins, and glucocorticorids), and the anti–inflammation drug indomethacin. Several drugs that are used to treat **mood disorders** (such as **anxiety** and depression) also can impair glucose absorption. These drugs include haloperidol, lithium carbonate, Zyprexa (olanzapine), Seroquel (quetiapine), phenothiazines, **tricyclic antidepressants**, and adrenergic agonists. Other medications that can cause diabetes symptoms include isoniazid, nicotinic acid, cimetidine, **protease inhibitors** used to treat HIV, and heparin. A 2004 study found that low levels of the essential mineral chromium in the body may be linked to increased risk for diseases associated with **insulin resistance**. Vitamin D deficiencies have also been linked with impaired glucose tolerance, and vitamin D deficient diabetics tend to have more difficulty in controlling their blood glucose levels.

Symptoms

Symptoms of diabetes can develop suddenly (over days or weeks) in previously healthy children or adolescents, or can develop gradually (over several years) in overweight adults over the age of 40. The classic symptoms include feeling tired and sick, frequent urination, excessive thirst, excessive hunger, and weight loss.

Ketoacidosis, a condition due to **starvation** or uncontrolled diabetes, is common in Type I diabetes. Ketones are acid compounds that form in the blood when the body breaks down fats and proteins. Symptoms include abdominal **pain**, **vomiting**, rapid breathing, weight loss, extreme lethargy, and drowsiness. Patients with ketoacidosis also have a sweet breath odor. Left untreated, this condition can lead to coma and death.

With Type II diabetes, the condition may not become evident until the patient presents for medical treatment for some other condition. A patient may have heart disease, chronic infections of the gums and urinary tract, blurred vision, **numbness** in the feet and legs, or slow-healing **wounds**. Women may experience genital **itching**.

Diagnosis

Diabetes is suspected based on symptoms. Urine tests can confirm a diagnosis of diabetes based on the amount of glucose found. Urine tests can also detect ketones and protein in the urine that may help diagnose diabetes and assess how well the kidneys are functioning. These tests also can be used to monitor the disease once the patient is on a standardized diet, oral medications, or insulin.

Urine tests

Clinistix and Diastix are paper strips or dipsticks that change color when dipped in urine. The test strip is compared to a chart that shows the amount of glucose in the urine based on the change in color. The level of glucose in the urine lags behind the level of glucose in the blood. Testing the urine with a test stick, paper strip, or tablet that changes color when sugar is present is not as accurate as blood testing. However it can give a fast and simple reading. It is no longer considered appropriate for use by diabetics as a means to assess glucose control.

Ketones in the urine can be detected using similar types of dipstick tests (Acetest or Ketostix). Ketoacidosis can be a life–threatening situation in Type I diabetics, so having a quick and simple test to detect ketones can assist in establishing a diagnosis sooner.

Another dipstick test can determine the presence of protein or albumin in the urine. Protein in the urine can indicate problems with kidney function and can be used to track the development of renal failure. A more sensitive test for urine protein uses radioactively tagged chemicals to detect microalbuminuria, small amounts of protein in the urine, that may not show up on dipstick tests.

Blood tests

FASTING GLUCOSE TEST. Blood is drawn from a vein in the patient's arm after a period at least eight hours after the patient has last eaten, usually in the morning before breakfast. Red blood cells are separated from the sample and the amount of glucose is measured in the remaining plasma. A plasma level of seven mmol/L (126 mg/L) or greater can indicate diabetes. The **fasting** glucose test is usually repeated on another day to confirm the results.

GLYCATED HEMOGLOBIN (A1C) TEST. This blood test indicates the average blood glucose level for the previous 60–90 days. Blood is drawn from a vein after the patient has fasted for at least eight hours. An A1C level that equals or exceeds 6.5 percent or more on two separate test dates indicates diabetes. In 2009, the International Diabetes Federation recommended the A1C test as the preferred method for diagnosing diabetes and monitoring the effectiveness of treatment.

ORAL GLUCOSE TOLERANCE TEST. Blood samples are taken from a vein before and after a patient drinks a thick, sweet syrup of glucose. In a non-diabetic, the level of glucose in the blood goes up immediately after the drink and then decreases gradually as insulin is used by the body to metabolize, or absorb, the sugar. In a diabetic, the glucose in the blood goes up and stays high after drinking the sweetened liquid. A plasma glucose level of 11.1 mmol/L (200 mg/dL) or higher at two hours after drinking the syrup confirms the diagnosis of diabetes.

A diagnosis of diabetes is confirmed if there are symptoms of diabetes and a plasma glucose level of at least 11.1 mmol/L, a fasting plasma glucose level of at least seven mmol/L; or a two–hour plasma glucose level of at least 11.1 mmol/L during an oral glucose tolerance test.

Home blood glucose monitoring kits are available so patients with diabetes can monitor their own levels. A small needle or lancet is used to prick the finger and a drop of blood is collected and analyzed by a monitoring device. Some patients may test their blood glucose levels several times during a day and use this information to adjust their doses of insulin.

Treatment

A successful pancreas transplant currently offers the only cure for Type 1 diabetes. Diabetes is usually managed with medication and lifestyle changes so that patients can live a relatively normal life. Treatment of diabetes focuses on two goals: keeping blood glucose within normal range and preventing the development of long-term complications. Careful monitoring of diet, exercise, and blood glucose levels are as important as the use of insulin or oral medications in preventing complications of diabetes.

Dietary changes

Diet and moderate exercise are the first treatments implemented in diabetes. For many Type II diabetics, weight loss may be an important goal in helping them to control their diabetes. A well-balanced, nutritious diet provides approximately 50–60% of calories from carbohydrates, approximately 10–20% of calories from protein, and less than 30% of calories from fat. The number of calories required by an individual depends on age, weight, and activity level. The calorie intake also needs to be distributed over the course of the entire day, so surges of glucose entering the blood system are kept to a minimum. Carbohydrates such as grains, vegetables, legumes, and fruits are healthier than carbohydrates provided by sweets and snack foods.

Keeping track of the number of calories and carbohydrates provided by different foods can become complicated, so patients usually are advised to consult a nutritionist or dietitian. An individualized, easy to manage diet plan can be set up for each patient. Both the American Diabetes Association and the American Dietetic Association recommend **diets** based on the use of food exchange lists. Each food exchange contains a known amount of calories in the form of protein, fat, or carbohydrate. A patient's diet plan will consist of a certain number of exchanges from each food category (meat or protein, fruits, breads and starches, vegetables, and fats) to be eaten at meal times and as snacks. Patients have flexibility in choosing which foods they eat as long as they stick with the number of exchanges prescribed.

For many Type II diabetics, weight loss is an important factor in controlling their condition. The food exchange system, along with a plan of moderate exercise, can help them lose excess weight and improve their overall health.

Oral medications

Oral medications are available to lower blood glucose in Type II diabetics. In 1990, 23.4 million outpatient prescriptions for oral antidiabetic agents were dispensed. By 2005, the number had increased to more than 100 million prescriptions. Oral antidiabetic agents accounted for more than $8 billion dollars in worldwide retail sales in 2005 and were the fastest-growing segment of diabetes drugs. There are five distinct classes of hypoglycemic agents available, each class displaying unique pharmacologic properties. These classes are the sulfonylureas, meglitinides, biguanides, thiazolidinediones and alpha-glucosidase inhibitors. In patients for whom diet and exercise do not provide adequate glucose control, therapy with a single oral agent can be tried. The drugs first prescribed for Type II diabetes are in a class of compounds called sulfonylureas and include tolbutamide, tolazamide, acetohexamide, and chlorpropamide. Other drugs in the same class include glyburide, glimeperide, and glipizide. How these drugs work is not well understood. However, they seem to stimulate cells of the pancreas to produce more insulin. Newer medications that are available to treat diabetes include Glucophage (metformin), Precose (acarbose), Glycet (miglitol), Actos (pioglitazone), and Avandia (rosiglitazone). The choice of medication depends in part on the individual patient profile. All drugs have side effects that may make them inappropriate for particular patients. Some for example, may stimulate weight gain or cause stomach irritation, so they may not be the best treatment for someone who is already overweight or who has stomach ulcers. Others, like metformin, have been shown to have positive effects such as reduced cardiovascular mortality. While these medications are an important aspect of treatment for Type II diabetes, they are not a substitute for a well-planned diet and moderate exercise. Oral medications have not been shown effective for Type I diabetes, in which the patient produces little or no insulin.

Constant advances are being made in development of new oral medications for persons with diabetes. One drug called Metaglip combining glipizide and metformin was approved in a single tablet. Along with diet and exercise, the drug is used as initial therapy for Type II diabetes. Another drug approved by the U.S. Food and Drug Administration (FDA) combines metformin and rosiglitazone (Avandia), a medication that increases muscle cells' sensitivity to insulin. It is marketed under the name Avandamet. Other combination drugs include Avandaryl (rosiglitazone and glimepiride), and Duetact (pioglitazone and glimepiride). As of 2010, more combination drugs were under development. So many new drugs are in the pipeline, a record 235 as of mid-2010, with many nearing FDA approval, that it is best to stay in touch with a physician for the latest information. Physicians can find the best drug, diet and exercise program to fit an individual patient's need. In 2007, a study in the *New England Journal of Medicine* suggested the use of Avandia (rosiglitazone) increased the risk of a **heart attack** and death from **heart failure**. Other studies regarding Avandia and its effect on heart health were underway as of mid-2010, including a pending review by the FDA. An FDA ruling also required that Avandia, Actos, Avandaryl, and Duetact carry stronger warnings on their labels.

Byetta (exenatide) and Victoza (liraglutide) are the first compunds in a class of injectable medicines called incretin mimetics to improve blood sugar levels in Type II diabetes. Byetta usually requires two injections daily compared to one with Victoza. However, long-term studies are under way to access a possible relationship between Victoza and an increased incidence of **pancreatitis** and thyroid tumors.

Insulin

Persons with Type I diabetes need daily injections of insulin to help their bodies use glucose. The amount and type of insulin required depends on the height, weight, age, food intake, and activity level of the individual diabetic patient. Some patients with Type II diabetes may need to use insulin injections if their diabetes cannot be controlled with diet, exercise, and oral medication. Injections are given subcutaneously, that is, just under the skin, using a small needle and syringe, using an injection pen, or an insulin pump. Injection sites can be anywhere on the body where there is looser skin, including the upper arm, abdomen, or upper thigh.

Purified human insulin is most commonly used. Insulin from animal sources is no longer used. Insulin may be given as an injection of a single dose of one type of insulin once a day. Different types of insulin can be mixed and given in one dose or split into two or more doses during a day. Patients who require multiple injections over the course of a day may be able to use an insulin pump that administers small doses of insulin on demand. The small battery-operated pump is worn outside the body and is connected to a needle that is inserted into the abdomen. Pumps can be programmed to inject small doses of insulin at various times during the day, or the patient may be able to adjust the insulin doses to coincide with meals and exercise.

Regular insulin is fast–acting and starts to work within 15–30 minutes, with its peak glucose-lowering effect about two hours after it is injected. Its effects last for about four to six hours. NPH (neutral protamine Hagedorn) and Lente insulin are intermediate-acting, starting to work within one to three hours and lasting up to 18–26 hours. Ultra-lente is a long-acting form of insulin that starts to work within four to eight hours and lasts up to 24 hours.

Hypoglycemia, or low blood sugar, can be caused by too much insulin, too little food (or eating too late to coincide with the action of the insulin), alcohol consumption, or increased exercise. A patient with symptoms of hypoglycemia may be hungry, cranky, confused, and tired. The patient may become sweaty and shaky. Left untreated, the patient can lose consciousness or have a seizure. This condition is sometimes called an insulin reaction and should be treated by giving the patient something sweet to eat or drink like a candy, sugar cubes, fruit juice, or another high sugar snack.

Surgery

Transplantation of a healthy pancreas into a diabetic patient is a successful treatment, however, this transplant is usually done only if a kidney transplant is performed at the same time. Although a pancreas transplant is possible, it is often not clear if the potential benefits outweigh the risks of the surgery and drug therapy needed.

Alternative treatment

Since diabetes can be a life–threatening condition if not properly managed, persons should not attempt to treat this condition without medical supervision. A variety of alternative therapies can be helpful in managing the symptoms of diabetes and supporting patients with the disease. **Acupuncture** can help relieve the pain associated with **diabetic neuropathy** by stimulation of certain points. A qualified practitioner should be consulted. Herbal remedies also may be helpful in managing diabetes. Although there is no herbal substitute for insulin, some herbs may help adjust blood sugar levels or manage other diabetic symptoms. Some options include:

- fenugreek (*Trigonella foenum-graecum*) has been shown in some studies to reduce blood insulin and glucose levels while also lowering cholesterol
- bilberry (*Vaccinium myrtillus*) may lower blood glucose levels, as well as helping to maintain healthy blood vessels
- garlic (*Allium sativum*) may lower blood sugar and cholesterol levels
- onions (*Allium cepa*) may help lower blood glucose levels by freeing insulin to metabolize them
- cayenne pepper (*Capsicum frutescens*) can help relieve pain in the peripheral nerves (a type of diabetic neuropathy)
- gingko (*Gingko biloba*) may maintain blood flow to the retina, helping to prevent diabetic retinopathy

Other alternative medicine therapies for controlling blood sugar include chromium picolinate, alpha lipoic acid, cinnamon, evening primrose oil, and pygenol (pine bark extract). Any therapy that lowers stress levels also can be useful in treating diabetes by helping to reduce insulin requirements. Among the alternative treatments that aim to lower stress are **hypnotherapy**, **biofeedback**, and **meditation**.

Prognosis

Uncontrolled diabetes is a leading cause of blindness, end–stage renal disease, and limb amputations. It also doubles the risks of heart disease and increases the risk of stroke. Eye problems including **cataracts**, glaucoma, and diabetic retinopathy also are more common in diabetics.

Diabetic **peripheral neuropathy** is a condition where nerve endings, particularly in the legs and feet, become less sensitive. Diabetic foot ulcers are a particular problem since the patient does not feel the pain of a blister, callous, or other minor injury. Poor blood circulation in the legs and feet contribute to delayed wound healing. The inability to sense pain along with the complications of delayed wound healing can result in minor injuries, blisters, or **calluses** becoming infected and difficult to treat. In cases of severe infection, the infected tissue begins to break down and rot away. The most serious consequence of this condition is the need for amputation of toes, feet, or legs due to severe infection.

Heart disease and **kidney disease** are common complications of diabetes. Long-term complications may include the need for **kidney dialysis** or a kidney transplant due to kidney failure.

Babies born to diabetic mothers have an increased risk of **birth defects** and distress at birth.

Prevention

Research continues on diabetes prevention and improved detection of those at risk for developing diabetes. As of 2010, research was being conducted in a number of countries, including the United States, China, and Finland. While the onset of Type I diabetes is unpredictable, the risk of developing Type II diabetes can be reduced by maintaining ideal weight and exercising regularly. The physical and emotional stress of surgery, illness, pregnancy, and alcoholism can increase the risks of diabetes, so maintaining a healthy lifestyle is critical to preventing the onset of Type II diabetes and preventing further complications of the disease.

Resources

BOOKS

American Diabetes Association. *American Diabetes Association Complete Guide to Diabetes*New York: Bantam, 2006.

Bernstein, Richard K. *Dr. Bernstein's Diabetes Solution: The Complete Guide to Achieving Normal Blood Sugars* New York: Little, Brown and Co., 2007.

Remedios, David M. *The Great Physician's Rx for Diabetes* Nashville, TN: Thomas Nelson, 2006.

PERIODICALS

"Study Estimates 15,000 Children and Adolescents Diagnosed With Type 1 Diabetes Annually; Among Youth in U.S., Whites Have Highest Incidence of Diabetes." *Ascribe Higher Education News Service* (June 26, 2007).

Babbington, Gabrielle. "Metformin Tops Diabetes Trial." *Australian Doctor* (July 27, 2007): 3.

Buchanan, Thomas A., et al. "What is Gestational Diabetes?" *Diabetes Care* (July 2007): S105–S111.

Carmichael, Mary. "Diabetes: A 'Disease of Poverty'?" *Newsweek* (July 2, 2007): 57.

James–Enger, Kelly. "The Dangerous Diabetes–Obesity Connection: How to Reduce Your Risk Now." *Vibrant Life* (July–August 2007): 6–11.

OTHER

National Library of Medicine. "Diabetes–Introduction." MedlinePlus. http://www.nlm.nih.gov/medlineplus/ tutorials/diabetesintroduction/ht m/index.htm (accessed September 9, 2010).

World Health Organization. "WHO Diabetes Programme." http://www.who.int/diabete s/en/index.html (accessed September 9, 2010).

ORGANIZATIONS

American Diabetes Association, 1701 North Beauregard St., Alexandria, VA, 22311, (800) 342–2383, AskADA@ diabetes.org, http://www.diabetes.org.

American Dietetic Association, 120 South Riverside Plaza, Suite 2000, Chicago, IL, 60606–6995, (312) 899–0040, (800) 877–1600, knowledge@eatright.org, http://www. eatright.org.

Canadian Diabetes Association, National Life Building, 1400–522 University Ave., Toronto, ON, Canada, M5G 2R5, (800) 226–8464, info@diabetes.ca, http:// www .diabetes.ca.

Juvenile Diabetes Research Foundation International, 26 Broadway, 14th Floor, New York, NY, 10004, (800) 533–2873, info@jdrf.org, http://www.jdrf.org.

Altha Roberts Edgren
Ken R. Wells

Diabetic control index *see* **Glycosylated hemoglobin test**

Diabetic foot infections

Definition

Diabetic foot infections are infections that can develop in the skin, muscles, or bones of the foot as a result of the nerve damage and poor circulation that is associated with diabetes.

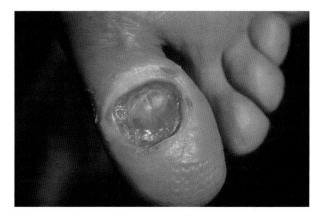

Persons with diabetes often suffer from foot ulcers, as shown above. (*Custom Medical Stock Photo, Inc. Reproduced by permission.*)

Description

People who have diabetes have a greater-than-average chance of developing foot infections. Because a person who has diabetes may not feel foot **pain** or discomfort, problems can remain undetected until **fever**, weakness, or other signs of systemic infection appear. As a result, even minor irritations occur more often, heal more slowly, and are more likely to result in serious health problems.

With diabetes, foot infections occur more frequently because the disease causes nervous system changes and poor circulation. Because the nerves that control sweating no longer work, the skin of the feet can become very dry and cracked, and **calluses** tend to occur more frequently and build up faster. If not trimmed regularly, these calluses can turn into open sores or ulcers. Because diabetic nerve damage can cause a loss of sensation (neuropathy), if the feet are not regularly inspected, an ulcer can quickly become infected and, if not treated, may result in the **death** of tissue (**gangrene**) or **amputation**.

The risk of infection is greatest for people who are over the age of 60 and for those who have one or more of the following:

- poorly controlled diabetes
- foot ulcers
- laser treatment for changes in the retina
- kidney or vascular disease
- loss of sensation (neuropathy)

Causes and symptoms

Bacteria can cause an infection through small cracks (fissures) that can develop in the dry skin around the heel and on other parts of the foot or through **corns**, calluses, blisters, hangnails, or ulcers. If not treated, the bacterial infection can destroy skin, tissue, and bone or spread throughout the body.

Common sites of diabetic foot infections include the following:

- blisters, corns, or callouses that bleed beneath the skin
- bunions, hammertoes, or other abnormalities in the bones of the foot
- scar tissue that has grown over the site of an earlier infection
- foot ulcers caused by pressure, nerve damage, or poor circulation (Ulcers occur most often over the ball of the foot, on the bottom of the big toe, or on the sides of the foot due to poorly fitting shoes.)
- injuries that tear or puncture the skin

Diagnosis

A physician who specializes in the treatment of the foot (podiatrist) or the doctor who normally treats the patient's diabetes will treat the infection. An x ray of the foot will be taken to determine whether the bone has become infected. A sample from the wound will be cultured to identify the organism that is causing the infection so that the appropriate antibiotic can be selected.

Treatment

From the results of the culture, the appropriate antibiotic will be prescribed. Any dead or infected tissue will be surgically removed and, if necessary, a cast and/or special shoes may be used to protect the area. In addition, the patient will be instructed to keep off their feet. If the ulcer does not heal, the physician may perform surgery to increase blood flow to the foot. It is also important for the patient to practice good diabetes control and keep blood glucose levels from getting too high.

Alternative treatment

Acupuncture and vitamin C can boost the body's infection-fighting ability. A variety of other **vitamins** and herbs may improve general health and diabetes control. Because diabetes is a potentially deadly disease, it can be dangerous to try alternative approaches without a doctor's approval or without consulting a trained practitioner of alternative medicine.

Prognosis

Without proper treatment, diabetic foot infections can lead to serious illness, gangrene, amputation, and even death if the infection spreads throughout the body. If treated properly and the patient practices good **foot care**, the prognosis is generally optimistic.

Prevention

There are many things that a diabetic individual can do to prevent the occurrence of foot infections, including the following:

- control blood glucose and do not allow it to get too high
- avoid smoking
- keep blood pressure and cholesterol under control
- exercise to stimulate blood flow
- keep feet clean, dry, and warm
- check your feet every day for blisters, scratches, and skin that is hard, broken, inflamed, or feels hot or cold when touched
- after bathing, carefully dry feet and apply thin coat of petroleum jelly or hand cream to prevent dry skin from cracking
- use a pumice stone and emery board to trim calluses
- do not neglect an ulcer, should one develop

ORGANIZATIONS

American Diabetes Association, 1701 North Beauregard Street, Alexandria, VA, 22311, (800) 342-2383, AskADA@diabetes.org, http://www.diabetes.org/.

Juvenile Diabetes Research Foundation International, 26 Broadway, 14th Floor, New York, NY, 10004, (212) 785-9595, (800) 533-2873, info@jdrf.org, http://www.jdf.org.

National Diabetes Information Clearinghouse (NDIC), 1 Information Way, Bethesda, MD, 20892-3560, (703) 738-4929, (800) 860-8747, ndic@info.niddk.nih.gov, http://diabetes.niddk.nih.gov/.

Maureen Haggerty

Diabetic ketoacidosis

Definition

Diabetic ketoacidosis is a dangerous complication of **diabetes mellitus** in which the chemical balance of the body becomes far too acidic.

Description

Diabetic ketoacidosis (DKA) always results from a severe insulin deficiency. Insulin is the hormone secreted by the body to lower the blood sugar levels when they become too high. Diabetes mellitus is the disease resulting from the inability of the body to produce or respond properly to insulin, required by the body to convert glucose to energy. In childhood diabetes, DKA complications represent the leading cause of **death**, mostly due to the accumulation of abnormally large amounts of fluid in the brain (cerebral **edema**). DKA combines three major features: hyperglycemia, meaning excessively high blood sugar kevels; hyperketonemia, meaning an overproduction of ketones by the body; and acidosis, meaning that the blood has become too acidic.

Insulin deficiency is responsible for all three conditions: the body glucose goes largely unused since most cells are unable to transport glucose into the cell without the presence of insulin; this condition makes the body use stored fat as an alternative source instead of the unavailable glucose for energy, a process that produces acidic ketones, which build up because they require insulin to be broken down. The presence of excess ketones in the bloodstream in turn causes the blood to become more acidic than the body tissues, which creates a toxic condition.

Causes and symptoms

DKA is most commonly seen in individuals with type I diabetes, under 19 years of age and is usually caused by the interruption of their insulin treatment or by acute infection or trauma. A small number of people with type II diabetes also experience ketoacidosis, but this is rare given the fact that type II diabetics still produce some insulin naturally. When DKA occurs in type II patients, it is usually caused by a decrease in food intake and an increased insulin deficiency due to hyperglycemia.

Some common DKA symptoms include:

- high blood sugar levels
- frequent urination (polyuria) and thirst
- fatigue and lethargy
- nausea
- vomiting
- abdominal pain
- fruity odor to breath
- rapid, deep breathing
- muscle stiffness or aching
- coma

Diagnosis

Diagnosis requires the demonstration of hyperglycemia, hyperketonemia, and acidosis. DKA is established if the patient's urine or blood is strongly positive for glucose and ketones. Normal glucose levels in a non-diabetic person on average range from 80–110 mg/dl. A person with diabetes will typically fluctuate outside those parameters. DKA glucose levels exceed 250 mg/dl and can reach 400 to 800 mg/dL. A low serum bicarbonate level (usually below 15 mEq/L) is also present, indicative of acidosis.

KEY TERMS

Acidosis—A condition that causes the pH of the blood to drop and become more acidic.

Diabetes mellitus—Disease characterized by the inability of the body to produce or respond properly to insulin, required by the body to convert glucose to energy.

Edema—The presence of abnormally large amounts of fluid in the intercellular tissue spaces of the body.

Glucose—The type of sugar found in the blood.

Hyperglycemia—Condition characterized by excessively high levels of glucose in the blood, and occurs when the body does not have enough insulin or cannot use the insulin it does have to turn glucose into energy. Hyperglycemia is often indicative of diabetes that is out of control.

Hyperketonemia—Condition characterized by an overproduction of ketones by the body.

Hypoglycemia—Lower than normal levels of glucose in the blood.

Hypokalemia—A deficiency of potassium in the blood.

Insulin—A hormone secreted by the pancreas in response to high blood sugar levels that induces hypoglycemia. Insulin regulates the body's use of glucose and the levels of glucose in the blood by acting to open the cells so that they can intake glucose.

Ketones—Poisonous acidic chemicals produced by the body when fat instead of glucose is burned for energy. Breakdown of fat occurs when not enough insulin is present to channel glucose into body cells.

Lactic acidosis—A serious condition caused by the build up of lactic acid in the blood, causing it to become excessively acidic. Lactic acid is a by-product of glucose metabolism.

Metabolism—The sum of all chemical reactions that occur in the body resulting in growth, transformation of foodstuffs into energy, waste elimination, and other bodily functions.

Polyuria—Excessive secretion of urine.

Type I diabetes—Also called juvenile diabetes. Type I diabetes typically begins early in life. Affected individuals have a primary insulin deficiency and must take insulin injections.

Type II diabetes—Type II diabetes is the most common form of diabetes and usually appears in middle aged adults. It is often associated with obesity and may be delayed or controlled with diet and exercise.

A blood test or **urinalysis** can quickly determine the concentration of glucose in the bloodstream. Test strips are available to patients commercially can submerge in urine to detect the presence or concentration of ketones.

Treatment

Ketoacidosis is treated under medical supervision and usually in a hospital setting.

Basic treatment includes:

- administering insulin to correct the hyperglycemia and hyperketonemia
- replacing fluids lost through excessive urination and vomiting intravenously
- balancing electrolytes to re-establish the chemical equilibrium of the blood and prevent potassium deficiency (hypokalemia) during treatment
- treatment for any associated bacterial infection

Prognosis

With proper medical attention, DKA is almost always successfully treated. The DKA mortality rate is about 10%. **Coma** on admission adversely affects the prognosis. The major causes of death are circulatory collapse, **hypokalemia**, infection, and cerebral edema.

Prevention

Once diabetes has been diagnosed, prevention measures to avoid DKA include regular monitoring of blood glucose, administration of insulin, and lifestyle maintenance. Glucose monitoring is especially important during periods of **stress**, infection, and trauma when glucose concentrations typically increase as a response to these situations. Ketone tests should also be performed during these periods or when glucose is elevated.

ORGANIZATIONS

American Diabetes Association, 1701 North Beauregard Street, Alexandria, VA, 22311, (800) 342-2383, AskADA@diabetes.org, http://www.diabetes.org/.

Juvenile Diabetes Research Foundation International, 26 Broadway, 14th Floor, New York, NY, 10004, (212) 785-9595, (800) 533-2873, info@jdrf.org, http://www.jdf.org.

National Institute of Diabetes and Digestive and Kidney Diseases, NIDDK, NIH Bldg 31, Rm 9A06 31 Center Drive, MSC 2560, Bethesda, MD, 20892-2560, (301) 496.3583, http://www2.niddk.nih.gov.

Gary Gilles

Diabetic neuropathy

Definition

Diabetic neuropathy is a nerve disorder caused by **diabetes mellitus**. Diabetic neuropathy may be diffuse, affecting several parts of the body, or focal, affecting a specific nerve and part of the body.

Demographics

The longer a person has diabetes, the more likely the development of one or more forms of neuropathy. Approximately 60–70% of patients with diabetes have neuropathy, but only about 5% experience painful symptoms.

Description

The nervous system consists of two major divisions: the central nervous systems (CNS), which includes the brain, the cranial nerves, and the spinal cord, and the peripheral nervous system (PNS), which includes the nerves that link the CNS with the sensory organs, muscles, blood vessels, and glands of the body. These peripheral nerves are either motor, meaning that they are involved in motor activity such as walking, or sensory, meaning that they carry sensory information back to the CNS. The PNS also works with the CNS to regulate involuntary (autonomic) processes such as breathing, heartbeat, blood pressure, etc.

There are two types of diffuse diabetic neuropathy that affect different nervous system functions. Diffuse **peripheral neuropathy** primarily affects the limbs, damaging the nerves of the feet and hands. Autonomic neuropathy is the other form of diffuse neuropathy and it affects the heart and other internal organs.

Focal—or localized—diabetic neuropathy affects specific nerves, most commonly in the torso, leg, or head.

Diabetic neuropathy can lead to muscular weakness, loss of feeling or sensation, and loss of autonomic functions such as digestion, erection, bladder control, and sweating among others.

Causes and symptoms

The exact cause of diabetic neuropathy is not known. Researchers believe that the process of nerve damage is related to high glucose concentrations in the blood that could cause chemical changes in nerves, disrupting their ability to effectively send messages. High blood glucose is also known to damage the blood vessels that carry oxygen and other nutrients to the nerves. In addition, some people may have a genetic predisposition to develop neuropathy.

There is a wide range of symptoms associated with diabetic neuropathy, and they depend on which nerves and parts of the body are affected, as well as the type of neuropathy present. Some patients have very mild symptoms, while others are severely disabled.

Common symptoms of diffuse peripheral neuropathy include:

- numbness and feelings of tingling or burning
- insensitivity to pain
- needle-like jabs of pain
- extreme sensitivity to touch
- loss of balance and coordination

Common symptoms of diffuse autonomic neuropathy include:

- impaired urination and sexual function
- bladder infections

- stomach disorders, due to the impaired ability of the stomach to empty (gastric stasis)
- nausea, vomiting, and bloating
- dizziness, lightheadedness, and fainting spells
- loss of appetite

Common symptoms of focal neuropathy include:

- pain in the front of a thigh
- severe pain in the lower back
- pain in the chest or stomach
- ache behind an eye
- double vision
- paralysis on one side of the face

In severe diabetic neuropathy loss of sensation can lead to injuries that are unnoticed, progressing to infections, ulceration and possibly **amputation**.

Diagnosis

Examination

The diagnosis of neuropathy is based on the symptoms that present during a physical exam. **Pain** assessment is usually the first step. Patients may have more than one type of pain, and the history helps the doctor determine whether a the pain has a neuropathic cause.

Tests

Based on finding during the physical exam, additional testing may be performed:

- screening tests for lost sensation
- nerve conduction studies to check the flow of electric current through a nerve
- electromyography (EMG) to see how well muscles respond to electrical impulses transmitted by nearby nerves
- ultrasound to show how the bladder and other parts of the urinary tract are functioning
- a nerve biopsy

Specialists who treat diabetic neuropathy include:

- neurologists: specialists in nervous system disorders
- urologists: specialists in urinary tract disorder
- gastroenterologists: specialists in digestive disorders
- podiatrists: specialists in caring for the feet

Treatment

Traditional

Treatment of diabetic neuropathy is usually focused on treating the symptoms associated with the neuropathy and addressing the underlying cause by improving the control of blood sugar levels, which may heal the early stages of neuropathy.

Drugs

There is no cure for the permanent nerve damage caused by neuropathy. To help control pain, drug therapy is normally used. The choice of proven drug therapies has broadened during the past decade. Pain medication, such as the topical skin cream capsaicin, is usually no stronger than codeine because of the potential for **addiction** with long-term use of such drugs.

Four main classes of drugs are available for **pain management**, alone or in combination: **tricyclic anti-depressants** (Imipramine, Nortriptyline), narcotic **analgesics** (Morphine), anticonvulsants (Carbamazepine, Gabapentin), and antiarrhythmics.

Prognosis

Early stage diabetic neuropathy can usually be reversed with good glucose control. Once nerve damage has occurred it cannot be reversed. The prognosis is largely dependent on the management of the underlying condition, diabetes, which may halt the progression of the neuropathy and improve symptoms. Recovery, if it occurs, is slow.

Prevention

Tight glucose control and the avoidance of alcohol and cigarettes help protect nerves from damage.

Resources

BOOKS

Colbert, Don. *The New Bible Cure for Diabetes.* Lake Mary, FL: Siloam Press, 2009.

Pierce, Dino Paul. *The Diabetes Handbook: Create Awareness and a New You.* Charleston, SC: CreateSpace, 2009.

Tesfaye, Solomin, and Andrew Boulton. *Diabetic Neuropathy.* New York: Oxford University Press, 2009.

Vaughn, Richard, A. *Beating The Odds: 64 Years of Diabetes Health.* Charleston, SC: CreateSpace, 2010.

ORGANIZATIONS

American Diabetes Association, 1701 North Beauregard Street, Alexandria, VA, 22311, (800) DIABETES (800-342-2383), http://www.diabetes.org.

Juvenile Diabetes Foundation, 120 Wall St., 19th Floor, New York, NY, 10005, (800) 533-CURE, http://www.jdf.org.

Gary Gilles
Ken R. Wells
Laura Jean Cataldo, RN, EdD

Dialysis, kidney

Definition

Dialysis treatment replaces the function of the kidneys, which normally serve as the body's natural filtration system. Through the use of a blood filter and a chemical solution known as dialysate, the treatment removes waste products and excess fluids from the bloodstream, while maintaining the proper chemical balance of the blood. There are two types of dialysis treatment: hemodialysis and peritoneal dialysis.

Purpose

Dialysis can be used in the treatment of patients suffering from poisoning or overdose, in order to quickly remove drugs from the bloodstream. Its most prevalent application, however, is for patients with temporary or permanent kidney failure. For patients with end-stage renal disease (ESRD), whose kidneys are no longer capable of adequately removing fluids and wastes from their body or of maintaining the proper level of certain kidney-regulated chemicals in the bloodstream, dialysis is the only treatment option available outside of **kidney transplantation**.

Demographics

In 1996 in the United States, over 200,000 people underwent regular dialysis treatments to manage their ESRD. As recently as 2007, the National Kidney and Urologic Diseases Information Clearinghouse (NKUDIC) reported that number increased to 368,544 residents receiving dialysis for ESRD. Of those individuals, 338,265 received in-center hemodialysis, 2,999 received home dialysis, and 26,364 received peritoneal dialysis.

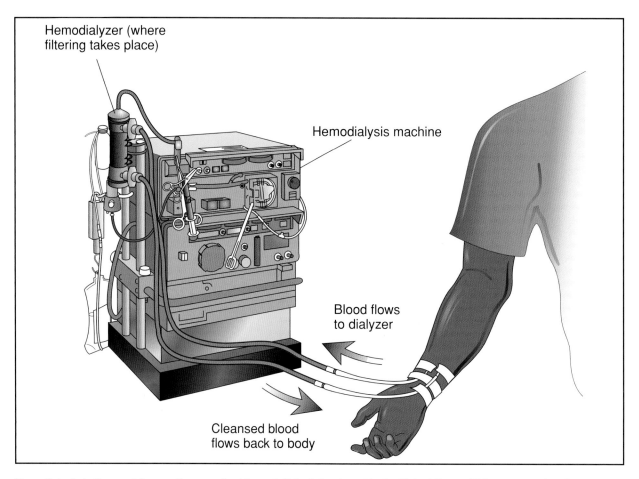

Hemodialysis is the most frequently prescribed type of dialysis treatment in the United States. This treatment involves circulating the patient's blood outside of the body through a dialysis circuit. The blood is filtered and cleansed inside the hemodialyzer and returned to the body. (Illustration by Electronic Illustrators Group. Reproduced by permission of Gale, a part of Cengage Learning.)

Description

There are two types of dialysis treatment: hemodialysis and peritoneal dialysis:

Hemodialysis

Hemodialysis is the most frequently prescribed type of dialysis treatment in the United States. The treatment involves circulating the patient's blood outside of the body through an extracorporeal circuit (ECC), or dialysis circuit. Two needles are inserted into the patient's vein, or access site, and are attached to the ECC, which consists of plastic blood tubing, a filter known as a dialyzer (artificial kidney), and a dialysis machine that monitors and maintains blood flow and administers dialysate. Dialysate is a chemical bath that is used to draw waste products out of the blood.

Since the 1980s, the majority of hemodialysis treatments in the United States have been performed with hollow fiber dialyzers. A hollow fiber dialyzer is composed of thousands of tube-like hollow fiber strands encased in a clear plastic cylinder several inches in diameter. There are two compartments within the dialyzer (the blood compartment and the dialysate compartment). The membrane that separates these two compartments is semipermeable. This means that it allows the passage of certain sized molecules across it, but prevents the passage of other, larger molecules. As blood is pushed through the blood compartment in one direction, suction or vacuum pressure pulls the dialysate through the dialysate compartment in a countercurrent, or opposite direction. These opposing pressures work to drain excess fluids out of the bloodstream and into the dialysate, a process called ultrafiltration.

A second process called diffusion moves waste products in the blood across the membrane into the dialysate compartment, where they are carried out of the body. At the same time, electrolytes and other chemicals in the dialysate solution cross the membrane into the blood compartment. The purified, chemically balanced blood is then returned to the body.

Most hemodialysis patients require treatment three times a week, for an average of three–four hours per dialysis "run." Specific treatment schedules depend on the type of dialyzer used and the patient's current physical condition. While the treatment prescription and regimen is usually overseen by a nephrologist (a doctor that specializes in the kidney), dialysis treatments are typically administered by a nurse or patient care technician in outpatient clinics known as dialysis centers, or in hospital-based dialysis units. In-home hemodialysis treatment is also an option for some patients, although access to this type of treatment may be limited by financial and lifestyle factors. An investment in equipment is required and another person in the household should be available for support and assistance with treatments.

Peritoneal dialysis

In peritoneal dialysis, the patient's peritoneum, or lining of the abdomen, acts as a blood filter. A catheter is surgically inserted into the patient's abdomen. During treatment, the catheter is used to fill the abdominal cavity with dialysate. Waste products and excess fluids move from the patient's bloodstream into the dialysate solution. After a waiting period of six to 24 hours, depending on the treatment method used, the waste-filled dialysate is drained from the abdomen, and replaced with clean dialysate.

There are three types of peritoneal dialysis:

- Continuous ambulatory peritoneal dialysis (CAPD). A continuous treatment that is self-administered and requires no machine. The patient inserts fresh dialysate solution into the abdominal cavity, waits four to six hours, and removes the used solution. The solution is immediately replaced with fresh dialysate. A bag attached to the catheter is worn under clothing.

- Continuous cyclic peritoneal dialysis (CCPD). An overnight treatment that uses a machine to drain and refill the abdominal cavity, CCPD takes 10–12 hours per session.

- Intermittent peritoneal dialysis (IPD). This hospital-based treatment is performed several times a week. A machine administers and drains the dialysate solution, and sessions can take up to 24 hours.

Peritoneal dialysis is often the treatment option of choice in infants and children, whose small size can make vascular (through a vein) access difficult to maintain. Peritoneal dialysis can also be done outside of a clinical setting, which is more conducive to regular school attendance.

Preparation

Patients are weighed immediately before and after each hemodialysis treatment to assess their fluid retention. Blood pressure and temperature are taken and the patient is assessed for physical changes since their last dialysis run. Regular blood tests monitor chemical and waste levels in the blood. Prior to treatment, patients are typically administered a dose of heparin, an anticoagulant that prevents blood clotting, to ensure the free flow of blood through the dialyzer and an uninterrupted dialysis run for the patient.

Aftercare

Both hemodialysis and peritoneal dialysis patients need to be vigilant about keeping their access sites and catheters clean and infection-free during and between dialysis runs.

Dialysis is just one facet of a comprehensive treatment approach for ESRD. Although dialysis treatment is very effective in removing toxins and fluids from the body, there are several functions of the kidney it cannot mimic, such as regulating high blood pressure and red blood cell production. Patients with ESRD need to watch their diet and fluid intake carefully and take medications as prescribed to manage their disease.

Risks

Many of the risks and side effects associated with dialysis are a combined result of both the treatment and the poor physical condition of the ESRD patient. Dialysis patients should always report side effects to their healthcare provider.

Anemia

Hematocrit (Hct) levels, a measure of red blood cells, are typically low in ESRD patients. This deficiency is caused by a lack of the hormone erythropoietin, which is normally produced by the kidneys. The problem is elevated in hemodialysis patients, who may incur blood loss during hemodialysis treatments. Epoetin alfa, or EPO (sold under the trade name Epogen), a hormone therapy, and intravenous or oral iron supplements are used to manage anemia in dialysis patients.

Cramps, nausea, vomiting, and headaches

Some hemodialysis patients experience cramps and flu-like symptoms during treatment. These can be caused by a number of factors, including the type of dialysate used, composition of the dialyzer membrane, water quality in the dialysis unit, and the ultrafiltration rate of the treatment. Adjustment of the dialysis prescription often helps alleviate many symptoms.

Hypotension

Because of the stress placed on the cardiovascular system with regular hemodialysis treatments, patients are at risk for **hypotension**, a sudden drop in blood pressure. This can often be controlled by medication and adjustment of the patient's dialysis prescription.

Infection

Both hemodialysis and peritoneal dialysis patients are at risk for infection. Hemodialysis patients should keep their access sites clean and watch for signs of redness and warmth that could indicate infection. Peritoneal dialysis patients must follow the same precautions with their catheter. **Peritonitis**, an infection of the peritoneum, causes flu-like symptoms and can disrupt dialysis treatments if not caught early.

Infectious diseases

Because there is a great deal of blood exposure involved in dialysis treatment, a slight risk of contracting **hepatitis B** and **hepatitis C** exists. The hepatitis B **vaccination** is recommended for most hemodialysis patients. There has only been one documented case of HIV being transmitted in a United States dialysis unit to a staff member, and no documented cases of HIV ever being transmitted between dialysis patients in the United States. The strict standards of **infection control** practiced in modern hemodialysis units makes the chance of contracting one of these diseases very small.

Normal results

Puffiness in the patient related to **edema**, or fluid retention, may be relieved after dialysis treatment. The patient's overall sense of physical well-being may also be improved. Because dialysis is an ongoing treatment process for many patients, a baseline for normalcy can be difficult to gauge.

Precautions

Blood pressure changes associated with hemodialysis may pose a risk for patients with heart problems. Peritoneal dialysis may be the preferred treatment option in these cases.

Peritoneal dialysis is not recommended for patients with abdominal **adhesions** or other abdominal defects, such as a **hernia**, that might compromise the efficiency of the treatment. It is also not recommended for patients who suffer frequent bouts of **diverticulitis**, an inflammation of small pouches in the intestinal tract.

Resources

BOOKS

Colbert, Don. *The New Bible Cure for Diabetes*. Lake Mary, FL: Siloam Press, 2009.

Gromko, Linda, and Jane C. McLure. *Arranging Your Life When Dialysis Comes Home*. Bellevue, WA: Arrange2-Live, 2009.

Pierce, Dino Paul. *The Diabetes Handbook: Create Awareness and a New You*. Charleston, SC: CreateSpace, 2009.

Stam, Lawrence, E. *100 Questions & Answers About Kidney Dialysis*.Sudbury, MA: Jones and Bartlett Publishers, 2009.

Vaughn, Richard, A. *Beating The Odds: 64 Years of Diabetes Health*. Charleston, SC: CreateSpace, 2010.

ORGANIZATIONS

American Association of Kidney Patients, 3505 E. Frontage Road, Suite 315, Tampa, FL, 33607, (813) 636-8122, (800) 749-2257, info@aakp.org, http://www.aakp.org.

American Urological Association Foundation, 1000 Corporate Blvd., Linthicum, MD, 21090, (410) 689-3700, (410) 689-3800, (866) 746-4282, auafoundation@auafoundation.org, http://www.urologyhealth.org/.

National Institute of Diabetes and Digestive and Kidney Diseases, NIDDK, NIH Bldg 31, Rm 9A06 31 Center Drive, MSC 2560, Bethesda, MD, 20892-2560, (301) 496-3583, http://www2.niddk.nih.gov/.

National Kidney Foundation, Inc. , 30 East 33rd Street, New York, NY, 10016, (212) 889-2210, (212) 689-9261, (800) 622-9010, http://www.kidney.org/.

United Network for Organ Sharing (UNOS), 700 N. 4th Street; PO Box 2484, Richmond, VA, 23218, (804) 782-4800, (804) 782-4817, (888) 894-6361, http://www.unos.org.

Paula Anne Ford-Martin
Gary Gilles
Ken R. Wells
Laura Jean Cataldo, RN, Ed.D.

Diaper rash

Definition

Dermatitis of the buttocks, genitals, lower abdomen, or thigh folds of an infant or toddler is commonly referred to as diaper rash.

Demographics

Diaper rash is believed to occur with the same frequency in infants who wear cloth or disposable diapers. It occurs most frequently in infants between eight and ten months of age, although it can occur in any child who wears diapers, generally from birth through about age three. It is estimated that about 10% of children will experience some significant diaper rash, although many more children will experience mild diaper rash at some time.

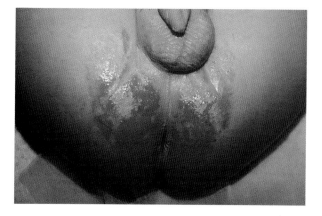

Baby with severe diaper rash. *(Custom Medical Stock Photo, Inc. Reproduced by permission.)*

Description

Diaper rash is a term that covers a broad variety of skin conditions that occur on the same area of the body. Some babies are more prone to diaper rash than others.

Frequently a flat, red rash is caused by simple chafing of the diaper against tender skin, initiating a friction rash. This type of rash is not seen in the skin folds. It may be more pronounced around the edges of the diaper, at the waist and leg bands. The baby generally does not appear to experience much discomfort. Sometimes the chemicals or detergents in the diaper are contributing factors and may result in **contact dermatitis**. These **rashes** should clear up easily with proper attention. Ignoring the condition may lead to a secondary infection that is more difficult to resolve.

Friction of skin against itself can cause a rash in the baby's skin folds, called intertrigo. This rash appears as reddened areas that may ooze and is often uncomfortable when the diaper is wet. Intertrigo can also be found on other areas of the body where there are deep skin folds that tend to trap moisture.

Seborrheic dermatitis is the diaper area equivalent of cradle cap. It is scaly and greasy in appearance and may be worse in the folds of the skin.

Yeast, or candidal dermatitis, is the most common infectious cause of diaper rash. The affected areas are raised and quite red with distinct borders, and satellite lesions may occur around the edges. Yeast is part of the normal skin flora, and is often an opportunistic invader when simple diaper rash is left untreated. It is particularly common after treatment with **antibiotics**, which kill the good bacteria that normally keep the yeast population in check. Usual treatments for diaper rash often are not sufficient to treat this rash. Repeated or difficult to resolve episodes of yeast infection may warrant further medical attention, since this is sometimes associated with diabetes or immune system problems.

Another infectious cause of diaper rash is **impetigo**. This bacterial infection is characterized by blisters that ooze and crust.

Causes and symptoms

The outside layer of skin normally forms a protective barrier that prevents infection. One of the primary causes of dermatitis in the diaper area is prolonged skin contact with wetness. Under these circumstances, natural oils are stripped away, the outer layer of skin is damaged, and there is increased susceptibility to infection by bacteria or yeast.

Diagnosis

The presence of red, blotchy skin or **skin lesions** in the diaper area means that the baby has diaper rash. However, there are several types of rash that may require specific treatment in order to heal. It is useful to be able to distinguish them by appearance as described above.

A baby with a rash that does not clear up within two to three days with home treatment or a rash with pustules, blisters, or bleeding should be seen by a healthcare professional for further evaluation. A rash accompanied by other symptoms such as a **fever**, rash on other areas of the body, or **vomiting** should also be seen quickly by the baby's doctor.

Treatment

Traditional

Antibiotics are generally prescribed for rashes caused by bacteria, particularly impetigo. This may be a topical or oral formulation, depending on the size of the area involved and the severity of the infection.

Over-the-counter antifungal creams, such as Lotrimin, are often recommended to treat a rash resulting from yeast. If topical treatment is not effective, an oral antifungal may be prescribed.

Mild steroid creams, such as 0.5–1% hydrocortisone, can be used for seborrheic dermatitis and sometimes intertrigo. Prescription strength creams may be needed for short-term treatment of more stubborn cases.

Alternative

In the event of suspected yeast, a tablespoon of cider vinegar can be added to a cup of warm water and used as a cleansing solution. This is dilute enough that it should not burn, but acidifies the skin pH enough to hamper yeast growth.

What the baby eats can make a difference in stool frequency and acidity. When adding a new food to the diet, the baby should be observed closely to see whether rashes are produced around the baby's mouth or anus. If this occurs, the new food should be discontinued.

Babies who are taking antibiotics are more likely to get rashes due to yeast. To help bring the good bacterial counts back to normal, *Lactobacillus bifidus* can be added to the diet. It is available in powder form from most health food stores.

Some herbal preparations can be useful for diaper rash. Calendula reduces inflammation, tightens tissues, and disinfects. It has been recommended for seborrheic dermatitis as well as for general inflammation of the skin. The ointment should be applied at each diaper change. Chickweed ointment can also be soothing for irritated skin and may be applied once or twice daily.

Home remedies

Good diaper hygiene will prevent or clear up many simple cases of diaper rash. Diapers should be checked very frequently and changed as soon as they are wet or soiled. Good air circulation is also important for healthy skin. Babies should have some time without wearing a diaper; a waterproof pad can be used to protect the bed or other surface. Rubber pants or other occlusive fabrics should not be used over the diaper area. There is no clear evidence that either cloth or disposable diapers are better at preventing diaper rash. It may be necessary for parents to experiment with diaper types to see if the baby's skin reacts better to cloth or disposable ones or if a particular brand works especially well. If the baby is wearing cloth diapers, they should be washed in a mild detergent and double rinsed. Using a larger size of diaper than normal until the rash heals can help speed healing and increase the baby's comfort.

The diaper area should be cleaned with something mild, even plain water. Some wipes contain alcohol or chemicals that can be irritating for some babies. Plain water may be the best cleansing substance when there is a rash. Using warm water in a spray bottle (or giving a quick bath) and then lightly patting the skin dry can produce less skin trauma than using wipes.

Barrier ointments can be valuable to treat rashes. Those that contain zinc oxide are especially effective. These creams and ointments protect already irritated skin from the additional insult of urine and stool, particularly if the baby has **diarrhea**. It is generally not recommended to use a talcum powder when changing the diaper, as inhaling the powder has been found to cause damage to infant's lungs.

Prognosis

Treated appropriately, diaper rash resolves fairly quickly if there is no underlying health problem or skin disease.

Prevention

Frequent diaper changes are important to keep the skin dry and healthy. Application of powders and ointments is not necessary when there is no rash. Finding the best combination of cleansing and diapering products for the individual baby will also help to prevent diaper rash.

Resources

BOOKS

Bremner, Gavin. J. and Theodore D. Wachs, editors. *The Wiley-Blackwell Handbook of Infant Development,* 2nd ed. Hoboken, NJ: Wiley-Blackwell, 2010.

Shelov, Steven P., and Tanya R. Altman, editors. *American Academy of Pediatrics, Caring for Your Baby and Young Child: Birth to Age 5,* 5th ed. New York: Bantam Books, 2009.

PERIODICALS

Adam, Ralf. "Skin Care of the Diaper Area." *Pediatric Dermatology* 25(4) (July–August 2008): 427–33.

Nield, Linda S., and Deepak Kamat. " Prevention, Diagnosis, and Management of Diaper Dermatitis." *Clinical Pediatrics.* 46(6) (July 2007): 480–486.

ORGANIZATIONS

American Academy of Dermatology (AAD), PO Box 4014, Schaumburg, IL, 60168–4014, (847) 330–0230, (866) 503–SKIN (7546), (847) 240–1859, MRC@aad.org, http://www.aad.org.

American Academy of Family Physicians (AAFP), PO Box 11210, Shawnee Mission, KS, 66207, (913) 906–6000, (800) 274–2237, (913) 906–6075, http://familydoctor.org.

American Academy of Pediatrics (AAP), 141 Northwest Point Blvd., Elk Grove Village, IL, 60007–1098, (847) 434–4000, (847) 434–8000, http://www.aap.org.

Judith Turner
Tish Davidson, AM

Diaphragm (birth control)

Definition

Diaphragms are dome-shaped barrier methods of **contraception** that block sperm from entering the uterus. They are made of latex (rubber) and formed like a shallow cup. Since vaginas vary in size, each patient will need to be fitted by a doctor or nurse with a diaphragm that conforms to the shape and contour of the vagina as well as the strength of the muscles in the vaginal walls. Diaphragms must be used with spermicidal cream or jelly. The device should cause no discomfort, and neither the woman nor her partner should feel that it is there.

Purpose

The purpose of a diaphragm is to prevent access to the womb (uterus) by the sperm and thus prevent conception. The level of effectiveness is about 95%.

Precautions

Each client will undergo a **physical examination** and a Pap smear. If these are normal, the physician will fit the patient for the device and give instructions on how to insert, remove, and clean the object. She will also be taught the signs and symptoms of potential complications.

Description

Prior to insertion, the inside of the dome and the rim are covered with a thick layer (perhaps a tablespoon) of a spermicide that is compatible with the diaphragm being used. The domed area covers the opening into the uterus (cervix) and keeps the spermicide in place. As a result, any sperm that might get under the diaphragm will be destroyed.

Diaphragms may be inserted two–three hours prior to intercourse, and must be left in place for six to eight hours following sexual relations. During this time the woman may not swim, bathe, or douche, but she may shower. If she desires to have intercourse again before the six to eight hours have passed, the diaphragm should not be removed. Instead, an applicator full of spermicide should be deposited into the vagina.

A diaphragm will last for a year or more. It should be examined weekly for holes. This can be done by holding it up to the light or filling it with water.

Preparation

Before inserting the diaphragm, the woman should empty her bladder and wash her hands with soap and water. The device should be checked for leaks by filling it with water or holding it up to the light. A spermicidal jelly is then applied to the inside and outside, and especially around the rim. While standing with one foot elevated on a chair or step, lying down, or squatting, the woman folds the diaphragm inward toward the middle and inserts it into the vagina as far as it will go.

Aftercare

When removed, the diaphragm should be washed with a mild soap and water. After being dried, it can be dusted with corn starch before being returned to its

---

KEY TERMS

Spermicide—A substance that kills sperm.

Toxic shock syndrome—An uncommon, but potentially fatal, disease that has been associated with the use of diaphragms and vaginal tampons. The symptoms include high fever, vomiting, and diarrhea.

---

container. The diaphragm should always be stored away from sunlight and heat in a cool, dry place. It should not be washed with harsh or perfumed soaps or used with perfumed powders because either of these substances can damage the diaphragm.

Risks

Although rare, wearing the diaphragm longer than the recommended time can result in **toxic shock syndrome**. The signs and symptoms of this serious illness include sudden onset of high **fever**, **vomiting**, **diarrhea**, **dizziness**, faintness, weakness, aching muscles and joints, and rash. The doctor must be notified immediately if any of these conditions appear. An allergic reaction to the spermicide or the material from which the device is made is also possible. Diaphragm use is also associated with an increased risk of bladder infections.

It should be noted that the diaphragm can become dislodged during intercourse, which could result in an unwanted **pregnancy**. To ensure a secure fit, a woman should be examined for a refitting if she gains or loses more than 10 lbs (4.5 kg), or after she gives birth.

Normal results

Consumers can expect an efficiency rate of about 95% in preventing pregnancy. Using a male condom in conjunction with the diaphragm decreases the potential for pregnancy. Diaphragms provide no protection against **AIDS** or other **sexually transmitted diseases**.

Resources

OTHER

"Guide to Safer Sex." *Sexual Health InfoCenter*. http://www.sexhealth.org/infocenter/GuideSS/diaphragm.htm.

ORGANIZATIONS

Planned Parenthood Federation of America, 434 West 33rd St., New York, NY, 10001, (212) 541-7800, (212) 245-1845, (800) 230-7526, http://www.plannedparenthood.org.

Donald G. Barstow, RN

Diaphragmatic hernia *see* **Hernia**

Diarrhea

Definition

To most individuals, diarrhea means an increased frequency or decreased consistency of bowel movements; however, the medical definition is more exact than this. In many developed countries, the average number of bowel movements is three per day. However, researchers have found that diarrhea best correlates with an increase in stool weight; stool weights above 10oz (300 gs) per day generally indicates diarrhea. This is mainly due to excess water, which normally makes up 60–85% of fecal matter. In this way, true diarrhea is distinguished from diseases that cause only an increase in the number of bowel movements (hyperdefecation) or incontinence (involuntary loss of bowel contents).

Diarrhea is also classified by physicians into acute, which lasts one or two weeks, and chronic, which continues for longer than 2 or 3 weeks. Viral and bacterial infections are the most common causes of acute diarrhea.

Description

In many cases, acute infectious diarrhea is a mild, limited annoyance. However, worldwide acute infectious diarrhea has a huge impact, causing over five million deaths per year. While most deaths are among children under five years of age in developing nations, the impact, even in developed countries, is considerable. For example, over 250,000 individuals are admitted to hospitals in the United States each year because of one of these episodes. Rapid diagnosis and proper treatment can prevent much of the suffering associated with these devastating illnesses.

Chronic diarrhea also has a considerable effect on health, as well as on social and economic well being. Patients with **celiac disease**, inflammatory bowel disease, and other prolonged diarrheal illnesses develop nutritional deficiencies that diminish growth and immunity. They affect social interaction and result in the loss of many working hours.

Causes and symptoms

Diarrhea occurs because more fluid passes through the large intestine (colon) than that organ can absorb. As a rule, the colon can absorb several times more fluid than is required on a daily basis. However, when this reserve capacity is overwhelmed, diarrhea occurs.

Diarrhea is caused by infections or illnesses that either lead to excess production of fluids or prevent absorption of fluids. Also, certain substances in the colon, such as fats and bile acids, can interfere with water absorption and cause diarrhea. In addition, rapid passage of material through the colon can also do the same.

Symptoms related to any diarrheal illness are often those associated with any injury to the gastrointestinal tract, such as **fever, nausea, vomiting**, and abdominal **pain**. All or none of these may be present depending on the disease causing the diarrhea. The number of bowel movements can vary—up to 20 or more per day. In some patients, blood or pus is present in the stool. Bowel movements may be difficult to flush (float) or contain undigested food material.

The most common causes of acute diarrhea are infections (the cause of **traveler's diarrhea**), **food poisoning**, and medications. Medications are a frequent and often over-looked cause, especially **antibiotics** and **antacids**. Less often, various sugar free foods, which sometimes contain poorly absorbable materials, cause diarrhea.

Chronic diarrhea is frequently due to many of the same things that cause the shorter episodes (infections, medications, etc.); symptoms just last longer. Some infections can become chronic. This occurs mainly with parasitic infections (such as *Giardia*) or when patients have altered immunity (**AIDS**).

The following are the more usual causes of chronic diarrhea:

- AIDS
- colon cancer and other bowel tumors
- endocrine or hormonal abnormalities (thyroid, diabetes mellitus, etc.)
- food allergy
- inflammatory bowel disease (**Crohn's disease** and ulcerative colitis)
- lactose intolerance
- malabsorption syndromes (celiac and Whipple's disease)
- other (alcohol, microscopic colitis, radiation, surgery)

Complications

The major effects of diarrhea are **dehydration, malnutrition**, and weight loss. Signs of dehydration can be hard to notice, but increasing thirst, **dry mouth**, weakness or lightheadedness (particularly if worsening on standing), or a darkening/decrease in urination are suggestive. Severe dehydration leads to changes in the body's chemistry and could become life-threatening. Dehydration from diarrhea can result in kidney failure, neurological symptoms, arthritis, and skin problems.

Diagnosis

Most cases of acute diarrhea never need diagnosis or treatment, as many are mild and produce few problems. But patients with fever over 102 °F (38.9 °C), signs of dehydration, bloody bowel movements, severe abdominal pain, known immune disease, or prior use of antibiotics need prompt medical evaluation.

When diagnostic studies are needed, the most useful are **stool culture** and examination for parasites; however these are often negative and a cause cannot be found in a large number of patients. The earlier cultures are performed, the greater the chance of obtaining a positive result. For those with a history of antibiotic use in the preceding two months, stool samples need to be examined for the toxins that cause **antibiotic-associated colitis**. Tests are also available to check stool samples for microscopic amounts of blood and for cells that indicate severe inflammation of the colon. Examination with an endoscope is sometimes helpful in determining severity and extent of inflammation. Tests to check changes in blood chemistry (potassium, magnesium, etc.) and a **complete blood count** (CBC) are also often performed.

Chronic diarrhea is quite different, and most patients with this condition will receive some degree of testing. Many exams are the same as for an acute episode, as some infections and parasites cause both types of diarrhea. A careful history to evaluate medication use, dietary changes, family history of illnesses, and other symptoms is necessary. Key points in determining the seriousness of symptoms are weight loss of over 10 lb (4.5 kg), blood in the stool, and nocturnal diarrhea (symptoms that awaken the patient from sleep).

Both prescription and over-the-counter medications can contain additives, such as lactose and sorbitol, that will produce diarrhea in sensitive individuals. Review of **allergies** or skin changes may also point to a cause. Social history may indicate if **stress** is playing a role or identify activities which can be associated with diarrhea (for example, diarrhea that occurs in runners).

A combination of stool, blood, and urine tests may be needed in the evaluation of chronic diarrhea; in addition a number of endoscopic and x-ray studies are frequently required.

Treatment

Treatment is ideally directed toward correcting the cause; however, the first aim should be to prevent or treat dehydration and nutritional deficiencies. The type of fluid and nutrient replacement will depend on whether oral feedings can be taken and the severity of fluid losses. Oral rehydration solution (ORS) or intravenous fluids are the choices; ORS is preferred if possible.

A physician should be notified if the patient is dehydrated, and if oral replacement is suggested then commercial (Pedialyte and others) or homemade preparations can be used. The World Health Organization (WHO) has provided this easy recipe for home preparation, which can be taken in small frequent sips:

- Table salt—3/4 tsp
- Baking powder—1 tsp
- Orange juice—1 c
- Water—1 qt (1l)

When feasible, food intake should be continued even in those with acute diarrhea. A physician should be consulted as to what type and how much food is permitted.

Anti-motility agents (loperamide, diphenoxylate) are useful for those with chronic symptoms; their use is limited or even contraindicated in most individuals with acute diarrhea, especially in those with high fever or bloody bowel movements. They should not be taken without the advice of a physician.

Other treatments are available, depending on the cause of symptoms. For example, the bulk agent psyllium helps some patients by absorbing excess fluid and solidifying stools; cholestyramine, which binds bile acids, is effective in treating bile salt induced diarrhea. Low fat **diets** or more easily digestible fat is useful in some patients. New **antidiarrheal drugs** that decrease excessive secretion of fluid by the intestinal tract is another approach for some diseases. Avoidance of medications or other products that are known to cause diarrhea (such as lactose) is curative in some, but should be discussed with a physician.

Alternative treatment

It is especially important to find the cause of diarrhea, since stopping diarrhea when it is the body's way of eliminating something foreign is not helpful and can be harmful in the long run.

One effective alternative approach to preventing and treating diarrhea involves oral supplementation of aspects of the normal flora in the colon with the yeasts *Lactobacillus acidophilus*, *L. bifidus*, or *Saccharomyces boulardii*. In clinical settings, these "biotherapeutic" agents have repeatedly been helpful in the resolution of diarrhea, especially antibiotic-associated diarrhea. Their effectiveness is also supported by the results of a research study published in the *Journal of the American Medical Association* in 1996.

KEY TERMS

Anti-motiltiy medications—Medications such as loperamide (Imodium), diphenoxylate (Lomotil), or medications containing codeine or narcotics that decrease the ability of the intestine to contract. These can worsen the condition of a patient with dysentery or colitis.

Colitis—Inflammation of the colon.

Endoscope—An endoscope, as used in the field of gastroenterology, is a thin flexible tube that uses a lens or miniature camera to view various areas of the gastrointestinal tract. Both diagnosis, through biopsies or other means, and therapeutic procedures can be done with this instrument.

Endoscopy—The performance of an exam using an endoscope is known generally as endoscopy.

Lactose intolerance—An inability to properly digest milk and dairy products.

Oral rehydration solution (ORS)—A liquid preparation developed by the World Health Organization that can decrease fluid loss in persons with diarrhea. Originally developed to be prepared with materials available in the home, commercial preparations have recently come into use.

Steatorrhea—Excessive amounts of fat in the feces.

Nutrient replacement also plays a role in preventing and treating episodes of diarrhea. Zinc especially appears to have an effect on the immune system, and deficiency of this mineral can lead to chronic diarrhea. Also, zinc replacement improves growth in young patients. Plenty of fluids, especially water, should be taken by individuals suffering from diarrhea to prevent dehydration. The BRAT diet also can be useful in helping to resolve diarrhea. This diet limits food intake to bananas, rice, applesauce, and toast. These foods provide soluble and insoluble fiber without irritation. If the toast is slightly burnt, the charcoal can help sequester toxins and pull them from the body.

Acute homeopathic remedies can be very effective for treating diarrhea especially in infants and young children.

Prognosis

Prognosis is related to the cause of the diarrhea; for most individuals in developed countries, a bout of acute, infectious diarrhea is at best uncomfortable.

However, in both industrialized and developing areas, serious complications and **death** can occur.

For those with chronic symptoms, an extensive number of tests are usually necessary to make a proper diagnosis and begin treatment; a specific diagnosis is found in 90% of patients. In some, however, no specific cause is found and only treatment with bulk agents or anti-motility agents is indicated.

Prevention

Proper hygiene and food handling techniques will prevent many cases. Traveler's diarrhea can be avoided by use of Pepto-Bismol and/or antibiotics, if necessary. The most important action is to prevent the complications of dehydration.

Resources

OTHER

"Directory of Digestive Diseases Organizations for Patients." *National Institute of Diabetes and Digestive and Kidney Disease.* http://www.niddk.nih.gov.
"A Neglected Modality for the Treatment and Prevention of Selected Intestinal and Vaginal Infections." *JAMA.* http://pubs.ama-assn.org.
Selected publications and documents on diarrhoeal diseases (including cholera). *World Health Organization (WHO).* http://www.who.ch/chd/pub/cdd/cddpub.htm.

ORGANIZATIONS

World Health Organization (WHO), Avenue Appia 201211, Geneva, Switzerland, 27, 4122791-2111, info@who.int, http://www.who.int.

David Kaminstein, MD

Diazep *see* **Benzodiazepines**

Diclofenac *see* **Nonsteroidal anti-inflammatory drugs**

Dicyclomine *see* **Antispasmodic drugs**

Didanosine *see* **Antiretroviral drugs**

Diets

Definition

Humans may alter their usual eating habits for many reasons, including weight loss, disease prevention or treatment, removing toxins from the body, or to achieve a general improvement in physical and mental health. Others adopt special diets for religious reasons. In the case of some vegetarians and vegans,

USDA MyPyramid food recommendations												
Daily caloric intake	1,000	1,200	1,400	1,600	1,800	2,000	2,200	2,400	2,600	2,800	3,000	3,200
Fruits	1 cup	1 cup	1.5 cups	1.5 cups	1.5 cups	2 cups	2 cups	2 cups	2 cups	2.5 cups	2.5 cups	2.5 cups
Vegetables	1 cup	1.5 cups	1.5 cups	2 cups	2.5 cups	2.5 cups	3 cups	3 cups	3.5 cups	3.5 cups	4 cups	4 cups
Grains	3 oz-eq	4 oz-eq	5 oz-eq	5 oz-eq	6 oz-eq	6 oz-eq	7 oz-eq	8 oz-eq	9 oz-eq	10 oz-eq	10 oz-eq	10 oz-eq
Meat and beans	2 oz-eq	3 oz-eq	4 oz-eq	5 oz-eq	5 oz-eq	5.5 oz-eq	6 oz-eq	6.5 oz-eq	6.5 oz-eq	7 oz-eq	7 oz-eq	7 oz-eq
Milk	2 cups	2 cups	2 cups	3 cups	3 cups	3 cups	3 cups	3 cups	3 cups	3 cups	3 cups	3 cups
Oils	3 tsp	4 tsp	4 tsp	5 tsp	5 tsp	6 tsp	6 tsp	7 tsp	8 tsp	8 tsp	10 tsp	11 tsp
Discretionary calorie allowance	165	171	171	132	195	267	290	362	410	426	512	648

SOURCE: U.S. Department of Agriculture, Center for Nutrition Policy and Promotion.

(Table by PreMediaGlobal. Reproduced by permission of Gale, a part of Cengage Learning.)

dietary changes are made out of ethical concerns for the rights of animals.

Purpose

People who are moderately to severely overweight can derive substantial health benefits from a weight-loss diet. A weight reduction of just 10–20 pounds can result in reduced cholesterol levels and lower blood pressure. Weight-related health problems include heart disease, diabetes, high blood pressure, and high levels of blood sugar and cholesterol.

In individuals who are not overweight, dietary changes also may be useful in the prevention or treatment of a range of ailments including acquired immuno deficiency syndrome (**AIDS**), **cancer**, **osteoporosis**, inflammatory bowel disease, chronic pulmonary disease, renal disease, **Parkinson's disease**, seizure disorders, and **food allergies** and intolerances.

Description

Origins

The practice of altering diet for special reasons has existed since antiquity. For example, Judaism has included numerous dietary restrictions for thousands of years. One ancient Jewish sect, the Essenes, is said to have developed a primitive **detoxification** diet aimed at preparing the bodies, minds, and spirits of its members for the coming of a "messiah" who would deliver them from their Roman captors. Preventive and therapeutic diets became popular during the late twentieth century. Books promoting the latest dietary plan continue to make the bestseller lists, although not all of the information given is considered authoritative.

The idea of a healthful diet is to provide all of the calories and nutrients needed by the body for optimal performance, at the same time ensuring that neither nutritional deficiencies nor excesses occur. Diet plans that claim to accomplish those objectives are so numerous they are virtually uncountable. These diets employ a variety of approaches, including the following:

- Fixed-menu: Offers little choice to the dieter. Specifies exactly which foods will be consumed. Easy to follow, but may be considered boring to some dieters.
- Formula: Replaces some or all meals with a nutritionally balanced liquid formula or powder.
- Exchange-type: Allows the dieter to choose between selected foods from each food group.
- Flexible: Doesn't concern itself with the overall diet, simply with one aspect such as fat or energy.

Diets also may be classified according to the types of foods they allow. For example, an omnivorous diet consists of both animal and plant foods, whereas a lacto-ovo-vegetarian diet permits no animal flesh, but includes eggs, milk, and dairy products. A vegan diet is a stricter form of **vegetarianism** in which eggs, cheese, and other milk products are prohibited.

A third way of classifying diets is according to their purpose: religious, weight-loss, detoxification, lifestyle-related, or aimed at prevention or treatment of a specific disease.

Precautions

Dieters should be cautious about plans that severely restrict the size of food portions, or that eliminate entire food groups from the diet. It is highly probable that they will become discouraged and drop out of such programs. The best diet is one that can be maintained indefinitely without ill effects, that offers sufficient variety and balance to provide everything needed for good health, and that is considerate of personal food preferences. Many controversies have arisen in the past over the benefits and risks of high-protein, low carbohydrate diets such as the **Atkins diet**. Most physician groups and health organizations have spoken out negatively against the program. In 2003, these statements were largely supported. Though clinical trials showed that these types of diets worked in lowering weight without raising cholesterol for the short-term, many of the participants gained a percentage of the weight back after only one year. A physician group also spoke out about high protein diets' dangers for people with decreased kidney function and the risk of bone loss due to decreased **calcium** intake.

Low-fat diets are not recommended for children under the age of two. Young children need extra fat to maintain their active, growing bodies. Fat intake may be gradually reduced between the ages of two and five, after which it should be limited to a maximum of 30% of total calories through adulthood. Saturated fat should be restricted to no more than 10% of total calories.

Weight-loss dieters should be wary of the "yo-yo" effect that occurs when numerous attempts are made to reduce weight using high-risk, quick-fix diets. This continued "cycling" between weight loss and weight gain can slow the basal metabolic rate and can sometimes lead to **eating disorders**. The dieter may become discouraged and frustrated by this success/failure cycle. The end result of yo-yo dieting is that it becomes more difficult to maintain a healthy weight.

Caution also should be exercised about weight loss diets that require continued purchases of special pre-packaged foods. Not only do these tend to be costly and over-processed, they also may prevent dieters from learning the food-selection and preparation skills essential to maintenance of weight loss. Further, dieters should consider whether they want to carry these special foods to work, restaurants, or homes of friends.

Concern has been expressed about weight-loss diet plans that do not include **exercise**, considered essential to long-term weight management. Some diets and supplements may be inadvisable for patients with special conditions or situations. In fact, use of the weight loss supplement ephedra was found to cause serious conditions such as **heart attack** and **stroke**. In 2003, the U.S. Food and Drug Administration (FDA) was considering controlling or banning the supplement. In short, most physician organizations see fad diets as distracting from learning how to achieve weight control over the long term through healthy lifestyle changes such as eating smaller, more balanced meals and exercising regularly.

Certain fad diets purporting to be official diets of groups such as the American Heart Association and the Mayo Clinic are in no way endorsed by those institutions. People thinking of starting such a diet should check with the institution to ensure its name has not been misappropriated by an unscrupulous practitioner.

Side effects

A wide range of side effects (some quite serious) can result from special diets, especially those that are nutritionally unbalanced. Further problems can arise if the dieter is taking high doses of dietary supplements. Food is essential to life, and improper **nutrition** can result in serious illness or **death**.

Research and general acceptance

It is agreed among traditional and complementary practitioners that many patients could substantially benefit from improved eating habits. Specialized diets have proved effective against a wide variety of conditions and diseases. However, dozens of unproved but widely publicized fad diets emerge each year, prompting widespread concerns about their usefulness, cost to the consumer, and their safety.

Resources

PERIODICALS

"American College of Preventive Medicine Weighs in Against Fad Diets." *Obesity and Diabetes Week*, March 17, 2003: 7.

"Atkins Diet Vindicated But Long-term Success Questionable." *Obesity, Fitness and Wellness Week*, June 14, 2003: 25.

"High-protein Diets Risky for Bones and Kidneys." *Health Science*, Spring 2003: 9.

Kirn, Timothy F. "FDA Probes Ephedra, Proposes Warning Label (Risk of Heart Attack, Seizure, Stroke)." *Clinical Psychiatry News*, April 2003: 49.

ORGANIZATIONS

American Dietetic Association, 120 S. Riverside Plaza, Suite 2000, Chicago, IL, 60606-6995, (312) 899-0040, (800) 877-1600, http://www.eatright.org/.

David Helwig
Teresa G. Odle

Diffuse esophageal spasm

Definition

Diffuse esophageal spasm is a term used to define an uncoordinated or spastic esophagus.

Description

The esophagus is a muscular tube that actively transports food from the throat to the stomach by rhythmic contractions known as peristalsis. The actual mechanism and anatomy are quite complex, involving three distinct segments and allowing a person to swallow even when upside-down. Diffuse esophageal spasm describes a condition where the entire esophagus is spastic—along its entire length, the muscular activity is increased and uncoordinated. The name corkscrew esophagus describes perfectly the appearance of this disorder on x rays.

X rays may reveal a slightly different appearance and result in the designation rosary bead esophagus, but the cause is still diffuse spasm, and the two entities behave in the same way.

Causes and symptoms

The cause appears to be disruption of the complex system of nerves that coordinates the muscular activity. The result is difficulty swallowing (dysphagia) and **pain** that feels like a **heart attack** and can involve the entire chest, jaw, and arms.

Diagnosis

Swallowing problems usually call for esophagograms. In the x-ray department, the patient is given a contrast agent to drink. During swallowing, x rays record the passage of the agent down the esophagus and into the stomach. Instead of a straight tube with well-coordinated waves of contraction, the resulting x rays show a writhing organ resembling a giant corkscrew.

Another test that is used in many disorders of esophageal motility is manometry. Pressures inside the esophagus are measured every inch or so using a balloon device that is passed all the way down to the stomach. The result is a precise record of its activity that yields a specific diagnosis.

Treatment

Soft and liquid foods pass more easily than solid pieces. Medications of several types are helpful—nifedipine, hydralazine, isoproterenol, and nitrates being the most successful. Several other treatments have uncertain results. For severe cases, relief is obtained two-thirds of the time by cutting the muscles along the entire length of the esophagus. This is a major surgical procedure.

Prognosis

This condition does not go away, nor is treatment entirely satisfactory. Patients need to be careful of

---

what they eat and continue on medication if a beneficial one is found. Fortunately, the condition does not get progressively worse as time passes.

Resources

BOOKS

Fauci, Anthony S., et al., eds. *Harrison's Principles of Internal Medicine.* 17th ed. New York: McGraw-Hill Professional, 2008.

J. Ricker Polsdorfer, MD

DiGeorge syndrome

Definition

DiGeorge syndrome (also called 22q11 deletion syndrome, congenital thymic hypoplasia, or third and fourth pharyngeal pouch syndrome) is a birth defect that is caused by an abnormality in chromosome 22 and affects the baby's immune system. The disorder is marked by absence or underdevelopment of the thymus and parathyroid glands. It is named for Angelo DiGeorge, the pediatrician who first described it in 1965. Some researchers prefer to call it DiGeorge anomaly, or DGA, rather than DiGeorge syndrome, on the grounds that the defects associated with the disorder represent the failure of a part of the human embryo to develop normally rather than a collection of symptoms caused by a single disease.

Description

The prevalence of DiGeorge syndrome is debated; the estimates range from 1:4000 to 1:6395. Because the symptoms caused by the chromosomal abnormality vary somewhat from patient to patient, the syndrome probably occurs much more often than was previously thought. DiGeorge syndrome is sometimes described as one of the "CATCH 22" disorders, so named because of their characteristics—cardiac defects, abnormal facial features, thymus underdevelopment, **cleft palate**, and

---

hypocalcemia—caused by a deletion of several genes in chromosome 22. The specific facial features associated with DiGeorge syndrome include low-set ears, wide-set eyes, a small jaw, and a short groove in the upper lip. The male/female ratio is 1:1. The syndrome appears to be equally common in all racial and ethnic groups.

Causes and symptoms

DiGeorge syndrome is caused either by inheritance of a defective chromosome 22 or by a new defect in chromosome 22 in the fetus. The type of defect that is involved is called deletion. A deletion occurs when the genetic material in the chromosomes does not recombine properly during the formation of sperm or egg cells. The deletion means that several genes from chromosome 22 are missing in DiGeorge syndrome patients. Although efforts have been made in the early 2000s to identify individual candidate genes for DGA, it appears that a combination of several genes in the deleted area is responsible for the disorder. Detailed genetic mapping of chromosome 22 has, however, identified a so-called DiGeorge critical region (DGCR), which has been completely sequenced.

According to a 1999 study, 6% of children with DiGeorge syndrome inherited the deletion from a parent, while 94% had a new deletion. Other conditions that are associated with DiGeorge syndrome are diabetes (a condition where the pancreas no longer produces enough insulin) in the mother and **fetal alcohol syndrome** (a pattern of **birth defects**, and learning and behavioral problems affecting individuals whose mothers consumed alcohol during **pregnancy**). Other chromosomal abnormalities that have been found in patients diagnosed with DGA include deletions on chromosomes 10p13, 17p13, and 18q21.

The loss of the genes in the deleted material means that the baby's third and fourth pharyngeal pouches fail to develop normally during the twelfth week of pregnancy. This developmental failure results in a completely or partially absent thymus gland and parathyroid glands. In addition, 74% of fetuses with DiGeorge syndrome have severe heart defects. The child is born with a defective immune system and an abnormally low level of **calcium** in the blood. Some children with DGA are also born with malformations of the genitals or urinary tract.

These defects usually become apparent within 48 hours of birth. The infant's heart defects may lead to **heart failure**, or there may be seizures and other evidence of a low level of calcium in the blood (**hypocalcemia**).

DiGeorge syndrome is also associated with an increased risk of **autoimmune disorders**. Cases have been reported of DGA in association with Graves' disease, immune thrombocytopenic purpura, juvenile **rheumatoid arthritis**, and severe **eczema**.

Diagnosis

Diagnosis of DiGeorge syndrome can be made by ultrasound examination around the eighteenth week of pregnancy, when abnormalities in the development of the heart or the palate can be detected. Another technique that is used to diagnose the syndrome before birth is called fluorescence in situ hybridization, or FISH. This technique uses DNA probes from the DiGeorge region on chromosome 22. FISH can be performed on cell samples obtained by **amniocentesis** as early as the fourteenth week of pregnancy. It confirms about 95% of cases of DiGeorge syndrome.

If the mother has not had prenatal testing, the diagnosis of DiGeorge syndrome is sometimes suggested by the child's facial features at birth. In other cases, the doctor makes the diagnosis during heart surgery when he or she notices the absence or abnormal location of the thymus gland. The diagnosis can be confirmed by blood tests for calcium, phosphorus, and parathyroid hormone levels, and by the sheep cell test for immune function.

Treatment

Hypocalcemia

Hypocalcemia in DiGeorge patients is unusually difficult to treat. Infants are usually given calcium and vitamin D by mouth. Severe cases have been treated by transplantation of fetal thymus tissue or bone marrow.

Heart defects

Infants with life-threatening heart defects are treated surgically.

Defective immune function

Children with DiGeorge syndrome should be kept on low-phosphorus **diets** and kept away from crowds or other sources of infection. They should not be immunized with vaccines made from live viruses or given **corticosteroids**.

Prognosis

The prognosis is variable; many infants with DiGeorge syndrome die from overwhelming infection, seizures, or heart failure within the first year. One study of a series of 558 patients reported 8% mortality within six months of birth, with heart defects accounting for all but one of the deaths. Infections resulting from severe immune deficiency are the second most common cause

KEY TERMS

Deletion—A genetic abnormality in which a segment of a chromosome is lost. DiGeorge syndrome is caused by a deletion on human chromosome 22.

Fetal alcohol syndrome—A cluster of birth defects that includes abnormal facial features and mental retardation, caused by the mother's consumption of alcoholic beverages during pregnancy.

Fluorescence in situ hybridization (FISH)—A technique for diagnosing DiGeorge syndrome before birth by analyzing cells obtained by amniocentesis with DNA probes. FISH is about 95% accurate.

Hypocalcemia—An abnormally low level of calcium in the blood.

Hypoplasia—A deficiency or underdevelopment of a tissue or body structure.

T cells—A type of white blood cell produced in the thymus gland. T cells are an important part of the immune system. Infants born with an underdeveloped or absent thymus do not have a normal level of T cells in their blood.

of **death** in patients with DGA. Advances in heart surgery indicate that the prognosis is most closely linked to the severity of the heart defects and the partial presence of the thymus gland. In most children who survive, the number of T cells, a type of white blood cell, in the blood rises spontaneously as they mature. Survivors are likely to be mentally retarded, however, and to have other developmental difficulties, including seizures or other psychiatric and neurological problems in later life.

Prevention

Genetic counseling is recommended for parents of children with DiGeorge syndrome because the disorder can be detected prior to birth. Although most children with DiGeorge syndrome did not inherit the chromosome deletion from their parents, they have a 50% chance of passing the deletion on to their own children.

Because of the association between DiGeorge syndrome and fetal alcohol syndrome, pregnant women should avoid drinking alcoholic beverages.

Resources

BOOKS

Beers, Mark H., Robert S. Porter, and Thomas V. Jones, eds. *The Merck Manual of Diagnosis and Therapy.* 18th ed. Whitehouse Station, NJ: Merck Research Laboratories, 2006.

DiGeorge Syndrome—A Medical Dictionary, Bibliography, and Annotated Research Guide to Internet References. San Diego: ICON Health Publications, 2004.

PERIODICALS

Verri, A., P. Maraschio, K. Devriendt, et al. "Chromosome 10p Deletion in a Patient with Hypoparathyroidism, Severe Mental Retardation, Autism and Basal Ganglia Calcifications." *Annales de génétique* 47 (July-September 2004): 281–287.

Yatsenko, S. A., A. N. Yatsenko, K. Szigeti, et al. "Interstitial Deletion of 10p and Atrial Septal Defect in DiGeorge 2 Syndrome." *Clinical Genetics* 66 (August 2004): 128–136.

ORGANIZATIONS

Canadian 22q Central, 338 Spruce Street North, Timmins, CanadaOntario, P4N 6N5 , (705) 268-3099, steph. stpierre@c22c.org, http://www.c22c.org.

Chromosome Disorder Outreach, P.O. Box 724, Boca Raton, FL, 33429-0724, (561) 395-4252, info@chromodisorder.org, http://www.chromodisorder.org.

National Organization for Rare Disorders, P.O. Box 8923, New Fairfield, CT, 06812-8923, (800) 999-6673, http://www.rarediseases.org.

Velo-Cardio-Facial Syndrome Educational Foundation, Inc., P.O. Box 874, Milltown, NJ, 08850, (214) 360-4740, info@vcfsef.org, http://www.vcfsef.org/.

Rebecca J. Frey, PhD

Digital rectal examination

Definition

The digital **rectal examination** (DRE) is a routine part of the **physical examination** and includes manual examination of the rectum, anus and, in men, the prostate.

Purpose

The purpose of the digital rectal examination is to identify lesions within the rectum and the prostate. It is the most widely used and oldest technique for the detection of **prostate cancer** and is used in screening for **colon cancer** and for the detection of **rectal polyps**.

Description

Usually the patient is positioned on the left side with the knees close to the chest. Sometimes the patient is asked to stand up and lean over the examination table. For women, sometimes this examination is part of the routine gynecological exam, and it may be done in a different manner than described here.

KEY TERMS

Fissure—Any cleft or groove, normal or otherwise, especially a deep fold in the anus.

Lesion—Any pathological or traumatic discontinuity of tissues or loss of function of a part.

Palpation—A simple technique in which a doctor presses lightly on the surface of the body to feel the organs or tissues underneath.

Peritonitis—Inflammation of the peritoneum. It may be accompanied by abdominal pain and tenderness, constipation, vomiting and moderate fever.

Polyp—Growth, usually benign, protruding from a mucous membrane.

Rectal prolapse—Protrusion of the rectal mucous membrane through the anus.

Skin tag—A small outgrowth of skin tissue that may be smooth or irregular, flesh-colored and benign.

During the examination, the health care practitioner examines the anus and the surrounding skin for **hemorrhoids**, tags, fissures and abscesses. After lubricating the gloved finger and anus, the examiner gently slides the finger into the anus and follows the contours of the rectum. The examiner notes the tone of the anus and feels the walls and the edges for texture, tenderness and masses as far as the examining finger can reach. The examiner evaluates the prostate for nodules and tenderness. Stool on the finger should be examined for blood, color, texture and tested for fecal occult blood.

The examination takes less than two minutes and can be uncomfortable when the patient is not relaxed or is anxious. Occasionally, when the DRE is performed on a man the penis may become erect. A gentle reminder and reassurance helps to relieve the embarrassment associated with the unexpected erection.

Preparation

The patient must be carefully positioned and the doctor should take care to explain the examination to the patient and to explain to the patient what to expect. The digital rectal examination may be uncomfortable and embarrassing. Much of the discomfort can be reduced by an understanding, unhurried and gentle examiner.

Precautions

When there are infections of the anus and of the rectum, the digital rectal examination should not be performed. Manipulation of the anal and rectal tissues increases the risk of infection and of bleeding.

Results

In the normal anus and rectum, there are no hemorrhoids or bleeding about the anus. The anal tone is not loose. The rectum is smooth and non-tender. No masses should be palpated, or felt.

The digital rectal examination is helpful in identifying areas of **peritonitis** or tender areas that can be felt through the wall of the rectum. It is used to identify perineal disease or deformity, abnormal location of the anus, **rectal prolapse** and atrophy of the gluteal muscle. Digital examination can detect a stenosis (or narrowing) of the anal canal, assess the tone and strength of the anal muscles or detect the presence of a rectal mass or fecal impaction.

Any masses, including hard stool, blood or tenderness is considered abnormal. **Cancer** masses may be flattened, nodular, cauliflower-like or ring-shaped. Polyps can be felt, but must be visualized using **anoscopy** or flexible **sigmoidoscopy** to be distinguished from other lesions, such as internal hemorrhoids or malignant growths. Hard masses of feces may be felt and may be removed.

Aftercare

Aftercare of the digital rectal examination is minimal. It requires removal of the lubricating jelly residue from around the anus. The lubricating jelly dissolves easily in water and may be washed off in bathing after the examination. It can be removed with toilet paper immediately after the examination.

Resources

BOOKS

Cheifetz, Adam S. *Oxford American Handbook of Gastroenterology and Hepatology.* Oxford, UK: Oxford University Press, 2010.

LeBlond, Richard, Donald Brown, and Richard DeGowin. *DeGowin's Diagnostic Examination*, 9th ed. New York: McGraw-Hill, 2009.

ORGANIZATIONS

American College of Gastroenterology, P.O. Box 342260, Bethesda, MD, 20827-2260, (301) 263-9000, http://www.acg.gi.org.

Cheryl L. Branche, MD
Brenda W. Lerner

Digoxin

Definition

Digitalis occurs naturally in the foxglove plant, (*Digitalis purpurea*), was used for centuries to treat heart disease. Currently, its active ingredient, digoxin (Lanoxin), is manufactured synthetically.

Purpose

Digoxin increase the strength and speed of heart muscle contractions and is used to treat congestive **heart failure**, where the heart is unable to pump all of the blood it receives.

Digoxin is used to slow the heart rate and improve the efficiency of the ventricles (main pumping chambers) when there are rapid or irregular heart beats, like **atrial flutter** or fibrillation.

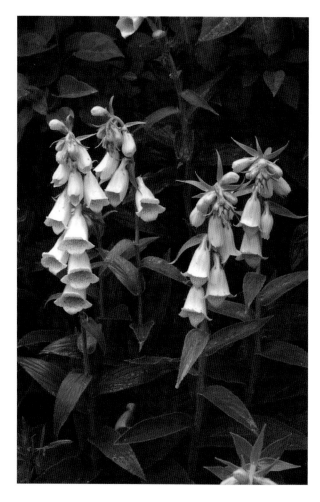

Digitalis purpurea. (Photo Researchers, Inc.)

The drug is also used to strengthen the heart in some cases of **shock**, like from **heart attack** or **sepsis** (overwhelming infection).

Description

Digoxin is available in tablet, capsule, liquid, and injectable forms.

Recommended dosage

The dose of digoxin is individualized for each patient. Physicians can tailor the dose based on patient response and laboratory measures of blood levels of the drug.

Precautions

This drug should be taken exactly as directed.

Digoxin is used with caution, or not given, in patients who have a number of serious heart diseases, like recent heart attack, subaortic ventricular stenosis and second or third degree **heart block**.

The elderly, newborns, and people with reduced kidney function are more sensitive to the effects of digoxin,

There is a narrow therapeutic range between effective and toxic doses of digoxin.

People taking digoxin should regularly check their pulse rate and rhythm; changes can signify side effects and should be reported to treating physicians.

Digitalis drugs are responsible for many accidental poisonings in children. Keep this medicine out of the reach of children.

Be alert to the signs and symptoms of digoxin overdose. If any of these signs occur, check with your physician soon:

- loss of appetite
- nausea
- vomiting
- pain in the lower stomach
- diarrhea
- tiredness or weakness
- extremely slow or irregular heartbeat (or fast heartbeat in children)
- blurred vision or other vision changes
- drowsiness
- confusion, unusual fatigue or depression
- headache
- fainting

Before taking digoxin, people with any of the following the medical problems should make sure their physicians are aware of their conditions:

- heart disease
- heart rhythm problems
- severe lung disease
- kidney disease
- liver disease
- thyroid disease

Side effects

In therapeutic doses, side effects are rare with digoxin. If skin rash, **hives**, or any other unusual or troublesome symptoms occur, check with your physician.

Interactions

Many drugs, foods and herbs can increase or decrease the effectiveness of digoxin. For example:

- Taking digoxin with other heart medicines or stimulant drugs like diet pills, amphetamines, or ephedra can increase the risk of heart rhythm problems.
- Calcium channel blocking drugs, like Procardia and Norvasc, used to treat high blood pressure, may cause higher than usual levels of digoxin.
- Many diuretics, like Hydrodiuril, cause the body to lose potassium and increase the risk of side effects from digoxin.
- Potassium supplements, like K-Dur, used to replentish potassium supplies in patients taking diuretics, can increase the risk of digoxin toxicity.
- Cholesterol-lowering drugs like Lipitor may increase digoxin levels in the blood.
- Cholestyramine, Questran, may reduce the absorption of digoxin. To reduce this possible problem, digoxin should be taken several hours before or after taking these medicines.
- Anti-diarrhea medicines may decrease the absorption of digoxin.
- St. Johns wort and natural licorice can decrease the effect of digoxin.

Check with a pharmacist on the possible interactions of all of the medications you take with digoxin.

James Waun, MD, RPh

▌Dilatation and curettage

Definition

Dilatation and curettage (D & C) is a gynecological procedure in which the lining of the uterus (endometrium) is scraped away.

Purpose

D & C is commonly used to obtain tissue for microscopic evaluation to rule out **cancer**. D & C may also be used to diagnose and treat heavy menstrual bleeding, and to diagnose endometrial polyps and **uterine fibroids**. A D & C can be used as a treatment as well, to remove **pregnancy** tissue after a **miscarriage**, incomplete abortion, or **childbirth**. Endometrial polyps may be removed, and sometimes benign uterine tumors (fibroids) may be scraped away. D & C can also be used as an early abortion technique up to 16 weeks.

Description

D & C is usually performed under **general anesthesia**, although local or epidural anesthesia can also be used. A local lessens risk and costs, but the woman will feel cramping during the procedure. The type of anesthesia used often depends upon the reason for the D & C.

In the procedure (which takes only minutes to perform), the doctor inserts an instrument to hold open the vaginal walls, and then stretches the opening of the uterus to the vagina (the cervix) by inserting a series of tapering rods, each thicker than the previous one, or by using other specialized instruments. This process of opening the cervix is called dilation.

Once the cervix is dilated, the physician inserts a spoon-shaped surgical device called a curette into the uterus. The curette is used to scrape away the uterine lining. One or more small tissue samples from the lining of the uterus or the cervical canal are sent for analysis by microscope to check for abnormal cells.

Although simpler, less expensive techniques such as a vacuum aspiration are quickly replacing the D & C as a diagnostic method, it is still often used to diagnose and treat a number of conditions.

Preparation

Because opening the cervix can be painful, sedatives may be given before the procedure begins. Deep breathing and other relaxation techniques may help ease cramping during cervical dilation.

Aftercare

A woman who has had a D & C performed in a hospital can usually go home the same day or the next day. Many women experience backache and mild cramps after the procedure, and may pass small **blood clots** for a day or so. Vaginal staining or bleeding may continue for several weeks.

Most women can resume normal activities almost immediately. Patients should avoid sexual intercourse, douching, and tampon use for at least two weeks to prevent infection while the cervix is closing and to allow the endometrium to heal completely.

Risks

The primary risk after the procedure is infection. Signs of infection include:

- fever
- heavy bleeding
- severe cramps
- foul-smelling vaginal discharge

A woman should report any of these symptoms to her doctor, who can treat the infection with **antibiotics** before it becomes serious.

D & C is a surgical operation, which carries certain risks associated with general anesthesia. Rare complications include puncture of the uterus (which usually heals on its own) or puncture of the bowel or bladder (which require further surgery to repair).

Normal results

Removal of the uterine lining causes no side effects, and may be beneficial if the lining has thickened so

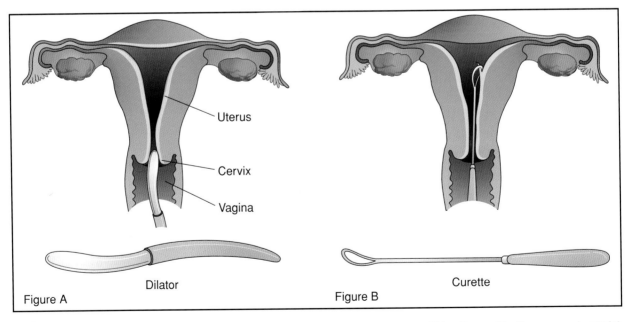

Uterus

Cervix

Vagina

Dilator

Figure A

Curette

Figure B

Dilatation and curettage (D & C) is used primarily to diagnose and treat heavy menstrual bleeding and to diagnose endometrial polyps, uterine fibroids, uterine cancer and cervical cancer. When performing a D & C, the physician inserts a speculum to separate and hold the vaginal walls, then stretches open the cervix with a dilator. Once the cervix is dilated, the physician will insert a curette into the uterus and scrape away small portions of the uterine lining for laboratory analysis. *(Illustration by Electronic Illustrators Group. Reproduced by permission of Gale, a part of Cengage Learning.)*

much that it causes heavy periods. The uterine lining soon grows again normally, as part of the menstrual cycle.

Resources

BOOKS

Carlson, Karen J., Stephanie A. Eisenstat, and Terra Ziporyn. *The New Harvard Guide to Women's Health.* Cambridge, MA: Harvard University Press, 2004.

Carol A. Turkington

Dilated cardiomyopathy *see* **Congestive cardiomyopathy**
Diltiazem *see* **Calcium channel blockers**
Dilution test *see* **Kidney function tests**
Diphenhydramine *see* **Antihistamines**

Diphtheria

Definition

Diphtheria is a potentially fatal, contagious disease that usually involves the nose, throat, and air passages, but may also infect the skin. Its most striking feature is the formation of a grayish membrane covering the tonsils and upper part of the throat.

Demographics

Before 1920 when the diphtheria toxoid was introduced, diphtheria was a major childhood killer, with 200,000 cases reported annually in the United States. In the twenty first century, diphtheria is rare and sporadic in the developed world because of widespread immunization. In countries that do not have routine immunization against this infection, periodic outbreaks occur. The largest recent outbreak occurred in the countries comprising the former Soviet Union and the Baltic States. From 1990–1995, 157,000 cases and 5,000 deaths were reported in this region, accounting for more than 80% of all diphtheria cases reported during those years. Other, smaller outbreaks have been reported in sub-Saharan Africa, India, and France. Like many other upper respiratory diseases, diphtheria is most likely to occur during the cold months. Individuals who have not been immunized may get diphtheria at any age; mortality rates are highest in those under five years or over 40 years of age.

Description

Diphtheria is spread most often by droplets from the coughing or sneezing of an infected person or carrier. The incubation period is two to seven days, with an average of three days. It is vital to seek medical help at once when diphtheria is suspected, because treatment requires emergency measures for adults as well as children.

Risk factors for developing diphtheria include:

- failure to immunize or incomplete immunization
- living in crowded, unhygienic conditions
- having a compromised immune system
- traveling to developing regions of the world where diphtheria is more common

Causes and symptoms

The symptoms of diphtheria are caused by toxins produced by the diphtheria bacillus, *Corynebacterium diphtheriae* (from the Greek for "rubber membrane"). In fact, toxin production is related to infections of the bacillus itself with a particular bacterial virus called a phage (from bacteriophage; a virus that infects bacteria). The infection destroys healthy tissue in the upper area of the throat around the tonsils, or in open **wounds** in the skin. Fluid from dying cells then coagulates to form the telltale gray or grayish-green membrane. Inside the membrane, the bacteria produce an exotoxin, which is a poisonous secretion that causes the life-threatening symptoms of diphtheria. The exotoxin is carried throughout the body in the bloodstream, destroying healthy tissue in other parts of the body.

The most serious complications caused by the exotoxin are inflammations of the heart muscle (**myocarditis**) and damage to the nervous system. The risk of serious complications is increased as the time between onset of symptoms and the administration of antitoxin increases and as the size of the membrane formed increases. Myocarditis may cause disturbances in the heart rhythm (**arrhythmias**) and may result in **heart failure**. Symptoms of nervous system involvement can include seeing double vision (diplopia), painful or difficult swallowing (dysphagia), and slurred speech or loss of voice, which are all indications of the exotoxin's effect on nerve functions. The exotoxin may also cause severe swelling in the neck ("bull neck").

The signs and symptoms of diphtheria vary according to the location of the infection.

Nasal

Nasal diphtheria produces few symptoms other than a watery or bloody discharge. On examination, there may be a small visible membrane in the nasal passages. Nasal infection rarely causes complications by itself, but it is a public health problem because it spreads the disease more rapidly than other forms of diphtheria.

Pharyngeal

Pharyngeal diphtheria gets its name from the pharynx, which is the part of the upper throat that connects the mouth and nasal passages with the voice box (larynx). This is the most common form of diphtheria, causing the characteristic grayish throat membrane. The membrane often bleeds if it is scraped or cut. It is important not to try to remove the membrane because the trauma may increase the body's absorption of the exotoxin. Other signs and symptoms of pharyngeal diphtheria include mild **sore throat**, **fever** of 101–102 °F (38.3–38.9 °C), a rapid pulse, and general body weakness.

Laryngeal

Laryngeal diphtheria, which involves the voice box or larynx, is the form most likely to produce serious complications. The fever is usually higher in this form of diphtheria (103–104 °F or 39.4–40 °C) and the patient is very weak. Patients may have a severe **cough**, have difficulty breathing, or lose their voice completely. The development of a "bull neck" indicates a high level of exotoxin in the bloodstream. Obstruction of the airway may result in difficulty breathing, respiratory compromise, and **death**.

Skin

This form of diphtheria, which is sometimes called cutaneous diphtheria, accounts for about 33% of diphtheria cases. It is found chiefly among people with poor hygiene, and is more common in tropical climates. Any break in the skin can become infected with diphtheria. The infected tissue develops an ulcerated area and a diphtheria membrane may form over the wound but is not always present. The wound or ulcer is slow to heal and may be numb or insensitive when touched.

Diagnosis

Because diphtheria must be treated as quickly as possible, doctors usually make the diagnosis on the

---

KEY TERMS

Antitoxin—An antibody against an exotoxin, usually derived from horse serum.

Bacillus—A rod–shaped bacterium, such as the diphtheria bacterium.

Carrier—A person who may harbor an organism without symptoms and may transmit it to others.

Cutaneous—Located in the skin.

Diphtheria–tetanus–pertussis (DTP)—The standard preparation used to immunize children against diphtheria, tetanus, and whooping cough. A so-called "acellular pertussis" vaccine (aP) is usually used since its release in the mid-1990s in a combined vaccine known as DTaP.

Exotoxin—A poisonous secretion produced by bacilli which is carried in the bloodstream to other parts of the body.

Gram's stain—A dye staining technique used in laboratory tests to determine the presence and type of bacteria.

Loeffler's medium—A special substance used to grow diphtheria bacilli to confirm a diagnosis.

Myocarditis—Inflammation of the heart tissue.

Toxoid—A preparation made from inactivated exotoxin, used in immunization.

---

basis of the visible symptoms without waiting for test results.

Examination

In making the diagnosis, the doctor examines the patient's eyes, ears, nose, and throat in order to rule out other diseases that may cause fever and sore throat, such as **infectious mononucleosis**, a sinus infection, or **strep throat**. The most important single symptom that suggests diphtheria is the membrane. When a patient develops skin infections during an outbreak of diphtheria, the doctor will consider the possibility of cutaneous diphtheria and take a smear to confirm the diagnosis.

Tests

The diagnosis of diphtheria can be confirmed by the results of a culture obtained from the infected area. Material from the swab is put on a microscope slide and stained using a procedure called Gram's stain. The diphtheria bacillus is called Gram-positive because it holds the dye after the slide is rinsed with alcohol. Under the microscope, diphtheria bacilli look like beaded rod-shaped cells, grouped in patterns that resemble Chinese characters. Another laboratory test involves growing the diphtheria bacillus on a special material called Loeffler's medium.

Treatment

Diphtheria is a serious disease requiring hospital treatment in an intensive care unit if the patient has developed respiratory symptoms. Treatment includes a combination of medications and supportive care:

Antitoxin

The most important step is prompt administration of diphtheria antitoxin, without waiting for laboratory results. The antitoxin is made from horse serum and works by neutralizing any circulating exotoxin. The doctor must first test the patient for sensitivity to animal serum. Patients who are sensitive (about 10%) must be desensitized with diluted antitoxin, since the antitoxin is the only specific substance that will counteract diphtheria exotoxin. No other type if antitoxin is available for the treatment of diphtheria.

The dose of antitoxin ranges from 20,000–100,000 units, depending on the severity and length of time of symptoms occurring before treatment. Diphtheria antitoxin is usually given intravenously. It must be obtained from the United States Centers for Disease Control and Prevention (CDC) and may not be available in some parts of the world.

Antibiotics

Antibiotics are given to kill the bacteria, to prevent the spread of the disease, and to protect the patient from developing **pneumonia**. They are not a substitute for treatment with antitoxin. Both adults and children may be given penicillin, ampicillin, or erythromycin. Erythromycin appears to be more effective than penicillin in treating people who are carriers because of better penetration into the infected area.

Cutaneous diphtheria is usually treated by cleansing the wound thoroughly with soap and water, and giving the patient antibiotics for 10 days.

Supportive care

Diphtheria patients need bed rest with intensive nursing care, including extra fluids, oxygenation, and monitoring for possible heart problems, airway blockage, or involvement of the nervous system. Patients with laryngeal diphtheria are kept in a **croup** tent or high-humidity environment; they may also need throat suctioning or emergency surgery if their airway is blocked.

Patients recovering from diphtheria should rest at home for a minimum of two to three weeks, especially if they have heart complications. In addition, patients should be immunized against diphtheria after recovery, because having the disease does not always induce antitoxin formation and protect them from re-infection.

Prevention of complications

Diphtheria patients who develop myocarditis may be treated with oxygen and with medications to prevent irregular heart rhythms. An artificial pacemaker may be needed. Patients with difficulty swallowing can be fed through a tube inserted into the stomach through the nose. Patients who cannot breathe are usually put on mechanical respirators.

Prognosis

The prognosis depends on the size and location of the membrane and on early treatment with antitoxin; the longer the delay, the higher the death rate. The most vulnerable patients are children under age five and those who develop pneumonia or myocarditis. Death rates generally range from five to 10 percent and may reach as high as 20% in young children and older adults. Nasal and cutaneous diphtheria are rarely fatal.

Prevention

Prevention of diphtheria has four aspects:

Immunization

Universal immunization is the most effective means of preventing diphtheria. The standard course of immunization for healthy children is three doses of DTaP (diphtheria-tetanus-acellular pertussis) preparation given between two months and six months of age, with booster doses given at 18 months and again between the ages of four and six years. At 12 years a booster shot of is given. Adults should be immunized at 10-year intervals with Td (tetanus-diphtheria) toxoid. A toxoid is a bacterial toxin that is treated to make it harmless but still can induce immunity to the disease.

Isolation of patients

Diphtheria patients must be isolated for one to seven days or until two successive cultures show that they are no longer contagious (up to six weeks). Children placed in **isolation** are usually assigned a primary nurse for emotional support.

Identification and treatment of contacts

Because diphtheria is highly contagious and has a short incubation period, family members and other contacts of diphtheria patients must be watched for symptoms and tested to see if they are carriers. They are usually given antibiotics for seven days and a booster shot of diphtheria/tetanus toxoid.

Reporting cases to public health authorities

Reporting is necessary to track potential epidemics, to help doctors identify the specific strain of diphtheria, and to see if resistance to penicillin or erythromycin has developed.

Resources

BOOKS

Guilfoile, Patrick. *Diphtheria.* New York: Chelsea House, 2009.
Sears, Robert. *The Vaccine Book: Making The Right Decision for Your Child.* New York: Little, Brown, 2007.

OTHER

"Diphtheria." Mayo Foundation for Education and Research. (April 7, 2009). http://www.mayoclinic.com/health/diphtheria/DS00495 (accessed September 17, 2010).
"Diphtheria." World Health Organization. (2010). http://www.who.int/topics/diphtheria/en (accessed September 17, 2010).
"Diphtheria." MedlinePlus. (March 27, 2010). http://www.nlm.nih.gov/medlineplus/diphtheria.html (accessed September 17, 2010).
"Vaccines." United States Centers for Disease Control and Prevention (CDC). (March 30, 2010). http://www.cdc.gov/vaccines (accessed September 17, 2010).

ORGANIZATIONS

Centers for Disease Control and Prevention (CDC), 1600 Clifton Rd., Atlanta, GA, 30333, (404) 639–3534, (800) CDC–INFO (800–232–4636). TTY: (888) 232–6348, inquiry@cdc.gov, http://www.cdc.gov.
World Health Organization (WHO), Avenue Appia 20, 1211 Geneva 27, Switzerland, + 22 41 791 21 11, + 22 41 791 31 11, info@who.int, http://www.who.int.

Rebecca J. Frey, PhD
Tish Davidson, A.M.

Diplegia *see* **Paralysis**
Direct Coombs' test *see* **Coombs' tests**
Direct laryngoscopy *see* **Laryngoscopy**

Discoid lupus erythematosus

Definition

Discoid lupus erythematosus (DLE) is a disease in which coin-shaped (discoid) red bumps appear on the skin.

Description

The disease called discoid lupus erythematosus only affects the skin, although similar discoid **skin lesions** can occur in the serious disease called **systemic lupus erythematosus** (SLE). Only about 10% of all patients with DLE will go on to develop the multi-organ disease SLE.

The tendency to develop DLE seems to run in families. Although men or women of any age can develop DLE, it occurs in women three times more frequently than in men. The typical DLE patient is a woman in her 30s.

Causes and symptoms

The cause of DLE is unknown. It is thought that DLE (like SLE) may be an autoimmune disorder. **Autoimmune disorders** are those that occur when cells of the immune system are misdirected against the body. Normally, immune cells work to recognize and help destroy foreign invaders like bacteria, viruses, and fungi. In autoimmune disorders, these cells mistakenly recognize various tissues of the body as foreign invaders, and attack and destroy these tissues. In SLE, the misdirected immune cells are antibodies. In DLE, the damaging cells are believed to be a type of white blood cell called a T lymphocyte. The injury to the skin results in inflammation and the characteristic discoid lesions.

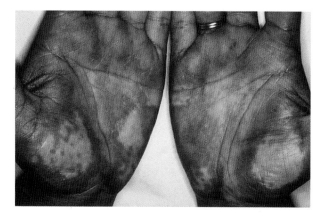

Discoloration of the hands is one characteristic of discoid lupus erythematosus. *(Custom Medical Stock Photo, Inc. Reproduced by permission.)*

In DLE, the characteristic skin lesion is circular and raised. The reddish rash is about 5–10 mm in diameter, with the center often somewhat scaly and lighter in color than the darker outer ring. The surface of these lesions is sometimes described as "warty." There is rarely any **itching** or **pain** associated with discoid lesions. They tend to appear on the face, ears, neck, scalp, chest, back, and arms. As DLE lesions heal, they leave thickened, scarred areas of skin. When the scalp is severely affected, there may be associated hair loss (**alopecia**).

People with DLE tend to be quite sensitive to the sun. They are more likely to get a **sunburn**, and the sun is likely to worsen their discoid lesions.

Diagnosis

Diagnosis of DLE usually requires a **skin biopsy**. A small sample of a discoid lesion is removed, specially prepared, and examined under a microscope. Usually, the lesion has certain microscopic characteristics that allow it to be identified as a DLE lesion. Blood tests will not reveal the type of antibodies present in SLE, and **physical examination** usually does not reveal anything other than the skin lesions. If antibodies exist in the blood, or if other symptoms or physical signs are found, it is possible that the discoid lesions are a sign of SLE rather than DLE.

Treatment

Treatment of DLE primarily involves the use of a variety of skin creams. **Sunscreens** are used for protection. Steroid creams can be applied to decrease inflammation. Occasionally, small amounts of a steroid preparation will be injected with a needle into a specific lesion. Because of their long list of side effects, steroid preparations taken by mouth are avoided. Sometimes, short-term treatment with oral **steroids** will be used for particularly severe DLE outbreaks. Medications used to treat the **infectious diseasemalaria** are often used to treat DLE.

Alternative treatment

Alternative treatments for DLE include eating a healthy diet, low in red meat and dairy products and high in fish containing **omega-3 fatty acids**. These types of fish include mackerel, sardines, and salmon. Following a healthy diet is thought to decrease inflammation. Dietary supplements believed to be helpful include **vitamins** B, C, E, and selenium. Vitamin A is also recommended to improve DLE lesions. Constitutional homeopathic treatment can help heal DLE as well as help prevent it developing into SLE.

KEY TERMS

Antibody—Specialized cells of the immune system that can recognize organisms invading the body (like bacteria, viruses, and fungi). The antibodies are then able to start a complex chain of events designed to kill these foreign invaders.

Autoimmune disorder—A disorder in which the body's antibodies mistake the body's own tissues for foreign invaders. The immune system then attacks and causes damage to these tissues.

Immune system—The system of specialized organs, lymph nodes, and blood cells throughout the body that work together to defend the body against foreign invaders (bacteria, viruses, fungi, etc.).

Prognosis

For the most part, the prognosis for people with DLE is excellent. While the lesions may be cosmetically unsightly, they are not life threatening and usually do not cause a patient to change his or her lifestyle. Only about 10% of patients with DLE will go on to develop SLE.

Prevention

DLE cannot be prevented. Recommendations to prevent flares of DLE in patients with the disease include avoiding exposure to sun and consistently using sunscreen.

ORGANIZATIONS

American College of Rheumatology, 2200 Lake Boulevard NE, Atlanta, GA, 30319, (404) 633-3777, (404) 633-1870, acr@rheumatology.org, http://www.rheumatology.org/.

Lupus Foundation of America, 2000 L Street, N.W., Suite 710, Washington, DC, 20036, (202) 349-1155, (202) 349-1156, (800) 558-0121, http://www.lupus.org.

Rosalyn Carson-DeWitt, MD

Disk removal

Definition

One of the most common types of back surgery is disk removal (diskectomy), the removal of an intervertebral disk, the flexible plate that connects any two

KEY TERMS

Diskectomy—The surgical removal of a portion of an intervertebral disk.

Dura—The strongest and outermost of three membranes that protect the brain, spinal cord, and nerves of the cauda equina.

Herniated disk—A blisterlike bulging or protrusion of the contents of the disk out through the fibers that normally hold them in place. It is also called a ruptured disk, slipped disk, or displaced disk.

Intervertebral disk—Cylindrical elastic-like gel pads that separate and join each pair of vertebrae in the spine.

Laminectomy—An operation in which the surgeon cuts through the covering of a vertebra to reach a herniated disk in order to remove it.

Vertebra—The bones that make up the back bone (spine).

adjacent vertebrae in the spine. Intervertebral disks act as shock absorbers, protecting the brain and spinal cord from the impact produced by the body's movements.

Purpose

About 150,000 Americans undergo disk removal each year in the United States. Removing the invertebral disk is performed to treat back **pain** that has lasted at least six weeks as a result of an abnormal disk and that has not responded to conservative treatment. Surgery is also performed if there is pressure on the lumbosacral nerve roots that causes weakness or bowel or bladder disfunction.

As a person ages, the disks between the vertebrae degenerate and dry out, and the fibers holding them in place tear. Eventually, the disk can form a blister-like bulge, compressing nerves in the spine and causing pain. This is called a "prolapsed" (or herniated) disk. If such a disk causes muscle weakness or interferes with bladder or bowel function because it is pressing on a nerve root, immediate surgery to remove the disk may be needed.

The aim of the surgery is to try to relieve all pressure on nerve roots by removing the pulpy material from the disk, or the disk itself. If it is necessary to remove material from several nearby vertebrae, the spine may become unsteady. In this case, the surgeon will perform a spinal fusion, removing all the disks between two or more vertebrae and roughening the bones so that the vertebrae heal together. Bone strips taken from the patient's leg or hip may be used to help hold the vertebrae together. Spinal fusion decreases pain but it also decreases spinal mobility.

Precautions

The doctor will obtain x rays, neuroimaging studies, including computed tomography scan (CT scan)

myelogram and **magnetic resonance imaging** (MRI), and clinical exams to determine the precise location of the affected disk.

Description

The surgery is done under general anaesthesia, which puts the patient to sleep and affects the whole body. Operating on the patient's back, the neurosurgeon or orthopedic surgeon makes an opening into the vertebral canal, and then moves the dura and the bundle of nerves called the "cauda equina" (horse's tail) aside, which exposes the disk. If a portion of the disk has moved from between the vertebrae out into the nerve canal, it is simply removed. If the disk itself has become fragmented and partially displaced, or not fragmented but bulging extensively, the surgeon will remove the bulging or displaced part of the disk and the part that lies in the space between the vertebrae.

Preparation

The patient is given an injection an hour before the surgery to dry up internal fluids and encourage drowsiness.

Aftercare

After the operation, the patient will awaken lying flat and face down, and must remain this way for several days, changing position only to avoid **bedsores**. There maybe slight pain or stiffness in the back area.

Patients should sleep on a firm mattress and avoid bending at the waist, lifting heavy weights, or sitting in one spot for a long time (such as riding in a car).

After surgery, patients can usually leave the hospital on the fourth or fifth day. They must:

- avoid sitting for more than 15–20 minutes
- use a reclined chair

- avoid bending, twisting, or lifting
- begin gentle walking (indoors or outdoors), gradually increasing
- begin stationary biking or gentle swimming after two weeks
- continue exercise for the next four weeks
- slow down if they experience more than minor pain in the back or leg

Risks

All surgery carries some risk due to heart and lung problems or the anesthesia itself, but this risk is generally extremely small. (The risk of **death** from **general anesthesia** for all types of surgery, for example, is only about 1 in 1,600.)

The most common risk of the surgery is infection, which occurs in 1–2% of cases. Rarely, the surgery can damage nerves in the lower back or major blood vessels in front of the disk. Occasionally, there may be some residual **paralysis** of a particular leg or bladder muscle after surgery, but this is the result of the disk problem that necessitated the surgery, not the operation itself.

While disk removals can relieve pain in 90% of cases, there are some people who do not get pain relief, depending on how long they had the condition requiring surgery and other factors.

Normal results

After about five days, most patients can leave the hospital. They can resume all normal activities, including work, after four to six weeks of recuperation at home.

In properly evaluated patients, there is a very good chance that disk removal will be successful in easing pain. Even in patients over age 60, disk surgery has a "good to excellent" result for 87% of patients. Disk surgery can relieve both back and leg pain, but the greatest pain relief will occur with the leg pain.

Resources

BOOKS

Sabiston, David C., et al. *Sabiston Textbook of Surgery: The Biological Basis of Modern Surgical Practice.* Philadelphia: Saunders/Elsevier, 2008.

Carol A. Turkington

Diskectomy *see* **Disk removal**

Dislocations and subluxations

Definition

In medicine, the terms dislocation and subluxation refer to the displacement of bones that form a joint. These conditions affecting the joint most often result from trauma that causes adjoining bones to no longer align with each other. A partial or incomplete dislocation is called a subluxation.

Description

In a healthy joint, the bones are normally held together with tough, fibrous bands called ligaments. These ligaments are attached to each bone along with a fibrous sac surrounding the joint called the articular capsule or joint capsule. The ligaments and joint capsule are relatively strong and nonelastic but permit movement within normal limits for each particular joint. In

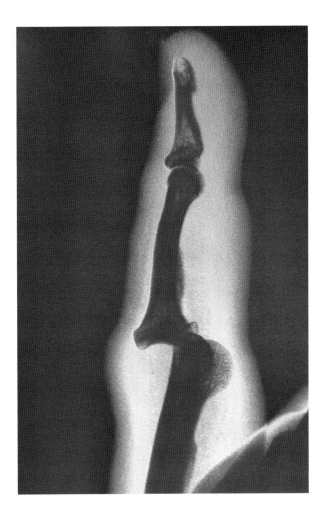

This x ray shows the dislocation between two bones in a finger. *(Photo Researchers, Inc.)*

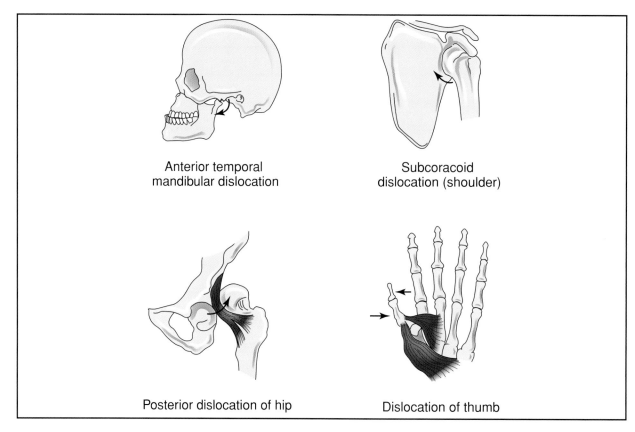

Anterior temporal
mandibular dislocation

Subcoracoid
dislocation (shoulder)

Posterior dislocation of hip

Dislocation of thumb

Dislocations and subluxations refer to the displacement of bones that form a joint. Such conditions most often result from trauma causing adjoining bones to no longer touch each other. A partial or incomplete dislocation is called a subluxation. The illustrations above indicate dislocation of the jaw bone, shoulder blade, hip bone, and the thumb. *(Illustration by Electronic Illustrators Group. Reproduced by permission of Gale, a part of Cengage Learning.)*

the event of a dislocation, one of the bones making up the joint is forced out of its natural alignment from excessive stretching and tearing of the joint ligaments and capsule. Muscles and tendons surrounding the joint are usually stretched and injured to some degree.

Causes and symptoms

A violent movement at the joint that exceeds normal limits usually causes a joint dislocation. Although dislocations often result from trauma, they sometimes occur as a result of disease affecting the joint structures. In the process of the dislocation, there is tearing of the ligaments and the articular capsule, which are vital structures for connecting the bone. Following a dislocation, the bones affected are often immobile and the affected limb may be locked in an abnormal position; **fractures** are also a concern with severe dislocations.

Important factors in recognizing a dislocation or subluxation include a history of experiencing a fall or receiving a blow in a particular joint followed by the sudden onset of loss of function to the involved limb. Immediately after the dislocation, the joint almost always swells significantly and feels painful when pressure is applied (point tenderness). If trauma to the joint causing the dislocation or subluxation is violent in nature, small chips of bone can be torn away with the supporting structures. Chronic recurrent dislocations may take place without severe **pain** because of the somewhat slack condition of the surrounding muscles and other supporting tissues. A first-time dislocation is considered and treated as a possible fracture. Risk factors that can increase susceptibility of joint dislocation and subluxation are shallow or abnormally formed joint surfaces present at birth (congenital) and/or other diseases of ligaments and tissue around a joint. Some infants are born with a hip dislocation. Both sexes and all ages are affected.

Diagnosis

A thorough medical history and physical exam by a physician is the first step in the correct diagnosis of dislocations and subluxations. X rays of the joint and adjacent bones can locate and help determine the extent of dislocated joints.

Treatment

Immediately after the dislocation, the application of ice is helpful to control swelling and decrease pain. If the patient needs to be transported, it is important to prevent the joint from moving (**immobilization**). At times, a cast or splint may be used to immobilize the joint and ensure proper alignment and healing. The treatment of realigning bones following a dislocation is called reduction. This may include simple maneuvers that manipulate the joint to reposition the bones or surgical procedures to restore the joint to its normal position. A **general anesthesia** or muscle relaxant may be used to help make joint reduction possible by relaxing surrounding muscles in spasm. **Acetaminophen** or **aspirin** are sometimes used to control moderate pain, and **narcotics** may be prescribed by the physician if the pain is severe. Recurring dislocation may require surgical reconstruction or replacement of the joint. It is not recommended to attempt to reset a dislocated joint outside of a medical environment with experienced medical personnel, because a fracture may be present.

Alternative treatment

Chiropractic care has been shown to be effective for joint subluxation and dislocation, especially in the spine. Swelling can be addressed using botanical therapies. Bromelain, a pineapple enzyme, and turmeric (*Curcuma longa*) are the most potent botanical remedies for this purpose. Acute homeopathic care with *arnica* (*Arnica montana*) can reduce the trauma to the body. Ligament and tendon strengthening can be assisted both botanically and homeopathically.

Prognosis

Joint ligaments have poor blood supply and, therefore, heal slowly. This healing process continues long after the symptoms of the dislocation injury have diminished. Once a joint has been either subluxated or completely dislocated, the connective tissue binding or holding it in correct alignment is stretched to such an extent that the joint becomes extremely vulnerable to repeated dislocations. However, this chance of recurrent dislocation and subluxation will decrease if a proper **rehabilitation** program is implemented to strengthen surrounding muscles of the joint. Most joint dislocations are curable with prompt treatment. After the dislocation has been corrected, the joint may require immobilization with a cast or sling for two to eight weeks.

Prevention

When an individual is involved in strenuous sports or heavy work, involved joints may be protected by elastic bandage wraps, tape wraps, knee and shoulder pads, or special support stockings. Keeping the muscles surrounding the joint strong will also help prevent dislocations. Long-term problems may also be prevented by allowing an adequate amount of time for an injured joint to rest and heal prior to resuming full activity.

Resources

OTHER

"Dislocation." MayoClinic.com. December 30, 2008 (accessed November 22, 2010). http://www.mayoclinic.com/health/dislocation/DS00239.

"Dislocation." MedlinePlus Medical Encyclopedia. November 15, 2010 (accessed November 22, 2010). http://www.nlm.nih.gov/medlineplus/ency/article/000014.htm.

Jeffrey P. Larson, RPT

Disopyramide *see* **Antiarrhythmic drugs**

Disproportionate dwarfism *see* **Achondroplasia**

Dissecting aneurysm *see* **Aortic dissection**

Dissecting hematoma *see* **Aortic dissection**

Disseminated lupus erythematosus *see* **Systemic lupus erythematosus**

Dissociative disorders

Definition

The dissociative disorders are a group of mental disorders that affect consciousness defined as causing significant interference with the patient's general functioning, including social relationships and employment.

Demographics

The dissociative disorders vary in their severity and the suddenness of onset. It is difficult to give statistics for their frequency in the United States because they are a relatively new category and are often misdiagnosed. Criteria for diagnosis require significant impairment in social or vocational functioning.

Description

In order to have a clear picture of these disorders, dissociation should first be understood. Dissociation is a mechanism that allows the mind to separate or compartmentalize certain memories or thoughts from normal consciousness. These split-off mental contents are not erased. They may resurface spontaneously or be triggered by objects or events in the person's environment.

Dissociation is a process that occurs along a spectrum of severity. It does not necessarily mean that a person has a dissociative disorder or other mental illness. A mild degree of dissociation occurs with some physical stressors; people who have gone without sleep for a long period of time, have had "laughing gas" for dental surgery, or have been in a minor accident often have brief dissociative experiences. Another example of dissociation is a person becoming involved in a book or movie so completely that the surroundings or the passage of time are not noticed. Another example might be driving on the highway and taking several exits without noticing or remembering. Dissociation is related to hypnosis in that hypnotic trance also involves a temporarily altered state of consciousness. Most patients with dissociative disorders are highly hypnotizable.

People in other cultures sometimes have dissociative experiences in the course of religious (in certain trance states) or other group activities. These occurrences should not be judged in terms of what is considered "normal" in the United States.

Moderate or severe forms of dissociation are caused by such traumatic experiences as childhood **abuse**, combat, criminal attacks, brainwashing in hostage situations, or involvement in a natural or transportation disaster. Patients with **acute stress disorder**, **post-traumatic stress disorder** (PTSD), or conversion disorder and somatization disorder may develop dissociative symptoms. Recent studies of trauma indicate that the human brain stores traumatic memories in a different way than normal memories. Traumatic memories are not processed or integrated into a person's ongoing life in the same fashion as normal memories. Instead, they are dissociated, or split off, and may erupt into consciousness from time to time without warning. The affected person cannot control or "edit" these memories. Over a period of time, these two sets of memories, the normal and the traumatic, may coexist as parallel sets without being combined or blended. In extreme cases, different sets of dissociated memories may alter subpersonalities of patients with dissociative identity disorder (**multiple personality disorder**).

Dissociative amnesia

Dissociative **amnesia** is a disorder in which the distinctive feature is the patient's inability to remember important personal information to a degree that cannot be explained by normal forgetfulness. In many cases, it is a reaction to a traumatic accident or witnessing a violent crime. Patients with dissociative amnesia may develop depersonalization or trance states as part of the disorder, but they do not experience a change in identity.

Dissociative fugue

Dissociative fugue is a disorder in which a person temporarily loses his or her sense of personal identity and travels to another location where he or she may assume a new identity. Again, this condition usually follows a major stressor or trauma. Apart from inability to recall their past or personal information, patients with dissociative fugue do not behave strangely or appear disturbed to others. Cases of dissociative fugue are more common in wartime or in communities disrupted by a natural disaster.

Depersonalization disorder

Depersonalization disorder is a disturbance in which the patient's primary symptom is a sense of detachment from the self. Depersonalization as a symptom (not as a disorder) is quite common in college-age populations. It is often associated with **sleep deprivation** or recreational drug use. It may be accompanied by derealization (where objects in an environment appear altered). Patients sometimes describe depersonalization as feeling like a robot or watching themselves from the outside. Depersonalization disorder may also involve feelings of **numbness** or loss of emotional "aliveness."

Dissociative identity disorder (DID)

Dissociative identity disorder (DID) is the newer name for multiple personality disorder (MPD). DID is considered the most severe dissociative disorder and involves all of the major dissociative symptoms.

Dissociative disorder not otherwise specified (DDNOS)

DDNOS is a diagnostic category ascribed to patients with dissociative symptoms that do not meet the full criteria for a specific dissociative disorder.

Causes and symptoms

The moderate to severe dissociation that occurs in patients with dissociative disorders is understood to result from a set of causes:

- an innate ability to dissociate easily
- repeated episodes of severe physical or sexual abuse in childhood
- lack of a supportive or comforting person to counteract abusive relative(s)
- the influence of other relatives with dissociative symptoms or disorders

The relationship of dissociative disorders to childhood abuse has led to intense controversy and lawsuits concerning the accuracy of childhood memories. The brain's storage, retrieval, and interpretation of memories are still not fully understood. Controversy also exists regarding how much individuals presenting dissociative disorders have been influenced by books and movies to describe a certain set of symptoms (scripting).

Amnesia

Amnesia in a dissociative disorder is marked by gaps in a patient's memory for long periods of time or for traumatic events. Doctors can distinguish this type of amnesia from loss of memory caused by head injuries or drug intoxication, because the amnesia is "spotty" and related to highly charged events and feelings.

Depersonalization

Depersonalization is a dissociative symptom in which the patient feels that his or her body is unreal, is changing, or is dissolving. Some patients experience depersonalization as being outside their bodies or watching a movie of themselves.

Derealization

Derealization is a dissociative symptom in which the external environment is perceived as unreal. The patient may see walls, buildings, or other objects as changing in shape, size, or color. In some cases, the patient may feel that other persons are machines or robots, though the patient is able to acknowledge the unreality of this feeling.

Identity disturbances

Patients with dissociative fugue, DDNOS, or DID often experience confusion about their identities or even assume new identities. Identity disturbances result from the patient having split off entire personality traits or characteristics as well as memories. When a stressful or traumatic experience triggers the reemergence of these dissociated parts, the patient may act differently, answer to a different name, or appear confused by his or her surroundings.

Diagnosis

Examination

When a doctor is evaluating a patient with dissociative symptoms, he or she will first rule out physical conditions that sometimes produce amnesia, depersonalization, or derealization. These physical conditions include **epilepsy**, head injuries, brain disease, side effects of medications, **substance abuse**, intoxication, **AIDS**, **dementia** complex, or recent periods of extreme physical **stress** and sleeplessness. In some cases, the doctor may give the patient an electroencephalogram (EEG) to exclude epilepsy or other seizure disorders.

Tests

If the patient appears to be physically normal, the doctor will rule out psychotic disturbances, including **schizophrenia**. In addition, doctors can use some **psychological tests** to narrow the diagnosis. One is a screener, the Dissociative Experiences Scale (DES). If the patient has a high score on this test, he or she can be evaluated further with the Dissociative Disorders Interview Schedule (DDIS) or the Structured Clinical Interview for *DSM-IV* Dissociative Disorders (SCID-D). It is also possible for doctors to measure a patient's hypnotizability as part of a diagnostic evaluation.

Treatment

Treatment of the dissociative disorders often combines several methods.

Drugs

Some doctors prescribe tranquilizers or antidepressants for the **anxiety** and/or depression that often accompany dissociative disorders. Patients with dissociative disorders are at risk for abusing or becoming dependent on medications.

Alternative

Patients with dissociative disorders often require treatment by a therapist with some specialized

KEY TERMS

Amnesia—A general medical term for loss of memory that is not due to ordinary forgetfulness. Amnesia can be caused by head injuries, brain disease, or epilepsy, as well as by dissociation.

Depersonalization—A dissociative symptom in which the patient feels that his or her body is unreal, is changing, or is dissolving.

Derealization—A dissociative symptom in which the external environment is perceived as unreal.

Dissociation—A psychological mechanism that allows the mind to split off traumatic memories or disturbing ideas from conscious awareness.

Fugue—A dissociative experience during which a person travels away from home, has amnesia for their past, and may be confused about their identity but otherwise appear normal.

Hypnosis—The means by which a state of extreme relaxation and suggestibility is induced: used to treat amnesia and identity disturbances that occur in dissociative disorders.

Multiple personality disorder (MPD)—An older term for dissociative identity disorder (DID).

Trauma—A disastrous or life-threatening event that can cause severe emotional distress, including dissociative symptoms and disorders.

understanding of dissociation. This background is particularly important if the patient's symptoms include identity problems. Many patients with dissociative disorders are helped by both group and individual treatment.

Hypnosis is frequently recommended as a method of treatment for dissociative disorders, partly because hypnosis is related to the process of dissociation. Hypnosis may help patients recover repressed ideas and memories. Therapists treating patients with DID sometimes use hypnosis in the process of "fusing" the patient's alternate personalities.

Prognosis

Prognoses for dissociative disorders vary. Recovery from dissociative fugue is usually rapid. Dissociative amnesia may resolve quickly, but can become a chronic disorder in some patients. Depersonalization disorder, DDNOS, and DID are usually chronic conditions. DID often requires five or more years of treatment for recovery.

Prevention

Since the primary cause of dissociative disorders is thought to involve extended periods of humanly inflicted trauma, prevention depends on the elimination of **child abuse** and psychological abuse of adult prisoners or hostages.

Resources

BOOKS

Courtois, Christine A., and Julian D. Ford, eds. *Treating Complex Traumatic Stress Disorders: An Evidence-Based Guide.* New York: The Guilford Press, 2009.

Graham, George. *The Disordered Mind: An Introduction to Philosophy of Mind and Mental Illness.* New York: Routledge, 2010.

North, Carol, and Sean Yutzy. *Goodwin and Guze's Psychiatric Diagnosis.* New York: Oxford University Press, 2010.

Shams, K. *Human Relation and Personified Relational Disorders.* Raleigh, NC: lulu.com, 2009.

ORGANIZATIONS

American Psychiatric Association, 1000 Wilson Boulevard, Suite 1825, Arlington, VA, 22209, (703) 907-7300, apa@psych.org, http://www.psych.org.

American Psychological Association (APA) , 750 First St. NE, Washington, DC, 20002-4242, (202) 336-5700, http://www.apa.org.

National Alliance on Mental Illness (NAMI), Colonial Place Three, 2107 Wilson Blvd., Suite 300, Arlington, VA, 22201, (703) 524-7600, (800) 950-NAMI (6264), (703) 524-9094, http://www.nami.org.

National Institute of Mental Health (NIMH), 6001 Executive Boulevard, Room 8184, MSC 9663, Bethesda, MD, 20892, (301) 443-4513, (866) 615-6464, (301) 443-4279, nimhinfo@nih.gov, http://www.nimh.nih.gov.

National Mental Health Association (NMHA), 2000 N. Beauregard Street, 6th Floor, Alexandria, VA, 22311, (703) 684-7722, (800) 969-NMHA, (703) 684-5968, http://www1.nmha.org.

Rebecca J. Frey, Ph.D.
Laura Jean Cataldo, RN, EdD

Dissociative identity disorder *see* **Multiple personality disorder**

Distal pancreatectomy

Definition

A distal **pancreatectomy** is the partial surgical removal of the pancreas, meaning that only the body and tail of the pancreas are removed and the head of the organ is left attached. A total pancreatectomy is the

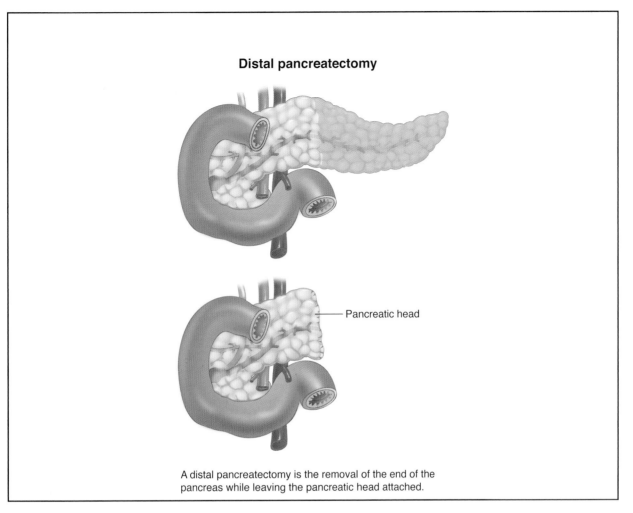

Distal pancreatectomy

Pancreatic head

A distal pancreatectomy is the removal of the end of the
pancreas while leaving the pancreatic head attached.

(Illustration by Electronic Illustrators Group. Reproduced by permission of Gale, a part of Cengage Learning.)

removal of the entire organ, usually along with the
spleen, gallbladder, common bile duct, and portions
of the small intestine and stomach. When the duodenum is removed along with all or part of the pancreas,
the procedure is called a pancreaticoduodenectomy,
which surgeons sometimes refer to as "Whipple's procedure." Pancreaticoduodenectomies are increasingly
used to treat a variety of malignant and benign diseases
of the pancreas. This procedure often involves removal
of the regional lymph nodes as well.

Purpose

A distal pancreatectomy is the most effective treatment for a cancerous tumor of the tail or bottom half of
the pancreas (islet cell tumors), an abdominal organ
that secretes digestive enzymes, insulin, and other hormones. The thickest part of the pancreas near the

duodenum (a part of the small intestine) is called the
head, the middle part is called the body, and the thinnest part adjacent to the spleen is called the tail.

While surgical removal of tumors in the pancreas
is the preferred treatment, it is only possible in the 10–
15% of patients who are diagnosed early enough for a
potential cure. Patients who are considered suitable
for surgery usually have small tumors in the head of
the pancreas (close to the duodenum, or first part of
the small intestine), have **jaundice** as their initial
symptom, and have no evidence of metastatic disease
(spread of **cancer** to other sites). The stage of the
cancer will determine whether the pancreatectomy to
be performed should be total or distal.

A distal pancreatectomy may be indicated when
the pancreas has been severely injured by trauma,
especially injury to the body and tail of the pancreas.

KEY TERMS

Chemotherapy—A cancer treatment that uses synthetic drugs to destroy the tumor either by inhibiting the growth of the cancerous cells or by killing the cancer cells.

Computed tomography (CT) scan—An imaging technique that creates a series of pictures of areas inside the body, taken from different angles. The pictures are created by a computer linked to an x-ray machine.

Endoscopic retrograde cholangiopancreatography (ERCP)—A procedure to x ray the ducts (tubes) that carry bile from the liver to the gallbladder and from the gallbladder to the small intestine.

Laparoscopy—In this procedure, a laparoscope (a thin, lighted tube) is inserted through an incision in the abdominal wall to determine if the cancer is within the pancreas only or has spread to nearby tissues and if it can be removed by surgery later. Tissue samples may be removed for biopsy.

Magnetic resonance imaging (MRI)—A procedure in which a magnet linked to a computer is used to create detailed pictures of areas inside the body.

Pancreas—A large gland located on the back wall of the abdomen, extending from the duodenum (first part of the small intestine) to the spleen. The pancreas produces enzymes essential for digestion, and

the hormones insulin and glucagon, which play a role in diabetes.

Pancreaticoduodenectomy—Removal of all or part of the pancreas along with the duodenum. Also known as "Whipple's procedure" or "Whipple's operation."

Pancreatitis—Inflammation of the pancreas, either acute (sudden and episodic) or chronic, usually caused by excessive alcohol intake or gallbladder disease.

Positron emission tomography (PET) scan—An imaging system that creates a picture showing the location of tumor cells in the body. A substance called radionuclide dye is injected into a vein, and the PET scanner rotates around the body to create the picture. Malignant tumor cells show up brighter in the picture because they are more active and take up more dye than normal cells.

Radiation therapy—A treatment using high energy radiation from x-ray machines, cobalt, radium, or other sources.

Ultrasonogram—A procedure where high-frequency sound waves that cannot be heard by human ears are bounced off internal organs and tissues. These sound waves produce a pattern of echoes which are then used by the computer to create sonograms, or pictures of areas inside the body.

While such surgery removes normal pancreatic tissue as well, the long-term consequences of this surgery are minimal, with virtually no effects on the production of insulin, digestive enzymes, and other hormones.

Description

A distal pancreatectomy can be performed through an open surgery technique, in which case one large incision is made, or it can be performed laparoscopically, in which case the surgeon makes four small incisions to insert tube-like surgical instruments. The abdomen is filled with gas, usually carbon dioxide, to help the surgeon view the abdominal cavity. A camera is inserted through one of the tubes and displays images on a monitor in the operating room. Other instruments are placed through the additional tubes. The laparoscopic approach allows the surgeon to work inside the patient's abdomen without making a large incision.

In a distal pancreatectomy, the surgeon clamps and cuts the blood vessels, and the pancreas is stapled

and divided for removal. If the disease affects the splenic artery or vein, the spleen is also removed.

During the procedure, several tubes are also inserted for postoperative care. To prevent tissue fluid from accumulating in the operated site, a temporary drain leading out of the body is inserted, as well as a **gastrostomy** or g-tube leading out of the stomach in order to help prevent **nausea and vomiting**. A jejunostomy or j-tube may also be inserted into the small intestine as a pathway for supplementary feeding.

Diagnosis/Preparation

Patients with symptoms of a pancreatic disorder undergo a number of tests before surgery is even considered. These can include ultrasonography, x-ray examinations, **computed tomography scans** (CT scan), and **endoscopic retrograde cholangiopancreatography** (ERCP), a specialized imaging technique to visualize the ducts that carry bile from the liver to the gallbladder. Tests may also include **angiography**, another imaging technique used to visualize the arteries feeding the pancreas, and needle aspiration cytology, in which cells are drawn from areas suspected to contain cancer. Such tests are required to establish a correct diagnosis for the pancreatic disorder and in the planning the surgery.

Since many patients with pancreatic cancer are undernourished, appropriate nutritional support, sometimes by **tube feedings**, may be required prior to surgery.

Some patients with pancreatic cancer deemed suitable for a distal pancreatectomy will also undergo **chemotherapy** and/or **radiation therapy**. This treatment is aimed at shrinking the tumor, which will improve the chances for successful surgical removal. Sometimes, patients who are not initially considered surgical candidates may respond so well to chemoradiation that surgical treatment becomes possible. Radiation therapy may also be applied during the surgery (intraoperatively) to improve the patient's chances of survival, but this treatment is not yet in routine use. Some studies have shown that intraoperative radiation therapy extends survival by several months.

Patients undergoing distal pancreatectomy that involves removal of the spleen may receive preoperative medication to decrease the risk of infection.

Aftercare

Extended hospitalization is usually required for an open distal pancreatectomy, with an average hospital stay of one to two weeks. Recovery time is much quicker with laparoscopic distal pancreatectomy.

Some pancreatic cancer patients may also receive combined chemotherapy and radiation therapy after surgery. This additional treatment has been clearly shown to enhance survival rates.

After surgery, patients experience **pain** in the abdomen and are prescribed pain medication. Follow-up exams are required to monitor the patient's recovery and remove implanted tubes.

In some cases of distal pancreatectomies, pancreatic insufficiency may arise. This is a condition caused because food can no longer be normally processed with the enzymes normally produced by the pancreas. Insulin secretion is likewise no longer possible. These conditions are treated with pancreatic enzyme replacement therapy, which supplies digestive enzymes; and with insulin injections. The occurrence of pancreatic insufficiency after distal pancreatectomy is dependent upon the patient's general health condition before surgery and on the extent of pancreatic tissue removal.

Risks

The most common complication is pancreatic fluid leak at the site of the cut.

Normal results

Patients usually resume normal activities within a month after surgery, although they are asked to avoid heavy lifting for six to eight weeks and not to drive as long as they take narcotic medication.

When a distal pancreatectomy is performed for chronic **pancreatitis**, the majority of patients obtain some relief from pain. Some studies report that one-half to three-quarters of patients become free of pain.

Morbidity and mortality rates

The mortality rate for pancreatectomy has decreased in recent years to 5–10%, depending on the extent of the surgery and the experience of the surgeon. A study of 650 patients at Johns Hopkins Medical Institution, Baltimore, found that only nine patients, or 1.4%, died from complications related to surgery.

Unfortunately, pancreatic cancer is the most lethal form of gastrointestinal malignancy. However, for a highly selective group of patients, a pancreatectomy offers a chance for cure, especially when performed by experienced surgeons. The risk for tumor recurrence is increased when the tumor is larger than 1.2 in (3 cm) and the cancer has spread to the lymph nodes or surrounding tissue.

Alternatives

Depending on the medical condition, a **pancreas transplantation** may be considered as an alternative for some patients.

Resources

BOOKS

Beger, Hans-Gunther, et al., eds. *The Pancreas: An Integrated Textbook of Basic Science, Medicine, and Surgery.* Oxford, UK: Blackwell, 2008.

Lowy, Andrew M., et al., eds. *Pancreatic Cancer.* (M.D. Anderson Solid Tumor Oncology Series). New York: Springer, 2008.

O'Reilly, Eileen. *100 Questions & Answers about Pancreatic Cancer.* 2nd ed. Sudbury, MA: Jones and Bartlett, 2010.

OTHER

"Pancreatic Carcinoma." Medline Plus, July 9, 2009. http://www.nlm.nih.gov/medlineplus/ency/article/000236.htm.

ORGANIZATIONS

American College of Gastroenterology, P.O. Box 342260, Bethesda, MD, 20827-2260, (301) 263-9000, http://www.acg.gi.org.

American Gastroenterological Association (AGA), 4930 Del Ray Avenue, Bethesda, MD, 20814, (301) 654-2055, (301) 654-5920, member@gastro.org, http://www.gastro.org.

National Cancer Institute, NCI Public Inquiries Office, 6116 Executive Boulevard, Bethesda, MD, 20892-8322, (800) 422-6237, http://www.cancer.gov.

Caroline A. Helwick
Monique Laberge, PhD
Brenda W. Lerner

Diuretics

Definition

Diuretics are medicines that help reduce the amount of water in the body.

Purpose

Diuretics are used to treat the buildup of excess fluid in the body that occurs with some medical conditions such as congestive **heart failure**, **liver disease**, and **kidney disease**. Some diuretics are also prescribed to treat high blood pressure. These drugs act on the kidneys to increase urine output. This reduces the amount of fluid in the bloodstream, which in turn lowers blood pressure.

Description

There are several types of diuretics, also called water pills:

- Loop diuretics, such as bumetanide (Bumex) and furosemide (Lasix), get their name from the loop-shaped part of the kidneys where they have their effect.
- Thiazide diuretics include such commonly used diuretics as hydrochlorothiazide (HydroDIURIL, Esidrix), chlorothiazide (Diuril), and chlorthalidone (Hygroton).
- Potassium-sparing diuretics prevent the loss of potassium, which is a problem with other types of diuretics. Examples of potassium-sparing diuretics are amiloride (Midamor) and triamterene (Dyrenium).

In addition, some medicines contain combinations of two diuretics. The brands Dyazide and Maxzide, for example, contain the thiazide diuretic hydrochlorothiazide with the potassium-sparing diuretic triamterene.

Some nonprescription (over-the-counter) medicines contain diuretics. However, the medicines described here cannot be bought without a physician's prescription. They are available in tablet, capsule, liquid, and injectable forms.

Recommended dosage

The recommended dosage depends on the type of diuretic and may be different for different patients. Check with the physician who prescribed the drug or the pharmacist who filled the prescription for the correct dosage, and take the medicine exactly as directed.

Precautions

Seeing a physician regularly while taking a diuretic is important. The physician will check to make sure the medicine is working as it should and will watch for unwanted side effects.

Some people feel unusually tired when they first start taking diuretics. This effect usually becomes less noticeable over time, as the body adjusts to the medicine.

Because diuretics increase urine output, people who take this medicine may need to urinate more often, even during the night. Health care professionals can help patients schedule their doses to avoid interfering with their sleep or regular activities.

For patients taking the kinds of diuretics that rob potassium from the body, physicians may recommend adding potassium-rich foods or drinks, such as citrus fruits and juices, to the diet. Or they may suggest taking a potassium supplement or taking another medicine that keeps the body from losing too much potassium. If the physician recommends any of these measures, be sure to closely follow his or her directions. Do not make other diet changes without checking with the physician. People who are taking potassium-sparing diuretics should not add potassium to their **diets**, as too much potassium may be harmful.

People who take diuretics may lose too much water or potassium when they get sick, especially if they have severe **vomiting** and **diarrhea**. They should check with their physicians if they become ill.

These medicines make some people feel light-headed, dizzy, or faint when they get up after sitting or lying down. Older people are especially likely to have this problem. Drinking alcohol, exercising, standing for long periods, or being in hot weather may make the problem worse. To lessen the problem, get up gradually and hold onto something for support if possible. Avoid drinking too much alcohol and be careful in hot weather or when exercising or standing for a long time.

Anyone who is taking a diuretic should be sure to tell the health care professional in charge before having surgical or dental procedures, medical tests, or emergency treatment.

Some diuretics make the skin more sensitive to sunlight. Even brief exposure to sun can cause a severe **sunburn**, **itching**, a rash, redness, or other changes in skin color. While being treated with this medicine, avoid being in direct sunlight, especially between 10 a.m. and 3 p.m.; wear a hat and tightly woven clothing that covers the arms and legs; use a sunscreen with a skin protection factor (SPF) of at least 15; protect the lips with a sun block lipstick; and do not use **tanning** beds, tanning booths, or sunlamps. People with fair skin may need to use a sunscreen with a higher skin protection factor.

Special conditions

People who have certain medical conditions or who are taking certain other medicines may have problems if they take diuretics. Before taking these drugs, be sure to let the physician know about any of these conditions:

ALLERGIES. Anyone who has had unusual reactions to diuretics or **sulfonamides** (sulfa drugs) in the past should let his or her physician know before using a diuretic. The physician should also be told about any **allergies** to foods, dyes, preservatives, or other substances.

PREGNANCY. Diuretics will not help the swelling of hands and feet that some women have during **pregnancy**. In general, pregnant women should not use diuretics unless a physician recommends their use. Although studies have not been done on pregnant women, studies of laboratory animals show that some diuretics can cause harmful effects when taken during pregnancy.

BREASTFEEDING. Some diuretics pass into breast milk, but no reports exist of problems in nursing babies whose mothers use this medicine. However, thiazide diuretics may decrease the flow of breast milk. Women who are **breastfeeding** and need to use a diuretic should check with their physicians.

OTHER MEDICAL CONDITIONS. Side effects of some diuretics may be more likely in people who have had a recent **heart attack** or who have liver disease or severe kidney disease. Other diuretics may not work properly in people with liver disease or severe kidney disease. Diuretics may worsen certain medical conditions, such as **gout**, **kidney stones**, **pancreatitis**, lupus erythematosus,

and hearing problems. In addition, people with diabetes should be aware that diuretics may increase blood sugar levels. People with heart or blood vessel disease should know that some diuretics increase cholesterol or triglyceride levels. The risk of an allergic reaction to certain diuretics is greater in people with bronchial **asthma**. Before using diuretics, people with any of these medical problems should make sure their physicians are aware of their conditions. Also, people who have trouble urinating or who have high potassium levels in their blood may not be able to take diuretics and should check with a physician before using them.

USE OF CERTAIN MEDICINES. Taking diuretics with certain other drugs may affect the way the drugs work or may increase the chance of side effects.

Side effects

Some side effects, such as loss of appetite, **nausea and vomiting**, stomach cramps, diarrhea, and **dizziness**, usually lessen or go away as the body adjusts to the medicine. These problems do not need medical attention unless they continue or interfere with normal activities.

Patients taking potassium-sparing diuretics should know the signs of too much potassium and should check with a physician as soon as possible if any of these symptoms occur:

- irregular heartbeat
- breathing problems
- numbness or tingling in the hands, feet, or lips
- confusion or nervousness
- unusual tiredness or weakness
- weak or heavy feeling in the legs

Patients taking diuretics that cause potassium loss should know the signs of too little potassium and should check with a physician as soon as possible if they have any of these symptoms:

- fast or irregular heartbeat
- weak pulse
- nausea or vomiting
- dry mouth
- excessive thirst
- muscle cramps or pain
- unusual tiredness or weakness
- mental or mood changes

Interactions

Diuretics may interact with other medicines. When this happens, the effects of one or both of the drugs may change or the risk of side effects may be

KEY TERMS

Inflammation—Pain, redness, swelling, and heat that usually develop in response to injury or illness.

Lupus erythematosus—A chronic disease that affects the skin, joints, and certain internal organs.

Pancreas—A gland located beneath the stomach. The pancreas produces juices that help break down food.

Potassium—A mineral found in whole grains, meat, legumes, and some fruits and vegetables. Potassium is important for many body processes, including proper functioning of the nerves and muscles.

Triglyceride—A substance formed in the body from fat in the diet. Triglycerides are the main fatty materials in the blood. Together with protein, they make up high- and low-density lipoproteins (HDLs and LDLs). Triglyceride levels are important in the diagnosis and treatment of many diseases including high blood pressure, diabetes, and heart disease.

---

greater. Anyone who takes a diuretic should let the physician know all other medicines he or she is taking and should ask whether the possible interactions can interfere with drug therapy. Among the drugs that may interact with diuretics are:

• Angiotensin-converting enzyme (ACE) inhibitors, such as benazepril (Lotensin), captopril (Capoten), and enalapril (Vasotec), used to treat high blood pressure. Taking these drugs with potassium-sparing diuretics may cause levels of potassium in the blood to be too high, increasing the chance of side effects.

• Cholesterol-lowering drugs such as cholestyramine (Questran) and colestipol (Colestid). Taking these drugs with combination diuretics such as Dyazide and Maxzide may keep the diuretic from working. Take the diuretic at least one hour before or four hours after the cholesterol-lowering drug.

• Cyclosporine (Sandimmune), a medicine that suppresses the immune system. Taking this medicine with potassium-sparing diuretics may increase the chance of side effects by causing levels of potassium in the blood to be too high.

• Potassium supplements, other medicines containing potassium, or salt substitutes that contain potassium. Taking these with potassium-sparing diuretics may lead to too much potassium in the blood, increasing the chance of side effects.

• Lithium, used to treat bipolar disorder (manic-depressive illness). Using this medicine with potassium-sparing diuretics may allow lithium to build up to poisonous levels in the body.

• Digitalis heart drugs, such as digoxin (Lanoxin). Using this medicine with combination diuretics such as triamterene-hydrocholorthiazide (Dyazide, Maxzide) may cause blood levels of the heart medicine to be too high, making side effects such as changes in heartbeat more likely.

The list above does not include every drug that may interact with diuretics. Check with a physician or pharmacist before combining diuretics with any other prescription or nonprescription (over-the-counter) medicine.

Nancy Ross-Flanigan

Diverticulitis *see* **Diverticulosis and diverticulitis**

Diverticulosis and diverticulitis

Definition

Diverticulosis refers to a condition in which the inner, lining layer of the large intestine (colon) bulges out (herniates) through the outer, muscular layer. These outpouchings are called diverticula. Diverticulitis refers to the development of inflammation and infection in one or more diverticula.

Description

Diverticula tend to occur most frequently in the last segment of the large intestine, the sigmoid colon. They occur with decreasing frequency as one examines further back toward the beginning of the large intestine. The chance of developing diverticula increases with age, so that by the age of 50, about 20–50% of all people will have some diverticula. By the age of 90, virtually everyone will have developed some diverticula. Most diverticula measure about 3 mm to just over 3 cm in diameter. Larger diverticula, termed giant diverticula, are quite infrequent, but may measure as large as 15 cm in diameter.

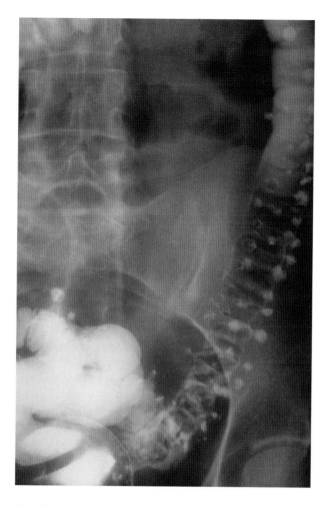

A barium study x ray showing colonic diverticulosis. *(Custom Medical Stock Photo, Inc. Reproduced by permission.)*

Causes and symptoms

Diverticula are believed to be caused by overly forceful contractions of the muscular wall of the large intestine. As areas of this wall spasm, they become weaker and weaker, allowing the inner lining to bulge through. The anatomically weakest areas of the intestinal wall occur next to blood vessels which course through the wall, so diverticula commonly occur in this location.

Diverticula are most common in the developed countries of the West (North America, Great Britain, northern and western Europe). This is thought to be due to the diet of these countries, which tends to be quite low in fiber. A diet low in fiber results in the production of smaller volumes of stool. In order to move this smaller stool along the colon and out of the rectum, the colon must narrow itself significantly, and does so by contracting down forcefully. This causes an increase in pressure, which, over time, weakens the

muscular wall of the intestine and allows diverticular pockets to develop.

The origin of giant diverticula development is not completely understood, although one theory involves gas repeatedly entering and becoming trapped in an already-existing diverticulum, causing stretching and expansion of that diverticulum.

The great majority of people with diverticulosis will remain symptom-free. Many diverticula are quite accidentally discovered during examinations for other conditions of the intestinal tract.

Some people with diverticulosis have symptoms such as **constipation**, cramping, and bloating. It is unclear whether these symptoms are actually caused by the diverticula themselves, or whether some other gastro-intestinal condition (such as **irritable bowel syndrome**) might be responsible. A complication of diverticulosis occurs because many diverticula develop in areas very near blood vessels. Therefore, one serious risk of diverticulosis involves bleeding. Although an infrequent complication, the bleeding can be quite severe. Seventy-five percent of such bleeding episodes occur due to diverticula located on the right side of the colon. About 50% of the time, such bleeding will stop on its own.

One of the most common and potentially serious complications of diverticulosis is inflammation and infection of a particular diverticulum, called diverticulitis.

Diverticulitis is three times more likely to occur in the left side of the large intestine. Since most diverticula are located in the sigmoid colon (the final segment of the large intestine which empties into the rectum), most diverticulitis also takes place in the sigmoid. The elderly have the most serious complications from diverticulitis, although very severe infections can also occur in patients under the age of 50. Men are three times as likely as women to be stricken with diverticulitis.

Diverticulitis is believed to occur when a hardened piece of stool, undigested food, and bacteria (called a fecalith) becomes lodged in a diverticulum. This blockage interferes with the blood supply to the area, and infection sets in.

An individual with diverticulitis will experience **pain** (especially in the lower left side of the abdomen) and **fever**. In response to the infection and the irritation of nearby tissues within the abdomen, the abdominal muscles may begin to spasm. About 25% of all patients with diverticulitis will have some rectal bleeding, although this rarely becomes severe. Walled-off pockets of infection, called abscesses, may appear within the wall of the intestine, or even on the exterior surface of

Diverticulosis and diverticulitis

the intestine. When a diverticulum weakens sufficiently, and is filled to bulging with infected pus, a perforation in the intestinal wall may develop. When the infected contents of the intestine spill out into the abdomen, the severe infection called **peritonitis** may occur. Peritonitis is an infection and inflammation of the lining of the abdominal cavity, the peritoneum. Other complications of diverticulitis include the formation of abnormal connections between two organs that normally do not connect (fistulas; for example, the intestine and the bladder), and scarring outside of the intestine which squeezes off a portion of the intestine, obstructing it.

Diagnosis

As mentioned, the majority of diverticula do not cause any symptoms, and are often found by coincidence during an examination being performed for some other medical condition.

When diverticula are suspected because a patient begins to have sudden rectal bleeding, the location of the bleeding can be studied by performing an **angiography**. Angiography involves inserting a tiny tube through an artery in the leg, and moving it up into one of the major arteries of the gastrointestinal system. A particular chemical (contrast medium) which will show up on x-ray films is injected, and the area of bleeding is located by looking for an area where the contrast is leaking into the interior (lumen) of the intestine.

A procedure called **endoscopy** provides another method for examining the colon and locating the site of bleeding. In endoscopy, a small, flexible scope (endoscope) is inserted through the rectum and into the intestine. The scope usually bears a fiber-optic camera, which allows the view through this endoscope to be projected onto a television screen. The operator can introduce the endoscope further and further through the intestine to find the location of the bleeding.

Diagnosis of diverticulitis is not difficult in patients with previously diagnosed diverticulosis. The presence of abdominal pain and fever in such an individual would make the suspicion of diverticulitis quite high. Examination of the abdomen will usually reveal tenderness to touch, with the patient's abdominal muscles contracting strongly to protect the tender area. During a rectal exam (performed by inserting a finger into the rectum), a doctor may be able to feel an abnormal mass. Touching this mass may prove painful to the patient.

When a practitioner is suspicious of diverticulitis as the cause for the patient's symptoms, he or she will most likely avoid the types of tests usually used to diagnose gastrointestinal disorders. These include **barium enema** and endoscopy. The concern is that the increased pressure exerted on the intestine during these exams may increase the likelihood of intestinal perforation. After medical treatment for the diverticulitis, these examinations may be performed in order to learn the extent of the patient's disease.

Treatment

Only about 20% of patients with diverticulosis ever have symptoms which lead them to seek medical help. Most people never know that they have diverticula. For those individuals who have cramping pain and constipation believed to be due to diverticulosis, the usual prescription involves increasing the fiber in the diet. This can be done by adding special diet supplements of bran or psyllium seed, which increase stool volume. Bleeding diverticula can usually be treated by bed rest, with blood **transfusion** needed for more severe bleeding (hemorrhaging). In cases of very heavy hemorrhaging, medications which encourage clotting can be injected during the course of a diagnostic angiography.

While there are almost no situations when uncomplicated diverticulosis requires surgery, giant diverticula always require removal. This is due to the very high chance of infection and perforation of these diverticula. When giant diverticula are diagnosed, the usual treatment involves removing that portion of the intestine.

Treatment for uncomplicated diverticulitis usually requires hospitalization. "Resting the bowel" is a mainstay of treatment, and involves keeping the patient from eating or sometimes even drinking anything by mouth. Therefore, the patient will need to receive fluids through a needle in the vein (intravenous or IV fluids). **Antibiotics** will also be administered through the IV. Some physicians will agree to try treatment at home for very mildly ill patients. These patients will be put on a liquid diet and receive oral antibiotics.

The various complications of diverticulitis need to be treated aggressively, because the **death** rate from such things as perforation and peritonitis is quite high. Abscesses can be drained of their infected contents by inserting a needle through the skin of the abdomen and into the **abscess**. When this is unsuccessful, open abdominal surgery will be required to remove the piece of the intestine containing the abscess. Fistulas require surgical repair, including the removal of the length of intestine containing the origin of the **fistula**, followed by immediate reconnection of the two free ends of intestine. Peritonitis requires open surgery. The entire abdominal cavity is cleaned by being irrigated (washed) with a warmed sterile saltwater

KEY TERMS

Angiography—An x-ray study of the arteries in a particular part of the body. Angiography is often performed in order to localize internal bleeding.

Bowel obstruction—A blockage in the intestine which prevents the normal flow of waste down the length of the intestine.

Colostomy—A procedure performed when a large quantity of intestine is removed. The end piece of the intestine leading to the rectum is closed.

Diverticula—Outpouchings in the large intestine caused when the inner, lining layer of the large

intestine (colon) bulges out (herniates) through the outer, muscular layer.

Endoscopy—Examination of an area of the gastrointestinal tract by putting a lighted scope, usually bearing a fiber-optic camera, into the rectum, and passing it through the intestine.

Fistula—An abnormal connection formed between two organs that usually have no connection whatsoever.

Sigmoid colon—The final portion of the large intestine that empties into the rectum.

---

solution, and the damaged piece of intestine is removed. Obstructions require immediate surgery to prevent perforation. Massive, uncontrollable bleeding, while rare, may require removal of part or all of the large intestine.

During any of these types of operations, the surgeon must make an important decision regarding the quantity of intestine which must be removed. When the amount of intestine removed is great, it may be necessary to perform a **colostomy**. A colostomy involves pulling the end of the remaining intestine through the abdominal wall, to the outside. This bit of intestine is then fashioned so that a bag can be fit over it. The patient's waste (feces) collect in the bag, because the intestine no longer connects with the rectum. This colostomy may be temporary, in which case another operation will be required to reconnect the intestine, after some months of substantial healing has occurred. Other times, the colostomy will need to be permanent, and the patient will have to adjust to living permanently with the colostomy bag. Most people with colostomies are able to go on with a very active life.

Occasionally, a patient will have such severe diverticular disease that a surgeon recommends planning ahead, and schedules removal of a portion of the colon. This is done to avoid the high risk of surgery performed after a complication has set in. Certain developments in a patient will identify those patients who are at very high risk of experiencing dangerous complications. Such elective surgery may be recommended:

- when an older individual has had several attacks of diverticulitis
- when someone under the age of 50 has had even one attack

- when treatment does not get rid of a painful mass
- when the intestine appears to be narrowing on x-ray examination (this could suggest the presence of cancer)
- when certain patients begin to regularly experience painful urination or urinary infections (this suggests that there may be a connection between the intestine and the bladder)
- when there is any question of cancer
- when the diverticular disease appears to be progressing rapidly

Prognosis

The prognosis for people with diverticula is excellent, with only 20% of such patients ever seeking any medical help for their condition.

While diverticulitis can be a difficult and painful disease, it is usually quite treatable. Prognosis is worse for individuals who have other medical problems, particularly those requiring the use of steroid medications, which increase the chances of developing a serious infection. Prognosis is also worse in the elderly.

Prevention

While there is no absolutely certain way to prevent the development of diverticula, it is believed that high-fiber **diets** are of help. Foods that are recommended for their high fiber content include whole grain breads and cereals, and all types of fruits and vegetables. Most experts suggest that individuals take in about 0.71–1.23 oz (20–35 g) of fiber daily. If this is not possible to achieve through a person's diet, there are fiber products which can be mixed into 8 oz (237 mL) of water or juice, and which provide about 0.13–19 oz (4–6 g) of fiber.

ORGANIZATIONS

National Digestive Diseases Information Clearinghouse (NDDIC), 2 Information Way, Bethesda, MD, 20892-3570, (703) 738-4929, (800) 891-5389, http://digestive.niddk.nih.gov.

Rosalyn Carson-DeWitt, MD

Dizziness

Definition

As a disorder, dizziness is classified into three categories—vertigo, syncope, and nonsyncope nonvertigo. Each category has a characteristic set of symptoms, all related to the sense of balance. In general, syncope is defined by a brief loss of consciousness (**fainting**) or by dimmed vision and feeling uncoordinated, confused, and lightheaded. Many people experience a sensation like syncope when they stand up too fast. Vertigo is the feeling that either the individual or the surroundings are spinning. This sensation is like being on a spinning amusement park ride. Individuals with nonsyncope nonvertigo dizziness feel as though they cannot keep their balance. This feeling may become worse with movement.

Description

The brain coordinates information from the eyes, the inner ear, and the body's senses to maintain balance. If any of these information sources is disrupted, the brain may not be able to compensate. For example, people sometimes experience **motion sickness** because the information from their body tells the brain that they are sitting still, but information from the eyes indicates that they are moving. The messages do not correspond and dizziness results.

Vision and the body's senses are the most important systems for maintaining balance, but problems in the inner ear are the most frequent cause of dizziness. The inner ear, also called the vestibular system, contains fluid that helps fine tune the information the brain receives from the eyes and the body. When fluid volume or pressure in one inner ear changes, information about balance is altered. The discrepancy gives conflicting messages to the brain about balance and induces dizziness.

Certain medical conditions can cause dizziness, because they affect the systems that maintain balance. For example, the inner ear is very sensitive to changes in blood flow. Because medical conditions such as high blood pressure or low blood sugar can affect blood flow, these conditions are frequently accompanied by dizziness. Circulation disorders are the most common causes of dizziness. Other causes are **head injury**, ear infection, **allergies**, and nervous system disorders.

Dizziness often disappears without treatment or with treatment of the underlying problem, but it can be long term or chronic. According to the National Institutes of Health, 42% of Americans will seek medical help for dizziness at some point in their lives. The costs may exceed a billion dollars and account for five million doctor visits annually. Episodes of dizziness increase with age. Among people aged 75 or older, dizziness is the most frequent reason for seeing a doctor.

Causes and symptoms

Careful attention to symptoms can help determine the underlying cause of the dizziness. Underlying problems may be benign and easily treated or they may be dangerous and in need of intensive therapy. Not all cases of dizziness can be linked to a specific cause. More than one type of dizziness can be experienced at the same time and symptoms may be mixed. Episodes of dizziness may last for a few seconds or for days. The length of an episode is related to the underlying cause.

The symptoms of syncope include dimmed vision, loss of coordination, confusion, lightheadedness, and sweating. These symptoms can lead to a brief loss of consciousness or fainting. They are related to a reduced flow of blood to the brain; they often occur when a person is standing up and can be relieved by sitting or lying down. Vertigo is characterized by a sensation of spinning or turning, accompanied by **nausea**, **vomiting**, ringing in the ears, **headache**, or **fatigue**. An individual may have trouble walking, remaining coordinated, or keeping balance. Nonsyncope nonvertigo dizziness is characterized by a feeling of being off balance that becomes worse if the individual tries moving or performing detail-intense tasks.

A person may experience dizziness for many reasons. Syncope is associated with low blood pressure, heart problems, and disorders in the autonomic nervous system, the system of involuntary functions such as breathing. Syncope may also arise from emotional distress, **pain**, and other reactions to outside stressors. Nonsyncope nonvertigo dizziness may be caused by rapid breathing, low blood sugar, or **migraine headache**, as well as by more serious medical conditions.

Vertigo is often associated with inner ear problems called vestibular disorders. A particularly intense vestibular disorder, Ménière's disease, interferes with the volume of fluid in the inner ear. This disease, which affects approximately one in every 1,000 people, causes intermittent vertigo over the course of weeks, months, or years. Ménière's disease is often accompanied by ringing or buzzing in the ear, **hearing loss**, and a feeling that the ear is blocked. Damage to the nerve that leads from the ear to the brain can also cause vertigo. Such damage can result from head injury or a tumor. An **acoustic neuroma**, for example, is a benign tumor that wraps around the nerve. Vertigo can also be caused by disorders of the central nervous system and the cirulatory system, such as hardening of the arteries (arteriosclerosis), **stroke**, or **multiple sclerosis**.

Some medications cause changes in blood pressure or blood flow. These medications can cause dizziness in some people. Prescription medications carry warnings of such side effects, but common drugs, such as **caffeine** or nicotine, can also cause dizziness. Certain **antibiotics** can damage the inner ear and cause hearing loss and dizziness.

Diet may cause dizziness. The role of diet may be direct, as through alcohol intake. It may be also be indirect, as through arteriosclerosis caused by a high-fat diet. Some people experience a slight dip in blood sugar and mild dizziness if they miss a meal, but this condition is rarely dangerous unless the person is diabetic. Food sensitivities or allergies can also be a cause of dizziness. Chronic conditions, such as heart disease, and serious acute problems, such as seizures and strokes, can cause dizziness. However, such conditions usually exhibit other characteristic symptoms.

Diagnosis

During the initial medical examination, an individual with dizziness should provide a detailed description of the type of dizziness experienced, when it occurs, and how often each episode lasts. A diary of symptoms may help track this information. Report any symptoms that accompany the dizziness, such as a ringing in the ear or nausea, any recent injury or infection, and any medication taken.

Blood pressure, pulse, respiration, and body temperature are checked, and the ear, nose, and throat are scrutinized. The sense of balance is assessed by moving the individual's head to various positions or by tilt-table testing. In tilt-table testing, the person lies on a table that can be shifted into different positions and reports any dizziness that occurs.

Further tests may be indicated by the initial examination. Hearing tests help assess ear damage. X rays, computed tomography scan (CT scan), and **magnetic resonance imaging** (MRI) can pinpoint evidence of nerve damage, tumor, or other structural problems. If a vestibular disorder is suspected, a technique called electronystagmography (ENG) may be used. ENG measures the electrical impulses generated by eye movements. Blood tests can determine diabetes, high cholesterol, and other diseases. In some cases, a heart evaluation may be useful. Despite thorough testing, an underlying cause cannot always be determined.

Treatment

Treatment is determined by the underlying cause. If an individual has a cold or **influenza**, a few days of bed rest is usually adequate to resolve dizziness. Other causes of dizziness, such as mild vestibular system damage, may resolve without medical treatment.

If dizziness continues, drug therapy may prove helpful. Because circulatory problems often cause dizziness, medication may be prescribed to control blood pressure or to treat arteriosclerosis. Sedatives may be useful to relieve the tension that can trigger or aggravate dizziness. Low blood sugar associated with diabetes sometimes causes dizziness and is treated by controlling blood sugar levels. An individual may be asked to avoid caffeine, nicotine, alcohol, and any substances that cause allergic reactions. A low-salt diet may also help some people.

When other measures have failed, surgery may be suggested to relieve pressure on the inner ear. If the dizziness is not treatable by drugs, surgery, or other means, **physical therapy** may be used and the patient may be taught coping mechanisms for the problem.

Alternative treatment

Because dizziness may arise from serious conditions, it is advisable to seek medical treatment. Alternative treatments can often be used alongside conventional medicine without conflict. Relaxation techniques, such as **yoga** and **massage therapy** that focus on relieving tension, are popularly recommended methods for reducing **stress**. Aromatherapists recommend a warm bath scented with essential oils of lavender, geranium, and sandalwood.

Homeopathic therapies can work very effectively for dizziness, and are especially applicable when no organic cause can be identified. An osteopath or

KEY TERMS

Acoustic neuroma—A benign tumor that grows on the nerve leading from the inner ear to the brain. As the tumor grows, it exerts pressure on the inner ear and causes severe vertigo.

Arteriosclerosis—Hardening of the arteries caused by high blood cholesterol and high blood pressure.

Autonomic nervous system—The part of the nervous system that controls involuntary functions such as breathing and heart beat.

Computed tomography (CT)—An imaging technique in which cross-sectional x rays of the body are compiled to create a three-dimensional image of the body's internal structures.

Electronystagmography—A method for measuring the electricity generated by eye movements. Electrodes are placed on the skin around the eye and the individual is subjected to a variety of stimuli so that the quality of eye movements can be assessed.

Magnetic resonance imaging (MRI)—An imaging technique that uses a large circular magnet and radio waves to generate signals from atoms in the body. These signals are used to construct images of internal structures.

Vestibular system—The area of the inner ear that helps maintain balance.

---

chiropractor may suggest adjustments of the head, jaw, neck, and lower back to relieve pressure on the inner ear. Acupuncturists also offer some treatment options for acute and chronic cases of dizziness. Nutritionists may be able to offer advice and guidance in choosing dietary supplements, identifying foods to avoid, and balancing nutritional needs.

Prognosis

Outcome depends on the cause of dizziness. Controlling or curing the underlying factors usually relieves dizziness. In some cases, dizziness disappears without treatment. In a few cases, dizziness can become a permanent disabling condition and a person's options are limited.

Prevention

Most people learn through experience that certain activities will make them dizzy and they learn to avoid them. For example, if reading in a car produces motion sickness, an individual leaves reading materials for after the trip. Changes to the diet can also cut down on episodes of dizziness in susceptible people. Relaxation techniques can help ward off tension and **anxiety** that can cause dizziness.

These techniques can help minimize or even prevent dizziness for people with chronic diseases. For example, persons with Méniére's disease may avoid episodes of vertigo by leaving salt, alcohol, and caffeine out of their **diets**. Reducing blood cholesterol can help diminish arteriosclerosis and indirectly treat dizziness.

Some cases of dizziness cannot be prevented. Acoustic neuromas, for example, are not predictable or preventable. When the underlying cause of dizziness cannot be discovered, it may be difficult to recommend preventive measures. Alternative approaches designed to rebalance the body's energy flow, such as **acupuncture** and constitutional homeopathy, may be helpful in cases where the cause of dizziness cannot be pinpointed.

ORGANIZATIONS

EAR Foundation of Arizona, 668 North 44th Street, Suite 300, Phoenix, AZ, 85008 , (602) 685-1050, (602) 239-5117, melissa@earfoundationaz.com, http://www.ear-foun dationaz.com.

Vestibular Disorders Association (VEDA), P.O. Box 4467, Portland, OR, 97208-4467, (503) 229-8064, (800) 837-8428, http://www.vestibular.og.

Julia Barrett

DKA *see* **Diabetic ketoacidosis**

DLE *see* **Discoid lupus erythematosus**

Domestic violence *see* **Abuse**

Donovanosis *see* **Granuloma inguinale**

Doppler echocardiography *see* **Echocardiography**

Doppler ultrasonography

Definition

Doppler ultrasonography is a non-invasive diagnostic procedure that changes sound waves into an image that can be viewed on a monitor.

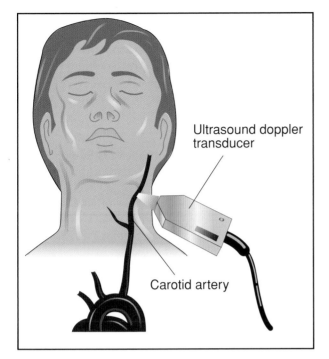

Doppler ultrasonography can detect the direction, velocity, and turbulence of blood flow. Because it is non-invasive and uses no x rays, Doppler ultrasonography is widely used for numerous diagnostic procedures. *(Illustration by Electronic Illustrators Group. Reproduced by permission of Gale, a part of Cengage Learning.)*

Purpose

Doppler ultrasonography can detect the direction, velocity, and turbulence of blood flow. It is frequently used to detect problems with heart valves or to measure blood flow through the arteries. Specifically, it is useful in the work up of **stroke** patients, in assessing blood flow in the abdomen or legs, and in viewing the heart to monitor carotid artery diseases.

Precautions

The test is widely used because it is noninvasive, uses no x rays, and gives excellent images. It is harmless, painless, and widely available.

Description

Doppler ultrasonography makes use of two different principles. The ultrasound principle is this: when a high-frequency sound is produced and aimed at a target, it will be reflected by its target and the reflected sound can be detected back at its origin. In addition, it is known that certain crystals (called piezoelectric crystals) produce an electrical pulse when vibrated by a returning sound.

The Doppler principle is simply that sound pitch increases as the source moves toward the listener and decreases as it moves away.

Medical science utilizes these two principles in the following way. A transducer (sometimes called a probe) containing piezoelectric crystals sends a series of short sound pulses into the body and pauses between each pulse to listen for the returning sounds. The machine then determines the direction and depth of each returning sound and coverts this into a point of light on a television monitor. Thousands of these pulses are computed and displayed every second to produce an image of the organ being studied. The image allows the doctor to see the organ functioning in real time.

The newest addition to this test is the addition of color. Adding color to the image shows the direction and rate of blood flow more clearly.

During a Doppler ultrasonography procedure the technician will apply a gel to the skin, then place the transducer against the skin at various angles. The transducer sends the information it receives to a television monitor that shows a moving image of the organ being studied. The technician can save these images either on video tape, paper, or x-ray film for further study.

Preparation

There is no special preparation needed for this test. The ultrasound technician may apply a clear gel to the skin in order to help the transducer more freely over the body.

Aftercare

No aftercare is necessary.

Normal results

A Doppler ultrasonography test showing no restricted blood flow is a normal finding.

Abnormal results

Disrupted or obstructed blood flow through the neck arteries may indicate the person is a risk of having a stroke. (Narrowed arterial flow in the legs does not necessarily indicate a risk of stroke.)

Resources

BOOKS

Allan, Paul L. P., et al. *Clinical Doppler Ultrasound*, Philadelphia: Churchill Livingstone Elsevier, 2006.

Dorothy Elinor Stonely

Down syndrome

Definition

Down syndrome is the most common chromosome disorder and genetic cause of intellectual disability. It occurs because of the presence of an extra copy of chromosome 21. For this reason, it is also called trisomy 21.

Demographics

As of 2009, the Centers for Disease Control (CDC) estimate that each year about 3,357 babies in the United States are born with Down syndrome. In other words, about 13 of every 10,000 babies born in the United States each year is born with Down syndrome. It affects an equal number of male and female babies. The majority of cases of Down syndrome occur due to an extra chromosome 21 within the egg cell supplied by the mother (nondisjunction).

Down syndrome occurs with equal frequency across all ethnic groups and subpopulations.

Description

Named after John Langdon Down, the first physician to identify the syndrome, Down syndrome is the result of genetic variations. When the reproductive cells, the sperm and ovum, combine at fertilization, the fertilized egg that results contains 23 chromosome pairs. A normal fertilized egg that will develop into a female contains chromosome pairs 1 through 22, and the XX pair. A normal fertilized egg that will develop into a male contains chromosome pairs 1 through 22, and the XY pair. When the fertilized egg contains extra material from chromosome number 21, this results in Down syndrome. This event is called nondisjunction and it occurs in 95% of Down syndrome cases. The baby therefore receives an extra chromosome at conception. Because of this extra chromosome 21, individuals affected with Down syndrome have 47 instead of 46 chromosomes. This additional genetic material disrupts the normal course of development, causing the characteristic features of Down syndrome.

Risk factors

Parents who have already have a baby with Down syndrome or who have abnormalities in their own chromosome 21 are at higher risk for having a baby with Down Syndrome. The chance of having a baby with Down syndrome also increases as a woman gets older. As a woman's age (maternal age) increases, the risk of having a Down syndrome baby increases significantly. By the time the woman is age 35, the risk increases to one in 400; by age 40 the risk increases to one in 110; and, by age 45, the risk becomes one in 35. There is no increased risk of either mosaicism or translocation with increased maternal age.

Causes and symptoms

Down syndrome is a chromosomal disorder caused by an error in cell division that results in the presence of an additional third chromosome 21. In approximately one to two percent of Down syndrome cases, the original egg and sperm cells contain the correct number of chromosomes, 23 each. The problem occurs sometime shortly after fertilization—during the phase when cells are dividing rapidly. One cell divides abnormally, creating a line of cells with an extra copy of chromosome 21. This form of genetic disorder is called mosaicism. The individual with this type of Down syndrome has two types of cells: those with 46 chromosomes (the normal number), and those with 47 chromosomes (as occurs in Down syndrome). Individuals affected with this mosaic form of Down syndrome generally have less severe signs and symptoms of the disorder.

Another relatively rare genetic accident that causes Down syndrome is called translocation. During cell division, chromosome 21 somehow breaks. The broken off piece of this chromosome then becomes attached to another chromosome. Each cell still has 46 chromosomes, but the extra piece of chromosome 21 results in the signs and symptoms of Down syndrome. Translocations occur in about 3–4% of cases of Down syndrome.

While Down syndrome is a chromosomal disorder, a baby is usually identified at birth through observation of a set of common physical characteristics. Not all affected babies will exhibit all of the symptoms discussed. There is a large variability in the number and severity of these characteristics from one affected individual to the next. Babies with Down syndrome tend to be overly quiet, less responsive to stimuli, and have weak, floppy muscles. A number of physical signs may also be present. These include: a flat appearing face; a small head; a flat bridge of the nose; a smaller than normal, low-set nose; small mouth, which causes the tongue to stick out and to appear overly large; upward slanting eyes; bright speckles on the iris of the eye (Brushfield spots); extra folds of skin located at the inside corner of each eye near the nose (epicanthal folds); rounded cheeks; small, misshapen ears; small, wide hands; an unusual deep crease across the center of the palm (simian crease); an inwardly curved little finger; a wide space between the great and the second toes; unusual creases on the soles of the feet; overly flexible joints (sometimes referred to as being double-jointed); and shorter-than-normal stature.

Other types of defects often accompany Down syndrome. Approximately 30–50% of all children with Down syndrome are found to have heart defects. A number of different heart defects are common in Down syndrome. All of these result in abnormal patterns of blood flow within the heart. Abnormal blood flow within the heart often means that less oxygen is sent into circulation throughout the body, which can cause **fatigue**, a lack of energy, and poor muscle tone.

Malformations of the gastrointestinal tract are present in about 5–7% of children with Down syndrome. The most common malformation is a narrowed, obstructed duodenum (the part of the intestine into which the stomach empties). This disorder, called duodenal atresia, interferes with the baby's milk or formula leaving the stomach and entering the intestine for digestion. The baby often vomits forcibly after feeding, and cannot gain weight appropriately until the defect is repaired.

Another malformation of the gastrointestinal tract that is seen in patients with Down syndrome is an abnormal connection between the windpipe (trachea) and the digestive tube of the throat (esophagus) called a tracheo-esophageal **fistula** (T-E fistula). This connection interferes with eating and/or breathing because it allows air to enter the digestive system and/or food to enter the airway.

Other medical conditions occurring in patients with Down syndrome include an increased chance of developing infections, especially ear infections and **pneumonia**; certain kidney disorders; thyroid disease (especially low or hypothyroid); **hearing loss**; vision impairment requiring glasses (corrective lenses); and a 20 times greater chance than the population as a whole of developing leukemia.

Development in a baby and child affected with Down syndrome occurs at a much slower than normal rate. Because of weak, floppy muscles (hypotonia), babies learn to sit up, crawl, and walk much later than their unaffected peers. Talking is also quite delayed. The level of **mental retardation** is considered to be mild-to-moderate in Down syndrome. The degree of mental retardation varies a great deal from one child to the next. While it is impossible to predict the severity of Down syndrome at birth, with proper education, children who have Down syndrome are capable of learning. Most children affected with Down syndrome can read and write and are placed in special education classes in school. The majority of individuals with Down syndrome become semi-independent adults, meaning that they can take care of their own needs with some assistance.

As people with Down syndrome age, they face an increased chance of developing the brain disease called Alzheimer's (sometimes referred to as **dementia** or senility). Most people have a 12% chance of developing Alzheimer's, but almost all people with Down syndrome will have either **Alzheimer's disease** or a similar type of dementia by the age of 50. Alzheimer disease causes the brain to shrink and to break down. The number of brain cells decreases, and abnormal deposits and structural arrangements occur. This process results in a loss of brain functioning. People with Alzheimer's have strikingly faulty memories. Over time, people with Alzheimer's disease will lapse into an increasingly unresponsive state.

As people with Down syndrome age, they also have an increased chance of developing a number of other illnesses, including **cataracts**, thyroid problems, diabetes, and seizure disorders.

Diagnosis

Examination

Diagnosis is usually suspected at birth, when the characteristic physical signs of Down syndrome are observed.

Tests

Once Down syndrome is suspected, **genetic testing** (chromosome analysis) can be undertaken in order to verify the presence of the disorder. This testing is usually done on a blood sample, although chromosome analysis can also be done on other types of tissue, including the skin. The cells to be studied are prepared

KEY TERMS

Chromosome—A microscopic thread-like structure found within each cell of the body and consists of a complex of proteins and DNA. Humans have 46 chromosomes arranged into 23 pairs. Changes in either the total number of chromosomes or their shape and size (structure) may lead to physical or mental abnormalities.

Karyotype—A standard arrangement of photographic or computer-generated images of chromosome pairs from a cell in ascending numerical order, from largest to smallest.

Mental retardation—Significant impairment in intellectual function and adaptation in society. Usually associated an intelligence quotient (IQ) below 70.

Mosaic—A term referring to a genetic situation in which an individual's cells do not have the exact same composition of chromosomes. In Down syndrome, this may mean that some of the individual's cells have a normal 46 chromosomes, while other cells have an abnormal 47 chromosomes.

Nondisjunction—Non-separation of a chromosome pair, during either meiosis or mitosis.

Translocation—The transfer of one part of a chromosome to another chromosome during cell division. A balanced translocation occurs when pieces from two different chromosomes exchange places without loss or gain of any chromosome material. An unbalanced translocation involves the unequal loss or gain of genetic information between two chromosomes.

Trisomy—The condition of having three identical chromosomes, instead of the normal two, in a cell.

in a laboratory. Chemical stain is added to make the characteristics of the cells and the chromosomes stand out. Chemicals are added to prompt the cells to go through normal development, up to the point where the chromosomes are most visible, prior to cell division. At this point, they are examined under a microscope and photographed. The photograph is used to sort the different sizes and shapes of chromosomes into pairs. In most cases of Down syndrome, one extra chromosome 21 will be revealed. The final result of such testing, with the photographed chromosomes paired and organized by shape and size, is called the individual's karyotype. An individual with Down syndrome will have a 47 XX + 21 karyotype if they are female and a 47 XY + 21 karyotype if they are male.

Women who become pregnant after the age of 35 are offered prenatal tests to determine whether or not their developing baby is affected with Down syndrome. A genetic counselor meets with these families to inform them of the risks and to discuss the types of tests available to make a diagnosis prior to delivery. Because there is a slight risk of **miscarriage** following some prenatal tests, all testing is optional, and couples need to decide whether or not they desire to take this risk in order to learn the status of their unborn baby.

Screening tests are used to estimate the chance that an individual woman will have a baby with Down syndrome. A test called the maternal serum alpha-fetoprotein test (MSAFP) is offered to all pregnant women under the age of 35. If the mother decides to have this test, it is performed between 15 and 22 weeks of **pregnancy**. The MSAFP screen measures a protein and two hormones that are normally found in maternal blood during pregnancy. A specific pattern of these hormones and protein can indicate an increased risk for having a baby born with Down syndrome. However, this is only a risk and MSAFP cannot diagnose Down syndrome directly. Women found to have an increased risk of their babies being affected with Down syndrome are offered **amniocentesis**. The MSAFP test can detect up to 60% of all babies who will be born with Down syndrome.

Ultrasound screening for Down syndrome is also available. This is generally performed in the mid-trimester of pregnancy. Abnormal growth patterns characteristic of Down syndrome such as growth retardation, heart defects, duodenal atresia, T-E fistula, shorter than normal long-bone lengths, and extra folds of skin along the back of the neck of the developing fetus may all be observed via ultrasonic imaging.

The only way to definitively establish (with about 99% accuracy) the presence or absence of Down syndrome in a developing baby is to test tissue during the pregnancy itself. This is usually done either by amniocentesis, or **chorionic villus sampling** (CVS). All women under the age of 35 who show a high risk for having a baby affected with Down syndrome via an MSAFP screen and all mothers over the age of 35 are offered either CVS or amniocentesis. In CVS, a tiny tube is inserted into the opening of the uterus to retrieve a small sample of the placenta (the organ that attaches the growing baby to the mother via the umbilical cord, and provides oxygen and **nutrition**). In amniocentesis, a small amount of the fluid in which the baby is floating is withdrawn with a long, thin needle. CVS may be performed as early as 10 to 12 weeks into a pregnancy. Amniocentesis is generally not performed until at least the fifteenth week. Both CVS and amniocentesis carry small risks of miscarriage. Approximately 1% of women miscarry after undergoing CVS testing, while approximately one-half of one percent miscarry after undergoing amniocentesis. Both amniocentesis and CVS allow the baby's own karyotype to be determined.

Approximately 75% of all babies diagnosed prenatally as affected with Down syndrome do not survive to term and spontaneously miscarry. In addition, these prenatal tests can only diagnose Down syndrome, not the severity of the symptoms that the unborn child will experience. For this reason, a couple might use this information to begin to prepare for the arrival of a baby with Down syndrome, to terminate the pregnancy, or in the case of miscarriage or termination, decide whether to consider adoption as an alternative.

Treatment

Traditional

No treatment is available to cure Down syndrome. Treatment is directed at addressing the individual concerns of a particular patient. For example, heart defects may require surgical repair, as will duodenal atresia and T-E fistula. Many Down syndrome patients will need to wear glasses to correct vision. Patients with hearing impairment benefit from **hearing aids**.

While some decades ago all children with Down syndrome were quickly placed into institutions for lifelong care, research shows very clearly that the best outlook for children with Down syndrome is a normal family life in their own home. This requires careful support and education of the parents and the siblings. It is a life-changing event to learn that a new baby has a permanent condition that will affect essentially all aspects of his or her development. Some community groups help families deal with the emotional effects of raising a child with Down syndrome. Schools are required to provide services to children with Down syndrome, sometimes in separate special education classrooms, and sometimes in regular classrooms (this is called mainstreaming or inclusion).

As of May 2000, the genetic sequence for chromosome 21 was fully determined, which opens the door to new approaches to the treatment of Down syndrome through the development of gene-specific therapies.

Alternative

Clinical trials for the treatment of Down syndrome are currently sponsored by the National Institutes of Health (NIH) and other agencies. In 2009, NIH reported 20 ongoing or recently completed studies.

A few examples include:

- The evaluation of a new prenatal blood test for Down syndrome. (NCT00877292)
- The evaluation of the efficacy on language and cognitive function in Down syndrome patients who take Rivastigmine. (NCT00748007)
- The evaluation of the efficacy and tolerability of Continuous Positive Pressure in case of SAOS by Down Syndrome patients. (NCT00394290)
- A study to assess whether memantine is effective and safe in preventing age related cognitive deterioration in people with Down's syndrome (DS) age 40 and over. (NCT00240760)

Clinical trial information is constantly updated by NIH and the most recent information on Down syndrome trials can be found at: http://clinicaltrials.gov/search/open/condition = %22Down + Syndrome%22

Prognosis

The prognosis for an individual with Down syndrome is quite variable, depending on the types of complications (heart defects, susceptibility to infections, development of leukemia, etc.). The severity of the retardation can also vary significantly. Without the presence of heart defects, about 90% of children with Down syndrome live into their teens. People with Down syndrome appear to go through the normal physical changes of **aging** more rapidly, however. The average age of **death** for an individual with Down syndrome is about 50 to 55 years.

Still, the prognosis for a baby born with Down syndrome is better than ever before. Because of modern medical treatments, including **antibiotics** to treat infections, and surgery to treat heart defects and duodenal atresia, life expectancy has greatly increased. Community and family support allows people with Down syndrome to have rich, meaningful relationships. Because of educational programs, some people with Down syndrome are able to hold jobs.

Prevention

There is no known way to prevent the Down syndrome. Women expecting to give birth however, can take steps before and during pregnancy to have a healthy pregnancy. Steps include taking a daily multivitamin with **folic acid** (400 micrograms), not **smoking**, and not drinking alcohol during pregnancy. Once a couple has had one baby with Down syndrome, they are often concerned about the likelihood of future offspring also being born with the disorder.

When a baby with Down syndrome has the type that results from a translocation, it is possible that one of the two parents is a carrier of a balanced translocation. A carrier has rearranged chromosomal information and can pass it on, but he or she does not have an extra chromosome and therefore is not affected with the disorder. When one parent is a carrier of a translocation, the chance of future offspring having Down syndrome is greatly increased. The specific risk will have to be assessed by a genetic counsellor. Approximately 60% of women with Down syndrome are fully capable of having children. The risk of a woman with trisomy 21 having a child affected with Down syndrome is 50%.

Resources

BOOKS

Groneberg, Jennifer Graf. *Road Map to Holland: How I Found My Way Through My Son's First Two Years With Down Syndrome*. New York, NY: New American Library (Penguin), 2008.

Kumin, Libby. *Helping Children with Down Syndrome Communicate Better: Speech and Language Skills for Ages 6–14*. Bethesda, MD: Woodbine House, 2008.

McGuire, Dennis, and Brian Chicoine. *Mental Wellness in Adults with Down Syndrome: A Guide to Emotional and Behavioral Strengths and Challenges*. Bethesda, MD: Woodbine House, 2006.

Moore-Mallinos, Jennifer. *My Friend Has Down Syndrome*. Hauppauge, NY: Barron's Educational Series, 2008.

Selikowitz, Mark. *Down Syndrome*. New York, NY: Oxford University Press, 2008.

Skallerup, Susan J., editor. *Babies with Down Syndrome: A New Parents' Guide*. Bethesda, MD: Woodbine House, 2008.

PERIODICALS

Creavin, A. L., and R. D. Brown. "Ophthalmic abnormalities in children with Down syndrome." *Journal of Pediatric Ophthalmology and Strabismus* 46, no. 2 (March–April 2009): 76–82.

Hartway, S. "A parent's guide to the genetics of Down syndrome." *Advances in Neonatal Care* 9, no. 1 (February 2009): 27–30.

Kusters, M. A., et al. "Intrinsic defect of the immune system in children with Down syndrome: a review." *Clinical and Experimental Immunology* 156, no. 2 (May 2009): 189–193.

Mégarbané, A., et al. "The 50th anniversary of the discovery of trisomy 21: the past, present, and future of research and treatment of Down syndrome." *Genetics in Medicine* 11, no. 9 (September 2009): 611–616.

Park, J., et al. "Function and regulation of Dyrk1A: towards understanding Down syndrome." *Cellular and Molecular Life Sciences* 66, no. 20 (October 2009): 3235–3240.

Patterson, D. "Molecular genetic analysis of Down syndrome." *Human Genetics* 126, no. 1 (July 2009): 195–214.

Ranweiler, R. "Assessment and care of the newborn with Down syndrome." *Advances in Neonatal Care* 9, no. 1 (February 2009): 17–24.

Wiseman, F. K., et al. "Down syndrome—recent progress and future prospects." *Human Molecular Genetics* 18, no. R1 (April 2009): R75–R83.

OTHER

"Chromosome 21." *Genetics Home Reference*. Information Page. http://ghr.nlm.nih.gov/chromosome=21 (accessed December 14, 2009).

"Down Syndrome." *CDC*. Information Page. http://www.cdc.gov/ncbddd/birthdefects/DownSyndrome.htm (accessed December 14, 2009).

"Down Syndrome." *Genetics Home Reference*. Information Page. http://ghr.nlm.nih.gov/condition=downsyndrome (accessed December 14, 2009).

"Down Syndrome." *March of Dimes*. Information Page. http://www.marchofdimes.com/professionals/14332_1214.asp (accessed December 14, 2009).

"Down Syndrome." *Medline Plus*. Health Topics. http://www.nlm.nih.gov/medlineplus/downsyndrome.html (accessed December 14, 2009).

"Down Syndrome." *NICHD*. Information Page. http://www.nichd.nih.gov/health/topics/Down_Syndrome.cfm (accessed December 14, 2009).

ORGANIZATIONS

March of Dimes Foundation, 1275 Mamaroneck Avenue, White Plains, NY, 10605, (914) 428-7100, (888) MOD-IMES, (914) 428-8203, askus@marchofdimes.com, http://www.marchofdimes.com.

National Association for Down Syndrome (NADS), PO Box 206, Wilmette, IL, 60091, (630) 325-9112, info@nads.org, http://www.nads.org.

National Center on Birth Defects and Developmental Disabilities, Centers for Disease Control and Prevention, 1600 Clifton Rd., Atlanta, GA, 75231, (800) 232-4636, http://www.cdc.gov/ncbddd/index.html.

National Down Syndrome Society, 666 Broadway, 8th Floor, New York, NY, 10012, (800) 221-4602, (212) 979-2873, info@ndss.org, http://www.ndss.org.

National Institute of Child Health and Human Development (NICHD), 31 Center Drive, Rm. 2A32, MSC 2425, Bethesda, MD, 20892-2425, (301) 496-5133, (301) 496-7101, http://www.nichd.nih.gov.

Paul A. Johnson
Monique Laberge, PhD

Down's syndrome *see* **Down syndrome**

Doxazosin *see* **Alpha₁-adrenergic blockers**

Doxepin *see* **Antidepressants, tricyclic**

Doxycycline *see* **Tetracyclines**

Dracontiasis *see* **Guinea worm infection**

Dracunculiasis *see* **Guinea worm infection**

Drooping eyelid *see* **Ptosis**

Drowning *see* **Near-drowning**

Drug abuse *see* **Substance abuse and dependence**

Drug addiction *see* **Substance abuse and dependence**

Drug dependence *see* **Substance abuse and dependence**

Drug metabolism/interactions

Definition

Drug metabolism is the process by which the body breaks down and converts medication into active chemical substances.

Precautions

Drugs can interact with other drugs, foods, and beverages. Interactions can lessen or magnify the desired therapeutic effect of a drug, or may cause unwanted or unexpected side effects. There are thousands of possible drug-to-drug and drug-to-food interactions, and many medications and supplements are contraindicated (not recommended) under certain conditions or in patients with specific diseases and disorders. This is why it is imperative that patients always keep their physician fully informed about all drugs and dietary supplements (including herbal remedies) they are taking.

Description

The primary site of drug metabolism is the liver, the organ that plays a major role in metabolism, digestion, **detoxification**, and elimination of substances from the body. Enzymes in the liver are responsible for chemically changing drug components into substances known as metabolites. Metabolites are then bound to other substances for excretion through the lungs, or bodily fluids such as saliva, sweat, breast milk, and urine, or through reabsorption by the intestines. The primary mode of excretion is through the kidneys.

The family of liver isoenzymes known as cytochrome P-450 are crucial to drug metabolism. These enzymes (labeled CYP1A2, CYP2C9, CYP2C19, CYP2D6, and CYP3A4) have a catabolic action on substances, breaking them down into metabolites. Consequently, they also act to lower the concentration of medication in the bloodstream.

Drug interactions can occur when one drug inhibits or induces a P-450 that acts on another drug. An example is nicotine, a drug contained in tobacco, and

known to induce P-450s. Individuals with **liver disease** (e.g., **cirrhosis**) may also have insufficient levels of P-450 enzymes. As a result, the concentration of drugs metabolized by these enzymes (e.g., amprenavir and other **protease inhibitors**) remains high and can build up to toxic levels in the bloodstream. In addition, certain medications and foods, such as grapefruit juice, can inactivate or lessen the metabolic activity of P-450s. Changing the drug dosage can alleviate the problem in some cases.

The metabolic rate can vary significantly from person to person, and drug dosages that work quickly and effectively in one individual may not work well for another. Factors such as genetics, environment, **nutrition**, and age also influence drug metabolism; infants and elderly patients may have a reduced capacity to metabolize certain drugs, and may require adjustments in dosage.

Causes and symptoms

Drugs that commonly interact with other medications include:

- Diuretics. Diuretics such as hydrochlorothiazide can reduce serum potassium and sodium electrolyte levels when taken with digoxin and lithium, respectively.

- Monoamine oxidase inhibitors (MAOIs). MAOI antidepressants can cause convulsions and other serious side effects when used with tricyclic antidepressants (e.g., Imipramine, Nortriptyline), selective serotonin reuptake inhibitors (SSRIs), or sympathomimetic drugs (e.g., amphetamines).

- Antibiotics. Antibiotics may reduce the efficiency of oral contraceptives.

- Metals. Medications containing metals, such as antacids with aluminum additives and iron supplements, can reduce the absorption of tetracyclines and fluoroquinolones.

- Drugs that inhibit liver enzyme function. Drugs that slow drug metabolism include ciprofloxacin, erythromycin, fluoxetine, nefazodone, paroxetine, and ritonavir. The therapeutic effect of other medications taken with these drugs may be amplified. Warfarin, a blood thinner, should be used with great caution in individuals taking these drugs.

Foods and beverages that may interact with drugs include:

- Grapefruit juice. Grapefruit juice inhibits the metabolism of many medications, including cyclosporine, felodipine, nifedipine, nitrendipine, nisoldipine, carbamazepine, triazolam, and midazolam.

- Foods and beverages with tyramines. Red wine, malted beers, smoked foods (e.g., fish and meats), dried fruits, and aged cheeses may contain tyramines, and can cause a severe and dangerous elevation in blood pressure when taken with MAOI inhibitors (a class of antidepressants).

- Dairy products. Milk, cream, and other dairy products containing calcium can prevention the absorption of antibiotics such as tetracycline, doxycycline, and ciprofloxacin when they are taken with the drug. In addition, whole milk with vitamin D can cause milk-alkali syndrome in patients taking aluminum hydroxide antacids.

- Caffeinated beverages. The caffeine contained in coffee and colas can influence drug metabolism.

- Alcohol. Alcohol is a central nervous system depressant, and should not be taken with other CNS depressants (e.g., antipsychotics, antihistamines). In addition, certain fermented beverages may contain tyramines.

This list is not all-inclusive and individuals should always let their doctor and pharmacist know when they are taking other medications, herbal remedies, or dietary supplements. Anyone who experiences a serious reaction to a drug that is not consistent with its product labeling should report the event to their doctor and/or the MedWatch adverse event reporting system of the United States Food and Drug Administration (FDA).

Alternative treatment

The growing use of herbal supplements has also increased the opportunity for adverse drug and herbal interactions. In 2000, the FDA issued a warning on the popular herb **St. John's wort** (*Hypericum perforatum*). The supplement was found to inhibit the effect of indinavir, a protease inhibitor used in the treatment of HIV. It may also affect the action of cyclosporine and other protease inhibitors (e.g., amprenavir, ritonavir). Further clinical studies are still necessary to determine the full metabolic effects of the herb.

Other herbs which may interact with allopathic medications include gingko bilboa, **ginseng**, and garlic, which may all heighten the blood thinning effect of the anticoagulant warfarin. Because herbs are regulated by the FDA as dietary supplements, they do not require the same extensive clinical trials and premarket testing as drugs do before they are cleared for sale in the United States. As such, there is still much to learn about the potential interactions and adverse effects associated with herbal supplements. Individuals who experience serious side effects from dietary supplements should report them to FDA's MedWatch program.

KEY TERMS

Catabolism—A process of metabolism that breaks down complex substances into simple ones.

Cirrhosis—Liver disease characterized by the widespread disruption of the normal liver structure and function.

CNS depressant—Anything that depresses, or slows, the sympathetic impulses of the central nervous system (i.e., respiratory rate, heart rate).

Drug interaction—A chemical or physiological reaction that can occur when two different drugs are taken together.

Enzymes—Organic substances (proteins) composed of amino acids that trigger and regulate chemical reactions in the body. There are over 700 identified human enzymes.

Liver—A solid organ located on the right in the upper abdomen. It plays a major role in metabolism, digestion, detoxification, and elimination of substances from the body.

Metabolism—The sum of all the physical and chemical processes occurring in the body to organize and maintain life.

Metabolites—Substances produced by metabolism or by a metabolic process.

Milk-alkali syndrome—Elevated blood calcium levels and alkalosis caused by excessive intake of milk and alkalis. Usually occurs in the treatment of peptic ulcer.

Diagnosis

Drug interactions can be difficult to detect. In some cases, adverse reactions may closely resemble the symptoms of the disease or condition the medication was prescribed to treat. Patients who take a number of medications or self-treat with over-the-counter drugs and/or herbal remedies may not be able to determine which drug actually triggered the interaction. A 2001 study by University of Florida researchers found that less than half of the women participating disclosed their use of herbal therapies to their healthcare providers. In cases where a serious drug or herb interaction occurs, withholding this information can delay diagnosis and put the patient at increased risk.

Treatment

Treatment of a drug interaction is dependant on a number of factors, including the medication(s) or

---

supplements used and the medical history of the patient. A dosage adjustment may reverse the effects of some interactions. Serious or life-threatening interactions will require more aggressive therapies.

Prevention

Patients with chronic health conditions, particularly those with liver disorders, should always inform their healthcare professional before taking any over-the-counter (OTC) medications or dietary supplements. Because of the risk for a drug-to-drug interaction, individuals should also let their doctor know if they are taking drugs prescribed by other physicians. Individuals should closely follow instructions for use and package directions on both prescription and over-the-counter drugs. Consulting with a pharmacist and/or physician may be beneficial if package directions are unclear to the patient.

As a rule, grapefruit juice should not be taken with medication unless recommended by a doctor. Patients taking MAOI inhibitors should always check food and beverage labels to ensure tyramines are not included, and should avoid all fermented drinks.

Resources

BOOKS

Beers, Mark H., Robert S. Porter, and Thomas V. Jones, eds. *The Merck Manual of Diagnosis and Therapy.* 18th ed. Whitehouse Station, NJ: Merck Research Laboratories, 2006.

The Physicians Desk Reference (PDR). 63rd ed. Montvale, NJ: Physicians' Desk Reference, 2008.

PERIODICALS

Hardy, Mary L. "Herb-Drug Interactions: An Evidence-Based Table." *Internal Medicine Alert* 23 (January 29, 2001): 1.

ORGANIZATIONS

United States Food and Drug Administration (FDA). MedWatch Adverse Events Reporting Program, 5600 Fishers Lane, Rockville, MD, 20857, (800) 332-0178, (800) 332-1088, http://www.fda.gov/medwatch/.

Paula Anne Ford-Martin

Drug overdose

Definition

A drug overdose is the accidental or intentional use of a drug or medicine in an amount that is higher than is normally used.

Drug-related emergency department (ED) visits, by selected drugs, 2008[1]

Drug	Number of visits
Alternative medicines	1,952
Analgesics	528,566
Antidepressants	99,037
Antihistamines	9,261
Anxiolytics, sedatives, and hypnotics	394,874
Cocaine	482,188
Heroin	200,666
Marijuana	374,435
Methamphetamine	66,308
Muscle relaxants	58,702
PCP	37,266
Topical agents	4,478
Total ED visits	**1,999,861[2]**

[1]Most recent year for which estimates were available.
[2]Includes drugs not listed in this chart.

SOURCE: Office of Applied Studies, SAMHSA, Drug Abuse Warning Network, 2008 (December 2009 update).

(Table by PreMediaGlobal. Reproduced by permission of Gale, a part of Cengage Learning.)

Description

All drugs have the potential to be misused, whether legally prescribed by a doctor, purchased over-the-counter at the local drug store, or bought illegally on the street. Taken in combination with other drugs or with alcohol, even drugs normally considered safe can cause **death** or serious long term consequences. Children are particularly at risk for accidental overdose, accounting for over one million poisonings each year from drugs, alcohol, and other chemicals and toxic substances. People who suffer from depression and who have suicidal thoughts are also at high risk for drug overdose.

Causes and symptoms

Accidental drug overdose may be the result of misuse of prescription medicines or commonly used medications like **pain** relievers and cold remedies. Symptoms differ depending on the drug taken. Some of the drugs commonly involved in overdoses are listed below along with symptoms and outcomes.

Acetaminophen is the generic name for the commonly used pain reliever Tylenol. Overdose of this drug causes liver damage with symptoms that include loss of appetite, tiredness, **nausea and vomiting**, paleness, and sweating. The next stage of symptoms indicates liver failure and includes abdominal pain and tenderness, swelling of the liver, and abnormal blood tests for liver enzymes. In the last stage of this poisoning, liver failure advances and the patient becomes jaundiced, with yellowing of the skin and whites of the eyes. They may also experience kidney failure, bleeding disorders, and encephalopathy (swelling of the brain).

Anticholinergic drugs (drugs that block the action of acetylcholine, a neurotransmitter) like atropine, scopolamine, belladonna, **antihistamines**, and antipsychotic agents cause the skin and moist tissues (like in the mouth and nose) to become dry and flushed. Dilated pupils, an inability to urinate, and mental disturbances are also symptoms. Severe toxicity can lead to seizures, abnormal heart rhythms, extremely high blood pressure, and **coma**.

Antidepressant drugs like amitriptyline, desipramine, and nortriptyline can cause irregular heart rate, **vomiting**, low blood pressure, confusion, and seizures. An overdose of antidepressants also causes symptoms similar to those seen with anticholinergic drug overdoses.

Cholinergic drugs (drugs that stimulate the parasympathetic nervous system) like carbamate and pilocarpine cause **nausea**, **diarrhea**, increased secretion of body fluids (sweat, tears, saliva, and urine), **fatigue**, and muscle weakness. Convulsions are possible. Death can occur due to **respiratory failure** and **heart failure**.

Cocaine and crack cocaine overdoses cause seizures, high blood pressure, increased heart rate, **paranoia**, and other changes in behavior. **Heart attack** or **stroke** are serious risks within three days after cocaine overdose.

Depressant drugs (tranquilizers, **antianxiety drugs**, sleeping pills) cause sleepiness, slowed or slurred speech, difficulty walking or standing, blurred vision, impaired ability to think, disorientation, and mood changes. Overdose symptoms can include slowed breathing, very low blood pressure, stupor, coma, **shock**, and death.

Digoxin, a drug used to regulate the heart, can cause irregular heart beats, nausea, confusion, loss of appetite, and blurred vision.

Narcotics or opiates are drugs like heroin, morphine, and codeine. Clonidine and diphenoxylate (Lomotil) are also in this category. Overdose with opiate drugs causes **sedation** (sleepiness), low blood pressure, slowed heart rate, and slowed breathing. Pinpoint pupils, where the black centers of the eyes become smaller than normal, are common in opiate overdose. However, if other drugs are taken at the same time as the opiates, they may counteract this effect on the pupils. A serious risk is that the patient will stop breathing.

Salicylates are found in **aspirin** and some creams or ointments used for muscle and joint pain (like Ben-Gay), and creams for **psoriasis**, a skin condition. Initial symptoms are gastrointestinal irritation, **fever**, and **vomiting**, possibly with blood in the vomit. This overdose will cause **metabolic acidosis** and **respiratory alkalosis**, conditions where the body's acid/base balance is malfunctioning. Symptoms include rapid heart beat and fast breathing. Nervous system symptoms include confusion, **hallucinations**, tiredness, and ringing in the ears. An increased tendency to bleed is also common. Serious complications include acute renal failure, coma, and heart failure. Acute salicylate poisoning can lead to death.

Diagnosis

Diagnosis of a drug overdose may be based on the symptoms that develop, however, the drug may do extensive damage to the body before significant symptoms develop. If the patient is conscious, he or she may be able to tell what drugs were taken and in what amounts. The patient's recent medical and social history may also help in a diagnosis. For example, a list of medications that the patient takes, whether or not alcohol was consumed recently, even if the patient has eaten in the last few hours before the overdose, can be valuable in determining what was taken and how fast it will be absorbed into the system.

Different drugs have varying effects on the body's acid/base balance and on certain elements in the blood like potassium and **calcium**. Blood tests can be used to detect changes in body chemistry that may give clues to what drugs were taken. Blood can also be screened for various drugs in the system. Once the overdose drug is identified, blood tests can be used to monitor how fast the drug is being cleared out of the body. Urine tests can also be used to screen for some drugs and to detect changes in the body's chemistry. Blood and urine tests may show if there is damage to the liver or kidneys as a result of the overdose.

Treatment

Immediate care

If a drug overdose is discovered or suspected, and the person is unconscious, having convulsions, or is not breathing, call for emergency help immediately. If the person who took the drug is not having symptoms, do not wait to see if symptoms develop; call a poison control center immediately. Providing as much information as possible to the poison control center can help determine what the next course of action should be.

The poison control center, paramedics, and emergency room staff will want to know:

- What drug(s) were taken? (Try to locate the drug's container.)
- How much of the drug was taken?
- When was the drug taken?
- Was the drug taken with alcohol or any other drugs or chemicals?
- What is the age of the patient?
- What symptoms are the patient experiencing?
- Is the patient conscious?
- Is the patient breathing?

The poison control center may recommend trying to get the patient to vomit. A liquid called **ipecac** syrup, which is used to induce vomiting, is available from pharmacies without a prescription. Pediatricians may recommend that families keep ipecac syrup on hand in households with children. This medication should be used only on the advice of a medical professional. Vomiting should not be induced if the patient is unconscious.

Emergency care

Emergency medical treatment may include:

- Assessment of the patient's airway and breathing to making sure that the trachea, the passage to the lungs, is not blocked. If needed, a tube may be inserted through the mouth and into the trachea to help the patient breath. This procedure is called intubation.
- Assessment of the patient's heart rate, blood pressure, body temperature, and other physical signs that might indicate the effects of the drug.
- Blood and urine samples may be collected to test for the presence of the suspected overdose drug, and any other drugs or alcohol that might be present.
- Elimination of the drug that has not yet been absorbed is attempted. Vomiting may be induced using ipecac syrup or other drugs that cause vomiting. Ipecac syrup should not be given to patients who overdosed with tricyclic antidepressants, theophylline, or any drug that causes a significant change in mental status. If a patient vomits while unconscious, there is a serious risk of choking.
- Gastric lavage, or washing out the stomach, may be attempted. For this procedure a tube flexible tube is inserted through the nose, down the throat, and into the stomach. The contents of the stomach are then suctioned out through the tube. A solution of saline (salt water) is injected into the tube to rinse out the stomach. This solution is then suctioned out. This is

the process used when someone has his/her stomach pumped.

- Activated charcoal is sometimes given to absorb the drug.
- Medication to stimulate urination or defecation may be given to try to flush the excess drug out of the body faster.
- Intravenous (IV) fluids may be given. An intravenous line, a needle inserted into a vein, may be put into the arm or back of the hand. Fluids, either sterile saline (salt water solution) or dextrose (sugar water solution), can be administered through this line. Increasing fluids can help to flush the drug out of the system and to reestablish balance of fluids and minerals in the body. The pH (acid/base balance) of the body may need to be corrected by administering electrolytes like sodium, potassium, and bicarbonate through this IV line. If drugs need to be administered quickly, they can also be injected directly into the IV line.
- Hemodialysis is a procedure where blood is circulated out of the body, pumped through a dialysis machine, then reintroduced back into the body. This process can be used to filter some drugs out of the blood. It may also be used temporarily or long term if the kidneys are damaged due to the overdose.
- Antidotes are available for some drug overdoses. An antidote is another drug that counteracts or blocks the overdose drug. For example, acetaminophen overdose can be treated with an oral medication, N-acetylcysteine (Mucomyst), if the level of acetaminophen found in the blood is extremely high. Naloxone is an anti-narcotic drug that is given to counteract narcotic poisoning. Nalmefen or methadone may also be used.
- Psychiatric evaluation may be recommended if the drug overdose was taken deliberately.

Prognosis

While many victims of drug overdose recover without long term effects, there can be serious consequences. Some drug overdoses cause the failure of major organs like the kidneys or liver, or failure of whole systems like the respiratory or circulatory systems. Patients who survive drug overdose may need **kidney dialysis**, kidney or liver transplant, or ongoing care as a result of heart failure, stroke, or coma. Death can occur in almost any drug overdose situation, particularly if treatment is not started immediately.

Prevention

To protect children from accidental drug overdose, all medications should be stored in containers with child resistant caps. All drugs should be out of sight and out of reach of children, preferably in a locked cabinet. Prescription medications should be used according to directions and only by the person whose name is on the label. Threats of **suicide** need to be taken seriously and appropriate help sought for people with depression or other mental illness that may lead to suicide.

Resources

OTHER

"Drug abuse first aid." MedlinePlus Medical Encyclopedia. June 29, 2010. http://www.nlm.nih.gov/medlineplus/ency/article/000016.htm6/29/2010 (accessed November 23, 2010).

"Drug abuse first aid." University of Maryland Medical Center (UMMC). July 23, 2008. http://www.umm.edu/ency/article/000016.htm (accessed November 23, 2010).

Altha Roberts Edgren

Drug therapy monitoring

Definition

Drug therapy monitoring, also known as Therapeutic Drug Monitoring (TDM), is a means of monitoring drug levels in the blood.

Purpose

TDM is employed to measure blood drug levels so that the most effective dosage can be determined, with toxicity prevented. TDM is also utilized to identify noncompliant patients (those patients who, for whatever reason, either cannot or will not comply with drug dosages as prescribed by the physician).

Therapeutic Drug Monitoring: Therapeutic and toxic ranges

Drug name	Use	Therapeutic level*	Toxic level
Acetaminophen	Analgesic, antipyretic	Depends on use	>250 mcg/mL
Amikacin	Antibiotic	12–25 mcg/mL**	>25
Aminophylline	Bronchodilator	10–20 mg/mL	>20
Amitriptyline	Antidepressant	120–150 ng/mL	>500
Carbamazepine	Anticonvulsant	5–12 mg/mL	>12
Chloramphenicol	Antibiotic	10–20 mcg/mL	>25
Digoxin	Cardiotonic	0.8–2.0 ng/mL	>2.4
Gentamicin	Antibiotic	5–10 mcg/mL	>12
Lidocaine	Antiarrhythmic	1.5–5.0 mcg/mL	>5
Lithium	Antimanic	0.8–1.2 mEq/L	>2.0
Nortriptyline	Antidepressant	50–150 ng/mL	>500
Phenobarbital	Anticonvulsant	10–30 mcg/mL	>40
Phenytoin	Anticonvulsant	10–20 mcg/mL	>30
Procainamide	Antiarrhythmic	4–10 mcg/mL	>16
Propranolol	Antiarrhythmic	50–100 ng/mL	>150
Quinidine	Antiarrhythmic	2–5 mcg/mL	>10
Salicylate	Analgesic	100–250 mcg/mL	>300
Theophylline	Bronchodilator	10–20 mg/mL	>20
Tobramycin	Antibiotic	5–10 mcg/mL**	>12
Valproic acid	Anticonvulsant	50–100 mcg/mL	>100

*Values are laboratory-specific.
**Concentration obtained 30 minutes after the end of a 30-minute infusion.

SOURCE: National Institutes of Health, U.S. National Library of Medicine.

(Table by PreMediaGlobal. Reproduced by permission of Gale, a part of Cengage Learning.)

Precautions

Because so many different factors influence blood drug levels, the following points should be taken into consideration during TDM: the age and weight of the patient; the route of administration of the drug; the drug's absorption rate, excretion rate, delivery rate, and dosage; other medications the patient is taking; other diseases the patient has; the patient's compliance regarding the drug treatment regimen; and the laboratory methods used to test for the drug.

Description

TDM is a practical tool that can help the physician provide effective and safe drug therapy in patients who need medication. Monitoring can be used to confirm a blood drug concentration level that is above or below the therapeutic range, or if the desired therapeutic effect of the drug is not as expected. If this is the case, and dosages beyond normal then have to be prescribed, TDM can minimize the time that elapses.

TDM is important for patients who have other diseases that can affect drug levels, or who take other medicines that may affect drug levels by interacting with the drug being tested. As an example, without drug monitoring, the physician cannot be sure if a patient's lack of response to an antibiotic reflects bacterial resistance, or is the result of failure to reach the proper therapeutic range of antibiotic concentration in the blood. In cases of life-threatening infections, timing of effective antibiotic therapy is critical to success. It is equally crucial to avoid toxicity in a seriously ill patient. Therefore, if toxic symptoms appear with standard dosages, TDM can be used to determine changes in dosing.

Drawn blood, used for TDM, demonstrates a drug action in the body at any specific time, whereas drug levels examined from urine samples reflect the presence of a drug over many days (depending on the rate of excretion). Therefore, blood testing is the procedure of choice when definite data are required. However, for adequate absorption and therapeutic levels to be accurate, it is important to allow for sufficient time to pass between the administration of the medication and the collection of the blood sample.

Blood specimens for drug monitoring can be taken at two different times: during the drug's highest therapeutic concentration ("peak" level), or its lowest ("trough" level). Occasionally called residual levels, trough levels show sufficient therapeutic levels; whereas peak levels show **poisoning** (toxicity). Peak and trough levels should fall within the therapeutic range.

Preparation

In preparing for this test, the following guidelines should be observed:

- Depending on the drug to be tested, the physician should decide if the patient is to be fasting (nothing to eat or drink for a specified period of hours) before the test.

- For patients suspected of symptoms of drug toxicity, the best time to draw the blood specimen is when the symptoms are occurring.

- If there is a question as to whether an adequate dose of the drug is being achieved, it is best to obtain trough (lowest therapeutic concentration) levels.

- Peak (highest concentration) levels are usually obtained one to two hours after oral intake, approximately one hour after intramuscular (IM) administration (a shot in the muscle), and approximately 30 minutes after intravenous (IV) administration. Residual, or trough, levels are usually obtained within 15 minutes of the next scheduled dose.

Risks

Risks for this test are minimal, but may include slight bleeding from the blood-drawing site, **fainting** or feeling lightheaded after blood is drawn, or accumulation of blood under the puncture site (hematoma).

Resources

BOOKS

Pagana, Kathleen Deska, and Timothy J. Pagana. *Mosby's Manual of Diagnostic and Laboratory Tests.* 4th ed. St. Louis: Mosby, 2009.

Janis O. Flores

Drugs used in labor

Definition

These drugs are used to induce (start) or continue labor.

Purpose

The drug decribed here, oxytocin, makes the uterus (womb) contract. Physicians use it to deliberately start labor. Because there are some risks with using oxytocin, this should be done only when there are good medical reasons. Any woman who is being given oxytocin should make sure she has discussed the benefits and risks with her physician.

Oxytocin also may be used to control bleeding after delivery or to help make the milk flow in women who are **breastfeeding** their babies.

Description

Oxytocin is a hormone and is available only with a physician's prescription. When used to start or continue labor, it is slowly injected into a vein. A nasal spray form is used to increase milk flow in breastfeeding. Some commonly used brand names are Pitocin and Syntocinon.

Recommended dosage

The dosages given here are average doses. However, doses may be different for different patients. Follow the orders of the physician who prescribed the drug.

For increasing milk production:

One spray into one or both nostrils, two–three minutes before nursing or using a breast pump.

For starting or continuing labor:

The physician in charge will determine the appropriate dose.

Precautions

Oxytocin does not help increase or continue labor in all patients. When it does not help, the physician may deliver the baby by **cesarean section**.

In women who are especially sensitive to oxytocin, the drug may cause contractions to become too strong. This could tear the uterus or deprive the fetus of blood and oxygen during labor.

Oxytocin does not help improve milk flow in all women who are breastfeeding. Check with a physician if the drug does not seem to be working.

Women with heart disease, high blood pressure, or **kidney disease** should let their physicians know about these conditions before taking oxytocin. Also, anyone who has had an unusual reaction to oxytocin in the past should inform their physician.

Side effects

Oxytocin has caused irregular heartbeat and increased bleeding in some women after delivery. It may also cause **jaundice** (yellowing of the eyes and skin) in newborns.

Other side effects are rare, but may include **nausea**, **vomiting**, confusion, **dizziness**, convulsions, breathing problems, **headache**, **hives**, skin rash, **itching**, pelvic or abdominal **pain**, and weakness. The nasal spray form may cause watery eyes or irritation of the nose.

Interactions

Anyone who takes oxytocin should let the physician know all other medicines she is taking.

Nancy Ross-Flanigan

Dry mouth

Definition

Dry mouth, known medically as xerostomia, is the abnormal reduction of saliva due to medication, disease, or medical therapy.

Description

Dry mouth due to the lack of saliva can be a serious medical problem. Decreased salivation can make swallowing difficult, can decrease taste sensation, and can promote **tooth decay**.

Causes and symptoms

Dry mouth, resulting from thickened or reduced saliva flow, can be caused by a number of factors: medications, both prescription and over-the-counter; such systemic diseases as anemia, HIV infection, or diabetes, manifestations of **Sjögren's syndrome** (as **rheumatoid arthritis**, lupus, chronic hardening and thickening of the skin, or chronic and progressive inflammation of skeletal muscles); infections of the salivary glands; blockage of the salivary ducts caused by stones or tumors forming in the ducts through which the saliva passes; **dehydration**; such medical therapies as local surgery or radiation; secretion reduction normally involved in the **aging** process; and emotional **stress**.

Diagnosis

The diagnosis of dry mouth is not difficult. The patient will state that his or her saliva is very thick or nonexistent. Finding the cause of dry mouth may be more difficult and require some laboratory testing. Salivary gland biopsy for stones or tumors should be performed if indicated.

Treatment

The treatment of dry mouth involves the management of the condition causing it. If dry mouth is caused by medication, the medication should be changed. If dry mouth is caused by blockage of the salivary ducts, the cause of the blockage should be investigated. When systemic diseases, such as diabetes and anemia, are brought under control dry mouth problems may decrease.

The use of caffeine-containing beverages, alcoholic beverages, and mouthwashes containing alcohol should be minimized. The drinking of water and fruit juices will decrease dry mouth problems. Chewing gum and lemon drops can be used to stimulate saliva flow. Bitters also can initiate salivary flow as long as the salivary glands

KEY TERMS

Salivary duct—Tube through which saliva is carried from the salivary gland to the mouth.

Salivary gland—Gland in which saliva forms.

Sialogogue—A medication given to increase the flow of saliva.

Xerostomia—The medical term for dry mouth.

and ducts are functional. Commercial saliva substitutes are available without prescription and can be used as frequently as needed. Use of a humidifier in the bedroom reduces nighttime oral dryness.

Dry mouth caused by the aging process or **radiation therapy** for **cancer** can be treated by such oral medications as pilocarpine (Salagen). Drugs that are given to increase the flow of saliva are known as sialogogues.

Prognosis

The prognosis for patients with xerostomia due to medication problems is good, if the offending agent can be changed. Dry mouth due to systemic problems may be eliminated or improved once the disease causing the dry mouth is under control. Persistent xerostomia can be managed well with saliva substitutes.

Prevention

A patient needs to ask his or her health care provider if any medication to be prescribed will cause dry mouth. Patients with persistent xerostomia need to practice good **oral hygiene** and visit a dentist on a regular basis; the lack of adequate saliva can cause severe dental decay. The salivary glands are very sensitive to radiation, so any patient scheduled for radiation therapy of the head and neck needs to discuss with the radiation therapist ways to minimize exposure of the salivary glands to radiation.

Resources

BOOKS

Beers, Mark H., Robert S. Porter, and Thomas V. Jones, eds. *The Merck Manual of Diagnosis and Therapy*. 18th ed. Whitehouse Station, NJ: Merck Research Laboratories, 2006.

PERIODICALS

Bruce, S. D. "Radiation-Induced Xerostomia: How Dry Is Your Patient?" *Clinical Journal of Oncology Nursing* 8 (February 2004): 61–67.

Nagler, R. M. "Salivary Glands and the Aging Process: Mechanistic Aspects, Health-Status and Medicinal-Efficacy Monitoring." *Biogerontology* 5 (March 2004): 223–233.

Pinto, A., and S. S. De Rossi. "Salivary Gland Disease in Pediatric HIV Patients: An Update." *Journal of Dentistry for Children (Chicago)* 71 (January-April 2004): 33–37.

Porter, S. R., C. Scully, and A. M. Hegarty. "An Update of the Etiology and Management of Xerostomia." *Oral Surgery, Oral Medicine, Oral Pathology, Oral Radiology, and Endodontics* 97 (January 2004): 28–46.

ORGANIZATIONS

American Dental Association, 211 E. Chicago Ave., Chicago, IL, 60611-2678, (312) 440-2500, http://www.ada.org.

American Medical Association, 515 N. State St., Chicago, IL, 60654, (800) 621-8335, http://www.ama-assn.org/.

Joseph Knight, PA
Rebecca J. Frey, PhD

Dry skin *see* **Ichthyosis**

Dual energy x-ray absorptiometry (DXA) scan *see* **Bone density test**

DUB *see* **Dysfunctional uterine bleeding**

Duchenne muscular dystrophy *see* **Muscular dystrophy**

Duodenal atresia *see* **Duodenal obstruction**

Duodenal obstruction

Definition

Duodenal obstruction is a failure of food to pass out of the stomach either from a complete or partial obstruction.

Description

The duodenum is the first part of the intestine, into which the stomach, the gall bladder, and the pancreas empty their contents. The pylorus connects the duodenum with the stomach and contains the valve that regulates stomach emptying. Obstruction usually occurs right at this outlet, so that the gall bladder and pancreas are unable to drain their secretions without hindrance.

Causes and symptoms

Obstruction of the duodenum occurs in adults and infants, each for a different set of reasons. In adults, the usual cause is a peptic ulcer of such antiquity that repeated cycles of injury and scarring have narrowed the passageway. Medical treatment of ulcers has progressed to the point where such obstinate ulcer disease is rarely seen any more. In infants, the conditions are congenital—either the channel is underdeveloped or the pylorus is overdeveloped. The first type is called duodenal hypoplasia and the second is termed hypertrophic **pyloric stenosis**. In rare cases, the channel may be missing altogether, a condition called duodenal atresia. To say that these anomalies are congenital is not to say their cause is understood. As with most **birth defects**, the specific cause is not known.

Food that cannot exit the stomach in the forward direction will return whence it came. **Vomiting** is the constant symptom of duodenal obstruction. It may be preceded by **indigestion** and **nausea** as the stomach attempts to squeeze its contents through an ever narrowing outlet.

Hypertrophic pyloric stenosis appears soon after birth. The infant will vomit feedings, lose weight, and be restless and irritable.

Diagnosis

X rays taken with contrast material in the stomach readily demonstrate the site of the blockage and often the ulcer that caused it. Gastroscopy is another way to evaluate the problem. In infants, x rays may not be necessary to detect pyloric stenosis. It is often possible to feel the enlarged pylorus, like an olive, deep under the ribs and see the stomach rippling as it labors to force food through.

Treatment

Bowel obstruction requires a surgeon, sometimes immediately. Newer surgical techniques constantly improve the outcome, but obstruction is a mechanical problem that needs a mechanical solution. Most adults who come to surgery for obstruction have suffered for years from peptic ulcer disease. They will usually benefit from **ulcer surgery** at the same time their obstruction is relieved. The surgeon will therefore select a procedure that combines relief of obstruction with remedy for ulcer disease. There are many choices. In fact, even without obstruction, functional considerations require ulcer surgery to include enhancement of stomach emptying.

To treat an infant with hypertrophic pyloric stenosis, some surgeons have had success with forceful balloon dilation of the pylorus done through a gastroscope, but the standard procedure is to cut across the overdeveloped circular muscle that is constricting the stomach outlet. There are reports of infant hypertrophic pyloric stenosis remitting without surgery

---

KEY TERMS

Atresia—Failure to develop; complete absence.

Contrast agent—A substance that produces shadows on an x ray so that hollow structures can be more easily seen.

Gastroscopy—Looking into the stomach with a flexible viewing instrument called a gastroscope.

Hypoplasia—Incomplete development.

Peptic ulcer—A wound in the lower stomach and duodenum caused by stomach acid and a newly discovered germ called *Helicobacter pylori*.

---

following a very careful feeding schedule, but mortality is unacceptably high.

Prognosis

A functioning and unrestricted intestine is a prerequisite for living independent of the most advanced and continuous medical care available. Achieving this desirable goal is the rule with surgery for duodenal obstructions of all types. The bowel is so malleable that there is a rearrangement to suit every occasion. The variety of possible configurations is limited only by the surgeon's imagination.

Prevention

Prompt and effective treatment of peptic ulcers will prevent chronic scarring and narrowing. Drugs developed over the past few decades have all but eliminated the need for ulcer surgery.

Resources

BOOKS

Sleisenger, Marvin H., et al. *Sleisenger & Fordtran's Gastrointestinal and Liver Disease: Pathophysiology, Diagnosis, Management.* 9th ed. St. Louis: MD Consult, 2009.

J. Ricker Polsdorfer, MD

Duodenal stenosis *see* **Duodenal obstruction**

Duodenal ulcers *see* **Ulcers (digestive)**

Duodenum x rays *see* **Hypotonic duodenography**

Duplicated ureter *see* **Congenital ureter anomalies**

Dwarfism *see* **Achondroplasia; Pituitary dwarfism**

Dysentery

Definition

Dysentery is a general term for a group of gastrointestinal disorders characterized by inflammation of the intestines, particularly the colon. Characteristic features include abdominal **pain** and cramps, straining at stool (tenesmus), and frequent passage of watery **diarrhea** or stools containing blood and mucus. The English word dysentery comes from two Greek words meaning "ill" or "bad" and "intestine."

It should be noted that some doctors use the word "dysentery" to refer only to the first two major types of dysentery discussed below, while others use the term in a broader sense. For example, some doctors speak of **schistosomiasis**, a disease caused by a parasitic worm, as bilharzial dysentery, while others refer to acute diarrhea caused by viruses as viral dysentery.

Description

Dysentery is a common but potentially serious disorder of the digestive tract that occurs throughout the world. It can be caused by a number of infectious agents ranging from viruses and bacteria to protozoa and parasitic worms; it may also result from chemical irritation of the intestines. Dysentery is one of the oldest known gastrointestinal disorders, having been described as early as the Peloponnesian War in the fifth century B.C. Epidemics of dysentery were frequent occurrences aboard sailing vessels as well as in army camps, walled cities, and other places in the ancient world where large groups of human beings lived together in close quarters with poor sanitation. As late as the eighteenth and nineteenth centuries, sailors and soldiers were more likely to die from the "bloody flux" than from injuries received in battle. It was not until 1897 that a bacillus (rod-shaped bacterium) was identified as the cause of one major type of dysentery.

Dysentery in the modern world is most likely to affect people in the less developed countries and travelers who visit these areas. According to the Centers for Disease Control and Prevention (CDC), most cases of dysentery in the United States occur in immigrants from the developing countries and in persons who live in inner-city housing with poor sanitation. Other groups of people at increased risk of dysentery are military personnel stationed in developing countries, frequent travelers, children in day care centers, people in nursing homes, and men who have sex with other men.

Causes and symptoms

Causes

The most common types of dysentery and their causal agents are as follows:

- Bacillary dysentery. Bacillary dysentery, which is also known as shigellosis, is caused by four species of the genus *Shigella*: *S. dysenteriae*, the most virulent species and the one most likely to cause epidemics; *S. sonnei*, the mildest species and the most common form of *Shigella* found in the United States; *S. boydii*; and *S. flexneri*. *S. flexneri* is the species that causes Reiter's syndrome, a type of arthritis that develops as a late complication of shigellosis. About 15,000 cases of shigellosis are reported to the CDC each year for the United States; however, the CDC maintains that the true number of annual cases may be as high as 450,000, since the disease is vastly underreported. About 85 percent of cases in the United States are caused by *S. sonnei*. The *Shigella* organisms cause the diarrhea and pain associated with dysentery by invading the tissues that line the colon and secreting an enterotoxin, or harmful protein that attacks the intestinal lining.

- Amebic dysentery. Amebic dysentery, which is also called intestinal amebiasis and amebic colitis, is caused by a protozoon, *Entamoeba histolytica*. *E. histolytica*, whose scientific name means "tissue-dissolving," is second only to the organism that causes malaria as a protozoal cause of death. *E. histolytica* usually enters the body during the cyst stage of its life cycle. The cysts may be found in food or water contaminated by human feces. Once in the digestive tract, the cysts break down, releasing an active form of the organism called a trophozoite. The trophozoites invade the tissues lining the intestine, where they are usually excreted in the patient's feces. They sometimes penetrate the lining itself, however, and enter the bloodstream. If that happens, the trophozoites may be carried to the liver, lung, or other organs. Involvement of the liver or other organs is sometimes called metastatic amebiasis.

- Balantidiasis, giardiasis, and cryptosporidiosis. These three intestinal infections are all caused by protozoa, *Balantidium coli*, *Giardia lamblia*, and *Cryptosporidium parvum* respectively. Although most people infected with these protozoa do not become severely ill, the disease agents may cause dysentery in children or immunocompromised individuals. There are about 3,500 cases of cryptosporidiosis reported to the CDC each year in the United States, and about 22,000 cases of giardiasis.

- Viral dysentery. Viral dysentery, which is sometimes called traveler's diarrhea or viral gastroenteritis, is caused by several families of viruses, including rotaviruses, caliciviruses, astroviruses, noroviruses, and adenoviruses. There are about 3.5 million cases of viral dysentery in infants in the United States each year, and about 23 million cases each year in adults. The CDC estimates that viruses are responsible for 9.2 million cases of dysentery related to food poisoning in the United States each year. Whereas most cases of viral dysentery in infants are caused by rotaviruses, caliciviruses are the most common disease agents in adults. Noroviruses were responsible for about half of the outbreaks of dysentery on cruise ships reported to the CDC in 2002.

- Dysentery caused by parasitic worms. Both whipworm (trichuriasis) and flatworm or fluke (schistosomiasis) infestations may produce the violent diarrhea and abdominal cramps associated with dysentery. Schistosomiasis is the second most widespread tropical disease after malaria. Although the disease is rare in the United States, travelers to countries where it is endemic may contract it. The World Health Organization (WHO) estimates that about 200 million people around the world carry the parasite in their bodies, with 20 million having severe disease.

Symptoms

In addition to the characteristic bloody and/or watery diarrhea and abdominal cramps of dysentery, the various types have somewhat different symptom profiles:

- Bacillary dysentery. The symptoms of shigellosis may range from the classical bloody diarrhea and tenesmus characteristic of dysentery to the passage of nonbloody diarrhea that resembles the loose stools caused by other intestinal disorders. The high fever associated with shigellosis begins within one to three days after exposure to the organism. The patient may also have pain in the rectum as well as abdominal cramping. The acute symptoms last for three to seven days, occasionally for as long as a month. Bacillary dysentery may lead to two potentially fatal complications outside the digestive tract: bacteremia (bacteria in the bloodstream), which is most likely to occur in malnourished children; and hemolytic uremic syndrome, a type of kidney failure that has a mortality rate above 50 percent.

- Amebic dysentery. Amebic dysentery often has a slow and gradual onset; most patients with amebiasis visit the doctor after several weeks of diarrhea and bloody stools. Fever is unusual with amebiasis unless the patient has developed a liver abscess as a complication of the infection. The most serious complication of amebic dysentery, however, is fulminant or necrotizing colitis, which is a severe inflammation of the colon characterized by dehydration, severe abdominal pain, and the risk of perforation (rupture) of the colon.

- Dysentery caused by other protozoa. Dysentery associated with giardiasis begins about 1–3 weeks after infection with the organism. It is characterized by bloating and foul-smelling flatus, nausea and vomiting, headaches, and low-grade fever. These acute symptoms usually last for three or four days. The symptoms of cryptosporidiosis are mild in most patients but are typically severe in patients with AIDS. Diarrhea usually starts between seven and 10 days after exposure to the organism and may be copious. The patient may have pain in the upper right abdomen, nausea, and vomiting, but fever is unusual.

- Viral dysentery. Viral dysentery has a relatively rapid onset; symptoms may begin within hours of infection. The patient may be severely dehydrated from the diarrhea but usually has only a low-grade fever. The diarrhea itself may be preceded by one to three days of nausea and vomiting. The patient's abdomen may be slightly tender but is not usually severely painful.

- Dysentery caused by parasitic worms. Patients with intestinal schistosomiasis typically have a gradual onset of symptoms. In addition to bloody diarrhea and abdominal pain, these patients usually have fatigue. An examination of the patient's colon will usually reveal areas of ulcerated tissue, which is the source of the bloody diarrhea.

Diagnosis

Patient history and physical examination

The **physical examination** in the primary care doctor's office will not usually allow the doctor to determine the specific parasite or other disease agent that is causing the bloody diarrhea and other symptoms of dysentery, although the presence or absence of **fever** may help to narrow the diagnostic possibilities. The patient's age and history are usually better sources of information. The doctor may ask about such matters as the household water supply and food preparation habits, recent contact with or employment in a nursing home or day care center, recent visits to tropical countries, and similar questions. The doctor will also need to know when the patient first noticed the symptoms.

The doctor will also evaluate the patient for signs of **dehydration** resulting from the loss of fluid through the intestines. **Fatigue**, drowsiness, dryness of the mucous membranes lining the mouth, low blood pressure, loss of normal skin tone, and rapid heartbeat (above 100 beats per minute) may indicate that the patient is dehydrated.

Laboratory tests

The most common laboratory test to determine the cause of dysentery is a stool sample. The patient should be asked to avoid using over-the-counter **antacids** or antidiarrheal medications until the sample has been collected, as these preparations can interfere with the test results. The organisms that cause **cryptosporidiosis**, bacillary dysentery, amebic dysentery, and **giardiasis** can be seen under the microscope, as can the eggs produced by parasitic worms. In some cases repeated stool samples, a sample of mucus from the intestinal lining obtained through a proctoscope, or a tissue sample from the patient's colon may be necessary to confirm the diagnosis. Antigen testing of a stool sample can be used to diagnose a rotavirus infection as well as parasitic worm infestations.

The doctor will also usually order a blood test to evaluate the electrolyte levels in the patient's blood in order to assess the need for rehydration.

Imaging studies

Imaging studies (usually CT scans, x rays, or ultrasound) may be performed in patients with amebic dysentery to determine whether the lungs or liver have been affected. They may also be used to diagnose schistosomiasis, as the eggs produced by the worms will show up on ultrasound or MRI studies of the liver, intestinal wall, or bladder.

Treatment

Medications are the primary form of treatment for dysentery:

- Bacillary dysentery. Dysentery caused by *Shigella* is usually treated with such antibiotics as trimethoprim-sulfamethoxazole (Bactrim, Septra), nalidixic acid (NegGram), or ciprofloxacin (Cipro, Ciloxan). Because the various species of *Shigella* are becoming resistant to these drugs, however, the doctor may prescribe one of the newer drugs described below. Patients with bacillary dysentery should not be given antidiarrheal medications, including loperamide (Imodium), paregoric, and diphenolate (Lomotil), because they may make the illness worse.

- Amebic dysentery. The most common drugs given for amebiasis are diloxanide furoate (Diloxide), iodoquinol (Diquinol, Yodoxin), and metronidazole (Flagyl). Metronidazole should not be given to pregnant women but paromomycin (Humatin) may be used instead. Patients with very severe symptoms may be given emetine dihydrochloride or dehydroemetine, but these drugs should be stopped once the patient's symptoms are controlled.

- Dysentery caused by other protozoa. Balantidiasis, giardiasis, and cryptosporidiosis are treated with the same drugs as amebic dysentery; patients with giardiasis resistant to treatment may be given albendazole (Zentel) or furazolidone (Furoxone).

- Viral dysentery. The primary concern in treating viral dysentery, particularly in small children, is to prevent dehydration. Antinausea and antidiarrhea medications should not be given to small children. Probiotics, including *Lactobacillus casei* and *Saccharomyces boulardii*, have been shown to reduce the duration and severity of viral diarrhea in small children by 30–70 percent.

- Dysentery caused by parasitic worms. Whipworm infestations are usually treated with anthelminthic medications, most commonly mebendazole (Vermox). Schistosomiasis may be treated with praziquantel (Biltricide), metrifonate (Trichlorfon), or oxamniquine, depending on the species causing the infestation.

Newer drugs that have been developed to treat dysentery include tinidazole (Tindamax, Fasigyn), an antiprotozoal drug approved by the Food and Drug Administration (FDA) in 2004 to treat giardiasis and **amebiasis** in adults and children over the age of three years. This drug should not be given to women in the first three months of **pregnancy**. In addition, adults taking tinidazole should not drink alcoholic beverages while using it, or for three days after the end of treatment. The other new drug is nitazoxanide (Alinia), another antiprotozoal medication that has the advantage of lacking the bitter taste of metronidazole and tinidazole.

Fluid replacement is given if the patient has shown signs of dehydration. The most common treatment is an oral rehydration fluid containing a precise amount of salt and a smaller amount of sugar to replace electrolytes as well as water lost through the intestines. Infalyte and Pedialyte are oral rehydration fluids formulated for the special replacement needs of infants and young children.

Surgery

Surgery is rarely necessary in treating dysentery, but may be required in cases of fulminant **colitis**, particularly if the patient's colon has perforated. Patients with liver abscesses resulting from amebic dysentery may also require emergency surgery if the **abscess** ruptures. In some cases exploratory surgery may be needed to determine whether severe abdominal pain is caused by schistosomiasis, amebic dysentery, or **appendicitis**.

Alternative treatments

There are a number of alternative treatments for dysentery, most of which are derived from plants used by healers for centuries. Because dysentery was known to ancient civilizations as well as modern societies, such alternative systems as **traditional Chinese medicine** (TCM) and **Ayurvedic medicine** developed treatments for it.

Ayurvedic medicine

Ayurvedic medicine recommends fruits and herbs, specifically cumin seed, bael fruit (*Aegle marmelos*, also known as Bengal quince), and arjuna (*Terminalia arjuna*) bark for the treatment of dysentery. Ayurvedic practitioners may also give the patient dietary supplements known as Isabbael, Lashunadi Bati, and Bhuwaneshar Ras. To rehydrate the body, adult patients may be given a combination of slippery elm water and barley to drink, at least a pint per day.

Traditional Chinese medicine

To treat dysentery, traditional Chinese doctors use astringent drugs, which are intended to constrict or tighten mucous membranes and other body tissues to slow down fluid loss. Myrobalan fruit (*Terminalia chebula*), nut galls (swellings produced on the leaves and stems of oak trees by the secretions of certain insects), and opium extracted from the opium poppy (*Papaver somniferum*) are the natural materials most commonly used. Paregoric, a water-based solution of morphine that is still used in the West to treat diarrhea, is derived from the opium poppy.

Other plant-based remedies

Researchers in Mexico reported in early 2005 that the roots of *Geranium mexicanum*, a plant that produces a sap traditionally used to treat coughs or diarrhea, contains compounds that are active against both *Giardia lamblia* and *Entamoeba histolytica*. Plant biologists in Africa are studying the effectiveness of African mistletoe (*Tapinanthus dodoneifolius*), a traditional remedy for dysentery among the Hausa and Fulani tribes of Nigeria.

Dietary supplements

A study published in the *American Journal of Clinical Nutrition* in early 2005 reported that supplemental zinc (twice the recommended daily dietary allowance) boosts the body's immune response during acute **shigellosis**.

Homeopathy

There are at least ten different homeopathic remedies used to treat diarrhea. Contemporary homeopaths, however, distinguish between diarrhea that can be safely treated at home with such homeopathic remedies as *Podophyllum*, *Veratrum album*, *Bryonia*, and *Arsenicum*, and diarrhea that indicates dysentery and should be referred to a physician. Signs of dehydration (loss of normal skin texture, **dry mouth**, sunken eyes), severe abdominal pain, blood in the stool, and unrelieved **vomiting** are all indications that mainstream medical care is required.

Prognosis

Most adults in developed countries recover completely from an episode of dysentery. Children are at greater risk of becoming dehydrated, however; bacillary dysentery in particular can lead to a child's **death** from dehydration in as little as 12–24 hours.

- Bacillary dysentery. Most patients recover completely from shigellosis, although their bowel habits may not become completely normal for several months. About 3 percent of people infected by *S. flexneri* will develop Reiter's syndrome, which may lead to a chronic form of arthritis that is difficult to treat. Elderly patients or those with weakened immune systems sometimes develop secondary bacterial infections after an episode of shigellosis.

- Amebic dysentery. Most people in North America who become infected with *E. histolytica* do not become severely ill. Patients who develop a severe case of amebic dysentery, however, are at increased risk for such complications as fulminant colitis or liver abscess. About 0.5 percent of patients with amebic dysentery develop fulminant colitis, but almost half of these patients die. Between 2 and 7 percent of cases of amebic liver abscess result in rupture of the abscess with a high mortality rate. Men are 7–12 times more likely to develop a liver abscess than women. Any patient diagnosed with amebic dysentery should have stool samples examined for relapse 1, 3, and 6 months after treatment with medications whether or not they have developed complications.

KEY TERMS

Anthelminthic (also spelled anthelmintic)—A type of drug or herbal preparation given to destroy parasitic worms or expel them from the body.

Bacillus—A rod-shaped bacterium. One common type of dysentery is known as bacillary dysentery because it is caused by a bacillus.

Enterotoxin—A type of harmful protein released by bacteria and other disease agents that affects the tissues lining the intestines.

Fulminant—Occurring or flaring up suddenly and with great severity. A potentially fatal complication of amebic dysentery is an inflammation of the colon known as fulminant colitis.

Probiotics—Food supplements containing live bacteria or other microbes intended to improve or restore the normal balance of microorganisms in the digestive tract.

Proctoscope—An instrument consisting of a thin tube with a light source, used to examine the inside of the rectum.

Protozoan (plural, protozoa)—A member of the simplest form of animal life, a one-celled organism. Amebic dysentery is caused by a protozoan.

Reiter's syndrome—A group of symptoms that includes arthritis, inflammation of the urethra, and conjunctivitis, and develops as a late complication of infection with *Shigella flexneri*. The syndrome was first described by a German doctor named Hans Reiter in 1918.

Tenesmus—Straining to urinate or defecate without being able to do so. Tenesmus is a characteristic feature of bacillary dysentery.

Trophozoite—The active feeding stage of a protozoal parasite, as distinct from its encysted stage.

- Dysentery caused by other protozoa. Cryptosporidiosis may lead to respiratory infections or pancreatitis in patients with AIDS. The risk of these complications, however, is reduced in AIDS patients who are receiving highly active antiretroviral therapy (HAART).

- Viral dysentery. Most people in North America recover completely without complications unless they become severely dehydrated. Viral dysentery in children in developing countries, however, is a major cause of mortality.

- Dysentery caused by parasitic worms. Untreated whipworm infections can lead to loss of appetite, chronic diarrhea, and retarded growth in children. Untreated schistosomiasis can develop into a chronic intestinal disorder in which fibrous tissue, small growths, or strictures (abnormal narrowing) may form inside the intestine. Patients treated for schistosomiasis should have stool samples checked for the presence of worm eggs 3 and 6 months after the end of treatment.

Prevention

The disease agents that cause dysentery do not confer immunity against reinfection at a later date. There are no vaccines for bacillary dysentery or amebic dysentery; however, a vaccine against schistosomiasis is under investigation. An oral vaccine against **rotavirus**

infections was developed for small children but was withdrawn in 2004 because it was associated with an increased risk of small-bowel disorders. Newer vaccines against rotaviruses and caliciviruses are being developed.

Public health measures

Public health measures to control the spread of dysentery include the following:

- Requiring doctors to report cases of disease caused by *Shigella*, *Entamoeba histolytica*, and other parasites that cause dysentery. Careful reporting allows the CDC and state public health agencies to investigate local outbreaks and plan prevention efforts.

- Posting advisories for travelers about outbreaks of dysentery and other health risks in foreign countries. The Travelers' Health section of the CDC website (http://wwwnc.cdc.gov/travel/) is a good source of up-to-date information.

- Instructing restaurant workers and other food handlers about proper methods of hand washing, food storage, and food preparation.

- Instructing workers in day care centers and nursing homes about the proper methods for changing and cleaning soiled diapers or bedding.

- Inspecting wells, other sources of drinking water, and swimming pools for evidence of fecal contamination.

Personal precautions

Individuals can lower their risk of contracting dysentery by the following measures:

- Not allowing anyone in the household who has been diagnosed with amebic or bacillary dysentery to prepare food or pour water for others until their doctor confirms that they are no longer carrying the disease agent.

- Avoiding anal sex or oral-genital contacts.

- Washing the hands carefully with soap and water after using the bathroom, and supervising the hand-washing of children in day care centers or those at home who are not completely toilet-trained.

- When traveling, drinking only boiled or treated water, and eating only cooked hot foods or fruits that can be peeled by the traveler.

- Avoiding swimming in fresh water in areas known to have outbreaks of schistosomiasis.

Resources

BOOKS

Beers, Mark H., Robert S. Porter, and Thomas V. Jones, eds. *The Merck Manual of Diagnosis and Therapy*. 18th ed. Whitehouse Station, NJ: Merck Research Laboratories, 2006.

PERIODICALS

Calzada, F., J. A. Cervantes-Martinez, and L. Yepez-Mulia. "In vitro Antiprotozoal Activity from the Roots of *Geranium mexicanum* and Its Constituents on *Entamoeba histolytica* and *Giardia lamblia*." *Journal of Ethnopharmacology* 98 (April 8, 2005): 191–193.

Deeni, Y. Y., and N. M. Sadiq. "Antimicrobial Properties and Phytochemical Constituents of the Leaves of African Mistletoe (*Tapinanthus dodoneifolius* (DC) Danser) (Loranthaceae): An Ethnomedicinal Plant of Hausalan, Northern Nigeria." *Journal of Ethnopharmacology* 83 (December 2002): 235–240.

Hlavsa, M. C., J. C. Watson, and M. J. Beach. "Cryptosporidiosis Surveillance—United States 1999–2002." *Morbidity and Mortality Weekly Report, Surveillance Summaries* 54 (January 28, 2005): 1–8.

Hlavsa, M. C., J. C. Watson, and M. J. Beach. "Giardiasis Surveillance—United States, 1998–2002." *Morbidity and Mortality Weekly Report, Surveillance Summaries* 54 (January 28, 2005): 9–16.

Hu, F., R. Lu, B. Huang, and M. Liang. "Free Radical Scavenging Activity of Extracts Prepared from Fresh Leaves of Selected Chinese Medicinal Plants." *Fitoterapia* 75 (January 2004): 14–23.

Rahman, M. J., P. Sarker, S. K. Roy, et al. "Effects of Zinc Supplementation as Adjunct Therapy on the Systemic Immune Responses in Shigellosis." *American Journal of Clinical Nutrition* 81 (February 2005): 495–502.

White, C. A. Jr. "Nitazoxanide: A New Broad-Spectrum Antiparasitic Agent." *Expert Review of Anti-Infective Therapy* 2 (February 2004): 43–49.

Wingate, D., S. F. Phillips, S. J. Lewis, et al. "Guidelines for Adults on Self-Medication for the Treatment of Acute Diarrhea." *Alimentary Pharmacology and Therapeutics* 15 (June 2001): 773–782.

OTHER

Centers for Disease Control and Prevention. Disease Information. "Shigellosis." http://www.cdc.gov/ncidod/dbmd/diseaseinfo/shigellosis_t.htm.

Centers for Disease Control and Prevention, Division of Parasitic Diseases. Fact Sheet. "Amebiasis." http://www.cdc.gov/ncidod/dpd/parasites/amebiasis/factsht_amebiasis.htm.

Centers for Disease Control and Prevention, National Center for Infectious Diseases, Travelers' Health. "New Medication Approved for Treatment of Giardiasis and Amebiasis." http://www.cdc.gov/travel/other/tinidazole_approval_2004.htm.

World Health Organization. "Shigella." http://www.who.int/topics/shigella/en/.

ORGANIZATIONS

Centers for Disease Control and Prevention (CDC), 1600 Clifton Road, Atlanta, GA, 30333, (800) 232-4636, cdcinfo@cdc.gov, http://www.cdc.gov.

Infectious Diseases Society of America (IDSA), 1300 Wilson Blvd., Suite 300, Arlington, VA, 22209, (703) 299-0200, (703) 299-0204, http://www.idsociety.org/.

World Health Organization (WHO), Avenue Appia 201211, Geneva, Switzerland, 27, 4122791-2111, info@who.int, http://www.who.int.

Rebecca Frey, PhD

Dysfunctional uterine bleeding

Definition

Dysfunctional uterine bleeding is irregular, abnormal uterine bleeding that is not caused by a tumor, infection, or **pregnancy**.

Description

Dysfunctional uterine bleeding (DUB) is a disorder that occurs most frequently in women at the beginning and end of their reproductive lives. About half the cases occur in women over 45 years of age, and about one fifth occur in women under age 20.

Dysfunctional uterine bleeding is diagnosed when other causes of uterine bleeding have been eliminated. Failure of the ovary to release an egg during the menstrual cycle occurs in about 70% of women with DUB. This is probably related to a hormonal imbalance.

DUB is common in women who have **polycystic ovary syndrome** (cysts on the ovaries). Women who are on dialysis may also have heavy or prolonged periods. So do some women who use an intrauterine device (**IUD**) for birth control.

DUB is similar to several other types of uterine bleeding disorders and sometimes overlaps these conditions.

Menorrhagia

Menorrhagia, sometimes called hypermenorrhea, is another term for abnormally long, heavy periods. This type of period can be a symptom of DUB, or many other diseases or disorders. In menorrhagia, menstrual periods occur regularly, but last more than seven days, and blood loss exceeds 3 oz (88.7 mL). Passing **blood clots** is common. Between 15–20% of healthy women experience debilitating menorrhagia that interferes with their normal activities. Menorrhagia may or may not signify a serious underlying problem.

Metrorrhagia

Metrorrhagia is bleeding between menstrual periods. Bleeding is heavy and irregular as opposed to ovulatory spotting which is light bleeding, in mid-cycle, at the time of ovulation.

Polymenorrhea

Polymenorrhea describes the condition of having too frequent periods. Periods occur more often than every 21 days, and ovulation usually does not occur during the cycle.

Causes and symptoms

Dysfunctional uterine bleeding often occurs when the endometrium, or lining of the uterus, is stimulated to grow by the hormone estrogen. When exposure to estrogen is extended, or not balanced by the presence of progesterone, the endometrium continues to grow until it outgrows its blood supply. Then it sloughs off, causing irregular bleeding. If the bleeding is heavy enough and frequent enough, anemia can result.

Menorrhagia is representative of DUB. It is caused by many conditions including some outside the reproductive system. Causes of menorrhagia include:

- adenomyosis (a benign condition characterized by growths in the area of the uterus)

- imbalance between the hormones estrogen and progesterone
- fibroid tumors
- pelvic infection
- endometrial cancer (cancer of the inner mucous membrane of the uterus)
- endometrial polyps
- endometriosis (a condition in which endometrial or endrometrial-like tissue appears outside of its normal place in the uterus)
- use of an intrauterine device (IUD) for contraception
- hypothyroidism
- blood clotting problems (rare)
- lupus erythematosus
- pelvic inflammatory disease
- steroid therapy
- advanced liver disease
- renal (kidney) disease
- chemotherapy (cancer treatment with chemicals)

To diagnose dysfunctional uterine bleeding, many of the potential causes mentioned above must be eliminated. When all potential causes connected with pregnancy, infection, and tumors (benign or malignant) are eliminated, then menorrhagia is presumed to be caused by dysfunctional uterine bleeding.

Diagnosis

Diagnosis of any menstrual irregularity begins with the patient herself. The doctor will ask for a detailed description of the problem, and take a history of how long it has existed, and any patterns the patient has observed. A woman can assist the doctor in diagnosing the cause of abnormal uterine bleeding by keeping a record of the time, frequency, length, and quantity of bleeding. She should also tell the doctor about any illnesses, including long-standing conditions, like **diabetes mellitus**. The doctor will also inquire about sexual activity, use of contraceptives, current medications, and past surgical procedures.

Laboratory tests

After taking the woman's history, the gynecologist or family practitioner does a pelvic examination and Pap smear. To rule out specific causes of abnormal bleeding, the doctor may also do a pregnancy test and blood tests to check the level of thyroid hormone. Based on the initial test results, the doctor may want to do tests to determine the level of other hormones that play a role in reproduction. A test of blood clotting time and an adrenal function test are also commonly done.

Imaging

Imaging tests are important diagnostic tools for evaluating abnormal uterine bleeding. Ultrasound examination of the pelvic and abdominal area is used to help locate **uterine fibroids**, also called uterine leiomyoma, a type of tumor. Visual examination through hysterscopy—where a camera inside a thin tube is inserted directly into the uterus so that the doctor can see the uterine lining—is also used to assess the condition of the uterus.

Hystersalpingography can help outline endometrial polyps and fibroids and help detect **endometrial cancer**. In this procedure an x ray is taken after contrast media has been injected into the cervix. **Magnetic resonance imaging** (MRI) of the pelvic region can also be used to locate fibroids and tumors.

Invasive procedures

Endometrial biopsy (the removal and examination of endometrial tissue) is the most important testing procedure. It allows the doctor to sample small areas of the uterine lining, while cervical biopsy allows the cervix to be sampled. Tissues are then examined for any abnormalities.

Dilatation and curettage (D & C), once common is rarely done today for diagnosis of DUB. It is done while the patient is under either general or regional anesthesia. Women over 30 are more likely to need a D & C, as part of the diagnostic procedure, than younger women.

Because DUB is diagnosed by eliminating other possible disorders, diagnosis can take a long time and involve many tests and procedures. Older women are likely to need more extensive tests than adolescents because the likelihood of reproductive cancers is greater in this age group, and therefore must be definitively eliminated before treating bleeding symptoms.

Treatment

Treatment of DUB depends on the cause of the bleeding and the age of the patient. When the underlying cause of the disorder is known, that disorder is treated. Otherwise the goal of treatment is to relieve the symptoms to a degree that uterine bleeding does not interfere with a woman's normal activities or cause anemia.

Generally the first approach to controlling DUB is to use **oral contraceptives** that provide a balance between the hormones estrogen and progesterone. Oral contraceptives are often very effective in adolescents and young women in their twenties. NSAIDs (**nonsteroidal anti-inflammatory drugs**), like Naprosyn and Motrin, are also used to treat DUB.

When bleeding cannot be controlled by hormone treatment, surgery may be necessary. Dilatation and curettage sometimes relieves the symptoms of DUB. If that fails, endometrial ablation removes the uterine lining, but preserves a woman's uterus. This procedure is sometimes be used instead of **hysterectomy**. However, as it affects the uterus, it can only be used when a woman has completed her childbearing years. The prescription of iron is also important to decrease the risk of enemia.

Until the 1980s, hysterectomy often was used to treat heavy uterine bleeding. Today hysterectomy is used less frequently to treat DUB, and then only after other methods of controlling the symptoms have failed. A hysterectomy leaves a woman unable to bear children, and, therefore, is limited largely to women who are unable to, or uninterested in, bearing children. Still, hysterectomy is a common treatment for long-standing DUB in women done with childbearing.

Alternative treatment

Alternative practitioners concentrate on good **nutrition** as a way to prevent heavy periods that are not caused by uterine fibroids, endometrial polyps, **endometriosis**, or **cancer**. Iron supplementation (100 mg per day) not only helps prevent anemia, but also appears to reduce menorrhagia in many women. Other recommended dietary supplements include **vitamins** A and C. Vitamin C improves capillary fragility and enhances iron uptake.

Vitamin E and bioflavonoid supplements are also recommended. Vitamin E can help reduce blood flow, and bioflavonoids help strengthen the capillaries. Vitamin K is known to play a role in clotting and is helpful in situations where heavy bleeding may be due to clotting abnormalities.

Botanical medicines used to assist in treating abnormal bleeding include spotted cranesbill (*Geranium maculatum*), birthroot (*Trillium pendulum*), blue cohosh (*Caulophyllum thalictroides*), witch hazel (*Hamamelis virginiana*), shepherd's purse (*Capsella bursa-pastoris*), and yarrow (*Achillea millifolia*). These are all stiptic herbs that act to tighten blood vessels and tissue. Hormonal balance can also be addressed with herbal formulations containing phytoestrogens and phytoprogesterone.

Prognosis

Response to treatment for DUB is highly individual and is not easy to predict. The outcome depends largely on the woman's medical condition and her age. Many women, especially adolescents, are successfully treated with hormones (usually oral contraceptives). As

KEY TERMS

Dilatation and curettage (D & C)—A procedure performed under anesthesia during which the cervix is dilated, and tissue lining the uterus is scraped out with a metal spoon-shaped instrument or a suction tube. The procedure can be either diagnostic, or to remove polyps.

Endometrial biopsy—The removal of tissue either by suction or scraping of samples of tissue from the uterus. The cervix is not dilated. The procedure has a lower rate of diagnostic accuracy than a D & C, but can be done as an office procedure under local anesthesia.

Endometrial cancer—Cancer of the inner mucous membrane of the uterus.

Fibroids, or fibroid tumors—Fibroid tumors are non-cancerous (benign) growths in the uterus. They occur in 30–40% of women over age 40, and do not need

to be removed unless they are causing symptoms that interfere with a woman's normal activities.

Hypothyroidism—A disorder in which the thyroid gland produces too little thyroid hormone causing a decrease in the rate of metabolism with associated effects on the reproductive system.

Lupus erythematosus—A chronic inflammatory disease in which inappropriate immune system reactions cause abnormalities in the blood vessels and connective tissue.

Progesterone—A hormone naturally secreted by the ovary, or manufactured synthetically, that prepares the uterus for implantation of a fertilized egg.

Prostaglandins—A group of chemicals that mediate, or determine the actions of other chemicals in the cell or body.

a last resort, hysterectomy removes the source of the problem by removing the uterus, but this operation is not without risk, or the possibility of complications.

Prevention

Dysfunctional uterine bleeding is not a preventable disorder.

Resources

OTHER

"Dysfunctional uterine bleeding (DUB)." MedlinePlus Medical Encyclopedia. September 2, 2009. http://www.nlm.nih.gov/medlineplus/ency/article/000903.htm (accessed November 23, 2010).

"Dysfunctional Uterine Bleeding: Menstrual Disorders and Abnormal Vaginal Bleeding." Merck Manual Home Edition. December 2008. http://www.merckmanuals.com/home/sec22/ch244/ch244e.html (accessed November 23, 2010).

Tish Davidson, A.M.

Dyslexia

Definition

Dyslexia is a learning disability noted for spatial reversals and shifts. It is characterized by problems in reading, spelling, writing, and sometimes math. In many cases, dyslexia appears to be inherited.

Demographics

Estimates of people with dyslexia range from 2–15% of the United States population. Most research studies give a figure of 5%. Originally it was thought that dyslexia affected more boys than girls (in a ratio of 5:1), but later studies found boys to be only slightly more likely than girls to be dyslexic. Figures for diagnosed child dyslexics are skewed because for various reasons boys tend to be referred more frequently for special education. Diagnosis is complicated by the fact that anywhere from 20–55% of dyslexics also suffer from attention deficit/hyperactivity disorder (**ADHD**), a behavioral disorder that may aggravate reading problems.

Description

Dyslexia is a specific learning disability characterized by a significant disparity between an individual's general intelligence and his or her language skills, usually reflected in school performance. The word dyslexia is derived from the Greek word, *dys* (meaning poor or inadequate) and the word *lexis* (meaning words or language). The term was coined in 1887 by German physician Rudolf Berlin who published a case study of a young boy who had difficulties with reading and writing in spite of having normal intelligence. In 1896, W. Pringle Morgan, a British doctor, published the first English-language case study of dyslexia. It concerned a 14-year-old boy who had not yet learned to read, even though his other intellectual abilities were well within the normal range.

A student with dyslexia has difficulty copying words. *(Will & Deni McIntyre/Science Source/Photo Researchers, Inc.)*

Most individuals with dyslexia have average or above average intelligence, and it is speculated that they have heightened visual-spatial and motor awareness. Many famous inventors, artists, and other creative people have had dyslexia; Thomas Edison, Albert Einstein, Winston Churchill, Michael Faraday, Woodrow Wilson, Guglielmo Marconi, General George Patton, and Auguste Rodin are all thought to have been dyslexic.

Risk factors

Dyslexia is believed to be strongly familial. About 40% of boys and 20% of girls with a dyslexic parent develop the disorder. Dyslexia is believed to occur equally in all races.

Causes and symptoms

There are many different theories about the causes and classifications of different types of dyslexia, but few hard conclusions. It is generally agreed that there is a strong hereditary component of dyslexia. Several genetic studies have found gene linkages on chromosomes 1 and 6 that demonstrate heterogeneous (multiple methods of) transmission. As of 2009, four specific genes linked to

dyslexia have been identified, and all four participate in brain development. **Positron emission tomography (PET)** studies have shown that dyslexics assigned reading tasks show a lower level of activity than children with normal reading skills in a part of the brain known as the left inferior parietal cortex, a region that is necessary for the rapid perception of word forms. Studies using functional **magnetic resonance imaging** (fMRI) pinpointed the left inferior frontal gyrus, the left inferior parietal lobule, and the left middle temporal gyrus as areas of low activation in dyslexic children given word tests to complete. Another indication that specific areas of the brain are involved in dyslexia comes from case studies of children who have suffered **stroke**. In one study reported in 2006, a six-year-old boy had suffered a stroke affecting the left hemisphere of his brain. He was able to read words that he had learned prior to the stroke, but attempts to read unfamiliar words were unsuccessful until he received special training.

The most obvious symptoms of the dyslexic show up in reading and writing; however, listening, speaking, and general organizational skills are also affected. The individual with dyslexia may have trouble transferring information across modalities, for example from verbal to written forms. The dyslexic's characteristic reversal of letters, confusion between such similar letters as "b" and "d," omission of words when reading aloud, trouble sounding out words, and difficulty following written instructions were first thought to be the result of vision and perceptual problems—that is, a failure of taking in the stimulus. Only a small percentage of dyslexics have vision disorders, however, and it is now generally agreed by physicians, researchers, and educators that dyslexia is primarily a language disorder. Whereas the non-dyslexic intuitively learns phonic (sound) rules while learning to read, the dyslexic needs specific and methodical drills and practice to learn the visual-auditory associations necessary for reading comprehension and written expression.

The most common symptoms of dyslexia include:

- lack of awareness of sounds
- delayed speech
- difficulty understanding spoken words
- difficulty reading single words
- extreme difficulty spelling words
- extreme difficulty with handwriting
- difficulty with locational and time indicators: up/down, right/left, yesterday/tomorrow
- lack of enjoyment in reading
- difficulty transferring information across modalities: writing down thoughts or speech, reading out loud

Diagnosis

Anyone who is suspected to have dyslexia should have a comprehensive evaluation, including hearing, vision, and intelligence testing. The test should include all areas of learning and learning processes, not just reading.

Currently, children and adults are usually referred for testing for dyslexia because of repeated problems in school or work settings. As further research pinpoints the genes responsible for some cases of dyslexia, there is a possibility that earlier testing will be established to allow for early interventions. Earlier interventions could help to prevent the negative educational outcomes that can be associated with dyslexia.

Tests

Children who demonstrate a reading level greater than two SEs below expected level for their age, intelligence, and education are generally diagnosed as dyslexic. Once reading problems are identified, a comprehensive series of tests of neuropsychological function (vision, hearing, and speech), intelligence, and achievement (word and letter recognition) will

determine the existence of visual and auditory problems, behavior problems, or subnormal intelligence, all of which may have symptoms similar to dyslexia. Because children of different ages have different levels of normal language skill, the specific tests used will differ by age group.

A child normally develops phonological awareness—the ability to differentiate between speech sounds and recognize their written symbols—while learning to read. The ability to sound out nonsense words (for example, the lines from Lewis Carroll's poem "Jabberwocky": "Twas brillig and the slithy toves/ Did gyre and gimble in the wabe") is a strong indicator of phonological awareness. In cases in which the dyslexic has compensated for the disability by paying special attention to context or simply by rote memorization, a nonsense-word test may reveal the reader's underlying phonological disability despite his academic success.

While teachers and physicians are trained to recognize some language problems, many symptoms of dyslexia will be noticeable to parents. Contrary to popular thought, a child's mirror writing (writing backwards), reversal of letters, and confusion over which hand to use are not definitively signs of dyslexia, and may only indicate lack of development.

Treatment

If caught early, especially before the third grade, dyslexia is highly treatable through special education. Dyslexia is categorized as a learning disability under the national Education for All Handicapped Children Act passed in 1975. Dyslexic children are entitled to a comprehensive evaluation by a team of educational specialists, to an individualized education plan (IEP), and to ongoing evaluation under the terms of the federal Individuals with Disabilities Education Act (IDEA), first passed in 1990 and amended in 2004. Parents or caretakers may request the initial evaluation, may participate in all levels of the process, and must give their consent before the treatment plan begins.

Traditional

There are many treatment approaches available to the public, ranging from visual stimulation to **diets** to enhancement of regular language education. But it is generally agreed that specialized education is the only successful remedy, and the American Academy of Ophthalmology, the American Academy of Pediatrics, and the American Association for Pediatric Ophthalmology and **Strabismus** have issued a policy statement warning against visual treatments and recommending

KEY TERMS

Attention deficit disorder (ADD)—A learning disability characterized by an inability to pay attention. It may be different from dyslexia in that dyslexic individuals are highly aware and able to pay attention, but unable to make sense of their perceptions.

Attention deficit hyperactivity disorder (ADHD)—A learning disability characterized by an inability to sit still or concentrate well. It has been demonstrated to be diagnostically different from dyslexia by speech and vocalization patterns.

Monoamine oxidase (MAO) inhibitors—A group of anti-depressant drugs.

Neurotransmitter—A chemical substance which facilitates the passing of messages along nerve pathways. There are several different neurotransmitters used in the human nervous system, each with distinct effects on mood, movement and perception.

Point of view—In a person with dyslexia, this term is used to describe the angle from which their mind's eye views an object. This point of view may be unanchored and moving about, as if several different people were telling what they see all at the same time.

a cross-disciplinary educational approach. In fact, the first researcher to identify and study dyslexia, Dr. Samuel Torrey Orton, developed the core principles of such an approach in the 1920s. The work of three of his followers—Bessie Stillman, Anna Gillingham, and Beth Slingerland—underlies many of the programs in wide use today such as project READ, the Wilson Reading System, and programs based on the Herman method. These and other successful programs have three characteristics in common. They are:

- Sound/symbol based. They break words down into their smallest visual components: letters and the sounds associated with them.

- Multisensory. They attempt to form and strengthen mental associations among visual, auditory, and kinesthetic channels of stimulation. The student simultaneously sees, feels, and says the sound-symbol association; for example, a child may trace the letter or letter combination with his finger while pronouncing a word out loud.

- Highly structured. Remediation begins at the level of the single letter-sound, works up to digraphs, then syllables, then into words and sentences in a very systematic fashion. Repetitive drill and practice serve to form necessary sound-symbol associations.

Whatever remediation program is used, the IEP itself should define the student's specific problems and learning objectives, rather than make vague or general recommendations such as "John needs more support in reading comprehension." A good example of a specific learning objective would be "Max will be able to identify the following sound/symbol association in nonsense words: consonants, short and long vowels, and blends." When ADD is co-diagnosed with dyslexia, special care should be taken to identify

specific reading problems and to define cognitive as well as behavioral learning objectives.

Drugs

Treatment for dyslexia can sometimes include use of anti-motion drugs, addressing the symptoms of balance and coordination which results from visual perception alterations; stimulant drugs, such as pemoline (Cylert) or methylphenidate (Ritalin), to address symptoms of low self esteem, restlessness, and distractibility, and 'nootropics' drugs, a class of drugs believed to improve cognitive function. The stimulant drugs may be more effective for **learning disorders** related to ADHD or ADD than for dyslexia. The drug piracetam (Nootropil), a nootropic, although reported as a possible treatment for dyslexia, is also reported to have legal issues because it has not been approved for use in the United States by the Food and Drug Administration (FDA).

Reported potential side effects of the stimulants include nervousness and **insomnia**, and are contra-indicated with **epilepsy**, **allergies**, blood pressure problems, or with use of monoamine oxidase (MAO) inhibitors. Long-term use of stimulants in children are reported to adversely affect growth, may ironically depress the nervous system or lead to loss of consciousness. By reducing natural levels of stimulants in the brain, they may also cause dependence. The stimulants and nootropics are said to increase the effects of alcohol and amphetamines. Other possible interactions include use of anti-convulsants or anti-epileptics; tricyclic anti-depressants; anti-coagulants, like Coumadin; and "atropine-like drugs" that blocks the neurotransmitter acetylcholine.

Alternative

Ronald D. Davis, writing in *The Gift of Dyslexia* outlines an alternative and complementary treatment consistent with the "moving point of view" model. According to this model, and the reason why letters seem to change shape and float, why lines of print appear to move, and why words appear to be other than they are is that the dyslexic individual sees the world predominantly through his or her "mind's eye," rather than through his or her physiologic eye. In other words, people with dyslexia more than all others, sees what they 'think' they see, rather than what their eyeballs see. To further complicate matters, they do this so quickly that they easily become confused when the multiple facets do not produce a solid view.

The object of treatment proposed by Ronald Davis, a dyslexic individual himself, is to train the mind's eye to return to a learned, anchored, viewpoint when they realize they are seeing with their mind, and not with their eyeballs. This is accomplished with assessment testing, followed by one-on-one exercises that retrain mental perception pathways. Using the gifts of the dyslexic individual—their imagination and curiosity—these exercises involve creative physical activities, including the use of modeling clay, "koosh" balls, and movement training. Davis founded the Reading Research Council's Dyslexia Correction Center in 1982, and the Davis Dyslexia Association International, which trains educators and therapists, in 1995.

Prognosis

If left unaddressed, a person with dyslexia may become "functionally illiterate," able to function limited by their ability to read, spell, have their handwriting understood, or do arithmetic. Recognizing that dyslexia is a developed learning disorder affecting people of extraordinary curiosity, imagination and intelligence—people of genius, often— from a productive or functional point of view, dyslexia may contribute significantly, positively or negatively, to performance levels. From an emotional or psychological point of view, dyslexia affects self esteem, and promotes confusion and frustration, that may contribute to under achievement.

Many people with dyslexia becoming very successful. The eventual outcome for an individual with dyslexia depends on a wide variety of factors, including severity of the disorder, age of diagnosis, and achievement level in other non-language areas. Early diagnosis and intervention are important in improving long-term outcomes.

Prevention

There is no known way to prevent dyslexia.

Resources

BOOKS

Berninger, Virginia W., and Beverly Wolf. *Teaching Students with Dyslexia and Dysgraphia: Lessons From Teaching and Science.* Baltimore: Paul H. Brooks Publishing, 2009.

Brunswick, Nicola. *Dyslexia: A Beginner's Guide.* Oxford: Oneworld, 2009.

Pugh, Ken, and Peggy McCardle, eds. *How Children Learn to Read: Current Issues and New Directions in the Integration of Cognition, Neurobiology, and Genetics of Reading and Dyslexia Research and Practice.* New York: Psychology Press, 2009.

Reid, Gavin, ed. *The Routledge Companion to Dyslexia.* New York: Routledge, 2009.

PERIODICALS

American Academy of Pediatrics, Section on Ophthalmology, Council on Children with Disabilities. American Academy of Ophthalmology. American Association for Pediatric Ophthalmology and Strabismus. American Association of Certified Orthoptists "Joint Statement-Learning Disabilities, Dyslexia, and Vision." *Pediatrics,* (August 2009), 837-844.

Gabriele, J.D. "Dyslexia: A New Synergy Between Education and Cognitive Neuroscience." *Science* (July 17, 2009), 325.

ORGANIZATIONS

Council for Learning Disabilities, 11184 Antioch Road, Box 405, Overland Park, KS, 66210, (913) 491-1011, (913)491-1012, http://www.cldinternational.org.

International Dyslexia Association, 40 York Road, 4th Floor, Baltimore, MD, 21204, (410) 296-0232, (410) 321-5069, http://www.interdys.org.

Katy Nelson, N.D.
Tish Davidson, A.M.

Dyslipidemia *see* **Hyperlipoproteinemia**

Dysmenorrhea

Definition

Dysmenorrhea is the occurrence of painful cramps during a woman's menstrual period. The English word comes from three Greek words that mean "painful," "month," and "flow." Most women experience some discomfort during their periods; however, dysmenorrhea is diagnosed when the **pain** is so severe as to limit the woman's normal activities or require medical or surgical treatment.

Demographics

Dysmenorrhea is by definition a disorder that affects only females of childbearing age. Some studies indicate that the rate of dysmenorrhea is highest among adolescents and young adults, and declines with age. Survey results are highly variable, ranging from 29% in one family practice setting to 90% in a group of Swedish adolescents. One group of researchers reported that 67% of teenagers in their sample reported dysmenorrhea, compared to 27% of women in their 30s. Primary dysmenorrhea is the leading cause of recurrent short-term absence from school among adolescent American girls. In the workplace, dysmenorrhea causes 600 million missed work hours in the United States each year and an economic loss of $2 billion.

Secondary dysmenorrhea is more common in older women than in teenagers; in general, women who experience dysmenorrhea for the first time after age 25 have secondary dysmenorrhea.

As far as is known as of 2010, race or ethnicity is not a risk factor for dysmenorrhea.

Description

Women with dysmenorrhea describe the pain in their abdomens as variously shooting, stabbing, burning, sharp, throbbing, or nauseating. Dysmenorrhea may precede the onset of the woman's period by several days, or accompany it. It usually subsides as the woman's flow tapers off.

In some women, dysmenorrhea is accompanied by unusually heavy blood loss—a condition known as menorrhagia.

Risk factors

The likelihood that a woman will have painful cramps increases if she:

- has a family history of painful periods
- leads a stressful life
- smokes
- has never borne a child
- is below 20 years of age
- began puberty before age 11
- has heavy periods
- doesn't get enough exercise
- drinks large quantities of beverages containing caffeine (coffee, tea, cola, energy drinks)
- has attempted to lose weight rapidly

- has pelvic inflammatory disease (PID)
- has a history of sexual abuse

Causes and symptoms

Dysmenorrhea is called "primary" when there is no specific abnormality, and "secondary" when the pain is caused by an underlying gynecological problem. It is believed that primary dysmenorrhea occurs when prostaglandins, hormone-like substances produced by uterine tissue, trigger strong muscle contractions in the uterus during menstruation. However, the level of prostaglandins does not seem to correlate with how strong a woman's cramps are. Some women have high levels of prostaglandins and no cramps, whereas other women with low levels have severe cramps. This is why experts assume that cramps must also be related to other causes, such as **diets**, genetics, **stress**, and different body types, in addition to prostaglandins. The first year or two of a girl's periods are not usually very painful. However, once ovulation begins, the blood levels of the prostaglandins rise, leading to stronger contractions.

Secondary dysmenorrhea may be caused by **endometriosis**, fibroids, **ovarian cysts**, an **ectopic pregnancy**, or an infection in the pelvis.

Symptoms of dysmenorrhea include a dull, throbbing cramping in the lower abdomen that may radiate to the lower back and thighs. In addition, some women may experience **nausea and vomiting**; **diarrhea** or **constipation**; hypersensitivity to lights, sounds, or odors; general irritability and **fatigue**; heavy sweating; or **dizziness**. Cramps usually last for two or three days at the beginning of each menstrual period. Many women often notice their painful periods disappear after they have their first child, probably due to the stretching of the opening of the uterus or because the birth improves the uterine blood supply and muscle activity, although other women do not notice a change in their level of menstrual discomfort after **childbirth**.

Diagnosis

A doctor should perform a thorough **pelvic exam** and take a patient history to rule out any underlying condition that could cause unusually painful cramps. The patient history will include such information as the patient's age at the time of her first period, family history of painful periods, sexual activity (if any), method of **contraception** used (if any), number of children, the regularity of the menstrual cycle, the cycle's length, date of the last menstrual period, and duration and amount of menstrual flow.

KEY TERMS

Cervix—The neck or lower narrow portion of the uterus that opens into the upper end of the vagina.

Ectopic pregnancy—A pregnancy in which the fertilized egg has implanted outside the uterus, most often in the Fallopian tubes, although in some cases the pregnancy implants in the ovary or in the abdomen. A ruptured ectopic pregnancy is a medical emergency.

Endometrioma—A type of cyst formed when endometrial tissue grows within the ovary.

Endometriosis—The growth of uterine tissue outside the uterus.

Fibroids—Benign (noncancerous) growths that arise from the smooth muscle layer and connective tissue of the uterus. They sometimes cause secondary dysmenorrhea.

Hormone—A chemical messenger secreted by a gland and released into the blood, where it travels to distant cells to exert an effect.

Hysterectomy—Surgical removal of the entire uterus.

Menorrhagia—Unusually heavy or prolonged menstrual period. It may or may not be associated with dysmenorrhea.

Ovary—One of the two almond-shaped glands in the female body that produces the hormones estrogen and progesterone.

Ovulation—The monthly release of an egg from an ovary.

Progesterone—The hormone produced by the ovary after ovulation that prepares the uterine lining for a fertilized egg.

Uterus—The female reproductive organ that contains and nourishes a fetus from implantation of the fertilized egg until birth.

Examination

An office examination of the patient's abdomen is usually sufficient in adolescents who have not been sexually active. Women who are sexually active should have a pelvic examination.

Tests

There are no laboratory tests that can be used to diagnose primary dysmenorrhea; however, the doctor may order a blood test to rule out a systemic infection, or take a smear of the cervix to evaluate the patient for a sexually transmitted disease.

If the abdominal and pelvic examinations suggest secondary dysmenorrhea, an ultrasound of the pelvis is the next step in evaluating endometriosis or ovarian cysts as possible causes of the dysmenorrhea. Other imaging studies that can be used include CT scans and MRIs.

Procedures

The doctor may recommend either a **hysteroscopy** or a **laparoscopy** to check for such causes of secondary dysmenorrhea as fibroids, ovarian cysts, endometriosis, or an ectopic **pregnancy**. In a hysteroscopy, the doctor inserts a thin lighted tube called an endoscope into the uterine cavity. The doctor can remove a small sample of uterine tissue for biopsy as well as examining the interior of the uterus visually. In a laparoscopy, the doctor makes small incisions in the skin of the abdomen and inserts an endoscope with a small camera lens. Laparoscopy can also be used for surgical removal of endometriomas, which are a type of cyst formed when endometrial tissue grows inside the ovaries rather than in the uterus. In extreme cases, the doctor may recommend a hysterectomy—surgical removal of the entire uterus.

A qualified physician is required in order to fit a woman with the Mirena (an intrauterine device described below). The woman's cervix must be dilated before insertion; the process is uncomfortable, and some doctors use a local anesthetic to reduce discomfort.

Treatment

Traditional

Drugs

Several over-the-counter medications can lessen or completely eliminate the pain of primary dysmenorrhea. Most popular are the **nonsteroidal anti-inflammatory drugs** (NSAIDs), which prevent or decrease the formation of prostaglandins. These include **aspirin**, ibuprofen (Advil), and naproxen (Aleve). For more severe pain, prescription-strength ibuprofen (Motrin) is available. These drugs are usually begun at the first sign of the period and taken for a day or two. Although NSAIDs are effective in providing short-term relief from cramps, some researchers think that long-term use of these medications increases the risk of side effects, particularly diarrhea and peptic ulcer.

If an NSAID is not available, **acetaminophen** (Tylenol) may also help ease the pain. Heat applied to the painful area may bring relief, and a warm bath twice a day also may help.

Hormonal therapy is another approach to dysmenorrhea that works for many women, although it involves prescription medications rather than over-the-counter pain relievers. Birth control pills and **Depo-Provera**, an injected contraceptive that must be given every 3 months, work by preventing ovulation. Depo-Provera is also given as a treatment for endometriosis as well as contraception.

Studies of a drug patch containing glyceryl trinitrate to treat dysmenorrhea suggest that it also may help ease pain. This drug has been used in the past to ease preterm contractions in pregnant women. One common side effect of the patch, however, is **headache**.

In 2002, an intrauterine device (**IUD**) was introduced to help eliminate the pain of menstrual cramps related to endometriosis. The IUD, known as Mirena, is approved for use in the United States as a contraceptive. The device works by releasing small amounts of progestin (a hormone) as well as preventing a fertilized egg from implanting in the lining of the uterus. Mirena cannot, however, be used by women with a history of **pelvic inflammatory disease**, current **gonorrhea** or chlamydia infection, or cervical or **breast cancer**.

There are two drugs that can be given to completely suppress menstrual periods—danazol (Danocrine) and leuprolide acetate (Lupron). These are generally regarded as treatments of last resort for secondary dysmenorrhea that is not helped by other medications. Both Danocrine and Lupron are expensive drugs with severe side effects.

Alternative

There are a variety of alternative therapies for dysmenorrhea. As of 2010, however, most of these have not been well studied.

NUTRITIONAL THERAPY. The following dietary changes may help prevent or treat menstrual pain:

- Increased dietary intake of foods such as fiber, calcium, soy foods, fruits and vegetables.
- Decreased consumption of foods that exacerbate PMS. They include caffeine, salt and sugar.
- Quitting smoking. Smoking has been found to worsen cramps.

- Taking daily multi-vitamin and mineral supplements that contain high doses of magnesium and vitamin B_6 (pyridoxine), and flaxseed or fish oil supplements. Recent research suggests that vitamin B supplements, primarily vitamin B_6 in complex, magnesium, calcium, zinc, vitamin E, and fish oil supplements (omega-3 fatty acids) also may help relieve cramps.

HERBAL THERAPY. An herbalist may recommend one of the following herbal remedies for menstrual pain:

- Chasteberry (*Vitex agnus-castus*) for women who also experience breast pain, irregular periods, and ovarian cysts.
- Dong quai (*Angelica sinensis*) for women with typical menstrual pain.
- Licorice (*Glycyrrhiza glabra*) for abdominal bloating and cramping.
- Black cohosh (*Cimifuga racemosa*) for relief of menstrual pain as well as mood swing and depression.

PHYSICAL EXERCISE. Several **yoga** positions are popular as methods to ease menstrual pain. In the "cat stretch" position, the woman rests on her hands and knees, slowly arching the back. The pelvic tilt is another popular yoga position, in which the woman lies with knees bent, and then lifts the pelvis and buttocks.

Exercise may be a way to reduce the pain of menstrual cramps through the brain's production of endorphins, the body's own painkillers.

OTHER REMEDIES. Acupuncture and Chinese herbs are other popular alternative treatments for cramps. There are particular formulas depending on the pattern of imbalance. **Aromatherapy** and massage may ease pain for some women. Transcutaneous **electrical nerve stimulation** (TENS) has been touted as a safe and practical way to relieve the pain of dysmenorrhea. It works by using electrodes to stimulate nerve fibers. Some women find relief through visualization, concentrating on the pain as a particular color and gaining control of the sensations. Others find that imagining a white light hovering over the painful area can actually lessen the pain for brief periods. Simply changing the position of the body can help ease cramps. The simplest technique is assuming the fetal position with knee pulled up to the chest while hugging a heating pad or pillow to the abdomen. Also, orgasm can make a woman feel more comfortable by releasing tension in the pelvic muscles.

Prognosis

Dysmenorrhea is a treatable condition with a good-to-excellent prognosis in most women. As noted above, most adolescents with primary dysmenorrhea outgrow their painful cramps as they enter their 20s and 30s. Older women with secondary dysmenorrhea usually do well after surgery to remove fibroids or endometriomas; some of these procedures can be done in outpatient surgical clinics. A complete **hysterectomy** is usually done as an inpatient procedure, but most women recover without complications.

Prevention

Most of the causes of secondary dysmenorrhea cannot be prevented as of 2010. However, avoidance of **caffeine**, alcohol, and sugar prior to the onset of the period, and NSAIDs taken a day before the period begins may eliminate cramps for some women with primary dysmenorrhea.

Resources

BOOKS

Emans, S. Jean Herriot, Marc R. Laufer, and Donald P. Goldstein. *Pediatric and Adolescent Gynecology*, 5th ed. Philiadelphia: Lippincott Williams and Wilkins, 2005.

Goodwin, T. Murphy, et al., eds. *Management of Common Problems in Obstetrics and Gynecology*, 5th ed. Chichester, West Sussex: Wiley-Blackwell, 2010.

Gordon, Catherine M., et al., eds. *The Menstrual Cycle and Adolescent Health*. Boston, MA: Blackwell, 2008.

PERIODICALS

Cho, S.H., and E.W. Hwang. "Acupuncture for Primary Dysmenorrhoea: A Systematic Review." *BJOG* 117 (April 2010): 509–21.

Guerrera, M.P., et al. "Therapeutic Uses of Magnesium." *American Family Physician* 80 (July 15, 2009): 157–62.

Lloyd, K.B., and L.B. Hornsby. "Complementary and Alternative Medications for Women's Health Issues." *Nutrition in Clinical Practice* 24 (October-November 2009): 589–608.

Morrow, C., and E.H. Naumburg. "Dysmenorrhea." *Primary Care* 36 (March 2009): 19–32.

Quinn, M. "Endometriosis: The Elusive Epiphenomenon." *Journal of Obstetrics and Gynecology* 29 (October 2009): 590–93.

Rose, S., et al. "Mirena (Levonorgestrel Intrauterine System): A Successful Novel Drug Delivery Option in Contraception." *Advanced Drug Delivery Reviews* 61 (August 10, 2009): 808–12.

Zahradnik, H.P., et al. "Nonsteroidal Anti-inflammatory Drugs and Hormonal Contraceptives for Pain Relief from Dysmenorrhea: A Review." *Contraception* 81 (March 2010): 185–96.

OTHER

American Congress of Obstetricians and Gynecologists (ACOG). *Dysmenorrhea*. http://www.acog.org/publications/patient_education/bp046.cfm

Calis, Karim Anton, et al. "Dysmenorrhea." *eMedicine*, January 28, 2009. http://emedicine.medscape.com/article/253812-overview

French, Linda. "Dysmenorrhea." *American Family Physician* 71 (January 15, 2005): 285–91. http://www.aafp.org/afp/2005/0115/p285.html

Mayo Clinic. *Menstrual Cramps*. http://www.mayoclinic.com/health/menstrual-cramps/DS00506

MedlinePlus Medical Encyclopedia. *Painful Menstrual Periods*. http://www.nlm.nih.gov/medlineplus/ency/article/003150.htm

ORGANIZATIONS

American Congress of Obstetricians and Gynecologists (ACOG), 409 12th St., S.W., P.O. Box 96920, Washington, DC, 20090-6920, (202) 638-5577, resources@acog.org, http://www.acog.org/.

Society for Adolescent Health and Medicine (SAHM), 111 Deer Lake Road, Suite 100, Deerfield, IL, 60015, (847) 753-5226, (847) 480-9282, info@adolescenthealth.org, http://www.adolescenthealth.org.

Mai Tran
Teresa G. Odle
Rebecca J. Frey, PhD

Dysmetria *see* **Movement disorders**

Dyspareunia

Definition

Dyspareunia is painful sexual intercourse in women. It is **pain** in the genitals or pelvis that is persistent or recurrent and is experienced at any time before, during, or following sexual intercourse. Dyspareunia usually results from a physical problem but can also stem from psychological difficulties.

Demographics

About 20% of women experience pain with intercourse at some point in their lives and it is estimated that one to two percent of women suffer from dyspareunia. However the true incidence may be higher since many women with dyspareunia do not seek help. The incidence of dyspareunia is significantly higher in women who have been raped or otherwise sexually abused.

Description

There are two types of dyspareunia. Primary dyspareunia begins with the onset of sexual activity and persists. Acquired or secondary dyspareunia occurs after some period of normal sexual function. Occasional discomfort or pain during intercourse is not unusual and is not considered to be dyspareunia.

The American Psychiatric Association's *Diagnostic and Statistical Manual of Mental Disorders*, fourth edition, text revised (*DSM-IV-TR*), classifies dyspareunia as a **sexual dysfunction**. However this listing is controversial, and some practitioners argue that it should be reclassified as a pain disorder in *DSM-V*.

The pain associated with dyspareunia may be confined to the genitals or can be located anywhere within the pelvis. Women with dyspareunia often have **vaginismus**, an involuntary tightening or spasm of the vaginal muscles in response to penetration, which can make intercourse painful or impossible.

Dyspareunia can cause embarrassment or shame. It can lead to relationship problems and may cause a woman to avoid sexual relationships altogether.

Risk factors

Risk factors for dyspareunia include:

- infection or another medical problem
- certain medications, such as antidepressants or high blood pressure medicines
- depression or anxiety
- emotional or psychological stress, especially with regard to a woman's relationship with her sexual partner
- a history of sexual abuse

Causes and symptoms

Primary dyspareunia can result from psychosocial as well as physical factors. Once a woman associates sex with pain, she may find it difficult to relax and become aroused, leading to dyspareunia:

- Prior sexual trauma—such as rape or childhood sexual abuse—can cause dyspareunia. Even when a woman later desires sex, the act of intercourse may trigger memories of the trauma and interfere with her enjoyment. Vaginismus is common in such situations.
- Misinformation or lack of information about sex, a belief that sex is wrong or evil, or fear of sex can lead to dyspareunia.
- A painful initial sexual experience can cause a woman to associate sex with pain.

- Guilt, anxiety, tension, or fear of pregnancy can prevent sexual arousal and cause the vaginal muscles to tense.

Secondary dyspareunia also can have both physical and psychological causes. A clear physical cause for dyspareunia can be identified in about 30–40% of women who consult a sex counselor for this condition. Dyspareunia in postmenopausal women usually results from lack of natural lubrication due to low estrogen levels. Estrogen deficiency can also cause dyspareunia after **childbirth** or while **breastfeeding**. Conditions that affect the skin around the vagina may cause pain during the insertion of a tampon, or even while sitting or wearing pants, as well as during sexual intercourse. Other physical causes of secondary dyspareunia include:

- lack of foreplay, causing vaginal dryness
- a yeast, vaginal, or urinary tract infection
- herpes sores, genital warts, or other sexually transmitted infections (STIs)
- inflammation of the vagina
- vulvar vestibulitis, an unexplained stinging or burning around the opening of the vagina
- eczema or other skin problems in the genital area
- genital irritation from soaps, detergents, douches, or feminine hygiene products
- injury to the vagina and/or surrounding tissues from an accident, pelvic surgery, female circumcision, or episiotomy, which can also cause vaginismus
- intercourse too soon after surgery or childbirth
- an improperly fitted diaphragm or cervical cap for birth control
- an allergic or other reaction to a birth control product such as foams, jellies, or a latex diaphragm or condom
- certain medications that may decrease sexual desire or arousal and natural lubrication, including antidepressants, high blood pressure medications, sedatives, antihistamines, or certain birth control pills

Pain that is felt deep in the pelvis, that occurs with deep penetration, that occurs only in certain positions, or that occurs with orgasm can result from lack of arousal or tension, but is much more likely to be indicative of a medical problem such as:

- fibroid growths in the uterus
- a tipped uterus
- a prolapsed uterus—a uterus that has slipped into the vagina—or a retroverted uterus
- infections in the cervix, uterus, or fallopian tubes

• an ovarian infection or certain other ovarian conditions such as cysts, especially if the pain is experienced only in certain sexual positions

• past surgery resulting in scar tissue, such as a hysterectomy

• endometriosis

• pelvic inflammatory disease

• cystitis

• irritable bowel syndrome

• hemorrhoids

• radiation or chemotherapy treatments for cancer

Vasocongestion—the unrelieved accumulation of blood in the dilated blood vessels—can cause dyspareunia. The pelvic area normally becomes congested with blood during sexual arousal. Orgasm quickly relieves this congestion. Dyspareunia from vasocongestion can occur when frequent arousal does not result in orgasm.

Psychological factors that can interfere with arousal and lead to painful intercourse include:

• anxiety or depression that leads to loss of interest in sex

• concerns about one's physical appearance

• fear of intimacy

• stress, which can affect the muscles of the pelvic floor

• relationship problems, including an abusive or emotionally distant sexual partner, loss of attraction to a partner, or fear that a partner has lost interest

Like the causes of dyspareunia, symptoms can vary greatly. The most common symptom of dyspareunia is pain at the vaginal opening as the penis enters the vagina. Entry may be difficult and the pain may be sharp or burning. The vagina may feel very dry; however the pain often occurs only upon initial penetration. Pain deep within the pelvis can resemble menstrual cramps. The pain may eventually ease or may continue throughout intercourse or as long as thrusting continues. Vasocongestion can cause an aching pain in the pelvic region that persists for hours after intercourse. Some women experience pain only with particular partners or under certain circumstances.

Diagnosis

Examination

A complete medical and sexual history and a gynecological exam including a **pelvic exam** may be necessary to determine the physical cause of dyspareunia. The type and location of the pain and the circumstances under which it occurs can be important clues as to the underlying cause. The examination

---

KEY TERMS

Estrogen—A female hormone produced by the ovaries that stimulates the growth of the lining of the uterus.

Sexually transmitted infection (STI)—An infectious disease that is transmitted through sexual activity.

Vaginismus—A painful spasmodic vaginal contraction.

Vulvar vestibulitis—A localized inflammation of the vestibule—the region immediately surrounding the opening of the vagina and the urethra.

---

should include questions about sexual activities as they relate to the pain. A psychological evaluation can help identify possible psychosocial causes for the disorder. Women who have been raped or abused may suffer from **post-traumatic stress disorder** (PTSD) or **generalized anxiety disorder** as well as dyspareunia.

Tests

Laboratory tests may be performed to test for yeast, bacterial, or other types of infection, including STIs. Urine or **allergy tests** may also be performed.

Procedures

In some cases a **pelvic ultrasound** or **laparoscopy** may be necessary to determine the physical cause underlying dyspareunia. Laparoscopy is a procedure in which a slender instrument called a laparoscope is used to view the pelvic organs.

Treatment

Traditional

Treatment of dyspareunia involves addressing the underlying problem, whether it is physical, psychological, or emotional. Dyspareunia can usually be treated by personal changes or medications. Only rarely is surgery required to treat an underlying problem.

Women whose dyspareunia is accompanied by vaginismus may be given a set of devices to use at home to dilate the vaginal opening. These aides retrain the vaginal muscles and help prevent the involuntary muscle tightening that is characteristic of vaginismus. Starting with a very small device, the woman uses progressively larger devices as she overcomes her pain or fear, eventually working up to a penis-sized device.

Counseling can be helpful for identifying and reframing negative feelings about sex. Women who have been abused or raped may benefit from counseling techniques that are designed to help overcome the fears and issues resulting from traumatic experiences. Couples therapy can improve communication between partners and resolve problems that may be affecting their sexual relationship. **Sex therapy** can provide information about the physical aspects of arousal and orgasm. A sex therapist will offer suggestions for improving sexual techniques. For example increased foreplay and allowing the woman to control the timing and method of penetration may help her relax and become more easily aroused.

Drugs

There are no specific medications for treating dyspareunia:

- Antibiotics or antiviral drugs may be required for urinary tract infections, STIs, or vaginal infections.
- Over-the-counter or prescription estrogen creams, tablets, or a flexible vaginal ring can often relieve dyspareunia in postmenopausal women.
- A medication may need to be changed if it is interfering with natural lubrication.
- Medications that increase blood flow or relax muscles can be helpful in some situations.
- Stool softeners can relieve dyspareunia caused by hemorrhoids.

Alternative

Desensitization training can teach vaginal relaxation exercises to decrease pain during intercourse.

Home remedies

The use of a vaginal lubricant, even temporarily, can often relieve dyspareunia. Kegal or pelvic–floor exercises also can decrease dyspareunia.

Prognosis

With treatment dyspareunia can usually be overcome, allowing for satisfying sexual relationships. However treatment can take several months, particularly for survivors of violent trauma such as **rape**. Persistent dyspareunia can cause women to lose all interest in sex.

Prevention

Methods for preventing dyspareunia include:

- communicating with one's partner about what is sexually pleasurable or painful
- prolonging foreplay to stimulate arousal and lubrication
- using a water- or silicone-based lubricant
- avoiding scented bath products such as shower gel and body washes, which can irritate the genitals and interfere with natural lubrication
- avoiding douching
- waiting at least six weeks after childbirth before resuming intercourse
- changing sexual positions; for example a woman may be better able to control penetration if she is on top

Resources

BOOKS

American Psychiatric Association. *Diagnostic and Statistical Manual of Mental Disorders,* 4th ed., text rev. (*DSM-IV-TR.*) Arlington, VA: American Psychiatric Association, 2007.

Bilheimer, Susan, and Robert J. Echenberg. *Secret Suffering: How Women's Sexual and Pelvic Pain Affects Their Relationships.* Santa Barbara, CA: Praeger/ABC–CLIO, 2009.

Goldstein, Andrew, Caroline F. Pukall, and Irwin Goldstein. *Female Sexual Pain Disorders.* Hoboken, NJ: Wiley–Blackwell, 2009.

Meana, Marta. "Painful Intercourse: Dyspareunia and Vaginismus." In Katherine M. Hertlein, Gerald R. Weeks, and Nancy Gambescia. *Systemic Sex Therapy.* New York: Routledge, 2009.

Rosenfeld, Jo Ann. *Handbook of Women's Health,* 2nd ed. New York: Cambridge University Press, 2009.

PERIODICALS

Binik, Yitzchak. "The DSM Diagnostic Criteria for Dyspareunia." *Archives of Sexual Behavior* 39(2) (April 2010): 292.

Brauer, Marieke, et al. "Automatic and Deliberate Affective Associations with Sexual Stimuli in Women with Superficial Dyspareunia." *Archives of Sexual Behavior.* 38(4) (August 2009): 486–97.

Edwards, Anne, and Michael L. Bowen. "Dyspareunia." *Practice Nurse* 39(1) (January 15, 2010): 26–30.

Kellogg–Spadt, Susan, Jennifer Fariello, and Pegah Safaeian. "Clinical Update: Dyspareunia in Women" *Female Patient* 33(2) (February 2008): 26.

Meana, Marta, and Amy Lykins. "Negative Affect and Somatically Focused Anxiety in Young Women Reporting Pain With Intercourse." *Journal of Sex Research* 46(1) (January 2009): 80–8.

Steege J. F., et al. "Evaluation and Treatment of Dyspareunia." *Obstetrics and Gynecology* 113 (2009): 1124.

OTHER

Editorial Staff. "Dyspareunia: Painful Sex for Women." FamilyDoctor.org. http://familydoctor.org/online/famdocen/home/women/reproductive/sex-dys/669.html (accessed September 25, 2010).

Mayo Clinic Staff. "Painful Intercourse (Dyspareunia)." MayoClinic.com. http://www.mayoclinic.com/print/painful–intercourse/DS01044 (accessed September 25, 2010).

National Library of Medicine. "Female Sexual Dysfunction." MedlinePlus. http://www.nlm.nih.gov/medlineplus/femalesexualdysfunction.html (accessed September 25, 2010).

"Sexual Intercourse—Painful." MedlinePlus. http://www.nlm.nih.gov/medlineplus/ency/article/003157.htm (accessed September 25, 2010).

ORGANIZATIONS

American Academy of Family Physicians (AAFP), 11400 Tomahawk Creek Pkwy., Leawood, KS, 66211–2680, (913) 906–6000, (800) 274–6000, (913) 906–6075, http://www.aafp.org/online/en/home.html.

American College of Obstetricians and Gynecologists (ACOG), PO Box 96920, Washington, DC, 20090–6920, (202) 638–5577, (800) 673–8444, resources@acog.org, http://www.acog.org.

Jody Bower, MSW
Emily Jane Willingham, PhD
Margaret Alic, PhD

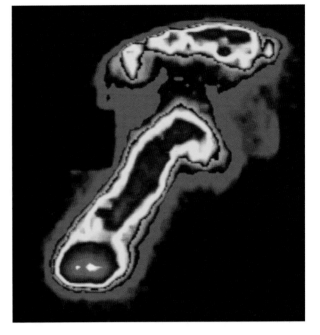

A false-color gamma scan of a human stomach with dyspepsia, or indigestion, during tests to study its rate of emptying. *(Custom Medical Stock Photo, Inc. Reproduced by permission.)*

Dyspepsia

Definition

Dyspepsia can be defined as painful, difficult, or disturbed digestion, which may be accompanied by symptoms such as **nausea and vomiting**, **heartburn**, bloating, and stomach discomfort.

Causes and symptoms

The digestive problems may have an identifiable cause, such as bacterial or viral infection, peptic ulcer, gallbladder, or **liver disease**. The bacteria *Helicobacter pylori* is often found in those individuals suffering from duodenal or gastric ulcers. Investigation of recurrent **indigestion** should rule out these possible causes.

Often, there is no organic cause for the problem, in which case dyspepsia is classified as functional or non-ulcer dyspepsia. There is evidence that functional dyspepsia may be related to abnormal motility of the upper gastrointestinal tract (a state known as dysmotility in which the esophagus, stomach, and upper intestine behave abnormally). These patients may respond to a group of drugs called prokinate agents. A review of eating habits (e.g., chewing with the mouth open, gulping food, or talking while chewing) may reveal a tendency to swallow air. This may contribute to feeling bloated, or to

excessive belching. **Smoking**, **caffeine**, alcohol, or carbonated beverages may contribute to the discomfort. When there is sensitivity or allergy to certain food substances, eating those foods may cause gastrointestinal distress. Some medications are associated with indigestion. Stomach problems may also be a response to **stress** or emotional unrest.

Diagnosis

A **physical examination** by a health care professional may reveal mid-abdominal **pain**. A **rectal examination** may be done to rule out bleeding. If blood is found on rectal exam, laboratory studies, including a blood count may be ordered. **Endoscopy** and barium studies may be used to rule out underlying gastrointestinal disease. Upper gastrointestinal x-ray studies using barium may allow for visualization of abnormalities. Endoscopy permits collection of tissue and culture specimens which may be used to further confirm a diagnosis.

Treatment

The treatment of dyspepsia is based on assessment of symptoms and suspected causative factors. Clinical evaluation is aimed at distinguishing those patients who require immediate diagnostic work-ups from those who can safely benefit from more conservative initial

KEY TERMS

Anemia—Diagnosed through laboratory study of the blood, a deficiency in hemoglobin or red blood cells, often associated with paleness or loss of energy.

Endoscopy—A diagnostic procedure using a lighted instrument to examine a body cavity or internal organ. Endoscopy permits collection of tissue and culture specimens.

treatment. Some of the latter may require only reassurance, dietary modifications, or antacid use. Medications to block production of stomach acids, prokinate agents, or antibiotic treatment may be considered. Further diagnostic investigation is indicated if there is severe abdominal pain, pain radiating to the back, unexplained weight loss, difficulty swallowing, a palpable mass, or anemia. Additional work-up is also indicated if a patient does not respond to prescribed medications.

Prognosis

Statistics show an average of 20% of patients with dyspepsia have duodenalor gastric ulcer disease, 20% have **irritable bowel syndrome**, fewer than 1% of patients had **cancer**, and the range for functional, or non-ulcer dyspepsia (**gastritis** or superficial erosions), was from 5–40%.

Resources

OTHER

"Dyspepsia—Diagnosis and Treatment Options." Mayo Clinic. http://www.mayoclinic.org/dyspepsia/ (accessed November 23, 2010).
"Dyspepsia: What It Is and What to Do About It." Family doctor.org. December 2009. http://familydoctor.org/online/famdocen/home/common/digestive/disorders/474.html (accessed November 23, 2010).

Kathleen D. Wright, RN

Dysphasia

Definition

Dysphasia is a language disorder in which there is a partial or complete impairment of the ability to communicate resulting from brain injury or degeneration. Because dysphasia is sometimes confused with the similar (but unrelated) medical word dysphagia (a problem with swallowing), the term **aphasia** is often used interchangeably with dysphasia. Conversely, aphasia is sometimes referred to as the "complete" inability to express oneself with verbal and written communications and the inability to comprehend such spoken and written means of communications. Further, dysphasia often denotes the "partial" inability to communicate in these ways—both resulting from an injury to, or degeneration of, the brain. Various amounts of disability can occur depending on the severity of the damage and to the portion of the brain affected. Dysphasia is derived from "dys" meaning difficult and "phasis" meaning speech. Aphasia is derived from "aphaatos", which means speechless.

Demographics

The acquired speech disorder called dysphasia can occur in any human. Men and women are affected equally from the condition. Because any human can be injured because of a blow or other such sudden impact to the brain or by degeneration of the brain (such as through a **stroke** or a tumor), dysphasia can occur in any person. However, people more at risk for dysphasia are those who are more likely to be involved in head injuries. These groups of people include males between the ages of 15 and 24 years of age. They are at increased risk because of their lifestyle, which frequently involves high-risk activities such as sports. In addition, young children and the elderly—those over the age of 75 years of age—are also at elevated risk for dysphasia because of their susceptibility to head injuries, such as from accidental falls. In addition, infants are sometimes shook violently, which can lead to brain trauma and, consequently, dysphasia.

Description

Approximately one million Americans suffer from one of the various forms of dysphasia, and an additional 80,000 new cases occur annually, as of statistics from 2007. However, by 2020, the number of current cases is estimated to increase to two million Americans and the number of annual new cases in the United States is projected to increase to 180,000, according to the National Aphasia Association. The term "dysphasia" is more frequently used by European health professionals, whereas in North American the term, "aphasia" is more commonly preferred. These two terms, however, can be and are used interchangeably. They both refer to the full or partial loss of verbal communication skills due to damage or degeneration of the brain's language centers. Developmental dysphasia is considered to be a learning disability, but will not be the focus of this article.

Verbal communication is derived from several regions located in the language-dominant hemisphere of the brain. These include the adjacent inferior parietal lobe, the inferolateral lobe, and the posterosuperior temporal lobe, as well as the subcortical connection between these areas. Disease, direct trauma, lesion, or infarction involving one or more of these regions can disrupt or prevent proper language function. Dysphasia does not necessarily prevent proper cognitive function, so the patient can think and feel with perfect clarity. This can be extremely frustrating for the patient, as they cannot express these thoughts and feelings to others.

Dysphasia can occur in a variety of forms, depending on how the communicative disruption manifests. Classically, dysphasia can affect one or more of the basic language functions: comprehension (understanding spoken language), naming (identifying items with words), repetition (repeating words or phrases), and speech. Although there are several sub-types of dysphasias, they most commonly manifest in one of three syndromes: expressive dysphasia, receptive dysphasia, or global dysphasia.

Expressive Dysphasia

Expressive dysphasia, also known as motor dysphasia, produces a conscious and recognizable disruption of a patient's speech production and language output. This includes the impairment of speech initiation, proper grammatical sequencing, and proper word forming and articulation. Although patients can perfectly understand what is said to them, they have great difficulty communicating their thoughts. They often express themselves with disjointed words and sentences. The problem is called agrammatism, which means the inability to speak in a grammatically correct manner. In the problem, sufferers omit many words within a sentence so that its meaning becomes disjointed and incomprehensible at times. In less severe cases, the sentence structure may become mixed up. For instance, the sentence "The tree is green." may become "The green is tree."

BROCA'S DYSPHASIA. Broca's dysphasia is the most common type of expressive dysphasia. It is caused by damage to the lower area of the premotor cortex, located just in front of the primary motor cortex. This region is most commonly referred to as the Broca's area. Speech for patients suffering from Broca's dysphasia may be completely impossible. Others may be able to form single words or full sentences, but only through great effort. "Telegraphing," the omission of articles and conjunctions, may also be exhibited.

TRANSCORTICAL DYSPHASIA. Also known as isolation syndrome, transcortical dysphasia is caused by damage to the language-dominant brain that separates all or parts of the central region from the rest of the brain. There are three sub-classes of transcortical dysphasia, which define the impairments to a patient's ability to repeat words, sentences, and phrases: transcortical motor dysphasia, transcortical sensory dysphasia, and mixed transcortical dysphasia. Additional impairments may occur depending on the extent and location of the damage.

Receptive Dysphasia

Receptive dysphasia, also known as sensory dysphasia, impairs the patient's comprehension and meaning of language. Unlike expressive dysphasia, the patient can speak fluently and articulately, but will utilize meaningless words, nonsensical grammar, and unnecessary phrases to the point of becoming incomprehensible. However, they will be completely unaware of their mistakes. Additionally, the patient will find it difficult to comprehend spoken language and/or word-object relation.

WERNICKE'S DYSPHASIA. Also known as semantic dysphasia, Wernicke's dysphasia is the most common of the receptive dysphasia. It is caused by damage to the Wernicke's area, located in the posterior superior temporal lobe of the language-dominant hemisphere. Although the patient can speak clearly and at length, many of their words, phases, and sentences will be nonsensical in nature. Additionally, they will experience difficulty in understanding spoken language, if not suffer a complete lack of comprehension. Semantic distinctions between words may become mixed up and jumbled, furthering confusion.

ANOMIC DYSPHASIA. Anomic dysphasia, also referred to as amnesic dysphasia, is caused by damage to the temporal parietal area and/or the angular gyrus region. Although very similar to Wernicke's dysphasia, anomic dysphasia is distinguished by its disruption of a patient's word-retrieval skills. They will be unable to correctly name people or objects, causing them to pause or substitute generalized words (like "thing"). Otherwise, the patient will exhibit few, if any, language impairments.

CONDUCTION DYSPHASIA. Also known as associative dysphasia, conduction dysphasia is a relatively uncommon disease (representing only 10% of the cases). Damage to the upper temporal lobe, lower parietal, or connection between the Wernicke's and Broca's areas can result in the inability to repeat words, phrases, or sentences. The patient may also suffer the inability to describe people or objects in the proper terms.

Global Dysphasia

Global dysphasia, the third most common form of dysphasia, results from damage to both the anterior and posterior regions of the language-dominant hemisphere. In global dysphasia, all of the patient's language skills are disrupted, along with the ability to comprehend language; however, some may be disrupted more severely than others. In global dysphasia, the symptoms of both expressive dysphasia and receptive dysphasia occurs, and in a severe form.

Causes and symptoms

As of the early 2010s, over one million people in the United States suffer a permanent type of dysphasia. Although dysphasia may manifest in several ways, the common cause for its onset is damage or trauma to the brain. Stroke, in particular, is the most common cause for dysphasia. A stroke is caused from a blockage or rupture of a blood vessel within the brain. This problem causes blood flow to be reduced or cut off to brain cells, which then die or are damaged. Of the half million stroke victims reported annually in the United States, approximately 100,000 will suffer some form of dysphasia. Infection, direct trauma, various injuries, **transient ischemic attack** (TIA), brain tumors, and degeneration (such as **dementia**) can also instigate the onset of dysphasia.

Symptoms of dysphasia will quickly manifest after damage to the brain has occurred, and will present in accordance to the particular type of dysphasia suffered. Due to the proximity to areas of the brain that control motor function, expressive dysphasias can be accompanied by noticeable motor impairment. The majority of symptoms will be language related, including:

- Difficulty remembering words
- Difficulty naming objects and/or people
- Difficulty speaking in complete and/or meaningful sentences
- Difficulty speaking in any fashion
- Using unrecognizable words
- Difficulty reading or writing
- Difficulty expressing thoughts and feelings
- Difficulty understanding spoken language
- Using incorrect or jumbled words
- Using words in the wrong order.

These symptoms may vary depending on the severity of the affliction, along with part of the brain that has been damaged. Some people with dysphasia may comprehend what other people say but have difficulty responding to such words or finding the correct words to say. Others may be able to understand the written word, but cannot speak them out loud.

Diagnosis

Dysphasia is frequently diagnosed while the patient is being treated for injury to the brain, be it from trauma or disease. The health professional, typically a neurologist, will conduct standard cognitive tests, including tests to determine whether the patient's language centers have been affected. If the patient exhibits signs of difficulty communicating, they will often be referred to a speech-language pathologist. In turn, the pathologist will conduct a comprehensive examination of the patient's ability language and comprehension skills. This examination may begin with evaluating the patient's ability to repeat words and phrases, recognize and describe objects, and comprehend what is said to them. More extensive and standardized language-based tests may be required, including the Porch Index of Speech Ability and the Boston Diagnostic Aphasia Examination. Based on the result of the examinations, the health professional will be able to determine the type of dysphasia inflicting the patient. More extensive damage may require the use of computed tomography (CT) or **magnetic resonance imaging** (MRI) for an effective diagnosis.

Treatment

A specific treatment is not available, due to the various forms of the condition, and its severity. Initially it is necessary to treat and stabilize the injury underlying the development of the patient's dysphasia. In some cases, such as with damage caused by TIA, a full recovery can be expedient and takes only a few days. Unfortunately, most dysphasias can take months, if not years, to recover from the problem. Even after prolonged therapy, many patients never achieve a full recovery. Efficacy of treatment greatly depends on the promptness with which it begins. **Speech therapy** is effective at promoting a full or partial recovery. For this reason, many medical facilities have speech-language pathologists on staff to begin the initial treatment process as quickly as possible.

There is not a medical or surgical cure for dysphasia. Treatment, instead, relies strongly upon the use of various speech therapies. Much like **physical therapy** strengthens muscles and bones back to normalcy, speech therapy allow the patient to regain language function, as well as rebuild their communications skills. Treatment is typically conducted with a trained speech therapist. However, group sessions are common and allow the patient to practice their language skills in a non-threatening environment with others sharing their disability. Although much of therapeutic work is conducted by a speech therapist, friends and family also play a vital role in the patient's recovery. They can help the patient continually practice and **exercise** language skills while outside the therapeutic setting. Many times, family members are included on therapy sessions to teach them how to communicate with and understand the patient.

There are several treatments available, which utilize the patient's remaining language abilities to rebuild and compensate for those that were lost. These include out-put focused therapy (stimulation-response), psycholinguistic therapy (cognitive), cognitive neurorehabilitation, and combinations thereof. Although these treatments approach aphasia differently, they all share a common thread by identifying the specific communication deficits and then targeting them with various modalities (computer-aided therapy, picture cards, reading and writing exercises, speech practice, etc.). These techniques stimulate the various parts of the brain associated with language, memory, and understanding, and thus allow it to heal. Therapies may frequently use computers to assist the patient in regaining the ability to communicate. In addition, patients who cannot recover from dysphasia can use communication devices, such as computers, to convey their thoughts back and forth between friends and family.

Medical researchers are also experimenting with and testing various drugs that may be used in the future to treat dysphasia, either in combination with speech therapy or not.

Prognosis

Fortunately, about half of patients will suffer from transient dysphasia, in which the symptoms fade completely after only a few days. However, a patient's prognosis will greatly depend on several factors, such as the cause and the location and extent of the underlying damage. Additional factors of importance are the patient's age, general health, and mental health and motivation. Children under the age of eight years usually regain their language skills even after serious damage to the brain. Handedness may also be an indicator for recovery, as left-handed individuals have language centers located in both hemispheres of the brain (not just the left). As such, left-handed patients have access to language skills from either side of the brain, which can expedite their recovery.

Even with speech therapy, dysphasia may take several years to overcome. Indeed, some patients will never regain their pre-trauma skill level of communication and speech. In such cases, alternative methods of communications may be necessary, such as sign language.

Prevention

Dysphasia can be prevented by avoiding the causes of brain injury and stroke, such as high blood pressure. In particular, eating a healthy diet and not **smoking** to maintain proper blood pressure will help prevent damaging strokes. Although it is impossible to predict head trauma, the use of head protection while participating in dangerous sports or activities can reduce the risk of serious brain damage.

Resources

BOOKS

Brookshire, Robert H. *Introduction to Neurogenic Communication Disorders (7th edition)*. St. Louis, MO: Mosby, 2007.

Brubaker, Susan Howell. *Basic Level Workbook for Aphasia*. Detroit: Wayne State University Press, 2010.

Helm-Estabrooks, Nancy, and Martin L. Albert. *Manual of Aphasia and Aphasia Therapy*. Austin, TX: Pro-Ed, 2004.

OTHER

Aphasia. Mayo Clinic. (March 6, 2010), http://www.mayoclinic.com/health/aphasia/DS00685 (accessed September 13, 2010).

Aphasia. Medline Plus, National Institutes of Health and National Library of Medicine. (July 6, 2010), http://www.nlm.nih.gov/medlineplus/aphasia.html (accessed September 13, 2010).

Aphasia. The Merck Manuals. Online Medical Library, Merck. (September 2008), http://www.merck.com/mmpe/sec16/ch210/ch210d.html (accessed September 13, 2010).

Aphasia. National Institute on Deafness and Other Communication Disorders. (October 2008), http://www.nidcd.nih.gov/health/voice/aphasia.asp (accessed September 13, 2010).

Aphasia Statistics for the US—Current. Aphasia.com (Lingraphica). (2007), http://www.aphasia.com/wordpdf/1.BasicStatistics.pdf (accessed September 13, 2010).

CMSD 336 Neuropathologies of Language and Cognition. The Neuroscience on the Web Series. (2007), http://www.csuchico.edu/~pmccaffrey/syllabi/SPPA336/index.html (accessed September 13, 2010).

ORGANIZATIONS

American Stroke Association, 7272 Greenville Avenue, Dallas, TX, 75231, (888) 478-7653, http://www.strokeassociation.org/STROKEORG/.

National Aphasia Association, 350 Seventh Avenue, New York City, NY, 10001, (800) 922-4622, http://www.aphasia.org/.

National Institute on Deafness and Other Communication Disorders, 31 Center Drive, MSC 2320, Bethesda, MD, 20892-2320, (800) 241-1044, nidcdinfo@nidcd.nih.gov, http://www.nidcd.nih.gov/.

Speakability, 1 Royal Street, London, United Kingdom, SE1 7LL, 030 7261 9572, 020 7928 9542, speakability@speakability.org.uk, http://www.speakability.org.uk/.

Jason Fryer

Dyspnea *see* **Shortness of breath**

Dysthymic disorder *see* **Depressive disorders**

Dystonia *see* **Movement disorders**

E

E. coli see *Escherichia coli*

E. coli infection *see* **Enterobacterial infections**

E. coli O157:H7 infection *see* ***Escherichia coli***

Ear canal infection *see* **Otitis externa**

Ear exam with an otoscope

Definition

An otoscope is a hand-held instrument with a tiny light and a cone-shaped attachment called an ear speculum, which is used to examine the ear canal. An ear examination is a normal part of most physical examinations by a doctor or nurse. It is also done when an ear infection or other type of ear problem is suspected.

Purpose

An otoscope is used to look into the ear canal to see the ear drum. Redness or fluid in the eardrum can indicate an ear infection. Some otoscopes can deliver a small puff of air to the eardrum to see if the eardrum will vibrate (which is normal). This type of ear examination with an otoscope can also detect a build up of wax in the ear canal, or a rupture or puncture of the eardrum.

Precautions

No special precautions are required. However, if an ear infection is present, an ear examination may cause some discomfort or **pain**.

Description

An ear examination with an otoscope is usually done by a doctor or a nurse as part of a complete **physical examination**. The ears may also be examined if an ear infection is suspected due to **fever**, ear pain, or **hearing loss**. The patient will often be asked to tip the head slightly toward the shoulder so the ear to be examined is pointing up. The doctor or nurse may hold the ear lobe as the speculum is inserted into the ear, and may adjust the position of the otoscope to get a better view of the ear canal and eardrum. Both ears are usually examined, even if there seems to be a problem with just one ear.

Preparation

No special preparation is required prior to an ear examination with an otoscope. The ear speculum, which is inserted into the ear, is cleaned and sanitized before it is used. The speculums come in various sizes, and the doctor or nurse will select the size that will be most comfortable for the patient's ear.

Aftercare

If an ear infection is diagnosed, the patient may require treatment with **antibiotics**. If there is a buildup of wax in the ear canal, it might be rinsed or scraped out.

Risks

This type of ear examination is simple and generally harmless. Caution should always be used any time an object is inserted into the ear. This process could irritate an infected external ear canal and could rupture an eardrum if performed improperly or if the patient moves.

Normal results

The ear canal is normally skin-colored and is covered with tiny hairs. It is normal for the ear canal to have some yellowish-brown earwax. The eardrum is typically thin, shiny, and pearly-white to light gray in color. The tiny bones in the middle ear can be seen pushing on the eardrum membrane like tent poles. The light from the otoscope will reflect off of the surface of the ear drum.

Abnormal results

An ear infection will cause the eardrum to look red and swollen. In cases where the eardrum has ruptured, there may be fluid draining from the middle ear. A doctor may also see scarring, retraction of the eardrum, or bulging of the eardrum.

ORGANIZATIONS

American Academy of Otolaryngology—Head and Neck Surgery, 1650 Diagonal Road, Alexandria, VA, 22314-2857, (703) 836-4444, http://www.entnet.org.

EAR Foundation of Arizona, 668 North 44th Street, Suite 300, Phoenix, AZ, 85008 , (602) 685-1050, (602) 239-5117, melissa@earfoundationaz.com, http://www.earfoundationaz.com.

Altha Roberts Edgren

Ear, nose, and throat surgery

Definition

Ear, nose, and throat surgery is the surgical treatment of diseases, injuries, or deformations of the ears, nose, throat, head, and neck areas.

Purpose

The purpose of surgery to the ears, nose, throat, head, and neck is to treat an abnormality, such as a defect or disease, in these anatomical areas. An anatomical deformity is a change that usually occurs during embryological development, leaving the affected person with the apparent defect. A disease in this area usually develops later in life, such as **head and neck cancer**. Additionally, the specialty known as otorhinolaryngology (ears [*oto*], nose [*rhino*], and throat [*laryn*], referring to the larynx or throat) also includes surgical intervention for diseases in the head and neck regions. Most ears, nose, and throat (ENT) surgeons in the United States are referred to as otolaryngologist and the specialty as otolaryngology. **Ear surgery** is usually performed to correct specific causes of **hearing loss**. Nose surgery can include different types of procedures necessary to treat sinus problems, like sinus surgery. Throat surgery can include complicated procedures such as **cancer** of the larynx resulting in a **laryngectomy**, or more simple procedures such as surgical removal of the adenoids, known as an **adenoidectomy**, or tonsils, known as a **tonsillectomy**. Head and neck surgery may be necessary to remove a tumor or reconstruct an area after disfigurement from trauma or injury.

Demographics

Ears, nose, and throat surgery comprises many different types of surgical procedures and spans over all age groups regardless of gender or ethnicity. Pediatric otolaryngology, a subspecialty, is the branch that treats ENT problems for infants and children.

Description

ENT surgery is the oldest surgical specialty in the United States, and it is one of the most elaborate fields of surgical specialty services, using advanced technology and a broad range of procedures that also includes major **reconstructive surgery** to correct deformity or injury. **Cosmetic surgery** can include surgical procedures to improve wrinkles in the face, contours of the nose and ears, chin augmentation, and **hair transplantation**.

Typically, ear surgery corrects defects causing hearing loss or impairment. Such procedures include **stapedectomy**, the removal of all or part of a bone in the middle ear called the stapes; tympanoplasty, or reconstruction of the ear drum; and **cochlear implants**, which is implantation of a device to stimulate nerve ends within the inner portion of the ear to enable hearing. Surgery of the ear also includes **myringotomy**, or insertion of **ear tubes** to drain fluid in persons with chronic ear infections.

Common surgical procedures of the throat include removal of tonsils (tonsillectomy) or adenoids (adenoidectomy). The tonsils, found on either side and in back

KEY TERMS

Cancer staging—A surgical procedure to remove a lymph node and examine the cells for cancer. It determines the extent of the cancer and how far it has spread.

of the throat, and adenoids, which are higher up the throat behind the nose, are masses of lymph tissue that play an active role in body defenses to fight infection. The tonsils and adenoids can get chronically infected, in which case surgical removal is usually indicated to relieve breathing problems and infection recurrence. Furthermore, chronic inflammation of the adenoids can cause repeated middle ear infections that can ultimately impair hearing.

Surgery of the nose can include procedures that treat sinus diseases. Advanced endoscopic surgery for sinus and nasal disorders can eliminate the need for external incisions and greater surgical precision. Other common surgical procedures include correction of a deviated nasal septum (**septoplasty**) and for chronic nasal obstruction (congestion).

Surgery of the neck region can commonly include **tracheotomy**, a surgical procedure in which an opening is made in the trachea or windpipe. Tracheotomy is indicated for a person who is unable to deliver enough oxygen to the lungs. ENT surgeons also perform complicated surgical procedures for the treatment of malignant head and neck cancers. In addition to **tumor removal**, when indicated, ENT surgeons may perform an operation called **radical neck dissection**, during which the ENT will remove cancer that has spread via lymphatic vessels to regional neck lymph nodes. Neck dissection is also useful since specimens can be removed for pathological examination, which can provide important information concerning metastasis, or spread, and can direct the treatment plan (i.e., **radiation therapy** and/or **chemotherapy** may be recommended for aggressive cancers). ENT surgeons also treat sleep-related disorders such as **sleep apnea** and excessive **snoring**; a procedure called laser-assisted uvula palatoplasty (LAUP) will remove tissue to allow for unobstructed airflow.

Other ENT procedures include surgical reconstruction of ear deformities (otoplasties), special surgery for diseases in the inner ear, and skull-based surgeries (neuro-otology). As well, ENT surgeons can surgically treat abnormalities near the eye, perform oral surgery for treatment of dental and jaw injury, and remove skin

cancer within the head and neck region. ENT surgeons also perform special surgical techniques that can preserve nerve and blood vessel function (microsurgery) and reconstruction of bone and soft tissue.

Diagnosis/Preparation

A careful history and **physical examination** of the ears, nose, throat, head, and neck is a standard approach during initial consultation. Different instruments with light sources, like an otoscope for ear examinations, enable ENT surgeons to quickly visualize the ears, nose, and throat. Visualization of these areas can reveal the severity of the disease or deformity. The head and neck area is inspected and the neck and throat area is typically felt with the surgeon's hands, a technique known as palpation. Special technological advancements have enabled ENT surgeons to further visualize deep internal anatomical structures. Nasal **endoscopy** allows visualization of the upper airway to detect anatomical problems related to sinuses. Videostroboscopy can be used to visualize the vocal cords, and triple endoscopy (**laryngoscopy**, esophagoscopy, and **bronchoscopy**) can diagnose and stage head and neck cancers. Preparation before surgery is fairly standardized and includes blood work-up and instructions to have nothing to eat or drink after midnight of the night before the procedure.

Aftercare

The aftercare for ENT surgery depends on the procedure and state of the health of the patient. The aftercare for a patient who is 60 years old with head/neck cancer is more extensive than a tonsillectomy performed in a young adolescent or child. Generally, aftercare should be directed toward wound care and knowledge gained from the surgeon specifically detailing the expected length of average convalescence. Wound care, such as cleansing and dressing changes, and postoperative follow-up with the ENT surgeon is essential. Medications for **pain** may be prescribed. Patients stay in the hospital for eight to 10 hours for the effects of anesthesia to subside for same-day surgical procedures like a tonsillectomy, or they may be admitted for a few days for more complicated procedures, such as those related to cancer treatment. Aftercare and convalescence may take longer for complicated procedures such as advanced cancer, temporal-bone surgery for nerve disorders that can affect balance, or for tumors.

Risks

The risk of ENT surgery depends on the procedure and the health status of the patient. Some procedures do not have much risk, while complications for other procedures can carry considerable risk. For example, the risk of a complicated operation such as neck dissection could result in loss of ear sensation, since the nerve that provides the feeling of sensation is commonly severed during the procedure.

Normal results

There will be a cure or an improvement of the primary disease. Ear surgery should help individuals hear well. Throat surgery can help remove chronically inflamed tonsils, adenoids, polyps, or cancer. Nose surgery for deviated septums or nasal congestion will improve breathing problems and help a person breath more easily and effectively through the nose. Neck surgery can help remove diseased tissue and prevent further spread of cancer. Surgery for sleep apnea will remove redundant tissue that blocks airways and obstructs normal airflow.

Morbidity and mortality rates

Outcome and disease progression vary for each disease state. There are no general statistics for all ENT procedures. Some procedures are generally correlated with excellent morbidity, such as over 90% success rates for all cases receiving tympanoplasty, and no mortality, while others may be associated with poor outcome and much illness, like advanced head/neck cancer.

Alternatives

Usually, surgery is indicated when benefit from surgery is a clear-cut primary intervention or when medical, or conservative treatment has failed to provide sustained symptomatic improvement. A person diagnosed with cancer may not have an alternative conservative treatment, depending on the stage of their cancer; however, a person with sinus problems may be treated conservatively with **antibiotics**, saline nasal spray wash, steroid nasal spray, and/or antihistamine spray before indication or necessity for surgery. There are many other services that the ENT surgeon uses to treat specific diseases, including audiology services for diagnostic and therapeutic purposes, like **hearing aids**, and services to treat disorders of speech and voice.

Resources

BOOKS

Corbridge, Rogan, and Nicholas Steventon. *Oxford Handbook of ENT and Head and Neck Surgery*. New York: Oxford University Press, 2006.

Stamm, Aldo C. and Wolfgang Craf. *Micro-endoscopic Surgery of the Paranasal Sinuses and the Skull Base*. New York: Springer, 2000.

ORGANIZATIONS

American Academy of Otolaryngology-Head and Neck Surgery, One Prince Street, Alexandria, VA, 22314-3357, (703) 836-4444, http://www.entnet.org.

American Hearing Research Foundation, 8 S. Michigan Avenue, Suite 814, Chicago, IL, 60603, (312) 726-9670, http://www.american-hearing.org/.

American Speech-Language-Hearing Association, 2200 Research Boulevard, Rockville, MD, 20850-3289, (800) 638-8255, http://www.asha.org.

Laith Farid Gulli, M.D., M.S.
Robert Ramirez, B.S.
Laura Jean Cataldo, R.N., Ed.D.

Ear surgery

Definition

Ear surgery is the treatment of diseases, injuries, or deformations of the ear by operation with instruments.

Purpose

Ear surgery is performed to correct certain types of **hearing loss**, and to treat diseases of, injuries to, or deformities of the ear's auditory tube, middle ear, inner ear, and auditory and vestibular systems. Ear surgery is commonly performed to treat conductive hearing loss, persistent ear infections, unhealed perforated eardrums, congenital ear defects, and tumors.

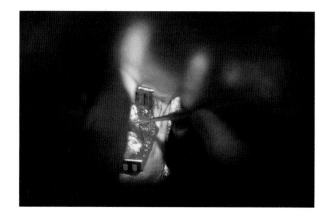

Microsurgery being performed in the inner ear.
(Hans Halberstadt/Photo Researchers, Inc.)

Ear surgery is performed on children and adults. In some cases, surgery is the only treatment; in others, it is used only when more conservative medical treatment fails.

Precautions

The precautions vary, depending on the type of ear surgery under consideration. For example, **stapedectomy** (removal of parts of the middle ear and insertion of prosthesis parts) should not be performed on people with external or middle ear infection or inner ear disease. For people with complete hearing loss in the other ear, it should be performed cautiously. Microsurgery for the removal of a cholesteatoma (a cyst-like mass of cells in the middle ear) should not be performed on patients who are extremely ill or have other medical conditions. Tympanoplasty (any surgical procedure on the eardrum or middle ear) should not be performed on patients with chronic sinus or nasal problems or with medical problems such as poorly controlled diabetes and heart disease. Surgery for congenital microtia and atresia (abscense of normal bodily openings, such as the outer ear canal) should not be performed if the middle ear space is totally or almost totally absent.

Description

Most ear surgery is microsurgery, performed with an operating microscope to enable the surgeon to view the very small structures of the ear. The use of minimally invasive **laser surgery** for middle ear procedures is growing. Laser surgery reduces the amount of trauma due to vibration, enhances coagulation, and enables surgeons to access hard to reach places in the middle ear. Laser surgery can be performed in an office operating suite. Types of ear surgery include stapedectomy, tympanoplasty, **myringotomy** and ear tube surgery, ear surgery to repair a **perforated eardrum**, **cochlear implants**, and **tumor removal**.

Stapedectomy

To restore hearing loss, which is usually due to **otosclerosis**, stapedectomy is performed. Stapedectomy is the removal of all or part of the stapes, one of the bones in the middle ear, and replacement with a tiny prosthesis. An incision is made in the middle ear, the small bones are identified, and the stapes is removed. The stainless steel wire and cellulose sponge prosthesis is inserted, blood and fluid are drained, and the wound is closed. Performed in a hospital or outpatient surgical facility under local or general anesthetic, full recovery takes about three weeks but hearing should improve immediately.

Tympanoplasty

Tympanoplasty is performed to reconstruct the eardrum after partial or total conductive hearing loss, usually caused by chronic middle ear infections, or perforations that do not heal. This is usually a same day surgery, performed under either local or **general anesthesia**. After making an incision in the ear to view the perforation, the ear drum is elevated away from the ear canal and lifted forward. If the bones of hearing (ossicular chain) are functioning, tissue is taken from the ear and grafted to the eardrum to close the perforation. A thin sheet of silastic and Gelfoam hold the graft in place. The ear is stitched together, and a sterile patch is placed on the outside of the ear canal. Tympanoplasty is successful in over 90% of all cases. The need for ossicular reconstruction (reconstruction of tiny bones of the middle ear) is sometimes known before surgery and even when identified during surgery, can usually be done while reconstructing the eardrum. If the gap between the anvil bone and the stapes is small, a small piece of bone or cartilage from the patient can be inserted; if is is large, the incus bone is removed, modelled into a prosthesis, and reinserted between the stapes and the malleus. Reconstruction could also be achieved by inserting a strut made from artificial bone. For tympanoplasty with ossicular reconstruction, the patient usually stays in the hospital overnight. The recovery period is about four weeks.

Myringotomy and ear tube surgery

Myringotomy and ear tube surgery is performed to drain ear fluid and prevent ear infections when **antibiotics** don't work or when ear infections are chronic. The process normalizes pressure in the middle ear and decreases fluid accumulation. It is most commonly performed on infants and children, in whom ear infections are most frequent, and may be done on one or both ears. The surgeon makes a small hole in the ear drum, then uses suction to remove fluid. A small ear tube of metal or plastic is inserted into the ear drum to allow continual drainage. The tube prevents infections as long as it stays in place, which varies from six months to three years. When the tube falls out, the hole grows over. As many of 25% of children under the age of two who need **ear tubes** may need them again. Myringotomy and ear tube surgery is performed in a hospital, using a general anesthetic for most children and a local anesthetic for older children or adults. No anesthetic may be used for infants. The procedure usually takes about two hours. Most patients can go home the same day; children under three years of age and those with chronic diseases usually stay overnight.

Ear surgery for a perforated eardrum

Ear surgery for a perforated eardrum is only performed in rare cases where it does not heal on its own. In most cases, this is performed in a surgeon's office using a topical anesthetic. The surgeon scratches the undersurface of the eardrum, stimulating the skin to heal and the eardrum to close. A thin patch placed on the eardrum's outer surface allows the skin under the eardrum to heal.

Cochlear implants

Cochlear implants stimulate nerve ends within the inner ear, enabling deaf children to hear. The device has a microphone that remains outside the ear, a processor that selects and codes speech sounds, and a receiver/stimulator to convert the coded sounds to electric signals that stimulate the hearing nerve and are recognized by the brain as sound. During surgery, an incision is made behind and slightly above the ear. A circular hole is drilled in the bone to receive the device's internal coil. The mastoid bone leading to the middle ear is opened to receive the electrodes. The internal coil is inserted and secured, followed by the electrodes. The wound is stitched up and when it heals, an external unit comprised of a stimulator with a microphone is worn behind the ear. Performed in a hospital under general anesthesia, the operation takes about two hours and usually requires a hospital stay overnight. The patient can resume normal activities in two to three weeks.

Ear surgery for tumors

Some ear tumors can be very serious and should be removed surgically. For a tumor on the skin of the ear canal, the skin is removed surgically, the bone beneath it is drilled away and a skin graft is placed in the ear canal. If the tumor is near the eardrum, the skin of the ear canal and the eardrum are removed along with the bone surrounding the ear canal. A skin graft is placed on the bare bone. For basal cell cancers and low grade glandular malignancies, surgical resection of the ear canal is adequate. Squamous cell carcinoma, a serious form of **cancer**, of the external ear canal requires radical surgery, followed by **radiation therapy**. Cholesteatoma, a benign tumor caused by an infection in a perforated eardrum that did not heal properly and can destroy the bones of hearing, is removed with microsurgery. **Mastoidectomy** is performed for **mastoiditis**, an inflammation of the middle ear, if medical therapy does not work. Petrous

apicectomy is performed to drain the petrous apicitis, the bone between the middle ear and the clivis.

Ear surgery for congenital ear defects

Congenital atresia, the absence of the external ear canal, and congenital microtia, abnormal growth of the external ear, often occur together, although atresia can occur without microtia. Surgery to reconstruct the ear usually takes place when the child is four or five years old and may require several operations. A facial plastic surgeon and an ear surgeon work together, repairing the microtia first and then the atresia. During surgery, a bony opening is created over the bones of hearing. The surfaces of the bony ear canal are then relined with a skin graft from the thigh or abdomen. Tissue from behind the eardrum is used to create a new eardrum. In many cases, the middle ear will also need to be reconstructed. Surgery is performed in a hospital under general anesthesia.

Other types of ear surgery

Surgery may also be appropriate to remove multiple bony overgrowths of the ear canal or in rare cases of compromised auditory tube function, to narrow the tube.

Preparation

The preparation depends upon the type of ear surgery performed. For many procedures, blood and urine studies and hearing tests are conducted.

Aftercare

The type of aftercare depends upon the type of surgery performed. In most cases, the ear(s) should be kept dry and warm. Non-prescription drugs such as **acetaminophen** can be used for **pain**.

Risks

The type of risk depends on the type of surgery performed. Total hearing loss is rare.

ORGANIZATIONS

American Academy of Otolaryngology—Head and Neck Surgery, 1650 Diagonal Road, Alexandria, VA, 22314-2857, (703) 836-4444, http://www.entnet.org.

American Hearing Research Organization, 8 South Michigan Avenue, Suite #1205, Chicago, IL, 60603-4539, (312) 726-9670, (312) 726-9695, http://www.american-hearing.org.

American Speech Language Hearing Association, 2200 Research Boulevard , Rockville, MD, 20850-3289, (301) 296-5700, (301) 296-8580, (800) 638-8255, actioncenter@asha.org, http://asha.org/.

Lori De Milto

Ear tubes *see* **Myringotomy and ear tubes**

Ear wax impaction *see* **Cerumen impaction**

Eardrum perforation *see* **Perforated eardrum**

Eastern equine encephalitis *see* **Arbovirus encephalitis**

Eating disorders

Definition

Eating disorders are psychiatric illnesses that result in abnormal eating patterns that have a negative effect on health.

Demographics

In general, more women have eating disorders than men. About 90% of people with **anorexia nervosa** and **bulimia nervosa** are female. Almost as many men as women develop binge-eating disorder. Anorexia athletica, muscle dysmorphic disorder, and orthorexia nervosa tend to be more common in men. Rumination, **pica**, and **Prader-Willi syndrome** affect men and women equally.

Anorexia can occur in people as young as age 7. However, the disorder most often begins during adolescence. It is most likely to start at one of two times, either age 14 or 18 and affects mainly white girls. There is a secondary peak of individuals who become anorexic in their 40s.

Bulimia is the most common eating disorder in the United States. Overall, about 3% of Americans are bulimic. Of these 85–90% are female. The rate is highest among adolescents and college women, averaging

---

Symptoms of eating disorders

Anorexia nervosa	Bulimia nervosa	Binge-eating disorder
Resistance to maintaining body weight at or above a minimally normal weight for age and height	Recurrent episodes of binge eating, characterized by eating an excessive amount of food within a discrete period of time and by a sense of lack of control over eating during the episode	Recurrent episodes of binge eating, characterized by eating an excessive amount of food within a discrete period of time and by a sense of lack of control over eating during the episode
Intense fear of gaining weight or becoming fat, even though underweight	Recurrent inappropriate compensatory behavior in order to prevent weight gain, such as self-induced vomiting or misuse of laxatives, diuretics, enemas, or other medications (purging); fasting; or excessive exercise	The binge-eating episodes are associated with at least 3 of the following: eating much more rapidly than normal; eating until feeling uncomfortably full; eating large amounts of food when not feeling physically hungry; eating alone because of being embarrassed by how much one is eating; feeling disgusted with oneself, depressed, or very guilty after overeating
Disturbance in the way in which one's body weight or shape is experienced, undue influence of body weight or shape on self-evaluation, or denial of the seriousness of the current low body weight	The binge eating and inappropriate compensatory behaviors both occur, on average, at least twice week for 3 months	Marked distress about the binge-eating behavior
Infrequent or absent menstrual periods (in females who have reached puberty)	Self-evaluation is unduly influenced by body shape and weight	The binge eating occurs, on average, at least 2 days a week for 6 months
		The binge eating is not associated with the regular use of inappropriate compensatory behaviors (e.g., purging, fasting, excessive exercise)

SOURCE: National Institute of Mental Health, National Institutes of Health, U.S. Department of Health and Human Services

(Table by PreMediaGlobal. Reproduced by permission of Gale, a part of Cengage Learning.)

5–6%. In men, the disorder is more often diagnosed in homosexuals than in heterosexuals. Bulimia usually develops in women the late teens and early twenties and in men around age 25 or later. It affects all racial, ethnic, and socioeconomic groups.

Estimates of the number of Americans who have binge-eating disorder range from less than 1% to 4%, with 2% being the most commonly cited figure. Although women with binge-eating disorder outnumber men three to two, **binge eating** is the most common male eating disorder. Binge-eating disorder is a problem of middle age and affects blacks and whites equally.

Prader-Willi syndrome begins in the toddler years. Not enough is known about the other disorders to determine when they are most likely to develop or which races or ethnic groups are most likely to be at risk.

Description

Eating disorders are mental disorders. They develop when a person has an unrealistic attitude toward or abnormal perception of his or her body. This causes behaviors that lead to destructive eating patterns that have negative physical and emotional consequences. Individuals with eating disorders often hide their symptoms and resist seeking treatment. Depression, **anxiety disorders**, and other mental illnesses often are present in people who have eating disorders, although it is not clear whether these cause the eating disorder or are a result of it.

The two best-known eating disorders, anorexia nervosa and bulimia nervosa, have formal diagnostic criteria and are recognized as psychiatric disorders in the *Diagnostic and Statistical Manual for Mental Disorders Fourth Edition (DSM-IV-TR)* published by the American Psychiatric Association (APA). Other eating disorders have recognized sets of symptoms, but have not been researched thoroughly enough to be considered separate psychiatric disorders as defined by the APA.

Anorexia nervosa

In the North America and Europe, anorexia nervosa is the most publicized of all eating disorders. It gained widespread public attention with the rise of the ultra-thin fashion model. People who have anorexia nervosa are obsessed with body weight. They constantly monitor their food intake and starve themselves to become thin. No matter how much weight they lose, they continue to restrict their calorie intake in an effort to become ever thinner. Some anorectics **exercise** to extreme or abuse drugs or herbal remedies that they believe will help them burn calories faster. A

few purge their body of the few calories they do eat by abusing **laxatives**, **enemas**, and **diuretics**. In time, they reach a point where their health is seriously, and potentially fatally, impaired.

People with anorexia nervosa have an abnormal perception of their body. They genuinely believe that they are fat, even when the clearly are life-threateningly thin. They will deny that they are too thin, or, if they admit they are thin, deny that their behavior will affect their health. People with anorexia will lie to family, friends, and healthcare providers about how much they eat. Many vigorously resist treatment and accuse the people trying to cure them of wanting to make them fat. Anorexia nervosa is the most difficult eating disorder to recover from.

Competitive athletes of all races have an increased risk of developing anorexia nervosa, especially in sports where weight is tied to performance. Jockeys, wrestlers, figure skaters, cross-country runners, and gymnasts (especially female gymnasts) have higher than average rates of anorexia. People such as actors, models, cheerleaders, and dancers (especially ballet dancers) who are judged mainly on their appearance are also at high risk of developing the disorder. This same group of people is also at higher risk for developing bulimia nervosa.

Bulimia nervosa

Bulimia nervosa is the only other eating disorder with specific diagnostic criteria defined by the *DSM-IV-TR*. People with bulimia often consume unreasonably large amounts of food in a short time. Afterwards, they purge their body of calories. This is done most often by self-induced **vomiting**, often accompanied by laxative abuse. A subset of people with bulimia does not vomit after eating, but fast and exercise obsessively to burn calories. Both behaviors result in impaired health.

People with bulimia feel out of control when they are binge eating. Unlike people with anorexia, they recognize that their behavior is abnormal. Often they are ashamed and feel guilty about their behavior and will go to great lengths to hide their binge/purge cycles from their family and friends. People with bulimia are often of normal weight. Although their behavior results in negative health consequences, because they are less likely to be ultra-thin, these consequences are less likely to be life-threatening.

Binge eating disorder

Binge eating is quite common, but it rises to the level of a disorder only when bingeing occurs at least twice a week for three months or more. People with binge-eating disorder may eat thousands of calories in an hour or two. While they are eating, they feel out of control and may continue to eat long after they feel full. Binge eaters do not purge or exercise to get rid of the calories they have eaten. As a result, many, but not all, people with binge-eating disorder, are obese, although not all obese people are binge eaters.

Binge eaters are usually ashamed of their behavior and try to hide it by eating in secret and hoarding food for future binges. After a binge, they usually feel disgusted with themselves and guilty about their eating behavior. They often promise themselves that they will never binge again, but are unable to keep this promise. Binge-eating disorder often takes the form of an endless cycle—rigorous dieting followed by an eating binge followed by guilt and rigorous dieting, followed by another eating binge. The main health consequences of binge eating are the development of obesity-related diseases such as type 2 diabetes, **sleep apnea**, **stroke**, and **heart attack**.

Lesser-known eating disorders

Quite a few eating problems are called disorders even though they do not have formal diagnostic criteria. They fall under the APA definition of eating disorders not otherwise specified. Many have only recently come to the attention of researchers and have been the subject of only a few small studies. Some have been known to the medical community for years but are rare.

Purge disorder is thought by some experts to be a separate disorder from bulimia. It is distinguished from bulimia by the fact that the individual maintains a normal or near normal weight despite purging by **vomiting** or laxative, enema, or diuretic abuse.

Anorexia athletica is a disorder of compulsive exercising. The individual places exercise above work, school, or relationships and defines his or her self-worth in terms of athletic performance. People with anorexia athletica also tend to be obsessed less with body weight than with maintaining an abnormally low percentage of body fat. This disorder is common among elite athletes.

Muscle dysmorphic disorder is the opposite of anorexia nervosa. Where the anorectic thinks she is always too fat, the person with muscle dysmorphic disorder believes he is always too small. This belief is maintained even when the person is clearly well muscled. Abnormal eating patterns are less of a problem in people with muscle dysmorphic disorder than damage from compulsive exercising (even when

injured) and the abuse of muscle-building drugs such as anabolic **steroids**.

Orthorexia nervosa is a term coined by Steven Bratman, a Colorado physician, to describe "a pathological fixation on eating 'proper,' 'pure,' or 'superior' foods." People with orthorexia allow their fixation with eating the correct amount of properly prepared healthy foods at the correct time of day to take over their lives. This obsession interferes with relationships and daily activities. For example, they may be unwilling to eat at restaurants or friends' homes because the food is "impure" or improperly prepared. The limitations they put on what they will eat can cause serious vitamin and mineral imbalances. Orthorectics are judgmental about what other people eat to the point where it interferes with personal relationships. They justify their fixation by claiming that their way of eating is healthy. Some experts believe orthorexia may be a variation of **obsessive-compulsive disorder**.

Rumination syndrome occurs when an individual, either voluntarily or involuntarily, regurgitates food almost immediately after swallowing it, chews it, and then either swallows it or spits it out. Regurgitation syndrome is the human equivalent of a cow chewing its cud. The behavior often lasts up to two hours after eating. It must continue for at least one month to be considered a disorder. Occasionally the behavior simply stops on its own, but it can last for years.

Pica is the eating of non-food substances by people developmentally past the stage where this is normal (usually around age 2). Earth and clay are the most common non-foods eaten, although people have been known to eat hair, feces, lead, laundry starch chalk, burnt matches, cigarette butts, light bulbs, and other equally bizarre non-foods. This disorder has been known to the medical community for years, and in some cultures (mainly tribes living in equatorial Africa) is considered normal. Pica is most common among people with **mental retardation** and developmental delays. It only rises to the level of a disorder when health complications require medical treatment.

Prader-Willi syndrome is a genetic defect that spontaneously arises in chromosome 15. It causes low muscle tone, short stature, incomplete sexual development, mental retardation, and an uncontrollable urge to eat. People with Prader-Willi syndrome never feel full. The only way to stop them from eating themselves to **death** is to keep them in environments where food is locked up and not available. Prader-

KEY TERMS

Body dysmorphic disorder—A psychiatric disorder marked by preoccupation with an imagined physical defect.

Diuretic—A substance that removes water from the body by increasing urine production.

Electrolyte—Ions in the body that participate in metabolic reactions. The major human electrolytes are sodium (Na+), potassium (K+), calcium (Ca 2+), magnesium (Mg2+), chloride (Cl-), phosphate (HPO4 2-), bicarbonate (HCO3-), and sulfate (SO4 2-).

Lanugos—A soft, downy body hair that develops on the chest and arms of anorexic women.

Neurotransmitter—One of a group of chemicals secreted by a nerve cell (neuron) to carry a chemical message to another nerve cell, often as a way of transmitting a nerve impulse. Examples of neurotransmitters include acetylcholine, dopamine, serotonin, and norepinephrine.

Purging—The use of vomiting, diuretics, or laxatives to clear the stomach and intestines after a binge.

Serotonin—5-Hydroxytryptamine; a substance that occurs throughout the body with numerous effects including neurotransmission. Inadequate amounts of serotonin are implicated in some forms of depression and obsessive-compulsive disorder.

Willi syndrome is a rare disease, and although it is caused by a genetic defect, tends not to run in families, but rather is an accident of development. Only 12,000–15,000 people in the United States have Prader-Willi syndrome.

Causes and symptoms

Eating disorders have multiple causes. There appears to be a genetic predisposition in some people toward developing an eating disorder. Biochemistry also seems to play a role. Neurotransmitters in the brain, such as serotonin, play a role in regulating appetite. Abnormalities in the amount of some neurotransmitters are thought to play a role in anorexia, bulimia, and binge-eating disorder. Other disorders have not been studied enough to draw any conclusions. Interestingly, serotonin also helps regulate mood, and low serotonin levels are thought to play a role in causing depression.

Personality type can also put people at risk for developing an eating disorder. Low self-worth is common among all people with eating disorders. Binge eaters and people with bulimia tend to have problems with impulse control and anger management. A tendency toward obsessive-compulsive behavior and black-or-white, all-or-nothing thinking also put people at higher risk.

Social and environmental factors also affect the development and maintenance of eating disorders and may trigger relapses during recovery. Relationship conflict, a disordered, unstructured home life, job or school **stress**, transition events such as moving or starting a new job all seems to act as triggers for some people to begin disordered eating behaviors. Dieting (nutritional and social stress) is the most common trigger of all. The United States in the early twenty-first century is a culture obsessed with thinness. The media constantly send the message through words and images that being not just thin, but ultra-thin, is fashionable and desirable. Magazines aimed mostly at women devote thousands of words every month to diet and exercise advice that creates a sense of dissatisfaction, unrealistic goals, and a distorted body image.

Signs and symptoms of anorexia and bulimia

Eating disorders have physical and psychological consequences. These include:

- excessive weight loss; loss of muscle
- stunted growth and delayed sexual maturation in preteens
- gastrointestinal complications: liver damage, diarrhea, constipation, bloating, stomach pain
- cardiovascular complications: irregular heartbeat, low pulse rate, cardiac arrest
- urinary system complications: kidney damage, kidney failure, incontinence, urinary tract infections
- skeletal system complications: loss of bone mass, increased risk of fractures, teeth eroded by stomach acid from repeat vomiting
- reproductive system complications (women): irregular menstrual periods, amenorhhea, infertility

- reproductive system complications (men): loss of sex drive, infertility
- fatigue, irritation, headaches, depression, anxiety, impaired judgment and thinking
- fainting, seizures, low blood sugar
- chronically cold hands and feet
- weakened immune system, swollen glands, increased susceptibility to infections
- development of fine hair called lanugos on the shoulders, back, arms, and face, head hair loss, blotchy, dry skin
- potentially life-threatening electrolyte imbalances
- coma
- increased risk of self-mutilation (cutting)
- increased risk of suicide
- death

Signs and symptoms of binge eating

Symptoms of binge eating may be difficult to detect. Binge eating is different from continuously snacking. Binge eaters are often secretive about food and their bingeing is often done in private. **Obesity** and obesity-related diseases such as **hypertension** (high blood pressure,) type 2 diabetes, and joint **pain** are signs that binge-eating disorder could be present, but not all obese people are binge-eaters. Behaviors such as secretive eating, constant dieting without losing weight, obsessive concern about weight, depression, **anxiety**, and **substance abuse** are all clues, but none of these signs are definitive. The individual may complain about symptoms related to obesity, such as **fatigue** and **shortness of breath**, or mention unsuccessful dieting, but again, these signs are not definitive.

Diagnosis

Diagnosis is based on several factors including a patient history, **physical examination**, laboratory tests, and a mental status evaluation. A patient history is less helpful in diagnosing eating disorders than in diagnosing many diseases because many people with an eating disorder lie repeatedly about how much they eat, purge, or use laxatives, enemas, and medications. The patient may, however, complain about related symptoms such as fatigue, headaches, **dizziness**, **constipation**, or frequent infections.

Tests

A physical examination begins with weight and blood pressure and moves through all the signs listed

above. Based on the physical exam, the physician will order laboratory tests. In general these tests will include a **complete blood count** (CBC), **urinalysis**, blood chemistries (to determine electrolyte levels), and **liver function tests**. The physician may also order an electrocardiogram to look for heart abnormalities. Other conditions including metabolic disorders, brain tumors (especially hypothalamus and pituitary gland lesions), diseases of the digestive tract, and a condition called superior mesenteric artery syndrome can cause weight loss or vomiting after eating. People with this condition sometimes vomit after meals because the blood supply to the intestine is blocked. The physician may perform tests needed to rule out the presence of these disorders and assess the patient's nutritional status.

The individual may be referred to a psychiatrist for a mental status evaluation. The physician will evaluate things such as whether the person is oriented in time and space, appearance, observable state of emotion (affect), attitude toward food and weight, delusional thinking, and thoughts of self-harm or **suicide**. This evaluation helps to distinguish between an eating disorder and other psychiatric disorders, including depression, **schizophrenia**, social phobia, obsessive-compulsive disorder, and **body dysmorphic disorder**. Two diagnostic tests that are often used are the Eating Attitudes Test (EAT) and the Eating Disorder Inventory (EDI).

Treatment

Treatment depends on the degree to which the individual's health is impaired.

Traditional medical treatment

Hospitalization is recommended for anorectics or bulimics with any of the following characteristics:

- weight of 40% or more below normal; or weight loss over a three-month period of more than 30 pounds
- severely disturbed metabolism
- severe bingeing and purging
- signs of psychosis
- severe depression or risk of suicide
- family in crisis

Hospital impatient care is first geared toward correcting problems that present as immediate medical crises, such as severe **malnutrition**, severe electrolyte imbalance, irregular heart beat, pulse below 45 beats per minute, or low body temperature. Patients are hospitalized if they are a high suicide risk, have severe clinical depression, or exhibit signs of an altered mental state. They may also need to be hospitalized to interrupt weight loss, stop the cycle of vomiting, exercising and/or laxative abuse, treat substance disorders, or for additional medical evaluation.

Individuals with eating disorders are treated with a variety of medications to address physical problems brought about by their eating disorder and to treat additional psychiatric problems such as depression, anxiety, and suicidal thoughts. The medications used will vary depending on the individual; however, depression is common among people with eating disorders and is most often treated with **antidepressant drugs**.

Psychotherapy

The mainstay of treatment is **psychotherapy**. An appropriate therapy is selected based on the type of eating disorder and the individual's psychological profile. Some of the common therapies used in treating eating disorders include:

- Cognitive behavior therapy (CBT) is designed to confront and then change the individual's thoughts and feelings about his or her body and behaviors toward food, but it does not address why those thoughts or feelings exist. Strategies to maintain self-control may be explored. This therapy is relatively short-term. CBT is often the therapy of choice for people with eating disorders.
- Psychodynamic therapy, also called psychoanalytic therapy, attempts to help the individual gain insight into the cause of the emotions that trigger their dysfunctional behavior. This therapy tends to be more long term than CBT.
- Interpersonal therapy is short-term therapy that helps the individual identify specific issues and problems in relationships. The individual may be asked to look back at his or her family history to try to recognize problem areas or stresses and work toward resolving them.
- Dialectical behavior therapy consists of structured private and group sessions in which the therapist and patient(s) work at reducing behaviors that interfere with quality of life, finding alternate solutions to current problem situations, and learning to regulate emotions.
- Family and couples therapy is helpful in dealing with conflict or disorder that may be a factor in perpetuating the eating disorder. Family therapy is especially useful in helping parents who are anorectics avoid passing on their attitudes and behaviors on to their children.

Nutrition education

A **nutrition** consultant or dietitian is an essential part of the team needed to successfully treat eating disorders. The first treatment concern is to get the individual medically stable by increasing calorie intake and balancing electrolytes. After that, nutritional therapy is needed to support the long process of recovery and stable weight gain. This is an intensive process involving nutrition education, meal planning, nutrition monitoring, and helping the anorectic develop a healthy relationship with food. However, nutritional counseling alone will not resolve an eating disorder.

Alternative and complementary treatment

Alternative treatments should serve as complements to a conventional treatment program. Alternative therapies for anorexia nervosa include diet and nutrition counseling, herbal therapy, **hydrotherapy**, **aromatherapy**, **Ayurvedic medicine**, and mind/body medicine.

The following herbs may help reduce anxiety and depression which are often associated with this disorder:

- chamomile (*Matricaria recutita*)
- lemon balm (*Melissa officinalis*)
- linden (*Tilia* spp.) flowers

Essential oils of herbs such as bergamot, basil, chamomile, sage, and lavender may help stimulate appetite, relax the body, and fight depression. They can be diffused into the air, inhaled, massaged, or put in bath water.

Relaxation techniques such as **yoga**, **meditation**, and t'ai chi can relax the body and release stress, anxiety, and depression.

Hypnotherapy may help resolve unconscious issues that contribute to anorexic behavior.

Other alternative treatments that may be helpful include hydrotherapy, **magnetic field therapy**, **acupuncture**, **biofeedback**, Ayurvedic medicine, and **traditional Chinese medicine**.

Prognosis

Recovery from eating disorders can be a long, difficult process interrupted by relapses. About half of all anorectics recover. Up to 20% die of complications of the disorder. The recovery rate for people with bulimia is slightly higher. Binge eaters experience many relapses and may have trouble controlling their weight even if they stop bingeing. Not enough is known about the other eating disorders to determine recovery rates. All eating disorders have serious social and emotional consequences. All except rumination disorder have serious health consequences. The sooner a person with an eating disorder gets professional help, the better the chance of recovery.

Prevention

Prevention involves both preventing and relieving stresses and enlisting professional help as soon as abnormal eating patterns develop. Some things that may help prevent an eating disorder from developing are listed below:

- Parents should not obsess about their weight, appearance, and diet in front of their children.
- Parents should not put their child on a diet unless instructed to by a pediatrician.
- Do not tease people about their body shapes or compare them to others.
- Make it clear that family members are loved and accepted as they are.
- Try to eat meals together as a family whenever possible; avoid eating alone.
- Avoid using food for comfort in times of stress.
- Monitoring negative self-talk; practice positive self-talk.
- Spend time doing something enjoyable every day.
- Stay busy, but not overly busy; get enough sleep every night.
- Become aware of the situations that are personal triggers for abnormal eating behaviors and look for ways to avoid or defuse them.
- Do not go on extreme diets.
- Be alert to signs of low self-worth, anxiety, depression, and drug or alcohol abuse and seek help as soon as these signs appear.

Resources

BOOKS

Carleton, Pamela and Deborah Ashin. *Take Charge of Your Child's Eating Disorder: A Physician's Step-By-Step Guide to Defeating Anorexia and Bulimia.* New York: Marlowe & Co., 2007.

Heaton, Jeanne A. and Claudia J. Strauss. *Talking to Eating Disorders: Simple Ways to Support Someone Who Has Anorexia, Bulimia, Binge Eating or Body Image Issues.* New York, NY: New American Library, 2005.

Liu, Aimee. *Gaining: The Truth About Life After Eating Disorders.* New York, NY: Warner Books, 2007.

Messinger, Lisa and Merle Goldberg. *My Thin Excuse: Understanding, Recognizing, and Overcoming Eating Disorders.* Garden City Park, NY: Square One Publishers, 2006.

Rubin, Jerome S., ed. *Eating Disorders and Weight Loss Research.* Hauppauge, NY: Nova Science Publishers, 2006.

Walsh, B. Timothy. *If Your Adolescent Has an Eating Disorder: An Essential Resource for Parents.* New York, NY: Oxford University Press, 2005.

OTHER

Eating Disorders. American Psychological Association. April 2009 [June 23, 2009]. http://www.apa.org/topics/topiceating.html.

Medline Plus. Eating Disorders. U. S. National Library of Medicine, May 15, 2009 [June 23, 2009] http://www.nlm.nih.gov/medlineplus/eatingdisorders.html

ORGANIZATIONS

American Psychological Association, 750 First Street, NE, Washington, DC, 20002-4242, (202) 336-5500; TDD/TTY: (202) 336-6123, (800) 374-2721, apa@psych.org, http://www.apa.org.

National Association of Anorexia Nervosa and Related Eating Disorders (ANAD), P.O. Box 7, Highland Park, IL, 60035, (847) 831-3438, (847) 433-3996, http://www.anad.org.

National Eating Disorders Association, 603 Stewart Street, Suite 803, Seattle, WA, 98101, (206) 382-3587, Help and Referral Line: (800) 931-2237, (206) 829-8501, info@NationalEatingDisorder.org, http://www.nationaleatingdisorders.org.

Tish Davidson, A.M.

Eaton agent pneumonia *see* **Mycoplasma infections**

Ebola virus infection *see* **Hemorrhagic fevers**

Ecchymosis *see* **Bruises**

ECG *see* **Electrocardiography**

Echinacea

Definition

Echinacea is the term given to several plants in the Asteraceae/Compositae family. It is known as the coneflower, narrow-leaf cone-flower, and black susan.

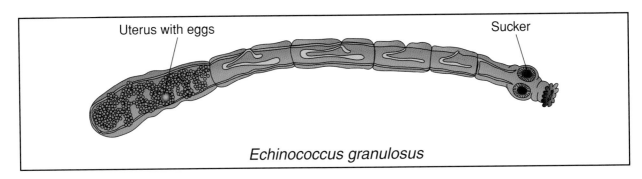

Uterus with eggs

Sucker

Echinococcus granulosus

Infection with the larva of *Echinococcus granulosus* (shown above) is responsible for the disease echinococcosis. *(Illustration by Electronic Illustrators Group. Reproduced by permission of Gale, a part of Cengage Learning.)*

Description

Echinacea is native to, and abundant in, the North American prairie. The plants are indigenous, perennial herbs in North America and thrive when planted in temperate climates in Europe and Asia.

Echinacea propagates easily from seed or root cuttings.

Purpose

Native Americans chewed Echinacea roots to relieve toothaches and inflamed gums. They used teas of the roots and leaves to relieve stomach pains, treat colds and infections, and heal skin **wounds** and infections.

European herbalists and physicians have used Echinacea for over a hundred years to treat colds and respiratory and urinary infections, and to treat wounds.

Echinacea is second only to Ginko in herbal sales in the U.S.

Preparations

The quality and potency of herbal supplements depends on the soil and weather conditions where the herb is grown, the timing and care in harvesting it, and the manner in which it is prepared and stored.

Echinacea has been clinically tested for a number of conditions, including preventing and treating colds and respiratory infections, **cancer**, boosting immune systems, increasing white blood counts after **radiation therapy**, inflammation of the eye, vaginal yeast infections, and **genital herpes**.

In all of those conditions, clinical Study results are, at best, inconclusive. It does not appear to prevent colds.

For treating colds, capsules containing from 300-1200mg can be taken per day for 7 days.

Precautions

Though used as medicines, herbal products like Echinacea are regulated like dietary supplements in the United States. Thus, manufacturers are responsible only for their production processes. Imported herbals may not meet U.S. manufacturing standards. Approval of herbals is based on traditional use, not demonstrated safety and effectiveness. Before an herbal can be forcefully withdrawn from the market, the FDA must prove that it is unsafe.

Many herbal products vary from stated label potency.

Side effects

People who are allergic to ragweed, mums, marigolds or daisies, or who have **asthma** may also react negatively to Echinaceae.

In therapeutic doses, Echinacea is generally safe. Approximately 1% of people taking the herb experience mild abdominal discomfort.

Interactions

Drug-herbal and herbal-herbal interactions are not well understood and have not been thoroughly tested. Patients must be careful observers of themselves for changes as they take new drugs or herbs, or as they take these products over many months.

Allergenic—A substance capable of causing an allergic reaction.

Cholangitis—Infection or inflammation of the bile ducts; often causes abdominal pain, fever, and jaundice.

Computed tomography (CT) scan—A specialized x-ray procedure in which cross-sections of the area in question can be examined in detail.

Cyst—A protective sac that includes either fluid or the cell of an organism. The cyst enables many organisms to survive in the environment for long periods of time without need for food or water.

Embryo—The very beginning stages of development of an organism.

Jaundice—The yellow-greenish coloring of the skin and eyes due to the presence of bile pigments. The presence of jaundice is usually, but not always, a sign of liver disease.

Tapeworm—An intestinal parasite that attaches to the intestine or travels to other organs such as the liver and lungs.

Ultrasound—A noninvasive procedure based on changes in sound waves of a frequency that cannot be heard, but respond to changes in tissue composition.

Resources

OTHER

"Herbs at a Glance." National Center for Complementary and Alternative Medicine. http://nccam.nih.gov/health/herbsataglance.html(accessed July 29, 2009).
Medline Plus. http://www.nlm.nih.gov/medlineplus/druginfo/natural/patient-echinacea.html.

James Waun, MD, RPh,

Echinococcosis

Definition

Echinococcosis (Hydatid disease) refers to human infection by the immature (larval) form of tapeworm, *Echinococcus*. One of three forms of the *Echinococcus* spp., *E. granulosus*, lives on dogs and livestock, and infects humans through contact with these animals. Allergic reactions and damage to various organs from cyst formation are the most common forms of disease in humans.

Description

E. granulosus is found in many areas of Africa, China, South America, Australia, New Zealand, and Mediterranean and eastern Europe, as well as in parts of the western United States. The parasite lives in regions where dogs and livestock cohabitate. Direct exposure to infectious dogs, as well as parasitic eggs released into the environment during shedding, are both sources of human infection.

In humans, cysts containing the larvae develop after ingestion of eggs. Cysts form primarily in the lungs and liver. Cysts developing in the liver are responsible for about two-thirds of echinococcosis cases. Echinococcosis is a significant public health problem in many areas of the world, but control programs have decreased the rate of infection in some regions. In Kenya alone, the numbers of persons infected each year is as high as 220 per 100,000 population.

Causes and symptoms

After ingestion, the eggs develop into embryos within the intestines and then travel to the liver and lungs through major blood vessels. The embryos then begin to form cysts within the liver and lungs, causing damage as they enlarge over a period of five to 20 years. Cysts may become over 8 in (20.3 cm) or more in size and contain a huge amount of highly allergenic fluid. Studies show that while the liver is most often targeted, lungs, brain, heart, and bone can also be affected.

The major symptoms are due to compression damage, blockage of vessels and ducts (such as the bile ducts), and leakage of fluid from cysts. The following symptoms are frequent.

- Liver involvement causes pain and eventually jaundice or cholangitis due to blockage of bile ducts. Infection of cysts leads to abscesses in up to 20%.
- Lung cysts cause cough and chest pain.
- Bone cysts cause fractures and damage to bone tissue.
- Heart involvement leads to irregularities of heart beat and inflammation of the covering of the heart (pericardium).
- Allergic reactions occur from leakage of cyst fluid that contains antigens. Itching, fever, and rashes are

frequent, and fatal allergic reactions (anaphylaxis) have been reported. Eosinophils, which are blood cells involved in allergic reactions, are increased in many patients.

Diagnosis

X rays, **computed tomography scans** (CT scans), and ultrasound are very helpful in detecting cysts. Some cysts will develop characteristic hardening of organ tissues from **calcium** deposits (calcifications). Blood tests to detect antibodies are useful when positive, but up to 50% of patients have negative results. Examination of aspirated cyst fluid for parasites can be diagnostic, but carries the danger of a fatal allergic reaction. Treatment with anti-parasitic medications before aspiration is reported to decrease allergic complications and decrease the risk of spread during the procedure.

Treatment

Treatment depends on the size and location of cysts, as well as the symptoms they are producing. Surgical removal of cysts and/or surrounding tissue is the accepted method of treatment, but carries a risk of cyst rupture with spread or allergic reactions. Recent studies using medication alongside aspiration and drainage of cysts instead of surgery are very encouraging.

The medication albenzadole can be taken before or after surgery or alone without surgery. However, its effectiveness as a single treatment is still not known. Multiple courses of medication are often necessary, with cure rates of only about 30%. Response to treatment is best monitored by serial CT scans or similar x-ray studies.

Prevention

Good hand washing, treating infected dogs, and preventing dogs' access to slaughter houses discourage spread of the disease. Limiting the population of stray dogs has also been helpful.

Resources

OTHER

"Percutaneous Drainage Compared with Surgery for HepaticHydatid Cysts." *New England Journal of Medicine Online.* http://content.nejm.org.

David Kaminstein, MD

Echinococcus granulosus infection *see* **Echinococcosis**

Echocardiography

Definition

Echocardiography is a noninvasive diagnostic test that uses ultrasound waves to produce an moving image of the heart.

Purpose

Echocardiography is one of the most widely used diagnostic tests for heart disease. Ultrasound waves generated by a device placed on the skin rebound or echo off the heart and are processed by a computer. The resulting image can show the size, shape, and movement of the heart's valves and chambers, as well as the flow of blood through the heart.

Echocardiography may reveal abnormalities such damage to the heart tissue from a **heart attack** or as a poorly functioning heart valve. Echocardiography is especially useful for assessing disorders of the heart valves. It not only allows doctors to evaluate the condition of the heart valves, but also can show abnormalities in the pattern of blood flow. For example, echocardiography can show the backward flow of blood through heart valves that remain partially open and should be fully closed.

By assessing the motion of the heart wall, echocardiography can help detect the presence and assess the severity of **coronary artery disease**, as well as help determine whether chest **pain** is related to heart disease. Additionally, echocardiography can help detect **hypertrophic cardiomyopathy**, a condition in which

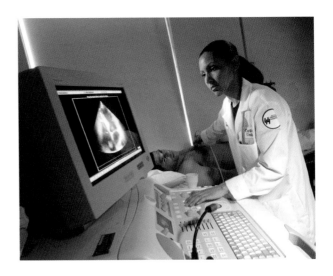

A patient during an echocardiography test. *(© Yoav Levy/ Phototake. — All rights reserved.)*

the walls of the heart thicken in an attempt to compensate for heart muscle weakness.

Echocardiography is also used to evaluate **heart murmurs** (abnormal heart sounds), determine the causes of congestive **heart failure**, assess enlarged hearts, hearts with septal defects (holes between pumping chambers), and to monitor the heart in patients with diseases that may affect heart function (e.g., lupus erythematosus, lung diseases). The biggest advantage to echocardiography is that it is noninvasive (it does not involve breaking the skin or entering body cavities), and it has no known risks or side effects. It also gives a more detailed picture of the heart than other imaging techniques. Echocardiography is often used in conjunction with other diagnostic tests for the heart such as **electrocardiography**.

Echocardiography is usually performed in the cardiology department at a hospital, but may also be performed in a cardiologist's office or an outpatient imaging center. Because the ultrasound scanners used to perform echocardiography are portable (handheld) or mobile, echocardiography can be performed in a hospital emergency department or at the bedside of patients who cannot be moved.

Description

Echocardiography creates an image of the heart using ultra-high-frequency sound waves—sound waves that are too high in frequency to be heard by the human ear. The technique is very similar to ultrasound scanning commonly used to visualize the fetus during **pregnancy**.

An echocardiography examination generally lasts 15–30 minutes. The patient lies bare-chested on an examination table. A special gel is spread over the chest to help the transducer make good contact and to slide smoothly over the skin. The transducer, also called a probe, is a small handheld device at the end of a flexible cable. The transducer is placed against the chest and directs ultrasound waves into the chest. Some of the waves get echoed (or reflected) back to the transducer. Since different tissues and blood reflect ultrasound waves differently, these returning sound waves can be translated into a meaningful image of the heart that is displayed on a monitor and recorded. The patient does not feel the sound waves, and the entire procedure is painless.

Occasionally, variations of the echocardiography test are used. For example, Doppler echocardiography employs a special transducer that allows technicians to measure and analyze the direction and speed of blood flow through blood vessels and heart valves. This makes it especially useful for detecting and evaluating

backflow through the heart valves. By assessing the speed of blood flow at different locations around an obstruction, it can also help to precisely locate the obstruction.

An **exercise** echocardiogram, or stress echo, is an echocardiogram performed during exercise, when the heart muscle must work harder to supply blood to the body. This allows doctors to detect heart problems that might not be evident when the body is at rest and needs less blood. For patients who are unable to exercise, certain drugs can be used to mimic the effects of exercise by dilating the blood vessels and making the heart beat faster.

A transesophageal is done when it is difficult to get a clear picture of the heart using standard electrocardiogram techniques (e.g., interference from internal scar tissue, **obesity**). A transducer is attached to an endoscope, a thin tube that is threaded down the throat after it has been numbed. This position allows a clearer picture of the heart.

During the examination, a trained sonographer takes measurements and, using the ultrasound scanner's computer, make calculations, including measuring blood flow speed. Most ultrasound scanners are equipped with videotape recorders or digital imaging/archiving devices to record the real-time examination, and with medical image printers to print out hard copies of still images. Information from the echocardiogram is then evaluated by a cardiologist.

Preparation

The patient removes any clothing and jewelry above the waist.

Aftercare

No special measures need to be taken following echocardiography. The procedure is painless.

Risks

There are no known complications associated with the use of echocardiography. There is a slight risk of having a heart attack during an exercise echocardiogram, due to the stress put on the heart during the test, mostly for patients with a history of heart attack or other risk factors.

Normal results

A normal echocardiogram shows a normal heart structure and the normal flow of blood through the heart chambers and heart valves. However, a normal echocardiogram does not rule out the possibility certain types of heart disease.

An echocardiogram may show a number of abnormalities in the structure and function of the heart, including:

- thickening of the wall of the heart muscle (especially the left ventricle)
- abnormal motion of the heart muscle
- blood leaking backward through the heart valves
- decreased blood flow through a heart valve due to narrowing of the valve (stenosis)

Resources

BOOKS

Baliga, Ragavendra R., and Kim A. Eagle. *Practical Cardiology: Evaluation and Treatment of Common Cardiovascular Disorders.* Phiadelphia: Lippincott Williams & Wilkins, 2008.

OTHER

"Echocardiogram." *Medline Plus* April 12, 2007 [cited January 4, 2008]. http://www.nlm.nih.gov/medlineplus/ency/article/003869.htm (accessed March 19, 2008).

"Echocardiogram: Sound Imaging of the Heart." *Mayo Clinic* July 14, 2006 [cited January 4, 2008]. http://www.mayoclinic.com/health/echocardiogram/HB00012 (accessed March 19, 2008).

ORGANIZATIONS

American College of Cardiology, Heart House, 2400 N Street NW, Washington, DC, 20037, (202) 375-6000, (202) 375-7000, resource@acc.org, http://www.acc.org.

American Heart Association, 7272 Greenville Avenue, Dallas, TX, 75231, (800) 242-8721, http://www.americanheart.org.

American Registry of Diagnostic Medical Sonographers, 51 Monroe Street, Plaza One East, Rockville, MD, 20850-2400, (301) 738-8401, (800) 541-9754, (301) 738-031, http://www.ardms.org.

American Society of Echocardiography, 2100 Gateway Centre Boulevard, Suite 310, Morrisville, NC, 27560, (919) 861-5574, (919) 882-9900, http://www.asecho.org.

Jennifer E. Sisk, MA
Lee Shratter, MD
Tish Davidson, AM
Brenda W. Lerner

Echovirus infections *see* **Enterovirus infections**

Eclampsia *see* **Preeclampsia and eclampsia**

ECT *see* **Electroconvulsive therapy**

Ectopic orifice of the ureter *see* **Congenital ureter anomalies**

Ectopic pregnancy

Definition

In an ectopic **pregnancy**, the fertilized egg implants in a location outside the uterus and tries to develop there. The word ectopic means "in an abnormal place or position." The most common site is the fallopian tube, the tube that normally carries eggs from the ovary to the uterus. However, ectopic pregnancy can also occur in the ovary, the abdomen, and the cervical canal (the opening from the uterus to the vaginal canal). The phrases tubal pregnancy, ovarian pregnancy, cervical pregnancy, and abdominal pregnancy refer to the specific area of an ectopic pregnancy.

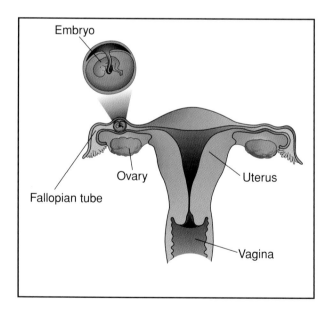

In an ectopic pregnancy, the fertilized egg implants in a location outside the uterus and attempts to develop at that site. The most common site of an ectopic pregnancy is the fallopian tube, but it can occur in the ovary, the abdomen, and the cervical wall. More than 95% of all ectopic pregnancies occur in the fallopian tube. *(Illustration by Electronic Illustrators Group. Reproduced by permission of Gale, a part of Cengage Learning.)*

Description

Once a month, an egg is produced in a woman's ovary and travels down the fallopian tube where it meets the male's sperm and is fertilized. In a normal pregnancy the fertilized egg, or zygote, continues on its passage down the fallopian tube and enters the uterus in three to five days. The zygote continues to grow, implanting itself securely in the wall of the uterus. The zygote's cells develop into the embryo (the organism in its first two months of development) and placenta (a spongy structure that lines the uterus and nourishes the developing organism).

In a tubal ectopic pregnancy, the fertilized egg cannot make it all the way down the tube because of scarring or obstruction. The fallopian tube is too narrow for the growing zygote. Eventually the thin walls of the tube stretch and may burst (rupture), resulting in severe bleeding and possibly the **death** of the mother. More than 95% percent of all ectopic pregnancies occur in the fallopian tube. Only 1.5% develop in the abdomen; less than 1% develop in the ovary or the cervix.

Causes and symptoms

As many as 50% of women with ectopic pregnancies have a history of **pelvic inflammatory disease** (PID). This is an infection of the fallopian tubes (salpingitis) that can spread to the uterus or ovaries. It is most commonly caused by the organisms *Gonorrhea* and *Chlamydia* and is usually transmitted by sexual intercourse.

Other conditions also increase the risk of ectopic pregnancy. They include:

- Endometriosis. A condition in which the tissue that normally lines the uterus is found outside the uterus, and can block a fallopian tube.
- Exposure to diethylsilbestrol (DES) as a fetus. If a woman's mother took DES (a synthetic version of the hormone estrogen) during pregnancy, the woman may have abnormalities in her fallopian tubes that can make ectopic pregnancy more likely.
- Taking hormones. Estrogen and progesterone are hormones that regulate the menstrual cycle and may be in medications prescribed by a doctor for birth control or other reasons. Taking these hormones can affect the interior lining of the fallopian tubes and slow the movement of the fertilized egg down the tube. Women who become pregnant in spite of taking some progesterone-only contraceptives have a greater chance of an ectopic pregnancy. Ectopic pregnancy is also more likely when the ovaries are artificially stimulated with hormones to produce eggs for in vitro fertilization (a procedure in which eggs are taken from a woman's body, fertilized, and then placed in the uterus in an attempt to conceive a child).

- Use of an intrauterine device (IUD). These contraceptive devices are designed to prevent fertilized eggs from becoming implanted in the uterus, but they have only a minimal effect on preventing ectopic pregnancies. Therefore, if a woman becomes pregnant while using an IUD for contraception, the fertilized egg is more likely to be implanted someplace other than the uterus. For example, among women who become pregnant while using a progesterone-bearing IUD, about 15% have ectopic pregnancies.
- Surgery on a fallopian tube. The risk of ectopic pregnancy can be as high as 60% after undergoing elective tubal sterilization, a procedure in which the fallopian tubes are severed to prevent pregnancy. Women who have successful surgery to reverse the procedure are also more likely to have an ectopic pregnancy.

Early symptoms

In an ectopic pregnancy all the hormonal changes associated with a normal pregnancy may occur. The early symptoms include: **fatigue**; **nausea**; a missed period; breast tenderness; **low back pain**; mild cramping on one side of the pelvis; and abnormal vaginal bleeding, usually spotting.

Later symptoms

As the embryo grows too large for the confined space in the tube, the first sign that something is wrong may be a stabbing **pain** in the pelvis or abdomen. If the tube has ruptured, blood may irritate the diaphragm and cause shoulder pain. Other warning signs are lightheadedness and **fainting**.

Diagnosis

To confirm an early diagnosis of ectopic pregnancy, the doctor must determine first that the patient is pregnant and that the location of the embryo is outside the uterus. If an ectopic pregnancy is suspected, the doctor will perform a pelvic examination to locate the source of pain and to detect a mass in the abdomen.

Several laboratory tests of the patient's blood provide information for diagnosis. Measurement of the human chorionic gonadotropin (hCG) level in the patient's blood serum is the most useful laboratory test in the early stages. In a normal pregnancy, the level of this hormone doubles about every two days during the first 10 weeks. In an ectopic pregnancy, the rate of the increase is much slower and the low hCG for the stage of the pregnancy is a strong indication that the pregnancy is abnormal. (It could also represent a **miscarriage** in progress.) The level is usually tested several times over a period of days to determine whether or not it is increasing at a normal rate.

Progesterone levels in the blood are also measured. Lower than expected levels can indicate that the pregnancy is not normal.

An ultrasound examination may provide information about whether or not the pregnancy is ectopic. A device called a transducer, which emits high frequency sound waves, is moved over the surface of the patient's abdomen or inserted into the vagina. The sound waves bounce off of the internal organs and create an image on a screen. The doctor should be able to see whether or not there is a fetus developing in the uterus after at least five weeks of gestation. Before that point, a normal pregnancy is too small to see.

A culdocentesis may also help confirm a diagnosis. In this procedure a needle is inserted into the space at the top of the vagina, behind the uterus and in front of the rectum. Blood in this area may indicate bleeding from a ruptured fallopian tube.

A **laparoscopy** will enable the doctor to see the patient's reproductive organs and examine an ectopic pregnancy. In this technique, a hollow tube with a light on one end is inserted through a small incision in the abdomen. Through this instrument the internal organs can be observed.

Treatment

Ectopic pregnancy requires immediate treatment. The earlier the condition is treated, the better the chance to preserve the fallopian tube intact for future normal pregnancies.

Medical

If the ectopic pregnancy is discovered in a very early stage of development, the drug methotrexate may be given. The best results are obtained when the pregnancy is less than six weeks old and the tubal mass is no more than 1.4 in (3.5 cm) in diameter. Methotrexate, which has been used successfully since 1987, works by inhibiting the growth of rapidly growing cells. (It is also used to treat some cancers.) Most side effects are mild and temporary, but the patient must be monitored after treatment. Usually the medication is injected into the muscle in a single dose, but may also be given intravenously or injected directly into the fallopian tube to dissolve the embryonic tissue. Methotrexate has also been used to treat ovarian, abdominal, and cervical pregnancies that are discovered in the early stages.

Surgical

When a laparoscopy is done to visualize the ectopic pregnancy, the scope can be fitted with surgical tools and used to remove the ectopic mass immediately after it is identified. The affected fallopian tube can be repaired or removed as necessary. This procedure can be done without requiring the patient to stay in the hospital overnight.

When the pregnancy has ruptured, a surgical incision into the abdomen, or laparotomy, is performed to stop the immediate loss of blood and to remove the embryo. This usually requires **general anesthesia** and a hospital stay. Every effort is made to preserve and repair the injured fallopian tube. However, if the fallopian tube has already ruptured, repair is extremely difficult and the tube is usually removed.

Alternative treatment

Ectopic pregnancy was first described in the eleventh century and was a potentially fatal condition until the advent of surgery and blood transfusions in the early twentieth century. The sophisticated diagnostic tools and surgical procedures developed since the 1970s have equipped modern medicine with the tools to not only save a woman's life, but also to preserve her future fertility.

Although there are herbal remedies for the temporary relief of the common symptoms of **anxiety** and abdominal discomfort, prompt medical treatment is the only sure remedy for ectopic pregnancy.

Prognosis

Ectopic pregnancies are the leading cause of pregnancy-related deaths in the first trimester and account for 9% of all pregnancy-related deaths in the United States. More than 1% of pregnancies are ectopic, and they are becoming more common. The reason for this increase is not clearly understood, though it is thought that the dramatic increase in **sexually transmitted diseases** (STD) is at least partly responsible.

The earlier an ectopic pregnancy is diagnosed and treated, the better the outcome. The chances of having a successful pregnancy are lower after an ectopic pregnancy, but depend on the extent of permanent

KEY TERMS

Embryo—In humans, the developing organism from conception until approximately the end of the second month.

Fallopian tube—The tube that carries the egg from the ovary to the uterus.

Human chorionic gonadotropin (hCG)—A hormone excreted during the development of an embryo or fetus.

Laparoscopy—Examination of the contents of the abdominal cavity with a fiberoptic tube inserted through a small incision.

Laparotomy—Surgical incision into the abdomen to locate, repair, and/or remove injured or diseased tissues.

Pelvic inflammatory disease (PID)—Acute or chronic inflammation in the pelvic cavity, particularly inflammation of the fallopian tubes (salpingitis) and its complications.

Rupture—A breaking apart of an organ or tissue.

Salpingitis—Inflammation of the fallopian tube.

Tubal pregnancy—Pregnancy in one of the fallopian tubes.

Zygote—The fertilized egg.

fallopian tube damage. If the tube has been spared, chances are as high as 60%. The chances of a successful pregnancy after the removal of one tube are 40%.

Prevention

Many forms of ectopic pregnancy cannot be prevented. However, tubal pregnancies, which make up the majority of ectopic pregnancies, may be prevented by avoiding conditions that cause damage to the fallopian tubes. Since half of all women who experience ectopic pregnancy have a history of PID, avoiding this infection or getting early diagnosis and treatment for sexually transmitted diseases will decrease the risk of a future problem.

ORGANIZATIONS

Resolve, 1760 Old Meadow Rd., Suite 500, McLean, VA, 22102, (703) 556-7172, (703) 506-3266, http://www.resolve.org.

Karen Ericson, RN

Eczema

Definition

Eczema, also called **atopic dermatitis** (AD), is a non-contagious inflammation of the skin characterized by dry, red, itchy, and oozing lesions that become scaly, crusty, or hardened. Various other types of **dermatitis** are sometimes referred to as eczema or eczematous, although AD is the most common type.

Demographics

Worldwide 10–20% of people develop atopic dermatitis at some point in their lives. Although eczema can affect anyone at any age, it is most common in children under age five. An estimated 65% of eczema cases begin during the first year of life and 90% develop before the age of five. The incidence of eczema and other allergic diseases appears to have increased in recent decades. As of 2009 it was estimated that almost one in ten American babies develop eczema.

Description

Eczema is sometimes described as "the itch that rashes," because scratching irritated areas sometimes initiates a rash. Eczema can be mild and intermittent or severe and chronic, disappearing as children grow up or lasting a lifetime. Eczema is frequently related to some form of allergy, including **allergies** to foods or inhalants.

The areas of the body affected by eczema tend to vary with age. Infants frequently have eczema on the face and other areas of the head. The stomach and limbs also may be affected. Older children commonly have more severe eczema on flexor surfaces—the inner wrists and elbows, backs of the knees, and tops of the ankles, as well as the hands and feet. The knees, elbows, hands, and feet may continue to be a problem into adulthood. Occasionally eczema becomes widespread throughout the body.

Other types of dermatitis that may be described as eczematous, but which usually affect older children and adults, include:

- contact dermatitis, which results from skin contact with an irritant or allergen

- nummular dermatitis, which usually affects people over the age of 55

- stasis dermatitis, which results from poor circulation in the legs

KEY TERMS

Allergic reaction—An immune system reaction to a substance in the environment; symptoms include rash, inflammation, sneezing, itchy watery eyes, runny nose, or skin irritations.

Antigen—A foreign protein or particle that causes the body to produce specific antibodies that bind to the antigen.

Atopy—Allergies, such as eczema, that are probably hereditary, with symptoms that develop upon exposure to specific environmental allergens.

Corticosteroids—A group of hormones produced by the adrenal glands or manufactured synthetically.

They are often used to treat inflammation. Examples include cortisone and prednisone.

Dermatitis—Inflammation of the skin.

Patch test—Scratch test; a test to identify allergens, in which the suspected substance is pricked or scratched into the skin and observed for the development of redness and swelling that are indicative of an allergic reaction.

Rash—Spotted, pink or red skin eruptions that may be accompanied by itching.

Risk factors

The major risk factor for eczema appears to be a family history of eczema and/or allergies.

Causes and symptoms

In many cases the exact cause of eczema is unknown, although it often appears to result from an interaction between an inherited genetic predisposition towards allergies and exposure to specific environmental allergens, especially those that are inhaled or ingested.

The hallmark sign of eczema is a red, itchy rash and skin that is abnormally dry. Chronic or severe cases of eczema can result in thick plaques (patches of slightly raised skin), serous (watery) exudates, or infection.

Diagnosis

Examination

Eczema is diagnosed by the appearance and location of the rash. An individual or family history of allergies, including **food allergies**, hay **fever**, or **asthma**, supports the diagnosis of eczema.

Tests

There are no laboratory tests for diagnosing eczema. Sometimes dermatologists conduct skin tests—scratch or patch tests or intradermal injections—to attempt to identify suspected allergens. A small amount of the suspected allergen is dabbed, scratched, or pricked into the skin, usually on the back. If no irritation develops within a few days, patch tests for other suspected allergens may be performed sequentially. Blood tests can measure the levels of immunoglobulin E (IgE)—the

antibodies involved in allergic reactions—and, in some cases, the levels of IgE that are specific for a given antigen.

Procedures

In rare cases a **skin biopsy** may be required to rule out certain diseases.

Treatment

Traditional

The best treatment for eczema is to identify the cause and eliminate it. Since this is often not possible, medications and home treatments for hydrating the skin are the best options. Since **itching** or scratching eczema can irritate and damage the skin and cause **rashes**, any treatment that reduces the itching is helpful.

Drugs

Drug treatments for eczema include:

- oral antihistamines to decrease itching
- calamine lotion
- mild topical corticosteroids containing at least 1% hydrocortisone
- rarely, oral corticosteroids for severe itching and inflammation
- topical antibiotics to prevent or treat infection
- oral antibiotics for widespread infection
- topical pimecrolimus (Elidel) and tacrolimus (Protopic)—immunomodulators that may be used in adults and children over age two when other treatments have failed

Alternative

Light therapy or **phototherapy** can effectively treat eczema, either by controlled exposure to natural sunlight or artificial ultraviolet A (UVA) and/or ultraviolet B (UVB) light. However a dermatologist should be consulted about the benefits and risks of phototherapy.

There are a number of alternative therapies that may prove helpful for treating eczema:

- acupuncture
- autogenic training, meditation, and self-hypnosis
- hypnotherapy—using the power of suggestion to relieve itching
- massage to reduce stress
- reflexology focusing on areas of the body corresponding to the eczema-affected patches, as well the solar plexus, adrenal glands, pituitary gland, liver, kidneys, gastrointestinal tract, and reproductive glands
- aromatherapy with small amounts of essential oils of lavender, bergamot, and geranium to decrease itching and inflammation; however improper dilutions of essential oils can worsen eczema
- evening primrose (*Oenothera biennis*) oil (EPO) diluted in a carrier oil and massaged into the skin

Herbal therapies that are often recommended for skin conditions such as eczema include:

- calendula (*Calendula officinalis*) ointment, for its anti-inflammatory and antiseptic properties
- chickweed (*Stellaria media*) ointment, to soothe itching
- evening primrose oil—topically to relieve itching and internally as a fatty acid supplement
- German chamomile (*Chamomilla recutita*) ointment, for its anti-inflammatory properties
- nettle (*Urtica dioica*) ointment, to relieve itching
- peppermint (*Menta piperita*) lotion, for its antibacterial and antiseptic properties
- traditional Chinese herbal formulas, both applied topically and taken internally, to moisten the skin, prevent itching, nourish the blood, and encourage healing Individuals vary in their responses to herbal treatments. Chronic, severe, or infected eczema requires the attention of a healthcare professional.

Various **nutritional supplements** may aid in treating eczema:

- Oral EPO, which contains gamma-linolenic acid, has been shown to significantly reduce itching from eczema at doses of approximately 6 grams (g) daily.

- Fish oil at a dose of about 1.8 g per day has been shown to improve AD.
- Vitamin C can promote both skin healing and the immune system. Doses of 50–75 milligrams per kilogram (mg/kg) of body weight have been shown to relieve symptoms of AD.
- Supplemental copper may be required with high doses of vitamin C.
- Vitamin E may be of use in treating eczema.

Home remedies

Home care for eczema focuses on keeping the skin clean and moist and avoiding irritants and known allergens as much as possible. Frequent long, tepid soaks help hydrate very dry skin; however soaking in plain water can be painful during severe episodes of eczema:

- Adding one-half cup of table salt to one-half tub of water creates a normal saline solution, similar to that present in the body tissues, and may relieve burning.
- Adding baking soda, a muslin bag filled with milled oats, or the commercial preparation Aveeno to the water can be soothing.
- Research has shown that dilute bleach baths—one-half cup (118 milliliters) of bleach in 40 gallons (151 liters) of warm water—can treat eczema by killing bacteria growing on the skin. The affected areas should be soaked for 5–10 minutes once or twice per week.
- Commercial Domeboro powder may be helpful.
- Bath water should cover as much of the skin as possible. Wet towels may be draped around the shoulders, upper trunk, and arms if they are above the water level.
- The face should be dabbed frequently during bathing to keep it moist.
- The use of soap should be minimized and limited to very mild agents such as Cetaphil.

Drying off should involve two–three minutes of gentle patting, followed by the thick application of a water-barrier ointment, such as Aquaphor, Unibase, or Vaseline. Oil or creams applied to damp skin can seal in moisture. However moisturizing lotions containing alcohol dry the skin and may burn when applied to eczema. Babies' skin should be kept lubricated with appropriate bath oils, lotions, creams, or ointments.

Soaking wraps are an alternative to bathing. Cotton towels or other cloths are soaked in tepid water, possibly containing table salt or Domeboro powder, and used to cover the bare skin as thoroughly as possible. The patient lies on a bed with a waterproof sheet and is covered by a second waterproof covering, such as vinyl sheeting or plastic wrap, to slow evaporation. The wraps are left in place for as long as possible, but for at least 30 minutes, followed by the application of a water barrier and any topical medications.

Environmental changes can provide relief for many eczema sufferers:

- Pet dander and cigarette smoke should be kept out of the home, or at least out of the room.
- Clothing should be loose fitting to prevent irritation from rubbing.
- Clothing and bedding should be 100% soft cotton.
- Clothing and bedding should be washed before initial use to rid them of potentially irritating residues.
- Laundry soap should by dye- and perfume-free.
- Laundry should be run through a double-rinse cycle to remove any vestiges of detergent.
- Bedding should be washed in hot water to kill dust mites, which can be major irritants to people with eczema.
- Fabric softener or dryer sheets are frequently scented and may be irritating.
- Clothes and bedding should not be dried outdoors where pollen and other potential allergens can cling to them.
- Mattresses and pillowcases can be covered by special casings that are impervious to microscopic dust mites.
- Dust-collecting items, such as curtains, carpeting, and stuffed animals, should be kept to a minimum.
- Vacuuming and dusting should be performed regularly when the patient is out of the room.

Temperature extremes can aggravate eczema, so heating and cooling should be employed appropriately, along with the use of a home humidifier. Eczema can interfere with normal body temperature regulation and can be aggravated by sweating. Central air-conditioning is preferable to evaporative cooling or open windows that can bring allergens into the house. Car air-conditioning is preferable to open windows. Electrostatic filters and vent covers can remove irritants from household air. These should be changed or cleaned frequently. A HEPA filter unit and a vacuum with a built-in HEPA filter can remove a high percentage of the dust and pollen.

It is difficult to keep children from scratching and damaging irritated and itchy skin:

- Fingernails should be kept short, using a nail file for a smoother edge.
- Pajamas and clothing with maximum coverage help to protect the bare skin from fingernails.
- Mittens or socks can be used to prevent scratching at night.
- Infant gowns with hand coverings are useful for very young children.

Prognosis

Although there is no cure for eczema, most children improve with age, often by age five. For others however, eczema is a lifelong problem. Diligent daily skin care and avoidance of known triggers can largely control most cases. However as many as 75% of children with eczema will develop other allergies, including hay fever, food allergies, or asthma.

Prevention

Breastfeeding an infant may help prevent eczema, particularly if there is a family history of eczema or allergies. It also may help for the breastfeeding mother to avoid foods that are common allergens. These include wheat, eggs, milk products, peanuts, and fish. If breastfeeding is not possible, a hypoallergenic formula should be used if there is family history of allergies.

Avoidance of known triggers and diligent skin care can minimize eczema flare-ups. A twice-daily emollient (moisturizing) routine should be followed even when the eczema appears to be under control. Eczematous skin is more susceptible to infection and patients should try to avoid contact with people infected with **chickenpox**, **cold sores**, and other contagious skin infections.

Resources

BOOKS

Balch, James F., Mark Stengler, and Robin Young-Balch. *Prescription for Drug Alternatives: All-Natural Options for Better Health Without the Side Effects.* Hoboken, NJ: John Wiley & Sons, 2008.

Joneja, Janice M. Vickerstaff. *Dealing with Food Allergies in Babies and Children.* Boulder, CO: Bull Publishing Co., 2007.

Sutton, Amy L. *Allergies Sourcebook.* Detroit: Omnigraphics, 2007.

PERIODICALS

Bieber, T. "Mechanisms of Disease: Atopic Dermatitis." *New England Journal of Medicine* 358 (2008): 1483.

Huang, J. T., et al. "Treatment of *Staphylococcus aureus* Colonization in Atopic Dermatitis Decreases Disease Severity." *Pediatrics* 123, no. 5 (May 1, 2009): e808-814.

Lawton, S. "Assessing and Treating Adult Patients with Eczema." *Nursing Standard* 23, no. 43 (July 1–7, 2009): 49-56.

Shrieves, Linda. "Childhood Eczema is a Growing Problem." *Connecticut Post* (April 20, 2009).

Van Bever, Hugo, Birgit Lane, and John Common. "Gene Defects and Allergy." *British Medical Journal* 339, no. 7712 (July 11, 2009): 58.

Watkins, Jean. "Eczema: Types, Presentation, Causes and Management." *Practice Nurse* 38, no. 4 (September 4, 2009): 11-16.

OTHER

"Atopic Dermatitis." *National Institute of Arthritis and Musculoskeletal and Skin Diseases.* http://www.niams.nih.gov/Health_Info/Atopic_Dermatitis/atopic_dermatitis_ff.asp

"Eczema." *MedlinePlus.* http://www.nlm.nih.gov/medlineplus/eczema.html

"Eczema/Atopic Dermatitis." *American Academy of Dermatology.* http://www.aad.org/public/publications/pamphlets/skin_eczema.html

"Eczema Quick Fact Sheet." *National Eczema Association.* http://www.nationaleczema.org/living/eczema_quick_fact_sheet.htm

"Evening Primrose Oil." *NCCAM Publication No. D341.* http://nccam.nih.gov/health/eveningprimrose/

Mayo Clinic Staff. "Atopic Dermatitis (Eczema)." *Mayo Clinic.com* http://www.mayoclinic.com/health/eczema/DS00986

Sampson, Hugh A. "Food Allergy Testing: When, Why, and What Does It Mean?" *Food Allergy & Anaphylaxis Network.* http://www.foodallergy.org/featuredtopic1.htm

"What is Eczema?" *American Academy of Dermatology.* http://www.skincarephysicians.com/eczemanet/whatis.html

ORGANIZATIONS

American Academy of Dermatology, PO Box 4014, Schaumburg, IL, 60168, (847) 240-1280, (866) 503-SKIN (7546), (847) 240-1859, http://www.aad.org.

American Academy of Family Physicians, 11400 Tomahawk Creek Parkway, Leawood, KS, 66211-2680, (913) 906-6000, (800) 274-6000, (913) 906-6075, http://www.aafp.org/online/en/home.html.

Food Allergy & Anaphylaxis Network, 11781 Lee Jackson Hwy., Suite 160, Fairfax, VA, 22033-3309, (800) 929-4040, (703) 691-2713, faan@foodallergy.org, http://www.foodallergy.org.

National Center for Complementary and Alternative Medicine, National Institutes of Health, 9000 Rockville Pike, Bethesda, MD, 20892, info@nccam.nih.gov, http://nccam.nih.gov.

National Eczema Association, 4460 Redwood Highway, Suite 16D, San Rafael, CA, 94903-1953, (415) 499-3474, (800) 818-7546, info@nationaleczema.org, http://www.nationaleczema.org.

National Institute of Arthritis and Musculoskeletal and Skin Diseases (NIAMS), Information Clearinghouse, National Institutes of Health, 1 AMS Circle, Bethesda, MD, 20892-3675, (301) 495-4484, (877) 22-NIAMS (226-4267), (301) 718-6366, NIAMSinfo@mail.nih.gov, http://www.niams.nih.gov.

Judith Turner
Teresa G. Odle
Margaret Alic, PhD

ED *see* **Impotence**

Edema

Definition

Edema is a condition of abnormally large fluid volume in the circulatory system or in tissues between the body's cells (interstitial spaces).

Description

Normally the body maintains a balance of fluid in tissues by ensuring that the same of amount of water entering the body also leaves it. The circulatory system transports fluid within the body via its network of blood vessels. The fluid, which contains oxygen and nutrients needed by the cells, moves from the walls of the blood vessels into the body's tissues. After its nutrients are used up, fluid moves back into the blood vessels and returns to the heart. The lymphatic system (a network of channels in the body that carry lymph, a colorless fluid containing white blood cells to fight infection) also absorbs and transports this fluid. In edema, either too much fluid moves from the blood vessels into the tissues, or not enough fluid moves from the tissues back into the blood vessels. This fluid imbalance can cause mild to severe swelling in one or more parts of the body.

Causes and symptoms

Many ordinary factors can upset the balance of fluid in the body to cause edema, including:

- Immobility. The leg muscles normally contract and compress blood vessels to promote blood flow with walking or running. When these muscles are not used, blood can collect in the veins, making it difficult for fluid to move from tissues back into the vessels.

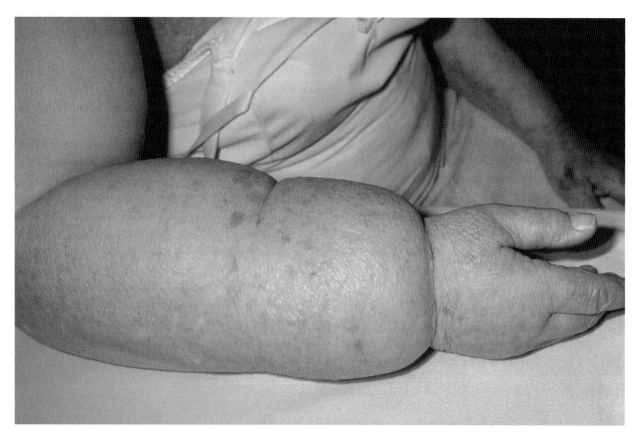

Gross lymphedema in the arm of an elderly woman following radiotherapy treatment for breast cancer. *(Dr. P. Marazzi/Photo Researchers, Inc.)*

- Heat. Warm temperatures cause the blood vessels to expand, making it easier for fluid to cross into surrounding tissues. High humidity also aggravates this situation.
- Medications. Certain drugs, such as steroids, hormone replacements, nonsteroidal anti-inflammatory drugs (NSAIDs), and some blood pressure medications may affect how fast fluid leaves blood vessels.
- Intake of salty foods. The body needs a constant concentration of salt in its tissues. When excess salt is taken in, the body dilutes it by retaining fluid.
- Menstruation and pregnancy. The changing levels of hormones affect the rate at which fluid enters and leaves the tissues.

Some medical conditions may also cause edema, including:

- Heart failure. When the heart is unable to maintain adequate blood flow throughout the circulatory system, the excess fluid pressure within the blood vessels can cause shifts into the interstitial spaces. Left-sided heart failure can cause pulmonary edema, as fluid shifts into the lungs. The patient may develop rapid, shallow respirations, shortness of breath, and a cough. Right-sided heart failure can cause pitting edema, a swelling in the tissue under the skin of the lower legs and feet. Pressing this tissue with a finger tip leads to a noticeable momentary indentation.
- Kidney disease. The decrease in sodium and water excretion can result in fluid retention and overload.
- Thyroid or liver disease. These conditions can change the concentration of protein in the blood, affecting fluid movement in and out of the tissues. In advanced liver disease, the liver is enlarged and fluid may build-up in the abdomen.
- Malnutrition. Protein levels are decreased in the blood, and in an effort to maintain a balance of concentrations, fluid shifts out of the vessels and causes edema in tissue spaces.

Some conditions that may cause swelling in just one leg include:

- Blood clots. Clots can cause pooling of fluid and may be accompanied by discoloration and pain. In some instances, clots may cause no pain.

- Weakened veins. Varicose veins, or veins whose walls or valves are weak, can allow blood to pool in the legs. This is a common condition.
- Infection and inflammation. Infection in leg tissues can cause inflammation and increasing blood flow to the area. Inflammatory diseases, such as gout or arthritis, can also result in swelling.
- Lymphedema. Blocked lymph channels may be caused by infection, scar tissue, or hereditary conditions. Lymph that can't drain properly results in edema. Lymphedema may also occur after cancer treatments, when the lymph system is impaired by surgery, radiation, or chemotherapy.
- Tumor. Abnormal masses can compress leg vessels and lymph channels, affecting the rate of fluid movement.

Symptoms vary depending on the cause of edema. In general, weight gain, puffy eyelids, and swelling of the legs may occur as a result of excess fluid volume. Pulse rate and blood pressure may be elevated. Hand and neck veins may be observed as fuller.

Diagnosis

Edema is a sign of an underlying problem, rather than a disease unto itself. A diagnostic explanation should be sought. Patient history and presenting symptoms, along with laboratory blood studies, if indicated, assist the health professional in determining the cause of the edema.

Treatment

Treatment of edema is based on the cause. Simple steps to lessen fluid build-up may include:

- Reducing sodium intake. A high sodium level causes or aggravates fluid retention.
- Maintaining proper weight. Being overweight slows body fluid circulation and puts extra pressure on the veins.
- Exercise. Regular exercise stimulates circulation.
- Elevation of the legs. Placing the legs at least 12 in (30.5 cm) above the level of the heart for 10–15 minutes, three to four times a day, stimulates excess fluid re-entry into the circulatory system.
- Use of support stocking. Elastic stockings, available at most medical supply or drug stores, will compress the leg vessels, promoting circulation and decreasing pooling of fluid due to gravity.
- Massage. Massaging the body part can help to stimulate the release of excess fluids, but should be avoided if the patient has blood clots in the veins.

KEY TERMS

Digitalis—A naturally occuring compound used in the preparation of the medication, digoxin, prescribed to increase the heart rate and strengthen the force of the heart's contractions.

Diuretics—Medications used in the treatment of fluid overload, to promote excretion of sodium and water.

Interstitial spaces—Areas of the body occuring outside the vessels or organs, between the cells.

Pitting edema—A swelling in the tissue under the skin, resulting from fluid accumulation, that is measured by the depth of indentation made by finger pressure over a boney prominence.

- Travel breaks. Sitting for long periods will increase swelling in the feet and ankles. Standing and/or walking at least every hour or two will help stimulate blood flow.

The three "Ds"–diuretics, digitalis, and diet–are frequently prescribed for medical conditions that result in excess fluid volume. **Diuretics** are medications that promote urination of **sodium** and water. **Digoxin** is a digitalis preparation that is sometimes needed to decrease heart rate and increase the strength of the heart's contractions. Dietary recommendations include less sodium in order to decrease fluid retention. Consideration of adequate protein intake is also made.

For patients with **lymphedema**, a combination of therapies may prove effective. Combined decongestive therapy includes the use of manual lymph drainage (MLD), compression bandaging, garments and pumps, and **physical therapy**. MLD involves the use of light massage of the subcutaneous tissue where the lymph vessels predominate. Massage begins in an area of the body trunk where there is normal lymph function and proceeds to areas of lymphatic insufficiency, in an effort to stimulate new drainage tract development. (MLD should not be used for patients with active **cancer**, deep vein clots, congestive **heart failure**, or cellulitis.) MLD sessions are followed by application of compression garments or pumps. Physical therapy is aimed at strengthening the affected limb and increasing joint mobility.

Alternative treatment

Dietary changes, in addition to cutting back the amount of sodium eaten, may also help reduce edema.

Foods that worsen edema, such as alcohol, **caffeine**, sugar, dairy products, soy sauce, animal protein, chocolate, olives, and pickles, should be avoided. Diuretic herbs can also help relieve edema. One of the best herbs for this purpose is dandelion (*Taraxacum mongolicum*), since, in addition to its diuretic action, it is a rich source of potassium. (Diuretics flush potassium from the body and it must be replaced to avoid potassium deficiency.) **Hydrotherapy** using daily contrast applications of hot and cold (either compresses or immersion) may also be helpful.

ORGANIZATIONS

Austin Wound and Lymphedema Center, 5750 Balcones Dr., Ste. 110, Austin, TX, 78731, (512) 453-1930, http://www.woundandlymphedemacare.com.

Kathleen D. Wright, RN

Edrophonium test *see* **Tensilon test**

Edwards' syndrome

Definition

Edwards' syndrome is caused by an extra copy of chromosome 18. For this reason, it is also called trisomy 18 syndrome. The extra chromosome is lethal for most babies born with this condition. It causes major physical abnormalities and severe **mental retardation**, and very few children afflicted with this disease survive beyond a year.

Description

Humans normally have 23 pairs of chromosomes. Chromosomes are numbered 1–22, and the 23rd pair is composed of the sex chromosomes, X and Y. A person inherits one set of 23 chromosomes from each parent. Occasionally, a genetic error occurs during egg or sperm cell formation. A child conceived with such an egg or sperm cell may inherit an incorrect number of chromosomes.

In the case of Edwards' syndrome, the child inherits three, rather than two, copies of chromosome 18. Trisomy 18 occurs in approximately one in every 3,000 newborns and affects girls more often than boys. Women older than their early thirties have a greater risk of conceiving a child with trisomy 18, but it can occur in younger women.

Causes and symptoms

A third copy of chromosome 18 causes numerous abnormalities. Most children born with Edwards' syndrome appear weak and fragile, and they are often underweight. The head is unusually small and the back of the head is prominent. The ears are malformed and low-set, and the mouth and jaw are small. The baby may also have a **cleft lip** or **cleft palate**. Frequently, the hands are clenched into fists, and the index finger overlaps the other fingers. The child may have clubfeet and toes may be webbed or fused.

Numerous problems involving the internal organs may be present. Abnormalities often occur in the lungs and diaphragm (the muscle that controls breathing), and heart defects and blood vessel malformations are common. The child may also have malformed kidneys and abnormalities of the urogenital system.

Diagnosis

Physical abnormalities point to Edwards' syndrome, but definitive diagnosis relies on karyotyping. Karyotyping involves drawing the baby's blood or bone marrow for a microscopic examination of the chromosomes. Using special stains and microscopy, individual chromosomes are identified, and the presence of an extra chromosome 18 is revealed.

Trisomy 18 can be detected before birth. If a pregnant woman is older than 35, has a family history of genetic abnormalities, has previously conceived a child with a genetic abnormality, or has suffered earlier miscarriages, she may undergo tests to determine whether her child carries genetic abnormalities. Potential tests include maternal serum analysis or screening, ultrasonography, **amniocentesis**, and **chorionic villus sampling**.

Treatment

There is no cure for Edwards' syndrome. Since trisomy 18 babies frequently have major physical abnormalities, doctors and parents face difficult choices regarding treatment. Abnormalities can be treated to a certain degree with surgery, but extreme invasive procedures may not be in the best interests of an infant whose lifespan is measured in days or weeks. Medical therapy often consists of supportive care with the goal of making the infant comfortable, rather than prolonging life.

Prognosis

Most children born with trisomy 18 die within their first year of life. The average lifespan is less than two months for 50% of the children, and 90–95% die before their first birthday. The 5–10% of children who survive

Aminocentesis—A procedure in which a needle is inserted through a pregnant woman's abdomen and into her uterus to withdraw a small sample of amniotic fluid. The amniotic fluid can be examined for signs of disease or other problems afflicting the fetus.

Chorionic villus sampling—A medical test that is best done during weeks 10–12 of a pregnancy. The procedure involves inserting a needle into the placenta and withdrawing a small amount of the chorionic membrane for analysis.

Chromosome—A structure composed of deoxyribonucleic acid (DNA) contained within a cell's nucleus (center) where genetic information is stored. Human have 23 pairs of chromosomes, each of which has recognizable characteristics (such as length and staining patterns) that allow individual chromosomes to be identified. Identification is assigned by number (1–22) or letter (X or Y).

Karyotyping—A laboratory test used to study an individual's chromosome make-up. Chromosomes are separated from cells, stained, and arranged

in order from largest to smallest so that their number and structure can be studied under a microscope.

Maternal serum analyte screening—A medical procedure in which a pregnant woman's blood is drawn and analyzed for the levels of certain hormones and proteins. These levels can indicate whether there may be an abnormality in the unborn child. This test is not a definitive indicator of a problem and is followed by more specific testing such as amniocentesis or chorionic villus sampling.

Trisomy—A condition in which a third copy of a chromosome is inherited. Normally only two copies should be inherited.

Ultrasound—A medical test that is also called ultrasonography. Sound waves are directed against internal structures in the body. As sound waves bounce off the internal structure, they create an image on a video screen. An ultrasound of a fetus at weeks 16–20 of a pregnancy can be used to determine structural abnormalities.

their first year are severely mentally retarded. They need support to walk, and learning is limited. Verbal communication is also limited, but they can learn to recognize and interact with others.

Prevention

Edwards' syndrome cannot be prevented.

ORGANIZATIONS

Chromosome 18 Registry & Research Society, 7155 Oakridge Drive, San Antonio, TX, 78229, (210) 657-4968, Office@Chromosome18.org, http://www.chromosome18.org.

Support Organization for Trisomy 18, 13, and Related Disorders (SOFT), 2982 South Union Street, Rochester, NY, 14624, (585) 594-4621, (800) 716-7638, barbsoft@ rochester.rr.com, http://www.trisomy.org.

Julia Barrett

EEG *see* **Electroencephalography**

Egyptian conjunctivitis *see* **Trachoma**

Ehlers-Danlos syndrome

Definition

The Ehlers-Danlos syndromes (EDS) refer to a group of inherited disorders that affect collagen structure and function. Genetic abnormalities in the manufacturing of collagen within the body affect connective tissues, causing them to be abnormally weak.

Description

Collagen is a strong, fibrous protein that lends strength and elasticity to connective tissues such as the skin, tendons, organ walls, cartilage, and blood vessels. Each of these connective tissues requires collagen tailored to meet its specific purposes. The many roles of collagen are reflected in the number of genes dedicated to its production. There are at least 28 genes in humans that encode at least 19 different types of collagen. Mutations in these genes can affect basic construction as well as the fine-tuned processing of the collagen.

EDS was originally described by Dr. Van Meekeren in 1682. Dr. Ehlers and Dr. Danlos further characterized

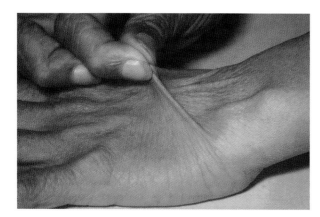

Elasticity of the skin is one characteristic of this rare disorder. *(© Biophoto Associates/Photo Researchers, Inc.)*

the disease in 1901 and 1908, respectively. Today, according to the Ehlers-Danlos National Foundation, one in 5,000 to one in 10,000 people are affected by some form of EDS.

EDS is a group of genetic disorders that usually affects the skin, ligaments, joints, and blood vessels. Classification of EDS types was revised in 1997. The new classification involves categorizing the different forms of EDS into six major sub-types, including classical, hypermobility, vascular, kyphoscoliosis, arthrochalasia, and dermatosparaxis, and a collection of rare or poorly defined varieties. This new classification is simpler and based more on descriptions of the actual symptoms.

Classical type

Under the old classification system, EDS classical type was divided into two separate types: type I and type II. The major symptoms involved in EDS classical type are the skin and joints. The skin has a smooth, velvety texture and **bruises** easily. Affected individuals typically have extensive scaring, particularly at the knees, elbows, forehead, and chin. The joints are hyperextensible, giving a tendency towards dislocation of the hip, shoulder, elbow, knee, or clavicle. Due to decreased muscle tone, affected infants may experience a delay in reaching motor milestones. Children may have a tendency to develop hernias or other organ shifts within the abdomen. Sprains and partial or complete joint dilocations are also common. Symptoms can range from mild to severe. EDS classical type is inherited in an autosomal dominant manner.

There are three major clinical diagnostic criteria for EDS classical type. These include skin hyperextensibility, unusually wide **scars**, and joint hypermobility. At this time there is no definitive test for the diagnosis

of classical EDS. Both DNA and biochemical studies have been used to help identify affected individuals. In some cases, a **skin biopsy** has been found to be useful in confirming a diagnosis. Unfortunately, these tests are not sensitive enough to identify all individuals with classical EDS. If there are multiple affected individuals in a family, it may be possible to perform prenatal diagnosis using a DNA information technique known as a linkage study.

Hypermobility type

Excessively loose joints are the hallmark of this EDS type, formerly known as EDS type III. Both large joints, such as the elbows and knees, and small joints, such as toes and fingers, are affected. Partial and total joint **dislocations** are common, and particularly involve the jaw, knee, and shoulder. Many individuals experience chronic limb and joint **pain**, although x rays of these joints appear normal. The skin may also bruise easily. **Osteoarthritis** is a common occurrence in adults. EDS hypermobility type is inherited in an autosomal dominant manner.

There are two major clinical diagnostic criteria for EDS hypermobility type. These include skin involvement (either hyperextensible skin or smooth and velvety skin) and generalized joint hypermobility. At this time there is no test for this form of EDS.

Vascular type

Formerly called EDS type IV, EDS vascular type is the most severe form. The connective tissue in the intestines, arteries, uterus, and other hollow organs may be unusually weak, leading to organ or blood vessel rupture. Such ruptures are most likely between ages 20 and 40, although they can occur any time, and may be life-threatening.

There is a classic facial appearance associated with EDS vascular type. Affected individuals tend to have large eyes, a thin pinched nose, thin lips, and a slim body. The skin is thin and translucent, with veins dramatically visible, particularly across the chest.

The large joints have normal stability, but small joints in the hands and feet are loose, showing hyperextensibility. The skin bruises easily. Other complications may include collapsed lungs, premature **aging** of the skin on the hands and feet, and ruptured arteries and veins. After surgery there tends to be poor wound healing, a complication that tends to be frequent and severe. **Pregnancy** also carries the risk complications. During and after pregnancy there is an increased risk of the uterus rupturing and of arterial bleeding. Due to the severe complications associated with EDS type IV,

death usually occurs before the fifth decade. A study of 419 individuals with EDS vascular type, completed in 2000, found that the median survival rate was 48 years, with a range of six to 73 years. EDS vascular type is inherited in an autosomal dominant manner.

There are four major clinical diagnostic criteria for EDS vascular type. These include thin translucent skin, arterial/intestinal/uterine fragility or rupture, extensive bruising, and characteristic facial appearance. EDS vascular type is caused by a change in the gene COL3A1, which codes for one of the collagen chains used to build Collage type III. Laboratory testing is available for this form of EDS. A skin biopsy may be used to demonstrate the structurally abnormal collagen. This type of biochemical test identifies more than 95% of individuals with EDS vascular type. Laboratory testing is recommended for individuals with two or more of the major criteria.

DNA analysis may als be used to identify the change within the COL3A1 gene. This information may be helpful for **genetic counseling** purposes. Prenatal testing is available for pregnancies in which an affected parent has been identified and their DNA mutation is known or their biochemical defect has been demonstrated.

Kyphoscoliosis type

The major symptoms of kyphoscoliosis type, formerly called EDS type VI, are general joint looseness. At birth, the muscle tone is poor, and motor skill development is subsequently delayed. Also, infants with this type of EDS have an abnormal curvature of the spine (**scoliosis**). The scoliosis becomes progressively worse with age, with affected individuals usually unable to walk by age 20. The eyes and skin are fragile and easily damaged, and blood vessel involvement is a possibility. The bones may also be affected as demonstrated by a decrease in bone mass. Kyphoscoliosis type is inherited in an autosomal recessive manner.

There are four major clinical diagnostic criteria for EDS kyphoscoliosis type. These include generaly loose joints, low muscle tone at birth, scoliosis at birth (which worsens with age), and a fragility of the eyes, which may give the white area of the eye a blue tint or cause the eye to rupture. This form of EDS is caused by a change in the PLOD gene on chromosome 1, which encodes the enzyme lysyl hydroxylase. A laboratory test is available in which urinary hydroxylysyl pryridinoline is measured. This test, performed on urine is extremely senstive and specific for EDS kyphoscolios type. Laboratory testing is recommended for infants with three or more of the major diagnostic criteria.

Prenatal testing is available if a pregnancy is known to be at risk and an identified affected family member has had positive laboratory testing. An **amniocentesis** may be performed in which fetal cells are removed from the amniotic fluid and enzyme activity is measured.

Arthrochalasia type

Dislocation of the hip joint typically accompanies arthrochalasia type EDS, formerly called EDS type VIIB. Other joints are also unusually loose, leading to recurrent partial and total dislocations. The skin has a high degree of stretchability and bruises easily. Individuals with this type of EDS may also experience mildly diminished bone mass, scoliosis, and poor muscle tone. Arthrochalasia type is inherited in an autosomal dominant manner.

There are two major clinical diagnostic criteria for EDS arthrochalasia type. These include sever generalized joing hypermobility and bilateral hip dislocation present at birth. This form of EDS is caused by a change in either of two components of Collage type I, called proa1(I) type A and proa2(I) type B. A skin biopsy may be preformed to demonstrate an abnormality in either components. Direct DNA testing is also available.

Dermatosparaxis type

Individuals with this type of EDS, once called type VIIC, have extremely fragile skin that bruises easily but does not scar excessively. The skin is soft and may sag, leading to an aged appearance even in young adults. Individuals may also experience hernias. Dermatosparaxis type is inherited in an autosomal recessive manner.

There are two major clinical diagnostic criteria for EDS dematosparaxis type. These include severe skin fragility and sagging or aged appearing skin. This form of EDS is caused by a change in the enzyme called procollagen I N-terminal peptidase. A skin biopsy may be preformed for a definitive diagnosis of Dermatosparaxis type.

Other types

There are several other forms of EDS that have not been as clearly defined as the aforementioned types. Forms of EDS within this category may present with soft, mildly stretchable skin, shortened bones, chronic **diarrhea**, joint hypermobility and dislocation, bladder rupture, or poor wound healing. Inheritance patterns within this group include X-linked recessive, autosomal dominant, and autosomal recessive.

Causes and symptoms

There are numerous types of EDS, all caused by changes in one of several genes. The manner in which EDS is inherited depends on the specific gene involved. There are three patterns of inheritance for EDS: autosomal dominant, autosomal recessive, and X-linked (extremely rare).

Chromosomes are made up of hundreds of small units known as genes, which contain the genetic material necessary for an individual to develop and function. Humans have 46 chromosomes, which are matched into 23 pairs. Because chromosomes are inherited in pairs, each individual receives two copies of each chromosome and likewise two copies of each gene.

Changes or mutations in genes can cause genetic diseases in several different ways, many of which are represented within the spectrum of EDS. In autosomal dominant EDS, only one copy of a specific gene must be changed for a person to have EDS. In autosomal recessive EDS, both copies of a specific gene must be changed for a person to have EDS. If only one copy of an autosomal recessive EDS gene is changed the person is referred to as a carrier, meaning they do not have any of the signs or symptoms of the disease itself, but carry the possibility of passing on the disorder to a future child. In X-linked EDS a specific gene on the X chromosome must be changed. However, this affects males and females differently because males and females have a different number of X chromosomes.

The few X-linked forms of EDS fall under the category of X-linked recessive. As with autosomal recessive, this implies that both copies of a specific gene must be changed for a person to be affected. However, because males only have one X-chromosome, they are affected if an X-linked recessive EDS gene is changed on their single X-chromosome. That is, they are affected even though they have only one changed copy. On the other hand, that same gene must be changed on both of the X-chromosomes in a female for her to be affected.

Although there is much information regarding the changes in genes that cause EDS and their various inheritance patterns, the exact gene mutation for all types of EDS is not known.

Diagnosis

Clinical symptoms such as extreme joint looseness and unusual skin qualities, along with family history, can lead to a diagnosis of EDS. Specific tests, such as skin biopsies are available for diagnosis of certain types of EDS, including vascular, arthrochalasia, and dermatosparaxis types. A skin biopsy involves removing a small sample of skin and examining its microscopic structure. A urine test is available for the Kyphoscoliosis type.

Management of all types of EDS may include genetic counseling to help the affected individual and their family understand the disorder and its impact on other family members and future children.

If a couple has had a child diagnosed with EDS the chance that they will have another child with the same disorder depends on with what form of EDS the child has been diagnosed and if either parent is affected by the same disease or not.

Individuals diagnosed with an autosomal dominant form of EDS have a 50% chance of passing the same disorder on to a child in each pregnancy. Individuals diagnosed with an autosomal recessive form of EDS have an extremely low risk of having a child with the same disorder.

X-linked recessive EDS is accompanied by a slightly more complicated pattern of inheritance. If a father with an X-linked recessive form of EDS passes a copy of his X chromosome to his children, the sons will be unaffected and the daughters will be carriers. If a mother is a carrier for an X-linked recessive form of EDS, she may have affected or unaffected sons, or carrier or unaffected daughters, depending on the second sex chromosome inherited from the father.

Prenatal diagnosis is available for specific forms of EDS, including kyphoscoliosis type and vascular type. However, prenatal testing is only a possibility in these types if the underlying defect has been found in another family member.

Treatment

Medical therapy relies on managing symptoms and trying to prevent further complications. There is no cure for EDS.

Braces may be prescribed to stabilize joints, although surgery is sometimes necessary to repair joint damage caused by repeated dislocations. **Physical therapy** teaches individuals how to strengthen muscles around joints and may help to prevent or limit damage. Elective surgery is discouraged due to the high possibility of complications.

Alternative treatment

There are anecdotal reports that large daily doses 0.04–0.14 oz (1–4 g) of vitamin C may help decrease

KEY TERMS

Arthrochalasia—Excessive loosness of the joints.

Blood vessels—General term for arteries, veins, and capillaries that transport blood throughout the body.

Cartilage—Supportive connective tissue that cushions bone at the joints or which connects muscle to bone.

Collagen—The main supportive protein of cartilage, connective tissue, tendon, skin, and bone.

Connective tissue—A group of tissues responsible for support throughout the body; includes cartilage, bone, fat, tissue underlying skin, and tissues that support organs, blood vessels, and nerves throughout the body.

Dermatosparaxis—Skin fragility caused by abnormal collagen.

Hernia—A rupture in the wall of a body cavity, through which an organ may protrude.

Homeopathic—A holistic and natural approach to healthcare.

Hyperextensibility—The ability to extend a joint beyond the normal range.

Hypermobility—Unusual flexibility of the joints, allowing them to be bent or moved beyond their normal range of motion.

Joint dislocation—The displacement of a bone.

Kyphoscoliosis—Abnormal front-to-back and side-to-side curvature of the spine.

Ligament—A type of connective tissue that connects bones or cartilage and provides support and strength to joints.

Osteoarthritis—A degenerative joint disease that causes pain and stiffness.

Scoliosis—An abnormal, side-to-side curvature of the spine.

Tendon—A strong connective tissue that connects muscle to bone.

Uterus—A muscular, hollow organ of the female reproductive tract. The uterus contains and nourishes the embryo and fetus from the time the fertilized egg is implanted until birth.

Vascular—Having to do with blood vessels.

---

bruising and aid in wound healing. Constitutional homeopathic treatment may be helpful in maintaining optimal health in persons with a diagnosis of EDS. An individual with EDS should discuss these types of therapies with their doctor before beginning them on their own. Therapy that does not require medical consultation involves protecting the skin with sunscreen and avoiding activities that place **stress** on the joints.

Prognosis

The outlook for individuals with EDS depends on the type of EDS with which they have been diagnosed. Symptoms vary in severity, even within one sub-type, and the frequency of complications changes on an individual basis. Some individuals have negligible symptoms while others are severely restricted in their daily life. Extreme joint instability and scoliosis may limit a person's mobility. Most individuals will have a normal lifespan. However, those with blood vessel involvement, particularly those with EDS vascular type, have an increased risk of fatal complications.

EDS is a lifelong condition. Affected individuals may face social obstacles related to their disease on a daily basis. Some people with EDS have reported living with fears of significant and painful skin ruptures, becoming pregnant (especially those with EDS vascular type), their condition worsening, becoming unemployed due to physical and emotional burdens, and social stigmatization in general.

Constant bruises, skin **wounds**, and trips to the hospital take their toll on both affected children and their parents. Prior to diagnosis parents of children with EDS have found themselves under suspicion of **child abuse**.

Some people with EDS are not diagnosed until well into adulthood and, in the case of EDS vascular type, occasionally not until after death due to complications of the disorder. Not only may the diagnosis itself be devastating to the family, but in many cases other family members find out for the first time they are at risk for being affected.

Although individuals with EDS face significant challenges, it is important to remember that each person is unique with their own distinguished qualities and potential. Persons with EDS go on to have families, to have careers, and to be accomplished citizens, surmounting the challenges of their disease.

Resources

OTHER

GeneClinics. http://www.geneclinics.org.

ORGANIZATIONS

Ehlers-Danlos Support Group - UK., P.O. Box 337, Aldershot, Surrey, GU12 6WZ, UK, 01252690940, http://www.ehlers-danlos.org/.

Elhers-Danlos National Foundation, 1760 Old Meadow Road, Suite 500, McLean, VA, 22102, (703) 506-2892, http://www.ednf.org/.

Java O. Solis, MS

Ehrlichiosis

Definition

Ehrlichiosis is a bacterial infection that is spread by ticks. Symptoms include **fever**, chills, **headache**, muscle aches, and tiredness.

Description

Ehrlichiosis is a tick-borne disease caused by infection with *Ehrlichia* bacteria. Ticks are small, blood-sucking arachnids. Although some ticks carry disease-causing organisms, most do not. When an animal or person is bitten by a tick that carries bacteria, the bacteria are passed to that person or animal during the tick's feeding process. It is believed that the tick must remain attached to the person or animal for at least 24 hours to spread the infection.

There are two forms of ehrlichiosis in the United States; human monocytic ehrlichiosis and human granulocytic ehrlichiosis. Monocytic ehrlichiosis is caused by *Ehrlichia chaffeensis*, which is spread by the Lone Star tick, *Amblyomma americanum*. As of 2006, about 600 cases of monocytic ehrlichiosis had been reported in 30 states, primarily in the southeastern and south central United States. The bacteria that causes granulocytic ehrlichiosis is not known, but suspected to be either *Ehrlichia equi* or *Ehrlichia phagocytophila*. Granulocytic ehrlichiosis is probably spread by the blacklegged tick *Ixodes scapularis* (which also spreads **Lyme disease**). About 100 cases of granulocytic ehrlichiosis have been reported in Connecticut, Massachusetts, Rhode Island, Minnesota, New York, and Wisconsin.

Causes and symptoms

Both forms of ehrlichiosis have similar symptoms, and the illnesses can range from mild to severe and life-threatening. Risk factors include old age and exposure to ticks through work or recreation. Symptoms occur seven to 21 days following a tick bite although patients may not recall being bitten. Fever, tiredness, headache, muscle aches, chills, loss of appetite, confusion, **nausea**, and **vomiting** are common to both diseases. A rash may occur.

Diagnosis

Ehrlichiosis may be diagnosed and treated by doctors who specialize in blood diseases (hematologists) or an **infectious disease** specialist. Because ehrlichiosis is not very common and the symptoms are not unique, it may be misdiagnosed. A recent history of a tick bite is helpful in the diagnosis. Blood tests will be done to look for antibodies to *Ehrlichia*. Staining and microscopic examination of the blood sample may show *Ehrlichia* bacteria inside white blood cells. Another test, called polymerase chain reaction (PCR), is a very sensitive assay to detect bacteria in the blood sample, but it is not always available.

Treatment

Antibiotic treatment should begin immediately if ehrlichiosis is suspected, even if laboratory results are not available. Treatment with either tetracycline (Sumycin, Achromycin V) or doxycycline (Monodox, Vibramycin) is recommended. Many patients with ehrlichiosis are admitted to the hospital for treatment.

Prognosis

For otherwise healthy people, a full recovery is expected following treatment for ehrlichiosis. Elderly patients are at a higher risk for severe disease, which may be fatal. Serious complications include lung or gastrointestinal bleeding. Two to 10 patients out of 100 die from the disease.

Prevention

The only prevention for ehrlichiosis is to minimize exposure to ticks by staying on the trail when walking through the woods, avoiding tall grasses, wearing long sleeves and tucking pant legs into socks, wearing insect repellent, and checking for ticks after an outing. Remove a tick as soon as possible by grasping the tick with tweezers and gently pulling.

Resources

BOOKS

Gorbach, Sherwood F., John S. Bartlett, and Neil R. Blacklow, eds.*Infectious Diseases*, 3rd ed. Philadelphia: W. B. Saunders Co., 2004.

Belinda Rowland, PhD

EKG *see* Electrocardiography

Elder abuse

Definition

Elder **abuse** is a general term used to describe harmful acts toward an elderly adult, such as physical abuse, **sexual abuse**, emotional or psychological abuse, financial exploitation, and neglect, including self-neglect.

Description

Results from the National Elder Abuse Incidence Study, funded in part by the Administration on **Aging**, suggest that over 500,000 people 60 years of age and older are abused or neglected each year in the United States. It was also found that four times as many incidents of abuse, neglect, or self-neglect are never reported, causing researchers to estimate that as many as two million elderly persons in the United States are abused each year. In 90% of the cases, the abusers were found to be family members and most often were the adult children or spouses of those abused. In addition, equal numbers of men and women have been identified as the abusers. However, women, especially those over 80 years of age, tend to be victimized more than men.

Elder abuse can take place anywhere, but the two main settings addressed by law are domestic settings, such as the elder's home or the caregiver's home, and institutional settings, such as a nursing home or group home. In general, there are five basic types of elderly abuse: physical, sexual, emotional or psychological, financial, and neglect. Data from National Center on Elder Abuse indicates that more than half of the cases reported involve some kind of neglect, whereas 1 in 7 cases involve physical abuse. It is considered neglect when a caretaker deprives an elderly person of the necessary care needed in order to avoid physical or mental harm. Sometimes the behavior of an elderly person threatens his or her own health; in those cases, the abuse is called self-neglect. Physical abuse refers to physical force that causes bodily harm to an elderly person, such as slapping, pushing, kicking, pinching, or burning.

About 1 in 8 cases of elderly abuse involve some form of financial exploitation, which is defined as the use of an elderly person's resources without his or her consent. The National Center on Elder Abuse defines emotional and psychological abuse of a senior as causing anguish, **pain**, or distress through verbal or nonverbal acts, such as verbal assaults, insults, intimidation, and humiliation, for example. Isolating elderly persons from their friends and family as well as giving them the silent treatment are two other forms of emotional and psychological abuse. Any kind of non-consensual sexual contact with an elderly person that takes place without his or her consent is considered sexual abuse.

Causes and symptoms

Elder abuse is a complex problem that can be caused by many factors. According to the National Center on Elder Abuse, social isolation and mental impairment are two factors of elder abuse. Studies show that people advanced in years, such as in their eighties, with a high level of frailty and dependency are more likely to be victims of elder abuse than people who are younger and better equipped to stand up for themselves. Because spouses make up a large percentage of elder abusers, at least 40% statistically, some research has been done in the area, which shows that a pattern of domestic violence is associated with many of the cases. The risk of elder abuse appears to be especially high when adult children live with their elderly parents for financial reasons or because they have personal problems, such as drug dependency or mental illness. Some experts have speculated that elderly people living in rural areas with their caretakers may have a higher risk of being abused than city dwellers. The idea behind this theory is that the opportunity exists for the abuse to occur, but there is less likelihood that the abuser will be caught. More research in this very important area is needed in order to illuminate the relationship between these factors.

The National Center on Elder Abuse identifies the following as signs of elder abuse:

- Bruises, pressure marks, broken bones, abrasions, and burns may indicate physical abuse or neglect.
- Unexplained withdrawal from normal activities and unusual depression may be indicators of emotional abuse.

- Bruises around the breasts or genital area, as well as unexplained bleeding around the genital area, may be signs of sexual abuse.
- Large withdrawals of money from an elder's bank account, sudden changes in a will, and the sudden disappearance of valuable items may be indications of financial exploitation.
- Bedsores, poor hygiene, unsanitary living conditions, and unattended medical needs may be signs of neglect.
- Failure to take necessary medicines, leaving a burning stove unattended, poor hygiene, confusion, unexplained weight loss, and dehydration may all be signs of self-neglect.

Diagnosis and Treatment

The National Committee for the Prevention of Elder Abuse notes that Adult Protective Services (APS) caseworkers are often on the front lines when it comes to elderly abuse. People being abused or those who believe abuse is taking place can turn to their local APS office for help. The APS routinely screens calls, keeps all information confidential, and, if necessary, sends a caseworker out to conduct an investigation. In the event that a crisis intervention is needed, the APS caseworker can arrange for any necessary emergency treatment. If it is unclear whether elder abuse has taken place, the APS caseworker can serve as a liaison between the elderly person and other community agencies.

According to the National Committee for the Prevention of Elder Abuse, "professionals in the field of aging are often the first to discover signs of elder abuse." Providing encouragement and advice, they play a critical role in educating others with regard to the needs of the elderly. They not only provide valuable support to the victims of abuse, but they also monitor high-risk situations and gather important information that can help validate that abuse has taken place.

Some people might think that a person who has cognitive impairment might be unable to describe mistreatment; however, that is not the case. In fact, guidelines set by the American Medical Association call for "routine questions about abuse and neglect even among patients with cognitive impairment in order to improve the identification of cases and implement appropriate treatment and referral." Rather than an inability to describe mistreatment, what might stop an elderly person from reporting abuse is a sense of embarrassment or fear of retaliation. To complicate matters, differences exist among cultural groups regarding what defines abuse.

Therefore, most states have established laws that define elder abuse and require health care providers to report any cases they encounter with penalties attached for failing to do so. Indeed, statistics show that health care providers, for example, report almost 25% of the known cases of elder abuse. Therefore, physicians play a very important role in identifying and treating elders who have been abused. And yet, in an article published by the *Journal of the American Geriatrics Society*, Dr. Conlin pointed out that only 1 of every 13 cases of elder abuse are reported by physicians. There may be several reasons for this. In some cases, the problem may simply go unnoticed, especially if the physician has no obvious reason to suspect any wrongdoing. In other cases, the patient may hide or deny the problem.

In recent years, much media attention has been focused on elderly abuse that takes place in institutional settings. Anyone who believes that a loved one is being abused while in a nursing home or other institutional setting should contact the authorities for assistance immediately.

Prognosis

The mortality rate of an elderly person who has been mistreated is higher than the mortality rate of an elderly person who has not experienced abuse. Nonetheless, numerous success stories exist regarding successful interventions. Social workers and health care professionals, as well as concerned citizens from a variety of backgrounds, have played a key role in identifying and obtaining treatment for abused elders.

Prevention

Planning for the future is one of the best ways to avoid elder abuse. Consider a variety of retirement options, ones that will encourage safety as well as independence. It is important to stay active in the community. Avoiding isolation minimizes the likelihood that abuse will occur. Seek professional counsel when necessary; it is important for everyone to know their rights and to be advocates on their own behalf.

Resources

OTHER

National Center on Elder Abuse "Elder Abuse: Frequently Asked questions." *National Center on Elder Abuse* May 25, 2010 National Center on Elder Abuse. http://www.ncea.aoa.gov/NCEAroot/Main_Site/FAQ/Questions.aspx.

Lee Ann Paradise,

Electric shock injuries

Definition

Electricity is a form of energy generated by the flow of electrons across a potential gradient from high to low concentration through a conductive material. Electrical injuries in humans are caused by contact with an electrical current, either natural lightning or mechanically generated.

Demographics

Electrical injuries were rare in industrialized societies until the 1870s and 1880s, when a series of inventions by Thomas Edison (1847–1931) and George Westinghouse (1846–1914) made it possible to transmit electricity over long-distance wires from one location to another for commercial and scientific purposes. The first fatal industrial accident involving an electric shock occurred in Lyon, France, in 1879.

As of 2010, electrical injuries are responsible for about 1,000 deaths in the United States each year, or about 1% of all accidental deaths. About a quarter of these fatalities are caused by natural lightning. Electric shocks are responsible for 5% of all admissions to specialized burn treatment units in North America.

In the United States, 80% of all electrical injuries occur in adult men, largely because of occupational choices. Among children, the male: female ratio is 3:1. Low-voltage injuries are most common among toddlers; high-voltage injuries primarily affect risk-taking adolescents and adults in high-risk occupations.

According to the Bureau of Labor Statistics, electric shocks are the second leading cause of **death** in the construction industry in North America. With regard to injuries caused by contact with overhead powerlines, between 27% and 60% of cases resulted in over 31 days lost from work—compared to 18%–20% for all other occupational injury and illness. Injuries caused by electric shocks are also costly to employers; a researcher at the Electric Power Research Institute in Palo Alto, California, estimates that the cost to American employers is approximately $15.75 million *per case* in direct and indirect costs.

Description

Accidental electrical injuries

Electrical injuries are classified according to three factors: power source (lightning or human-generated electricity; voltage (high or low); and type of current (alternating or direct). Each is associated with certain patterns of injury. Most electrical injuries are accidental.

The minimum current that humans can feel is 1 milliampere (abbreviated mA). An ampere, named for the French mathematician and physicist André-Marie Ampère (1775–1836), is a measure of the amount of electric charge passing a given point per unit time. One ampere represents 6.241×10^{18} electrons passing a given point in a wire in one second of time. In general, a current of 100 mA will be lethal if it passes through sensitive parts of the human body; a current as low as 60 mA can cause **ventricular fibrillation**, irregular contraction of the muscles in the two lower chambers of the heart.

Intentional use of electric shocks

Electric shocks have been used in medicine to treat mental illness, particularly depression (**electroconvulsive therapy** or ECT); to correct irregular heart rhythms (**defibrillation** and **cardioversion**); and to relieve **pain** by stimulating opioid receptors in the central nervous system (transcutaneous **electrical nerve stimulation** or TENS).

Electricity was used as a form of torture or punishment almost as soon as it was known to cause accidental workplace injuries. Since the 1930s, the Nazis and other tyrannical regimes used cattle prods and similar devices to torture people. The tasers currently used by some police departments are electroshock devices that cause strong involuntary contractions of the muscles controlling movement, thus temporarily incapacitating violent or intoxicated suspects.

Electrocution as a method of capital punishment was introduced in the late 1880s on the recommendation of a committee in New York State seeking a more humane method of execution than hanging. Thomas Edison recommended the use of alternating current to electrocute criminals, maintaining that it would cause instantaneous death. The first use of the electric chair in New York in 1890, however, was a disaster, requiring eight minutes to cause death. George Westinghouse is reported to have said that it would have been more humane to use an axe. As of 2010, only six states still use the electric chair as an option for execution.

Risk factors

Risk factors for electrical injuries include:

- Working or playing outside during an electrical storm.
- Employment in an occupation related to the generation of electricity or servicing of electrical equipment or power lines.

Alternating current (AC)—An electric current in which the flow of the electric charge periodically reverses direction. AC is the form in which electricity is usually delivered to homes. The usual household wall outlet (120 volts) provides a current with 120 reversals of the direction of flow occurring each second and is termed 60-cycle alternating current.

Amperage—A measurement of the amount of electric charge passing a given point per unit time. One ampere represents about 6.241 x 10^{18} electrons passing a given point in a wire in one second of time.

Antibiotics—Substances used against microorganisms that cause infection.

Arc flash—A type of electrical explosion resulting from electrical breakdown of the gases in air, which normally does not conduct electricity. Arc flashes can occur where there is sufficient voltage in an electrical system and a path to the ground or to lower voltage.

Cataract—Clouding of the lens of the eye or its capsule (surrounding membrane).

Computed tomography scan (CT scan)—A process that uses x rays to create three-dimensional images of structures inside the body.

Direct current (DC)—An electric current in which the electric charge moves in only one direction. It is the type of current produced by batteries and solar cells.

Electrolytes—Substances that conduct electric current within the body and are essential for sustaining life.

Magnetic resonance imaging (MRI)—The use of electromagnetic energy to create images of structures inside the body.

Skin grafting—A technique in which a piece of healthy skin from the patient's body (or a donor's) is used to cover another part of the patient's body that has lost its skin.

Taser—Also called a conducted electrical weapon or CEW, a taser is an electroshock device used by some police departments in various countries to subdue armed or otherwise dangerous suspects without having to use lethal force. Tasers work by interfering with the ' capacity to control voluntary muscles. The name *taser* is an acronym for *Thomas A. Swift's Electric Rifle*, an adventure novel about a fictional weapon published in 1911.

Voltage—The force necessary to drive an electric current between two specified points. A large voltage exerts a greater force, which moves more electrons through a wire at a given rate of time.

- Employment in the construction industry, mining, or public transportation.
- Natural disasters, including hurricanes, tornadoes, earthquakes, and ice storms, which bring down or disrupt high-voltage power lines.
- Theft of copper and other metals from construction sites and other areas close to high-voltage wires.

Causes and symptoms

Causes

Electricity damages the cells in human tissues in two basic ways: heating and blast force. The passage of electrical current through cell membranes causes their temperatures to rise, leading to disruption of the cell membrane itself (at 108°F); denaturation of protein molecules in the cell (at 113°F); and destruction of DNA (at 149°F or higher). In most cases of high-voltage electrical shock, heat damage occurs immediately at contact points but requires 1–3 seconds to injure deeper tissues. The blast force of electric current can cause significant blunt trauma injuries.

The overall severity of electrical injury depends on the current's pressure (voltage), the amount of current (amperage), the type of current (direct vs. alternating), the body's resistance to the current, the current's path through the body, and how long the body remains in contact with the current. The interplay of these factors can produce effects ranging from barely noticeable **tingling** to instant death; every part of the body is vulnerable. Although the severity of injury is determined primarily by the voltage, low voltage can be just as dangerous as high voltage under the right circumstances. People have been killed by shocks of just 50 volts. Electric voltage of 380 volts or less is considered low voltage. The United States national electric code defines high voltage as 600 volts or higher. High voltage is generated at power plants and is transformed down to approximately 120 volts for most wall outlets in homes.

Symptoms

Electric shocks can affect all the major organ systems in the human body. How electric shocks affect the skin is determined by the skin's resistance, which in turn is dependent upon the wetness, thickness, and cleanliness of the skin. Thin or wet skin is much less resistant than thick or dry skin. When skin resistance is low, the current may cause little or no skin damage but severely burn internal organs and tissues. Conversely, high skin resistance can produce severe skin **burns** but prevent the current from entering the body.

The nervous system (the brain, spinal cord, and nerves) is particularly vulnerable to injury. In fact, neurological problems are the most common kind of nonlethal harm suffered by electric shock victims. Some neurological damage is minor and clears up on its own or with medical treatment, but some is severe and permanent. Neurological problems may be apparent immediately after the accident, or gradually develop over a period of up to three years.

Damage to the respiratory and cardiovascular systems is most acute at the moment of injury. Electric shocks can paralyze the respiratory system or disrupt heart action, causing instant death. Also at risk are the smaller veins and arteries, which dissipate heat less easily than the larger blood vessels and can develop **blood clots**. Damage to the smaller vessels is probably one reason why **amputation** is often required following high-voltage injuries.

Many other sorts of injuries are possible after an electric shock, including **cataracts**, kidney failure, and substantial destruction of muscle tissue. The victim may suffer a fall or be hit by debris from exploding equipment. An electric arc flash may set clothing or nearby flammable substances on fire. Arc flashes can produce light intense enough to cause permanent blindness as well as heat intense enough (5000°F to 7000°F) to melt bone and vaporize the surfaces of nearby human beings and other objects. Strong shocks are often accompanied by violent **muscle spasms** that can break and dislocate bones. These spasms can also freeze the victim in place and prevent him or her from breaking away from the source of the current. Alternating current is considered three times as dangerous as direct current for this reason: high-voltage DC tends to cause one strong muscle spasm that throws the victim away from the source, whereas the cyclical flow of electrons in AC of the same voltage causes **paralysis** of the muscles that holds the victim in contact with the current.

Diagnosis

Diagnosis relies on gathering information about the circumstances of the accident, a thorough **physical examination**, and monitoring of cardiovascular and kidney activity. When at all possible, witnesses of the accident should be questioned about the circumstances of the event, particularly if the victim has lost consciousness or normal mental status. The victim's neurological condition can fluctuate rapidly and requires close observation. A computed tomography scan (CT scan) or **magnetic resonance imaging** (MRI) may be necessary to check for brain injury. Blood and urine samples may be taken. In some cases, the doctor may make a trial incision into burned muscle to assess the extent of tissue damage. The tissue sample is frozen and examined under a microscope to see whether the muscle tissue is still viable. If an arm or leg damaged by electricity is determined not to be viable, immediate amputation is necessary.

Treatment

Treatment of an electrical injury usually begins at the scene, although first responders will generally take the victim to an emergency department or specialized burn or trauma center as soon as possible. The victim of a severe electrical injury may be examined and treated by a variety of specialists, including emergency physicians, plastic surgeons, neurologists, ophthalmologists, and orthopedic surgeons.

Traditional

When an electric shock accident happens at home or in the workplace, the main power should immediately be shut off and 911 should be called. If that cannot be done, and current is still flowing through the victim, the alternative is to stand on a dry, nonconducting surface such as a folded newspaper, flattened cardboard carton, or plastic or rubber mat and use a nonconducting object such as a wooden broomstick (never a damp or metallic object) to push the victim away from the source of the current. The victim and the source of the current must not be touched while the current is still flowing, for this contact can electrocute the rescuer. Emergency medical help should be summoned as quickly as possible. Trained electricians must use lineman's gloves to separate the victim from the circuit by a specially insulated pole. Looping a polydacron rope around the injured patient is another method of pulling him or her from the electric power source. Ideally, the electrician or first responder should stand on a dry surface during the rescue. People who are trained to perform **cardiopulmonary resuscitation** (CPR) should, if appropriate, begin **first aid** while waiting for emergency medical help to arrive.

Burn victims usually require treatment at a specialized burn center. Fluid replacement therapy is necessary to restore lost fluids and electrolytes. Severely injured tissue is repaired surgically, which can involve **skin grafting** or amputation. **Antibiotics** and antibacterial creams are used to prevent infection. Victims may also require treatment for kidney failure. Following surgery, **physical therapy** to facilitate recovery, and psychological counseling to cope with disfigurement, may be necessary.

Prognosis

The mortality rate for electrical injuries in the United States as of 2010 is 3–5%. Many survivors, however, require amputation or are permanently disfigured by their burns. **Anxiety disorders** are common in survivors of high-voltage electrical injuries. About 73% of pregnant women injured by lightning or high-voltage electricity lose the baby. Injuries from household appliances and other low-voltage sources are less likely to produce extreme damage.

Prevention

Prevention of electrical injuries in the home or workplace begins with age-appropriate education about the nature of electricity and the importance of safety measures. The National Safety Council in the United States and Hydro-Québec (a power company) in Canada have handouts, videos, quizzes, and fact sheets about electrical safety on their websites (http://www.nsc.org/ and http://www.hydroquebec.com/security/index.html), some of which are listed under Resources below. These materials are written for the general public and are intended to help people recognize dangerous situations and take steps to protect themselves and their families before an electrical accident occurs.

People who are employed in workplaces with high-voltage electrical equipment or whose jobs require working with electricity should follow all safety precautions recommended by the National Safety Council:

- Those working near high-voltage lines should wear Class B helmets, which are designed to withstand 20,000 volts of AC for 3 minutes.
- Special insulated gloves should be worn, either Class 2 (provides protection against 20,000 volts) or Class 4 (protection against 40,000 volts), along with tinted eyewear to protect the eyes against arc flashes.
- Only employees with special training and authorization should work on high-voltage lines or equipment; other workers should not try to perform tasks for which they are not qualified or trained.
- Rubber-soled shoes or work boots must be worn on damp or wet surfaces.

- Workers should check that circuits, wiring, insulation, equipment, and cords or extension cords are in good repair.
- Hazards of any kind, including water or spills as well as damaged or defective equipment, should be reported to supervisors at once.

Parents and other adults need to be alert to possible electric dangers in the home. Damaged electric appliances, wiring, cords, and plugs should be repaired or replaced. Electrical repairs should be attempted only by people with the proper training. Hair dryers, radios, and other electric appliances should never be used in the bathroom or anywhere else they might accidentally come in contact with water. Young children need to be kept away from electric appliances and should be taught about the dangers of electricity as soon as they are old enough. Electric outlets require safety covers in homes with young children.

People should be particularly careful when using metal ladders outside or when installing outdoor television or CB radio base antennas, as accidental contact with an overhead power line can be fatal. In the late 1970s, there were about 100 deaths each year in the United States involving amateur installation of outdoor antennas.

During thunderstorms, people should go indoors immediately, even if no rain is falling, and boaters should return to shore as rapidly as possible. People who cannot reach indoor shelter should move away from such metallic objects as golf clubs and fishing rods and lie down in low-ground areas. Standing or lying under or next to tall or metallic structures is unsafe. An automobile is appropriate cover, as long as the radio is off. Telephones, computers, hair dryers, and other appliances that can act as conduits for lightning should not be used during thunderstorms.

Resources

BOOKS

Bledsoe, Bryan E., and Randall W. Benner. *Critical Care Paramedic.* Upper Saddle River, NJ: Pearson Prentice Hall, 2006.

Denegar, Craig R., et al. *Therapeutic Modalities for Musculoskeletal Injuries,* 3rd ed. Champaign, IL: Human Kinetics, 2010.

Fish, Raymond M., and Leslie A. Geddes, eds. *Electrical Injuries: Medical and Bioengineering Aspects,* 2nd ed. Tucson, AZ: Lawyers and Judges Publishing, 2009.

PERIODICALS

Chudasama, S., et al. "Does Voltage Predict Return to Work and Neuropsychiatric Sequelae Following Electrical

Burn Injury?" *Annals of Plastic Surgery* 64 (May 2010): 522–25.

Curinga, G., et al. "Electrical Injuries Due to Theft of Copper." *Journal of Burn Care and Research* 31 (March-April 2010): 341–46.

Fichet, J. "Left Ventricular Function and High-Voltage Electrical Injury." *Critical Care Medicine* 37 (November 2009): 2995.

Fish, R.M., and L.A. Geddes. "Conduction of Electrical Current to and through the Human Body: A Review." *Eplasty* 9 (October 12, 2009): e44.

Lakosha, H., et al. "High-Voltage Electrical Trauma to the Eye." *Canadian Journal of Ophthalmology* 44 (October 2009): 605–06.

Li, A.L., et al. "Effectiveness of Pain Management Following Electrical Injury." *Journal of Burn Care and Research* 31 (January-February 2010): 73–82.

Murphy, P., et al. "A Shocking Call: Prehospital Assessment and Management of Electrical Injuries and Lightning Strikes." *EMS Magazine* 39 (February 2010): 46–53.

Nagesh, K.R., et al. "Arcing Injuries in a Fatal Electrocution." *American Journal of Forensic Medicine and Pathology* 30 (June 2009): 183–85.

OTHER

Chicago Electrical Trauma Research Institute (CETRI). *Electrical Injury.* http://www.cetri.org/electrical_injury.html

Cushing, Tracy A., and Ronald K. Wright. "Electrical Injuries." *eMedicine,* April 10, 2010. http://emedicine.medscape.com/article/770179-overview

Edlich, Richard F., and David B. Drake. "Burns, Electrical." *eMedicine,* March 4, 2010. http://emedicine.medscape.com/article/1277496-overview

Hydro-Québec. *Effects of an Electric Current on the Body.* http://www.hydroquebec.com/security/effet_courant.html

Hydro-Québec. *The Four Shock Factors.* This is a pop-up animation about electrical safety that viewers can watch at their own pace. http://www.hydroquebec.com/security/pop_4acteurs.html

Hydro-Québec. *What to Do in Case of Electric Shock.* http://www.hydroquebec.com/security/que_faire_choc.html

National Safety Council (NSC). *Electrical Safety.* http://www.nsc.org/news_resources/Resources/Documents/Electrical_Safety.pdf

ORGANIZATIONS

American Burn Association, 625 N. Michigan Ave., Suite 2550, Chicago, IL, 60611, 312-642-9260, 312-642-9130, info@ameriburn.org, http://www.ameriburn.org/.

American College of Emergency Physicians (ACEP), 1125 Executive Circle, Irving, TX, 75038-2522, 972-550-0911, 800-798-1822, 972-580-2816, http://www. acep.org/.

American Society of Plastic Surgeons (ASPS), 444 East Algonquin Road, Arlington Heights, IL, 60005, 847-228-9900, http://www.plasticsurgery.org/.

Chicago Electrical Trauma Research Institute (CETRI), 4047 West 40th Street, Chicago, IL, 60632, 800-516-8709, info@cetri.org, http://www.cetri.org/.

National Safety Council (NSC), 1121 Spring Lake Drive, Itasca, IL, 60143, 630-285-1121, 800-621-7615, 630-285-1315, http://www.nsc.org/Pages/Home.aspx.

Howard Baker
Rebecca J. Frey, PhD

Electrical nerve stimulation

Definition

Electrical nerve stimulation, also called transcutaneous electrical nerve stimulation (TENS), is a noninvasive, drug-free **pain management** technique. By sending electrical signals to underlying nerves, the battery-powered TENS device can relieve a wide range of chronic and acute **pain**.

Purpose

TENS is used to relieve pain caused by a variety of chronic conditions, including:

- neck and lower back pain
- headache/migraine
- arthritis
- post-herpetic neuralgia (lingering chronic pain after an attack of shingles)
- sciatica (pain radiating from lower back, through the legs, to the foot)
- temporomandibular joint pain
- osteoarthritis
- amputation (phantom limb)
- fibromyalgia (a condition causing aching and stiffness throughout the body)

The device is also effective against short-term pain, such as:

- shingles (painful skin eruptions along the nerves)
- bursitis (inflammation of tissue surrounding a joint)
- childbirth
- post-surgical pain
- fractures
- muscle and joint pain
- sports injuries
- menstrual cramps

Precautions

Because TENS may interfere with pacemaker function, patients with **pacemakers** should consult a cardiologist before using a TENS unit. Patients should also avoid electrical stimulation in the front of the neck, which can be hazardous. The safety of the device during **pregnancy** has not been established.

TENS doesn't cure any condition; it simply eases pain. Patients who are not sure what is causing their pain should consult a physician before using TENS.

Description

The TENS device is a small battery-powered stimulator that produces low-intensity electrical signals through electrodes on or near a painful area, producing a **tingling** sensation that reduces pain. There is no dosage limitation, and the patient controls the amount of pain relief.

Some experts believe TENS works by blocking pain signals in the spinal cord, or by delivering electrical impulses to underlying nerve fibers that lessen the experience of pain. Others suspect that the electrical stimulation triggers the release of natural painkillers in the body.

Patients can rent a TENS unit before buying one, to see if it is effective against their pain.

Preparation

After TENS has been prescribed, a doctor will refer the patient to a TENS specialist, who will explain how to use the machine. The specialist works with the patient to determine the settings and electrode placements for the best pain relief.

Risks

TENS is nonaddictive and completely safe. The only side effect may be a slight skin irritation or redness in some people, which can be prevented by using different gels or electrodes.

Normal results

The amount of relief a person gets using TENS depends on the underlying cause of the pain, a person's mental state, and whether or not medication is also used. At least one study found that both a real TENS machine and a placebo were equally effective in reducing pain. This suggests that at least part of its effectiveness may be due to the patient's belief in its ability to ease pain.

Carol A. Turkington

Electrical stimulation of the brain

Definition

Electrical stimulation of the brain (ESB) is a relatively new technique used to treat chronic **pain** and **tremors** associated with **Parkinson's disease**. ESB is administered by passing an electrical current through an electrode implanted in the brain.

Purpose

While the implantation of electrodes in the brain is used to treat or diagnose several disorders, the term ESB is limited here to the treatment of tremors, and as a **pain management** tool for patients suffering from back problems and other chronic injuries and illnesses.

Precautions

An ESB tremor control device, used in treating **Parkinson's** patients, may interfere with or be affected by cardiac **pacemakers** and other medical equipment. As a result, patients with other implanted medical equipment may not be good candidates for the therapy.

Description

Electrical stimulation of the brain, or deep brain stimulation, is effective in treating tremor in up to 88% of **Parkinson's** disease patients. An electrode is implanted into the thalamus (part of the brain) of the patient, and attached to an electric pulse generator via an extension wire. The pulse generator is implanted into the patient's pectoral, or chest area, and the extension wire is tunneled under the skin. The pulse generator sends out intermittent electrical stimulation to the electrode in the thalamus, which inhibits or partially relieves the tremor. The generator can be turned on and off with a magnet, and needs to be replaced every three to five years.

Similar methods have been used to treat chronic pain that responded unfavorably to conventional therapies. A remote transmitter allows these patients to trigger electric stimulation to relieve their symptoms on an as-needed basis. Patients with failed back syndrome, trigeminal neuropathy (pertaining to the fifth cranial nerve), and **peripheral neuropathy** fared well for pain control with this treatment, while patients with **spinal cord injury** and postherpetic neuralagia (pain along the nerves following herpes) did poorly.

Preparation

The patient should be free of any type of infection before undergoing an ESB procedure. He or she may be advised to discontinue any medication for a prescribed period of time before surgery.

Aftercare

After **neurosurgery**, patients should undergo regular head dressing changes, minimize exposure to others, and practice good personal hygiene in order to prevent a brain infection. The head may also be kept elevated for a prescribed period of time in order to decrease swelling of the brain.

Risks

The implantation of electrodes into the brain carries risks of hemorrhage, infarction, infection, and cerebral **edema**. These complications could cause irreversible neurological damage.

Patients with an implanted ESB tremor control device may experience headaches, disequilibrium (a disturbance of the sense of balance), burning or **tingling** of the skin, or partial **paralysis**.

Normal results

ESB is effective in pain control for specific conditions. It can provide long-term pain relief with few side effects or complications.

For the control of tremors a deep brain stimulator does provide some relief. It is recommended for patients with tremors severe enough to affect their quality of life.

Resources

OTHER

Eskandar, Emand, et al. *Surgery for Parkinson's Disease.* May 11, 2005. http://neurosurgery.mgh.harvard.edu/functional/PDsurgery.htm.

Paula Anne Ford-Martin

Electrocardiography

Definition

Electrocardiography is a commonly used noninvasive procedure for recording electrical changes in the heart. The record, which is called an electrocardiogram

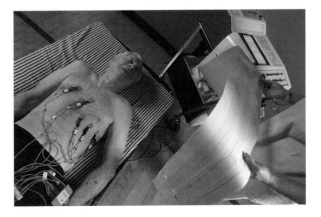

A patient undergoing electrocardiography. (Russell Curtis/ Photo Researchers, Inc.)

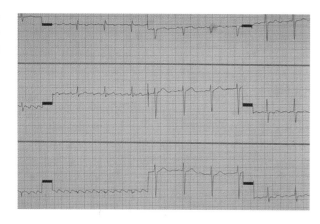

An EKG strip indicating atrial flutter. *(Custom Medical Stock Photo, Inc. Reproduced by permission.)*

(ECG or EKG), shows the series of waves related to the electrical impulses that occur during each beat of the heart. The results are printed on paper and/or displayed on a monitor to provide a visual representation of heart function. The waves in a normal record are named P, Q, R, S, and T, and follow in alphabetical order. The number of waves may vary, and other waves may be present.

Purpose

Electrocardiography is a starting point for detecting many cardiac problems, including **angina** pectoris, stable angina, ischemic heart disease, **arrhythmias** (irregular heartbeat), tachycardia (fast heartbeat), bradycardia (slow heartbeat), myocardial infarction (**heart attack**), and certain congenital heart conditions. It is used routinely in physical examinations and for monitoring a patient's condition during and after surgery, as well as in the intensive care setting. It is the basic measurement used in **exercise** tolerance tests (i.e., **stress** tests) and is also used to evaluate symptoms such as chest **pain**, **shortness of breath**, and **palpitations**.

Demographics

The ECG is a common diagnostic test, with about 30 million performed each year in the United States.

Men are more likely to experience heart attacks than women, although a woman's risk of heart attack rises after **menopause**. African-Americans, Hispanics, and Native Americans are all at greater risk for cardiovascular disease than Caucasians, in part because of the higher incidence of **diabetes mellitus** (a major risk factor for cardiovascular disease) in these populations.

Description

The patient disrobes from the waist up, and electrodes (tiny wires in adhesive pads) are applied to specific sites on the arms, legs, and chest. When attached, these electrodes are called leads; three to 12 leads may be employed for the procedure.

Muscle movement may interfere with the recording, which lasts for several beats of the heart. In cases where rhythm disturbances are suspected to be infrequent, the patient may wear a small Holter monitor in order to record continuously over a 24-hour period. This is known as ambulatory monitoring.

Special training is required for interpretation of the electrocardiogram. To summarize in the simplest manner the features used in interpretations, the P wave of the electrocardiogram is associated with the contraction of the atria—the two chambers of the heart that receive blood from the veins. The QRS series of waves, or QRS complex, is associated with ventricular contraction, with the T wave coming after the contraction. The ventricles are the two chambers of the heart that receive blood from the atria and that send the blood into the arteries. Finally, the P-Q or P-R interval gives a value for the time taken for the electrical impulse to travel from the atria to the ventricle (normally less than 0.2 seconds).

Newer developments in electrocardiography include the Open ECG Project, an online group of doctors and technical experts who aim to develop an open-source, low-cost 12-lead PC-based ECG with interpretive software. The first step toward that goal might be a 3-lead PC-based ECG. The project hopes to make ECGs affordable in the Third World and other areas lacking medical facilities with standard ECG equipment. Another new device is the AngelMed Guardian, an implantable device similar to a pacemaker that records cardiac data and detects shifts in the ST segment of the heart waves—an early warning sign of a heart attack. The Guardian has been implanted in 55 patients in the United States and Brazil as of late 2009 and is presently undergoing phase 2 clinical trials with the Food and Drug Administration (FDA).

In terms of telecommunications, software is now available that allows health care personnel to download ECG notes to tablet PCs or iPhones. This technology was introduced in January 2009 and is now widely used in telemedicine. It has already proved valuable in such countries as the Philippines and other island-based nations, where fixed telephone wiring is often difficult to construct and maintain.

Diagnosis/Preparation

Patients are asked not to eat for several hours before a **stress test**. Before the leads are attached, the skin is cleaned to obtain good electrical contact at the electrode positions and, occasionally, shaving the chest may be necessary. Patients should avoid using greasy or oily skin creams or lotions before the test. They should wear a shirt or blouse that can be easily removed. Women should avoid wearing full-length hosiery, as the legs must be bare for the test.

Heart problems are diagnosed by the pattern of electrical waves produced during the EKG, and an abnormal rhythm can be called dysrhythmia. The cause of dysrhythmia is ectopic beats. Ectopic beats are premature heartbeats that arise from a site other than the sinus node—commonly from the atria, atrioventricular node, or the ventricle. When these dysrhythmias are only occasional, they may produce no symptoms or simply a feeling that the heart is turning over or "flip-flopping." These occasional dysrhythmias are common in healthy people, but they also can be an indication of heart disease.

The varied sources of dysrhythmias provide a wide range of alterations in the form of the electrocardiogram. Ectopic beats display an abnormal QRS complex. This can indicate disease associated with insufficient blood supply to the heart muscle (myocardial **ischemia**). Multiple ectopic sites lead to rapid and uncoordinated contractions of the atria or ventricles. This condition is known as fibrillation. When the atrial impulse fails to reach the ventricle, a condition known as **heart block** results.

Aftercare

To avoid skin irritation from the salty gel used to obtain good electrical contact, the skin should be thoroughly cleaned after removal of the electrodes.

Risks

The EKG is a noninvasive procedure that is virtually risk-free for the patient. There is a slight risk of heart attack for individuals undergoing a stress test EKG, but patients are carefully screened for their suitability for this test before it is prescribed.

Risk factors for heart disease include **obesity**, **hypertension** (high blood pressure), high **triglycerides** and total blood cholesterol, low HDL ("good") cholesterol, tobacco **smoking**, and increased age. People who have diabetes mellitus (either type 1 or type 2) are also at increased risk for cardiovascular disease.

Normal results

When the heart is operating normally, each part contracts in a specific order. Contraction of the muscle is triggered by an electrical impulse. These electrical impulses travel through specialized cells that form a conduction system. Following this pathway ensures that contractions will occur in a coordinated manner.

When the presence of all waves is observed in the electrocardiogram, and these waves follow the order defined alphabetically, the heart is said to show a normal sinus rhythm, and impulses may be assumed to be following the regular conduction pathway.

In the normal heart, electrical impulses—at a rate of 60–100 times per minute—originate in the sinus node. The sinus node is located in the first chamber of the heart, known as the right atrium, where blood reenters the heart after circulating through the body. After traveling down to the junction between the upper and lower chambers, the signal stimulates the atrioventricular node. From here, after a delay, it passes by specialized routes through the lower chambers or ventricles. In many disease states, the passage of the electrical impulse can be interrupted in a variety of ways, causing the heart to perform less efficiently.

The heart is described as showing arrhythmia or dysrhythmia when time intervals between waves, or the order or the number of waves do not fit the normal pattern described above. Other features that may be altered include the direction of wave deflection and wave widths.

Morbidity and mortality rates

According to the American Heart Association, cardiovascular disease is the number one cause of **death** in the United States. It is also the leading cause of death among people with diabetes.

Alternatives

Electrocardiography is the gold standard for detecting heart conditions involving irregularities in electrical conduction and rhythm. Other tests that may be used in conjunction with an EKG include an echocardiogram (a sonogram of the heart's pumping action) and a stress test—an EKG that is done in conjunction with treadmill or other supervised exercise to observe the heart's function under stress—may also be performed.

Resources

BOOKS

Baltazar, Romulo F. *Basic and Bedside Electrocardiography*. Philadelphia: Lippincott Williams and Wilkins, 2009.

Booth, Kathryn A., Patricia DeiTos, and Thomas O'Brien. *Electrocardiography for Health Care Personnel*, 2nd ed. Boston: McGraw Hill Higher Education, 2008.

PERIODICALS

Alis, C., et al. "Lifelink: 3G-based Mobile Telemedicine System." *Telemedicine Journal and E-Health* 15 (April 2009): 241–47.

Hopenfeld, B., et al. "The Guardian: An Implantable System for Chronic Ambulatory Monitoring of Acute Myocardial Infarction." *Journal of Electrocardiology* 42 (November-December 2009): 481–86.

Hsieh, J.C., et al. "The Realization of Ubiquitous 12-lead ECG Diagnosis in Emergency Telemedicine." *Telemedicine Journal and E-Health* 15 (November 2009): 896–906.

Krucoff, M.W. "From ST-elevation Myocardial Infarction to ST Elevation with No Myocardial Infarction—Review and Overview of a New Horizon of Computerized Electrocardiographic Ischemia Detection Using High-fidelity Implantable Devices." *Journal of Electrocardiology* 42 (November-December 2009): 487–93.

Kumar, A., and C.P. Cannon. "Acute Coronary Syndromes: Diagnosis and Management, Part I." *Mayo Clinic Proceedings* 84 (October 2009): 917–38.

Ogawa, H., et al. "A Remote-access ECG Monitoring System—Biomed 2009." *Biomedical Sciences Instrumentation* 45 (2009): 430–35.

OTHER

American Heart Association. *Electrocardiogram (ECG) Animation*. http://www.americanheart.org/presenter.jhtml?identifier = 3057186

Cleveland Clinic. *Electrocardiogram*. http://my.clevelandclinic.org/heart/services/tests/electrocard/ecg.aspx

Mayo Clinic. *Electrocardiogram*. http://www.mayoclinic.com/health/electrocardiogram/MY00086

ORGANIZATIONS

American Heart Association, 7272 Greenville Ave., Dallas, TX, 75231, (301) 223-2307, (800) 242-8721, http://www.americanheart.org.

European Society of Cardiology, The European Heart House, 2035 Route des Colles, B.P. 179-Les Templiers, Sophia-Antipolis, France, 06903, 33 4 9294 7600, 33 4 9294 7601, http://www.escardio.org.

Heart Foundation, 80 William St., Level 3, SydneyNSW, Australia, 2011, 02 9219 2444, 300 36 27 87, http://www.heartfoundation.org.au.

National Heart, Lung, and Blood Institute, P.O. Box 30105, Bethesda, MD, 20824-0105, (301) 592-8573, (204) 629-3246, nhlbiinfo@nhlbi.nih.gov, http://www.nhlbi.nih.gov.

Maggie Boleyn, R.N., B.S.N.
Paula Ford-Martin
Rebecca J. Frey, PhD
Brenda W. Lerner

Electroconvulsive therapy

Definition

Electroconvulsive therapy (ECT) is a medical treatment for severe mental illness in which a small, carefully controlled amount of electricity is introduced into the brain. This electrical stimulation, used in conjunction with anesthesia and muscle relaxant medications, produces a mild generalized seizure or convulsion. While used to treat a variety of psychiatric disorders, it is most effective in the treatment of severe depression, and provides the most rapid relief currently available for this illness.

Purpose

The purpose of electroconvulsive therapy is to provide relief from the signs and symptoms of mental illnesses such as severe depression, **mania**, and **schizophrenia**. ECT is indicated when patients need rapid improvement because they are suicidal, self-injurious, refuse to eat or drink, cannot or will not take medication as prescribed, or present some other danger to themselves. Antidepressant medications, while effective in many cases, may take two–six weeks to produce a therapeutic effect. Antipsychotic medications used to treat mania and schizophrenia have many uncomfortable and sometimes dangerous side effects, limiting their use. In addition, some patients develop **allergies** and therefore are unable to take their medicine.

Precautions

The most common risks associated with ECT are disturbances in heart rhythm. Broken or dislocated bones occur very rarely.

Description

The treatment of severe mental illness, such as schizophrenia, using electroconvulsive therapy was introduced in 1938 by two Italian doctors named Cerletti and Bini. In those days many doctors believed that convulsions were incompatible with schizophrenia since, according to their obervations, this disease rarely occurred in individuals suffering from **epilepsy**. They concluded, therefore, that if convulsions could be artifically produced in patients with schizophrenia, the illness could be cured. Some doctors were already using a variety of chemicals to produce seizures, but many of their patients died or suffered severe injuries because the strength of the convulsions could not be well controlled.

Electroconvulsive therapy is among the most controversial of all procedures used to treat mental illness. When it was first introduced, many people were frightened simply because it was called "shock treatment." Many assumed the procedure would be painful, others thought it was a form of electrocution, and still others believed it would cause brain damage. Unfortunately, unfavorable publicity in newspapers, magazines, and movies added to these fears.

Indeed, in those early years, patients and families were rarely educated by doctors and nurses regarding this or other forms of psychiatric treatment. In addition, no anesthesia or **muscle relaxants** were used. As a result, patients had violent seizures, and even though they did not remember them, the procedure itself was frightening.

The way these treatments are given today is very different from the procedures used in the past. Currently, ECT is offered on both an inpatient and outpatient basis. Hospitals have specially equipped rooms with oxygen, suction, and **cardiopulmonary resuscitation** (CPR) in order to deal with the rare emergency.

The treatment is carried out as follows: approximately 30 minutes before the scheduled treatment time, the patient may receive an injection of a medication (such as atropine) that keeps the pulse rate from decreasing too much during the convulsion. Next, the patient is placed on a cot and hooked up to a machine that automatically takes and displays vital signs (temperature, pulse, respiration, and blood pressure) on a television-like monitor. A mild anesthetic is then injected into a vein, followed by a medication (such a Anectine) that relaxes all of the muscles in the body so that the seizure is mild, and the risk of broken bones is virtually eliminated.

When the patient is both relaxed and asleep, an airway is placed in the mouth to aid with breathing. Electrodes are placed on the sides of the head in the temple areas. An electric current is passed through the brain by means of a machine specifically designed for this purpose. The usual dose of electricity is 70–150 volts for 0.1–0.5 seconds. In the first stage of the seizure (tonic phase), the muscles in the body that have not been paralyzed by medication contract for a period of five to 15 seconds. This is followed by the second stage (clonic phase) that is characterized by twitching movements, usually visible only in the toes or in a non-paralyzed arm or leg. These are caused by alternating contraction and relaxation of these same muscles. This stage lasts approximately 10–60 seconds. The entire procedure, from beginning to end, lasts about 30 minutes.

The total number of treatments a patient will receive depends upon many factors such as age, diagnosis, the history of illness, family support, and response to therapy. Patients with depression, for example, usually require six to 12 treatments. Treatments are usually administered every other day, three times a week.

The electrodes may be placed on both sides of the head (bilateral) or one side (unilateral). While bilateral

ECT appears to be somewhat more effective, unilateral ECT is preferred for individuals who experience prolonged confusion or forgetfulness following treatment. Many doctors begin treatment with unilateral ECT, then change to bilateral if the patient is not improving.

Post-treatment confusion and forgetfulness are common, though disturbing symptoms associated with ECT. Doctors and nurses must be patient and supportive by providing patients with factual information about recovery. Elderly patients, for example, may become increasingly confused and forgetful as the treatments continue. These symptoms usually subside with time, but a small minority of patients state that they have never fully recovered from these effects.

With the introduction of antipsychotics in the 1950s, the use of ECT became less frequent. These new medications provided relief for untold thousands of patients who suffered greatly from their illness. However, there are a number of side effects associated with these drugs, some of which are irreversible. Another drawback is that some medications do not produce a therapeutic effect for two–six weeks. During this time the patient may present a danger to himself or others. In addition, there are patients who do not respond to medicine or who have severe allergic reactions. For these individuals, ECT may be the only treatment that will help.

Preparation

Patients and relatives are prepared for ECT by being shown video tapes that explain both the procedure and the risks involved. The physician then answers any questions these individuals may have, and the patient is asked to sign an "Informed Consent Form." This gives the doctor and the hospital permission to administer the treatment.

Once the form is signed, the doctor performs a complete **physical examination**, and orders a number of tests that can help identify any potential problem. These tests may include a **chest x ray**, an electrocardiogram (ECG), **urinalysis**, spinal x ray, brain wave (EEG), and **complete blood count** (CBC).

Some medications, such as lithium and a type of antidepressant known as **monoamine oxidase inhibitors**, should be discontinued for some time before treatment. Patients are instructed not to eat or drink for at least eight hours prior to the procedure in order to reduce the possibility of **vomiting** and **choking**.

Aftercare

After the treatment, patients are moved to a recovery area. Vital signs are recorded every five

---

KEY TERMS

Mania—A mood disorder in which a person experiences prolonged elation or irritability characterized by overactivity that can lead to exhaustion and medical emergencies.

Relapse—A return of the signs and symptoms of an illness.

Schizophrenia—A severe mental illness in which a person has difficulty distinguishing what is real from what is not real. It is often characterized by hallucinations, delusions, and withdrawal from people and social activities.

---

minutes until the patient is fully awake, which may take 15–30 minutes. Some initial confusion may be present but usually disappears in a matter of minutes. There may be complaints of **headache**, muscle **pain**, or back pain. Such discomfort is quickly relieved by mild medications such as **aspirin**.

Risks

Advanced medical technology has substantially reduced the complications associated with ECT. These include slow heart beat (bradycardia), rapid heart beat (tachycardia), **memory loss**, and confusion. Persons at high risk for ECT include those with recent **heart attack**, uncontrolled blood pressure, brain tumors, and previous spinal injuries.

Normal results

ECT often produces dramatic improvement in the signs and symptoms of major depression, especially in elderly individuals, sometimes during the first week of treatment. While it is estimated that 50% of these patients will experience a future return of symptoms, the prognosis for each episode of illness is good. Mania also often responds well to treatment. The picture is not as bright for schizophrenia, which is more difficult to treat and is characterized by frequent relapses.

A few patients are placed on maintenance ECT. This means they return to the hospital every one–two months, as needed, for an additional treatment. These individuals are thus able to keep their illness under control and lead a normal and productive life.

Resources

BOOKS

Stuart, Gail Wiscarz.*Principles and Practice of Psychiatric Nursing*. 9th ed. St. Louis: Mosby Elsevier, 2009.

ORGANIZATIONS

National Institutes of Health, 9000 Rockville Place, Bethesda, MD, 20892, (301) 496-4000, NIHinfo@od. nih.gov, http://www.nih.gov.

Donald G. Barstow, RN

Electrocution *see* **Electric shock injuries**

Electroencephalography

Definition

Electroencephalography, or EEG, is a neurological test that uses an electronic monitoring device to measure and record electrical activity in the brain.

Purpose

The EEG is a key tool in the diagnosis and management of **epilepsy** and other seizure disorders. It is also used to assist in the diagnosis of brain damage and disease (e.g., **stroke**, tumors, **encephalitis**), **mental retardation**, **sleep disorders**, degenerative diseases such as **Alzheimer's disease** and **Parkinson's disease**, and certain mental disorders (e.g., **alcoholism, schizophrenia, autism**).

An EEG may also be used to monitor brain activity during surgery and to determine brain **death**.

Precautions

Electroencephalography should be administered and interpreted by a trained medical professional only. Data from an EEG is only one element of a complete medical and/or psychological patient assessment, and should never be used alone as the sole basis for a diagnosis.

Description

Before the EEG begins, a nurse or technician attaches approximately 16–20 electrodes to the patient's scalp with a conductive, washable paste. Depending on

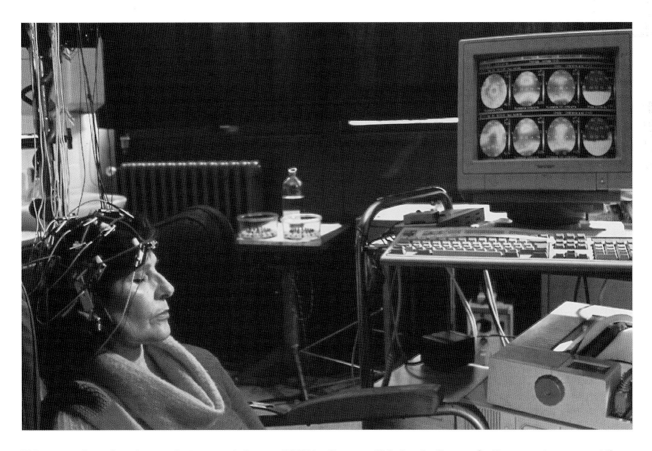

This woman is undergoing an electroencephalogram (EEG) to diagnose Alzheimer's disease. On the computer screen at the right are the colored scans of the electrical activity in her brain. Alzheimer's patients show a specific abnormality in their EEGs. *(Catherine Pouedras/Photo Researchers, Inc.)*

the purpose for the EEG, implantable or invasive electrodes are occasionally used. Implantable electrodes include sphenoidal electrodes, which are fine wires inserted under the zygomatic arch, or cheekbone; and depth electrodes, which are surgically-implanted into the brain. The EEG electrodes are painless, and are used to measure the electrical activity in various regions of the brain.

For the test, the patient lies on a bed, padded table, or comfortable chair and is asked to relax and remain still during the EEG testing period. An EEG usually takes no more than one hour. During the test procedure, the patient may be asked to breathe slowly or quickly; visual stimuli such as flashing lights or a patterned board may be used to stimulate certain types of brain activity. Throughout the procedure, the electroencephalograph machine makes a continuous graphic record of the patient's brain activity, or brainwaves, on a long strip of recording paper or on a computer screen. This graphic record is called an electroencephalogram.

The sleep EEG uses the same equipment and procedures as a regular EEG. Patients undergoing a sleep EEG are encouraged to fall asleep completely rather than just relax. They are typically provided a bed and a quiet room conducive to sleep. A sleep EEG lasts up to three hours.

In an ambulatory EEG, patients are hooked up to a portable cassette recorder. They then go about their normal activities, and take their normal rest and sleep for a period of up to 24 hours. During this period, the patient and patient's family record any symptoms or abnormal behaviors, which can later be correlated with the EEG to see if they represent seizures.

Many insurance plans provide reimbursement for EEG testing. Costs for an EEG range from $100 to more than $500, depending on the purpose and type of test (i.e., asleep or awake, and invasive or non-invasive electrodes). Because coverage may be dependent on the disorder or illness the EEG is evaluating, patients should check with their individual insurance plan.

Preparation

Full instructions should be given to EEG patients when they schedule their test. Typically, individuals on medications that affect the central nervous system, such as anticonvulsants, stimulants, or antidepressants, are told to discontinue their prescription for a short time prior to the test (usually one to two days). Patients may be asked to avoid food and beverages that contain **caffeine**, a central nervous system stimulant. However, any such request should be cleared by the treating physician. Patients may also be asked to

---

KEY TERMS

Epilepsy—A neurological disorder characterized by recurrent seizures with or without a loss of consciousness.

Ictal EEG—Used to measure brain activity during a seizure. May be useful in learning more about patients who aren't responding to conventional treatments.

---

arrive for the test with clean hair free of spray or other styling products.

Patients undergoing a sleep EEG may be asked to remain awake the night before their test. They may be given a sedative prior to the test to induce sleep.

Aftercare

If the patient has suspended regular medication for the test, the EEG nurse or technician should advise him when he can begin taking it again.

Risks

Being off medication for one–two days may trigger seizures. Certain procedures used during EEG may trigger seizures in patients with epilepsy. Those procedures include flashing lights and deep breathing. If the EEG is being used as a diagnostic for epilepsy (i.e., to determine the type of seizures an individual is suffering from), this may be a desired effect, although the patient needs to be monitored closely so that the seizure can be aborted if necessary. This type of test is known as an ictal EEG.

Normal results

In reading and interpreting brainwave patterns, a neurologist or other physician will evaluate the type of brainwaves and the symmetry, location, and consistency of brainwave patterns. He will also look at the brainwave response to certain stimuli presented during the EEG test (such as flashing lights or noise). There are four basic types of brainwaves: alpha, beta, theta, and delta. "Normal" brainwave patterns vary widely, depending on factors of age and activity. For example, awake and relaxed individuals typically register an alpha wave pattern of eight to 13 cycles per second. Young children and sleeping adults may have a delta wave pattern of under four cycles per second.

Abnormal results

The EEG readings of patients with epilepsy or other seizure disorders display bursts or spikes of electrical activity. In focal epilepsy, spikes are restricted to one hemisphere of the brain. If spikes are generalized to both hemispheres of the brain, multifocal epilepsy may be present.

The diagnostic brainwave patterns of other disorders varies widely. The appearance of excess theta waves (four to eight cycles per second) may indicate brain injury. Brain wave patterns in patients with brain disease, mental retardation, and brain injury show overall slowing. A trained medical specialist should interpret EEG results in the context of the patient's medical history, and other pertinent medical test results.

Resources

BOOKS

Libenson, Mark H. *Practical Approach to Electroencephalography.* Philadelphia: Elsevier/Saunders, 2010.

Paula Anne Ford-Martin

Electrolyte disorders

Definition

An electrolyte disorder is an imbalance of certain ionized components (i.e., bicarbonate, **calcium**, chloride, magnesium, phosphate, potassium, and **sodium**) in the blood.

Description

Electrolytes are ionized molecules found throughout the blood, tissues, and cells of the body. These molecules, which are either positive (cations) or negative (anions), conduct an electric current and help to balance pH and acid-base levels in the body. Electrolytes also facilitate the passage of fluid between and within cells through a process known as osmosis and play a part in regulating the function of the cardiovascular, neuromuscular, endocrine, and excretory systems.

The serum electrolytes include:

- Sodium (Na). A positively charged electrolyte that helps to balance fluid levels in the body and facilitates neuromuscular functioning.
- Potassium (K). A main component of cellular fluid, this positive electrolyte helps to regulate neuromuscular function and osmotic pressure.
- Calcium (Ca). A cation, or positive electrolyte, that affects neuromuscular performance and contributes to skeletal growth and blood coagulation.
- Magnesium (Mg). Influences muscle contractions and intracellular activity. A cation.
- Chloride (Cl). An anion, or negative electrolyte, that regulates blood pressure.
- Phosphate (HPO_4). Negative electrolyte that impacts metabolism and regulates acid-base balance and calcium levels.
- Bicarbonate (HCO_3). A negatively charged electrolyte that assists in the regulation of blood pH levels. Bicarbonate insufficiencies and elevations cause acid-base disorders (i.e., acidosis, alkalosis).

Risk factors

Medications, chronic diseases, and trauma (for example, **burns**, or **fractures**, etc.) may cause the concentration of certain electrolytes in the body to become too high (hyper-) or too low (hypo-). When this happens, an electrolyte imbalance, or disorder, results.

Causes and symptoms

Sodium

HYPERNATREMIA. Sodium helps the kidneys to regulate the amount of water the body retains or excretes. Consequently, individuals with elevated serum sodium levels experience a loss of fluids, or **dehydration. Hypernatremia** can be caused by inadequate water intake, excessive fluid loss (i.e., **diabetes insipidus**, **kidney disease**, severe burns, and prolonged **vomiting** or **diarrhea**), or sodium retention (caused by excessive sodium intake or aldosteronism). In addition, certain drugs, including loop **diuretics, corticosteroids**, and antihypertensive medications may cause elevated sodium levels.

Symptoms of hypernatremia include:

- thirst
- orthostatic hypotension
- dry mouth and mucous membranes
- dark, concentrated urine
- loss of elasticity in the skin
- irregular heartbeat (tachycardia)
- irritability
- fatigue
- lethargy
- heavy, labored breathing
- muscle twitching and/or seizures

HYPONATREMIA. Up to 1% of all hospitalized patients and as many as 18% of nursing home patients develop **hyponatremia**, making it one of the most common electrolyte disorders. Diuretics, certain psychoactive drugs (i.e., fluoxetine, sertraline, haloperidol), specific antipsychotics (lithium), vasopressin, chlorpropamide, the illicit drug ecstasy, and other pharmaceuticals can cause decreased sodium levels. Low sodium levels may also be triggered by inadequate dietary intake of sodium, excessive perspiration, water intoxication, and impairment of adrenal gland or kidney function.

Symptoms of hyponatremia include:

- nausea, abdominal cramping, and/or vomiting
- headache
- edema (swelling)
- muscle weakness and/or tremor
- paralysis
- disorientation
- slowed breathing
- seizures
- coma

Potassium

HYPERKALEMIA. **Hyperkalemia** may be caused by ketoacidosis (diabetic **coma**), myocardial infarction (**heart attack**), severe burns, kidney failure, **fasting, bulimia nervosa**, gastrointestinal bleeding, adrenal insufficiency, or **Addison's disease**. Diuretic drugs, cyclosporin, lithium, heparin, ACE inhibitors, **beta blockers**, and trimethoprim can increase serum potassium levels, as can heavy **exercise**. The condition may also be secondary to hypernatremia. Symptoms may include:

- weakness
- nausea and/or abdominal pain
- irregular heartbeat (arrhythmia)
- diarrhea
- muscle pain

HYPOKALEMIA. Severe dehydration, aldosteronism, **Cushing's syndrome**, kidney disease, long-term diuretic therapy, certain **penicillins**, laxative **abuse**, congestive **heart failure**, and adrenal gland impairments can all cause depletion of potassium levels in the bloodstream. A substance known as glycyrrhetinic acid, which is found in licorice and chewing tobacco, can also deplete potassium serum levels. Symptoms of **hypokalemia** include:

- weakness
- paralysis
- increased urination

- irregular heartbeat (arrhythmia)
- orthostatic hypotension
- muscle pain
- tetany

Calcium

HYPERCALCEMIA. Blood calcium levels may be elevated in cases of thyroid disorder, **multiple myeloma**, metastatic **cancer**, multiple bone fractures, milk-alkali syndrome, and Paget's disease. Excessive use of calcium-containing supplements and certain over-the-counter medications (i.e., **antacids**) may also cause **hypercalcemia**. In infants, lesser known causes may include blue diaper syndrome, Williams syndrome, secondary **hyperparathyroidism** from maternal **hypocalcemia**, and dietary phosphate deficiency. Symptoms include:

- fatigue
- constipation
- depression
- confusion
- muscle pain
- nausea and vomiting
- dehydration
- increased urination
- irregular heartbeat (arrhythmia)

HYPOCALCEMIA. Thyroid disorders, kidney failure, severe burns, **sepsis, vitamin D deficiency**, and medications such as heparin and glucogan can deplete blood calcium levels. Lowered levels cause:

- muscle cramps and spasms
- tetany and/or convulsions
- mood changes (depression, irritability)
- dry skin
- brittle nails
- facial twitching

Magnesium

HYPERMAGNESEMIA. Excessive magnesium levels may occur with end-stage renal disease, Addison's disease, or an overdose of magnesium salts. Hypermagnesemia is characterized by:

- lethargy
- hypotension
- decreased heart and respiratory rate
- muscle weakness
- diminished tendon reflexes

Acid-base balance—A balance of acidity and alkalinity of fluids in the body that keeps the pH level of blood around 7.35–7.45.

Aldosteronism—A condition defined by high serum levels of aldosterone, a hormone secreted by the adrenal gland that is responsible for increasing sodium reabsorption in the kidneys.

Addison's disease—A disease characterized by a deficiency in adrenocortical hormones due to destruction of the adrenal gland.

Bulimia nervosa—An eating disorder characterized by binging and purging (self-induced vomiting) behaviors.

Milk-alkali syndrome—Elevated blood calcium levels and alkalosis caused by excessive intake of milk

and alkalis. Usually occurs in the treatment of peptic ulcer.

Orthostatic hypotension—A drop in blood pressure that causes faintness or dizziness and occurs when one rises to a standing position. Also known as postural hypotension.

Osmotic pressure—Pressure that occurs when two solutions of differing concentrations are separated by a semipermeable membrane, such as a cellular wall, and the lower concentration solute is drawn across the membrane into the higher concentration solute (osmosis).

Tetany—A disorder of the nervous system characterized by muscle cramps, spasms of the arms and legs, and numbness of the extremities.

HYPOMAGNESEMIA. Inadequate dietary intake of magnesium, often caused by chronic **alcoholism** or **malnutrition**, is a common cause of hypomagnesemia. Other causes include malabsorption syndromes, **pancreatitis**, aldosteronism, burns, hyperparathyroidism, digestive system disorders, and diuretic use. Symptoms of low serum magnesium levels include:

- leg and foot cramps
- weight loss
- vomiting
- muscle spasms, twitching, and tremors
- seizures
- muscle weakness
- arrthymia

Chloride

HYPERCHLOREMIA. Severe dehydration, kidney failure, hemodialysis, traumatic brain injury, and aldosteronism can cause hyperchloremia. Drugs such as boric acid and ammonium chloride and the intravenous (IV) infusion of sodium chloride can also boost chloride levels, resulting in hyperchloremic **metabolic acidosis**. Symptoms include:

- weakness
- headache
- nausea
- cardiac arrest

HYPOCHLOREMIA. Hypochloremia usually occurs as a result of sodium and potassium depletion (i.e.,

hyponatremia, hypokalemia). Severe depletion of serum chloride levels causes **metabolic alkalosis**. This alkalization of the bloodstream is characterized by:

- mental confusion
- slowed breathing
- paralysis
- muscle tension or spasm

Phosphate

HYPERPHOSPHATEMIA. Skeletal fractures or disease, kidney failure, **hypoparathyroidism**, hemodialysis, **diabetic ketoacidosis**, acromegaly, systemic infection, and intestinal obstruction can all cause phosphate retention and build-up in the blood. The disorder occurs concurrently with hypocalcemia. Individuals with mild hyperphosphatemia are typically asymptomatic, but signs of severe hyperphosphatemia include:

- tingling in hands and fingers
- muscle spasms and cramps
- convulsions
- cardiac arrest

HYPOPHOSPHATEMIA. Serum phosphate levels of 2 mg/dL or below may be caused by hypomagnesemia and hypokalemia. Severe burns, alcoholism, diabetic ketoacidosis, kidney disease, hyperparathyroidism, **hypothyroidism**, Cushing's syndrome, malnutrition, hemodialysis, vitamin D deficiency, and prolonged diuretic therapy can also diminish blood phosphate levels. There are typically few physical signs of mild phosphate depletion. Symptoms of severe hypophosphatemia include:

- muscle weakness
- weight loss
- bone deformities (osteomalacia)

Diagnosis

Examination

Diagnosis is performed by a physician or other qualified healthcare provider who will take a medical history, discuss symptoms, perform a complete **physical examination**, and prescribe appropriate laboratory tests. Because electrolyte disorders commonly affect the neuromuscular system, the provider will test reflexes. If a calcium imbalance is suspected, the physician will also check for Chvostek's sign, a reflex test that triggers an involuntary facial twitch, and Trousseau's sign, a muscle spasm that occurs in response to pressure on the upper arm.

Tests

Serum electrolyte imbalances can be detected through blood tests. Blood is drawn from a vein on the back of the hand or inside of the elbow by a medical technician, or phlebotomist, and analyzed at a lab.

Normal levels of electrolytes are:

- Sodium: 135–145 mEq/L (serum)
- Potassium: 3.5–5.5 mEq/L (serum)
- Calcium: 8.8–10.4 mg/dL (total Ca; serum); 4.7–5.2 mg/dL (unbound Ca; serum)
- Magnesium: 1.4–2.1 mEq/L (plasma)
- Chloride: 100–108 mEq/L (serum)
- Phosphate: 2.5–4.5 mg/dL (plasma; adults)

Standard ranges for test results may vary due to differing laboratory standards and physiological variances (gender, age, and other factors). Other blood tests that determine pH levels and acid-base balance may be performed.

Treatment

Treatment of electrolyte disorders depends on the underlying cause of the problem and the type of electrolyte involved. If the disorder is caused by poor diet or improper fluid intake, nutritional changes may be prescribed. If medications such as diuretics triggered the imbalance, discontinuing or adjusting the drug therapy may effectively treat the condition. Fluid and electrolyte replacement therapy, either intravenously or by mouth, can reverse electrolyte depletion.

Hemodialysis treatment may be required to reduce serum potassium levels in hyperkalemic patients with impaired kidney function. It may also be recommended for renal patients with severe hypermagnesemia.

Prognosis

A patient's long-term prognosis depends upon the root cause of the electrolyte disorder. When treated quickly and appropriately, electrolyte imbalances in and of themselves are usually effectively reversed.

When they are mild, some electrolyte imbalances have few to no symptoms and may pass unnoticed. For example, transient hyperphosphatemia is usually fairly benign. However, long-term elevations of blood phosphate levels can lead to potentially fatal soft tissue and vascular calcifications and bone disease, and severe serum phosphate deficiencies (hypophosphatemia) can cause encephalopathy, coma, and **death**.

Severe hypernatremia has a mortality rate of 40–60%. Death is commonly due to cerebrovascular damage and hemorrhage resulting from dehydration and shrinkage of the brain cells.

Prevention

Physicians should use caution when prescribing drugs known to affect electrolyte levels and acid-base balance. Individuals with kidney disease, thyroid problems, and other conditions that may place them at risk for developing an electrolyte disorder should be educated on the signs and symptoms.

Resources

PERIODICALS

Ghali, J.K. "Mechanisms, Risks, and New Treatment Optons for Hyponatremia." *Cardiology* 111, no. 3 (April 2008): 147–57.

Lumachi, F., A. Brunello, A. Roma, and U. Basso. "Medical Treatment of Malignancy Associated Hypercalcemia." *Current Medicinal Chemistry* 15, no. 4 (2008): 415–21.

Shingarev, R., and M. Allon. "A Physiologic-Based Approach to the Treatment of Acute Hyperkalemia." *American Journal of Kidney Disease* (June 4, 2010): [E-Pub Ahead of Print].

Paula Anne Ford-Martin
Teresa G. Odle
Melinda Granger Oberleitner,
RN, DNS, APRN, CNS

Electrolyte supplements

Definition

Electrolyte supplements are a varied group of prescription and nonprescription preparations used to correct imbalances in the body's electrolyte levels. Electrolytes themselves are substances that dissociate into ions (electrically charged atoms or atom groups) when they melt or are dissolved, thus serving to conduct electricity. In the human body, electrolytes are critical to the proper distribution of water, muscle contraction and expansion, transmission of nerve impulses, delivery of oxygen to body tissues, heart rate and rhythm, acid-base balance, and other important functions or conditions.

The ions that are formed when electrolytes are dissolved in body fluids are either positively or negatively charged. Positively charged ions are called cations, and are formed when an atom or atom group loses electrons. The most important cations in the human body are **sodium**, potassium, magnesium, and **calcium** ions. Negatively charged ions are called anions, and are formed when an atom or atom group gains electrons. The principal anions in the body include bicarbonate, chloride, phosphate, and sulfate ions, as well as ions formed by certain protein compounds or organic acids.

About 60% of an adult human male's total body weight is water. In adult women, the figure is about 55%, and is even lower in the elderly and in obese people. Two-thirds of total body water (TBW) lies inside cells and is known as intracellular fluid or ICF. The remaining third of TBW lies outside the cells and is called extracellular fluid or ECF. About 75% of ECF lies in connective tissue or the spaces between tissues outside the blood vessels (interstitial spaces), while the remaining 25% is within the blood vessels. In addition to representing different proportions of TBW, ICF and ECF differ significantly in their electrolyte content. Whereas the major cation in ICF is potassium, the most important cation in ECF is sodium. These differences in electrolyte levels help to regulate the movement of water between ICF and ECF.

Children are more vulnerable than adults to fluid and electrolyte imbalances, in part because they have different ratios of TBW to total body weight, and of ICF to ECF. A newborn baby carried to full term has a TBW ratio between 75 and 80%. The baby's total body water ratio decreases by 4–5% during the first week after birth and reaches the adult level of 60% by twelve months of age. Similarly, a newborn has an ICF:ECF ratio of 55:45, which falls to the adult ratio of 70:30 during the first year of life. In addition to these different fluid ratios, children's kidneys are less efficient than adults in regulating water balance; children have smaller organ systems that dissipate body heat less efficiently; and their core body temperature rises faster than that of an adult when they become dehydrated. All these factors help to explain why some electrolyte supplements are formulated specifically for children.

Purpose

The purpose of electrolyte supplements is to restore the proper ratio of total body water to total body weight and the correct proportions of the various electrolytes in body fluids. Electrolyte imbalances may result from excessive intake or inadequate elimination of electrolytes on the one hand or by insufficient intake or excessive elimination on the other hand.

Body regulation of water and electrolytes

Under normal conditions, the water and electrolyte content of the body is regulated by the kidneys, the secretion of antidiuretic hormone, and the sensation of thirst. The average adult needs to take in about 700–800 mL (about 1.5–1.7 pints) of water per day in order to match the water lost through perspiration, breathing, and excretion of waste products (urine and feces). The water taken in by mouth is added to the 200–300 mL (0.42–0.63 pints) of water that are formed in the body each day through tissue breakdown.

The amount of water needed to match fluid losses may be considerably greater than the average during **exercise** or in patients with **fever**, severe **vomiting**, or **diarrhea**. Adults with fever typically lose an additional 0.75–1.0 oz of fluid per day for each degree that their temperature rises above normal. With regard to diarrhea, adults with **cholera** have been reported to lose as much as a quart of fluid per hour in their stools. The fluid lost in this way contains sodium, potassium, and chloride, resulting in electrolyte imbalances in cholera patients as well as **dehydration**.

Exercise raises the total metabolism of the body to 5–15 times the resting rate. Most of this energy (70–90%) is released as heat, which is partially dissipated by the evaporation of sweat. Depending on weather conditions, the type and weight of clothing being worn, and the intensity of exercise or physical work performed, adults may lose anywhere from 1 to 2.5 qt of fluid per hour through perspiration. Sweat contains sodium chloride as well as smaller amounts of potassium, calcium, and magnesium. In order to maintain the proper balance of electrolytes in the body as well as fluid, athletes or people employed in outdoor work during warm weather may need to replace the electrolytes lost in sweat by taking capsules or drinking beverages containing supplemental electrolytes.

With regard to the sense of thirst, it is not always an accurate indication of the body's need for water. Researchers have found that many people do not feel thirsty until they have already lost about 2% of their total body weight through fluid losses. As a result, most people do not replace enough fluid during exercise or hot weather simply by drinking water until they no longer feel thirsty. In addition, the **aging** process, certain mental disorders, or drugs may affect a person's sense of thirst.

At the other extreme of water intake, a person may drink excessive amounts of water due to misunderstandings about their need for extra fluid during exercise. This condition is known as water intoxication or hyperhydration. It leads to abnormally low levels of sodium in the blood, a condition known as **hyponatremia**. This condition is also known as exercise-associated hyponatremia (EAH). Water intoxication may lead to swelling of the brain, confusion, disorientation, and eventually **coma** or **death**. Several marathon runners have died from water intoxication, as have teenagers who consumed large amounts of water after taking doses of Ecstasy (MDMA), a so-called "club drug." Other persons at risk for water intoxication include people with **eating disorders** and children with **mental retardation**. Research reported in the *New England Journal of Medicine* revealed that as many as 13% of marathon runners developed hyponatremia during the course of a race as a result of drinking too much water, usually 3 qt or more. Female athletes appear to be at greater risk of water intoxication and hyponatremia than male athletes.

Conditions associated with fluid and electrolyte imbalance

Several common conditions can lead to fluid and electrolyte imbalance:

- Exposure to extended periods of extremely hot weather.
- High levels of athletic activity, military training, or outdoor work in such fields as construction, agriculture, forestry, fishing, and certain types of manufacturing.
- Extreme changes in diet.
- Reduced fluid intake.
- Medication side effects. Certain drugs, particularly diuretics, beta-blockers, and vasodilators, may increase the loss of electrolytes in urine and/or

interfere with the body's ability to regulate its temperature during exercise or in hot weather.
- Severe illnesses characterized by high fever, recurrent diarrhea, and/or frequent vomiting. Such illnesses include cholera, viral gastroenteritis (stomach flu), shigellosis, and amebic dysentery.
- Severe burns covering more than 10% of the body.
- Surgical creation of a stoma or urinary diversion. These operations sometimes lead to an increased loss of body fluids while the patient's body is adjusting to the changes in urination and excretion resulting from the surgery. In addition, some forms of weight loss surgery intended to bypass parts of the small intestine in which food absorption occurs have a 70% rate of electrolyte imbalances as a complication of the operation.
- Diseases affecting the kidneys. These include diabetes mellitus, diabetes insipidus, and syndrome of inappropriate antidiuretic hormone secretion (SIADH) as well as cancer or infections of the kidneys.
- In infants, premature birth.

Description

The various electrolyte supplements used in the United States and Canada are intended to prevent or treat electrolyte imbalances in very different situations or groups of patients. They range from sports drinks and other supplements used by amateur or professional athletes to prevent **muscle cramps** and improve athletic performance, to liquids used at home to prevent dehydration in children with diarrhea, to injections administered as part of enteral (feeding through a tube or stoma directly into the small intestine) or parenteral **nutrition** (intravenous feeding that bypasses the digestive tract).

The major categories of electrolyte supplements are:

- Sports drinks. Sports drinks are beverages specially formulated to contain appropriate amounts of electrolytes and carbohydrates as well as water to replace the fluid and sodium lost through sweat during athletic activities. These beverages are popular with athletes at the college level. According to the American College of Sports Medicine as well as American and Canadian dietitians' associations, sports drinks are effective in supplying food energy for the muscles, maintaining proper levels of blood sugar, maintaining the proper functioning of the thirst mechanism, and lowering the risk of dehydration or hyponatremia. Other researchers have noted that the flavoring added to sports drinks encourages athletes to drink more during periods of exercise and thus maintain

KEY TERMS

Anion—An ion carrying a negative charge owing to a surplus of electrons. Anions in the body include bicarbonate, chloride, phosphate, sulfate, certain organic acids, and certain protein compounds.

Cation—An ion carrying a positive charge due to a loss of electrons. Cations in the body include sodium, potassium, magnesium, and calcium ions.

Cholera—A severe bacterial infection of the small intestine characterized by profuse diarrhea and eventual dehydration. Cholera is still a frequent cause of death among children in developing countries.

Electron—An elementary particle carrying a negative charge. Electrons may exist either independently or as components of an atom outside its nucleus.

Enteral nutrition—Nourishment given through a tube or stoma directly into the small intestine, thus bypassing the upper digestive tract.

Hyponatremia—Insufficient sodium in the blood.

Interstitial spaces—Spaces within body tissues that are outside the blood vessels. Also known as interstitial compartments.

Ion—An atom or group of atoms that acquires an electrical charge by the gain or loss of electrons.

Metabolism—The sum of an organism's physical and chemical processes that produce and maintain living tissue, and make energy available to the organism. Insulin resistance is a disorder of metabolism.

Parenteral nutrition—Nutrition supplied intravenously, thus bypassing the patient's digestive tract entirely.

Stoma—A surgical opening made in the abdominal wall to allow waste products to pass directly to the outside.

Water intoxication—A potentially life-threatening condition caused by drinking too much water, which leads to hyponatremia and may result in seizures, coma, and death.

proper levels of hydration. Sports drinks can be purchased in supermarkets and health food stores; they include such well-known beverages as Gatorade and Powerade. Some of these supplements come in a semisolid form known as energy gels, which contain caffeine or various herbal compounds as well as carbohydrates and electrolytes.

- Over-the-counter powders and tablets. Some athletes–particularly those who participate in long-distance running or endurance cycling—prefer capsules or concentrated powders to maintain their electrolyte balance during exercise. The powders are mixed with 12 or 16 oz of cold water prior to drinking, while the capsules can be taken before, during, and after exercise. Most contain flavorings to mask the naturally salty or bitter taste of the electrolytes themselves. Common brand names include eForce, NutriBiotic, and Endurolytes;. These products are regarded by the Food and Drug Administration (FDA) as dietary supplements.

- Over-the-counter electrolyte replenishers for children. Infants and young children are more vulnerable to dehydration than adults, particularly from severe gastroenteritis or diarrhea. A child may become dehydrated in less than a day from recurrent vomiting or episodes of diarrhea. Some doctors recommend that parents keep oral rehydration fluids containing mixtures of carbohydrates and electrolytes specially formulated for children in the medicine chest at home in case the child becomes dehydrated from a stomach virus or similar illness. Common brand names for these products, which are regulated by the FDA as medical foods, include Pedialyte, Infalyte, Naturalyte, and Rehydralyte. Most come in a powdered form to be mixed with water as well as liquid forms; Pedialyte is also available as fruit-flavored freezer pops.

- Oral rehydration formulae for children and adults. Oral rehydration salts, also known as ORS, have been a staple of treatment for cholera and other diseases accompanied by severe diarrhea in developing countries for almost half a century. First researched in the 1940s, oral rehydration salts were adopted by the World Health Organization (WHO) in 1978 in order to reduce the risk of death from dehydration caused by cholera-related diarrhea. Since the introduction of ORS, the number of children around the world who die from acute diarrhea has been reduced from 5 million per year to 1.3 million. Reformulated by WHO in 2002, the ORS salts come in packets to be kept in the home and mixed with water as soon as a child (or adult) falls ill. The formula is a low-glucose and low-sodium mixture. If the WHO packets are unavailable, a comparable form of oral rehydration solution can be made by adding 8 tsp of table sugar, ½ tsp of salt, ½ tsp of baking soda (bicarbonate of soda), and $\frac{1}{3}$ tsp of potassium chloride to 1 L (1.05 qt) of water. In an emergency, a solution prepared from 1 tbsp of sugar and ½ tsp of salt added to 1 L of water can be used to treat diarrhea.

- Multiple electrolyte injections. Various mixtures of electrolytes are available by prescription in injectable form to be added to enteral or parenteral nutrition formulae. These forms of feeding are used in patients who require supplementation or complete replacement of feeding by mouth, including patients with various intestinal disorders, AIDS, or severe burns. Basic solutions for total parenteral nutrition, or TPN, contain the electrolytes sodium, potassium, chloride, phosphate, and magnesium, although the exact proportion of electrolytes can be tailored to an individual patient's needs. Some injectable formulae contain dextrose, a sugar, and acetate or lactate as well as the five major electrolytes. Common brand names include TPN Electrolytes, Lypholyte, Nutri-lyte, Plasma-Lyte 148, and others. Some patients are taught to use these injectable formulae at home.

Recommended dosage

Recommended dosages for electrolyte supplements are:

- Sports drinks. Since sports drinks and energy gels are not medications in the strict sense, the amount consumed will vary not only from person to person but also in a given individual from day to day depending on weather conditions, level of athletic conditioning, length of activity, and other factors. To lower the risk of dehydration in adults in hot weather, the American College of Sports Medicine recommends drinking approximately 2 to 3 mL/lb of body weight of water or sports drink four hours before exercising. Overhydration during this time period should be avoided. During exercise, enough fluid should be consumed to prevent a water deficit greater then 2% of body weight. Recommended beverages are those that contain electrolytes and carbohydrates. If the exercise event lasts longer than an hour, consumption of carbohydrate beverages that contain 6–8% carbohydrate is recommended. After exercise, rapid and complete recovery from exercise-induced dehydration can be accomplished by drinking at least 16–24 oz (450–675 mL) of fluid for every pound of weight lost during exercise. To replace fluids and electrolytes lost during endurance events lasting longer than two hours, the current recommendation is consumption of sports drinks that contain 0.5–0.7 g/L of sodium and 0.8–2.0 g/L of potassium and that also contain carbohydrate.

- Over-the-counter powders and tablets. The usual recommended dose of powdered electrolytes is one scoopful (or prepackaged envelope) of powder dissolved in 12–16 oz of water before exercising. Capsules

may be taken as follows: 1–3 capsules 30–60 minutes before exercising; 1–6 capsules per hour during the workout; and 1–3 capsules after exercising.

- Over-the-counter electrolyte replenishers for children. Dosages for Pedialyte and similar oral rehydration solutions for children are usually based on the child's age and weight. The child's doctor should determine the quantity to be given if the child is younger than 12 months of age. Children between the ages of one and two years are usually given 34 mL of electrolyte solution per pound of body weight during the first eight hours of treatment and 75 mL per pound of body weight during the next 16 hours, although the doctor may adjust the dose if the child is very thirsty. Children between the ages of two and ten are given 23 mL of electrolyte solution per pound of body weight for the first four to six hours of treatment, followed by 45 mL per pound taken over the next 18–24 hours. Freezer pops may be given to children older than one year as often as the child desires.

- Oral rehydration formulae. The WHO form of oral rehydration liquid is made by adding the full contents of one packet of powdered oral rehydration salts to a quart of drinking water. The solution should not be boiled. A fresh quart of solution should be mixed each day. Infants and young children should be given the solution in small amounts by spoon as often as possible. Adults and teenagers should take the WHO formula according to the doctor's directions.

- Multiple electrolyte injections. Basic TPN solutions are usually made up in liter batches and adjusted to each individual patient's needs. The standard adult dosage is 2 L per day, usually administered by drip through a needle or catheter placed in the patient's vein for a 10–12-hour period once a day or five days per week. The patient may be given several units of premixed TPN fluid to store at home in the refrigerator or freezer. Each dose should be taken from the refrigerator 4–6 hours prior to use to allow it to warm to room temperature. TPN solution stored in a freezer should be moved to a refrigerator 24 hours before use.

Precautions

Sports drinks should not be given to rehydrate children with **vomiting** or diarrhea, as they do not contain the proper balance of carbohydrates and electrolytes needed by children's bodies.

Over-the-counter powders and tablets should always be taken with adequate amounts of water and kept out of the reach of children.

Over-the-counter electrolyte replenishers for children should be stored out of the reach of children and away from heat and direct sunlight. In addition, they should not be given to patients with intestinal blockage.

WHO oral rehydration salts and packets of similar formulae should not be stored in damp places, as moisture can cause the contents to lose their effectiveness. These products should also be kept away from heat or direct sunlight. Unused oral rehydration solution should be discarded at the end of each day. As with electrolyte replenishers for children, oral rehydration formulae should not be given to patients with intestinal blockage.

Patients using multiple electrolyte injections as part of **total parenteral nutrition** should have their blood and urine checked at regular intervals while they are receiving these medicines. They should also be taught to recognize the signs of infection at the injection site (**pain**, swelling, redness, or a cold sensation). In addition, these patients should not use sports drinks, other electrolyte supplements, or over-the-counter medications (including herbal preparations) without consulting their doctor. The injections should not be used if the fluid looks cloudy, has solid particles floating in it, or has separated. The injections should be stored away from sunlight and moisture. In addition, patients receiving multiple electrolyte injections should not stop them suddenly without telling their doctor, as the dosage may need to be reduced slowly before the TPN is discontinued.

Side effects

Some persons do not like the salty taste of many sports drinks. They may wish to consider products containing glycine, which is an amino acid that neutralizes the salty taste of the electrolytes themselves. A more serious side effect of sports drinks is **tooth decay**. An article published by researchers at the University of Maryland Dental School showed that sports drinks erode tooth enamel at a rate three to 11 times faster than cola-based soft drinks.

No side effects have been reported for over-the-counter powders and tablets.

Side effects from children's electrolyte replenishers may include allergic reactions, including **hives**, swelling of the face or hands, trouble breathing, **tingling** in the mouth or throat. Other side effects may include signs of too much sodium in the body, such as **dizziness**, seizures, muscle twitching, or restlessness. The doctor should be notified immediately if any of these side effects occur. A less serious side effect that occurs in some children is mild vomiting.

Oral rehydration formulae may produce the same side effects as electrolyte replenishers for children.

Minor side effects from multiple electrolyte injections may include increased frequency of urination, **dry mouth**, increased thirst, or drowsiness. Serious side effects include rapid weight gain, yellowing of the skin or eyes, fruity odor on the breath, **numbness** or tingling in the hands or feet, uneven heartbeat, **shortness of breath**, confusion, or weakness with muscle twitching. Patients should notify their doctor immediately if they notice any of these side effects.

Interactions

Sports drinks may raise blood electrolyte levels in patients receiving total parenteral nutrition. They should not be consumed by patients receiving multiple electrolyte injections.

Children receiving premixed forms of electrolyte replenishers should not eat food with added salt or drink fruit juices until the diarrhea has stopped.

No interactions with other medications have been reported with oral rehydration formulae for adults or over-the-counter powders and tablets. However, the doctor should be informed of all other medications the patient is taking in case a dosage adjustment is necessary.

Resources

BOOKS

Beals, K., and M. Manore. "Nutritional Considerations for the Female Athlete." In *Advances in Sports and Exercise Science Series*. Philadelphia: Elsevier, 2007.

Otten, J., J. Hellwig, and L. Meyers, Eds. *Dietary Reference Intakes: The Essential Guide to Nutrient Requirements*. Washington, DC: The National Academies Press, 2006.

PERIODICALS

Almond, Christopher S. D., et al. "Hyponatremia among Runners in the Boston Marathon." *New England Journal of Medicine* 352 (April 14, 2005): 1550–1556.

Bender, B.J., P.O. Ozuah, and E.F. Crain. "Oral Rehydration Therapy: Is Anyone Drinking?" *Pediatric Emergency Care* 23, no. 9 (September 2007): 624–6.

Diggins, K.C. "Treatment of Mild to Moderate Dehydration in Children with Oral Replacement Therapy." *Journal of the American Academy of Nurse Practitioners* 20, no. 8 (August 2008): 402–6.

Messahel, S., and T. Hussain. "Oral Rehydration Therapy: A Lesson from the Developing World." *Archives of Disease in Childhood* 93, no. 2 (February 2008): 183–4.

Sawka, M.N., et al. "American College of Sports Medicine Position Stand: Exercise and Fluid Replacement." *Medicine & Science in Sports & Exercise* 39 (2007): 377–90.

von Frauenhofer, J. A., and M. M. Rogers. "Effects of Sports Drinks and Other Beverages on Dental Enamel." *General Dentistry* 53 (January-February 2005): 28–31.

Woolley, W.L., and J.H. Burton. "Pediatric Acute Gastroenteritis: Clinical Assessment, Oral Rehydration, and Antiemetic Therapy." *Pediatric Health* 3, no. 2 (2009): 191–7.

OTHER

Rodriguez, Nancy, Nancy DiMarco, and Susie Langley. "Nutrition and Athletic Performance." *Medscape Today*. March 1, 2010. http://www.medscape.com/viewarticle/717046 (accessed October 3, 2010).

ORGANIZATIONS

American College of Sports Medicine (ACSM), P.O. Box 1440, Indianapolis, IN, 46206-1440, (317) 637-9200, (317) 634-7817, http://www.acsm.org.

American Society of Health-System Pharmacists (ASHP), 7272 Wisconsin Avenue, Bethesda, MD, 20814, (301) 657-3000, (866) 279-0681, http://www.ashp.org.

Rebecca J. Frey, PhD
Melinda Granger Oberleitner,
RN, DNS, APRN, CNS

Electrolyte tests

Definition

Electrolytes are positively and negatively charged molecules, called ions, that are found within cells, between cells, in the bloodstream, and in other fluids throughout the body. Electrolytes with a positive charge include **sodium**, potassium, **calcium**, and magnesium; the negative ions are chloride, bicarbonate, and phosphate. The concentrations of these ions in the bloodstream remain fairly constant throughout the day in a healthy person. Changes in the concentration of one or more of these ions can occur during various acute and chronic disease states and can lead to serious consequences.

Purpose

Tests that measure the concentration of electrolytes are useful in the emergency room and to obtain clues for the diagnosis of specific diseases. Electrolyte tests are used for diagnosing dietary deficiencies, excess loss of nutrients due to urination, **vomiting**, and **diarrhea**, or abnormal shifts in the location of an electrolyte within the body. When an abnormal electrolyte value is detected, the physician may either act to immediately correct the imbalance directly (in the case of an emergency) or run further tests to determine the underlying cause of the abnormal electrolyte value. Electrolyte disturbances can occur with malfunctioning of the kidney (renal failure), infections that produce severe and continual diarrhea or vomiting, drugs that cause loss of electrolytes in the urine (**diuretics**), **poisoning** due to accidental consumption of electrolytes, or diseases involving hormones that regulate electrolyte concentrations.

Precautions

Electrolyte tests are performed from routine blood tests. The techniques are simple, automated, and fairly uniform throughout the United States. During the preparation of blood plasma or serum, health workers must take care not to break the red blood cells, especially when testing for serum potassium. Because the concentration of potassium within red blood cells is much higher than in the surrounding plasma or serum, broken cells would cause falsely elevated potassium levels.

Description

Electrolyte tests are typically conducted on blood plasma or serum, urine, and diarrheal fluids. Electrolytes can be classified in at least five different ways. One way is that some electrolytes tend to exist mostly inside cells, or are intracellular, while others tend to be outside cells, or are extracellular. Potassium, phosphate, and magnesium occur at much greater levels inside the cell than outside, while sodium and chloride occur at much greater levels extracellularly. A second classification distinguishes those electrolytes that participate directly in the transmission of nerve impulses and those that do not. Sodium, potassium, and calcium are the important electrolytes involved in nerve impulses, and disorders affecting them are most closely associated with neurological disorders. A third classification focuses on electrolytes that are able to form a tight union, or complex, with one another. Calcium and phosphate have the greatest tendency to form complexes with each other. Disorders that cause an increase in either plasma calcium or phosphate can result in the deposit of calcium-phosphate crystals in the soft tissues of the body. A fourth classification concerns those electrolytes that influence the acidity or alkalinity of the bloodstream, also known as the pH. The pH of the bloodstream is normally in the range of 7.35–7.45. A decrease below this range is called acidosis, while a pH above this range is called alkalosis. The electrolytes most closely associated with the pH of the bloodstream are bicarbonate, chloride, and phosphate.

Preparation

All electrolyte tests can be performed on plasma or serum. Plasma is prepared by withdrawing a blood sample and placing it in a test tube containing a chemical that prevents blood from clotting (an anticoagulant). Serum is prepared by withdrawing a blood sample, placing it in a test tube, and allowing it to clot. The blood spontaneously clots within a minute of withdrawing the blood from a vein. The serum or plasma is then rapidly spun with a centrifuge in order to remove the blood cells or clot.

Normal results

Electrolyte concentrations are similar whether measured in serum or plasma. Values can be expressed in terms of weight per unit volume (mg/deciliter; mg/dL) or in the number of molecules in a volume, or molarity (**moles** or millimoles/liter; M or mM). The range of normal values sometimes varies slightly between different age groups, for males and females, and between different analytical laboratories.

The normal level of serum sodium is in the range of 136–145 mM. The normal levels of serum potassium are 3.5–5.0 mM. Note that sodium occurs at a much higher concentration than potassium. The normal concentration of total serum calcium (bound calcium plus free calcium) is in the range of 8.8–10.4 mg/dL. About 40% of the total calcium in the plasma is loosely bound to proteins; this calcium is referred to as bound calcium. The normal range of free calcium is 4.8–5.2 mg/dL. The normal concentration of serum magnesium is in the range of 2.0–3.0 mg/dL.

The normal concentration range of chloride is 350–375 mg/dL or 98–106 mM. The normal level of phosphate, as expressed as the concentration of phosphorus, is 2.0–4.3 mg/dL. Bicarbonate is an electrolyte that is freely and spontaneously interconvertible with carbonic acid and carbon dioxide. The normal concentration of carbonic acid (H_2CO_3) is about 1.35 mM. The normal concentration of bicarbonate (HCO_3^-) is about 27 mM. The concentration of total carbon dioxide is the sum of carbonic acid and bicarbonate; this sum is normally in the range of 26–28 mM. The ratio of bicarbonate/carbonic acid is more significant than the actual concentrations of these two forms of carbon dioxide. Its normal value is 27/1.35 (equivalent to 20/1).

Abnormal results

Positively charged electrolytes

High serum sodium levels (**hypernatremia**) occur at sodium concentrations over 145 mM, with severe hypernatremia over 152 mM. Hypernatremia is usually caused by diseases that cause excessive urination. In these cases, water is lost, but sodium is still retained in the body. The symptoms include confusion and can lead to convulsions and **coma**. Low serum sodium levels (**hyponatremia**) are below 130 mM, with severe hyponatremia at or below 125 mM. Hyponatremia often occurs with severe diarrhea, with losses of both water and sodium, but with sodium loss exceeding water loss. Hyponatremia provokes clinical problems only if serum sodium falls below 125 mM, especially if this has occurred rapidly. The symptoms can be as mild as tiredness but may lead to convulsions and coma.

High serum potassium (**hyperkalemia**) occurs at potassium levels above 5.0 mM; it is considered severe over 8.0 mM. Hyperkalemia is relatively uncommon, but sometimes occurs in patients with kidney failure who take potassium supplements. Hyperkalemia can result in abnormal beating of the heart (cardiac **arrhythmias**). Low serum potassium (**hypokalemia**) occurs when serum potassium falls below 3.0 mM. It can result from low dietary potassium, as during **starvation** or in patients with **anorexia nervosa**; from excessive losses via the kidneys, as caused by diuretic drugs; or by diseases of the adrenal or pituitary glands. Mild hypokalemia causes muscle weakness, while severe hypokalemia can cause **paralysis**, the inability to breathe, and cardiac arrhythmias.

High levels of calcium ions (**hypercalcemia**) occur at free calcium ion concentrations over 5.2 mg/dL or total serum calcium above 10.4 mg/dL. Hypercalcemia usually occurs when the body dissolves bone at an abnormally fast rate, increasing both serum calcium and serum phosphate. Sudden hypercalcemia can cause vomiting and coma, while prolonged and moderate hypercalcemia results in the deposit of calcium phosphate crystals in the kidneys and eye. **Hypocalcemia** occurs when serum free calcium ions fall below 4.4 mg/dL, or when total serum calcium falls below 8.8 mg/dL. Hypocalcemia can result from **hypoparathyroidism** (low parathyroid hormone), from failure to produce 1,25-dihydroxyvitamin D, from low levels of plasma magnesium, and from phosphate poisoning (the phosphate enters the bloodstream and forms a complex with the free serum calcium). Hypocalcemia can cause depression and **muscle spasms**.

Hypermagnesemia occurs at serum magnesium levels over 25 mM (60 mg/dL). Hypermagnesemia is rare but can occur with the excessive consumption of magnesium salts. Hypomagnesemia occurs when serum magnesium levels fall below 0.8 mM, and can result from poor **nutrition**. Chronic **alcoholism** is the most common cause of hypomagnesemia, in part because of poor diet. Magnesium levels below 0.5 mM (1.2 mg/dL) cause serum calcium levels to decline. Some of the symptoms of hypomagnesemia, including twitching and convulsions, actually result from the concurrent hypocalcemia. Hypomagnesemia can also result in hypokalemia and thereby cause cardiac arrhythmias.

Negatively charged electrolytes

Serum chloride levels sometimes increase to abnormal levels as an undesirable side effect of medical treatment with sodium chloride or ammonium chloride. The toxicity of chloride results not from the chloride itself, but from the fact that the chloride occurs as the acid, hydrogen chloride (more commonly known as hydrochloric acid, or HCl). An overdose of chloride may cause the accumulation of hydrochloric acid in the bloodstream, with consequent acidosis. **Renal tubular acidosis**, one of many kidney diseases, involves the failure to release acid into the urine. The acidosis produces weakness, **headache**, **nausea**, and cardiac arrest. Low plasma chloride leads to the opposite situation: a decline in the acid content of the bloodstream. This is known as alkalization of the bloodstream, or alkalosis. Hydrochloric acid, originally from extracellular fluids, can be lost by vomiting. At its most severe, alkalosis results in paralysis (tetany).

Hyperphosphatemia occurs at serum phosphate levels above 5 mg/dL. It can result from the failure of the kidneys to excrete phosphate into the urine, causing phosphate to accumulate in the bloodstream. Hyperphosphatemia can also be caused by the impaired action of parathyroid hormone and by phosphate poisoning. Severe hyperphosphatemia can cause paralysis, convulsions, and cardiac arrest. These symptoms result because the phosphate, occurring in elevated levels, complexes with free serum calcium, resulting in hypocalcemia. Tests for heart function (an electrocardiogram) and parathyroid hormone levels are used in the diagnosis of hyperphosphatemia. Hypophosphatemia occurs if serum phosphorus falls to 2.0 mg/dL or lower. It often results from a shift of inorganic phosphate from the bloodstream to various organs and tissues. This shift can be caused by a rise in pH (alkalization) of the bloodstream, which can occur during hyperventilation, a reaction in various disease states. A shift in phosphate to intracellular tissues may draw calcium away from the bloodstream via the formation of insoluble calcium phosphate crystals within cells, with consequent hypocalcemia. Thus, tests for abnormalities in phosphate metabolism also involve tests for serum calcium.

Bicarbonate metabolism involves several compounds. When dietary starches, sugars, and fats are broken down for energy production, carbon dioxide is created. Much of this carbon dioxide (CO_2) spontaneously converts to carbonic acid (H_2CO_3), and some of the carbonic acid spontaneously converts to bicarbonate (HCO_3^-) plus a hydrogen ion (H^-). Eventually, almost every molecule of carbon dioxide produced in the body, whether in the form of carbon dioxide, carbonic acid, or bicarbonate, must convert back to carbon dioxide in order to leave via the lungs during normal breathing.

If one holds one's breath, carbon dioxide cannot escape from the lungs, but continues to be generated within the body. This results in an increase in production of carbonic acid. A portion of the carbonic acid breaks apart (dissociates), causing an increase in hydrogen ions in the plasma, with a resulting acidosis. Tests for serum bicarbonate levels are accompanied by tests for acidosis (pH test). Conversely, when one breathes too rapidly (hyperventilation), the carbon dioxide is drawn off from the bloodstream and expelled in the breath at an increased rate. This results in an increase in the rate of combination of bicarbonate with hydrogen ions, resulting in alkalosis. Acidosis and alkalosis can be produced by means other than by altering the rate of breathing. The carbonic acid and bicarbonate in the bloodstream minimize (or buffer) any trend to acidosis or alkalosis. Tests for bicarbonate are generally accompanied by tests for blood pH and possibly tests for kidney malfunction, abnormal hormone function, or gastrointestinal disorders.

Resources

PERIODICALS

Mayor, Susan. "UK report into acute kidney injury deaths urges electrolyte checks in all emergency admissions." *British Medical Journal* 338, no. 7708 (June 13, 2009): 1407.

Tom Brody, PhD

Electromyography

Definition

Electromyography (EMG) is a diagnostic procedure that is used to determine the health of muscles, along with the nerve cells that control these muscles, or what are called motor neurons. In purpose, the EMG is an electrical recording of muscle activity that aids in the diagnosis of neuromuscular disease. The EMG scan, sometimes also called a myogram, is used to identify the electrical signals that originate from these motor neurons (which cause the muscles to move). These electrical signals identified by the EMG allows the medical specialist to interpret such signals in order to diagnosis any problems within the muscles and the nerves that control them.

Purpose

Muscles are stimulated by signals from nerve cells called motor neurons. This stimulation causes electrical activity in the muscle, which in turn causes contraction. An electrode, which consists of a very small, solid needle (pin), is inserted through the skin and into the muscle. It is connected to a recording device that detects this electrical activity. When a needle is used the process is called a needle EMG, or simply an EMG. The needle electrode and recorder pair is called an electromyography machine, which includes a monitor called an oscilloscope. A speaker is included, which provides crackling sounds as the electrical intensity rises and falls.

EMG can determine whether a particular muscle is responding appropriately to stimulation, and whether a muscle remains inactive when not stimulated. Thus, during the test, the patient will be asked to contract particular muscles, such as those in the leg. The electrical wave produced on the EMG machine will determine the condition of the muscle and nerves as it responds to the contraction. Usually a nerve conduction velocity (NCV) test (or nerve conduction study) is also performed at the same time as an EMG. This test consists of two electrode being placed apart on the surface of the skin. One electrode is activated so that a muscle is electronically simulated. The second electrode senses the activity (electrical impulse) of the muscle as it moves. The NCV test measures the intensity and speed at which electrical signals pass between two points.

The EMG procedure is performed most often to help diagnose different diseases causing weakness. Although EMG is a test of the motor system, it may help identify abnormalities of nerves or spinal nerve roots that may be associated with **pain** or **numbness**. Other symptoms for which EMG may be useful include numbness, **tingling**, atrophy, stiffness, fasciculation (twitch), pain or cramping, deformity, and spasticity (abnormal muscle performance, such as muscle weakness). EMG results can help determine whether symptoms are due to a muscle disease or a neurological disorder, and, when combined with clinical findings, usually allow a confident diagnosis.

EMG can help diagnose many muscle and nerve disorders, including (but not restricted to) the following:

- muscular dystrophy or polymyositis
- congenital myopathies
- myasthenia gravis
- mitochondrial myopathies
- metabolic myopathies
- myotonias
- peripheral neuropathies
- radiculopathies
- nerve lesions
- amyotrophic lateral sclerosis
- polio
- spinal muscular atrophy
- Guillain-Barré syndrome
- ataxias
- myasthenias

Precautions

Only a few special precautions are needed for this test. Patients with a history of bleeding disorder should consult with their treating physician before the test. Any person taking blood-thinning medications should inform the neurologist or other medical professional conducting the EMG procedure. A person with a pacemaker or other electrical medical device should inform the medical team of this before the procedure. If a muscle biopsy is planned as part of the diagnostic work-up, the EMG should not be performed at the same site, as it may effect the appearance of the muscle.

Description

During an EMG test, a fine needle is inserted into the muscle to be tested. This may cause some discomfort, similar to that of an injection. Recordings are made while the muscle is at rest, and then during the contraction. The person performing the test may move the limb being tested, and direct the patient to move it with various levels of force. The needle may be repositioned in the same muscle for further recording. Other muscles may be tested as well.

A slightly different test, the *nerve conduction velocity* test, is often performed at the same time with the same equipment. In this test, stimulating and recording electrodes are used, and small electrical shocks are applied to measure the ability of the nerve to conduct electrical signals. This test may cause mild tingling and discomfort similar to a mild shock from static electricity. Evoked potentials may also be performed for additional diagnostic information. Nerve conduction velocity and evoked potential testing are especially helpful when pain or sensory complaints are more prominent than weakness.

The EMG procedure will take usually from thirty to sixty minutes to complete.

Preparation

Very few special preparations are needed before the EMG. Natural oils on the skin should be removed before the test. Therefore, take a shower or bath before the procedure. In addition, do not apply creams or lotions. The doctor supervising and interpreting the test should be given information about the symptoms, medical conditions, suspected diagnosis, neuroimaging studies, and other test results.

Aftercare

Minor bruising may occur after the procedure; it will fade over the next few days. Minor pain and bleeding may continue for several hours after the test. The muscle may be tender for a day or two. If any of these do not go away after several days, contact your family doctor or other medical professional. The doctor will not restrict activities after the test is completed under normal circumstances.

Risks

There are not significant risks in performing this procedure. The only minor risks occur when a needle is inserted under the skin. Such risks may include pain or discomfort, bleeding, bruising, or infection. Since medicine is not being injected under the skin, less pain is usually the case when compared to the insertion of a regular needle.

In addition, there is a minute risk for nerve injury when the needle is inserted under the skin. When such an electrode is inserted into the chest wall, a small risk is present that the puncture could cause air to leak into the cavity between the lungs and the chest wall. In such a case, a collapsed lung could result; although it is highly unlikely.

When the nerve conduction velocity test is performed, the patient will perceive a brief and very mild shock or tingling sensation.

Results

The results of the test are available immediately upon completion of the EMG. However, a trained medical specialist, such as a neurologist, is needed to analyze and interpret the results.

KEY TERMS

Motor neurons—Nerve cells that transmit signals from the brain or spinal cord to the muscles.

Motor unit action potentials—Spikes of electrical activity recorded during an EMG that reflect the number of motor units (motor neurons and the muscle fibers they transmit signals to) activated when the patient voluntarily contracts a muscle.

Normal results

There should be some brief EMG activity during needle insertion. This activity may be increased in diseases of the nerve and decreased in long-standing muscle disorders where muscle tissue is replaced by fibrous tissue or fat. Muscle tissue normally does not show EMG activity when at rest or when moved passively by the examiner. When the patient actively contracts the muscle, spikes (motor unit action potentials) should appear on the recording screen, reflecting the electrical activity within. As the muscle is contracted more forcefully, more groups of muscle fibers are recruited or activated, causing more EMG activity.

Abnormal results

The interpretation of EMG results is not a simple matter, requiring analysis of the onset, duration, amplitude, and other characteristics of the spike patterns.

Electrical activity at rest is abnormal; the particular pattern of firing may indicate denervation (for example, a nerve lesion, radiculopathy, or lower motor neuron degeneration), myotonia, or inflammatory myopathy.

Decreases in the amplitude and duration of spikes are associated with muscle diseases, which also show faster recruitment of other muscle fibers to compensate for weakness. Recruitment is reduced in nerve disorders.

Resources

BOOKS

Daube, Jasper R., and Devon I. Rubin, editors. *Clinical Neurophysiology*. New York: Oxford University Press, 2009.

Kamen, Gary, and David A. Gabriel. *Essentials of Electromyography*. Champaign, IL: Human Kinetics, 2010.

Pease, William S., Henry L. Lew, and Ernest W. Johnson. *Johnson's Practical Electromyography*. Philadelphia: Lippincott Williams and Wilkins, 2007.

OTHER

Electromyography. Medline Plus, National Library of Medicine and National Institutes of Health. (September 22, 2008), http://www.nlm.nih.gov/medlineplus/ency/article/003929.htm (accessed September 14, 2010).

Electromyography (EMG). Emedicinehealth.com, WebMD. http://www.emedicinehealth.com/electromyography_emg/article_em.htm (accessed September 14, 2010).

Electromyography (EMG). Mayo Clinic. (August 26, 2010), http://www.mayoclinic.com/health/emg/MY00107 (accessed September 14, 2010).

ORGANIZATIONS

American Association of Neuromuscular and Electrodiagnostic Medicine, 2621 Superior Drive NW, Rochester, MN, 55901, (507) 288-0100, (507) 288-1225, aanem@aanem.org, http://www.aanem.org/.

Richard Robinson

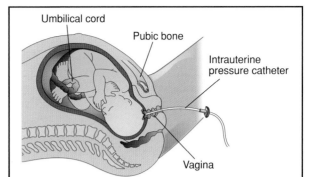

Electronic fetal monitoring (EFM) is performed late in pregnancy or continuously during labor to ensure normal delivery of a healthy baby. EFM can be utilized either externally or internally in the womb. The illustration above shows the internal procedure, in which an electrode is attached directly to the baby's scalp to monitor the heart rate. Uterine contractions are recorded using an intrauterine pressure catheter which is inserted through the cervix into the uterus. *(Illustration by Electronic Illustrators Group. Reproduced by permission of Gale, a part of Cengage Learning.)*

Electronic fetal monitoring

Definition

The electronic fetal monitor (EFM) is a device that records a fetus's heart rate and the presence or absence of the mother's uterine contractions.

Purpose

The EFM is used to assess fetal well being during routine prenatal visits. It is also used during labor and delivery when high-risk factors exist or when a clinical condition develops beforehand that places the fetus at risk. High-risk factors for EFM during labor include:

- low gestational age
- high maternal age
- placenta or cord problems
- meconium in the amniotic fluid
- maternal hypertension
- protein in the urine (proteinuria)

A fetus having trouble in labor often exhibits characteristic changes in heart rate after a contraction (late decelerations). Trouble also is indicated by significant slowing of the heart rate during a contraction (variable deceleration). If the fetus is not receiving enough oxygen to withstand the stress of labor, and delivery is many hours away, a **cesarean section** (C-section) may be necessary.

Description

The monitor produces a continuous paper record of the fetal heart rate (FHR) and records uterine contractions. FHR is captured on the top part of the paper printout; uterine activity, when monitored, appears on the lower part of the tracing.

Electronic fetal monitoring can be performed externally or internally. The external ultrasound approach is non-invasive and uses sensors (electrodes) placed on the mother's abdomen with an elastic belt. Another belt holds the contraction monitor.

External electronic fetal monitoring includes a non-stress test, which measures fetal heart rate (FHR) accelerations with normal movement of the fetus. Sometimes the fetal movement is encouraged by giving the mother a small meal or something to drink. Fetal acoustic stimulation and moving the fetus by rubbing the abdomen gently also may be used.

Two contraction stress tests, which measure the placenta's ability to provide enough oxygen to the fetus during pressure, are also used with electronic fetal monitoring. The nipple stimulation contractions **stress test** involves the mother self-stimulating her nipple while contractions and FHR are monitored. Another test, called oxytocin stimulation, involves the administration of the hormone oxytocin intravenously

KEY TERMS

Cesarean section—Also called a C-section; delivery of a baby through an incision in the mother's abdomen instead of through the vagina.

Late deceleration—Transient slowing of the fetal heart (brachycardia), which reaches its height more than 30 seconds after the peak of the uterine contraction and may indicate the fetus is not receiving enough oxygen (hypoxia).

Non-stress test—A record of the fetal heart rate in the absence of contractions (stress).

Reactive stress test—A positive sign of fetal well being. The FHR rises at least 20 beats per minute above the baseline heart rate for at least 20 seconds, occurring at least twice in a 20-minute period.

Variable deceleration—Fetal bradycardia below 100 beats per minute denoting compression of the umbilical cord at the height of a uterine contraction.

until three uterine contractions are observed within ten minutes, during which time the FHR is monitored.

Sometimes, it is difficult to hear the fetus's heartbeat with the monitoring device. Other times, the monitor may show subtle signs of a developing problem. In either case, the physician may recommend the use of an internal monitor, which provides a more accurate record of the fetus's heart rate. The internal monitor (or fetal scalp electrode) uses an electrode attached to the fetus's scalp through the cervix during an internal vaginal exam. The internal monitor can only be used when the cervix is dilated. In complicated pregnancies, continuous EFM is recommended during labor.

Benefits

Electronic fetal monitoring allows the physician to judge the well being of the fetus before and during delivery. Should the fetus appear to be in distress, the physician can recommend immediate delivery via cesarean section. EFM also allows an evaluation of the strength of the mother's contractions. Should labor not be progressing normally, medical intervention can be ordered.

Precautions

In general, no risks are associated with external fetal monitoring. However, the test can initiate labor and is generally not given to mothers at risk for preterm labor or with a condition that requires a cesarean section. Internal monitoring poses risks associated with improper placement of the electrodes. Some data suggest that EFM leads to unnecessary cesarean sections. Another drawback includes loss of maternal mobility when used during labor, which may slow labor.

Preparation

There are no special preparations required for external fetal monitoring. Preparation for placement of an internal scalp lead (ISL) is the same as for a routine vaginal exam.

Aftercare

No special preparations are required for electronic fetal monitoring.

Risks

Fetal monitoring is not a perfect test. Fetal assessment in labor is subject to differences in interpretation and consequent intervention; therefore, institutional policies and procedures should be followed.

Results

The normal fetal heart rate ranges from 120 to 160 beats per minute (bpm). Just as an adult's heart rate increases with movement, FHR increases when the fetus moves. A reactive heart rate tracing (also known as a reactive non-stress test, or NST) is considered a positive sign of fetal well being. A non-reactive NST may or may not imply fetal well being. The monitor strip is considered to be reactive when the FHR rises at least 15 to 20 bpm above the baseline heart rate for at least 20 seconds. This must occur at least twice in a 20-minute period.

Results are considered abnormal if the FHR drops below 120 or rises above 160 for sustained periods. In either of these cases the fetus may be exhibiting fetal distress. A mean FHR of less than 110 bpm may indicate bradycardia (slow heart beat). A mean FHR of over 160 bpm may indicate a tachycardia (rapid beating of the heart). However, some babies who are having problems may not exhibit such clear signs.

During a contraction, the flow of oxygen from the mother through the placenta to the fetus is temporarily stopped. It is as if the fetus has to hold its breath during each contraction. Both the placenta and the fetus are designed to withstand this condition. Between contractions, the fetus should be receiving more than enough oxygen to do well during the contraction.

One sign that a fetus is not getting enough oxygen between contractions is a drop in the FHR after the contraction (late deceleration). The heart rate recovers to a normal level between contractions, only to drop again after the next contraction. This is a subtler sign of distress. Trouble is also indicated by significant slowing during a contraction (variable decelerations).

Training and certification

Electronic fetal monitoring is primarily conducted by specialists in obstetrics and gynecology. Qualified registered nurses and advanced practice nurses may assist in or conduct electronic fetal monitoring.

Applying the external monitor is simple, but requires practice in the proper placement of the monitoring devices. The interpretation of the tracings, however, requires continued vigilance in education and clinical practice. Training should include instruction electronic FHR monitoring and evaluation of uterine activity.

Resources

OTHER

Fetal Heart Monitoring. MedlinePlus Encyclopedia. May 8, 2008. http://www.nlm.nih.gov/medlineplus/ency/article/003405.htm

Jocoy, Sandy. Electronic Fetal Monitoring. WebMD. June 28, 2008. http://www.webmd.com/baby/electronic-fetal-heart-monitoring

ORGANIZATIONS

American College of Nurse-Midwives, 8403 Colesville Rd, Suite 1550, Silver Spring, MD, 20919, (240) 485-1800, (240) 485-1818, http://www.midwife.org.

American College of Obstetricians and Gynecologists, P.O. Box 96920, Washington, DC, 20090-6920, (202) 638-5577, http://www.acog.org.

Association of Women's Health, Obstetric, and Neonatal Nurses, 2000 L St., NW, Suite. 740, Washington, DC, 20036, (202) 261-2400, (800) 673-8499. Toll free in Canada (800) 245-0231, (202) 728-0575, customerservice@awhonn.org, http://www.awhonn.org.

Society for Maternal-Fetal Medicine, 409 12th Street, SW, Washington, DC, 20024, (202) 863-2476, (202) 554-1132, smfm@smfm.org, https://www.smfm.org.

Maggie Boleyn, R.N., B.S.N.
Tish Davidson, A.M.

Electrophysiology study of the heart

Definition

An electrophysiology (EP) study of the heart is a nonsurgical analysis of the electrical conduction system (normal or abnormal) of the heart. The test employs cardiac catheters and sophisticated computers to generate electrocardiogram (EKG) tracings and electrical measurements with exquisite precision from within the heart chambers.

The EP study can be performed solely for diagnostic purposes. It also is performed to pinpoint the exact location of electrical signals (cardiac mapping) in conjunction with a therapeutic procedure called **catheter ablation**.

The test is simple, not painful, and performed in a special laboratory under controlled clinical circumstances by cardiologists and nurses who subspecialize in electrophysiology.

Purpose

A cardiologist may recommend an EP study when the standard EKG, Holter monitor, event recorder, **stress test**, echocardiogram, or angiogram cannot provide enough information to evaluate an abnormal heart rhythm, called an arrhythmia.

An EP study also may be beneficial in diagnosing a suspected arrhythmia in a patient who shows symptoms of an arrhythmia but in whom it could not be detected from other tests.

The purpose and great value of an EP study is that it offers more detailed information to the doctor about the electrical activity in the heart than the aforementioned noninvasive tests because electrodes are placed directly *on* heart tissue. This allows the electrophysiologist to determine the specific location of an arrhythmia and, oftentimes, correct it during the same procedure. This corrective treatment is permanent and considered a cure, and, in many cases, the patient may not need to take heart medications.

EP studies may be helpful in assessing:

- certain tachycardias or bradycardias of unknown cause
- patients who have been resuscitated after experiencing sudden cardiac death
- various symptoms of unknown cause, such as chest pain, shortness of breath, fatigue, or syncope (dizziness/fainting)
- response to anti-arrhythmic therapy

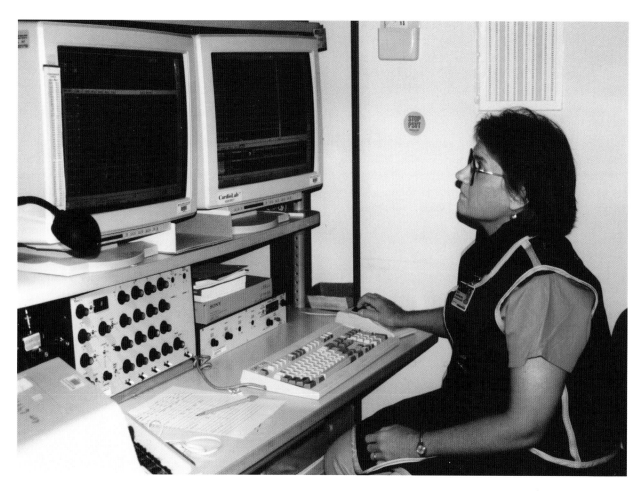

An electrophysiologist nurse monitors a patient's heart rhythm during an electrophysiology study for tachycardia. *(Collette Placek. Reproduced by permission.)*

Precautions

Pregnant patients should not undergo an EP study because of exposure to radiation during the study, which may be harmful to the growing baby.

Patients who have **coronary artery disease** may need to have that treated before having an EP study.

Description

The rhythmic pumping action of the heart, which is essentially a muscle, is the result of electrical impulses traveling throughout the walls of the four heart chambers. These impulses originate in the sinoatrial (SA) node, which are specialized cells situated in the top right chamber of the heart: the right atrium. Normally, the SA node, acting like a spark plug, spontaneously generates the impulses, which travel through specific pathways throughout the atria to the atrioventricular (AV) node. The AV node is a relay station, sending the impulses to more specialized muscle fibers throughout the bottom chambers of the heart: the ventricles. If these pathways become damaged or blocked or if extra (abnormal) pathways exist, the heart's rhythm may be altered (perhaps too slow, too fast, or irregular), which can seriously affect the heart's pumping ability.

The patient is transported to the x-ray table in the EP lab and connected to various monitors. Sterile sheets are placed over him or her. A minimum of two catheters are inserted into the right femoral (thigh) vein in the groin area. Depending on the type of arrhythmia, the number of catheters used in an EP test and their route to the heart may vary. For certain tachycardias, two more catheters may be inserted in the left groin and one in the internal jugular (neck) vein or in the subclavian (below the clavicle) vein. The catheters are about 0.08 in (2 mm) in diameter, about the size of a spaghetti noodle. The catheters used in catheter ablation are slightly larger.

With the help of fluoroscopy (x rays on a television screen), all the catheters are guided to several

Ablation—Remove or destroy, such as by burning or cutting.

Angiogram—X ray of a blood vessel after special x-ray dye has been injected into it.

Bradycardia—Slow heartbeat.

Cardiac catheter—Long, thin, flexible tube that is threaded into the heart through a blood vessel.

Cardiologist—Doctor who specializes in diagnosing and treating heart diseases.

Echocardiogram—Ultrasound image of the heart.

Electrocardiogram—Tracing of the electrical activity of the heart.

Electrode—Medium for conducting an electrical current–in this case, platinum wires.

Electrophysiology—Study of how electrical signals in the body relate to physiologic function.

Event recorder—A small machine, worn by a patient usually for several days or weeks, that is activated by the patient to record his or her EKG when a symptom is detected.

Fibrillation—Rapid, random contraction (quivering).

Holter monitor—A small machine, worn by a patient usually for 24 hours, that continuously records the patient's EKG during usual daily activity.

Stress test—Recording a patient's EKG during exercise.

Supraventricular tachycardia—A fast heart beat that originates above the ventricles.

Tachycardia—Fast heartbeat.

Vascular—Pertaining to blood vessels.

specific locations in the heart. Typically, four to 10 electrodes are located on the end of the catheters, which have the ability to send electrical signals to stimulate the heart (called pacing) and to receive electrical signals from the heart–but not at the same time (just as a walkie-talkie cannot send and receive messages at the same time).

First, the electrodes are positioned to receive signals from inside the heart chambers. This allows the doctor to measure how fast the electrical impulses travel currently in the patient's heart. These measurements are called the patient's baseline measurements. Next, the electrodes are positioned to pace: The EP team actually tries to induce (sometimes in combination with various heart drugs) the arrhythmia that the patient has previously experienced so the team can observe it in a controlled environment, compare it to the patient's clinical or spontaneous arrhythmia, and decide how to treat it.

Once the arrhythmia is induced and the team determines it can be treated with catheter ablation, cardiac mapping is performed to locate precisely the origin and route of the abnormal pathway. When this is accomplished, the ablating electrode catheter is positioned directly against the abnormal pathway, and high radio-frequency energy is delivered through the electrode to destroy (burn) the tissue in this area.

Preparation

The following preparations are made for an EP study:

- the patient may be advised to stop taking certain medications, especially heart drugs, that may interfere with the test results.
- blood tests usually are ordered the week before the test.
- the patient undergoes conscious sedation (awake but relaxed) during the test. This is accomplished quite often with the anesthetic drugs VersedR (Roche laboratories) and fentanyl.
- a local anesthetic is injected at the site of catheter insertion.

Aftercare

The patient needs to rest flat in bed for several hours after the procedure to allow healing at the catheter insertion sites.

The patient often returns home either the same day of the test or the next day. Someone should drive him or her home.

The doctor may prescribe drugs and/or insert an AFCD to treat the arrhythmia and may do a possible follow-up EP study.

Risks

The EP diagnostic study and catheter ablation are low-risk procedures. There is a small risk of bleeding and/or infection at the site of catheter insertion, but this occurs less than 1% of the time. Blood clot formation occurs only two in 1,000 instances and is minimized with blood thinner medications administered during the procedure. Vascular injuries causing hemorrhage or **thrombophlebitis** are possible but occur less than 0.7% of the time. Cardiac perforations occur only in one or two per 1,000 instances. If the right internal jugular vein is accessed, the small possibility of puncturing the lung with the catheter exists, which, at worst, could cause a collapsed lung.

Because **ventricular tachycardia** or fibrillation (lethal **arrhythmias**) may be induced in the patient, the EP lab personnel must be prepared to defibrillate the patient as necessary.

Normal results

The heart initiates and conducts electrical impulses normally.

Abnormal results

Confirmation of arrhythmias, such as:

- supraventricular tachycardias
- ventricular arrhythmias
- accessory (extra) pathways
- bradycardias

ORGANIZATIONS

Cardiac Arrhythmia Research and Education Foundation (C.A.R.E.), 427 Fulton Street; P.O. Box 69, Seymour, WI, 54165, (920) 833-7000, (920) 833-7005, (800) 404-9500, care@careforhearts.org, http://www.longqt.com/
.

Midwest Heart Specialists. , 1901 S. Meyers Road, Suite 350, Oak Brook Terrace, IL, 60181, (630) 932-2165, (630) 268-9609, http://www.midwestheart.com.

Collette L. Placek

Electroshock therapy *see* **Electroconvulsive therapy**

Elephantiasis

Definition

The word elephantiasis is a vivid and accurate term for the syndrome it describes: the gross (visible) enlargement of the arms, legs, or genitals to elephantoid size.

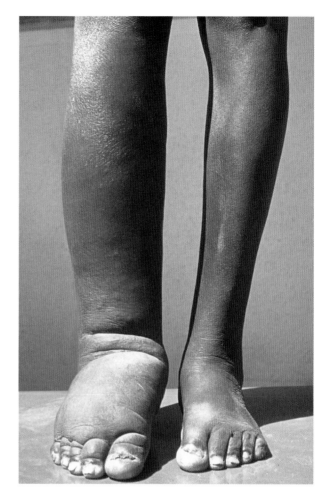

Man suffering from elephantiasis. *(© C. James Webb/ Phototake. — All rights reserved.)*

Description

True elephantiasis is the result of a parasitic infection caused by three specific kinds of round worms. The long, threadlike worms block the body's lymphatic system—a network of channels, lymph nodes, and organs that helps maintain proper fluid levels in the body by draining lymph from tissues into the bloodstream. This blockage causes fluids to collect in the tissues, which can lead to great swelling, called "lymphedema." Limbs can swell so enormously that they resemble an elephant's foreleg in size, texture, and color. This is the severely disfiguring and disabling condition of elephantiasis.

There are a few different causes of elephantiasis, but the agents responsible for most of the elephantiasis in the world are filarial worms: white, slender round worms found in most tropical and subtropical places. They are transmitted by particular kinds (species) of mosquitoes, that is, bloodsucking insects. Infection with these worms is called "lymphatic filariasis" and over a long period of time can cause elephantiasis.

Lymphatic **filariasis** is a disease of underdeveloped regions found in South America, Central Africa, Asia, the Pacific Islands, and the Caribbean. It is a disease that has been present for centuries, as ancient Persian and Indian writings clearly described elephant-like swellings of the arms, legs, and genitals. It is estimated that 120 million people in the world have lymphatic filariasis. The disease appears to be spreading, in spite of decades of research in this area.

Other terms for elephantiasis are Barbados leg, elephant leg, morbus herculeus, mal de Cayenne, and myelolymphangioma.

Other situations that can lead to elephantiasis are:
- a protozoan disease called leishmaniasis
- a repeated streptococcal infection
- the surgical removal of lymph nodes (usually to prevent the spread of cancer)
- a hereditary birth defect

Causes and symptoms

Three kinds of round worms cause elephantiasis filariasis: *Wuchereria bancrofti*, *Brugia malayi*, and *Brugia timori*. Of these three, *W. bancrofti* makes up about 90% of the cases. Man is the only known host of *W. bancrofti*.

Culex, *Aedes*, and *Anopheles* mosquitoes are the carriers of *W. bancrofti*. *Anopheles* and *Mansonia* mosquitoes are the carriers of *B. malayi*. In addition, *Anopheles* mosquitoes are the carriers of *B. timori*.

Infected female mosquitoes take a blood meal from a human, and in doing so, introduce larval forms of the particular parasite they carry to the person. These larvae migrate toward a lymphatic channel, then travel to various places within the lymphatic system, usually positioning themselves in or near lymph nodes throughout the body. During this time, they mature into more developed larvae and eventually into adult worms. Depending upon the species of round worm, this development can take a few months or more than a year. The adult worms grow to about 1 in (2.5 cm) to 4 in (10 cm) long.

The adult worms can live from about three to eight years. Some have been known to live to 20 years, and in one case 40 years. The adult worms begin reproducing numerous live embryos, called microfilariae. The microfilariae travel to the bloodstream, where they can be ingested by a mosquito when it takes a blood meal from the infected person.

If they are not ingested by a mosquito, the microfilariae die within about 12 months. If they are ingested by a mosquito, they continue to mature. They are totally dependent on their specific species of mosquito to develop further. The cycle continues when the mosquito takes another blood meal.

Most of the symptoms an infected person experiences are due to the blockage of the lymphatic system by the adult worms and due to the substances (excretions and secretions) produced by the worms.

The body's allergic reactions may include repeated episodes of **fever**, shaking chills, sweating, headaches, **vomiting**, and **pain**. Enlarged lymph nodes, swelling of the affected area, skin ulcers, bone and joint pain, tiredness, and red streaks along the arm or leg also may occur. Abscesses can form in lymph nodes or in the lymphatic vessels. They may appear at the surface of the skin as well.

Long-term infection with lymphatic filariasis can lead to **lymphedema**, hydrocele (a buildup of fluid in any saclike cavity or duct) in the scrotum, and elephantiasis of the legs, scrotum, arms, penis, breasts, and vulvae. The most common site of elephantiasis is the leg. It typically begins in the ankle and progresses to the foot and leg. At first the swollen leg may feel soft to the touch but eventually becomes hard and thick. The skin may appear darkened or warty and may even crack, allowing bacteria to infect the leg and complicate the disease. The microfilariae usually don't cause injury. In some instances, they cause "eosinophilia," an increased number of eosinophils (a type of white blood cells) in the blood.

This disease is more intense in people who never have been exposed to lymphatic filariasis than it is in the native people of tropical areas where the disease occurs. This is because many of the native people often are immunologically tolerant.

Diagnosis

The only sure way to diagnose lymphatic filariasis is by detecting the parasite itself, either the adult worms or the microfilariae.

Microscopic examination of the person's blood may reveal microfilariae. But many times, people who have been infected for a long time do not have microfilariae in their bloodstream. The absence of them, therefore, does not mean necessarily that the person is not infected. In these cases, examining the urine or hydrocele fluid or performing other clinical tests is necessary.

Collecting blood from the individual for microscopic examination should be done during the night

KEY TERMS

Antigen—Any substance (usually a protein) that causes an immune response by the body to produce antibodies.

Filarial—Threadlike. The word "filament" is formed from the same root word.

Host—A person or animal in which a parasite lives, is nourished, grows, and reproduces.

Lymph—A watery substance that collects in the tissues and organs of the body and eventually drains into the bloodstream.

Lymphatic system—A network composed of vessels, lymph nodes, the tonsils, the thymus gland, and the spleen. It is responsible for transporting fluid and nutrients to the bloodstream and for maturing certain blood cells that are part of the body's immune system.

Lymphedema—The unnatural accumulation of lymph in the tissues of the body, which results in swelling in that area.

Protozoa—(Plural form of protozoan) Single-celled organisms (not bacteria) of which about 30 kinds cause disease in humans.

Streptococcal—Pertaining to any of the *Streptococcus* bacteria. These organisms can cause pneumonia, skin infections, and many other diseases.

when the microfilariae are more numerous in the bloodstream. (Interestingly, this is when mosquitoes bite most frequently.) During the day microfilariae migrate to deeper blood vessels in the body, especially in the lung. If it is decided to perform the blood test during the day, the infected individual may be given a "provocative" dose of medication to provoke the microfilariae to enter the bloodstream. Blood then can be collected an hour later for examination.

Detecting the adult worms can be difficult because they are deep within the lymphatic system and difficult to get to. Biopsies usually are not performed because they usually don't reveal much information.

Treatment

The drug of choice in treating lymphatic filariasis is diethylcarbamazine (DEC). The trade name in the United States is Hetrazan.

The treatment schedule is typically 2 mg/kg per day, three times a day, for three weeks. The drug is taken in tablet form.

DEC kills the microfilariae quickly and injures or kills the adult worms slowly, if at all. If all the adult worms are not killed, remaining paired males and females may continue to produce more larvae. Therefore, several courses of DEC treatment over a long time period may be necessary to rid the individual of the parasites.

DEC has been shown to reduce the size of enlarged lymph nodes and, when taken long-term, to reduce elephantiasis. In India, DEC has been given in the form of a medicated salt, which helps prevent spread of the disease.

The side effects of DEC almost all are due to the body's natural allergic reactions to the dying parasites rather than to the DEC itself. For this reason, DEC must be given carefully to reduce the danger to the individual. Side effects may include fever, chills, **headache**, **dizziness**, **nausea and vomiting**, **itching**, and joint pain. These side effects usually occur within the first few days of treatment. These side effects usually subside as the individual continues taking the drug.

There is an alternate treatment plan for the use of DEC. This plan is designed to kill the parasites slowly (to reduce allergic reactions to the dead microfilariae and dying adult worms within the body). Lower doses of DEC are taken for the first few days, followed by the higher dose of 2 mg/kg per day for the remaining three weeks. In addition, **steroids** may be prescribed to prevent the individual's body from reacting severely to the dead worms.

Another drug used is Ivermectin. Early research studies of Ivermectin show that it is excellent in killing microfilariae, but the effects of this drug on the adult worms are still being investigated. It is probable that patients will need to continue using DEC to kill the adult worms. Mild side effects of Ivermectin include headache, fever, and myalgia.

Other means of managing lymphatic filariasis are pressure **bandages** to wrap the swollen limb and elastic stockings to help reduce the pressure. Exercising and elevating a bandaged limb also can help reduce its size.

Surgery can be performed to reduce elephantiasis by removing excess fatty and fibrous tissue, draining the swelled area, and removing the dead worms.

Prognosis

With DEC treatment, the prognosis is good for early and mild cases of lymphatic filariasis. The prognosis is poor, however, for heavy parasitic infestations.

Prevention

The two main ways to control this disease are to take DEC preventively, which has shown to be effective, and to reduce the number of carrier insects in a particular area.

Avoiding mosquito **bites** with insecticides and insect repellents is helpful, as is wearing protective clothing and using bed netting.

Much effort has been made in cleaning the breeding sites (stagnant water) of mosquitoes near people's homes in areas where filariasis is found.

Before visiting countries where lymphatic filariasis is found, it would be wise to consult a travel physician to learn about current preventative measures.

ORGANIZATIONS

National Lymphedema Network, 116 New Montgomery Street, Suite 235, San Francisco, CA, 94105, (415) 908-3681, (415) 908-3813, (800) 541-3259, nln@lymphnet.org, http://www.lymphnet.org.
National Organization for Rare Disorders, P.O. Box 8923, New Fairfield, CT, 06812-8923, (800) 999-6673, http://www.rarediseases.org.

Collette L. Placek

ELISA (Enzyme-linked immunosorbent assay) *see* **AIDS tests**

Embolism

Definition

An embolism is an obstruction in a blood vessel due to a blood clot or other foreign matter that gets stuck while traveling through the bloodstream. The plural of embolism is emboli.

Description

Emboli have moved from the place where they were formed through the bloodstream to another part of the body, where they obstruct an artery and block the flow of blood. The emboli are usually formed from **blood clots** but are occasionally comprised of air, fat, or tumor tissue. Embolic events can

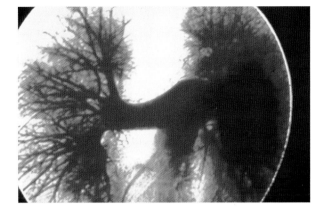

A close-up view of a pulmonary embolism. *(Custom Medical Stock Photo, Inc. Reproduced by permission.)*

be multiple and small, or single and massive. They can be life-threatening and require immediate emergency medical care. There are three general categories of emboli: arterial, gas, and pulmonary. Pulmonary emboli are the most common.

Arterial embolism

In arterial emboli, blood flow is blocked at the junction of major arteries, most often at the groin, knee, or thigh. Arterial emboli are generally a complication of heart disease. An **arterial embolism** in the brain (cerebral embolism) causes **stroke**, which can be fatal. An estimated 5–14% of all strokes are caused by cerebral emboli. Arterial emboli to the extremities can lead to tissue **death** and **amputation** of the affected limb if not treated effectively within hours. Intestines and kidneys can also suffer damage from emboli.

Gas embolism

Gas emboli result from the compression of respiratory gases into the blood and other tissues due to rapid changes in environmental pressure, for example, while flying or scuba diving. As external pressure decreases, gases (like nitrogen) that are dissolved in the blood and other tissues become small bubbles that can block blood flow and cause organ damage.

Pulmonary embolism

In a **pulmonary embolism**, a common illness, blood flow is blocked at a pulmonary artery. When emboli block the main pulmonary artery, and in cases where there are no initial symptoms, a pulmonary embolism can quickly become fatal. According to the American Heart Association, an estimated 600,000

Americans develop pulmonary emboli annually and 60,000 die from it.

A pulmonary embolism is difficult to diagnose. Less than 10% of patients who die from a pulmonary embolism were diagnosed with the condition. More than 90% of cases of pulmonary emboli are complications of **deep vein thrombosis**, blood clots in the deep vein of the leg or pelvis.

Causes and symptoms

Arterial emboli are usually a complication of heart disease where blood clots form in the heart's chambers. Gas emboli are caused by rapid changes in environmental pressure that could happen when flying or scuba diving. A pulmonary embolism is caused by blood clots that travel through the blood stream to the lungs and block a pulmonary artery. More than 90% of the cases of pulmonary embolism are a complication of deep vein thrombosis, which typically occurs in patients who have had **orthopedic surgery** and patients with **cancer** or other chronic illnesses like congestive **heart failure**.

Risk factors for arterial and pulmonary emboli include: prolonged bed rest, surgery, **childbirth**, **heart attack**, stroke, congestive heart failure, cancer, **obesity**, a broken hip or leg, **oral contraceptives**, sickle cell anemia, chest trauma, certain congenital heart defects, and old age. Risk factors for gas emboli include: scuba diving, amateur plane flight, **exercise**, injury, obesity, **dehydration**, excessive alcohol, colds, and medications such as **narcotics** and **antihistamines**.

Symptoms of an arterial embolism include:

- severe pain in the area of the embolism
- pale, bluish cool skin
- numbness
- tingling
- muscular weakness or paralysis

Common symptoms of a pulmonary embolism include:

- labored breathing, sometimes accompanied by chest pain
- a rapid pulse
- a cough that may produce sputum
- a low-grade fever
- fluid build-up in the lungs

Less common symptoms include:

- coughing up blood
- pain caused by movement or breathing
- leg swelling
- bluish skin
- fainting
- swollen neck veins

Diagnosis

An embolism can be diagnosed through the patient's history, a physical exam, and diagnostic tests. The use of various tests may change, as physicians and clinical guidelines evaluate the most effective test in terms of accuracy and cost. For arterial emboli, cardiac ultrasound and/or arteriography are ordered. For a pulmonary embolism, a **chest x ray**, lung scan, pulmonary **angiography**, **electrocardiography**, arterial blood gas measurements, and **venography** or venous ultrasound could be ordered.

Diagnosing an arterial embolism

Ultrasound uses sound waves to create an image of the heart, organs, or arteries. The technologist applies gel to a hand-held transducer, then presses it against the patient's body. The sound waves are converted into an image that can be displayed on a monitor. Performed in an outpatient diagnostic laboratory, the test takes 30–60 minutes.

An arteriogram is an x ray in which a contrast medium is injected to make the arteries visible. It can be performed in a radiology unit, outpatient clinic, or diagnostic center of a hospital.

Diagnosing a pulmonary embolism

A chest x ray can show fluid build-up and detect other respiratory diseases. The perfusion lung scan shows poor flow of blood in areas beyond blocked arteries. The patient inhales a small amount of radiopharmaceutical and pictures of airflow into the lungs are taken with a gamma camera. Then a different radiopharmaceutical is injected into an arm vein and lung blood flow is scanned. A normal result essentially rules out a pulmonary embolism. A lung scan can be performed in a hospital or an outpatient facility and takes about 45 minutes.

Pulmonary angiography is one of the most reliable tests for diagnosing a pulmonary embolism. Pulmonary angiography is a radiographic test that involves injection of a radio contrast agent to show the pulmonary arteries. A cinematic camera records the blood flow through the patient, who lies on a table. Pulmonary angiography is usually performed in a hospital's radiology department and takes 30–60 minutes.

An electrocardiograph shows the heart's electrical activity and helps distinguish a pulmonary embolism from a heart attack. Electrodes covered with conducting jelly are placed on the patient's chest, arms, and legs. Impulses of the heart's activity are traced on paper. The test takes about 10 minutes.

Arterial blood gas measurements are sometimes helpful but, alone, they are not diagnostic for pulmonary embolism. Blood is taken from an artery instead of a vein, usually in the wrist.

Venography is used to look for the most likely source of a pulmonary embolism, deep vein thrombosis. It is very accurate, but it is not used often, because it is painful, expensive, exposes the patient to a fairly high dose of radiation, and can cause complications. Venography identifies the location, extent, and degree of attachment of the blood clots and enables the condition of the deep leg veins to be assessed. A contrast solution is injected into a foot vein through a catheter. The physician observes the movement of the solution through the vein with a fluoroscope while a series of x rays are taken. Venography takes between 30–45 minutes and can be done in a physician's office, a laboratory, or a hospital. Radionuclide venography, in which a radioactive isotope is injected, is occasionally used, especially if a patient has had reactions to contrast solutions. Venous ultrasound is the preferred evaluation of leg veins.

As noninvasive methods such as high-speed computed tomography (CT) scanning improve, they may be used to diagnose emboli. For instance, spiral (also called helical) CT scans may be the preferred tool for diagnosing pulmonary embolism in pregnant women.

Treatment

Patients with emboli require immediate hospitalization. They are generally treated with clot-dissolving and/or clot-preventing drugs. **Thrombolytic therapy** to dissolve blood clots is the definitive treatment for a severe pulmonary embolism. Streptokinase, urokinase, and recombinant tissue plasminogen activator (TPA) are used. Heparin has been the anticoagulant drug of choice for preventing formation of blood clots. A new drug has been approved for treatment of acute pulmonary emboli. Called fondaparinux (Arixtra), it usually is administered with Warfarin, an oral anticoagulant. Warfarin is sometimes used with other drugs to treat acute embolism events and is usually continued after the hospitalization to help prevent future emboli. Arixtra also has been used on an ongoing basis to prevent pulmonary emboli.

In the case of an arterial embolism, the affected limb is placed in a dependent position and kept warm.

Embolectomy is the treatment of choice in the majority of early cases of arterial emboli in the extremities. In this procedure, a balloon-tipped catheter is inserted into the artery to remove thromboembolic matter.

With a pulmonary embolism, **oxygen therapy** is often used to maintain normal oxygen concentrations. For people who can't take anticoagulants and in some other cases, surgery may be needed to insert a device that filters blood returning to the heart and lungs.

Prognosis

Of patients hospitalized with an arterial embolism, 25–30% die, and 5–25% require amputation of a limb. About 10% of patients with a pulmonary embolism die suddenly within the first hour of onset of the condition. The outcome for all other patients is generally good; only 3% of patients die who are properly diagnosed early and treated. In cases of an undiagnosed pulmonary embolism, about 30% of patients die.

Prevention

Embolism can be prevented in high risk patients through antithrombotic drugs such as heparin, venous interruption, gradient elastic stockings, and intermittent pneumatic compression of the legs. The combination of graduated compression stockings and low-dose heparin is significantly more effective than low-dose heparin alone.

Gradient elastic stockings, also called anti-embolism stockings, decrease the risk of blood clots by compressing superficial leg veins and forcing blood into the deep veins. They can be knee-, thigh-, or waist-length. Many physicians order the use of stockings before surgery and until there is no longer an elevated risk of developing blood clots. The risk of deep vein thrombosis after surgery is reduced 50% with the use of these stockings. The American Heart Association recommends that the use of graduated compression stockings be considered for all high-risk surgical patients.

Intermittent pneumatic compression involves wrapping knee- or thigh-high cuffs around the legs to prevent blood clots. The cuffs are connected to a pump that inflates and deflates, mimicking the heart's normal pumping action and reducing the pooling of blood. Intermittent pneumatic compression can be used during surgery and recovery and continues until there is no longer an elevated risk of developing blood clots. The American Heart Association recommends the use of intermittent pneumatic compression for patients who cannot take anticoagulants, for example, spinal cord and brain trauma patients.

Resources

PERIODICALS

Doyle, Nora M., et al. "Diagnosis of Pulmonary Embolism: A Cost-effective Analysis." *American Journal of Obstetrics and Gynecology* September 2004: 1019–1024.

Truelove, Christiane. "First for Pulmonary Embolism." *Med Ad News* August 2004: 82.

ORGANIZATIONS

American Heart Association National Center, 7272 Greenville Avenue, Dallas, TX, 75231, (800) 242-8721, Review.personal.info@heart.org.

Lori De Milto
Teresa G. Odle

Emergency contraception

Definition

Emergency **contraception** or emergency birth control uses either emergency contraceptive pills (ECPs) or a Copper-T intrauterine device (**IUD**) to help prevent **pregnancy** following unprotected vaginal intercourse.

Purpose

Emergency contraception may be used to prevent pregnancy after vaginal intercourse when:

- A birth control method was not used. Young people, in particular, may not be prepared for their first experience of sexual intercourse.
- A condom broke or slipped and ejaculation occurred within the woman's vagina.
- The male failed to withdraw from the vagina before ejaculation.
- A woman failed to take her birth control pills.
- A diaphragm, cap, or shield slipped out of place, followed by ejaculation within the vagina.
- A woman's "safe days" were miscalculated.
- A woman was raped or otherwise forced to have unprotected intercourse.

Women who missed taking their **oral contraceptives** may consider emergency contraception if:

- A new packet of pills was started at least two days late.
- Two to four of the first seven active (hormone-containing) pills (days 1–7) were missed.
- Five or more active pills were missed consecutively.

On average eight out of every 100 fertile women will become pregnant after having one episode of unprotected vaginal intercourse during the second or third week of their menstrual cycle. Following treatment with combined ECPs, only two of those 100 women will become pregnant—a 75% reduction. Following treatment with progestin-only ECPs, only one woman out of the 100 will become pregnant—an 89% reduction. Following emergency insertion of an IUD there is a 99.9% reduction in the risk of pregnancy.

Precautions

Emergency contraception does not work after the onset of pregnancy; nor should it be used as a regular method of birth control. ECPs do not prevent pregnancy from intercourse that occurs following the treatment; another birth control method must be used to prevent pregnancy. Although ECPs will not affect an existing pregnancy and will not harm the fetus, emergency contraception should not be used if a woman is already pregnant.

Frequent use of ECPs can result in irregular or unpredictable menstrual periods. Additional doses of ECPs usually do not reduce the risk of pregnancy and they increase the risk of side effects including **nausea and vomiting**.

Almost all women can use emergency contraception safely, even those who cannot use oral contraceptives as a regular method of birth control because of heart disease, **blood clots**, **stroke**, or other cardio-vascular problems. The anti-convulsive medication Dilantin may reduce the effectiveness of ECPs. Some physicians recommend doubling the first of the two ECP doses if taken with Dilantin.

Progestin-only ECPs (POPs) are not recommended for women who:

- may be pregnant already
- have a hypersensitivity to any component of the medication
- have abnormal, undiagnosed genital bleeding.

Copper-T IUDs should not be used for emergency contraception if a woman:

- is pregnant
- has a history of pelvic inflammatory disease (PID) that has impaired her fertility
- has one of numerous other conditions affecting her reproductive system
- has—or is currently at risk for contracting—a sexually transmitted disease (STD) such as HIV/AIDS, chlamydia, or gonorrhea, since IUD insertion can introduce infectious agents into the sterile uterine cavity.

Those at risk for contracting an STD include women who:

- have been raped
- have had unprotected sex with a new partner
- are in a non-monogamous relationship
- use intravenous drugs
- have partners who use intravenous drugs

Description

Although emergency contraception—sometimes called post-coital or morning-after contraception—has been available for over a quarter of a century, almost one-half of the 6.3 million pregnancies in the United States each year are unintended. Among teen pregnancies 80% are unintentional. About one-half of unintended pregnancies are caused by contraceptive failure, either a failure of the method or a mistake by the user. The remainder of unintended pregnancies occurs because birth control was not employed. Emergency contraception could help prevent some of the 1.4 million abortions that take place in the United States every year.

Emergency contraception prevents pregnancy by one of the following methods:

- delaying or inhibiting ovulation—the release of eggs from the ovary
- altering the transport of the sperm or egg, thereby preventing fertilization of the egg by a sperm

- altering the endometrium or uterine lining, thereby preventing implantation—the attachment of the fertilized egg to the wall of the uterus

The mechanism by which ECPs prevent pregnancy depends on the stage of the woman's menstrual cycle. In most cases ECPs delay or inhibit ovulation and have no effect on implantation. IUDs used as emergency contraception appear to interfere with implantation of the fertilized egg; although they also may prevent fertilization, as they are thought to do when they are used as a regular method of birth control.

Emergency contraceptive pills (ECPs)

ECPs contain synthetic hormones that mimic the hormones produced by a woman's body. Many common brands of birth control pills can be used for emergency contraception even though they are not labeled for that use. Any of the first 21 pills in a regular 28-pill package of oral contraceptives can be used for emergency contraception. The last seven pills in 28-pill packs do not contain hormones. The number of pills that constitute an emergency contraceptive dose depends on the brand of pill. The same brand should be used for both doses of ECPs. Many ECPs are available outside of the United States, where they are packaged, labeled, and sold for emergency contraceptive purposes.

COMBINED ECPs. Combined ECPs available in the United States contain 100 micrograms of the synthetic estrogen, ethinyl estradiol, and 0.5–0.6 mg of the synthetic progestin levonorgestrel per dose. Combined ECPs are taken according to the Yuzpe Regimen, named after A. Albert Yuzpe, the Canadian researcher who first demonstrated their safety and effectiveness in 1974. With the Yuzpe Regimen, the first dose of combined ECPs is taken as soon as possible after unprotected intercourse and the second dose is taken 12 hours later. However the timing of the second dose can vary by a few hours without diminishing its effectiveness. The Preven Emergency Contraceptive Kit—the first product to be specifically labeled and marketed for emergency contraception—is no longer available.

Combined ECPs available in the United States include:

- Alesse, manufactured by Wyeth-Ayerst; five pink pills per dose
- Aviane, manufactured by Duramed; five orange pills per dose
- Cryselle, manufactured by Barr; four white pills per dose

- Enpresse from Barr; four orange pills per dose
- Lessina from Barr; five pink pills per dose
- Levlen from Berlex; four light orange pills per dose
- Levlite from Berlex; five pink pills per dose
- Levora from Watson; four white pills per dose
- Lo/Ovral from Wyeth-Ayerst; four white pills per dose
- Low-Ogestrel from Watson; four white pills per dose
- Lutera from Watson; five white pills per dose
- Nordette from Wyeth-Ayerst; four light orange pills per dose
- Ogestrel from Watson; two white pills per dose
- Ovral from Wyeth-Ayerst; two white pills per dose
- Portia from Barr; four pink pills per dose
- Seasonale from Barr; four pink pills per dose
- Tri-Levlen from Berlex; four yellow pills per dose
- Triphasil from Wyeth-Ayerst; four yellow pills per dose
- Trivora from Watson; four pink pills per dose

PROGESTIN-ONLY ECPs. Progestin-only ECPs (POPs) are prescribed frequently, particularly for women who cannot take estrogen or who are **breastfeeding**. POPs contain 0.75 mg of levonorgestrel per dose. They are equally effective regardless of whether the two doses are taken simultaneously or 12–24 hours apart. POPs are most effective if taken within 72 hours of unprotected intercourse; however they reduce the risk of pregnancy if taken within 120 hours.

Progestin-only pills include:

- Plan B from Barr is the only drug available in the United States that is specifically designed and designated as an ECP—one white pill per dose.
- Ovrette from Wyeth-Ayerth requires swallowing 20 yellow pills for each dose.

The Copper-T IUD

The Copper-T 380A IUD (ParaGard) is a T-shaped device that provides emergency contraception if inserted into the uterus by a healthcare provider within seven days after unprotected intercourse. It can be removed by the healthcare provider after the woman's next menstrual period begins or it can remain in place for up to 10–12 years as an effective method of birth control.

Availability

In most of the United States, emergency contraception requires a special prescription or a prescription for a monthly supply of an appropriate oral contraceptive. Most physicians do not routinely discuss the use of emergency contraception with their patients and some pharmacies refuse to carry ECPs.

Emergency contraception is available from:

- public and college health clinics
- women's health centers
- Planned Parenthood clinics
- private doctors
- hospital emergency rooms, except those affiliated with a religion that opposes the use of birth control
- pharmacists directly, in a small number of states.

Some healthcare providers may prescribe ECPs over the telephone. **Sexual assault** victims may be offered ECPs in the hospital emergency room.

In many countries ECPs are available without a prescription. However in the United States emergency contraception remains controversial. In September of 2004, the U. S. Department of Justice released guidelines for the treatment of sexual assault victims without mentioning the option of emergency contraception. As of early 2005, the U.S. Food and Drug Administration (FDA) had delayed approval of over-the-counter (OTC) status for Plan B. However many professional healthcare organizations and advocacy groups for women's reproductive rights were working to make ECPs available without a prescription in the United States.

Costs

The cost of emergency contraception varies greatly according to region and location and any additional required services. Family-planning clinics and public healthcare centers may provide lower-cost emergency contraception or charge according to an income-based sliding scale.

Estimated costs for emergency contraception are:

- $8–$35 for Plan B
- $20–$50 for combined ECPs
- $50–$70 for other progestin-only ECPs
- $35–$150 for a visit to a healthcare provider
- $10–$20 for a pregnancy test
- about $400 for an exam, IUD, and insertion; however the IUD can remain in place for up to 12 years.

Preparation

For emergency contraception to be effective, it must be used as soon as possible following unprotected intercourse. Some healthcare providers and **women's health** centers prescribe or supply packets of ECPs—called EC-to-Go—so that they are available immediately if required. Supplies of ECPs are particularly important for women who are at high risk for having unprotected intercourse. EC-to-Go also avoids the cost of an extra visit to a healthcare provider.

Studies have found that neither the use of ECPs, nor having a supply of ECPs on hand, reduce the likelihood that women, including teenagers, will use conventional contraceptive methods. In fact it has been shown that the use of ECPs often increases the likelihood that a regular birth control method will be employed.

If an office visit is required, a healthcare provider may take a medical history, perform a pregnancy test on a urine sample, and—provided that pregnancy has not occurred—discuss the appropriate type of emergency contraception.

Aftercare

For about 10–15% of women who take ECPs, the timing, duration, and/or amount of bleeding for their next menstrual period may be different than usual. About 50% of women have their first post-ECP menstrual period one to three days earlier or later than expected. Most often it is earlier than expected. Bleeding may be normal or heavier, lighter, or more spotty than usual.

Following IUD insertion, a woman may need to be escorted or driven home and she may require rest.

Risks

Emergency contraception is considered to be both safe and effective for teenagers as well as adult women. However emergency contraception may not prevent an ectopic pregnancy—a pregnancy outside of the uterus, in the fallopian tubes or abdomen. Ectopic pregnancies are medical emergencies and can be fatal.

Side effects of ECPs

About 50% of women feel sick to their stomachs for approximately 24 hours after taking combined ECPs. **Nausea** occurs in 30–50% of women and 15–25% of women experience **vomiting**. Only 23% of women who take progestin-only ECPs experience nausea and only 6% have **vomiting**.

If vomiting occurs within one hour of taking ECPs, the dose may have to be repeated. OTC medications such as Dramamine II, Bonine, or their generic equivalents, taken one hour before the ECPs, reduce the risk of nausea and vomiting, although they may cause drowsiness. Two 25-mg tablets of Meclizine, taken one hour before the ECPs, reduce the risk of

nausea by 27% and the risk of vomiting by 64%; however there is about a 30% risk of drowsiness. If vomiting occurs after the first dose of an ECP, anti-nausea medication should be taken one hour before the second dose. The second dose also may be taken as a vaginal suppository by placing the pills as far as possible into the vagina for absorption through the vaginal tissue.

Other side effects of ECPs can include:

• breast tenderness
• abdominal pain
• irregular bleeding
• dizziness
• headaches
• fatigue.

Side effects usually last only one to two days and are far less frequent with progestin-only ECPs as compared with combined ECPs.

Side effects of IUD insertion

Side effects of IUD insertion may include:

• abdominal discomfort
• vaginal bleeding or spotting
• infection.

However the risk of pelvic infection is very small among women who are not at risk for STDs.

Other possible side effects of IUD insertion include:

• heavy menstrual flow
• cramping
• infertility
• uterine puncture.

Normal results

The effectiveness of emergency contraception depends both on the stage of the woman's menstrual cycle and on how soon the emergency contraception is used following unprotected vaginal intercourse. The closer a woman is to ovulation—her fertile period during which eggs are released from the ovary—the less effective emergency contraception will be.

ECPs are less effective than the most popular birth control methods:

• If taken within 72 hours of unprotected intercourse, combined ECPs are about 75% effective for preventing pregnancy.

KEY TERMS

Emergency contraceptive pills; ECPs—Medication containing synthetic hormones for preventing pregnancy after unprotected vaginal intercourse.

Endometrium—The lining of the uterus.

Ethinyl estradiol—A semi-synthetic derivative of estradiol—an estrogen or female sex hormone—used in birth control pills and combined ECPs.

Implantation—The embedding of a fertilized egg in the inner wall of the uterus.

Intrauterine device; IUD—A device inserted into the uterus to prevent pregnancy.

Levonorgestrel—A synthetic progestin used in ECPs.

Ovulation—The discharge of an ovum (egg) from the mature follicle of the ovary.

Progestin—A synthetic or natural drug that acts on the uterine lining.

Yuzpe Regimen—A two-dose treatment with combined ECPs to prevent pregnancy after unprotected intercourse; the first dose is taken as soon as possible and the second dose is taken 12 hours after the first.

- Progestin-only ECPs are 95% effective if taken within 24 hours of unprotected intercourse and about 89% effective if taken within 72 hours.
- A Copper-T IUD is 99.9% effective if inserted within seven days of unprotected intercourse.

If a normal menstrual period does not begin within three weeks after taking ECPs, or if signs of pregnancy develop, a healthcare provider should be consulted immediately.

Signs of pregnancy include:

- a missed menstrual period
- nausea
- unexplained fatigue
- enlarged or sore breasts
- headaches
- frequent urination

The majority of women express satisfaction with emergency contraception. One study of 235 women who had used ECPs found that 91% were satisfied with the method and 97% would recommend it to others.

Resources

BOOKS

Emergency Contraception: A Medical Dictionary, Bibliography, and Annotated Research Guide to Internet References. San Diego: ICON Health Publications, 2004.

The Essential Guide for Emergency Contraception. Atlanta, GA: American Healthcare Consultants, 2004.

PERIODICALS

Brody, Jane E. "The Politics of Emergency Contraception." *New York Times* August 24, 2004: F.7.

Cantor, Julie, and Ken Baum. "The Limits of Conscientious Objection—May Pharmacists Refuse to Fill

Prescriptions for Emergency Contraception?" *New England Journal of Medicine* 351, no. 19 (November 4, 2004): 2008–12.

Raine, Tina R., et al. "Direct Access to Emergency Contraception Through Pharmacies and Effect on Unintended Pregnancy and STIs." *Journal of the American Medical Association* 293, no. 1 (January 5, 2005): 54–62.

Weismiller, David G. "Emergency Contraception." *American Family Physician* 70, no. 4 (August 15, 2004): 707–14.

OTHER

Emergency Contraception. Planned Parenthood. February 2005 [cited March 6, 2005]. http://www.plannedparenthood.org/pp2/portal/medicalinfo/ec/pub-emergency-contraception.xml.

Emergency Contraception. Planned Parenthood. June 2004 [cited March 6, 2005]. http://www.plannedparenthood.org/pp2/portal/medicalinfo/ec/fact-emergency-contraception.xml.

Frequently Asked Questions About Emergency Contraception. The National Women's Health Information Center. November 2002 [cited March 6, 2005]. http://www.4woman.gov/faq/econtracep.htm.

Not-2-Late.com. The Emergency Contraception Website. Office of Population Research, Princeton University and the Association of Reproductive Health Professionals. [Cited March 6, 2005]. http://ec.princeton.edu.

ORGANIZATIONS

American College of Obstetricians and Gynecologists, PO Box 96920, Washington, DC, 20090-6920, (202) 638-5577, http://www.acog.org.

Association of Reproductive Health Professionals, 1901 L Street, NW, Suite 300, Washington, DC, 20036, (202) 466-3825, http://arhp.org.

Office of Population Research, Princeton University, Wallace Hall, Princeton, NJ, 08544, (609) 258-4870, (609) 258-1039, http://opr.princeton.edu.

PATH, PO Box 900922, Seattle, WA, 98109, (206) 285-3500, (206) 285-6619, info@path.org, http://www.path.org.

Planned Parenthood Federation of America, Inc., 434 West 33rd St., New York, NY, 10001, (212) 541-7800, (212) 245-1845, (800) 230-7526, http://search. plannedparenthood.org.

United States Food and Drug Administration (FDA), 10903 New Hampshire Ave, Silver Spring, MD, 02993-0002, (888) 463-6332, http://www.fda.gov.

Margaret Alic, Ph.D.

EMG *see* **Electromyography**

Emollient bath *see* **Therapeutic baths**

Emphysema

Definition

Emphysema is a chronic respiratory disease in which there is progressive overinflation of the air sacs (alveoli) in the lungs, causing a loss of lung function and often breathlessness. Its name comes from a Greek word meaning "to blow into," hence "air-containing" or "air-inflated." Emphysema is sometimes grouped together with chronic **bronchitis** under the name of **chronic obstructive**

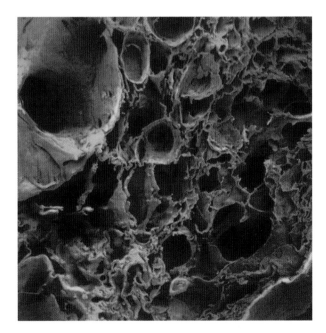

A scanning electron microscopy (SEM) of lung tissue indicating emphysema. *(Custom Medical Stock Photo, Inc. Reproduced by permission.)*

X ray showing emphysema in the lungs. *(Photo Researchers, Inc.)*

pulmonary disease, or COPD. Many people who are diagnosed with emphysema also have chronic bronchitis.

Demographics

Emphysema is increasing in the United States, Canada, and other developed countries primarily because of cigarette **smoking**. It is almost entirely a disease of adults. About 12 million adults in the United States have been diagnosed with the disease as of 2009; however, many doctors believe emphysema is underdiagnosed. Between 4 and 6 percent of male adults and 1–3 percent of female adults in North America are estimated to have emphysema. The number of women diagnosed with the disease is rising rapidly; the year 2000 was the first year that more women than men were identified as having emphysema. In 2005, almost 66,000 females died compared to 61,000 males. According to the American Lung Association, the cost to the United States for COPD each year is approximately $42.6 billion, including $26.7 billion in direct health care expenditures, $8.0 billion in indirect morbidity costs and $7.9 billion in indirect mortality costs.

Rates of emphysema are rising worldwide as more people in the developing countries take up cigarette smoking. The Global Initiative for Chronic Obstructive Lung Disease (GOLD) estimates that 9–10 percent of adults around the world have either chronic bronchitis or emphysema.

People who develop emphysema as a result of smoking generally start to have symptoms in their late 40s or early 50s. Those who have emphysema because of a genetic condition (described below) may begin to have symptoms in their 30s. This genetic condition, discovered by a Swedish doctor in 1963 and known as alpha 1-antitrypsin deficiency (A1AT), is more common in Caucasians than in members of other races and accounts for about 2 percent of all emphysema cases in the United States. Current estimates suggest that between 60,000 and 100,000 Americans have severe A1AT deficiency, but only 4% of these patients have been identified.

Worldwide, people of Spanish, Portuguese, Scandinavian, and Saudi Arabian ancestry are at increased risk of emphysema associated with A1AT deficiency. The genetic disorder is thought to affect as many as 4 percent of these populations. Newborns in Sweden are routinely screened for A1AT deficiency as of 2009.

Description

Emphysema is a lung disease in which a person's ability to breathe easily and deeply is steadily weakened over time by the destruction of lung tissue. The human lung consists of tissue containing millions of tiny air sacs called alveoli, which are arranged like bunches of grapes around very small air tubes called bronchioles. There are about 300 million alveoli in each lung. When a person breathes in air, the air travels from the nose and mouth through the windpipe and then into the right and left bronchi, which are the main air passages into each of the two lungs. The bronchi divide and subdivide repeatedly into smaller and smaller air passages, finally ending in the bronchioles and alveoli. In a normal person, oxygen from the air that has been taken in is exchanged in the walls of the alveoli for carbon dioxide in the person's blood. When the person breathes out, the carbon dioxide leaves the body in the air that travels out from the lungs and through the upper airway to the nose and mouth.

To perform their function effectively, the tissue in the lungs that separates the alveoli from one another needs to be as elastic as possible. The alveoli contain tiny elastic fibers in their cell walls that allow them to act like miniature balloons. What happens in emphysema is that tobacco smoke or other irritants causes the alveoli to become inflamed and lose their elasticity. The bronchioles start to collapse, which traps air inside the alveoli and overstretches them. In time the alveoli rupture, leading to the formation of fewer but larger air sacs in the lungs. The smaller areas of alveoli destruction are known as blebs and the larger ones are called bullae. These larger and less flexible sacs are less

efficient in forcing air out of the lungs when the person breathes out. As a result, the person has to breathe more frequently or breathe harder in order to get enough oxygen and get rid of carbon dioxide.

In addition to the loss of elasticity in the alveoli, the cells in the airways secrete more mucus than usual, which collects in the airways and clogs them, making breathing even more difficult.

Risk factors

Cigarette smoking is the biggest single risk factor for emphysema. Some people who do not smoke cigarettes, however, are at increased risk of emphysema. They include:

- People who work in occupations that expose them to high levels of dust from grain or cotton, or chemical irritants. These occupations include mining, certain types of agricultural work, and lumbering. Most miners suffer from emphysema to some degree after a lifetime in the mining pit. In fact, emphysema is sometimes referred to as miner's lung or black lung.
- People exposed to high levels of automobile exhaust or secondhand smoke.
- People who are HIV-positive.
- People who abuse intravenous drugs. The cotton fibers and other materials used as fillers in these drugs can irritate and eventually destroy lung tissue.
- People who smoke marijuana. Marijuana smoke may be even more damaging to some people than tobacco because it is inhaled deeply and held in by the smoker.
- People with certain diseases that affect connective tissue, such as Marfan syndrome and Ehlers-Danlos syndrome.
- People whose occupations require heavy use of the lungs for blowing, such as trumpet players, woodwind players, and glassblowers.

Causes and symptoms

Causes

Emphysema is caused by a weakening of the tissues in the lungs as a result of inflammation due to tobacco smoke or other chemical irritants in the air, or a hereditary deficiency of a protein that protects the elasticity of lung tissue. As the bronchioles in the lungs collapse and the alveoli become enlarged, the lungs become less efficient in getting rid of carbon dioxide and the person has to breathe more frequently in order to get enough oxygen. In addition, the person has to use their chest muscles to expel air from the lungs forcefully rather than being able to rely on the normal movement of

Alveolus (plural: alveoli)—The medical term for one of the tiny air sacs in the lungs where oxygen is transferred from the lungs to the blood and carbon dioxide is removed.

Arterial blood gases test—A test to analyze blood for oxygen, carbon dioxide, and bicarbonate content, as well as blood pH (acidity level). Used to test the effectiveness of respiration.

Bronchiole—A very small thin-walled air passage in the lungs that branches off from a bronchus.

Bronchus (plural: bronchi)—One of the two major divisions of the airway that lead into the right and left lungs.

Cor pulmonale—Enlargement and structural change of the right ventricle of the heart as a result of emphysema or other respiratory disorder.

Diaphragm—A sheet of muscle tissue that divides the chest cavity from the abdominal cavity.

Peak flow measurement—Measurement of the maximum rate of airflow attained during a forced vital capacity determination.

Progressive—A term that refers to a disease that gets worse over time.

Pulmonary—Related to or associated with the lungs.

Pulse oximetry—The noninvasive monitoring or determination of oxygen-hemoglobin saturation of the blood.

Spirometer—A device that is used to test the air capacity of a person's lungs and the amount of air that enters and leaves the lungs during breathing.

Ventricle—One of the two lower chambers of the heart.

the diaphragm during breathing. This need to use muscular force leads to the development of a so-called barrel chest; that is, the person's chest is almost the same size from front to back as from side to side.

About 2 percent of cases of emphysema are caused by a deficiency of a liver enzyme known as alpha 1-antitrypsin, or A1AT. The enzyme ordinarily protects the alveoli in the lungs from damage by another enzyme that harms connective tissue. In people with A1AT deficiency, there is not enough of the protective enzyme to keep the alveoli in good working condition. A1AT is an inherited condition caused by a mutation in a gene on the long arm of chromosome 14.

Symptoms

The most noticeable symptoms of emphysema are breathlessness, coughing, and **wheezing**. These symptoms typically develop gradually over many years. It is a common occurrence for many emphysema patients to have lost over half of their functioning lung tissue before they become aware that something is wrong. The **cough**, which is often dismissed as "smoker's cough," may be productive of large amounts of dark, thick sputum.

In addition to **shortness of breath**, coughing, and wheezing, people with emphysema often develop the following symptoms:

- Pursed-lips breathing. This is a way of partially closing the lips that allows the person to fully exhale.

When the mouth opening is smaller, the airways that have been weakened by the disease open wide and allow the person to expel more air from the lungs.

- Greater difficulty exercising or doing work that requires physical activity.
- Loss of appetite and weight loss. Eating can make it harder to breathe because the stomach expands during a meal and pushes upward against the diaphragm.
- Fatigue. Emphysema leads to a lower level of oxygen in the blood, which in turn causes people to feel tired easily.
- Swelling of the feet, ankles, or legs.
- Slow recovery from such upper respiratory infections as colds and flu. Those with emphysema are at risk for a variety of other complications resulting from weakened lung function, including pneumonia, pulmonary hypertension, cor pulmonale, and chronic respiratory failure.

Diagnosis

Many patients are diagnosed with emphysema in the course of seeking treatment for chronic bronchitis. The first step in diagnosing emphysema is a careful patient history, particularly a history of smoking.

Examination

A history of heavy smoking alone, however, is not enough for a physician to differentiate emphysema from other respiratory diseases. A physician will combine information on symptoms, medical history, **physical examination**, lung function tests, and **chest x ray** results to make a diagnosis of emphysema. One of the first clues may be a hollow sound heard through a stethoscope as the patient's chest is being tapped. The hollow sound is the result of the enlargement or rupture of the lungs' alveoli.

Tests

A variety of **pulmonary function tests** may be ordered. In the early stages of emphysema, the only result may be dysfunction of the small airways. Patients with emphysema may show an increase in the total amount of air that is in the lungs (total lung capacity), but a decrease in the amount of air that can be breathed out after taking a deep breath (vital capacity). With severe emphysema, vital capacity is substantially below normal. **Spirometry**, a procedure that measures air flow and lung volume, helps in the diagnosis of emphysema.

A chest x ray is often ordered to aid in the diagnosis of emphysema, though patients in the early stages of the disease may have normal findings. Abnormal findings on the chest x ray include overinflation of the lungs and an abnormally increased chest diameter. The diaphragm may appear depressed or flattened. In addition, patients with advanced emphysema may show a smaller or vertical heart. The physician may observe blisters in the lungs and bulging of the accessory muscles of the respiratory system. Late in the disease, an EKG will show signs of right ventricular failure in the heart and increased hemoglobin due to lower levels of oxygen in the patient's blood.

Other tests that may be performed include peak flow measurements, arterial blood gases, and pulse oximetry.

A1AT deficiency can be diagnosed by a simple fingerstick blood test. Individuals with symptoms of emphysema or COPD should ask their doctor whether this test is appropriate for them. Their doctor can order the test, or they can choose to be tested on a confidential basis through the Alpha-1 Foundation's Alpha-1 Coded Testing (ACT) study. The foundation's contact information is listed below.

Treatment

There is no cure for emphysema as of 2009. Treatment is focused on slowing the progress of the disease and easing the patient's symptoms. The first part of treatment for patients who smoke is quitting the habit.

Smoking cessation programs may be effective. Consistent encouragement along with the help of health care professionals as well as family and friends can help increase the success rate of someone attempting to quit smoking.

Traditional

Drugs

The next stage in treatment is the use of medications. The doctor may prescribe one or more of the following types of drugs:

- Bronchodilators. Bronchodilators are drugs that work by opening up the airways, which allows for more efficient exchange of carbon dioxide and oxygen. Some are taken in tablet form while others are dispensed in inhalers. Depending on the severity of the patient's emphysema, they may use the inhaler only when needed for shortness of breath or they may take a dose of the medication at prescribed regular intervals. There are three primary categories of bronchodilators: sympathomimetics (isoproterenol, metaproterenol, terbutaline, albuterol), which can be inhaled, taken by mouth, or injected; parasympathomimetics (atropine); and methylxanthines (theophylline), which may be administered intravenously, orally, or rectally.

- Steroids (beclomethasone, dexamethasone, triamcinolone, flunisolide). This type of medication works by lowering the inflammation in the tissues lining the airways. These drugs can also be taken in pill form or through inhalers. Some patients' lung function improves with corticosteroids, and inhaled steroids may be beneficial to patients with few side effects.

- Antibiotics. People who have infections in the lungs as well as emphysema may be given antibiotics to treat the infections.

- Expectorants. These are drugs that can help to loosen respiratory secretions, enabling the patient to more easily expel them from the airways.

Many of the medications prescribed for emphysema involve the use of a metered dose inhaler (MDI) that may require special instruction to be used correctly. MDIs are a convenient and safe method of delivering medication to the lungs. If they are used incorrectly, however, the medication will not get to the right place. Proper technique is essential for inhaled medication to be effective.

Among all other treatments for emphysema, only **oxygen therapy** has shown an increase in the survival rate.

Home oxygen therapy may improve the survival times in those patients with advanced emphysema who also have low blood oxygen levels. It may improve the patient's tolerance of **exercise**, as well as improve their performance in certain aspects of brain function and muscle coordination. The functioning of the heart may also improve with an increased concentration of oxygen in the blood. Oxygen may also decrease **insomnia** and headaches. Some patients may receive oxygen only at night, but studies have illustrated that it is most effective when administered at least 18 but preferably 24 hours per day. Portable oxygen tanks prescribed to patients carry a limited supply and must be refilled on a regular basis by a home health provider. Medicare and most insurance companies cover a large proportion of the cost of home oxygen therapy. Patients should be instructed regarding special safety issues involving the transport and presence of oxygen in the home.

Surgery

Emphysema is sometimes treated surgically. In some cases, part of the diseased lung is removed. This procedure, which is called lung volume reduction, creates space for the remaining portions of the lungs; it does improve breathing and quality of life for some patients. Another surgical option is **lung transplantation**. This is a risky procedure, however, and requires the patient to take medications to prevent the rejection of the transplanted lung. In addition, not everyone qualifies for transplantation, and those who do are limited by the short supply of available organs. Up through 2006, emphysema was the single most common diagnosis of American patients awaiting lung transplantation.

Other interventions

For those patients with advanced emphysema, keeping the air passages reasonably clear of secretions can prove difficult. Some common methods for mobilizing and removing secretions include:

- Postural drainage. This helps to remove secretions from the airways. The patient lies in a position that allows gravity to aid in draining different parts of the lung. This is often done after the patient inhales an aerosol medication. The basic position involves the patient lying on the bed with his chest and head over the side and the forearms resting on the floor.

- Chest percussion. This technique involves lightly clapping the back and chest, and may help to loosen thick secretions.

- Coughing and deep breathing. These techniques may aid the patient in bringing up secretions.

- Aerosol treatments. These treatments may involve solutions of saline, often mixed with a bronchodilator, which are then inhaled as an aerosol. The aerosols thin and loosen secretions. A treatment normally takes 10 to 15 minutes, and is given three or four times a day.

Another important part of treatment for emphysema is called pulmonary **rehabilitation**. This approach is aimed at educating patients about their disease and helping them with lifestyle changes that will slow the progression of the disease and improve quality of life. Pulmonary rehabilitation includes a physical exercise program designed to improve the patient's physical endurance and energy level. Many patients are also encouraged to lose weight in order to reduce the burden on their lungs. One important benefit of pulmonary rehabilitation is psychological: patients report that their self-esteem and sense of control over their life improve when they start to see benefits from the rehabilitation program.

Patients with emphysema can learn to perform a variety of self-help measures that may help improve their symptoms and their ability to participate in everyday activities. These measures include:

- Avoiding any exposure to dust and fumes.

- Avoiding air pollution, including secondhand cigarette smoke.

- Avoiding other people who have infections like colds or flu, and getting a pneumonia vaccination and a yearly flu shot.

- Drinking plenty of fluids. This helps to loosen respiratory secretions so they can be brought up more easily through coughing.

- Avoiding extreme temperatures of heat or cold, and also avoiding high altitudes. Special precautions can be taken that may enable the emphysema patient to fly on a plane.

- Maintaining adequate nutritional intake. Normally a high-protein diet taken in many small feedings is recommended.

Treatment for A1AT deficiency

Emphysema related to A1AT deficiency can be treated by intravenous infusions of the A1AT protein as well as by avoiding breathing substances that irritate the lungs and by lung transplantation if needed. The intravenous protein infusions are derived from donated human blood plasma. This type of treatment is called augmentation therapy; present recommendations are that patients should not begin this treatment before the symptoms of emphysema appear. Augmentation therapy is not a cure for emphysema but can slow its progression.

Alternative

There are several alternative approaches to relieving the symptoms of emphysema. As with mainstream treatments, these are not cures for the disease.

HERBALISM. Herbs can be beneficial in helping the body to ward off infection, and easing the asthmatic symptoms that often accompany emphysema.

Some beneficial herbs are:

- Lobelia. This is a mild sedative, also having strong expectorant properties. It is widely used for chest complaints, including emphysema and bronchitis, and can help to shorten an asthma attack.
- Thyme. A tea made with thyme is recommended for overcoming shortness of breath. It is also a powerful antiseptic.
- Mullein. This is another traditional remedy for chest complaints. To make a tea, one boils two tablespoons of the dried leaves with a glass of milk and drinks the mixture.
- Echinacea. Echinacea is a powerful immune system stimulant and strengthens the body in general, warding off colds and infections.
- Lungwort. A member of the borage family, this herb is very healing for the lungs. It should be taken as an infusion.
- Black cohosh. This herb is an expectorant and astringent. It relieves coughing.
- Sage. This is one of the most useful of all herbs and is said to be good for whatever it is taken for. It is antiviral and bactericidal.
- Garlic. A very powerful antiviral, garlic can be of real help to those trying to avoid infections and lung congestion.

CHINESE HERBAL MEDICINE. Qing Qi Hua Tan Wan (Pinellia expectorant pills) are the Chinese herbalists' treatment for chronic lung complaints, particularly bronchitis and **asthma**.

JUICE THERAPY. Kitty Campion, a British naturopathic herbalist expert, recommends the following juices for the treatment of emphysema: equal parts of carrot juice, parsnip juice, watercress juice, and potato juice, or equal parts of orange juice and lemon juice, diluted half and half with a strong decoction of rosehip tea.

AROMATHERAPY. Aromatherapy involves massaging the patient with potent plant essential oils, which have been proven to enter the circulation through the skin. The constituents of the oils can have a powerful effect on a variety of illnesses, but since their beneficial qualities are also transported through the air, they are considered to be doubly beneficial to those who suffer from respiratory ailments.

Aromatherapy oils for respiratory disease:

- *Canada balsam* may alleviate respiratory symptoms and is an expectorant. It is also a bactericide and recommended for those suffering from chronic chest ailments.
- *Tolu balsam* is an excellent treatment for chest infections.
- *Frankincense* is good for infection and catarrhal discharge.
- *Niaouli* is a very strong antiseptic and beneficial for pulmonary trouble.
- *Rose damascena* is recommended for bronchial complaints, and it also lifts the spirits.
- *Tea tree oil* is one of the most potent anti-viral, anti-bacterial and anti-fungal agents known to herbal medicine, therefore, highly beneficial as a preventative measure against chest infection.

ACUPUNCTURE. This ancient Chinese system of holistic treatment works on the principle that illness is the result of blockage in the flow of life force. The practitioner aims to stimulate relevant meridians in the body and thus release trapped life force, returning bodily functions to normal. The treatment is virtually painless.

Treatment can be expected to improve blood circulation and the capacity of the body to restore itself. Research has indicated that **acupuncture** can produce changes in the electrical fields of body cells, which promote a return to the body's normal state. Consequently, few negative side effects are associated with acupuncture treatment.

Prognosis

Emphysema is known to shorten a patient's life span. It is the fourth most common cause of **death** in the United States as of 2009, being responsible for 4.5 percent of all deaths and a contributing factor in another 4.3 percent. Some patients, however, live longer than others depending on the cause of their emphysema and the measurement of their lung capacity at diagnosis. Complications of emphysema include higher risks for **pneumonia** and acute bronchitis. In general, men have worse prognoses than women. Patients who have smoked 20 cigarettes per day for 20 years or longer with a severely reduced breathing capacity have the worst prognosis; only 5 percent survive for 12 years after diagnosis. Smoking has been estimated to speed up the appearance of emphysema in patients with A1AT deficiency by 19 years.

The prognosis for emphysema associated with A1AT deficiency is poor. Long-term studies of the efficacy of augmentation therapy have not been carried out as of 2009 although the therapy has been used for about 20 years and is considered safe. Most patients with this form of emphysema suffer some degree of disability and a shortened life expectancy.

Prevention

Most cases of emphysema can be prevented by simply not smoking or by quitting smoking as soon as possible and avoiding secondhand smoke. Emphysema related to genetic factors cannot always be prevented, but its development can be postponed in people who inherited the defective gene by avoiding smoking.

Health care team roles

Many members of the health care team may treat a patient with emphysema. The patient usually seeks help from a physician first, who will make the diagnosis. In the course of the diagnostic workup, x-ray technicians and respiratory therapists may treat the patient. The nurse plays an important role in assessing the patient, administering medications, in teaching the patient how best to cope with and understand the disease, and—in some cases—provides home care. The physical therapist may assist the patient to find ways of increasing their strength and activity tolerance.

Resources

BOOKS

Green, Robert J., Jr. *Natural Therapies for Emphysema and COPD: Relief and Healing for Chronic Pulmonary Disorders*. Rochester, VT: Healing Arts Press, 2007.

Hedrick, Hannah L., and Austin Kutcher. *The Quiet Killer: Emphysema, Chronic Obstructive Pulmonary Disease*. Lanham, MD: Scarecrow Press, 2002.

Matthews, Dawn D. *Lung Disorders Sourcebook: Basic Information for Consumers*. Detroit, MI: Omnigraphics, 2002.

Quinn, Campion E. *100 Questions and Answers about Chronic Obstructive Pulmonary Disease (COPD)*. Sudbury, MA: Jones and Bartlett Publishers, 2006.

PERIODICALS

Bernspång, E., et al. "Lung Function in 30-year-old Alpha-1-Antitrypsin-deficient Individuals." *Respiratory Medicine* 103 (June 2009): 861–65.

Fregonese, L., and J. Stolk. "Hereditary Alpha-1-Antitrypsin Deficiency and Its Clinical Consequences." *Orphanet Journal of Rare Diseases*, June 19, 2008; 3:16.

Lee, G., et al. "Chronic Inflammation, Chronic Obstructive Pulmonary Disease, and Lung Cancer." *Current Opinion in Pulmonary Medicine* 15 (July 2009): 303–307.

McCurry, K. R., et al. "Lung Transplantation in the United States, 1998–2007." *American Journal of Transplantation* 9 (April 2009): 942–58.

Rennard, S. I., and J. Vestbo. "Natural Histories of Chronic Obstructive Pulmonary Disease." *Proceedings of the American Thoracic Society* 5 (December 15, 2008): 878–83.

Schwartz, A. G., et al. "Chronic Obstructive Lung Diseases and Risk of Non-Small-Cell Lung Cancer in Women." *Journal of Thoracic Oncology* 4 (March 2009): 291–99.

Shah, A. A., and T. A. D'Amico. "Lung Volume Reduction Surgery for the Management of Refractory Dyspnea in Chronic Obstructive Pulmonary Disease." *Current Opinion in Supportive and Palliative Care* 3 (June 2009): 107–111.

OTHER

Alpha-1 Foundation. *Alpha-1 Lung Disease*. http://www.alphaone.org/alphas/?c = 03-Alpha-1-Lung-Disease

American Lung Association. *Chronic Obstructive Pulmonary Disease (COPD) Fact Sheet*. http://www.lungusa.org/site/apps/nlnet/content3.aspx?c = dvLUK9O0E&b = 2060053&content_id = {EE451F66-996B-4C23-874D-BF66586196FF}notoc = 1

National Emphysema Foundation. *COPD*. http://www.emphysemafoundation.org/?page_id = 28

National Heart, Lung, and Blood Institute (NHLBI). *COPD: Are You at Risk?*http://www.nhlbi.nih.gov/health/public/lung/copd/campaign-materials/html/copd-atrisk.htm

National Heart, Lung, and Blood Institute (NHLBI). *COPD: Breathing Better with a COPD Diagnosis*. http://www.nhlbi.nih.gov/health/public/lung/copd/campaign-materials/pub/copd-patient.pdf

Sharma, Sat. "Emphysema." *eMedicine*, June 14, 2006. http://emedicine.medscape.com/article/298283-overview

ORGANIZATIONS

Alpha-1 Foundation, 2937 S.W. 27th Avenue, Suite 302, Miami, FL, 33133, 305-567-9888, 877-228-7321, 305-567-1317, http://www.alphaone.org/.

American Lung Association, 1301 Pennsylvania Ave., NW, Suite 800, Washington, DC, 20004, 212-315-8700, 800-548-8252, http://www.lungusa.org/site/c.dvLU-K9O0E/b.22542/k.CA6A/Home.htm.

National Emphysema Foundation, 128 East Avenue, Norwalk, CT, 06851, 203-866-5000, 203-286-1105, http://www.emphysemafoundation.org/.

National Heart, Lung, and Blood Institute (NHLBI),
Health Information Center, P.O. Box 30105, Bethesda,
MD, 20824-0105, 301-592-8573, 240-629-3246,
nhlbiinfo@nhlbi.nih.gov, http://www.nhlbi.nih.gov/.
Global Initiative for Chronic Obstructive Lung Disease
(GOLD), http://www.goldcopd.com/.

Deanna M. Swartout-Corbeil, RN
Patricia Skinner
Rebecca J. Frey, PhD

Empyema

Definition

Empyema is a condition in which pus and fluid from infected tissue collects in a body cavity. The name comes from the Greek word *empyein* meaning pus-producing (suppurate). Empyema is most often used to refer to collections of pus in the space around the lungs (pleural cavity), but sometimes refers to similar collections in the gall bladder or the pelvic cavity. Empyema in the pleural cavity is sometimes called empyema thoracis, or empyema of the chest, to distinguish it from empyema elsewhere in the body.

Description

Empyema may have a number of causes but is most frequently a complication of **pneumonia**. Its development can be divided into three phases: an acute phase in which the body cavity fills with a thin fluid containing some pus; a second stage in which the fluid thickens and a fibrous, coagulation protein (fibrin) begins to accumulate within the cavity; and a third or chronic stage in which the lung or other organ is encased within a thick covering of fibrous material.

Causes and symptoms

Empyema thoracis can be caused by a number of different organisms, including bacteria, fungi, and amebas, in connection with pneumonia, chest **wounds**, chest surgery, lung abscesses, or a ruptured esophagus. The infective organism can get into the pleural cavity either through the bloodstream or other circulatory system, in secretions from lung tissue, or on the surfaces of surgical instruments or objects that cause open chest wounds. The most common organisms that cause empyema are the following bacteria: *Streptococcus pneumoniae*, *Haemophilus influenzae*, and *Staphylococcus aureus*. *S. aureus* is the most common cause in all age groups, accounting for 90% of cases of empyema in infants and children. Pelvic empyema in women is most often caused by *Bacteroides* strains or *Pseudomonas aeruginosa*. In elderly, chronically ill, or alcoholic patients, empyema is often caused by *Klebsiella pneumoniae* species of bacteria.

When the disease organisms arrive in the cavity surrounding the lungs, they infect the tissues that cover the lungs and line the chest wall. As the body attempts to fight off the infection, the cavity fills up with tissue fluid, pus, and dead tissue cells. Empyema of the gall bladder or pelvis results from similar reactions to infection in those parts of the body.

The signs and symptoms of empyema vary somewhat according to the location of the infection and its severity. In empyema thoracis, patients usually exhibit symptoms of pneumonia, including **fever**, **cough**, **fatigue**, **shortness of breath**, and chest **pain**. They may prefer to lie on the side of the body affected by the empyema. Family members may notice **bad breath**. In severe cases, the patient may become dehydrated, cough up blood or greenish-brown sputum, run a fever as high as 105°F (40.6°C), or fall into a **coma**.

Patients with thoracic empyema may develop potentially life-threatening complications if the condition is not treated. The infected tissues may develop large collections of pus (abscesses) that can rupture into the patient's airway, or the infection may spread to the tissues surrounding the heart. In extreme cases the empyema may spread to the brain by means of bacteria carried in the bloodstream.

In pelvic empyema, the infection produces large amounts of thick, foul-smelling pus that is rapidly replaced even after drainage. Empyema of the gall-bladder is marked by intense pain on the upper right side of the abdomen, high fever, and rigidity of the muscles over the infected area.

Diagnosis

A physician may consider the possibility of empyema thoracis in patients with pneumonia or other symptoms of lung infection. When listening to sounds within the patient's chest with a stethoscope, the sounds of breathing will be partly muffled and harder to hear in the patients with empyema. The area of the chest over the infection will sound dull when tapped or thumped (percussed). On an x ray, empyema thoracis will appear as a cloudy or opaque area. The amount of fluid present in the pleural cavity can be estimated using an ultrasound imaging procedure. The diagnosis of empyema, however, has to be confirmed with laboratory tests because its symptoms can be caused by other disease conditions.

Abscess—An area of inflamed and injured body tissue that fills with pus.

Decortication—Surgical removal of the fibrous peel that covers the lungs in third-stage empyema.

Empyema—The collection of pus in a body cavity, particularly the lung or pleural cavity.

Fibrin—A fibrous blood protein vital to coagulation and blood clot formation.

Percussion—A diagnostic technique in which the back, chest, or abdomen is tapped to determine whether body cavities contain abnormal fluid.

Pleural cavity—The space surrounding the lungs, including the membranes covering the lungs and lining the inside of the chest wall.

Pneumonia—Inflammation of the lungs usually caused by a virus, bacteria, or other organism.

Resection—The surgical removal of part of an organ or body structure, as in rib resection.

Suppurate—To produce or discharge pus.

Thoracentesis—A procedure in which fluid is withdrawn from the pleural cavity through a needle inserted between the ribs. The fluid may be withdrawn either for diagnostic tests or to drain the cavity.

Video-assisted thoracic surgery (VATS)—A technique used to aid in the placement of chest tubes or when performing decortications when treating advanced empyema.

The diagnosis of empyema is usually confirmed by analyzing a sample of fluid taken from the pleural cavity. The sample is obtained by a procedure called **thoracentesis**. In this procedure, the patient is given a local anesthetic, a needle is inserted into the pleural cavity through the back between the ribs on the infected side, and a sample of fluid is withdrawn. If the patient has empyema, there will be a very high level of one particular kind of immune cell (white blood cells), a high level of protein, and a very low level of blood sugar. The fluid can also be tested for the specific disease organism by staining or tissue cultures. In some cases, the color, smell, or consistency of the tissue fluid also helps to confirm the diagnosis.

Treatment

Empyema is treated using a combination of medications and surgical techniques. Treatment with medication involves intravenously administering a two-week course of **antibiotics**. It is important to give antibiotics as soon as possible to prevent first-stage empyema from progressing to its later stages. The antibiotics most commonly used are penicillin and vancomycin. Patients experiencing difficulty breathing are also given **oxygen therapy**.

Surgical treatment of empyema has two goals: drainage of the infected fluid and closing up of the space left in the pleural cavity. If the infection is still in its early stages, the fluid can be drained by thoracentesis. In second-stage empyema, the surgeon will insert a chest tube in the patient's rib cage or remove part of a rib (rib resection) in order to drain the fluid. In third-stage empyema, the surgeon may cut or peel away the thick fibrous layer coating the lung. This procedure is called decortication. When the fibrous covering is removed, the lung will expand to fill the space in the chest cavity. The doctor can use video-assisted **thoracic surgery** (VATS) techniques to position the chest tube or to perform a limited decortication. The VATS technique allows a physician to see within the body during certain surgical procedures. Empyema of the gallbladder is a serious condition that is treated with intravenous antibiotics and surgical removal of the gallbladder.

Prognosis

The prognosis for recovery is generally good, except in those cases with complications, such as a **brain abscess** or blood poisoning, or cases caused by certain types of streptococci.

Resources

BOOKS

McPhee, Stephen, and Maxine Papadakis.*Current Medical Diagnosis and Treatment, 2010*, 49th ed. New York: McGraw–Hill Medical, 2009.

Rebecca J. Frey, PhD

Enalapril *see* **Angiotensin-converting enzyme inhibitors**

Encephalitis

Definition

Encephalitis is an inflammation of the brain, usually caused by a direct viral infection or a hypersensitivity reaction to a virus or foreign protein. Brain inflammation caused by a bacterial infection is sometimes called cerebritis. When both the brain and spinal cord are involved, the disorder is called encephalomyelitis. An inflammation of the brain's covering, or meninges, is called **meningitis**.

Description

Encephalitis is an inflammation of the brain. The inflammation is a reaction of the body's immune system to infection or invasion. During the inflammation, the brain's tissues become swollen. The combination of the infection and the immune reaction to it can cause **headache** and a **fever**, as well as more severe symptoms in some cases.

Approximately 2,000 cases of encephalitis are reported to the Centers for Disease Control in Atlanta, GA each year. The viruses causing primary encephalitis can be epidemic or sporadic. The **polio** virus is an epidemic cause. Arthropod-borne viral encephalitis is responsible for most epidemic viral encephalitis. The viruses live in animal hosts and mosquitos that transmit the disease. The most common form of non-epidemic or sporadic encephalitis is caused by the herpes simplex virus, type 1 (HSV-1) and has a high rate of **death. Mumps** is another example of a sporadic cause.

Causes and symptoms

Causes

There are more than a dozen viruses that can cause encephalitis, spread by either human-to human contact or by animal **bites**. Encephalitis may occur with several common viral infections of childhood. Viruses and viral diseases that may cause encephalitis include:

- chickenpox
- measles
- mumps
- Epstein-Barr virus (EBV)
- cytomegalovirus infection
- HIV
- herpes simplex
- herpes zoster (shingles)
- herpes B
- polio
- rabies
- mosquito-borne viruses (arboviruses)

Primary encephalitis is caused by direct infection by the virus, while secondary encephalitis is due to a post-infectious immune reaction to viral infection elsewhere in the body. Secondary encephalitis may occur with **measles**, **chickenpox**, mumps, **rubella**, and EBV. In secondary encephalitis, symptoms usually begin five to 10 days after the onset of the disease itself and are related to the breakdown of the myelin sheath that covers nerve fibers.

In rare cases, encephalitis may follow **vaccination** against some of the viral diseases listed above. **Creutzfeldt-Jakob disease**, a very rare brain disorder caused by an infectious particle called a prion, may also cause encephalitis.

Mosquitoes spread viruses responsible for equine encephalitis (eastern and western types), St. Louis encephalitis, California encephalitis, and **Japanese encephalitis**. **Lyme disease**, spread by ticks, can cause encephalitis, as can Colorado tick fever. **Rabies** is most often spread by animal bites from dogs, cats, mice, raccoons, squirrels, and bats and may cause encephalitis.

Equine encephalitis is carried by mosquitoes that do not normally bite humans but do bite horses and birds. It is occasionally picked up from these animals by mosquitoes that do bite humans. Japanese encephalitis and St. Louis encephalitis are also carried by mosquitoes. The risk of contracting a mosquito-borne virus is greatest in mid- to late summer, when mosquitoes are most active, in those rural areas where these viruses are known to exist. Eastern equine encephalitis occurs in eastern and southeastern United States; western equine and California encephalitis occur throughout the West; and St. Louis encephalitis occurs throughout the country. Japanese encephalitis does not occur in the United States, but is found throughout much of Asia. The viruses responsible for these diseases are classified as arbovirus and these diseases are collectively called **arbovirus encephalitis**.

Herpes simplex encephalitis, the most common form of sporadic encephalitis in western countries, is a disease with significantly high mortality. It occurs in children and adults and both sides of the brain are affected. It is theorized that brain infection is caused by the virus moving from a peripheral location to the brain via two nerves, the olfactory and the trigeminal (largest nerves in the skull).

Cerebrospinal fluid analysis—A analysis that is important in diagnosing diseases of the central nervous system. The fluid within the spine will indicate the presence of viruses, bacteria, and blood. Infections such as encephalitis will be indicated by an increase of cell count and total protein in the fluid.

Computerized tomography (CT) Scan—A test to examine organs within the body and detect evidence of tumors, blood clots, and accumulation of fluids.

Electroencephalagram (EEG)—A chart of the brain waves picked up by the electrodes placed on the scalp. Changes in brain wave activity can be an indication of nervous system disorders.

Inflammation—A response from the immune system to an injury. The signs are redness, heat, swelling, and pain.

Magnetic resonance imaging (MRI)—MRI is diagnostic radiography using electromagnetic energy to create an image of the central nervous system (CNS), blood system, and musculoskeletal system.

Vaccine—A prepartation containing killed or weakened microorganisms used to build immunity against infection from that microorganism.

Virus—A very small organism that can only live within a cell. They are unable to reproduce outside that cell.

Herpes simplex encephalitis is responsible for 10% of all encephalitis cases and is the main cause of sporadic, fatal encephalitis. In untreated patients, the rate of death is 70% while the mortality is 15–20% in patients who have been treated with acyclovir. The symptoms of herpes simplex encephalitis are fever, rapidly disintegrating mental state, headache, and behavioral changes.

Symptoms

The symptoms of encephalitis range from very mild to very severe and may include:

- headache
- fever
- lethargy (sleepiness, decreased alertness, and fatigue)
- malaise
- nausea and vomiting
- visual disturbances
- tremor
- decreased consciousness (drowsiness, confusion, delirium, and unconsciousness)
- stiff neck
- seizures

Symptoms may progress rapidly, changing from mild to severe within several days or even several hours.

Diagnosis

Diagnosis of encephalitis includes careful questioning to determine possible exposure to viral sources. Tests that can help confirm the diagnosis and rule out other disorders include:

- Blood tests. These are to detect antibodies to viral antigens, and foreign proteins.
- Cerebrospinal fluid analysis (spinal tap). This detects viral antigens, and provides culture specimens for the virus or bacteria that may be present in the cerebrospinal fluid.
- Electroencephalogram (EEG).
- CT and MRI scans.

A **brain biopsy** (surgical gathering of a small tissue sample) may be recommended in some cases where treatment to date has been ineffective and the cause of the encephalitis is unclear. Definite diagnosis by biopsy may allow specific treatment that would otherwise be too risky.

Treatment

Choice of treatment for encephalitis will depend on the cause. Bacterial encephalitis is treated with **antibiotics**. Viral encephalitis is usually treated with **antiviral drugs** including acyclovir, ganciclovir, foscarnet, ribovarin, and AZT. Viruses that respond to acyclovir include herpes simplex, the most common cause of sporadic (non-epidemic) encephalitis in the United States.

The symptoms of encephalitis may be treated with a number of different drugs. **Corticosteroids**, including prednisone and dexamethasone, are sometimes prescribed to reduce inflammation and brain swelling. **Anticonvulsant drugs**, including dilantin and phenytoin, are used to control seizures. Fever may be reduced with **acetaminophen** or other fever-reducing drugs.

A person with encephalitis must be monitored carefully, since symptoms may change rapidly. Blood tests may be required regularly to track levels of fluids and salts in the blood.

Prognosis

Encephalitis symptoms may last several weeks. Most cases of encephalitis are mild, and recovery is usually quick. Mild encephalitis usually leaves no residual neurological problems. Overall, approximately 10% of those with encephalitis die from their infections or complications such as secondary infection. Some forms of encephalitis have more severe courses, including herpes encephalitis, in which mortality is 15–20% with treatment, and 70–80% without. Antiviral treatment is ineffective for eastern equine encephalitis, and mortality is approximately 30%.

Permanent neurological consequences may follow recovery in some cases. Consequences may include personality changes, **memory loss**, language difficulties, seizures, and partial **paralysis**.

Prevention

Because encephalitis is due to infection, it may be prevented by avoiding the infection. Minimizing contact with others who have any of the viral illnesses listed above may reduce the chances of becoming infected. Most infections are spread by hand-to-hand or hand-to-mouth contact; frequent hand washing may reduce the likelihood of infection if contact cannot be avoided.

Mosquito-borne viruses may be avoided by preventing mosquito bites. Mosquitoes are most active at dawn and dusk, and are most common in moist areas with standing water. Minimizing exposed skin and use of mosquito repellents on other areas can reduce the chances of being bitten.

Vaccines are available against some viruses, including polio, herpes B, Japanese encephalitis, and equine encephalitis. Rabies vaccine is available for animals; it is also given to people after exposure. Japanese encephalitis vaccine is recommended for those traveling to Asia and staying in affected rural areas during transmission season.

ORGANIZATIONS
Centers for Disease Control and Prevention (CDC), 1600 Clifton Road, Atlanta, GA, 30333, (800) 232-4636, cdcinfo@cdc.gov, http://www.cdc.gov.

Richard Robinson

Encephalocele *see* **Congenital brain defects**

Encopresis

Definition

Encopresis is repeatedly having bowel movements in places other than the toilet after the age when bowel control can normally be expected.

Description

Most children have established bowel control by the time they are four years old. After that age, when they repeatedly have bowel movements in inappropriate places, they may have encopresis. In the United States, encopresis affects 1–2% of children under age 10. About 80% of these are boys.

Encopresis can be either involuntary or voluntary. Involuntary encopresis is related to **constipation**, passing hard painful feces, and difficult bowel movements. Often children with involuntary encopresis stain their underpants with liquid feces. They are usually unaware that this has happened. Voluntary encopresis is much less common and is associated with behavioral or psychological problems. Both types of encopresis occur most often when the child is awake, rather than at night.

Causes and symptoms

Although a few children experience encopresis because of malformations of the lower bowel and anus or irritable bowel disease, most have no physical problems to explain this disorder. Constipation is present in about 80% of children who experience involuntary encopresis. As feces moves through the large intestine, water is removed. The longer the feces stays in the large intestine, the more water is removed, and the harder the feces becomes. The result can be hard or painful bowel movements. In response, children may start to hold back when they feel the urge to eliminate in order to avoid **pain**. This starts a cycle of constipation that results in retentive encopresis.

Once elimination is avoided, the bowel becomes full of hard feces. This stretches the large intestine. Eventually the intestine becomes so stretched that liquid feces backed up behind the blockage is able to leak around the hard feces. Children with this type of encopresis do not feel the urge to have a bowel movement and are often surprised when their pants are stained with foul smelling liquid feces. This leakage of feces is called overflow incontinence. Parents sometimes mistake this soiling for **diarrhea**, because the feces expelled is liquid. Every so often, children with involuntary encopresis may pass large stools, sometimes with volumes big enough to clog the toilet, but the relief this brings is temporary.

Although about 95% of encopresis is involuntary, some children intentionally withhold bowel movements. The American Psychiatric Association (APA) recognizes voluntary encopresis without constipation as a psychological disorder. This disorder is said to occur when a child who has control over his bowel movements chooses to have them in an inappropriate place. The feces is a normal consistency, not hard. Sometimes it is smeared in an obvious place, but it may also be hidden from adults.

Voluntary encopresis may result from a power struggle between caregivers and the child during toilet training, or the child may have developed an unusual fear of the toilet. It is also associated with **oppositional defiant disorder** (ODD), **conduct disorder**, **sexual abuse**, and high levels of psychological **stress**. For example, children who were separated from their parents during World War II were reported to have a high rate of encopresis. However, parents and caregivers should be aware that very few children soil intentionally and most do not have a behavioral or psychological problem and should not be punished for their soiling accidents.

Diagnosis

Diagnosis is based primarily on the child's history of inappropriate bowel movements. Physical examinations are almost always normal, except for a mass of hard feces blocking the lower intestine. Other physical causes of soiling, such as illness, reaction to medication, **food allergies**, and physical disabilities, may also be ruled out through history and a **physical examination**. In addition, to be diagnosed with encopresis the child must be old enough to establish regular bowel control—usually chronologically and developmentally at least four years of age.

Treatment

The goal of treatment is to establish regular, soft, pain free bowel movements in the toilet. First the physician tries to determine the cause of encopresis, whether physical or psychological. Regardless of the cause, the bowel must be emptied of hard, impacted feces This can be done using an enema, **laxatives**, and/or stool softeners such as mineral oil. **Enemas** and laxatives should be used only at a doctor's recommendation.

Next, the child is given stool softeners to keep feces soft and to give the stretched intestine time to shrink back to its normal size. This shrinking process may take several months, during which time stool softeners may need to be used regularly. Children also need two or three regularly scheduled toilet sits daily in an effort to

> ### KEY TERMS
>
> **Feces**—Waste products eliminated from the large intestine; excrement.
>
> **Incontinence**—The inability to control the release of urine or feces.
>
> **Laxative**—Material that encourages a bowel movement.
>
> **Stools**—Feces; bowel movements.

establish consistent bowel habits. These toilet sits are often more effective if done after meals. Maintaining soft, easy-to-pass stools is also important if the child is afraid of the toilet because of past painful bowel movements. A child psychologist or psychiatrist can suggest treatment for the rare child with serious behavioral problems such as smearing or hiding feces.

Alternative treatment

Many herbal stool softeners and laxatives are available as both tablets and liquids. Psyllium, the seed of several plants of the genus *Plantago* is one of the most effective. Other natural remedies for constipation include castor seed oil (*Ricinus communis*), senna (*Cassia senna* or *Senna alexandrina*), and dong quai *Angelica polymorpha* or *Angelica sinensis*).

Prognosis

For almost all children, once constipation is controlled, the problem of soiling disappears. This make take several months, and relapses may occur, but with effective prevention strategies, encopresis can be eliminated. Children who are in a power struggle over toileting usually outgrow their desire to have bowel movements in inappropriate places. The prognosis for children with serious behavioral and psychological problems that result in smearing or hiding feces depends largely on resolving the underlying problems.

Prevention

The best way to prevent encopresis is to prevent constipation. Methods of preventing constipation include:

- increasing the amount of liquids, especially water, the child drinks
- adding high fiber foods to the diet (e.g. dried beans, fresh fruits and vegetables, whole wheat bread and pasta, popcorn)

- establishing regular bowel habits
- limiting the child's intake of dairy products (e.g. milk, cheese, yogurt, ice cream) that promote constipation.
- treating constipation promptly with stool softeners, so that it does not become worse.

Resources

BOOKS

Christophersen, Edward R., and Patrick C Friman.*Elimination Disorders in Children and Adolescents*, Cambridge, MA; Toronto: Hogrefe, 2010.

OTHER

Borowitz, Stephen. *Encopresis,*March 8, 2010 [cited October 16, 2010]. http://emedicine.medscape.com/article/928795-overview.

ORGANIZATIONS

American Academy of Child and Adolescent Psychiatry (AACAP), 3615 Wisconsin Ave. NW, Washington, DC, 20013-3007, (202) 966-7300, (202) 966-2891, communications@aacap.org, http://www.aacap.org.

Tish Davidson, A.M.

Endarterectomy

Definition

Endarterectomy is an operation to remove or bypass the fatty deposits, or blockage, in an artery narrowed by the buildup of fatty tissue (**atherosclerosis**).

Purpose

Removing the fatty deposits restores normal blood flow to the part of the body supplied by the artery. An endarterectomy is performed to treat cerebrovascular disease in which there is a serious reduction of blood supply to the brain (carotid endarterectomy), or to treat **peripheral vascular disease** (impaired blood supply to the legs).

Endarterectomy is most often performed on one of the two main arteries in the neck (the carotids) opening the narrowed arteries leading to the brain. When performed by an experienced surgeon, the practice is extremely effective, reducing the risk of **stroke** by up to 70%. Recent studies indicate it is effective in preventing stroke, even among those patients who had no warning signs except narrowed arteries detected by their doctors on a routine exam.

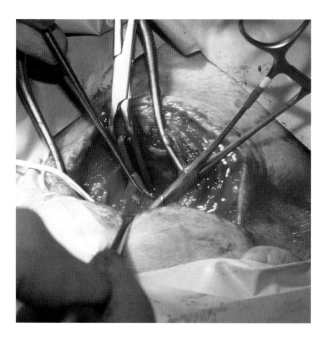

In this procedure, surgeons are removing plaque from the carotid artery. *(Custom Medical Stock Photo, Inc. Reproduced by permission.)*

Precautions

Before the surgery, a full medical exam is usually done to assess any specific health problems, such as diabetes, high blood pressure, heart disease, or stroke. If possible, reversible health problems, such as cigarette **smoking** or being overweight, should be corrected.

Description

Carotid artery disease

Every person has four carotid arteries (the internal and external carotids on each side of the neck) through which blood from the heart moves into the brain. If one of these arteries becomes blocked by fat and cholesterol, the patient may have a range of symptoms, including:

- weakness in one arm, leg, half of the face, or one entire side of the body
- numbness or tingling
- paralysis of an arm, leg, or face
- slurred speech
- dizziness
- confusion, fainting, or coma
- stroke

Removing this fatty buildup, or bypassing a blocked segment, may restore blood flow to the brain, eliminate or decrease the symptoms, and lessen the risk of a stroke.

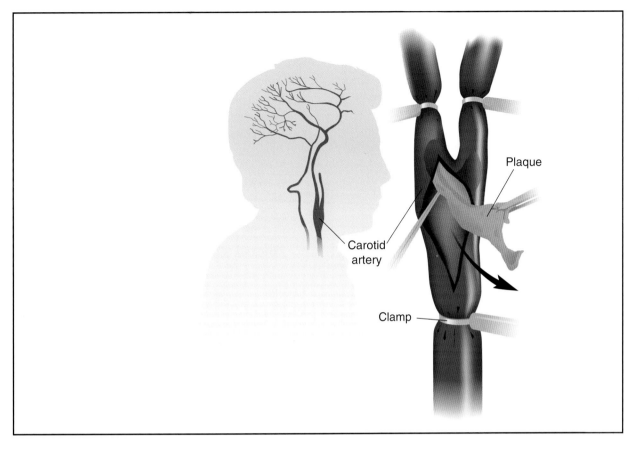

Plaque is removed from the carotid artery by clamping the artery, cutting the plaque out, and closing the opening back up.
(Illustration by Argosy, Inc. Reproduced by permission of Gale, a part of Cengage Learning.)

Peripheral vascular disease

When the blood vessels in the legs (and sometimes the arms) become narrowed, this can restrict blood flow and cause **pain** in the affected area. In severe cases, the tissue may die, requiring **amputation**.

The narrowing is usually caused by buildup of fatty plaques in the vessels, often as the result of smoking, high blood pressure, or poorly-controlled **diabetes mellitus**. The vessels usually narrow slowly, but it's possible for a blood clot to form quickly, causing sudden severe pain in the affected leg or arm.

Procedure

Endarterectomy is a delicate operation that may require several hours. The surgeon begins by making an incision over the blocked artery and inserting a tube above and below the blockage to redirect the blood flow while the artery is opened.

Next, the surgeon removes the fat and cholesterol buildup, along with any **blood clots** that have formed, with a blunt dissecting instrument. Then the surgeon

bathes the clean wall in salt solution combined with heparin, an anticoagulant. Then the surgeon stitches the artery just enough so that the bypass shunt tube can be removed, and then he/she stitches the artery completely closed. After checking to make sure no blood is leaking, the surgeon next closes the skin incision with stitches.

The operation should improve symptoms, although its long-term effects may be more limited, since arterial narrowing is rarely confined to one area of one artery. If narrowing is a problem throughout the body, arterial **reconstructive surgery** may be required.

The total cost of an endarterectomy, including diagnostic tests, surgery, hospitalization, and follow-up care, will vary according to hospital, doctor, and area of the country where the operation is performed, but a patient can expect to pay in the range of $15,000. Patients who are very young, very old, or very ill, or who need more extensive surgery, may require more expensive treatment.

Preparation

Before surgery, the doctor pinpoints the location of the narrowed artery with an x-ray procedure called

Carotid arteries—The four principal arteries of the neck and head. There are two common carotid arteries, each of which divides into the two main branches (internal and external).

Diabetes mellitus—A disorder in which the pancreas doesn't produce enough (or any) insulin. As a result, the blood levels of sugar become very high. Among other things, diabetes can lead to the breakdown of small

blood vessels and a high risk of atherosclerosis and high blood pressure.

Stroke—Damage to the part of the brain caused by an interruption of the blood supply. In some cases, small pieces of plaque in the carotid artery may break loose and block an artery in the brain. A narrowed carotid artery also can be the source of blood clots travelling to the brain, or the artery can become completely clogged, blocking all blood flow to the brain.

angiography. For surgery to be effective, the degree of narrowing should be at least 70%, but it should not be total. Patients undergoing angiography are given a local anesthetic, but the endarterectomy itself requires the use of a **general anesthesia**.

Aftercare

After the surgery, the patient spends the first two days lying flat in bed. Patients who have had carotid endarterectomy should not bend the neck sharply during this time. Because the blood flow to the brain is now greatly increased, patients may experience a brief but severe **headache**, or lightheadedness. There may be a slight loss of sensation in the skin, or maybe a droop in the mouth, if any of the nerves in the neck were lightly bruised during surgery. In time, this should correct itself.

Risks

The amount of risk depends on the hospital, the skill of the surgeon, and the severity of underlying disease. Patients who have just had an acute stroke are at greatest risk. During carotid artery surgery, blood flow is interrupted through the artery, so that **paralysis** and other stroke symptoms may occur. These may resolve after surgery, or may result in permanent stroke. Paralysis is usually one-sided; other stroke symptoms may include loss of half the field of vision, loss of sensation, double vision, speech problems, and personality changes. Risks of endarterectomy to treat either carotid artery or peripheral **vascular disease** include:

- reactions to anesthesia
- bleeding
- infection
- blood clots

Normal results

The results after successful surgery are usually striking. The newly opened artery should help to restore normal blood flow. In carotid endarterectomy, surgery should prevent the risk of brain damage and stroke. However, the buildup of fat and cholesterol usually affects all arteries, not just the one that was operated on. Affected arteries in other parts of the body may be equally clogged and potentially dangerous. Even arteries that were operated electively will likely begin to clog up again after the surgery.

For this reason, lifestyle changes (no smoking, low fat, low cholesterol diet) are important, especially if diet and lifestyle contributed to the development of the problem in the first place.

ORGANIZATIONS

National Institute of Neurological Disorders and Stroke (NINDS), NIH Neurological Institute, P. O. Box 5801, Bethesda, MD, 20824, (301) 496-5751, (800) 352-9424, http://www.ninds.nih.gov/.

Carol A. Turkington

Endemic syphilis *see* **Bejel**
Endocardial resection *see* **Myocardial resection**

Endocarditis

Definition

The endocardium is the inner lining of the heart muscle, which also covers the heart valves. When the endocardium becomes damaged, bacteria from the

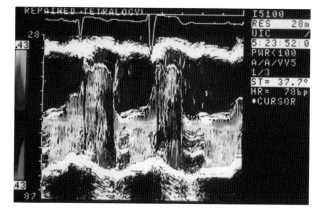

This echocardiogram shows an aortic regurgitation due to endocarditis, an infection of the lining membrane of the cardiac chambers. *(Custom Medical Stock Photo, Inc. Reproduced by permission.)*

blood stream can become lodged on the heart valves or heart lining. The resulting infection is known as endocarditis.

Description

The endocardium lines all four chambers of the heart–two at the top (the right and left atria) and two at the bottom (the right and left ventricles)–through which blood passes as the heart beats. It also covers the four valves (the tricuspid valve, the pulmonary valve, the mitral valve, and the aortic valve), which normally open and close to allow the blood to flow in

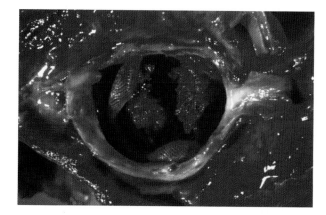

A close-up view of an infected artificial heart valve showing bacterial endocarditis (the granulated tissue at center of image). When infection occurs early after surgery, it is likely that organisms have gained entry during the operative period. This type of infection is usually caused by *Staphylococcus epidermidis* and *S. aureus* and is treated with antibiotic drugs. *(Dr. E. Walker/Photo Researchers, Inc.)*

only one direction through the heart during each contraction.

For the heart to pump blood efficiently, the four chambers must contract and relax, and the four valves must open and close, in a well coordinated fashion. By damaging the valves or the walls of the heart chambers, endocarditis can interfere with the ability of the heart to do its job.

Endocarditis rarely occurs in people with healthy, normal hearts. Rather, it most commonly occurs when there is damage to the endocardium. The endocardium may be affected by a congenital heart defect, such as **mitral valve prolapse**, in which blood leaks through a poorly functioning mitral valve back into the heart. It may also be damaged by a prior scarring of the heart muscle, such as **rheumatic fever**, or replacement of a heart valve. Any of these conditions can damage the endocardium and make it more susceptible to infection.

Bacteria can get into the blood stream (a condition known as **bacteremia**) in a number of different ways: It may spread from a localized infection such as a **urinary tract infection**, **pneumonia**, or skin infection or get into the blood stream as a result of certain medical conditions, such as severe **periodontal disease**, **colon cancer**, or inflammatory bowel disease. It can enter the blood stream during minor procedures, such as periodontal surgery, tooth extractions, teeth cleaning, tonsil removal, prostate removal, or endoscopic examination. It can also be introduced through in-dwelling catheters, which are used for intravenous medications, intravenous feeding, or dialysis. In people who use intravenous drugs, the bacteria can enter the blood stream through unsterilized, contaminated needles and syringes. (People who are prone to endocarditis generally need to take prescribed **antibiotics** before certain surgical or dental procedures to help prevent this infection.)

If not discovered and treated, infective endocarditis can permanently damage the heart muscle, especially the valves. For the heart to work properly, all four valves must be functioning well, opening at the right time to let blood flow in the right direction and closing at the right time to keep the blood from flowing in the wrong direction. If the valve is damaged, this may allow blood to flow backward–a condition known as regurgitation. As a result of a poorly functioning valve, the heart muscle has to work harder to pump blood and may become weakened, leading to **heart failure**. Heart failure is a chronic condition in which the heart is unable to pump blood well enough to supply blood adequately to the body.

Another danger associated with endocarditis is that the vegetation formed by bacteria colonizing on

KEY TERMS

Aortic valve—The valve between the left ventricle of the heart and the aorta.

Bacteremia—An infection caused by bacteria in the blood.

Congestive heart failure—A condition in which the heart muscle cannot pump blood as efficiently as it should.

Echocardiography—A diagnostic test using reflected sound waves to study the structure and motion of the heart muscle.

Embolus—A bit of foreign material, such as gas, a piece of tissue, or tiny clot, that travels in the circulation until it becomes lodged in a blood vessel.

Endocardium—The inner wall of the heart muscle, which also covers the heart valves.

Mitral valve—The valve between the left atrium and the left ventricle of the heart.

Osler's nodes—Small, raised, reddish, tender areas associated with endocarditis, commonly found inside the fingers or toes.

Petechiae—Tiny purple or red spots on the skin associated with endocarditis, resulting from hemorrhages under the skin's surface.

Pulmonary valve—The valve between the right ventricle of the heart and the pulmonary artery.

Transducer—A device that converts electrical signals into ultrasound waves and ultrasound waves back into electrical impulses.

Transesophageal echocardiography—A diagnostic test using an ultrasound device, passed into the esophagus of the patient, to create a clear image of the heart muscle.

Tricuspid valve—The valve between the right atrium and the right ventricle of the heart.

Vegetation—An abnormal growth of tissue around a valve, composed of blood platelets, bacteria, and a protein involved in clotting.

heart valves may break off, forming emboli. These emboli may travel through the circulation and become lodged in blood vessels. By blocking the flow of blood, emboli can starve various tissues of nutrients and oxygen, damaging them. For instance, an embolus lodged in the blood vessels of the lungs may cause pneumonia-like symptoms. An embolus may also affect the brain, damaging nerve tissue, or the kidneys, causing **kidney disease**. Emboli may also weaken the tiny blood vessels called capillaries, causing hemorrhages (leaking blood vessels) throughout the body.

Causes and symptoms

Most cases of infective endocarditis occur in people between the ages of 15 and 60, with a median age at onset of about 50 years. Men are affected about twice as often as women are. Other factors that put people at increased risk for endocarditis are congenital heart problems, heart surgery, previous episodes of endocarditis, and intravenous drug use.

While there is no single specific symptom of endocarditis, a number of symptoms may be present. The most common symptom is a mild **fever**, which rarely goes above 102°F (38.9°C). Other symptoms include chills, weakness, **cough**, trouble breathing, headaches, aching joints, and loss of appetite.

Emboli may also cause a variety of symptoms, depending on their location. Emboli throughout the body may cause Osler's nodes, small, reddish, painful bumps most commonly found on the inside of fingers and toes. Emboli may also cause petechiae, tiny purple or red spots on the skin, resulting from hemorrhages under the skin's surface. Tiny hemorrhages resembling splinters may also appear under the fingernails or toenails. If emboli become lodged in the blood vessels of the lungs, they may cause coughing or **shortness of breath**. Emboli lodged in the brain may cause symptoms of a mini-stroke, such as **numbness**, weakness, or **paralysis** on one side of the body or sudden vision loss or double vision. Emboli may also damage the kidneys, causing blood to appear in the urine. Sometimes the capillaries on the surface of the spleen rupture, causing the spleen to become enlarged and tender to the touch. Anyone experiencing any of these symptoms should seek medical help immediately.

Diagnosis

Doctors begin the diagnosis by taking a history, asking the patient about the symptoms mentioned above. During a **physical examination**, the doctor may also uncover signs such as fever, an enlarged spleen, signs of kidney disease, or hemorrhaging. Listening to the patient's chest with a stethoscope, the doctor may also hear a heart murmur. A heart murmur may indicate abnormal flow of blood through one of the heart chambers or valves.

Doctors take a sample of the patient's blood to test it for bacteria and other microorganisms that may be causing the infection. They usually also use a test called **echocardiography**, which uses ultrasound waves to make images of the heart, to check for abnormalities in the structure of the heart wall or valves. One of the tell-tale signs they look for in echocardiography is vegetation, the abnormal growth of tissue around a valve composed of blood platelets, bacteria, and a clotting protein called fibrin. Another tell-tale sign is regurgitation, or the backward flow of blood, through one of the heart valves. A normal echocardiogram does not exclude the possibility of endocarditis, but an abnormal echocardiogram can confirm its presence. If an echocardiogram cannot be done or its results are inconclusive, a modified technique called **transesophageal echocardiography** is sometimes performed. Transesophageal echocardiography involves passing an ultrasound device into the esophagus to get a clearer image of the heart.

Treatment

When doctors suspect infective endocarditis, they will admit the patient to a hospital and begin treating the infection before they even have the results of the **blood culture**. Their choice of antibiotics depends on what the most likely infecting microorganism is. Once the results of the blood culture become available, the doctor can adjust the medications, using specific antibiotics known to be effective against the specific microorganism involved.

Unfortunately, in recent years, the treatment of endocarditis has become more complicated as a result of antibiotic resistance. Over the past few years, especially as antibiotics have been overprescribed, more and more strains of bacteria have become increasingly resistant to a wider range of antibiotics. For this reason, doctors may need to try a few different types of antibiotics–or even a combination of antibiotics–to successfully treat the infection. Antibiotics are usually given for about one month, but may need to be given for an even longer period of time if the infection is resistant to treatment.

Once the fever and the worst of the symptoms have gone away, the patient may be able to continue antibiotic therapy at home. During this time, the patient should make regular visits to the health care team for further testing and physical examination to make sure that the antibiotic therapy is working, that

it is not causing adverse side effects, and that there are no complications such as emboli or heart failure. The patient should alert the health-care team to any symptoms that could indicate serious complications: For instance, trouble breathing or swelling in the legs could indicate congestive heart failure. **Headache**, joint **pain**, blood in the urine, or **stroke** symptoms could indicate an embolus, and fever and chills could indicate that the treatment is not working and the infection is worsening. Finally, **diarrhea**, rash, **itching**, or joint pain may suggest a bad reaction to the antibiotics. Anyone experiencing any of these symptoms should alert the health care team immediately.

In some cases, surgery may be needed. These include cases of congestive heart failure, recurring emboli, infection that doesn't respond to treatment, poorly functioning heart valves, and endocarditis involving prosthetic (artificial) valves. The most common surgical treatment involves cutting away (debriding) damaged tissue and replacing the damaged valve.

Prognosis

If left untreated, infective endocarditis continues to progress and is always fatal. However, if it is diagnosed and properly treated within the first six weeks of infection, the infection can be completely cured in about 90% of the cases. The prognosis depends on a number of factors, such as the patient's age and overall physical condition, the severity of the diseases involved, the exact site of the infection, how vulnerable the microorganisms are to antibiotics, and what kind of complications the endocarditis may be causing.

Prevention

Some people are especially prone to endocarditis. These include people with past episodes of endocarditis, those with congenital heart problems or heart damage from rheumatic fever, and those with artificial heart valves. Intravenous drug users are also at increased risk. Anyone who falls into a high-risk category should alert his or her health-care professionals before undergoing any surgical or dental procedures. High-risk patients must be treated in advance with antibiotics before these procedures to minimize the risk of infection.

Resources

BOOKS

Brusch, John L.*Endocarditis Essentials 2011.* Sudbury, MA: Jones & Bartlett Learning, 2011.

ORGANIZATIONS

American Heart Association National Center, 7272 Greenville Avenue, Dallas, TX, 75231, (800) 242-8721, Review.personal.info@heart.org.

National Heart Lung and Blood Institute Health Information Center, P.O. Box 30105, Bethesda, MD, 20824-0105, (301) 592-8573, (240) 629-3246, http://www.nhlbi.nih.gov.

Robert Scott Dinsmoor

Endocrine pancreatic cancer *see* **Pancreatic cancer, endocrine**

Endometrial biopsy

Definition

Endometrial biopsy is a procedure in which a sample of the endometrium (tissue lining the inside of the uterus) is removed for microscopic examination.

Purpose

The test is most often performed to find out the cause of abnormal uterine bleeding. Abnormal bleeding includes bleeding between menstrual periods, excessive bleeding during a menstrual period, or bleeding after **menopause**. Since abnormal uterine bleeding can indicate **cancer**, an endometrial biopsy is done to rule out **endometrial cancer** or hyperplasia (a potentially precancerous condition).

Endometrial biopsies are also done as a screening test for endometrial cancer in postmenopausal women on **hormone replacement therapy**. Hormone replacement therapy usually requires a woman to take estrogen and progesterone. An endometrial biopsy is particularly useful in cases where postmenopausal women take estrogen, but cannot take progesterone. Estrogen in the system without the balancing effect of progesterone has been linked to an increased risk of endometrial cancer.

An endometrial biopsy can be used as part of an **infertility** exam to rule out problems with the

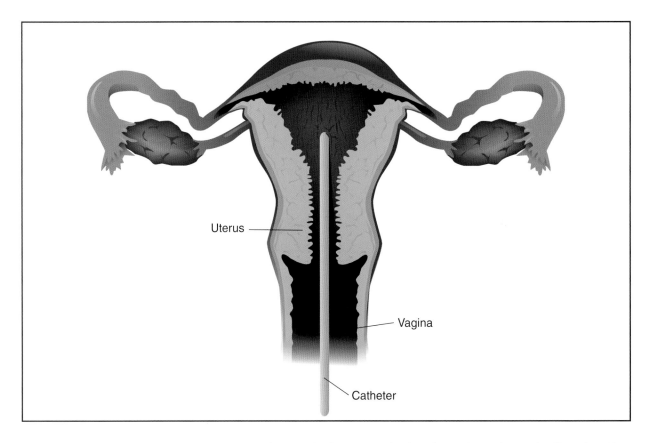

A catheter is inserted into the uterus to remove uterine cells for further examination. *(Illustration by Argosy, Inc. Reproduced by permission of Gale, a part of Cengage Learning.)*

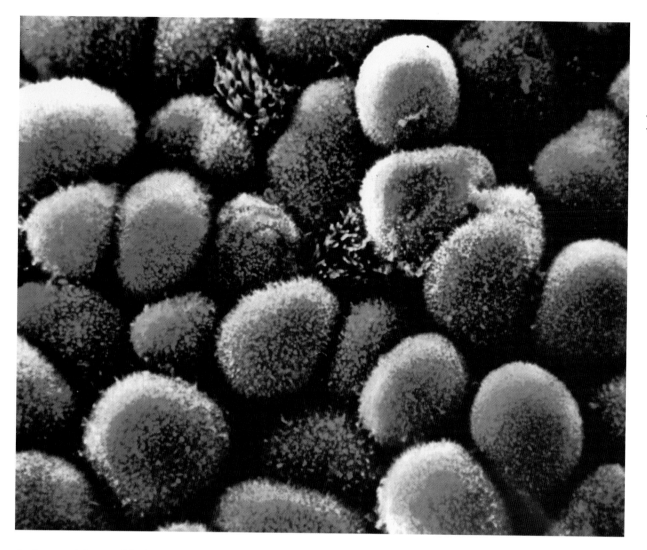

A micrograph image of the internal human uterine wall depicting the mucosa, or endometrium. *(Custom Medical Stock Photo, Inc. Reproduced by permission.)*

development of the endometrium. This condition is called luteal phase defect and can cause the endometrium to not support a **pregnancy**. An endometrial biopsy can also be used to evaluate the problem of repeated early miscarriages.

Description

The test is performed by a doctor who specializes in women's reproductive health (an obstetrician/gynecologist). The test is performed either in the doctor's office or in a local hospital. The patient may be asked to take **pain** medication (like ibuprofen) an hour or so before the procedure. A local anesthetic may be injected into the cervix in order to decrease pain and discomfort during the procedure.

The woman is asked to lie on her back with knees apart and feet in stirrups. The doctor first conducts a thorough exam of the pelvic region, including the vulva (the external genitals), vagina, and uterus. A speculum (an instrument that is used to hold the walls of the vagina open) is inserted into the vagina and then a small, hollow plastic tube is passed into the uterine cavity. A small piece of the uterine lining is evacuated with a plunger attached to the tube. Once the sample is obtained, the instruments are removed. The sample is sent to the laboratory for microscopic examination.

The patient may experience some pain when the cervix is grasped. The patient may also feel some cramping, pressure, and discomfort when the instruments are inserted into the uterus and the tissue sample is collected.

Preparation

For the small number of endometrial biopsies that are done as part of infertility testing, a pregnancy test is often performed before the procedure. Since the biopsy is performed late in the menstrual cycle, it is possible that the woman may be pregnant.

Aftercare

The biopsy may cause a small amount of bleeding (spotting). The woman can resume normal activities right away. If cramping becomes severe, heavy bleeding occurs, or the woman develops a high temperature, the doctor should be notified immediately.

If the test is being done to determine the cause of infertility, the onset of the menstrual period following the biopsy should be reported to the doctor. This will allow the doctor to correctly predict if the endometrium has been developing at the expected rate.

Risks

The risks of an endometrial biopsy are very small. There is a possibility that prolonged bleeding may occur after the procedure. There is also a slight chance of infection. Very rarely, there are instances when the uterus is pierced (perforated) or the cervix is torn because of the biopsy.

Results

Most biopsies are done to rule out endometrial cancer or endometrial hyperplasia. A normal result shows no cancerous or precancerous cells. Normal results also show that the uterine lining is changing at the proper rate. If it is, then the results of the biopsy are said to be "in-phase" because the tissue looks appropriate and has developed normally for the late phase of the menstrual cycle.

If the endometrium is not developing at the appropriate rate, the results are said to be "out-of-phase" or abnormal. The endometrium has not developed appropriately and cannot support a pregnancy. This condition is called luteal phase defect and may need to be treated with progesterone.

Abnormal appearance of the cells forming the uterine tissue could indicate uterine cancer, or the presence of fibroids or polyps in the uterus.

Resources

BOOKS

Katz, V.L. "Diagnostic Procedures: Imaging, Endometrial Sampling, Endoscopy: Indications and Contraindications." In Katz, V.L., Lentz, G.M., Lobo, R.A., Gershenson, D.M. Eds. *Comprehensive Gynecology.* 5th ed. Philadelphia: Mosby, 2007.

OTHER

"Endometrial Biopsy." *MedlinePlus.* September 2, 2009. http://www.nlm.nih.gov/medlineplus/ency/article/003917.htm (accessed October 3, 2010).

ORGANIZATIONS

American Cancer Society, (800) 227-2345, http://www.cancer.org.
Cancer Research Institute, One Exchange Plaza, 55 Broadway, Suite 1802, New York, NY, 10006, (800) 992-2623, http://www.cancerresearch.org.
Gynecologic Cancer Foundation, 230 W. Monroe, Suite 2528, Chicago, IL, 60606, (800) 444-4441, http://www.thegcf.org.
National Cancer Institute, Building 31, Room 10A31, 31 Center Drive, MSC 2580, Bethesda, MD, 20892-2580, (800) 422-6237, http://www.cancer.gov.

Lata Cherath, PhD
Melinda Granger Oberleitner
RN, DNS, APRN, CNS

Endometrial cancer

Definition

Endometrial **cancer** develops when the cells that make up the inner lining of the uterus (the endometrium) become abnormal and grow uncontrollably.

Description

Endometrial cancer (also called uterine cancer) is the fourth most common type of cancer among

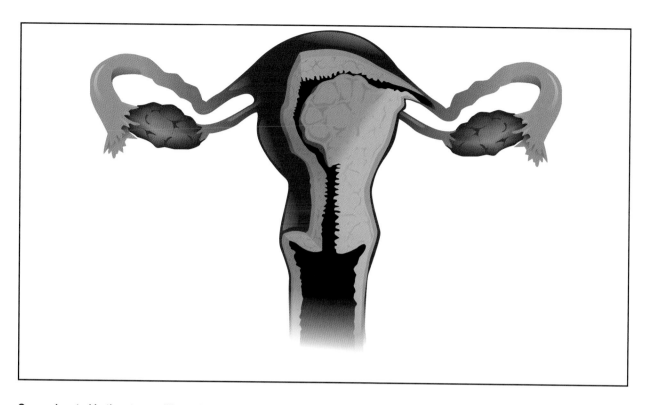

Cancer located in the uterus. *(Illustration by Argosy, Inc. Reproduced by permission of Gale, a part of Cengage Learning.)*

women and the most common gynecologic cancer. Approximately 34,000 women are diagnosed with endometrial cancer each year. In 2010, approximately 7,950 women died from this cancer. Although endometrial cancer generally occurs in women who have gone through **menopause** and are 45 years of age or older, 30% of the women with endometrial cancer are younger than 40 years of age. The average age at diagnosis is 60 years old.

The uterus, or womb, is the hollow female organ that supports the development of the unborn baby during **pregnancy**. The uterus has a thick muscular wall and an inner lining called the endometrium. The endometrium is very sensitive to hormones and it changes daily during the menstrual cycle. The endometrium is designed to provide an ideal environment for the fertilized egg to implant and begin to grow. If pregnancy does not occur, the endometrium is shed causing the menstrual period.

More than 95% of uterine cancers arise in the endometrium. The most common type of uterine cancer is adenocarcinoma. It arises from an abnormal multiplication of endometrial cells (atypical adenomatous hyperplasia) and is made up of mature, specialized cells (well-differentiated). Less commonly,

endometrial cancer arises without a preceding hyperplasia and is made up of poorly differentiated cells. The more common of these types are the papillary serous and clear cell carcinomas. Poorly differentiated endometrial cancers are often associated with a less promising prognosis.

The highest incidence of endometrial cancer in the United States is in Caucasians, Hawaiians, Japanese, and African Americans. American Indians, Koreans, and Vietnamese have the lowest incidence. African American and Hawaiian women are more likely to be diagnosed with advanced cancer and, therefore, have a higher risk of dying from the disease.

Causes and symptoms

Although the exact cause of endometrial cancer is unknown, it is clear that high levels of estrogen, when not balanced by progesterone, can lead to abnormal growth of the endometrium. Factors that increase a woman's risk of developing endometrial cancer are:

- Age. The risk is considerably higher in women who are over the age of 50 and have gone through menopause.
- Obesity. Being overweight is a very strong risk factor for this cancer. Fatty tissue can change other normal

body chemicals into estrogen, which can promote endometrial cancer.

- Estrogen replacement therapy. Women receiving estrogen supplements after menopause have a 12 times higher risk of getting endometrial cancer if progesterone is not taken simultaneously.

- Diabetes. Diabetics have twice the risk of getting this cancer as nondiabetic women. It is not clear if this risk is due to the fact that many diabetics are also obese and hypertensive. One 1998 study found that women who were obese and diabetic were three times more likely to develop endometrial cancer than women who were obese but nondiabetic. This study also found that nonobese diabetics were not at risk of developing endometrial cancer.

- Hypertension. High blood pressure (or hypertension) is also considered a risk factor for uterine cancer.

- Irregular menstrual periods. During the menstrual cycle, there is interaction between the hormones estrogen and progesterone. Women who do not ovulate regularly are exposed to high estrogen levels for longer periods of time. If a woman does not ovulate regularly, this delicate balance is upset and may increase her chances of getting uterine cancer.

- Early first menstruation or late menopause. Having the first period at a young age (the mean age of menses is 12.16 years in African American girls and 12.88 years in caucasian girls) or going through menopause at a late age (over age 51) seem to put women at a slightly higher risk for developing endometrial cancer.

- Tamoxifen. This drug, which is used to treat or prevent breast cancer, increases a woman's chance of developing endometrial cancer. Tamoxifen users tend to have more advanced endometrial cancer with an associated poorer survival rate than those who do not take the drug. In many cases, however, the value of tamoxifen for treating breast cancer and for preventing the cancer from spreading far outweighs the small risk of getting endometrial cancer.

- Family history. Some studies suggest that endometrial cancer runs in certain families. Women with inherited mutations in the BRCA1 and BRCA2 genes are at a higher risk of developing breast, ovarian, and other gynecologic cancers. Those with the hereditary nonpolyposis colorectal cancer gene have a higher risk of developing endometrial cancer.

- Breast, ovarian, or colon cancer. Women who have a history of these other types of cancer are at an increased risk of developing endometrial cancer.

- Low parity or nulliparity. Endometrial cancer is more common in women who have born few (low parity) or no (nulliparity) children. The high levels of progesterone produced during pregnancy has a protective effect against endometrial cancer. The results of one study suggest that nulliparity is associated with a lower survival rate.

- Infertility. Risk is increased due to nulliparity or the use of fertility drugs.

- Polycystic ovary syndrome. The increased level of estrogen associated with this abnormality raises the risk of cancers of the breast and endometrium.

The most common symptom of endometrial cancer is unusual vaginal spotting, bleeding, or discharge. In women who are near menopause (perimenopausal), symptoms of endometrial cancer could include bleeding between periods (intermenstrual bleeding), heavy bleeding that lasts for more than seven days, or short menstrual cycles (fewer than 21 days). For women who have gone through menopause, any vaginal bleeding or abnormal discharge is suspect. **Pain** in the pelvic region and the presence of a lump (mass) are symptoms that occur late in the disease.

Diagnosis

If endometrial cancer is suspected, a series of tests will be conducted to confirm the diagnosis. The first step will involve taking a complete personal and family medical history. A **physical examination**, which will include a thorough pelvic examination, will also be done.

The doctor may order an **endometrial biopsy**. This is generally performed in the doctor's office and does not require anesthesia. A thin, flexible tube is inserted through the cervix and into the uterus. A small piece of endometrial tissue is removed. The patient may experience some discomfort, which can be minimized by taking an anti-inflammatory medication (like Advil or Motrin) an hour before the procedure.

If an adequate amount of tissue was not obtained by the endometrial biopsy, or if the biopsy tissue looks abnormal but confirmation is needed, the doctor may perform a **dilatation and curettage** (D & C). This procedure is done in the outpatient surgery department of a hospital and takes about an hour. The patient may be given **general anesthesia**. The doctor dilates the cervix and uses a special instrument to scrape tissue from inside the uterus.

The tissue that is obtained from the biopsy or the D & C is sent to a laboratory for examination. If cancer is found, then the type of cancer will be determined. The treatment and prognosis depends on the type and stage of the cancer.

Trans-vaginal ultrasound may be used to measure the thickness of the endometrium. For this painless procedure, a wand-like ultrasound transducer is inserted into the vagina to enable visualization and measurement of the uterus, the thickness of the uterine lining, and other pelvic organs.

Other possible diagnostic procedures include sonohysterography and **hysteroscopy**. For sonohysteroscopy, a small tube is passed through the cervix and into the uterus. A small amount of a salt water (saline) solution is injected through the tube to open the space within the uterus and allow ultrasound visualization of the endometrium. For hysteroscopy, a wand-like camera is passed through the cervix to allow direct visualization of the endometrium. Both of these procedures cause discomfort, which may be reduced by taking an anti-inflammatory medication prior to the procedure.

Treatment

Clinical staging

The International Federation of Gynecology and Obstetrics (FIGO) has adopted a staging system for endometrial cancer. The stage of cancer is determined after surgery. Endometrial cancer is categorized into four stages (I, II, III, and IV) that are subdivided (A, B, and possibly C) based on the depth or spread of cancerous tissue. Seventy percent of all uterine cancers are stage I, 10–15% are stage II, and the remainder are stages III and IV. The cancer is also graded (G1, G2, and G3) based upon microscopic analysis of the aggressiveness of the cancer cells.

The FIGO stages for endometrial cancer are:

- Stage I. Cancer is limited to the uterus.

- Stage II. Cancer involves the uterus and cervix.

- Stage III. Cancer has spread out of the uterus but is restricted to the pelvic region.

- Stage IV. Cancer has spread to the bladder, bowel, or other distant locations.

The mainstay of treatment for most stages of endometrial cancer is surgery. **Radiation therapy**, hormonal therapy, and **chemotherapy** are additional treatments (called adjuvant therapy). The necessity of adjuvant therapy is a controversial topic which should be discussed with the patient's treatment team.

Surgery

Most women with endometrial cancer, except those with stage IV disease, are treated with a **hysterectomy**. A simple hysterectomy involves the removal of the uterus. In a bilateral **salpingo-oophorectomy** with total hysterectomy, the ovaries, fallopian tubes, and uterus are removed. This may be necessary because endometrial cancer often spreads to the ovaries first. The lymph nodes in the pelvic region may also be biopsied or removed to check for metastasis. Hysterectomy is traditionally performed through an incision in the abdomen (laparotomy), however, endoscopic surgery (**laparoscopy**) with vaginal hysterectomy is also being used. Women with stage I disease may require no further treatment. However, those with higher grade disease will receive adjuvant therapy.

Radiation therapy

The decision to use radiation therapy depends on the stage of the disease. Radiation therapy may be used before surgery (preoperatively) and/or after surgery (postoperatively). Radiation given from a machine that is outside the body is called external radiation therapy. Sometimes applicators containing radioactive compounds are placed inside the vagina or uterus. This is called internal radiation therapy or brachytherapy and requires hospitalization.

Side effects are common with radiation therapy. The skin in the treated area may become red and dry. **Fatigue**, upset stomach, **diarrhea**, and **nausea** are also common complaints. Radiation therapy in the pelvic area may cause the vagina to become narrow (vaginal stenosis), making intercourse painful. **Premature menopause** and some problems with urination may also occur.

Chemotherapy

Chemotherapy is usually reserved for women with stage IV or recurrent disease because this therapy is not a very effective treatment for endometrial cancer. The **anticancer drugs** are given by mouth or intravenously. Side effects include stomach upset, **vomiting**, appetite loss, hair loss, mouth or vaginal sores, fatigue, menstrual cycle changes, and premature menopause. There is also an increased chance of infections.

Hormonal therapy

Hormonal therapy uses drugs like progesterone to slow the growth of endometrial cells. These drugs are usually available as pills. This therapy is usually reserved for women with advanced or recurrent

KEY TERMS

Adjuvant therapy—A treatment done when there is no evidence of residual cancer in order to aid the primary treatment. Adjuvant treatments for endometrial cancer are radiation therapy, chemotherapy, and hormone therapy.

Atypical adenomatous hyperplasia—The overgrowth of the endometrium. This precancerous condition is estimated to progress to cancer in one third of the cases.

Dilatation and curettage (D & C)—A procedure in which the doctor opens the cervix and uses a special instrument to scrape tissue from the inside of the uterus.

Endometrial biopsy—A procedure in which a sample of the endometrium is removed and examined under a microscope.

Endometrium—The mucosal layer lining the inner cavity of the uterus. The endometrium's structure changes with age and with the menstrual cycle.

Estrogen—A female hormone responsible for stimulating the development and maintenance of female secondary sexual characteristics.

Estrogen replacement therapy (ERT)—A treatment in which estrogen is used therapeutically during menopause to alleviate certain symptoms such as hot flashes. ERT has also been shown to reduce the risk of osteoporosis and heart disease in women.

Progesterone—A female hormone that acts on the inner lining of the uterus and prepares it for implantation of the fertilized egg.

Progestins—A female hormone, like progesterone, that acts on the inner lining of the uterus.

disease. Side effects include fatigue, fluid retention, and appetite and weight changes.

Alternative treatment

Although alternative and complementary therapies are used by many cancer patients, very few controlled studies on the effectiveness of such therapies exist. Mind-body techniques, such as prayer, **biofeedback**, visualization, **meditation**, and **yoga**, have not shown any effect in reducing cancer, but they can reduce **stress** and lessen some of the side effects of cancer treatments. Clinical studies of hydrazine sulfate found that it had no effect on cancer and even worsened the health and well-being of the study subjects. One clinical study of the drug amygdalin (Laetrile) found that it had no effect on cancer. Laetrile can be toxic and has caused deaths. Shark cartilage, although highly touted as an effective cancer treatment, is an improbable therapy that has not been the subject of clinical study.

The American Cancer Society has found that the "metabolic diets" pose serious risk to the patient. The effectiveness of the macrobiotic, Gerson, and Kelley **diets** and the Manner metabolic therapy has not been scientifically proven. The FDA was unable to substantiate the anticancer claims made about the popular Cancell treatment.

There is no evidence for the effectiveness of most over-the-counter herbal cancer remedies. Some herbals have shown an anticancer effect. As shown in clinical studies, Polysaccharide krestin, from the mushroom

Coriolus versicolor, has significant effectiveness against cancer. In a small study, the green alga *Chlorella pyrenoidosa* has been shown to have anticancer activity. In a few small studies, evening primrose oil has shown some benefit in the treatment of cancer.

Prognosis

Because it is possible to detect endometrial cancer early, the chances of curing it are excellent. The five year survival rates for endometrial cancer by stage are: 90%, stage I; 60%, stage II; 40%, stage III; and 5%, stage IV. Endometrial cancer most often spreads to the lungs, liver, bones, brain, vagina, and certain lymph nodes.

Prevention

Women (especially postmenopausal women) should report any abnormal vaginal bleeding or discharge to the doctor. Controlling **obesity**, blood pressure, and diabetes can help to reduce the risk of this disease. Women on estrogen replacement therapy have a substantially reduced risk of endometrial cancer if progestins are taken simultaneously. Long term use of birth control pills has been shown to reduce the risk of this cancer. Women who have irregular periods may be prescribed birth control pills to help prevent endometrial cancer. Women who are taking tamoxifen and those who carry the hereditary nonpolyposis colorectal cancer gene should be screened regularly, receiving annual pelvic examinations.

Resources

BOOKS

DeVita, Vincent T., Samuel Hellman, and Steven A Rosenberg.*Cancer: Principles and Practice of Oncology*. 7th ed. Philadelphia: Lippincott, Williams & Wilkins, 2005.

Diaz–Montes, Teresa, Lillie Shockney, and Gary R Shapiro*Johns Hopkins Medicine Patients' Guide to Uterine Cancer*. Sudbury, MA: Jones and Bartlett Publishers, 2010.

Hartmann, Lynn C., Charles L. Loprinzi, and Bobbie S Gostout.*Mayo Clinic Guide to Women's Cancers*.

Muggia, Franco M., and Esther Oliva*Uterine Cancer: Screening, Diagnosis, and Treatment*. Dordrecht, Nethelands; New York: Humana Press, 2009.

ORGANIZATIONS

American Cancer Society, 1599 Clifton Rd. NE, Atlanta, GA, 30329, (800) 227-2345, http://www.cancer.org.

Cancer Research Institute (National Headquarters), One Exchange Plaza, 55 Broadway, Suite 1802, New York, NY, (212) 688-7515, (212) 832-9376, (800) 992-2623, http://www.cancerresearch.org/.

Gynecologic Cancer Foundation, 230 W. Monroe, Suite 2528, Chicago, IL, 60606, (312) 578-1439, (312) 578-9769, info@thegcf.org, http://www.wcn.org/.

National Cancer Institute (National Institutes of Health), NCI Office of Communications and Education, 6116 Executive Blvd. Suite 300, Bethesda, MD, 20892-8322, (800) 4-CANCER (422-6237), cancergovstaff@mail. nih.gov, http://www.cancer.gov/.

Lata Cherath, PhD
Belinda Rowland, PhD

Endometriosis

Definition

Endometriosis is a condition in which bits of the tissue similar to the tissue lining the uterus (endometrium) grow in other parts of the body

Demographics

It is difficult to determine the exact number of women who have endometriosis because some never show symptoms, but estimates suggest that 6–8% of women of childbearing age in the United States have the condition. It most commonly is diagnosed in women between the ages of 25 and 40. Endometriosis can appear in the teenage girls, but rarely before the start of menstruation. It is seldom seen in postmenopausal women and occurs independent of race or

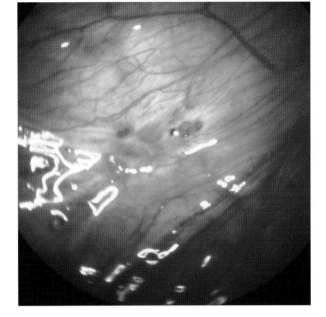

An endoscopic view of endometriosis on pelvic wall.
(Custom Medical Stock Photo, Inc. Reproduced by permission.)

ethnicity. The prevalence of endometriosis in the United States has remained stable since the early 1980s.

Description

Endometrial tissue like that lining the uterus sometimes develops in other parts of the body. These patches of misplaced endometrial tissue are called implants. Like the endometrial lining the uterus, this tissue builds up and sheds in response to monthly hormonal cycles (menstruation). However, there is no natural outlet for the material from these implants. Instead, it moves onto surrounding tissues, causing swelling, inflammation, and often **pain**. Repeated irritation leads to the development of scar tissue and **adhesions** in the area of the endometrial implants. Depending on their location, these **scars** may interfere with a woman's ability to conceive a child.

Endometrial implants are found most often on the pelvic organs—the ovaries, Fallopian tubes, and in the cavity behind the uterus. They can also be found on organs in the abdominal cavity such as the bladder and large intestine (colon). Occasionally, this tissue grows in distant parts of the body such as the lungs, arms, and kidneys.

Endometriosis is a progressive condition that usually advances slowly, over the course of many years. Doctors rank cases from minimal to severe based on factors such as the number and size of the endometrial implants, their appearance and location, and the extent of the scar tissue and adhesions in the vicinity of the growths.

Risk factors

If a first-degree female relative (mother, sister) has endometriosis, a woman has a higher risk of also developing the disorder. Another possible risk factor is the length of a woman's menstrual cycle. Women whose periods last longer than a week with an interval of less than 27 days between them seem to be more prone to the condition. This corresponds with studies that show that women with the most stable hormone levels are less likely to develop endometriosis. In addition, some studies have found that women who are tall and thin with a lower than average body mass index (BMI) are more likely to develop endometriosis, although there is no understanding of why this occurs.

Causes and symptoms

Endometriosis was once called the "career woman's disease" because it was thought to be a product of delayed childbearing. The statistics defy such a narrow generalization; however, the hormonal changes that accompany **pregnancy** may slow the progress of the condition.

Although the exact cause of endometriosis is unknown, several theories have been put forward to explain the origins of the disorder. These include:

• Retrograde (reverse) menstruation theory. Originally proposed in the 1920s, this theory states that a partial reversal in the direction of menstrual flow (a common event) sends discarded endometrial cells into the Fallopian tubes and then into the body cavity where they attach to internal organs and seed endometrial implants. There is considerable evidence to support this explanation. Reversed menstrual flow occurs in 70–90% of women and is thought to be more common in women with endometriosis. However, this does not explain why many women with retrograde menstrual flow do not develop endometriosis.

• Vascular-lymphatic theory. This theory suggests that the lymph system or blood vessels (vascular system) is the vehicle for the distribution of endometrial cells out of the uterus.

• Coelomic metaplasia theory. The endometrium and the peritoneal mesothelium arise from the same embryonic cells called coelomic wall epithelium. According to this hypothesis, some cells in the peritoneal mesothelium retain their embryonic ability to transform into endometrium, either spontaneously or after chronic irritation caused by exposure to retrograde menstrual flow.

• Iatrogenic theory. Iatrogenic disorders are those caused by the action of a physician. This theory suggests that surgery or procedures in the region of the woman's reproductive organs either deposits endometrial cells in inappropriate places where they grow or in some stimulates other cells to develop into endometrium.

In addition to these theories, the following factors are thought to influence the development of endometriosis:

• Heredity. A woman's chance of developing endometriosis is seven times greater if her mother or sisters have the disease.

• Immune system function. Women with endometriosis may have lower functioning immune systems that have trouble eliminating stray endometrial cells. This would explain why a high percentage of women experience reversed menstrual flow while relatively few develop endometriosis.

• Dioxin exposure. Some research suggests a link between the exposure to dioxin (TCCD), a toxic chemical found in weed killers, and the development of endometriosis.

While many women with endometriosis suffer debilitating chronic or acute pain symptom, others have none and are unaware they have the disorder. There does not, however, seem to be any relation between the severity of the symptoms and the extent of the disorder.

The most common symptoms of endometriosis are:

• Menstrual pain (dysmenorrhea). Pain in the lower abdomen that begins a day or two before the menstrual period starts and continues through to the end is typical of endometriosis. Some women also report lower back aches and pain during urination and bowel movement, especially during their periods.

• Painful sexual intercourse. Pressure on the vagina and cervix causes severe pain for some women.

• Abnormal bleeding. Heavy menstrual periods, irregular bleeding, and spotting are common features of endometriosis.

• Infertility. There is a strong association between endometriosis and infertility, although the reasons for this have not been fully explained. It is thought that the build up of scar tissue and adhesions blocks the Fallopian tubes and prevents the ovaries from

KEY TERMS

Adhesions—Web-like scar tissue that may develop as a result of surgery or a disease such as endometriosis and bind organs to one another.

Endometrial implants—Growths of endometrial tissue that attach to organs, primarily in the pelvic cavity.

Endometrium—The tissue lining the uterus that grows and sheds each month during a woman's menstrual cycle.

Estrogen—Any of several steroid hormones, produced mainly in the ovaries, that stimulate the development of the endometrium and the development of female secondary sexual characteristics.

Hormonal therapy—Use of hormone medications to inhibit menstruation and relieve the symptoms of endometriosis.

Iatrogenic—Resulting from the activity of the physician.

Laparoscopy—A diagnostic procedure, which when performed for endometriosis performed by inserting a slender, wand-like instrument through a small incision in the woman's abdomen.

Menopause—The end of a woman's menstrual periods when a woman no longer can conceive a child.

Retrograde menstruation—Menstrual flow that travels into the body cavity rather than being expelled through the uterus.

releasing eggs. Endometriosis may also affect fertility by causing hormonal irregularities and a higher rate of early miscarriage.

Diagnosis

If a doctor suspects endometriosis, the first step will be to perform a **pelvic exam** to try to feel if implants are present. Very often there is no strong evidence of endometriosis from a physical exam.

Tests

The only way to make a definitive diagnosis is through minor surgery called a **laparoscopy**. A laparoscope, a slender scope with a light on the end, is inserted into the woman's abdomen through a small incision near her belly button. This allows the doctor to examine the internal organs for endometriotic growths. Often, a sample of tissue (biopsy) is taken for later examination in the laboratory. Endometriosis is sometimes unintentionally discovered when a woman has abdominal surgery for another reason such as **tubal ligation** or **hysterectomy**.

Various imaging techniques such as transvaginal ultrasonography or endorectal ultrasonography, computed tomography scan (CT scan), **magnetic resonance imaging** (MRI) can offer some additional information but are not useful in making the initial diagnosis. They may be done, however, to rule out other conditions with similar symptoms. Various other tests such as a pregnancy test, may also be done to rule out other conditions. A test for the blood protein CA125 is not useful in making the initial diagnosis, but testing for this

substance before and after treatment can predict a recurrence of the disease.

Treatment

How endometriosis is treated depends on the woman's symptoms, her age, the extent of the disease, and her personal preferences. The condition cannot be fully eradicated without surgery. Conservative treatment focuses on managing the pain, preserving fertility, and delaying the progress of the condition.

Drugs

Over-the-counter pain relievers such as **aspirin** and **acetaminophen** (Tylenol) are useful for mild cramping and menstrual pain.)ver-the-counter or prescription-strength **nonsteroidal anti-inflammatory drugs** (NSAIDs), such as ibuprofen (Motrin, Advil) and naproxen (Aleve, Naprosyn), may be effective. If pain is severe, a doctor may prescribe narcotic pain medications, although these can be addicting and are rarely used.

Hormonal therapies may effectively treat symptoms of endometriosis, but they also act as contraceptives. Before beginning hormone treatment, a woman should discuss her reproductive plans with her physician.

The following hormonal treatments may be used to treat endometriosis:

- Oral contraceptives. Continuously taking estrogen-progestin pills tricks the body into thinking it is pregnant. This state of pseudo pregnancy may result in pelvic pain and a temporary withering of endometrial implants.

- Danazol (Danocrine) and gestrinone are synthetic male hormones that lower estrogen levels, prevent menstruation, and shrink endometrial tissues. Negative side effects include weight gain and menopause-like symptoms and cause some women to develop masculine characteristics.

- Progestins. Medroxyprogesterone (Depo-Provera) and related drugs also may be used in treating endometriosis. They have been proven effective in minimizing pain and halting the progress of the condition but are rarely used because of the high rate of side effects.

- Gonadotropin-releasing hormone (GnHR) agonists. These estrogen-inhibiting drugs successfully limit pain and prevent the growth of endometrial implants. They can cause menopause symptoms, however, and doses have to be closely regulated to prevent bone loss associated with low estrogen levels.

Surgery

Removing the uterus, ovaries, and Fallopian tubes is the only permanent method of eliminating endometriosis. This is an extreme measure that deprives a woman of her ability to bear children and forces her body into early **menopause**. In some cases, endometrial implants can be removed with **laser surgery** performed through a laparoscope. For women with minimal endometriosis, this technique usually is successful in reducing pain and slowing the condition's progress. It may help infertile women increase their chances of becoming pregnant.

Alternative therapies

Although severe endometriosis should not be self-treated, many women find they can help relieve symptoms through alternative therapies. In a survey conducted by the Endometriosis Association, 40% to 60% of the women who used alternative medicines reported relief of pain and other symptoms.

DIET. A high-fiber diet, particularly from grains and beans, may decrease cramping and inflammation. The oils in seeds, nuts, and certain fish (cod, salmon, mackerel, and sardines) may help to relieve cramping. Carrots, beets, lemons, cauliflower, Brussels sprouts, cabbage, onions, garlic, citrus fruits, vegetables, chicory, radicchio, and yogurt may help to reduce symptoms Sugar and animal fats can increase inflammation and aggravate pain. Milk and meat may contain hormones, so these should be avoided. Vegetarian or vegan **diets** may be recommended for those with

endometriosis. Occasionally, an allergy elimination diet may be recommended.

SUPPLEMENTS. The following supplements can be used to treat endometriosis:

- vitamin B complex to help the liver break down excess estrogen
- vitamin C to reduce heavy menstrual bleeding
- calcium
- bioflavonoids to help reduce heavy menstrual bleeding
- magnesium to relieve pain and flush out toxins
- vitamin E to heal inflamed tissues
- iron for anemia resulting from heavy bleeding
- lipotropic factors (Choline, methionine, and inositol enhance liver function)
- fish oil capsules, flax oil, or any essential fatty acid to reduce cramping

HERBAL REMEDIES. Several herbal remedies for endometriosis exist. The first four in this list are the most commonly used remedies:

- Genistein (soy/isoflavone) helps the body excrete excess estrogen and possibly blocks estrogen's effect.
- Cramp bark *(Viburnum opulus)* helps ease cramping
- Dong quai *(Angelica sinensis)* balances hormone levels and reduces inflammation.
- Black cohosh *Cimicifuga racemosa)* helps the body excrete excess estrogen and improves the health of pelvic organs.
- Red clover *(Trifolium pratense)* balances hormone levels.
- Milk thistle *(Silybum marianum)* may improve liver function.
- Life root *(Senecio aureus)* may improve the health of pelvic organs
- Feverfew *(Chrysanthemum parthenium)* eases pain and cramping.
- Dandelion eases pain and cramping and supports the liver.
- Yarrow *(Archillea millefolium)* eases cramping and restores hormonal balance.
- Evening primrose *(Oenothera biennis)* oil relieved endometriosis symptoms in 90% of patients in one study.
- Shepherd's purse *(Capsella bursa-pastoris)* reduces heavy menstrual bleeding and tones the uterus.
- Meadowsweet *(Filipendula ulmaria)* reduces pain.

OTHER THERAPIES. Other remedies for endometriosis include **acupuncture** or **acupressure** to relieve pain, visualization, **guided imagery**, naturopathy, homeopathy (Lilium tigrum, sepia, and belladonna), **hydrotherapy**, **exercise**, and **meditation**.

Home remedies

Studies have shown that by gradually increasing their level of physical activity some women are able to reduce their level of pelvic pain. However, for unknown reasons, this does not work for all women.

Prognosis

Most women who have endometriosis have minimal symptoms and do well with conservative treatment. Overall, endometriosis symptoms recur in an average of 40% of women over the five years following treatment. With hormonal therapy, pain returned after five years in 37% of patients with minimal symptoms and 74% of those with severe cases. The highest success rate followed complete removal of implants using laser surgery. Eighty percent of these women were still pain-free five years later. In cases that do not respond to these treatments, a woman and her doctor may consider surgery to remove her reproductive organs. The most serious complication from endometriosis is reduced fertility or complete **infertility**.

Prevention

There is no proven way to prevent endometriosis.

Resources

BOOKS

Krotec, Joseph, and Sharon Perkins. *Endometriosis for Dummies.* Hoboken, NJ: Wiley, 2007.

Redwine, David B. *100 Questions & Answers About Endometriosis.* Sudbury, MA: Jones and Bartlett, 2009.

Worwood, Valerie Ann, and Julia Stonehouse. *The Endometriosis Natural Treatment Program: A Complete Self-Help Plan for Improving Health and Well-Being.* Novato, CA: New World Library, 2007.

PERIODICALS

Rodgers, Allison K., and Tommaso Falcone. "Treatment Strategies for Endometriosis." *Expert Opinion on Pharmacotherapy* (February 2008): 243–255.

OTHER

"Endometriosis." MedlinePlus September 21, 2009 [September 25, 2009]. http://www.nlm.nih.gov/medlineplus/endometriosis.html

Stoppler, Melissa C. and Robert M. McNamara "Endometriosis." eMedicineHealth August 5, 2009 [September 25, 2009]. http://www.emedicinehealth.com/endometriosis/article_em.htm

ORGANIZATIONS

American College of Obstetricians and Gynecologists, P.O. Box 96920, Washington, DC, 20090-6920, (202) 638-5577, http://www.acog.org.

Endometriosis Association, 8585 N. 76th Place, Milwaukee, WI, 53223, (414) 355-2200, (414) 355-6065, http://endometriosisassn.org.

Stephanie Slon
Tish Davidson, A.M.

Endometritis *see* **Pelvic inflammatory disease**

Endorectal ultrasound

Definition

Endorectal ultrasound (ERUS) is a procedure where a probe is inserted into the rectum and high frequency sound waves (ultrasound waves) are generated. The pattern of echoes as they bounce off tissues is converted into a picture (sonogram) on a television screen.

Purpose

ERUS is used as a diagnostic procedure in **rectal cancer** to determine stage of the tumor and as a post-radiation, presurgical examination to assess extent of tumor shrinkage. ERUS can also be used in cases of anal **fistula** (an abnormal passage) and problems with the anal sphincter muscles (muscles that control the opening and closing of the anus).

Precautions

Normal precautions should be taken with any diagnostic procedure. Since the population in which this procedure is normally done is elderly, the imaging staff should be extra cautious about stressing the patient. The procedure is invasive and may be embarrassing to some. Other patients may be anxious about their medical condition since endorectal ultrasounds are not routine. This places an added burden on already stressed hearts and nervous systems. Physicians, nurses, and technicians may need to be prepared for **stress** reactions that could include the heart, **asthma**, or anxious behaviors.

Description

ERUS has been used as a means to determine the depth of rectal cancers and to assess whether the tumor has affected surrounding tissues. This pre-

KEY TERMS

Anal sphincter muscles—Muscles that control the opening and closing of the anus.

Fistula—An abnormal passage.

Sonogram—The picture formed by the pattern of echoes from an ultra sound.

Ultrasound waves—High-frequency sound waves.

treatment procedure has proven to be an accurate tool for tailoring surgery for patients.

Problems with interpretation of the sonograms after radiation and before surgery have resulted in tumors being identified that were merely the formation of fibrous tissues that remained after the tumors had been eliminated by the radiation. Yet, some of the fibrous areas actually hid residual tumors. Rectal anatomy itself can affect the accuracy of ultrasound reading. This makes ERUS problematic in determining the amount of tumor reduction a patient has after **radiation therapy**.

Preparation

The patient must evacuate the bowels completely before the procedure is done. This usually is assisted though the use of several **enemas**. The patient may be told to adhere to a liquid diet the day prior to doing this procedure. The probe is inserted, usually with little discomfort for the patient since it will only be examining the first few inches of the colon.

Aftercare

Since ERUS is a minor invasive procedure, there is no aftercare.

Risks

There are no risks to having an ultrasound.

Normal results

Normal results after an endorectal ultrasound are normal, healthy tissues.

Abnormal results

Abnormal results range from any number of congenital deformities in the lining of the rectum to serious rectal cancers.

Resources

BOOKS

Rosen, L. S., and A. J. Bilchik, eds. *New Aproaches to Assessing and Treating Early–stage Colon and Rectal Cancers*. Philadelphia: American Association for Cancer Research, 2007.

Santoro, Giulio Aniello, et al. *Atlas of Endoanal and Endorectal Ultrasonography: Staging and Treatment Options for Anorectal Cancer*. Milan; New York: Springer, 2004.

OTHER

National Cancer Institute. "NCI/PDQ Patient Statement: Rectal Cancer Updated 11/2000." *OncoLink*. May 9, 2001. http://www.oncolink.upenn.edu/pdq_html/2/engl/200076.html.

Janie F. Franz

Endoscopic retrograde cholangiopancreatography

Definition

Endoscopic retrograde cholangiopancreatography (ERCP) is an imaging technique used to diagnose diseases of the pancreas, liver, gallbladder, and bile ducts. It combines **endoscopy** and x-ray imaging.

Purpose

ERCP is used in the management of diseases that affect the gastrointestinal tract, specifically the pancreas, liver, gall bladder, and bile ducts. The pancreas is an organ that secretes pancreatic juice into the upper part of the intestine. Pancreatic juice is composed of specialized proteins that help to digest fats, proteins, and carbohydrates. Bile is a substance that helps to digest fats; it is produced by the liver, secreted through the bile ducts, and stored in the gallbladder. Bile is released into the small intestine after a person has eaten a meal containing fat.

A doctor may recommend ERCP if a patient is experiencing abdominal **pain** of unknown origin, weight loss, or **jaundice**. These may be symptoms of biliary disease. For instance, **gallstones** that form in the gallbladder or bile ducts may become stuck there, causing cramping or dull pain in the upper right area of the abdomen, **fever**, and/or jaundice. Other causes of biliary obstruction include tumors, injury from gallbladder surgery, or inflammation. The bile ducts may also become narrowed (called a biliary stricture)

KEY TERMS

Bile—A bitter yellowish-brown fluid secreted by the liver that contains bile salts, bile pigments, cholesterol, and other substances. It helps the body to digest and absorb fats.

Congenital—Present at birth.

Endoscope—An instrument with a light source attached that allows the doctor to examine the inside of the digestive tract or other hollow organ.

Gastrointestinal tract—A group of organs and related structures that includes the esophagus, stomach, liver, gallbladder, pancreas, small intestine, large intestine, rectum, and anus.

Jaundice—A condition characterized by deposits of bile pigments in the skin, mucous membranes, and the whites of the eyes. It is also known as icterus.

Magnetic resonance imaging—A technique that uses a strong magnetic field and pulses of radio waves to produce cross-sectional images of the body.

Stent—A thin rod-like or tube-like device made of wire mesh, inserted into a blood vessel or duct to keep it open.

Stricture—An abnormal narrowing of a duct or canal.

as a result of **cancer**, blunt trauma to the abdomen, **pancreatitis** (inflammation of the pancreas), or **primary biliary cirrhosis** (PBC). PBC may be caused by a condition called primary sclerosing **cholangitis**, an inflammation of the bile ducts that may cause pain, jaundice, **itching**, or other symptoms. These symptoms may also be experienced by a patient with cholangitis, or with infection of the bile ducts caused by bacteria or parasites.

ERCP can also be used to diagnose a number of pancreatic disorders. Pancreatitis is an inflammation of the pancreas, caused by chronic alcohol **abuse**, injury, obstruction of the pancreatic ducts (e.g., by gallstones), or other factors. The condition may be either acute (having a severe but short course) or chronic (persistent). Symptoms of pancreatitis include abdominal pain, weight loss, **nausea**, and **vomiting**. ERCP may be used to diagnose cancer of the pancreas; pancreatic pseudocysts (collections of pancreatic fluid); or strictures of the pancreatic ducts. Certain

congenital disorders may also be identified by ERCP, such as pancreas divisum, a condition in which parts of the pancreas fail to fuse during fetal development.

Demographics

Diseases of the pancreas and biliary tract affect millions of Americans each year. According to the National Health and **Nutrition** Survey, gallbladder disease affects approximately 6.3 million men and 14.2 million women in the United States between the ages of 24 and 74. Approximately one million new cases of gallstones are diagnosed each year. The incidence of gallstones is higher among women; adults over the age of 40; and people who are overweight. Primary sclerosing cholangitis occurs at a rate of two to seven cases per 100,000 persons. The rate of **gallbladder cancer** is approximately 2.5 out of 100,000 persons. In addition, approximately 87,000 cases of pancreatitis and 30,000 cases of pancreatic cancer are diagnosed each year in the United States.

Description

ERCP is performed with the patient given either a sedative or **general anesthesia**. The physician then sprays the back of the patient's throat with a local anesthetic. The endoscope (a thin, hollow tube attached to a viewing screen) is then inserted into the mouth. It is threaded down the esophagus, through the stomach, and into the duodenum (upper part of the small intestine) until it reaches the spot where the bile and pancreatic ducts empty into the duodenum. At this point a small tube called a cannula is inserted through the endoscope and used to inject a contrast dye into the ducts. The term "retrograde" in the name of the procedure refers to the backward direction of the dye as it is injected through the ducts. A series of x-rays are then taken as the dye moves through the ducts.

If the x-rays show that a problem exists, ERCP may be used as a therapeutic tool. Special instruments can be inserted into the endoscope to remove gallstones, take samples of tissue for further examination (e.g., in the case of suspected cancer), or place a special tube called a stent into a duct to relieve an obstruction.

Diagnosis/Preparation

ERCP is generally not performed unless other less invasive diagnostic tests have first been used to determine the cause of a patient's symptoms. Such tests include:

- complete medical history and physical examination
- blood tests (certain diseases can be diagnosed by abnormal levels of blood components)

- ultrasound imaging (a procedure that uses high-frequency sound waves to visualize structures in the human body)
- computed tomography (CT) scan (an imaging device that uses x-rays to produce two-dimensional cross-sections on a viewing screen)

Before undergoing ERCP, the patient will be instructed to refrain from eating or drinking for at least six hours to ensure that the stomach and upper part of the intestine are empty. Arrangements should be made for someone to take the patient home after the procedure, as he or she will not be able to drive. The physician should also be given a complete list of all prescription, over-the-counter, and alternative medications or preparations that the patient is taking. The patient should also notify the doctor if he or she is allergic to iodine because the contrast dye contains it.

Aftercare

After the procedure, the patient will remain at the hospital or outpatient facility until the effects of the sedative wear off and no signs of any complications have appeared. A longer stay may be warranted if the patient experiences complications or if other procedures were performed.

Risks

Complications that have been reported with ERCP include pancreatitis; cholangitis (inflammation of the bile ducts); **cholecystitis** (inflammation of the gallbladder); injury to the duodenum; pain; bleeding; infection; and formation of **blood clots**. Factors that increase the risk of complications include liver damage, bleeding disorders, a history of post-ERCP complications, and a less experienced endoscopist.

Normal results

Following ERCP, the patient's biliary and pancreatic ducts should be free of stones and show no strictures, obstructions, or evidence of infection or inflammation.

Morbidity and mortality rates

The overall complication rate associated with ERCP is approximately 11%. Pancreatitis may occur in up to 7% of patients. Cholangitis and cholecystitis occur in less than 1% of patients. Infection, injury, bleeding, and blot clot formation also occur in less than 1%. The mortality rate for ERCP is approximately 0.1%.

Alternatives

Although less invasive techniques exist (such as computed tomography and ultrasonography) to help to diagnose gastrointestinal diseases, these imaging studies are often not precise enough to allow for definite diagnosis of certain conditions. **Percutaneous transhepatic cholangiography** (PTCA) is an alternative to ERCP that involves the insertion of a long, flexible needle through the skin to the bile ducts; contrast dye is then injected into the ducts so that they may be visualized by x-ray. PTCA may be recommended if ERCP fails or cannot be performed. Magnetic resonance cholangiopancreatography (MRCP) is an imaging technology that allows for non-invasive examination of the biliary and pancreatic ducts. Its disadvantage, however, is that unlike ERCP, it cannot be used for therapeutic procedures as well as imaging.

Resources

OTHER

Endoscopic Retrograde Cholangiopancreatography. [cited June 21, 2004]. http://www.asge.org.
Measuring Procedural Skills. [cited June 21, 2004]. http://www.acponline.org/journals/annals/15dec96/procskil.htm.
Treatment of Acute Biliary Pancreatitis. [cited June 21, 2004]. http://content.nejm.org.

ORGANIZATIONS

American College of Gastroenterology, P.O. Box 342260, Bethesda, MD, 20827-2260, (301) 263-9000, http://www.acg.gi.org.
American Gastroenterological Association, 4930 Del Ray Avenue, Bethesda, MD, 20814, (301) 654-2055, (301) 654-5920, member@gastro.org, http://www.gastro.org.
American Society for Gastrointestinal Endoscopy, 1520 Kensington Road, Suite 202, Oak Brook, IL, 60523, (630) 573-0600, (866) 353-2743, (630) 573-0691, info@asge.org, http://www.asge.org.

Stephanie Dionne Sherk
Brenda W. Lerner

Endoscopic sclerotherapy *see* **Sclerotherapy for esophageal varices**

Endoscopic sphincterotomy

Definition

Endoscopic sphincterotomy or endoscopic retrograde sphincterotomy (ERS) is a relatively new endoscopic technique developed to examine and treat abnormalities of the bile ducts, pancreas and

Endoscope, Endoscopy—An endoscope as used in the field of gastroenterology is a thin flexible tube which uses a lens or miniature camera to view various areas of the gastrointestinal tract. When the procedure is performed to examine certain organs such as the bile ducts or pancreas, the organs are not viewed directly, but rather indirectly through the injection of x-ray dye. The performance of an exam using an endoscope is referred by the general term endoscopy. Diagnosis through biopsies or other means and therapeutic procedures can be done with these instruments.

NSAIDS—This abbreviation stands for non-steroidal anti-inflammatory drugs, which are medications such as Ibufprofen that are used to control pain and inflammation. Most may be purchased over the counter. One of their major side effects is that they decrease the effect of the normal blood clotting factors in blood. In patients undergoing surgical or endoscopic procedures, this can lead to an increased risk of bleeding.

gallbladder. The procedure was developed as an extension to the diagnostic examination, ERCP (**endoscopic retrograde cholangiopancreatography**); with the addition of "sphincterotomy," abnormalities found during the study could be treated at the same time without the need for invasive surgery.

The term ERS has three parts to its definition:

- endoscopic refers to the use of an endoscope
- retrograde refers to the insertion of the endoscope *up* into the ducts in a direction opposite to or against the normal flow of bile *down* the ducts
- sphincterotomy, which means cutting of the sphincter or muscle that lies at the juncture of the intestine with both the bile and pancreatic ducts.

Purpose

Until the 1970s, patients with symptoms related to disease of the bile ducts or pancreas frequently needed surgery to diagnose the cause and treat any abnormalities. ERCP allowed physicians for the first time to obtain high quality x rays of the common bile and pancreatic ducts, and detect areas of narrowing (strictures), stones, and tumors. ERCP was not initially designed for treatment. ERS was developed shortly after and enabled physicians to treat the abnormalities identified by the injection of dye and x rays.

The revolutionary technique made possible the endoscopic removal of stones and stretching of areas of narrowing (strictures). It has since been expanded to include drainage of bile from blocked ducts and treatment of various abnormalities of the pancreas.

Precautions

The most important precaution related to both ERCP and ERS is to have the procedure performed by an experienced physician. ERS is technically more difficult than many other gastrointestinal endoscopic studies, including ERCP. Patients should inquire as to the physician's experience with the procedure. The physician should also be informed of any **allergies**, medication use, and medical problems.

Description

ERS is generally performed only after ERCP has been successfully accomplished and detail of the anatomy and abnormalities is known. During ERS, a number of various instruments are inserted through the endoscope in order to "cut" or stretch the sphincter. Once this is done, additional instruments are passed that enable the removal of stones and the stretching of narrowed regions of the ducts. Drains (stents) can also be used to prevent a narrowed area from rapidly returning to its previously narrowed state.

Preparation

The upper intestinal tract must be empty for the procedure, so patients must not eat or drink for at least six to 12 hours before the exam. Patients need to inquire about taking their medications before the procedure. Some patients may require **antibiotics** before and/or after the procedure. When possible, **aspirin** or NSAIDS should not be taken within several days before the procedure, because they interfere with blood clotting.

Aftercare

When ERS is performed, physicians will usually want to observe the patient closely for several hours to ensure that there are no signs of complications. **Pain** or any other unusual symptoms should be reported. Admission to the hospital may be advised.

Risks

ERS complications are related either to the drugs used during the procedure, or the results of dye injection or cutting of tissue. The overall complication rate is 5–10%. During the exam, the endoscopist can cut or stretch structures (such as the muscle leading to the bile duct) to treat the cause of the patient's symptoms. Cutting or stretching of these structures can sometimes cause a hole or perforation. The use of sedatives also carries a risk of decreasing cardiac and respiratory function, however, it is very difficult to perform these procedures without these drugs.

Other major complications related to ERCP or ERS are **pancreatitis** (inflammation of the pancreas) and **cholangitis** (inflammation of the bile ducts). **Bacteremia** (the passage of bacteria into the blood stream) and bleeding are also risks.

Normal results

Certain standards have been set for the diameter or width of the pancreatic and bile ducts. Measurements by x ray are used to determine if the ducts are too large (dilated) or too narrow (strictured). Lastly, the ducts and gallbladder should be free of any solid particles, such as stones, and free of areas of narrowing.

Resources

OTHER

"Endoscopic Retrograde Cholangiopancreatography." *American Society for Gastrointestinal Endoscopy.* http://www.asge.org.
"Treatment of Acute Biliary Pancreatitis." *New England Journal of Medicine Online.* http://content.nejm.org.

David Kaminstein, MD

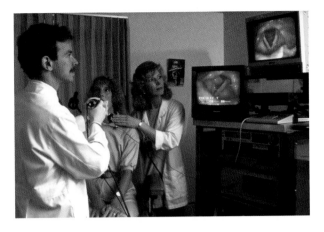

Patient undergoing an endoscopic exam. *(© National Audubon Society Collection/Photo Researchers, Inc.)*

time view with true colors. It also is sometimes used to remove polyps, cauterize bleeding, or remove samples for examination under the microscope.

Endoscopy is used in a variety of settings. It is often used to help diagnose the cause of **pain** or other symptoms that are of unclear origin. It can also be used during minimally invasive surgery, when an endoscopy is passed through a very small incision so that the surgeon is able to view the inside of the patient and perform the surgery.

Description

During endoscopy, a small camera or viewer attached to the end of a thin, usually flexible tube, is passed into the individual. This device is called an endoscope. The endoscope is usually introduced into the patient through the mouth, rectum, ureter, or a small incision. The place of endoscope entry is determined by the are of the body the doctor wishes to view.

Some endoscopes have a view piece that allows the doctor to see directly into the patient. Others have camera at the end, which sends video signals through fiber optic wires in the endoscope to a television monitor in the procedure room. This allows the doctor and others to get a clear, enlarged view of the area of interest, and can allow for recording the procedure to review later if there are any questions.

In most cases the patient is mildly or heavily sedated during the procedure. Many patients actual sleep through the majority of the procedure. The area under investigation may also receive **local anesthesia** if discomfort from the procedure is expected.

Many endoscopes allow the doctor not only to see the inside of the patient, but also to perform some

Endoscopy

Definition

An endoscopy is a procedure that uses a small camera mounted on a thin, flexible tube called an endoscope to allow a doctor to see inside the body.

Purpose

Endoscopy is used to provide the doctor or surgeon with the ability to see inside the patient's body. Unlike many other forms of imaging, such as x-ray and ultrasound, endoscopy can provide the doctor with a real-

KEY TERMS

Biopsy—Removal of a small tissue sample from the body to examine for evidence of disease.

Gastroenterologist—A doctor who specializes in diagnosing and treating conditions of the gastrointestinal system, including the mouth, pharynx, esophagus, diaphragm, stomach, gall bladder, bile duct, liver, small intestine, large intestine, and anus.

Polyp—An abnormal growth of tissue arising from and protruding from a mucous membrane.

additional procedures. Some endoscopes have a device for cauterizing as an available attachment, which can be sued to stop internal bleeding in the area being investigated. Other endoscopes allow the doctor to cut and remove polyps during the procedure. Some endoscopes allows for the biopsy of suspicious tissue during the procedure, removing the need for an additional, usually more invasive procedure later.

One of the newest endoscopy technologies, capsule endoscopy, allows the physician to examine the esophagus, stomach, and small intestine. For this procedure, the patient swallows a capsule (slightly larger than a large vitamin) containing video chips, lights, and a transmitter. Rapid photos are made as the capsule travels through the digestive tract, and are transmitted to a receiver worn around the patient's waist. The capsule eventually passes in the stool, and images are downloaded from the receiver for the physician to evaluate. Limitations of capsule endoscopy include the inability to gather samples or remove polyps, and the fact the capsule battery sometimes fades before the capsule travels to the area targeted for inspection.

Precautions

The precautions for endoscopy vary depending on the type of endoscopy performed. Individuals who have conditions that require regular consumption of food or liquids may not be good candidates for endoscopy. Individuals who are allergic to one or more sedatives or anesthesia products should alert their doctor and health care team so that alternative medications can be found and special precautions can be taken.

Preparation

The preparation for an endoscopy depends heavily on the type of endoscopy being performed. The patient is generally instructed not to eat or drink for a certain amount of time before the procedure. If there is food in the upper digestive system this can reduce visibility, and **vomiting** can occur causing complications. If an endoscopy is being performed on the lower digestive tract the patient may be prescribed **laxatives** or one or more **enemas** before the procedure so that the area of interest is clearly visible.

The patient may be required to stop taking, or reduce the dosage of, some medications, supplements, or herbs before the procedure. Blood thinners can increase the risk of bleeding as a complication of the procedure, so individuals taking blood thinners may be asked to stop for a few days before the procedure. The patient is given specific instructions for his or her case, usually when the endoscopy is scheduled.

Aftercare

After the endoscopy the patient is often brought to a special recovery room to wait until the effects of any sedatives administered wear off, and to ensure there were no complications from the procedure. The patient should arrange for transportation home after the procedure because he or she will not be able to drive after **sedation**. Generally, patients can begin to eat and drink again as desired after the procedure is over. The patient will generally begin to feel better quickly as any medication administered wears off, although some soreness may occur. The patient should usually allow the remainder of the day to rest after the procedure.

Risks

An endoscopy can result in soreness in the area in which the endoscopy was performed. Bloating and gas sometimes occur after endoscopies performed on the gastrointestinal tract. In rare cases endoscopy can cause bleeding, and in extremely rare cases can cause rupture or tearing of the intestinal wall. If anesthesia or sedatives were used these can have their own risks of complications. In most cases no serious complications result from endoscopy.

Results

An endoscopy produces pictures of the area being looked at so that the doctor can use them to assist in making a diagnosis. In some cases the endoscopy will also produce samples that can be examined under the microscope. The results of the endoscopy will vary depending on the reason it was performed, the area examined, and whether any biopsies were taken. A normal endoscopy will produce images that show healthy, normally functioning organs and tissues with no tears, growths, or bleeding. An abnormal endoscopy may show growths, bleeding, tearing of the intestinal wall, abnormal coloration, or a variety of other problems.

Caregiver concerns

A doctor determines the need for an endoscopy based on a **physical examination** of the patient, the patient's self-reported symptoms, a health history, and the results of any other diagnostic imaging, blood, or urine tests. The endoscopy may be performed in a doctor's office, in a clinic, or in a hospital. In general, an endoscopy is performed by a doctor who specializes in the area being imaged. For example, an endoscopy of the upper digestive system is performed by a gastroenterologist, a doctor who specializes in the gastrointestinal system. A surgeon may perform an endoscopy if the endoscopy is being used to visualize the surgery site during minimally invasive surgery.

During the procedure, a variety of other health care team members may assist the doctor or surgeon who is performing the endoscopy. Technologists may help to set up and monitor video and other equipment. One or more nurses may supervise the administration of any medications or sedatives, and may help to monitor the patient's vital signs during the procedure. If the patient is going to be under **general anesthesia** during the procedure, an anesthesiologist will administer the anesthesia and be present during the procedure to monitor the patient. If the endoscopy is being performed doing a surgery a variety of operating room nurses, technologists, and technicians may be present to assist. If any material is removed during the procedure for a biopsy, a laboratory technician may examine the sample to determine if it is cancerous.

Resources

BOOKS

Faigel, Douglas O. and Michael L. Kochman, eds. *Endoscopic Oncology: Gastrointestinal Endoscopy and Cancer Management.* Totowa, NJ: Humana Press, 2006.

Nahai, Foadand Renato Saltz, eds. *Endoscopic Plastic Surgery,* 2nd ed. St. Louis, MO: Quality Medical Pub. 2007.

Ogilvie, Jeanette, Lisa M. Hicks, and Anthony N. Kallo. *John Hopkins Manual for Gastrointestinal Endoscopy Nursing,* 2nd ed. Thorofare, NJ: Slack, 2008.

PERIODICALS

Misra, Sri Prakash, and Manisha Dwivedi. "Colonoscopy and Colonscopic Polypectomy Using Side-Viewing Endoscope: A Useful, Effective, and Safe Procedure." *Digestive Disease and Sciences* 53.5 (May 2008): 1285–1289.

Pedersen, Amanda. "Study: Endoscopy Found Safe for Gastric Bypass Complication." *Medical Device Week* (August 20, 2007).

OTHER

National Institutes of Health. "Endoscopy." *Medline Plus.*http://www.nlm.nih.gov/medlineplus/ency/article/003338.htm

ORGANIZATIONS

American Gastroenterological Association, 4930 Del Ray Avenue, Bethesda, MD, 20814, (310) 654-2055, (310) 654-5920, www.gastro.org.

Robert Bockstiegel
Brenda W. Lerner

Enemas

Definition

An enema is the insertion of a solution into the rectum and lower intestine.

Purpose

Enemas may be given for the following purposes:

- to remove feces when an individual is constipated or impacted,

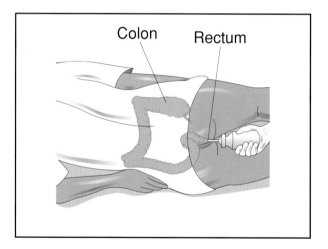

Enemas may be given for the following purposes: to remove feces when an individual is constipated, or to remove feces and cleanse the rectum in preparation for an examination, or prior to surgery to prevent contamination. There are two types of enemas: the high enema, given to cleanse the large bowel, and the low enema, to cleanse only the lower bowel. *(Illustration by Electronic Illustrators Group. Reproduced by permission of Gale, a part of Cengage Learning.)*

- to remove feces and cleanse the rectum in preparation for an examination,
- to remove feces prior to a surgical procedure to prevent contamination of the surgical area,
- to administer drugs or anesthetic agents.

Precautions

The rectal tube used for infusion of the enema solution should be smooth and flexible to decrease the possibility of damage to the mucous membrane that lines the rectum. Tap water is commonly used for adults but should not be used for infants because of the danger of electrolyte (substance that conducts electric current within the body and is essential for sustaining life) imbalance. The colon absorbs water, and repeated tap water enemas can cause cardiovascular overload and electrolyte imbalance. Similarly, repeated saline enemas can cause increased absorption of fluid and electrolytes into the bloodstream, resulting in overload. Individuals receiving frequent enemas should be observed for overload symptoms that include **dizziness**, sweating, or **vomiting**.

Soap suds and saline used for cleansing enemas can cause irritation of the lining of the bowel, with repeated use or a solution that is too strong. Only white soap should be used; the bar should not have been previously used, to prevent infusing undesirable organisms into the individual receiving the enema. Common household detergents are considered too strong for the rectum and bowel. The commercially prepared castile soap is preferred, and should be used in concentration no greater than 5 cc soap to 1,000 cc of water.

Description

Cleansing enemas act by stimulation of bowel activity through irritation of the lower bowel, and by distention with the volume of fluid instilled. When the enema is administered, the individual is usually lying on the left side, which places the sigmoid colon (lower portion of bowel) below the rectum and facilitates infusion of fluid. The length of time it takes to administer an enema depends on the amount of fluid to be infused. The amount of fluid administered will vary depending on the age and size of the person receiving the enema, however general guidelines would be:

- Infant: 250 cc or less
- Toddler and preschooler: 500 cc or less
- School-aged child: 500–1,000 cc
- Adult: 750–1,000 cc

KEY TERMS

Electrolyte—A substance that conducts electric current within the body and is essential for sustaining life.

Intestine—Also called the bowels and divided into large and small intestine, they extend from the stomach to the anus, where waste products exit the body. The small intestine is about 20 ft (6.1m) long and the large intestine, about 5 ft (1.5m) long.

Rectum—The portion of bowel just before the anus. The prefix *recto* is used with a variety of words in relation to conditions that affect the rectum.

Some may differentiate between high and low enemas. A high enema, given to cleanse as much of the large bowel as possible, is usually administered at higher pressure and with larger volume (1,000 cc), and the individual changes position several times in order for the fluid to flow up into the bowel. A low enema, intended to cleanse only the lower bowel, is administered at lower pressure, using about 500 cc of fluid.

Oil retention enemas serve to lubricate the rectum and lower bowel, and soften the stool. For adults, about 150–200 cc of oil is instilled, while in small children, 75–150 cc of oil is considered adequate. Salad oil or liquid petrolatum are commonly used at a temperature of 91°F (32.8°C). There are also commercially prepared oil retention enemas. The oil is usually retained for one to three hours before it is expelled.

The rectal tube used for infusion of the solution, usually made of rubber or plastic, has two or more openings at the end through which the solution can flow into the bowel. The distance to which the tube must be inserted is dependent upon the age and size of the patient. For adult, insertion is usually 3–4 in (7.5–10 cm); for children, approximately 2–3 in (5–7.5 cm); and for infants, only 1–1.5 in (2.5–3.75 cm). The rectal tube is lubricated before insertion with a water soluble lubricant to ease insertion and decrease irritation to the rectal tissues.

The higher the container of solution is placed, the greater the force in which the fluid flows into the patient. Routinely, the container should be no higher than 12 in (30 cm) above the level of the bed; for a high cleansing enema, the container may be 12–18 in (30–45 cm) above the bed level, because the fluid is to be instilled higher into the bowel.

Preparation

The solution used in the procedure is measured, mixed, and warmed before administration of the enema.

Aftercare

If necessary, a specimen will be collected for diagnostic evaluation. If the enema was given to alleviate **constipation**, the better approach to combatting constipation in the future is with a high fiber diet (five to six servings of whole grain foods) and adequate fluid intake (seven to eight glasses of water per day). Regular **exercise** and going to the bathroom when necessary will also help. If constipation is a chronic problem, medical help should be consulted to determine if there is underlying disorder.

Risks

Habitual use of enemas as a means to combat constipation can make the problem even more severe when their use is discontinued. Enemas should be used only as a last resort for treatment of constipation and with a doctor's recommendation. Enemas should not be administered to individuals who have recently had colon or rectal surgery, a **heart attack**, or who suffer from an unknown abdominal condition or an irregular heartbeat.

Resources

OTHER

"The urge to purge. (The risks of colonic irrigation and enemas)." *The University of California, Berkeley Wellness Letter.* Jan 2010, 1.

Kathleen D. Wright, RN

Enhanced external counterpulsation

Definition

Enhanced external counterpulsation (EECP) is a noninvasive procedure in which a set of inflatable cuffs (much like blood pressure cuffs) mechanically compress the blood vessels in the patient's lower limbs to increase blood flow in the coronary arteries of the heart. The blood pressure cuffs (also called stockings) are wrapped around the patient's calves, lower thighs, and upper thighs. Computer technology, **electrocardiography**, and blood pressure monitors enable the pressure cuffs to be inflated and deflated in time with the patient's heartbeat and blood pressure.

Purpose

EECP is performed to restore blood flow to the heart and to relieve chest **pain** (**angina** pectoris) and **ischemia**. The goals of the procedure are to relieve the symptoms of **coronary artery disease**, enable the patient to resume a normal lifestyle, and lower the risk of a **heart attack** or other heart problems. EECP may encourage blood vessels to open small channels (called collateral blood vessels) to eventually bypass blocked vessels and improve blood flow to the heart.

Demographics

The concept of counterpulsation is not new; it was first introduced in 1953 at Harvard, and refined in the late 1950s. Early models of EECP, however, used non-sequenced pulsation; that is, compression of the patient's blood vessels was performed simultaneously along the full length of the body. In the 1970s, researchers in China reported on a sequential compression system in which four sets of pressure cuffs were applied to the patient's legs, buttocks, and arms. Favorable reports about the effectiveness of sequential compression encouraged a research team at SUNY Stony Brook to develop the three-cuff EECP model in use in the early 2000s. The computerized technology currently available with EECP makes it a relatively new procedure compared to the systems used in the 1960s and early 1970s. As of 2008, it was available in about 200 centers across the United States.

EECP is used to treat patients with chronic stable angina, coronary artery disease, or high blood pressure. The Food and Drug Administration (FDA) approved EECP for the treatment of congestive **heart failure** (CHF) in the early 2000s. Researchers at the Ohio Heart and Vascular Center reported in 2006 that EECP improved **exercise** duration as well as quality of life in patients with CHF. The treatment may be appropriate for patients who are not eligible for such non-surgical interventional procedures as balloon **angioplasty**, stent placement, rotablation, **atherectomy**, or brachytherapy. It may also be used for patients who do not qualify for such surgical treatments as **coronary artery bypass graft surgery**.

EECP is not the first-line treatment for angina. Rather, it is reserved for patients who have not achieved good results from medication or interventional management of their symptoms. To be eligible for EECP, a patient must have coronary artery disease that includes at least one heart vessel with at least 70% obstruction. In addition, the patient must have evidence of either an infarction or significant ischemia on a **stress test** with nuclear or echocardiographic imaging.

KEY TERMS

Angina—Also called angina pectoris; chest pain or discomfort that occurs when diseased blood vessels restrict blood flow to the heart.

Aorta—The main artery that carries blood from the heart to the rest of the body; the largest artery in the body.

Artery—A vessel that carries oxygen-rich blood to the body.

Atherectomy—A nonsurgical technique for treating diseased arteries with a rotating device that cuts or shaves away obstructing material inside the artery.

Atria (singular, atrium)—The right and left upper chambers of the heart.

Balloon angioplasty—A nonsurgical technique for treating diseased arteries by temporarily inflating a tiny balloon inside an artery.

Beta blocker—An antihypertensive drug that limits the activity of epinephrine, a hormone that increases blood pressure.

Brachytherapy—The use of radiation during angioplasty to prevent the artery from narrowing again (a process called restenosis).

Calcium channel blocker—A drug that lowers blood pressure by regulating calcium-related electrical activity in the heart.

Cardiac catheterization—An invasive procedure used to create x rays of the coronary arteries, heart chambers and valves.

Collateral vessel—A side branch or network of side branches of a large blood vessel.

Coronary artery disease—Also called atherosclerosis, it is a buildup of fatty matter and debris in the coronary artery wall that causes narrowing of the artery.

Echocardiogram—An imaging procedure used to create a picture of the heart's movement, valves and chambers.

Electrocardiogram (ECG, EKG)—A test that records the electrical activity of the heart, using small electrode patches attached to the skin on the chest.

Infarction—An area of dead tissue caused by obstruction of the blood supply to that tissue.

Ischemia—Decreased blood flow to an organ, usually caused by constriction or obstruction of an artery.

Rotablation—A nonsurgical technique for treating diseased arteries in which a special catheter with a diamond-coated tip is guided to the point of narrowing in the artery. The catheter tip spins at high speed and grinds away the blockage or plaque on the artery walls.

Stent—A device made of expandable metal mesh that is placed (by using a balloon catheter) at the site of a narrowing artery. The stent remains in place to keep the artery open.

Stress test—A test that determines how the heart responds to stress.

Vein—A blood vessel that returns oxygen-depleted blood from various parts of the body to the heart.

Ventricles—The lower pumping chambers of the heart that propel blood to the lungs and the rest of the body.

EECP may benefit patients with such other medical conditions as **erectile dysfunction**, **kidney disease**, eye disease, **diabetic neuropathy**, **restless legs syndrome**, and other circulatory disorders. More research is needed to evaluate the outcomes of EECP for these patients.

Many insurance providers and Medicare have approved EECP treatment for reimbursement. Medicare pays about $5,500 for the full series of 35 treatments.

Contraindications

EECP is not recommended for patients who have certain types of valve disease, uncontrolled **arrhythmias** (irregular heart rhythms), severe **hypertension**, uncontrolled congestive heart failure, significant blockages or **blood clots** in the leg arteries, or those who have had a recent **cardiac catheterization**, angioplasty, or bypass surgery. It should also not be given to pregnant women.

Description

While the patient lies on a bed, the leg cuffs are deflated and inflated with each heartbeat. A computer synchronizes the compression of the cuffs with the heartbeat. The electrocardiogram indicates when each heartbeat begins, triggering the cuffs to be mechanically deflated. As each heartbeat ends, the cuffs are mechanically inflated in sequential order, starting with the cuffs on the calves and working upward to the cuffs on the lower and then the upper thighs. The pressure produced by the inflation of the cuffs when the heart is at rest pushes the blood in the legs upward toward the heart. The deflating action that occurs just when the heart begins to beat reduces the work of the heart as it pumps blood to other parts of the body. Inflation is controlled by a pressure monitor that inflates the cuffs to about 300 mm Hg. When timed correctly, the procedure increases the cardiac output.

EECP treatments are performed on an outpatient basis and generally last one to two hours. Treatments must be repeated about five times a week for up to seven weeks to achieve improved circulation. This 35-hour regimen is generally followed because it was used in the first multicenter study of EECP in 1999.

Diagnosis/Preparation

Preparation

The patient is usually instructed to wear tight-fitting seamless cycling pants or athletic tights to prevent chafing, one of the main adverse side effects.

Before the procedure, the patient's weight, blood pressure, pulse, and breathing rate are measured and recorded. The patient's legs are examined for areas of redness and signs of potential vascular problems.

The patient is asked to record his or her symptoms during the course of treatment to determine whether and how symptoms improve over time. The patient should record the severity and duration of troublesome symptoms, the time the symptoms occurred, and any activities that may have triggered the symptoms. This patient record is reviewed before each treatment session.

PATIENT EDUCATION. The healthcare team will ensure that the patient understands the potential benefits and risks of the procedure. Informative and instructional handouts are usually provided to explain the procedure. Because the procedure requires multiple outpatient visits (generally 35 visits over a seven-week period), the patient must be able to meet the treatment schedule.

INFORMED CONSENT. Informed consent is an educational process between healthcare providers and patients. Before any procedure is performed, the patient is asked to sign a consent form. Before signing the form, the patient should understand the nature and purpose of the diagnostic procedure or treatment; the risks and benefits of the procedure; and alternatives, including the option of not proceeding with the test or treatment. During the discussion about the procedure, the healthcare providers are available to answer all of the patient's questions.

SMOKING CESSATION. Patients who will undergo any procedure to treat cardiovascular disease are encouraged to stop **smoking** and using any tobacco products before the procedure, and to make a commitment to be a nonsmoker after the procedure. There are several smoking cessation programs available in the community. The patient should ask a healthcare provider for more information if he or she needs help quitting smoking.

Aftercare

Discomfort

Patients report little or no discomfort during the procedure. Some people may feel tired after the first few treatments, but this loss of energy improves over time.

Lifestyle changes

To manage heart disease, the patient needs to make several lifestyle changes before and after the procedure, including:

- Quitting smoking. Smoking causes damage to blood vessels, increases the patient's blood pressure and heart rate, and decreases the amount of oxygen available in the blood.
- Managing weight. Maintaining a healthy weight, by watching portion sizes and exercising, is important. Being overweight increases the work of the heart.
- Participating in an exercise program. The cardiac rehabilitation exercise program is usually tailored for the patient, who will be supervised by professionals.
- Making dietary changes. Patients should eat a lot of fruits, vegetables, grains, and nonfat or low-fat dairy products, and reduce fats to less than 30% of all calories. Alcoholic beverages should be limited or avoided.
- Taking medications as prescribed. Aspirin and other heart medications may be prescribed, and the patient may need to take these medications for life.
- Following up with healthcare providers. The patient should visit the physician regularly for follow-up visits to control risk factors.

Risks

EECP is a relatively safe and effective treatment, and few adverse side effects have been reported. The main adverse side effect is chafing (skin irritation from the compression of the cuffs). To reduce or prevent this side effect, patients are instructed to wear tight-fitting cycling pants or athletic tights. Leg pain is another adverse side effect.

Normal results

The benefits of EECP are comparable to the results of angioplasty and coronary artery bypass graft surgery: 70–80% of patients experience significant improvement after EECP treatment for as long as five years. The largest research study on EECP indicates that after receiving treatment, patients used less medication, had fewer angina attacks with less severe symptoms, and increased their capacity to exercise without experiencing symptoms. EECP improves the patient's sense of well-being and overall quality of life, and in some cases, prolongs the patient's life. Benefits five years after EECP treatment are comparable to surgical outcomes.

The effects of EECP treatment last from three to five years and sometimes longer.

EECP does not prevent coronary artery disease from recurring; therefore, lifestyle changes are strongly recommended and medications are prescribed to reduce the risk of recurrent disease.

Morbidity and mortality rates

Morbidity and mortality have not been reported with this procedure.

Alternatives

All patients with coronary artery disease can help improve their condition by making lifestyle changes such as quitting smoking, losing weight if they are overweight, eating healthful foods, reducing blood cholesterol, exercising regularly, and controlling diabetes and high blood pressure.

All patients with coronary artery disease should be prescribed medications to treat their condition. Such antiplatelet medications as **aspirin** or clopidogrel (Plavix) are usually recommended. Other medications used to treat angina may include **beta blockers**, nitrates, and angiotensin-converting enzyme (ACE) inhibitors. Medications may also be prescribed to lower lipoprotein levels, since elevated lipoprotein levels have been associated with an increased risk of cardiovascular problems.

Treatment with vitamin E is not recommended because it does not lower the rate of cardiovascular events in people with coronary artery disease. Although such **antioxidants** as vitamin C, beta-carotene, and probucol show promising results, they are not recommended for routine use. Treatment with **folic acid** and **vitamins** B_6 and B_{12} lowers **homocysteine** levels (reducing the risk for cardiovascular problems), but more studies are needed to determine if lowered homocysteine levels correlate with a reduced rate of cardiovascular problems in treated patients.

Such nonsurgical interventional procedures as balloon angioplasty, stent placement, rotablation, atherectomy, or brachytherapy can be performed to open a blocked artery.

Coronary artery bypass graft surgery is a surgical procedure in which one or more blocked coronary arteries are bypassed by a blood vessel graft to restore normal blood flow to the heart. These grafts usually come from the patient's own arteries and veins located in the leg, arm, or chest.

Resources

BOOKS

Elefteriades, John A., and Lawrence S. Cohen. *Your Heart: An Owner's Guide: Answers to Your Questions about Heart Disease.* Amherst, NY: Prometheus Books, 2007.

McGoon, Michael D., and Bernard J. Gersh, eds. *Mayo Clinic Heart Book: The Ultimate Guide to Heart Health,* 2nd ed. New York: William Morrow, 2000.

Topol, Eric J., ed. *Textbook of Cardiovascular Medicine,* 3rd ed. Philadelphia: Lippincott Williams and Wilkins, 2007.

Trout, Darrell, and Ellen Welch. "Enhanced External Counterpulsation (EECP)." In *Surviving with Heart: Taking Charge of Your Heart Care,* Golden, CO: Fulcrum, 2002.

PERIODICALS

Abbottsmith, C. W., E. S. Chung, T. Varricchione, et al. "Enhanced External Counterpulsation Improves Exercise Duration and Peak Oxygen Consumption in Older Patients with Heart Failure: A Subgroup Analysis of the PEECH Trial." *Congestive Heart Failure* 12 (November–December 2006): 307–311.

Feldman, A. M., M. A. Silver, G. S. Francis, et al. "Enhanced External Counterpulsation Improves Exercise Tolerance in Patients with Chronic Heart Failure." *Journal of the American College of Cardiology* 48 (September 19, 2006): 1198–1205.

Feldman, A. M., M. A. Silver, G. S. Francis, et al. "Treating Heart Failure with Enhanced External Counterpulsation (EECP): Design of the Prospective Evaluation of EECP in Heart Failure (PEECH) Trial." *Journal of Cardiac Failure* 11 (April 2005): 240–245.

Lawson, W. E., J. C. Hui, E. D. Kennard, et al. "Effect of Enhanced External Counterpulsation on Medically Refractory Angina Patients with Erectile Dysfunction." *International Journal of Clinical Practice* 61 (May 2007): 757–762.

Machanda, A., and O. Soran. "Enhanced External Counterpulsation and Future Directions: Step beyond Medical Management for Patients with Angina and Heart
Failure." *Journal of the American College of Cardiology*
50 (October 16, 2007): 1523–1531.

OTHER

Heart Information Network. http://www.heartinfo.org
(accessed March 19, 2008).

ORGANIZATIONS

American College of Cardiology, Heart House, 2400 N.
Street NW, Washington, DC, 20037, (202) 375-6000,
(202) 375-7000, resource@acc.org, http://www.acc.org.

American Heart Association, 7272 Greenville Avenue, Dallas, TX, 75231, (214) 373-6300, (800) 242-8721, http://
www.americanheart.org.

Cleveland Clinic Heart and Vascular Institute, The Cleveland Clinic Foundation, 9500 Euclid Avenue, F25,
Cleveland, OH, 44195, (216) 445-9288, (800) 223-2273,
http://www.clevelandclinic.org/heartcenter.

International ECP Therapists Association, 1500 Sunday
Drive, Suite 102, Raleigh, NC, 27607, (877) 558-0409,
http://www.ietaonline.com.

National Heart, Lung, and Blood Institute (NHLBI),
NHLBI Health Information Center, P.O. Box 30105,
Bethesda, MD, 20824-0105, (301) 592-8573, (240) 629-
3246, http://www.nhlbi.nih.gov.

Texas Heart Institute, Heart Information Service, P.O. Box
20345, Houston, TX, 77225-0345, (832) 355-1000, (800)
292-2221, http://www.texasheartinstitute.org.

Angela M. Costello
Rebecca Frey, PhD
Brenda W. Lerner

Enlarged prostate

Definition

A non-cancerous condition that affects many men
past 50 years of age, enlarged prostate makes urinating
more difficult by narrowing the urethra, a tube running from the bladder through the prostate gland. It
can be effectively treated by surgery and, today, by
certain drugs.

Description

The common term for enlarged prostate is BPH,
which stands for benign (non-cancerous) prostatic
hyperplasia or hypertrophy. Hyperplasia means that
the prostate cells are dividing too rapidly, increasing
the total number of cells, and, therefore, the size of the
organ itself. Hypertrophy simply means "enlargement."

BPH is part of the **aging** process. The actual changes in
the prostate may start as early as the 30s but take place
very gradually, so that significant enlargement and
symptoms usually do not appear until after age 50.
Past this age the chances of the prostate enlarging and
causing urinary symptoms become progressively
greater. More than 40% of men in their 70s have an
enlarged prostate. Symptoms generally appear between
ages 55–75. About 10% of all men eventually will require
treatment for BPH.

BPH has been viewed as a rare condition in
African, Chinese, and other Asian peoples for reasons
that are not clear.

Causes and symptoms

The cause of BPH is a mystery, but age-related
changes in the levels of hormones circulating in the
blood may be a factor. Whatever the cause, an enlarging
prostate gradually narrows the urethra and obstructs the
flow of urine. Even though the muscle in the bladder wall
becomes stronger in an attempt to push urine through
the smaller urethra, in time, the bladder fails to empty
completely at each urination. The urine that collects in
the bladder can become infected and lead to stone formation. The kidneys themselves may be damaged by
infection or by urine constantly "backing up."

When the enlarging prostate gland narrows the urethra, a man will have increasing trouble starting the urine
stream. Because some urine remains behind in the bladder, he will have to urinate more often, perhaps two or
three times at night (nocturia). The need to urinate can
become very urgent and, in time, urine may dribble out
to stain a man's clothing. Other symptoms of BPH are a
weak and sometimes a split stream and general aching or
pain in the perineum (the area between the scrotum and
anus). Some men may have considerable enlargement of
the prostate before even mild symptoms develop.

If a man must strain hard to force out the urine,
small veins in the bladder wall and urethra may rupture,
causing blood to appear in the urine. If the urinary
stream becomes totally blocked, the urine collecting in
the bladder may cause severe discomfort, a condition
called acute urinary retention. Urine that stagnates in
the bladder can easily become infected. A burning feeling during urination and **fever** are clues that infection
may have developed. Finally, if urine backs up long
enough it may increase pressure in the kidneys, though
this rarely causes permanent kidney damage.

Diagnosis

When a man's symptoms point to BPH, the first
thing the physician will want to do is a **digital rectal**

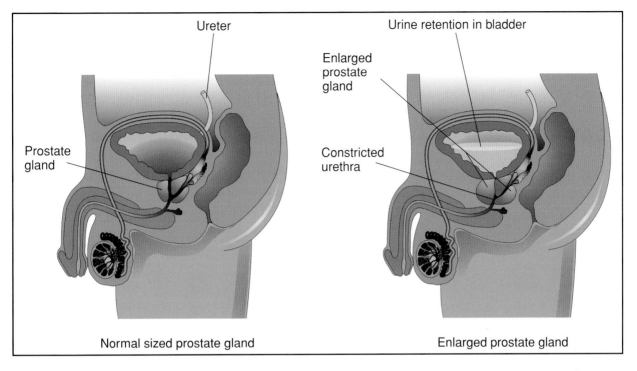

Ureter

Urine retention in bladder

Enlarged prostate gland

Prostate gland

Constricted urethra

Normal sized prostate gland

Enlarged prostate gland

An enlarged prostate is a non-cancerous condition in which the narrowing of the urethra makes the elimination of urine more difficult. It most often occurs in men over age 50. *(Illustration by Electronic Illustrators Group. Reproduced by permission of Gale, a part of Cengage Learning.)*

examination, inserting a finger into the anus to feel whether—and how much—the prostate is enlarged. A smooth prostate surface suggests BPH, whereas a distinct lump in the gland might mean **prostate cancer**. The next step is a blood test for a substance called prostate-specific antigen or PSA. Between 30–50% of men with BPH have an elevated PSA level. This does not mean **cancer** by any means, but other measures are needed to make sure that the prostate enlargement is in fact benign. An ultrasound exam of the prostate, which is entirely safe and delivers no radiation, can show whether it is enlarged and may show that cancer is present.

If digital or ultrasound examination of the prostate raises the suspicion of cancer, most urologists will recommend that a prostatic tissue biopsy be performed. This is usually done using a lance-like instrument that is inserted into the rectum. It pierces the rectal wall and, guided by the physcian's finger, obtains six to eight pieces of prostatic tissue that are sent to the laboratory for microscopic examination. If cancer is present, the prognosis and treatment are changed accordingly.

A catheter placed through the urethra and into the bladder can show how much urine remains in the bladder after the patient urinates—a measure of how severe the obstruction is. Another and very simple test for obstruction is to have the man urinate into a uroflowmeter, which measures the rate of urine flow. A very certain—though invasive—way of confirming obstruction from an enlarged prostate is to pass a special viewing instrument called a cystoscope into the bladder, but this is not often necessary.

It is routine to check a urine sample for an increased number of white blood cells, which may mean there is infection of the bladder or kidneys. The same sample may be cultured to show what type of bacterium is causing the infection, and which **antibiotics** will work best. The state of the kidneys may be checked in two ways: imaging by either ultrasound or injecting a dye (the intravenous urogram, or pyelogram); or a blood test for creatinine, which collects in the blood when the kidneys cannot eliminate it.

Treatment

Drugs

A class of drugs called alpha-adrenergic blockers, which includes phenoxybenzamine and doxazosin, relax the muscle tissue surrounding the bladder outlet and lining the wall of the urethra to permit urine to flow more freely. These drugs improve obstructive symptoms, but do not keep the prostate from enlarging. Other drugs (**finasteride** is a good example) do

KEY TERMS

Catheter—A rubber or plastic tube placed through the urethra into the bladder to remove excess urine when the flow of urine is cut off, or to prevent urinary infection.

Creatinine—One of the "waste" substances normally excreted by the kidneys into the urine. When urine flow is slowed, creatinine may collect in the blood and cause toxic effects.

Hyperplasia—A condition where cells, such as those making up the prostate gland, rapidly divide abnormally and cause the organ to become enlarged.

Hypertrophy—A technical term for enlargement, as in BPH (benign prostatic hypertrophy).

Urethra—In males, the tube that conducts urine from the bladder through the penis to the outside of the body. When narrowed by an enlarging prostate, symptoms of BPH develop.

Urinary retention—The result of progressive obstruction of the urethra by an enlarging prostate, causing urine to remain in the bladder even after urination.

shrink the prostate and may delay the need for surgery. Symptoms may not, however, improve until the drug has been used for three months or longer. Antibiotic drugs are given promptly whenever infection is diagnosed. Some medications, including **antihistamines** and some **decongestants**, can make the symptoms of BPH suddenly worse and even cause acute urinary retention, and therefore should be avoided.

Intermediate treatments

When drugs have failed to control symptoms of BPH but the physician does not believe that conventional surgery is yet needed, a procedure called transurethral needle ablation may be tried. In the office and using **local anesthesia**, a needle is inserted into the prostate and radiofrequency energy is applied to destroy the tissue that is obstructing urine flow. Another new approach is microwave hyperthermia, using a device called the Prostatron to deliver microwave energy to the prostate through a catheter. This procedure is done at an outpatient surgery center.

Surgery

For many years the standard operation for BPH has been transurethral resection (TUR) of the prostate. Under general or spinal anesthesia, a cystoscope is passed through the urethra and prostate tissue surrounding the urethra is removed using either a cutting instrument or a heated wire loop. The small pieces of prostate tissue are washed out through the scope. No incision is needed for TUR. There normally is some blood in the urine for a few days following the procedure. In a few men—less than 5% of all those having TUR—urine will continue to escape unintentionally. Other uncommon complications include a temporary rise in blood pressure with mental confusion, which is treated by giving salt solution. Impotence—the inability to achieve lasting penile erections—does occur, but probably in fewer than 10% of patients. A narrowing or stricture rarely develops in the urethra, but this can be treated fairly easily.

Alternatives to TUR, some only recently introduced, include:

- Laser ablation of the prostate. Laser energy is applied to the prostate through a special fiber passed through a cystoscope. The procedure is done in an operating room, and several patients have retained urine postoperatively.

- Transurethral incision of the prostate. Less invasive than standard TUR, an incision is made through the prostate to open up the part of the urethra passing through it. This may work well in men whose prostate is not grossly enlarged.

- Transurethral vaporization. A small roller ball is used to break up and vaporize the obstructing prostatic tissue, rather than cutting it away as in standard TUR. This is equally successful but patients usually can leave the hospital within 24 hours, and there is less blood loss.

- If the prostate is greatly enlarged—as is the case in about 5–10% of those diagnosed – an incision is made to perform an open prostatectomy, removing the entire gland under direct vision.

Alternative treatment

An extract of the **saw palmetto** (*Serenoa repens* or *S. serrulata*) has been shown to stop or decrease the hyperplasia of the prostate. Symptoms of BPH will improve after taking the herb for one to two months, but continued use is recommended.

Prognosis

In a man without symptoms whose prostate is enlarged, it is hard to predict when urinary symptoms will develop and how rapidly they will progress. For this reasons some specialists (urologists) advise a period of "watchful waiting." When BPH is treated by conventional TUR, there is a small risk of complications but, in the great majority of men, urinary symptoms will be relieved and their quality of life will be much enhanced. In the future, it is possible that the less invasive forms of surgical treatment will be increasingly used to achieve results as good as those of the standard operation. It also is possible that new medications will be developed that shrink the prostate and eliminate obstructive symptoms so that surgery can be avoided altogether.

Prevention

Whether or not BPH is caused by hormonal changes in aging men, there is no known way of preventing it. Once it does develop and symptoms are present that interfere seriously with the patient's life, timely medical or surgical treatment will reliably prevent symptoms from getting worse. Also, if the condition is treated before the prostate has become grossly enlarged, the risk of complications is minimal. One of the potentially most serious complications of BPH, urinary infection (and possible infection of the kidneys), can be prevented by using a catheter to drain excess urine out of the bladder so that it does not collect, stagnate, and become infected.

ORGANIZATIONS

American Urological Association Foundation, 1000 Corporate Blvd., Linthicum, MD, 21090, (410) 689-3700, (410) 689-3800, (866) 746-4282, auafoundation@auafoundation.org, http://www.urologyhealth.org/.

David A. Cramer, MD

Entamoeba histolytica infection *see* **Amebiasis**
Enteric fever *see* **Typhoid fever**
Enterically transmitted non-A non-B *see* **Hepatitis E**

Enterobacterial infections

Definition

Enterobacterial infections are disorders of the digestive tract and other organ systems produced by a group of gram-negative, rod-shaped bacteria called Enterobacteriaceae. Gram-negative means that the organisms do not retain the violet color of the dye used to make Gram stains. The most troublesome organism in this group is *Escherichia coli*. Other enterobacteria are species of *Salmonella*, *Shigella*, *Klebsiella*, *Enterobacter*, *Serratia*, *Proteus*, and *Yersinia*.

Description

Enterobacterial infections can be produced by bacteria that normally live in the human digestive tract without causing serious disease, or by bacteria that enter from the outside. In many cases these infections are nosocomial, which means that they can be acquired in the hospital. *Klebsiella* and *Proteus* sometimes cause **pneumonia**, ear and sinus infections, and urinary tract infections. *Enterobacter* and *Serratia* often cause bacterial infection of the blood (**bacteremia**), particularly in patients with weakened immune systems.

Diarrhea caused by enterobacteria is a common problem in the United States. It is estimated that each person in the general population has an average of 1.5 episodes of diarrhea each year, with higher rates in children, institutionalized people, and Native Americans. This type of enterobacterial infection can range from a minor nuisance to a life-threatening disorder, especially in infants, elderly persons, **AIDS** patients, and malnourished people. Enterobacterial infections are one of the two leading killers of children in developing countries.

Causes and symptoms

Causes

Enterobacterial infections in the digestive tract typically start when the organisms invade the mucous tissues that line the digestive tract. They may be bacteria that are already present in the stomach and intestines, or they may be transmitted by contaminated food and water. It is also possible for enterobacterial infections to spread by person-to-person contact. The usual incubation period is 12–72 hours.

***ESCHERICHIA COLI* INFECTIONS.** *E. coli* infections cause most of the enterobacterial infections in the United States. The organisms are categorized according to whether they are invasive or noninvasive. Noninvasive types of *E. coli* include what are called enteropathogenic *E. coli*, or EPEC, and enterotoxigenic *E. coli*, or ETEC. EPEC and ETEC types produce a bacterial poison (toxin) in the stomach that interacts with the digestive juices and causes the patient to lose large amounts of water through the intestines.

The invasive types of *E. coli* are called enterohemorrhagic *E. coli*, or EHEC, and enteroinvasive *E. coli,* or EIEC. These subtypes invade the stomach tissues directly, causing tissue destruction and bloody stools. EHEC can produce complications leading to **hemolytic-uremic syndrome** (HUS), a potentially fatal disorder marked by the destruction of red blood cells and kidney failure. EHEC has become a growing problem in the United States because of outbreaks caused by contaminated food. A particular type of EHEC known as O157:H7 has been identified since 1982 in undercooked hamburgers, unpasteurized milk, and apple juice. Between 2–7% of infections caused by O157:H7 develop into HUS.

Symptoms

The symptoms of enterobacterial infections are sometimes classified according to the type of diarrhea they produce.

WATERY DIARRHEA. Patients infected with ETEC, EPEC, some types of *Salmonella*, and some types of *Shigella* develop a watery diarrhea. These infections are located in the small intestine, result from bacterial toxins interacting with digestive juices, do not produce inflammation; and do not usually need treatment with **antibiotics**.

BLOODY DIARRHEA (DYSENTERY). Bloody diarrhea is sometimes called **dysentery**. It is produced by EHEC, EIEC, some types of *Salmonella*, some types of *Shigella*, and *Yersinia*. In dysentery, the infection is located in the colon, cells and tissues are destroyed, inflammation is present, and antibiotic therapy is usually required.

NECROTIZING ENTEROCOLITIS (NEC). Necrotizing enterocolitis (NEC) is a disorder that begins in newborn infants shortly after birth. Although NEC is not yet fully understood, it is thought that it results from a bacterial or viral invasion of damaged intestinal tissues. The disease organisms then cause the **death** (necrosis) of bowel tissue or **gangrene** of the bowel. NEC is primarily a disease of **prematurity**; 60–80% of cases occur in high-risk preterm infants. NEC is responsible for 2–5% of cases in newborn intensive care units (NICU). Enterobacteriaceae that have been identified in infants with NEC include *Salmonella, E. coli, Klebsiella,* and *Enterobacter.*

Diagnosis

Patient history

The diagnosis of enterobacterial infections is complicated by the fact that viruses, protozoa, and other types of bacteria can also cause diarrhea. In most cases of mild diarrhea, it is not critical to identify the organism because the disorder is self-limiting. Some groups of patients, however, should have stool tests. They include:

- patients with bloody diarrhea,
- patients with watery diarrhea who have become dehydrated,
- patients with watery diarrhea that has lasted longer than three days without decreasing in amount,
- patients with disorders of the immune system.

The patient history is useful for public health reasons as well as helping the doctor determine what type of enterobacterium may be causing the infection. The doctor will ask about the frequency and appearance of the diarrhea as well as other digestive symptoms. If the patient is nauseated and **vomiting**, the infection is more likely to be located in the small intestine. If the patient is running a **fever**, a diagnosis of dysentery is more likely. The doctor will also ask if anyone else in the patient's family or workplace is sick. Some types of enterobacteriaceae are more likely to cause group outbreaks than others. Other questions include the patient's food intake over the last few days and whether he or she has recently traveled to countries with **typhoid fever** or **cholera** outbreaks.

Physical examination

The most important parts of the **physical examination** are checking for signs of severe fluid loss and examining the abdomen to rule out typhoid fever. The doctor will look at the inside of the patient's mouth and evaluate the skin for signs of **dehydration**. The presence of a skin rash and an enlarged spleen suggests typhoid rather than a bacterial infection. If the patient's abdomen hurts when the doctor examines it, a diagnosis of dysentery is more likely.

Laboratory tests

The most common test that is used to identify the cause of diarrhea is the stool test. Examining a stool sample under a microscope can help to rule out parasitic and protozoal infections. Routine stool cultures, however, cannot be used to identify any of the four types of *E. coli* that cause intestinal infections. ETEC, EPEC, and EIEC are unusual in the United States and can usually be identified only by specialists in research laboratories. Because of concern about EHEC outbreaks, however, most laboratories in the United States can now screen for O157:H7 with a test that identifies its characteristic toxin. All patients with bloody diarrhea should have a stool sample tested for *E. coli* O157:H7.

KEY TERMS

Dysentery—A type of diarrhea caused by infection and characterized by mucus and blood in the stools.

Empirical treatment—Medical treatment that is given on the basis of the doctor's observations and experience.

Escherichia coli—A type of enterobacterium that is responsible for most cases of severe bacterial diarrhea in the United States.

Hemolytic-uremic syndrome (HUS)—A potentially fatal complication of *E. coli* infections characterized by kidney failure and destruction of red blood cells.

Necrotizing enterocolitis (NEC)—A disorder in newborns caused by bacterial or viral invasion of vulnerable intestinal tissues.

Nosocomial infections—Infections acquired in hospitals.

Toxin—A poison produced by certain types of bacteria.

Treatment

The initial treatment of enterobacterial diarrhea is usually empiric. Empiric means that the doctor treats the patient on the basis of the visible symptoms and professional experience in treating infections, without waiting for laboratory test results. Since the results of stool cultures can take as long as two days, it is important to prevent dehydration. The patient will be given fluids to restore the electrolyte balance and paregoric to relieve abdominal cramping.

Newborn infants and patients with immune system disorders will be given antibiotics intravenously once the organism has been identified. Gentamicin, tobramycin, and amikacin are being used more frequently to treat enterobacterial infections because many of the organisms are becoming resistant to ampicillin and cephalosporin antibiotics.

Alternative treatment

Alternative treatments for diarrhea are intended to relieve the discomfort of abdominal cramping. Most alternative practitioners advise consulting a medical doctor if the patient has sunken eyes, dry eyes or mouth, or other signs of dehydration.

Herbal medicine

Herbalists may recommend cloves taken as an infusion or ginger given in drop doses to control intestinal cramps, eliminate gas, and prevent **vomiting**. Peppermint (*Mentha piperita*) or chamomile (*Matricaria recutita*) tea may also ease cramps and intestinal spasms.

Homeopathy

Homeopathic practitioners frequently recommend *Arsenicum album* for diarrhea caused by contaminated food, and *Belladonna* for diarrhea that comes on suddenly with mucus in the stools. *Veratrum album* would be given for watery diarrhea, and *Podophyllum* for diarrhea with few other symptoms.

Prognosis

The prognosis for most enterobacterial infections is good; most patients recover in about a week or 10 days without needing antibiotics. HUS, on the other hand, has a mortality rate of 3–5% even with intensive care. About a third of the survivors have long-term problems with kidney function, and another 8% develop high blood pressure, seizure disorders, and blindness.

Prevention

The World Health Organization (WHO) offers the following suggestions for preventing enterobacterial infections, including *E. coli* O157:H7 dysentery:

- Cook ground beef or hamburgers until the meat is thoroughly done. Juices from the meat should be completely clear, not pink or red. All parts of the meat should reach a temperature of 70°C (158°F) or higher.

- Do not drink unpasteurized milk or use products made from raw milk.

- Wash hands thoroughly and frequently, especially after using the toilet.

- Wash fruits and vegetables carefully, or peel them. Keep all kitchen surfaces and serving utensils clean.

- If drinking water is not known to be safe, boil it or drink bottled water.

- Keep cooked foods separate from raw foods, and avoid touching cooked foods with knives or other utensils that have been used with raw meat.

ORGANIZATIONS

Centers for Disease Control and Prevention (CDC), 1600 Clifton Road, Atlanta, GA, 30333, (800) 232-4636, cdcinfo@cdc.gov, http://www.cdc.gov.

Rebecca J. Frey, PhD

Enterobiasis

Definition

Enterobiasis, or pinworm infection as it is commonly called, is an intestinal infection caused by the parasitic roundworm called *Enterobius vermicularis*. The most common symptom of this irritating, but not particularly dangerous, disease is **itching** around the anal area.

Description

Enterobiasis is also called seatworm infection or oxyuriasis. In the United States, enterobiasis is the most common worm infection, and some estimate that approximately 10% of the United States population is infected. Worldwide, approximately 200 million people are infected. Enterobiasis can affect people of any age, but is most common among children ages 5–14 and particularly affects those in the daycare setting.

Causes and symptoms

The disease is highly contagious and is caused by a parasitic worm called *Enterobius vermicularis*. The adult female worm is about the size of a staple (approximately 0.4 in [1 cm long] and 0.02 in [0.5 mm] wide) and

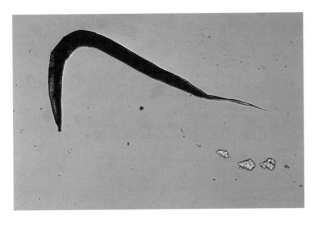

The pinworm of the genus *Enterobius* pictured above is the source of this infestation occurring in children. *(Photo Researchers, Inc.)*

has a pointed tip. The disease is transmitted by ingesting the eggs of the pinworm. These eggs travel to the small intestine where, after approximately one month, they hatch and mature into adult worms. During the night, the female adult worms travel to the area around the anus and deposit eggs in the folds of the anal area. A single female pinworm can lay 10,000 eggs and, after laying eggs, dies. The eggs are capable of causing infection after six hours at body temperature.

Significant itching in the anal region is caused by the movement of the adult worm as the eggs are deposited. When an individual scratches the anal region, the tiny eggs get under the finger nails and in the underwear and night clothes. Anything the individual touches with the contaminated fingers, for example, toys, bedding, blankets, bathroom door knobs, or sinks, becomes contaminated. The eggs are very hardy and can live on surfaces for two to three weeks. Anyone touching these contaminated surfaces can ingest the eggs and become infected. An individual can also become infected by inhaling and swallowing the eggs, for example, when the bedcovers are shaken.

Many individuals with enterobiasis exhibit no symptoms. When present, however, symptoms of the infection begin approximately two weeks after ingesting the pinworm eggs. The main symptom is itching around the anus. Because the itching intensifies at night, when the female worms comes to the anus to lay eggs, it often leads to disrupted sleep and irritability. Poor sleeping at night in small children can be related to pinworms. Occasionally, the itching causes some bleeding and bruising in the region, and secondary bacterial infections can occur. In females, the itching may spread to the vagina and sometimes causes an infection of the vaginal region (vaginitis). Enterobiasis usually lasts one to two months.

Diagnosis

First, a physician will rule out other potential causes of the itching, such as **hemorrhoids**, lice, or fungal or bacterial infection. Once these have been ruled out, an accurate diagnosis of enterobiasis will require that either the eggs or the adult worms are detected. Rarely, the adult worms are seen as thin, yellowish-white threads, about 0.4 in (1 cm) long, in the stools of the infected person. Usually, an hour or so after the individual goes to sleep, the adult female worms may be seen moving around laying eggs if a flashlight is shone at the rectal area.

An easier method is to observe the eggs under the microscope. In order to collect a specimen for laboratory diagnosis, the physician may provide a paddle with

KEY TERMS

Anus—The opening through which feces are eliminated.

Hemorrhoid—An area around the anus where veins become dilated and the tissue swells, causing itching and pain.

Rectum—The end of the large intestine in which feces collects for elimination through the anus.

Vaginitis—Inflammation of the vagina.

a sticky adhesive on one side, or an individual may be instructed to place a piece of shiny cellophane tape sticky side down against the anal opening. The best time to perform this test is at night or as soon as the individual wakes up in the morning, before having a bowel movement or taking a bath or shower. The pinworm eggs will stick to the tape, which can then be placed on a specimen slide. When under a microscope in the laboratory, the eggs will be clearly visible.

Treatment

In order to treat the disease, either mebendazole (Vermox) or pyrantel pamoate (Pin-X) will be given in two oral doses spaced two weeks apart. These medications eradicate the infection in approximately 90% of cases. Re-infection is common and several treatments may be required. Because the infection is easily spread through contact with contaminated clothing or surfaces, it is recommended that all family members receive the therapeutic dose. Sometimes a series of six treatments are given, each spaced two weeks apart. If family members continue to be infected, a source outside the house may be responsible.

To relieve the rectal itching, a shallow warm bath with either half a cup of table salt, or Epsom salts is recommended. Also, application of an ointment containing zinc oxide or regular petroleum jelly can be used to relieve rectal itching.

Prognosis

Pinworms cause little damage and can be easily eradicated with proper treatment. Full recovery is expected.

Prevention

The disease can be prevented by treating all the infected cases and thus eliminating the source of infection. Some ways to keep from catching or spreading the disease include the following recommendations:

- wash hands thoroughly before handling food and eating
- keep finger nails short and clean
- avoiding scratching the anal area
- take early morning showers to wash away eggs deposited overnight
- once the infection has been identified, and treatment is started, change the bed linen, night clothes, and underwear daily
- machine wash linens in hot water and dry with heat to kill any eggs
- open the blinds or curtains since eggs are sensitive to sunlight

Resources

BOOKS

Fauci, Anthony S., et al., eds. *Harrison's Principles of Internal Medicine*. 17th ed. New York: McGraw–Hill Professional, 2008.

Lata Cherath, PhD

Enterohemorrhagic *E. coli* see **Escherichia coli**

Enterostomy

Definition

An enterostomy is an operation in which the surgeon makes a passage into the patient's small intestine through the abdomen with an opening to allow for drainage or to insert a tube for feeding. The opening is called a stoma, from the Greek word for mouth. Enterostomies may be either temporary or permanent. They are classified according to the part of the intestine that is used to create the stoma. If the ileum, which is the lowest of the three sections of the small intestine, is used to make the stoma, the operation is called an ileostomy. If the jejunum, which is the middle section of the small intestine, is used, the operation is called a jejunostomy. Some people use the word *ostomy* as a word that covers all types of enterostomies.

Purpose

Enterostomies are performed in order to create a new opening for the passage of fecal matter when normal intestinal functioning is interrupted or when diseases of the intestines cannot be treated by medications or less radical surgery. Some situations that may require enterostomies include:

- Healing of inflamed bowel segments. Enterostomies performed for this reason are usually temporary.

- Emergency treatment of gunshot or other penetrating wounds of the abdomen. An enterostomy is needed to prevent the contents of the intestine from causing a serious inflammation of the inside of the abdominal cavity (peritonitis). These enterostomies are also often temporary.

- Placement of a tube for enteral feeding. Enteral feeding is a method for conveying nutritional solutions directly into the stomach or jejunum through a tube. Tube enterostomies may be long-term but are not permanent.

- Removal of diseased sections of the intestines. Ileostomies performed for this reason are permanent. The most common disorders requiring permanent ileostomy are Crohn's disease, familial polyposis, and ulcerative colitis. Familial polyposis and ulcerative colitis are serious health risks because they can develop into cancer.

- Treatment of advanced cancer or other causes of intestinal obstruction.

Precautions

Enterostomies are usually performed only as emergency treatments for traumatic injuries in the abdomen or as final measures for serious disorders of the intestines. Most patients do not refuse to have the operation performed when the need for it is explained to them. A small minority, however, refuse enterostomies because of strong psychological reactions to personal disfigurement and the need to relearn bowel habits.

Description

Ileostomy

Ileostomies represent about 25% of enterostomies. They are performed after the surgeon removes a diseased colon and sometimes the rectum as well. The most common ileostomy is called a Brooke ileostomy after the English surgeon who developed it. In a Brooke ileostomy, the surgeon makes the stoma in the lower right section of the abdomen. The ileum is pulled through an opening (incision) in the muscle layer. The surgeon then turns the cut end of the intestine inside out and sews it to the edges of the hole. He or she then positions an appliance for collecting the fecal material. The appliance consists of a plastic bag that fits over the stoma and lies flat against the abdomen. The patient is taught to drain the bag from time to time during the day. Ileostomies need to be emptied frequently because the digested food contains large amounts of water. Shortly after the operation, the ileostomy produces 1–2 qt.(0.9–1.9 l) of fluid per day; after a month or two of adjustment, the volume decreases to 1–2 pt (0.5–0.9) per day.

KOCK POUCH (CONTINENT ILEOSTOMY). The Kock pouch is a variation of the basic ileostomy and is named for its Swedish inventor. In the Kock technique, the surgeon forms a pouch inside the abdominal cavity behind the stoma that collects the fecal material. The stoma is shaped into a valve to prevent fluid from leaking onto the patient's abdomen. The patient then empties the pouch several times daily by inserting a tube (catheter) through the valve. The Kock technique is sometimes called a continent ileostomy because the fluid is contained inside the abdomen. It is successful in 70–90% of patients who have it done.

Jejunostomy

A jejunostomy is similar to an ileostomy except that the stoma is placed in the second section of the small intestine rather than the third. Jejunostomies are performed less frequently than ileostomies. They are almost always temporary procedures.

Tube enterostomies

Tube enterostomies are operations in which the surgeon makes a stoma into the stomach itself or the jejunum in order to insert a tube for liquid nutrients. Tube enterostomies are performed in patients who need tube feeding for longer than six weeks, or who have had recent mouth or nose surgery. As long as the patient's intestinal tract can function, **tube feedings** are considered preferable to intravenous feeding. Enteral **nutrition** is safer than intravenous fluids and helps to keep the patient's digestive tract functioning.

Preparation

Preoperative preparation includes both patient education and physical preparation.

Patient education

If the patient is going to have a permanent ileostomy, the doctor will explain what will happen during the operation and why it is necessary. Most patients are willing to accept an ostomy as an alternative to the chronic **pain** and **diarrhea** of ulcerative **colitis** or the risk of **cancer** from other intestinal disorders. The patient can also meet with an enterostomal therapist (ET) or a member of the United Ostomy Association, which is a support group for people with ostomies.

Crohn's disease—A disease of the intestines that causes inflammation leading to scarring, thickening of the walls of the intestine, and eventual obstruction.

Duodenum—The first of the three segments of the small intestine. The duodenum connects the stomach and the jejunum.

Enteral nutrition—A technique for feeding patients with liquid formulas conveyed directly into the stomach or jejunum through tubes.

Enterostomal therapist (ET)—A specialized counselor, usually a registered nurse, who provides ostomy patients with education and counseling before the operation. After surgery, the ET helps the patient learn to take care of the stoma and appliance, and offers long-term emotional support.

Familial polyposis—A disease that runs in families in which lumps of tissue (polyps) form inside the colon. Familial polyposis may develop into cancer.

Ileum—The third segment of the small intestine, connecting the jejunum and the large intestine.

Jejunum—The second of the three segments of the small intestine, connecting the duodenum and the ileum.

Kock pouch—A type of ileostomy in which the surgeon forms an artificial rectum from a section of the ileum. A Kock pouch is sometimes called a continent ileostomy because it is drained with a tube.

Ostomy—A common term for all types of enterostomies.

Stoma—The surgically constructed mouth or passage between the intestine and the outside of the patient's body.

Tube enterostomy—An enterostomy performed to allow the insertion of a feeding tube into the jejunum or stomach.

Ulcerative colitis—A disease of the colon characterized by inflammation of the mucous lining, ulcerated areas of tissue, and bloody diarrhea.

Medical preparation

The patient is prepared for surgery with an evaluation of his or her nutritional status, possible need for blood transfusions, and **antibiotics** if necessary. If the patient does not have an intestinal obstruction or severe inflammation, he or she may be given a large quantity of a polyethylene glycol (PEG) solution to cleanse the intestines before surgery.

Aftercare

Aftercare of an enterostomy is both psychological and medical.

Medical aftercare

If the enterostomy is temporary, aftercare consists of the usual monitoring of surgical **wounds** for infection or bleeding. If the patient has had a permanent ileostomy, aftercare includes learning to use the appliance or empty the Kock pouch; learning to keep the stoma clean; and readjusting bathroom habits. Recovery takes a long time because major surgery is a shock to the system and the intestines take several days to resume normal functioning. The patient's fluid intake and output will be checked frequently to minimize the risk of **dehydration**.

Patient education

Ileostomy patients must learn to watch their fluid and salt intake. They are at greater risk of becoming dehydrated in hot weather, from **exercise**, or from diarrhea. In some cases they may need extra bananas or orange juice in the diet to keep up the level of potassium in the blood.

Patient education includes social concerns as well as physical self-care. Many ileostomy patients are worried about the effects of the operation on their close relationships and employment. If the patient has not seen an ET before the operation, the aftercare period is a good time to find out about self-help and support groups. The ET can also evaluate the patient's emotional reactions to the ostomy.

Risks

Enterostomies are not considered high-risk operations by themselves. About 40% of ileostomy patients have complications afterward, however; about 15% require minor surgical corrections. Possible complications include:

• skin irritation caused by leakage of digestive fluids onto the skin around the stoma; Irritation is the most common complication of ileostomies

- diarrhea
- the development of abscesses
- gallstones or stones in the urinary tract
- inflammation of the ileum
- odors can often be prevented by a change in diet
- intestinal obstruction
- a section of the bowel pushing out of the body (prolapse)

Normal results

Normal results include recovery from the surgery with few or no complications. About 95% of people with ostomies recover completely, are able to return to work, and consider themselves to be in good health. Many ileostomy patients enjoy being able to eat a full range of foods rather than living on a restricted diet. Some patients, however, need to be referred to psychotherapists to deal with depression or other emotional problems after the operation.

ORGANIZATIONS

United Ostomy Association, Inc. (UOA), PO Box 512, Northfield, MN, 55057-0512, (800) 826-0826, info@ostomy.org, http://www.ostomy.org.

Rebecca J. Frey, PhD

Enterovirus infections

Definition

Enteroviruses are so named because they reproduce initially in the gastrointestinal tract after infection occurs. Despite, this, they usually do not lead to intestinal symptoms; rather it is their spread to organs, such as the nervous system, heart, skin, and others that causes disease. Enteroviruses are part of a larger group of viruses known as Picornaviruses. The word comes from the combination of "pico" (Spanish, meaning "a little bit"), and RNA (ribonucleic acid, an important component of genetic material).

Description

There are four groups of enteroviruses: Coxsackievirus, Echovirus, ungrouped Enterovirus, and Y Poliovirus.

Viruses are generally divided into those that use DNA (deoxyribonucleic acid) or RNA as their genetic material; all enteroviruses are RNA viruses. They are found worldwide, but infection is more common in areas of poor hygiene and overcrowding.

Although most cases of enterovirus do not produce symptoms, some five to 10 million individuals in the United States each year suffer from one of the enteroviral diseases. Illness is more common in the very young. While there are close to 70 different strains of enteroviruses, over 70% of infections are caused by only 10 types.

The virus is most commonly transmitted by the fecal-oral route (contamination of fingers or objects by human waste material); in some instances transmission is through contaminated food or water. Passage of some strains of virus by way of air droplets can lead to respiratory illness. Infection of fetuses by way of the placenta also has been documented. Breast milk contains antibodies which can protect newborns.

The incubation period for most enteroviruses ranges from two to 14 days. In areas of temperate climate, infections occur mainly in the summer and fall.

Causes and symptoms

Enteroviruses are believed to be the cause of at least 10 distinct illnesses. Once they enter the body, they multiply in the cells that line the gastrointestinal tract, and eventually reach sites of lymphatic tissue (such as the tonsils). While most of these diseases are of short duration and do not cause significant injury, some can produce severe illness. Each presents its own unique symptoms. And a 2003 report to the Infectious Diseases Society of America reminded physicians that infants with enteroviral infections often present early in their illnesses with no signs of **fever**, complicating diagnosis.

The main syndromes caused by the various enteroviruses are the following:

- Summer grippe (nonspecific febrile illness). This is the most common syndrome, and is characterized by flu-like symptoms of fever, headache, and weakness, that typically last three to four days. Many patients also develop upper respiratory symptoms and some nausea and vomiting. One of the major ways to distinguish this disease from influenza, is the fact that grippe most often occurs in the summer.
- Generalized disease of the newborn is a potentially serious infection in which infants from one week to three months of age develop a syndrome that can be difficult to distinguish from a severe bacterial

infection. Fever, irritability, and decreased responsiveness or excessive sleepiness are the major symptoms. Inflammation of heart muscle (myocarditis), low blood pressure, hepatitis, and meningitis sometimes complicate the illness.

- Aseptic meningitis encephalitis is a well known syndrome caused by this group of viruses. In fact, enteroviruses are responsible for over 90% of cases of aseptic meningitis, and most often hit children and young adults. Headache, fever, avoidance of light, and eye pain are characteristic. Drowsiness may be prominent, and other symptoms include sore throat, cough, muscle pain, and rash. Occasionally, not only the meninges—the covering around the brain and spinal cord—is infected, but also brain tissue itself, producing encephalitis. The illness resolves after about a week or so, and permanent damage is unusual. Enteroviruses can also produce the Guillian-Barré syndrome, which involves weakness and paralysis of the extremities and even the muscles of respiration.

- Pleurodynia (Bornholm's disease) is due to viral infection and inflammation of the chest and abdominal muscles used for breathing. Pain occurs as acute episodes, lasting 30 minutes or so. Coxsackie B virus is the usual cause of the illness.

- Myocarditis and/or pericarditis involves infection of the heart muscle (myocardium) and the covering around the heart (pericardium). Infants and young adults are the most susceptible, and for some reason, more than two-thirds of cases occur in males. The disease usually begins as an upper respiratory tract infection with cough, shortness of breath, and fever. Chest pain, increasing shortness of breath, irregularities of cardiac rhythm, and heart failure sometimes develop. Some patients wind up with long-term heart failure if the heart muscle is significantly affected.

- Exanthems is the medical term for rashes, and enterovirus is the number one cause of summer and fall rashes in children. They occur anywhere on the body, and often resemble diseases such as measles.

- Hand-foot-and-mouth disease occurs initially as a sore throat (often involving the tongue as well), and is followed by a rash on the hands, and sometimes the feet. The rash often forms small blisters, which lead to ulcers. Symptoms generally resolve within a week. A specific Coxsackievirus (A16) is the most frequent cause of this highly infectious disease.

- Herpangina is most often caused by one of the Coxsackie A viruses, and appears as the acute onset of fever and sore throat. This last symptom is particularly severe, as the virus produces multiple ulcers in the throat. Swallowing becomes very painful; symptoms can persist for several weeks.

KEY TERMS

Antibodies—Proteins that are formed by the body and play a role in defense against infection.

Antibiotic—A medication that is designed to kill or weaken bacteria.

Meninges—Outer covering of the spinal cord and brain. Infection is called meningitis, which can lead to damage to the brain or spinal cord and lead to death.

- Acute hemorrhagic conjunctivitis involves viral infection of the conjunctiva, which is a covering around the eye. Pain, blurred vision, aversion to light, and a discharge from the eye are the main symptoms. Headache and fever occur in about one in five patients. The disease runs its course in about 10 days.

A number of other illnesses have been attributed to enteroviruses, including **pneumonia** and other respiratory infections, **myositis** or muscle inflammation, arthritis, and acute inflammation of the kidneys. It is clear then that these viruses produce a number of various illnesses, most often in younger age groups.

Diagnosis

In the majority of cases, diagnosis is based on the characteristic symptoms that the virus produces (such as the chest **pain** in pleurodynia). Rarely is it necessary to identify a specific strain of virus causing the illness. It is more important to be certain that the infection is due to a virus that does not require treatment with **antibiotics**.

Culture, or growing the organism outside of the body, is helpful only when obtained from areas that tend to indicate recent infection, such as from swollen joints, cerebrospinal fluid, or blood. Cultures from other areas, such as the throat, can be misleading. This is because the virus may remain for long periods of time in places with a large amount of lymphatic tissue. As a rule, cultures done early in the illness are more likely to identify the virus.

New techniques that involve identification of viral genetic material (PCR) are useful in certain cases, but are not indicated for routine testing.

Treatment

As noted above, enterovirus is capable of attacking many different organs and producing a variety of symptoms. Most infections are mild and improve without complications, requiring no specific therapy.

When the virus attacks critical organs however, such as the heart, respiratory muscles, nervous system, etc., specialized care is often needed.

No effective antiviral medication for enterovirus has undergone investigation in patients, though some drugs appeared promising for the future. In some patients who are unable to produce antibodies (hypogammaglobunemia), administrating antibodies themselves is helpful.

Prognosis

The overall outlook for enterovirus infection depends on the organs involved, and the immune condition of the individual patient. Unless vital organs are involved or immunity is abnormal, infection causes few problems. On the other hand, patients who have diseases that affect antibody production can develop chronic infection of the brain or meninges. A 2003 study found that enterovirus infections can increase the risk of type 1 diabetes in children who are genetically predisposed to diabetes.

Prevention

In the hospital setting, the best means of avoiding transmission of infection is the use of good hand-washing practices and other appropriate precautions (gowns and gloves for hospital staff). The virus is found in feces for up to one week after infection; therefore precautions that isolate waste material (enteric precautions) will help decrease the chance of spreading the illness.

Resources

PERIODICALS

"Enterovirus Infections Increase Risk of Type 1 Diabetes in High-Risk Children." *Diabetes Week* June 16, 2003: 22.

Tucker, Miriam E. "Fever Often Absent in Early Enteroviral Illness (Severe Cases)." *Pediatric News* January 2003: 20–22.

OTHER

"Weekly Clinicopathological Exercises: Case 47- 1993: A 28-Year-Old Man with Recurrent Ventricular Tachycardia and Dysfunction of Multiple Organs." *New England Journal of Medicine Online.* http://content.nejm.org.

David Kaminstein, MD
Teresa G. Odle

Entropy *see* **Eyelid disorders**

Enuresis *see* **Bed-wetting**

Environmental medicine *see* **Wilderness medicine**

Enzyme therapy

Definition

Enyzme therapy is a plan of dietary supplements of plant and animal enzymes used to facilitate the digestive process and improve the body's ability to maintain balanced metabolism.

Purpose

In traditional medicine, enzyme supplements are often prescribed for patients suffering from disorders that affect the digestive process, such as **cystic fibrosis**, Gaucher's disease, and **celiac disease**. A program of enzyme supplementation is rarely recommended for healthy patients. However, proponents of enzyme therapy believe that such a program is beneficial for everyone. They point to enzymes' ability to purify the blood, strengthen the immune system, enhance mental capacity, cleanse the colon, and maintain proper pH balance in urine. They feel that by improving the digestive process, the body is better able to combat infection and disease.

Some evidence exists that pancreatic enzymes derived from animal sources are helpful in **cancer** treatment. The enzymes may be able to dissolve the coating on cancer cells and may make it easier for the immune system to attack the cancer.

A partial list of the wide variety of complaints and illnesses that can be treated by enzyme therapy includes:

- AIDS
- anemia
- alcohol consumption
- anxiety
- acute inflammation
- back pain
- cancer
- colds
- chronic fatigue syndrome
- colitis
- constipation
- diarrhea
- food allergies
- gastritis
- gastric duodenal ulcer
- gout
- headaches
- hepatitis

KEY TERMS

Celiac disease—A chronic disease characterized by defective digestion and use of fats.

Cystic fibrosis—A genetic disease that causes multiple digestive, excretion, and respiratory complications. Among the effects, the pancreas fails to provide secretions needed for the digestion of food.

Duodenum—The first part of the small intestine.

Gaucher's disease—A rare genetic disease caused by a deficiency of enzymes needed for the processing of fatty acids.

Metabolism—The system of chemical processes necessary for living cells to remain healthy.

- hypoglycemia
- infections
- mucous congestion
- multiple sclerosis
- nervous disorders
- nutritional disorders
- obesity
- premenstrual syndrome (PMS)
- stress

Description

Origins

Enzymes are protein molecules used by the body to perform all of its chemical actions and reactions. The body manufactures several thousands of enzymes. Among them are the digestive enzymes produced by the stomach, pancreas, small intestine, and the salivary glands of the mouth. Their energy-producing properties are responsible for not only the digestion of nutrients, but their absorption, transportation, metabolization, and elimination as well.

Enzyme therapy is based on the work of Dr. Edward Howell in the 1920s and 1930s. Howell proposed that enzymes from foods work in the stomach to pre-digest food. He advocated the consumption of large amounts of plant enzymes, theorizing that if the body had to use less of its own enzymes for digestion, it could store them for maintaining metabolic harmony. Four categories of plant enzymes are helpful in pre-digestion: protease, amylase, lipase, and cellulase. Cellulase is particularly helpful because the body is unable to produce it.

Animal enzymes, such as pepsin extracted from the stomach of pigs, work more effectively in the duodenum. They are typically used for the treatment of nondigestive ailments.

The seven categories of food enzymes and their activities

- amylase breaks down starches
- cellulase breaks down fibers
- lactase breaks down dairy products
- lipase breaks down fats
- maltase breaks down grains
- protease breaks down proteins
- sucrase breaks down sugars

Enzyme theory generated further interest as the human diet became more dependent on processed and cooked foods. Enzymes are extremely sensitive to heat, and temperatures above 118°F (48°C) destroy them. Modern processes of pasteurization, canning, and microwaving are particularly harmful to the enzymes in food.

Enzyme supplements are extracted from plants like pineapple and papaya and from the organs of cows and pigs. The supplements are typically given in tablet or capsule form. Pancreatic enzymes may also be given by injection. The dosage varies with the condition being treated. For nondigestive ailments, the supplements are taken in the hour before meals so that they can be quickly absorbed into the blood. For digestive ailments, the supplements are taken immediately before meals accompanied by a large glass of fluids. Pancreatic enzymes may be accompanied by doses of vitamin A.

Preparations

No special preparations are necessary before beginning enzyme therapy. However, it is always advisable to talk to a doctor or pharmacist before purchasing enzymes and beginning therapy.

Precautions

People with **allergies** to beef, pork, pineapples, and papaya may suffer allergic reactions to enzyme supplements. Tablets are often coated to prevent them from breaking down in the stomach, and usually shouldn't be chewed or crushed. People who have difficulty swallowing pills can request enzyme supplements in capsule form. The capsules can then be opened and the contents sprinkled onto soft foods like applesauce.

Side effects

Side effects associated with enzyme therapy include **heartburn**, **nausea and vomiting**, **diarrhea**, bloating, gas, and **acne**. According to the principles of therapy, these are temporary cleansing symptoms. Drinking eight to 10 glasses of water daily and getting regular **exercise** can reduce the discomfort of these side effects. Individuals may also experience an increase in bowel movements, perhaps one or two per day. This is also considered a positive effect.

Plant enzymes are safe for pregnant women, although they should always check with a doctor before using enzymes. Pregnant women should avoid animal enzymes. In rare cases, extremely high doses of enzymes can result in a build up of uric acid in the blood or urine and can cause a break down of proteins.

Research and general acceptance

In the United States, the Food and Drug Administration (FDA) has classified enzymes as a food. Therefore, they can be purchased without a prescription. However, insurance coverage is usually dependent upon the therapy resulting from a doctor's orders.

Resources

OTHER

Enzyme Therapy for Your Health. http://members.tripod.com/~colloid/enzyme.htm.
Questions and Answers about Food Enzymes and Nutrition. http://www.enzymes.com.
Therapies: Enzyme Therapy. http://library.thinkquest.org/24206/enzyme-therapy.html.

Mary McNulty

Eosinophilic granuloma *see* **Histiocytosis X**

Eosinophilic pneumonia

Definition

Eosinophilic **pneumonia** is a group of diseases in which there is an above normal number of eosinophils in the lungs and blood.

KEY TERMS

Infiltrates—Cells or body fluids that have passed into a tissue or body cavity.

Sputum—Material coughed up from the throat or lungs.

Description

Eosinophilia is an increase in the number of eosinophils. Eosinophilic pneumonia is characterized by a large number of eosinophils in the lungs, usually in the absence of an **infectious disease**. Eosinophils are one of the white blood cells and are classified as a granulocyte. They are part of the non-specific immune system and participate in inflammatory reactions. Eosinophils contain cationic molecules that are useful for destroying infectious agents, especially heiminthic parasites (worms). There are several types of eosinophilic pneumonia. Loffler's pneumonia is a temporary infiltration of eosinophils into the lungs. The patient will feel tired, have a **cough**, spasms of the bronchial airway, and difficulty breathing. Loffler's pneumonia will clear spontaneously, but slowly over the course of about a month. Another form of eosinophilic pneumonia, pulmonary infiltrates with eosinophilia (PIE), is a more serious and potentially fatal disease. In PIE, the patient experiences **asthma**, pulmonary infiltrates, disorders of the peripheral nervous system, central nervous systems symptoms, and periarteritis nodosa.

Causes and symptoms

Pneumonia with eosinophils occurs as part of a hypersensitivity reaction. A hypersensitivity reaction is an over-reaction of the immune system to a particular stimulus. As part of the hypersensitive reaction, cells of the immune system are produced in increased numbers and migrate into areas targeted by the hypersensitivity reaction. In the case of eosinophilic pneumonia, the lungs are the target. Generally, eosinophilia pneumonia is not a reaction to an infection. There is a correlation between asthma and eosinophilic pneumonia. Eosinophilic pneumonia can also be caused by drugs and, in some people, by polluted air. The symptoms range from mild (coughing, **wheezing**, and **shortness of breath**) to severe and life threatening (severe shortness of breath and difficulty getting enough oxygen). The symptoms may resolve spontaneously or can persist for long periods of time. In a few cases, the disease may rapidly produce life-threatening pneumonia.

Diagnosis

Since eosinophilia is common to a number of conditions, the physician must rule out asthma and infection by helminths when diagnosing eosinophilic pneumonia. A whole blood count will reveal an increased number of eosinophils in the blood. An x ray of the lungs may show the presence of infiltrates (the eosinophils and fluid). If sputum is produced in coughing, eosinophils will be seen instead of the more normal profile of granulocytes seen when an infectious agent is present.

Treatment

Eosinophilic pneumonia may not respond to drugs used to treat asthma. Eosinophilic pneumonia is usually treated with **steroids**, particularly glucocorticosteroids. Steroids are not effective against infectious agents, but the main disease process in eosinophilic pneumonia is an inflammatory reaction, not a response to infection. When eosinophilia is produced as a consequence of asthma or an infection by helminths, treatment of the asthma or helminths will reduce the eosinophilia.

Resources

BOOKS

Beers, Mark H., Robert S. Porter, and Thomas V. Jones, eds. *The Merck Manual of Diagnosis and Therapy.* 18th ed. Whitehouse Station, NJ: Merck Research Laboratories, 2006.

John T. Lohr, PhD

Ephedrine *see* **Bronchodilators**

Epicondylitis *see* **Tennis elbow**

Epidemic icterus *see* **Hepatitis A**

Epidemic typhus *see* **Typhus**

Epidemic viral gastroenteritis *see* **Rotavirus infections**

Epidermolysis bullosa

Definition

Epidermolysis bullosa (EB) is a group of rare inherited skin diseases that are characterized by the development of blisters following minimal pressure to the skin. Blistering often appears in infancy in response to simply being held or handled. In rarer forms of the disorder, EB can be life-threatening. There is no cure for the disorder. Treatment focuses on preventing and treating **wounds** and infection.

Description

Epidermolysis bullosa has three major forms and at least 16 subtypes. The three major forms are EB simplex, junctional EB, and dystrophic EB. These can range in severity from mild blistering to more disfiguring and life-threatening disease. Physicians diagnose the form of the disease based on where the blister forms in relation to the epidermis (the skin's outermost layer) and the deeper dermis layer.

The prevalence of epidermolysis varies among different populations. A study in Scotland estimated the prevalence to be one in 20,400. Researchers in other parts of the world estimate the prevalence to be one in 100,000. This variance is due to the variability of expression. Many cases of epidermolysis bullosa are often not accurately diagnosed and thus, are not reported.

Causes and symptoms

EB can be inherited as the result of a dominant genetic abnormality (only one parent carries the abnormal gene) or a recessive genetic abnormality (both parents carry the abnormal gene).

EB simplex results from mutations in genes responsible for keratin 5 and 14, which are proteins that give cells of the epidermis its structure. EB simplex is transmitted in an autosomal dominant fashion.

Dystrophic EB is caused by mutations in genes for type VII collagen, the protein contained in the fibers anchoring the epidermis to the deeper layers of the skin. The genetic mutations for junctional EB are found in the genes responsible for producing the protein Laminin-5. Dystrophic EB is an autosomal disorder and will only result if both parents transmit an abnormal gene during conception.

EB simplex, the most common form of EB, is the least serious form of the disease. In most affected individuals, the blisters are mild and do not scar after they heal. Some forms of EB simplex affect just the hands and feet. Other forms of EB simplex can lead to more widespread blistering, as well as hair loss and missing teeth. Recurrent blistering is annoying but not life threatening.

The second, or junctional, form of EB does not lead to scarring. However, skin on the areas prone to blistering, such as elbows and knees, often shrinks. In one variation of junctional EB, called gravis junctional EB of Herlitz, the blistering can be so severe that affected infants may not survive due to massive infection and **dehydration**.

The third form of EB, dystrophic EB, varies greatly in terms of severity, but more typically affects the arms and legs. In one variation, called Hallopeau-Siemens EB, repeated blistering and scarring of the hands and feet causes the fingers and toes to fuse, leaving them dysfunctional and with a mitten-like appearance.

Diagnosis

Physicians and researchers distinguish between the three major subtypes of EB based on which layer of the epidermis separates from the deeper dermis layer of the skin below. Patients suspected of having EB should have a fresh blister biopsied for review. This sample of tissue is examined under an electron microscope or under a conventional microscope using a technique called immunofluorescence, which helps to map the underlying structure.

Knowing that a family member has EB can help establish the diagnosis, but it is possible that parents or siblings will show no sign of the disease, either because it is caused by a new genetic mutation, or because the parents are carriers of the recessive trait and do not display the disease.

Treatment

The most important treatment for EB is daily wound care. Because the skin is very fragile, care must be taken to be certain that dressing changes do not cause further damage. Tape should not be applied directly to skin and **bandages** should be soaked off. Infection is a major concern, so a topical antibiotic, such as bacitracin, mupirocin, or sulfadiazine, should be routinely applied. Among persons with recessive dystrophic EB, the anticonvulsant phenytoin is sometimes effective because it decreases production of an enzyme that breaks down collagen.

Prognosis

The prognosis of EB varies depending on the subtype of the disease. Individuals with EB simplex can live long, fulfilling lives. The severity of the junctional and dystrophic forms of EB can vary greatly. Infants affected with some forms of the disease often do not survive infancy; other forms can lead to severe scarring and disfigurement.

Resources

BOOKS

Fine, Jo–David, and Helmut Hintner.*Life with Epidermolysis Bullosa (EB): Etiology, Diagnosis, Multidisciplinary Care, and Therapy*. Wien; New York: Springer, 2009.

Weinberg, Samuel, Neil S. Prose, and Leonard Kristal.*Color Atlas of Pediatric Dermatology*. 4th ed. New York : McGraw–Hill Medical, 2008.

Wolff, Klaus, and Richard Allen Johnson.*Fitzpatrick's Color Atlas and Synopsis of Clinical Dermatology*. 6th ed. NewYork: McGraw–Hill Medical, 2009.

OTHER

Dermatology Information System. http://www.dermis.net.

Dystrophic Epidermolysis Bullosa Research Association International. http://debra-international.org/index1.htm.

Epidermolysis Bullosa Medical Research Foundation. http://www.med.stanford.edu/school/dermatology/ebmrf/.

Oregon Health Sciences University. http://www.ohsu.edu.

University of Iowa College of Medicine. http://www.uihealthcare.com/depts/med/dermatology/index.html.

ORGANIZATIONS

American Academy of Dermatology, PO Box 4014, Schaumburg, IL, 60168-4014, (847) 240-1859, (866) 503-SKIN (7546), http://www.aad.org.

L. Fleming Fallon, Jr., MD, PhD, DrPH

Epididymitis

Definition

Epididymitis is an inflammation or infection of the epididymis—the long coiled tube at the back of each testicle that stores and transports sperm. Epididymitis causes swelling and **pain** in the testicle. There are many causes of epididymitis, but the most common cause is a sexually transmitted bacterial infection.

Demographics

Epididymitis is the most common cause of pain in the scrotum of adult males. It occurs most frequently in sexually active men between the ages of 18 and 40. Epididymitis is the second most common cause of scrotal pain in adolescent males, but seldom occurs in those who are not sexually active since most cases are caused by sexually transmitted infections (STIs). Boys, older men, and homosexual men are more likely to have epididymitis caused by a non-sexually transmitted bacterial **urinary tract infection**. These are particularly common among members of the military who **exercise** for extended periods without emptying their bladders. They are also more common in males with anatomical abnormalities of the urinary tract or who have undergone surgery for urinary tract problems.

Description

Epididymitis most often stems from an STI or other infection in the urethra (the tube that drains urine from the bladder) or other parts of the urinary tract that has spread to the epididymis. In prepubescent boys epididymitis usually begins with a bladder or kidney infection that spreads to the epididymis. Acute epididymitis is usually associated with the most severe pain and swelling. It comes on quickly and subsides with treatment. Chronic epididymitis continues for more than six weeks after treatment begins or recurs frequently. If the testicle as well as the epididymis is inflamed, the condition is known as epididymo-orchitis.

Risk factors

High-risk sexual behaviors put males at risk for epididymitis caused by an STI. High-risk behaviors include multiple sexual partners, a sexual partner with an STI, or sex without a condom. A previous STI increases the risk for future STIs.

Risk factors for epididymitis caused by a non-sexually transmitted infection include:

- infection of the urinary tract, bladder, kidney, or prostate
- previous or chronic urinary tract or prostate infections
- other recent illness
- an uncircumcised penis
- an anatomical abnormality of the urinary tract, such as narrowing of the urethra
- medical procedures that can introduce bacteria into the genitourinary tract, including surgery or urinary catheterization
- prostate enlargement

Risk factors for epididymitis in boys include:

- painful urination
- a history of urinary tract infections
- abnormal bladder function
- abnormalities of the genitals and/or urinary tract

Causes and symptoms

The most common causes of epididymitis among sexually active males under age 35 are the bacteria *Chlamydia trachomatis* and *Neisseria gonorrhoeae*, the causative organisms of the STIs chlamydia and **gonorrhea**, respectively. These infections begin in the urethra and spread to the testicle. The most common cause of epididymitis in prepubescent boys, homosexual men, and older men is a urinary tract infection that spreads to the testicle. Such infections are most often caused by *Escherichia coli* (*E. coli*). Other bacteria, such as *Ureaplasma*, can also cause epididymitis. In prepubescent boys epididymitis is usually associated with a congenital abnormality that predisposes them to urinary tract infections.

Other causes of epididymitis include:

- bacterial infection of the prostate (prostatitis)
- infection with *Mycobacterium tuberculosis*, which causes tuberculosis (TB)
- rarely, a fungal infection
- injury or infection of the scrotum
- irritation from urine that has accumulated in the vas deferens (the sperm duct leading from the epididymitis)
- urine that has flowed backwards into the epididymitis, as can occur with heavy lifting or strain
- an enlarged prostate that obstructs the bladder outlet
- partial blockage of the urethra
- urethral catheterization
- the heart arrhythmia medication amiodarone The cause of chronic epididymitis is sometimes difficult or impossible to determine.

Epididymitis is characterized by testicular pain. Usually only one testicle is affected. The pain of acute epididymitis generally develops gradually over several hours or days and is accompanied by a sudden redness and swelling of the testicle. The symptoms of chronic epididymitis generally come on much more gradually. The affected testicle is hard and sore and the other testicle may feel tender. Enlarged lymph nodes in the groin can cause pain in the scrotum, which intensifies throughout the day and may become so severe that it is impossible to walk normally. Bowel movements can

Acute—Sharp or severe, reaching a crisis rapidly.

Catheter—A hollow flexible tube that is inserted into a body cavity, duct, or vessel for the passage of fluids.

Chronic—Of long duration or frequent recurrence.

Epididymis—The duct between the testis and the vas deferens for the passage of sperm.

Prostate—The walnut-shaped gland that surrounds the urethra at the neck of the bladder in males and supplies fluid for semen.

Sexually transmitted infection (STI)—An infectious disease that is transmitted through sexual activity.

Testicle, testis—One of the pair of male sex glands, located in the scrotum, which produces hormones and sperm.

Urethra—The opening at the end of the penis that drains urine from the bladder.

Vas deferens—The duct that stores sperm and carries it from the epididymis to the ejaculatory duct.

increase the pain. Other symptoms of epididymitis include:

- chills
- a low-grade fever
- acute urethritis or inflammation of the urethra
- painful urination
- urgent or frequent need to urinate
- painful intercourse and/or ejaculation
- possibly a discharge from the urethra and blood in the semen
- a lump on the testicle
- pain or discomfort in the lower abdominal or pelvic region

Diagnosis

Examination

Diagnosis of epididymitis includes a medical history, sexual history, and a **physical examination**. The patient will be examined for enlarged lymph nodes in the groin, an enlarged testicle, tenderness in the area of the testicle where the epididymis attaches, and discharge from the penis. A **rectal examination** may reveal prostate tenderness or enlargement. Epididymitis may require consultation with a urologist.

Tests

Initial tests involve screening for an STI or other infection:

- urinalysis to check for the presence of bacteria and white blood cells, possibly including urine from an initial stream, mid-stream, and after a prostate massage
- urine cultures to identify the organism responsible for an infection

- tests of any discharge from the urethra and prostate gland
- a white blood cell count, which is usually elevated in the presence of infection

Procedures

Ultrasound or a nuclear scan of the testicles can reveal an enlarged epididymis and rule out conditions such as twisting of the spermatic cord (**testicular torsion**) or a testicular tumor. A nuclear scan involves injecting trace amounts of a radioactive material and using a special camera to detect areas of increased blood flow, indicating epididymitis, or decreased blood flow, indicating torsion.

Treatment

Traditional

Epididymitis is generally treated with **antibiotics** to rid the body of infection. If a pocket of pus (an **abscess**) has formed, it may need to be surgically drained. In some instances part or all of the epididymis or even the testicle must be surgically removed. An epididymectomy removes the inflamed section of the epididymis through a small incision in the scrotum. A **vasectomy** prevents fluid and sperm from passing through the epididymis. Surgery is usually performed only in cases of severe chronic epididymitis, on elderly patients undergoing prostate surgery, or when the epididymitis is caused by an underlying physical defect. However tuberculous epididymitis often requires surgical removal of a testicle.

Drugs

- Epididymitis caused by an STI or other bacterial infection is treated with antibiotics, usually for at least two weeks. Sexual partners must also be treated for an STI. The antibiotics must be taken exactly as prescribed, even if the symptoms disappear before the course of antibiotics is completed.

- If a second course of treatment does not completely eradicate symptoms, long-term anti-inflammatory therapy may be required.
- Tuberculous epididymitis is treated with anti-tuberculosis medications.
- Over-the-counter nonsteroidal anti-inflammatory drugs (NSAIDs), such as ibuprofen or naproxen, are used to reduce inflammation and relieve pain.
- For severe pain a local anesthetic such as lidocaine (Xylocaine) may be injected directly into the spermatic cord.
- Epididymitis caused by amiodarone is treated by temporarily discontinuing the drug or reducing the dosage.

Alternative

Although antibiotics are required to treat infections that cause epididymitis, alternative therapies can reduce inflammation and promote healing. **Fasting** is recommended for some patients, since digestion slows down the body's healing mechanisms. A water fast may be preferred, but if this is not possible, a fruit- and vegetable-juice fast or a light diet of fresh fruits and vegetables is recommended.

Traditional Chinese medicine prescribes herbal formulas designed for individuals and their particular symptoms. Herbs for treating epididymitis that are toxic and should be used only under the direct supervision of an experienced herbalist include:

- philodendron (Huang Bai) for inflammation in the lower torso
- pulsatilla for pain and swelling, especially in the genitals
- podophyllum

Other herbs for treating epididymitis include:

- echinacea
- horsetail
- saw palmetto berries
- cranberry extract
- chimaphilla

Other alternative treatments for epididymitis include:

- homeopathic remedies prescribed specifically for the individual by a homeopathic practitioner
- acupuncture, which may help ward off another infection

- aromatherapy, such as a hot sitz bath with drops of juniper berry or sandalwood to relieve symptoms of infection
- chiropractic manipulation to strengthen bladder muscles by adjusting the joints and bones in the pelvic area to help control infection

Home remedies

Epididymitis usually requires at least one or two days of bed rest until symptoms subside. Scrotal elevation is considered to be very important: the patient lies with a folded towel under the scrotum to position it above the level of the heart. This improves blood flow out of the testicle, reduces swelling and pain, and promotes healing. Other self-care for epididymitis includes:

- applying scrotal cold packs, which should be wrapped in a towel and removed every 30 minutes to avoid skin damage
- hydrotherapy—sitting in water as hot as can be tolerated for 15–30 minutes once or twice a day, to alleviate discomfort and speed recovery
- drinking plenty of fluids to treat infection
- avoiding caffeine
- using stool softeners or eating plenty of fruit, nuts, whole-grain cereals, and other foods with laxative properties to prevent constipation
- avoiding strenuous activities until symptoms disappear
- wearing an athletic supporter when resuming normal activities
- avoiding sexual activity until symptoms have disappeared and possibly for as long as one month afterward

Prognosis

Symptoms of epididymitis caused by an STI or other bacterial infection usually improve within a few days of beginning antibiotic treatment. However complete healing may take weeks or even months. Chronic epididymitis may require years of medication and ongoing treatment. Even an epididymectomy may not relieve scrotal pain.

Untreated epididymitis can lead to serious complications including:

- abscesses
- chronic epididymitis
- shrinkage (atrophy) of the affected testicle
- rarely, reduced fertility or infertility

Prevention

Many cases of epididymitis can be prevented through monogamy, the use of **condoms**, and avoiding sex with a partner who is infected with an STI. If the epididymitis is caused by an STI, all sexual partners must be treated to prevent re-infection. Drinking plenty of fluids to increase urine flow helps prevent urine retention, which can lead to infection and epididymitis.

Resources

BOOKS

Judd, Sandra J. *Men's Health Concerns Sourcebook*, 3rd ed. Detroit: Omnigraphics, 2009.

Larson, Laura. *Sexually Transmitted Diseases Sourcebook*, 4th ed. Detroit: Omnigraphics, 2009.

PERIODICALS

Tracy, C. R., et al. "Diagnosis and Management of Epididymitis." *Urologic Clinics of North America* 35 (2008): 101.

Trojian, Thomas H., Timothy S. Lishnak, and Diana Heiman. "Epididymitis and Orchitis: An Overview." *American Family Physician* 79, no. 7 (April 1, 2009): 583-587.

OTHER

American Urological Association Foundation. "Epididymitis and Orchidis." *UrologyHealth.org.* http://urologyhealth.org/adult/index.cfm?cat = 11&topic = 490

"Epididymitis." *MedlinePlus.* http://www.nlm.nih.gov/medlineplus/ency/article/001279.htm

Mayo Clinic Staff. "Epididymitis." *MayoClinic.com.* http://www.mayoclinic.com/print/epididymitis/DS00603/DSECTION = all&METHOD = print

ORGANIZATIONS

American Academy of Family Physicians, 11400 Tomahawk Creek Parkway, Leawood, KS, 66211-2680, (913) 906-6000, (800) 274-6000, (913) 906-6075, http://www.aafp.org/online/en/home.html.

American Urological Association, 1000 Corporate Boulevard, Linthicum, MD, 21090, (410) 689-3700, (866) RING-AUA (746-4282), (410) 689-3800, aua@AUAnet. org, http://www.auanet.org.

Lisa Frick
Margaret Alic, PhD

Epidural abscess *see* **Central nervous system infections**

Epidural anesthetic *see* **Anesthesia, local**

Epiglottitis

Definition

Epiglottitis is an infection of the epiglottis, which can lead to severe airway obstruction.

Description

When air is inhaled (inspired), it passes through the nose and the nasopharynx or through the mouth and the oropharynx. These are both connected to the larynx, a tube made of cartilage. The air continues down the larynx to the trachea. The trachea then splits into two branches, the left and right bronchi (bronchial tubes). These bronchi branch into smaller air tubes that run within the lungs, leading to the small air sacs of the lungs (alveoli).

Either food, liquid, or air may be taken in through the mouth. While air goes into the larynx and the respiratory system, food and liquid are directed into the tube leading to the stomach, the esophagus. Because food or liquid in the bronchial tubes or lungs could cause a blockage or lead to an infection, the airway is protected. The epiglottis is a leaf-like piece of cartilage extending upwards from the larynx. The epiglottis can close down over the larynx when someone is eating or drinking, preventing these food and liquids from entering the airway.

Epiglottitis is an infection and inflammation of the epiglottis. Because the epiglottis may swell considerably, there is a danger that the airway will be blocked off by the very structure designed to protect it. Air is then unable to reach the lungs. Without intervention, epiglottitis has the potential to be fatal.

Epiglottitis is primarily a disease of two to seven-year-old children, although older children and adults can also contract it. Boys are twice as likely as girls to develop this infection. Because epiglottitis involves swelling and infection of tissues, which are all located at or above the level of the epiglottis, it is sometimes referred to as supraglottitis (*supra,* meaning above). About 25% of all children with this infection also have **pneumonia**.

Causes and symptoms

The most common cause of epiglottitis is infection with the bacteria called *Haemophilus influenzae type b.* Other types of bacteria are also occasionally responsible for this infection, including some types of *Streptococcus* bacteria and the bacteria responsible for causing **diphtheria**.

KEY TERMS

Epiglottis—A leaf-like piece of cartilage extending upwards from the larynx, which can close like a lid over the trachea to prevent the airway from receiving any food or liquid being swallowed.

Extubation—Removal of a breathing tube.

Intubation—Putting a breathing tube into the airway.

Laryngospasm—Spasm of the larynx.

Larynx—The part of the airway lying between the pharynx and the trachea.

Nasopharynx—The part of the airway into which the nose leads.

Oropharynx—The part of the airway into which the mouth leads.

Supraglottitis—Another term for epiglottitis.

Trachea—The part of the airway that leads into the bronchial tubes.

Tracheostomy—A procedure in which a small opening is made in the neck and into the trachea. A breathing tube is then placed through this opening.

A patient with epiglottitis typically experiences a sudden **fever**, and begins having severe throat and neck **pain**. Because the swollen epiglottis interferes significantly with air movement, every breath creates a loud, harsh, high-pitched sound referred to as **stridor**. Because the vocal cords are located in the larynx just below the area of the epiglottis, the swollen epiglottis makes the patient's voice sound muffled and strained. Swallowing becomes difficult, and the patient may drool. The patient often leans forward and juts out his or her jaw, while struggling for breath.

Epiglottitis strikes suddenly and progresses quickly. A child may begin complaining of a **sore throat**, and within a few hours be suffering from extremely severe airway obstruction.

Diagnosis

Diagnosis begins with a high level of suspicion that a quickly progressing illness with fever, sore throat, and airway obstruction is very likely to be epiglottitis. If epiglottitis is suspected, no efforts should be made to look at the throat, or to swab the throat in order to obtain a culture for identification of the causative organism. These maneuvers may cause the larynx to go into spasm (laryngospasm), completely closing the airway. These procedures should only be performed in a fully-equipped operating room, so that if laryngospasm occurs, a breathing tube can be immediately placed in order to keep the airway open.

An instrument called a laryngoscope is often used in the operating room to view the epiglottis, which will appear cherry-red and quite swollen. An x-ray picture taken from the side of the neck should also be obtained. The swollen epiglottis has a characteristic appearance, called the "thumb sign."

Treatment

Treatment almost always involves the immediate establishment of an artificial airway: inserting a breathing tube into the throat (intubation); or making a tiny opening toward the base of the neck and putting a breathing tube into the trachea (tracheostomy). Because the patient's apparent level of distress may not match the actual severity of the situation, and because the disease's progression can be quite surprisingly rapid, it is preferable to go ahead and place the artificial airway, rather than adopting a wait-and-see approach.

Because epiglottitis is caused by a bacteria, **antibiotics** such as cefotaxime, ceftriaxone, or ampicillin with sulbactam should be given through a needle placed in a vein (intravenously). This prevents the bacteria that are circulating throughout the bloodstream from causing infection elsewhere in the body.

Prognosis

With treatment (including the establishment of an artificial airway), only about 1% of children with epiglottitis die. Without the artificial airway, this figure jumps to 6%. Most patients recover form the infection, and can have the breathing tube removed (extubation) within a few days.

Prevention

Prevention involves the use of a vaccine against *H. influenzae type b* (called the Hib vaccine). It is given to babies at two, four, six, and 15 months. Use of this vaccine has made epiglottitis a very rare occurrence.

ORGANIZATIONS

American Academy of Otolaryngology—Head and Neck Surgery, 1650 Diagonal Road, Alexandria, VA, 22314-2857, (703) 836-4444, http://www.entnet.org.

Rosalyn Carson-DeWitt, MD

Epilepsy

Definition

Epilepsy is a chronic (persistent) disorder of the nervous system. The primary symptoms of this disease are periodic or recurring seizures that are triggered by sudden episodes of abnormal electrical activity in the brain. The term "seizure" refers to any unusual body functions or activities that are under the control of the nervous system.

Demographics

Epilepsy affects about one percent of the population. Approximately 2.3 million Americans and 40 million people throughout the world have epilepsy. It is the second most common neurological disorder. According to the Epilepsy Foundation, about 30% of the 200,000 new cases reported every year begin in childhood, particularly in early childhood and around the time of adolescence. Another period of relatively high incidence is in people over the age of 65.

Description

The word epilepsy is derived from the Greek term for seizure. Seizures can involve a combination of sensations, muscle contractions, and other abnormal body functions. Seizures may appear spontaneously—without any apparent cause—or can be triggered by a specific type of stimulus such as a flashing light. Specific cases of epilepsy may result from known causes, such as brain injury, or may have no apparent cause (referred to as *idiopathic epilepsy*). Idiopathic epilepsy may be initiated by a combination of genetic and environmental factors.

An epileptic seizure involves a transient (temporary) episode of abnormal electrical activity in the brain. During a seizure, many nerve cells within a specific region of the brain may begin to fire at the same time. This activity may then spread out over other parts of the brain. In addition to abnormal physical symptoms, seizures can bring on emotions ranging from fear, anger, and rage, to joy or happiness. During a seizure, patients may experience disorientation, spontaneous sensations of sounds, smells, visions, and distorted visual perception—such as misshapen objects and places.

Epilepsy can be caused by some event or condition that results in damage to the brain such as strokes, tumors, abscesses, trauma (physical injury), or infections such as **meningitis**. Epilepsy can also be triggered by inherited (genetic) factors or some form of injury or trauma at birth. Epilepsy cases that seem to have no readily identifiable cause are referred to as "idiopathic" cases in medical terminology. Symptoms of this disease can appear at any age. Seizures can damage and destroy brain cells and scar tissue can develop in the section of brain tissue where seizures originate.

There are many forms of epileptic seizures. The parts of the body that are affected by a seizure and the distinctive characteristics, duration and severity of the symptoms can distinguish each type of epilepsy. Patients can experience more than one type of seizure. The nature of the symptoms depends on where in the brain the seizure originated and how much of the brain is involved. Seizures can be classified as either "generalized" or "partial." Partial seizures involve abnormal activity in a specific region of the brain.

Generalized (also called tonic–clonic) seizures last about two minutes and are the result of abnormal electrical activity that spreads out over both sides or hemispheres of the brain. They were formerly referred to as grand mal seizures. The patient will usually lose consciousness and fall during the episode. The term "tonic" refers to the first phase of a generalized seizure in which the body muscles become taunt or stiff. This is followed by strong, rhythmic muscular contractions (convulsions) of the "clonic" phase. Sometimes a patient's breathing may be hampered by a brief stoppage of the respiratory muscles, causing the skin to develop a bluish tinge due to lack of oxygen.

Epileptic seizures can also be classified as complex or simple. Complex seizures generally involve a loss of consciousness, whereas simple seizures do not. Simple partial seizures can begin as a localized (focal) seizure and then evolve into a secondary generalized episode in which the initial abnormal electrical activity spreads to involve other parts of the brain. Patients may actually remember the physical and psychological events that occur during a simple seizure, such as the types of movement, emotions, and sensations, but frequently are completely unaware of the event. Partial seizures are more common in adults.

An absence seizure (once called *petit mal*) typically results in brief periods of lack of awareness and some abnormal muscle movement. The patient generally remains conscious during the seizure episode, but may become absent–minded and unresponsive. They may also appear to be starring. Absence seizures last about 5–10 seconds.

How seizures affect a person's memory depends where in the brain seizures occur. Seizures can interfere with learning, storage, and retrieval of new information. For example, a form of epilepsy that produces seizures in the temporal lobe of the brain can cause a serious deterioration (loss) of memory function. Early treatment can help prevent or reduce **memory loss**.

In some forms of epilepsy, seizures can be triggered by a particular mental—or cognitive—activity. For example, the simple activity of reading aloud can trigger a seizure in patients with reading epilepsy. Symptoms include face **muscle spasms**. In medical terms, this type of epilepsy is referred to as idiopathic localization–related epilepsy. This means that seizures occur in one part of the brain (in this case, the temporal lobes) and that there is no apparent cause that brought on the disease.

Risk factors

Certain factors may increase the risk of epilepsy. The Mayo Clinic lists the following:

- Age: the onset of epilepsy is most common during early childhood and after age 65, but the condition can occur at any age.
- Sex: men are slightly more at risk of developing epilepsy than are women.
- Family history: a family history of epilepsy may increase the risk of developing a seizure disorder.
- Head injuries: head injuries injuries are responsible for many cases of epilepsy.
- Stroke and other vascular diseases: these conditions can lead to brain damage that may trigger epilepsy.
- Brain infections: infections like meningitis, which causes an inflammation in the brain or spinal cord, can increase the risk of epilepsy.
- Prolonged seizures in childhood: high fevers in childhood can sometimes be associated with prolonged seizures and subsequent epilepsy later in life.

Causes and symptoms

Epilepsy has many causes that have an effect on the clinical presentation of symptoms. In order for epilepsy to occur, there must be an underlying physical problem in the brain. The problem can be so mild that a person can be perfectly normal aside from having seizures. The brain has roughly 50–100 billion neurons. Each neuron can have up to 10,000 contacts with neighboring neurons. Hence, trillions of connections exist. However, only a very small area of dysfunctional brain tissue is necessary to create a persistent generator of seizures and, hence, epilepsy. The following are potential causes of epilepsy:

- genetic and/or hereditary
- perinatal neurological insults
- trauma with brain injury
- stroke
- brain tumors
- infections such as meningitis and encephalitis
- multiple sclerosis
- idiopathic (unknown or genetic)

Any of the above conditions has the potential for causing the brain or a portion of it to be dysfunctional and produce recurrent seizures. Regardless of the exact cause, epilepsy is a paroxysmal (sudden) condition. It involves the synchronous discharging of a population of neurons. This is an abnormal event that, depending on the location in the brain, will correspond to the particular symptoms of a seizure. The International League Against Epilepsy (ILAE) issued a classification of types of seizures. Individual seizure types are based on the clinical behavior (semiology) and electrophysiological characteristics as seen on an electroencephalogram (EEG). Generalized seizures included in the list include:

- tonic–clonic seizures (includes variations beginning with a clonic or myoclonic phase)
- clonic seizures, including without tonic features and with tonic features
- typical absence seizures
- atypical absence seizures
- myoclonic absence seizures
- tonic seizures
- spasms
- myoclonic seizures
- eyelid myoclonia, including without absences and with absences
- myoclonic atonic seizures
- negative myoclonus
- atonic seizures
- reflex seizures in generalized epilepsy syndromes

Partial (or focal) seizures included in the ILAE list are:

- focal sensory seizures with elementary sensory symptoms (e.g., occipital and parietal lobe seizures) and experiential sensory symptoms (e.g., temporo–parieto–occipital junction seizures)
- focal motor seizures with elementary clonic motor signs, asymmetrical tonic motor seizures (e.g., supplementary motor seizures), typical (temporal lobe) automatisms (e.g., mesial temporal lobe seizures), hyperkinetic automatisms, focal negative myoclonus, and inhibitory motor seizures
- gelastic seizures
- hemiclonic seizures
- secondarily generalized seizures
- reflex seizures in focal epilepsy syndromes

The International League Against Epilepsy has also issued the following classification of epilepsies and epileptic syndromes:

- benign familial neonatal seizures
- early myoclonic encephalopathy
- Ohtahara syndrome
- migrating partial seizures of infancy (syndrome in development)
- West syndrome
- benign myoclonic epilepsy in infancy
- benign familial and non–familial infantile seizures
- Dravet's syndrome
- HH syndrome
- myoclonic status in nonprogressive encephalopathies (syndrome in development)
- benign childhood epilepsy with centrotemporal spikes
- early onset benign childhood occipital epilepsy (Panayiotopoulos type)
- late–onset childhood occipital epilepsy (Gastaut type)
- epilepsy with myoclonic absences
- epilepsy with myoclonic–astatic seizures
- Lennox–Gastaut syndrome
- Landau–Kleffner syndrome (LKS)
- epilepsy with continuous spike–and–waves during slow–wave sleep (other than LKS)
- childhood absence epilepsy
- progressive myoclonus epilepsies
- idiopathic generalized epilepsies with variable phenotypes include juvenile absence epilepsy, juvenile myoclonic epilepsy, and epilepsy with generalized tonic–clonic seizures only
- reflex epilepsies
- idiopathic photosensitive occipital lobe epilepsy

- other visual sensitive epilepsies
- primary reading epilepsy
- startle epilepsy
- autosomal dominant nocturnal frontal lobe epilepsy
- familial temporal lobe epilepsies
- generalized epilepsies with febrile seizures plus (syndrome in development)
- familial focal epilepsy with variable foci (syndrome in development)
- symptomatic focal epilepsies
- limbic epilepsies
- mesial temporal lobe epilepsy with hippocampal sclerosis
- mesial temporal lobe epilepsy defined by specific etiologies
- neocortical epilepsies
- Rasmussen syndrome

Classifying epilepsy is used in the evaluation and management of patients with seizure disorders. The combination of seizure type(s), etiology (cause), age of onset, family history, and other medical or neurological conditions can help identify an epilepsy syndrome. Syndrome classification schemes are revised periodically as individual components of particular categories are better understood.

The term idiopathic refers to a cause that is unknown. Cryptogenic is a term that suggests that an underlying cause is suspected, but not yet fully understood. Symptomatic is a term that is applied to epilepsies that are a result of understood underlying pathologies.

The management and prognosis vary considerably among these differing syndromes. Epilepsies that have a genetic basis can be inherited or occur spontaneously. A detailed family history can often identify other family members who have had seizures. However, because seizures are common, it is possible to have more than one family member with epilepsy, though the causes may not be related. To say that a particular type of epilepsy is genetic does not mean that it is necessarily transmitted by heredity. Often, disorders can have a genetic cause, but may be spontaneously occurring in only one member of a family. In this case, there may simply be a random mutation in that particular person's genes.

Genetic factors contribute to about 40% of all epilepsy cases. Most of the generalized epilepsy syndromes and some of the partial epilepsy syndromes have an inherited component. Medical researchers suggest that at least 500 genes may somehow be

KEY TERMS

Aura—A sensation of a cold breeze or bright light that precedes the onset of a seizure.

Automatisms—Movements during a seizure that are semi–purposeful but involuntary.

Clonic—Referring to clonus, rapid contractions and relaxations of a muscle.

Convulsion—Involuntary contractions of body muscles that accompany a seizure episode.

Gelastic seizures—Seizures manifesting with brief involuntary laughter.

Gray matter—The portion of the brain that contains neurons, as opposed to white matter, which contains nerve tracts.

Infantile spasms—Clusters of rapid jerks followed by stiffening or jackknife movements. Usually starts in the first year of life and stops by age 4.

Idiopathic—Of unknown origin.

Lesion—A defective or injured section or region of the brain (or other body organ).

Magnetic resonance imaging (MRI)—A technique that employs magnetic fields and radio waves to create detailed images of internal body structures and organs, including the brain.

Myoclonic—A rapid, involuntary muscle contraction, particularly near the eye.

Myoclonus—Jerking, involuntary movements of the arms and legs. These may occur normally during sleep.

Neuron—A unique type of cell found in the brain and body that is specialized to process and transmit information.

Partial seizure—A seizure that starts in one particular part of the brain. The abnormal electrical activity may remain confined to that area, or may spread to the entire brain. Also called a focal seizure.

Reflex seizure—Seizure brought on by specific sensory stimuli.

Seizure—Any unusual body functions or activity that is under the control of the nervous system.

Spike wave discharge—Characteristic abnormal wave pattern in the electroencephalogram that is a hallmark of an area that has the potential of generating a seizure.

---

involved in the development of various forms of epilepsy. It is believed that some of these genes can make people with epilepsy more susceptible or sensitive to environmental factors that initiate or start seizures. Only a few types of epilepsy are thought to be caused by just one type of gene.

Gene mutations can cause a variety of nervous system abnormalities that are associated with epilepsy. Different mutations may lead to abnormal brain development or progressive degeneration of brain tissue. Some gene mutations make nerve cells hyperexcitable. These abnormal nerve cells can trigger outbursts of abnormal patterns of electrical activity that can initiate an epileptic seizure.

Specific gene locations (called gene markers) have been linked to various forms of the disease, such as juvenile myoclonic epilepsy. However, researchers have discovered that some individuals who possess this gene do not develop symptoms of this disease. In some pairs of identical twins with this gene, one twin may appear normal while the other develops typical symptoms of epilepsy. Thus, genetic inheritance seems to be just one of many factors that influence the possibility of developing epilepsy symptoms.

Some genetic mutations may also reduce the effectiveness of antiepileptic medication. One of the major goals of epilepsy research is to determine how a patient's genetic makeup can influence their drug therapy.

With epilepsy, symptoms vary considerably depending on the type. The common link among the epilepsies is, of course, seizures. The different epilepsies can sometimes be associated with more than one seizure type. This is the case with Lennox–Gastaut syndrome.

The specific symptoms of epilepsy accordingly depend in part on the particular seizures that occur and other medical problems that may be associated. Seizures, themselves, can take on a variety of features. A simple sustained twitching of an extremity could be a partial seizure. If a seizure arises in the occipital lobes of the brain, then a visual experience can occur. Aura is a term often used to describe symptoms that a person may feel prior to the loss of consciousness of a seizure. However, auras are, themselves, small partial seizures that have not spread in the brain to involve consciousness. Smells, well–formed **hallucinations**, **tingling** sensations, or **nausea** have all occurred in auras. The particular sensation can be a clue as to the location in the brain where a seizure starts. Partial seizures can then spread to involve other areas of the brain and lead to an alteration of consciousness, and possibly convulsions. In certain epilepsy syndromes such as Lennox–Gastaut, there can be more than one type of seizure experienced, such as atonic, atypical absence, and tonic–axial seizures.

Diagnosis

Examination

The diagnosis of epilepsy is relatively straightforward: when people suffer two or more seizures, they are considered to have epilepsy. However, diagnosing the specific epilepsy syndrome is much more complex. The first step in the evaluation process is to obtain a very detailed history of the illness, not only from the patient but from the family as well. In a child, this includes birth history, complications, if any, maternal history, and developmental milestones. At any age, other medical problems are also considered. Medications that have been taken or currently being prescribed are documented. Since seizures can impair consciousness, the patient may not be able to recall specifics. In these cases, family or friends that have witnessed the episodes can fill in the gaps about the particulars of the seizure. The description of the behaviors during a seizure helps to categorize the type of seizure and with the overall diagnosis.

A complete **physical examination** is performed, especially a **neurological exam**. Because seizures are an episodic disorder, abnormal neurological findings may not be present. Frequently, people with epilepsy have a normal exam. However, in some, there can be abnormal findings that can provide clues to the underlying cause of epilepsy. For example, if someone has had a **stroke** that subsequently caused seizures, then the neurological exam can be expected to reveal a focal neurological deficit such as weakness or language difficulties. In some children with seizures, there can be a variety of associated neurologic abnormalities such as **mental retardation** and **cerebral palsy** that are themselves non–specific but indicate that the brain has suffered, at some point in development, an injury or malformation. Also, subtle findings on examination can lead to a diagnosis of tuberous sclerosis. This is an autosomal dominantly inherited disorder associated with infantile spasms in 25% of cases. On examination, patients have so–called ash–leaf spots and adenoma sebaceum on the skin. There can also be a variety of systemic abnormalities that involve the kidneys, retina, heart, and gums, depending on severity.

Tests

In the course of evaluating epilepsy, a number of tests are typically ordered. Usually, **magnetic resonance imaging** (MRI) of the brain is performed. This is a scan that can help to find causes of epilepsy such as tumors, strokes, trauma, and congenital malformations. However, while MRI can reveal incredible brain details, it cannot image the presence of abnormalities in the microscopic neuronal environment. Another test that is routinely ordered is an electroencephalogram (EEG). Unlike the MRI scan, this can be considered a functional test of the brain. The EEG measures the electrical activity of the brain. Some seizure disorders or epilepsies have a characteristic EEG with particular abnormalities that can help in diagnosis. Blood tests are also frequently ordered to help screen for abnormalities that could be a factor in the cause of seizures. Occasionally, **genetic testing** is performed in those instances where a known genetic cause is suspected and can be tested. A major concern in the course of an evaluation of epilepsy is to identify the presence of life–threatening causes such as brain tumors, infections, and cerebrovascular disease.

Treatment

Traditional

Currently, no cure exists for epilepsy. However, a wide range of treatment programs are available that provide varying degrees of success in controlling the symptoms of epilepsy.

Drugs

Medication is the most effective and widely used treatment for the symptoms of epilepsy. Most medications work by interfering with or stopping the abnormal electrical activity in nerve cells that cause seizures. This form of treatment is generally referred to as anticonvulsant therapy. Medication is considered effective if the patient is free of seizures for at least one year.

As with any medication, individuals can have very different experiences with same drug. Consequently, it is difficult to predict the efficacy of treatment. A key concept of treatment is to first strive for monotherapy (or single drug therapy). This simplifies treatment and minimizes the chance of side effects. Sometimes, however, two or more drugs may be necessary to achieve satisfactory control of seizures. As with any treatment, potential side effects can be worse than the disease itself. Moreover, there is little point in controlling seizures if severe side effects limit quality of life. If a **seizure disorder** is characterized by mild, focal, or brief symptoms that do not interfere with routine activities, then aggressive treatments may not be advisable. Epilepsy medications do not cure epilepsy; the medications can only control the frequency and severity of seizures. A list of the most commonly used medications in the management of epilepsy includes:

- phenobarbital
- phenytoin (Dilantin, Phenytek)
- clonazepam (Klonipin)
- ethosuxamide (Zarontin)
- carbamazepine (Tegretol, Carbatrol)
- divalproex sodium (Depakote, Depakene)
- felbamate (Felbatol)
- gabapentin (Neurontin)
- lamotrigine (Lamictal)
- topiramate (Topamax)
- tiagabine (Gabatril)
- zonisamide (Zonegran)
- oxcarbazepine (Trileptal)
- leviteracetam (Keppra)

Anticonvulsants are powerful drugs that can produce a variety of side effects, including nausea, **fatigue**, **dizziness**, and weight change. They can also increase the risk of **birth defects**, especially involving the early stages of embryonic development of the nervous system if taken during **pregnancy**.

Doctors prefer to put their patients on just one type of anticonvulsant drug. Some patients, however, experience more effective relief from their epilepsy symptoms by taking a combination of two different but complementary forms of medication. The choice of medication depends on the type of seizure that affects a patient, the patient's medical history— including response to other drug therapies, their age, and gender. For example, the drug Carbamazepine is one of the most effective medications and has little impact on important cognitive functions such as thinking, memory and learning.

Newer medications generally produce fewer side effects than their predecessors. Research into **gene therapy** may ultimately be the most effective form of epilepsy treatment, but is still in the very early stages.

Unfortunately, medication is ineffective for more than one third of known cases of epilepsy. More than 30% of patients with epilepsy cannot maintain adequate control of their seizures. Some genetic mutations may reduce the effectiveness of antiepileptic medications.

Alternative

Surgery is recommended for some patients for whom medication cannot effectively control the frequency or severity of their seizures. Surgery is a treatment option only in extreme cases where doctors can identify the specific site in the brain where seizures originate. The most promising candidates for surgery are those with a single lesion on the temporal, frontal, or occipital lobes of the brain.

Prior to surgery, the patient must complete extensive testing to determine the precise patterns of seizures and to locate their point of origin in the brain. Patients spend extended stays in hospital during which their seizures are recorded on video and with the aid of EEGs. This machine records patterns of electrical activity in the brain using sensors (referred to as "electrodes") attached to various parts of the body.

The surgical procedure involves the removal of a small part of brain tissue in the "suspected" region. The anterior temporal lobe and hippocampus are the most common areas in which tissue is removed. In some studies, more than 83% of patients become free of seizures following surgery. Ninety–seven percent show significant improvement in their condition.

Vagus Nerve Stimulation (VNS) is another form of treatment for some cases of epilepsy that are unresponsive (referred to as refractory epilepsy) to other forms of medical therapy. VNS may also be recommended for patients who cannot tolerate the side effects of medication. This procedure involves implanting a device that stimulates the Vagus nerve, located in the left side of the neck. In one study, this treatment reduced seizures by 78%.

A special dietary program is another treatment option for patients who are not good candidates for surgery or who have had little success with anticonvulsant medication. This form of treatment called the Ketogenic Diet can be effective for many types of epilepsy. It is most appropriate for young children whose parents can follow the rigid requirements of the diet. Older children and adults tend to have greater difficulty in sticking to the dietary rules for an extended period of time. The Ketogenic Diet is a stringent diet that is very high in fat, but low in proteins, carbohydrates, and calories. The excessive fat produces high levels of a substance called ketones (which the body makes when it breaks down fat for energy). Somehow these ketones help reduce the incidence of epileptic seizures. The success of this form of treatment varies. For some patients, the high fat diet is the best form of treatment. For others, the diet is less effective.

As of 2009, 153 clinical trials for the study and treatment of epilepsy were being sponsored by the National Institutes of Health (NIH)and other agencies.

A few examples include:

- The effectiveness and safety of diazepam for patients with epilepsy who receive antiepileptic drugs. (NCT00319501)
- The role played by the brain chemical serotonin in seizures. (NCT00439387)
- The effectiveness and dose requirements of levetiracetam in subjects with newly diagnosed childhood absence epilepsy. (NCT00361010)
- The effectiveness of electrical brain stimulation to reduce epileptic seizures. (NCT00344877)
- The use of simultaneous EEG and functional magnetic resonance imaging (fMRI) to study the different brain regions involved in child absence seizures and how they are related to attention and cognition. (NCT00393666)
- The effectiveness and safety of seletracetam when it is used in addition to other anti–epileptic medications by patients with partial onset seizures. (NCT00422110)
- The evaluation of standard diagnostic tests and treatments for patients with epilepsy. (NCT00013845)
- The collection of brain tissue samples for research purposes from patients undergoing surgery to treat epilepsy. (NCT00025714)
- The use of functional magnetic resonance imaging (fMRI) and diffusion tensor imaging (DTI) to examine how the brain processes tasks involving language and emotion in normal volunteers and in patients with epilepsy. (NCT00081432)

Clinical trial information is constantly updated by NIH and the most recent information on epilepsy trials can be found at: http://clinicaltrials.gov.

Prognosis

The prognosis of epilepsy varies widely depending on the cause, severity, and patient's age. Even individuals with a similar diagnosis may have different experiences with treatment. For example, in benign epilepsy of childhood with centrotemporal spikes (also called benign rolandic epilepsy), the prognosis is excellent with nearly all children experiencing remission by their teens. With childhood absence epilepsy, the prognosis is variable. In this case, the absence seizures become less frequent with time, but almost half of patients may eventually develop generalized tonic–clonic seizures. Overall, the seizures are responsive to an appropriate anticonvulsant. On the other hand, the seizures in Lennox–Gastaut syndrome are very difficult to control. In this case, however, the ketogenic diet can help. In seizures that begin in adulthood, one can expect that medications will control seizures in up to 60–70% of cases. However, in some of the more than 30% of medically intractable cases, epilepsy surgery can improve or even cure the problem.

Overall, most patients have a good chance of controlling seizures with the available treatment options. The goal of treatment is complete cessation of seizures since a mere reduction in seizure frequency and/or severity may continue to limit patients' quality of life: for instance, they may not be able to drive, sustain employment, or be productive in school.

Prevention

Head injuries are associated with many epilepsy cases. The risk can be reduced by always wearing a seat belt while riding in a car and by wearing a helmet while bicycling, skiing, riding a motorcycle or engaging in other activities with a high risk of **head injury**. **Vascular disease** may also lead to epilepsy. Limiting alcohol intake, avoiding cigarettes, eating a healthy diet and exercising regularly can reduce the risk for these diseases.

Resources

BOOKS

Browne, Thomas R., and Gregory L. Holmes. *Handbook of Epilepsy,* 4th edition, Philadelphia, PA: Lippincott Williams & Wilkins, 2008.

Devinsky, Orrin. *Epilepsy: Patient and Family Guide.* 3rd edition, New York, NY: Demos Health, 2007.

Gay, Kathlyn. *Epilepsy: The Ultimate Teen Guide.* Lanham, MD: Scarecrow Press, 2007.

Karia, Roopal. *The Why and What of Epilepsy: A Book for Children and Teens.* Frederick, MD: PublishAmerica, 2008.

Reuber, Markus, et al. *Epilepsy Explained: A Book for People Who Want to Know More.* New York, NY: Oxford University Press, 2009.

Shorvon, Simon D., et al., editors. *The Treatment of Epilepsy,* 3rd edition, New York, NY: Wiley–Blackwell, 2009.

Wilner, Andrew N. *Epilepsy: 199 Answers: A Doctor Responds to His Patients' Questions,* 3rd edition, New York, NY: Demos Health, 2007.

Wyllie, Elaine, et al., editors. *The Treatment of Epilepsy: Principles and Practice,* 4th edition, Philadelphia, PA: Lippincott Williams & Wilkins, 2005.

Zelenka, Yvonne. *Let's Learn with Teddy about Epilepsy.* Leonia, NJ: Medicus Press, 2008.

PERIODICALS

Arts, W. F., and A. T. Geerts. "When to start drug treatment for childhood epilepsy: the clinical–epidemiological evidence." *European Journal of Paediatric Neurology* 13, no. 2 (March 2009): 93–101.

Beenhakker, M. P., and J. R. Huguenard. "Neurons that fire together also conspire together: is normal sleep circuitry hijacked to generate epilepsy?" *Neuron* 62, no. 5 (June 2009): 612–632.

Brodie, M. J., et al. "Epilepsy in later life." *Lancet Neurology* 8, no. 11 (November 2009): 1019–1030.

Fastenau, P. S., et al. "Neuropsychological status at seizure onset in children: risk factors for early cognitive deficits." *Neurology* 73, no. 7 (August 2009): 526–534.

Hamani, C., et al. "Deep brain stimulation for the treatment of epilepsy." *International Journal of Neural Systems* 19, no. 3 (June 2009): 213–226.

Hughes, J. R. "Absence seizures: a review of recent reports with new concepts." *Epilepsy & Behavior* 15, no. 4 (August 2009): 404–412.

McCagh, J., et al. "Epilepsy, psychosocial and cognitive functioning." *Epilepsy Research* 86, no. 1 (September 2009): 1–14.

McElroy–Cox, C. "Alternative approaches to epilepsy treatment." *Current Neurology and Neuroscience Reports* 9, no. 4 (July 2009): 313–318.

Rodin, E., et al. "Spikes and epilepsy." *Clinical EEG and Neuroscience* 40, no. 4 (October 2009): 288–299.

Sherman, E. M. "Maximizing quality of life in people living with epilepsy." *Canadian Journal of Neurological Sciences* 36, suppl. 2 (August 2009): S17–S24.

Vining, E. P. "Tonic and atonic seizures: medical therapy and ketogenic diet." *Epilepsia* 50, suppl. 8 (September 2009): 21–24.

Wheless, J. W. "Managing severe epilepsy syndromes of early childhood." *Journal of Child Neurology* 24, suppl. 8 (August 2009): 24S–32S.

OTHER

"Epilepsy." *Medline Plus.* Health Topics. http://www.nlm.nih.gov/medlineplus/epilepsy.html (accessed November 15, 2009)

"Epilepsy." *Mayo Clinic.* Information Page. http://www.mayoclinic.com/print/epilepsy/DS00342/DSECTION=all&METHOD=print (accessed November 15, 2009)

"Epilepsy." *FamilyDoctor.org.* Information Page. http://familydoctor.org/online/famdocen/home/common/brain/disorders/214.printerview.html (accessed November 15, 2009)

"Epilepsy." *NINDS.* Information Page. http://www.ninds.nih.gov/disorders/epilepsy/epilepsy.htm (accessed November 15, 2009)

"Facts about Epilepsy." *Epilepsy Institute.* Information Page. http://www.epilepsyinstitute.org/facts/index.htm (accessed November 15, 2009)

"Seizures and Epilepsy: Hope Through Research." *NINDS.* Information Page. http://www.ninds.nih.gov/disorders/epilepsy/detail_epilepsy.htm (accessed November 15, 2009)

"What is Epilepsy?" *Epilepsy Foundation.* Information Page. http://www.epilepsyfoundation.org/about (accessed November 15, 2009)

ORGANIZATIONS

Antiepileptic Drug Pregnancy Registry, MGH East, CNY-149, 10th Floor 149 13th Street, Charlestown, MA, 02129-2000, (800) 233-2334, (617) 724-8307, info@aedpregnancyregistry.org, http://www2.massgeneral.org/aed.

Charlie Foundation to Help Cure Pediatric Epilepsy, 1223 Wilshire Blvd., Suite 815, Santa Monica, CA, 90403, (310) 393-2347, (310) 453-4585, ketoman@aol.com, http://www.charliefoundation.org.

Citizens United for Research in Epilepsy (CURE), 730 North Franklin Street, Suite 404, Chicago, IL, 60654, (312) 255-1801, (312) 255-1809, info@CUREepilepsy.org, http://www.CUREepilepsy.org.

Epilepsy Foundation, 8301 Professional Place, Landover, MD, 20785-7223, (301) 459-3700, (800) 332-1000, (301) 577-2684, postmaster@efa.org, http://www.epilepsyfoundation.org.

Epilepsy Institute, 257 Park Avenue South, New York, NY, 10010, (212) 677-8550, (212) 677-5825, website@epilepsyinstitute.org, http://www.epilepsyinstitute.org.

Epilepsy Therapy Project, P.O. Box 742, Middleburg, VA, 20118, (540) 687-8077, (540) 687-8066, epilepsytherapy@epilepsytherapy.org, http://www.epilepsy.com.

National Institute of Neurological Disorders and Stroke (NINDS), PO Box 5801, Bethesda, MD, 20824, (301) 496-5751, (800) 352-9424, http://www.ninds.nih.gov.

People Against Childhood Epilepsy (PACE), 7 East 85th Street, Suite A3, New York, NY, 10028, (212) 665-PACE, (212) 327-3075, pacenyemail@aol.com, http://www.paceusa.org.

Monique Laberge, PhD
Marshall G. Letcher, MA
Roy Sucholeiki, MD

Epinephrine *see* **Bronchodilators**

Episiotomy

Definition

An episiotomy is a surgical incision made in the area between the vagina and anus (perineum). This is done during the last stages of labor and delivery to expand the opening of the vagina to prevent tearing during the delivery of the baby.

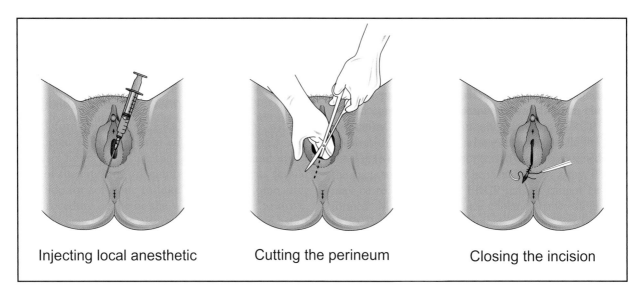

Injecting local anesthetic   Cutting the perineum   Closing the incision

An episiotomy is a surgical incision made in the perineum, the area of tissue between the vaginal opening and the anus, during the birthing process. This procedure may be used if the tissue around the vaginal opening begins to tear or is not stretching enough to allow the baby to be delivered vaginally. In the United States, the rate of episiotomies being performed is estimated at 65–95%. *(Illustration by Electronic Illustrators Group. Reproduced by permission of Gale, a part of Cengage Learning.)*

Purpose

This procedure is usually done during the delivery or birthing process when the vaginal opening does not stretch enough to allow the baby to be delivered without tearing the surrounding tissue.

Precautions

Prior to the onset of labor, pregnant women may want to discuss the use of episiotomy with their care providers. It is possible that, with adequate preparation and if the stages of labor and delivery are managed with adequate coaching and support, the need for an episiotomy may be reduced.

Description

An episiotomy is a surgical incision, usually made with sterile scissors, in the perineum as the baby's head is being delivered. This procedure may be used if the tissue around the vaginal opening begins tearing or does not seem to be stretching enough to allow the baby to be delivered.

In most cases, the physician makes a midline incision along a straight line from the lowest edge of the vaginal opening to toward the anus. In other cases, the episiotomy is performed by making a diagonal incision across the midline between the vagina and anus. This method is used much less often, may be more painful, and may require more healing time than the midline incision. After the baby is delivered through the extended vaginal opening, the incision is closed with stitches. A local anesthetic agent may be applied or injected to numb the area before it is sewn up (sutured).

Several reasons are cited for performing episiotomies. Some experts believe that an episiotomy speeds up the birthing process, making it easier for the baby to be delivered. This can be important if there is any sign of distress that may harm the mother or baby. Because tissues in this area may tear during the delivery, another reason for performing an episiotomy is that a clean incision is easier to repair than a jagged tear and may heal faster. Although the use of episiotomy is sometimes described as protecting the pelvic muscles and possibly preventing future problems with **urinary incontinence**, it is not clear that the procedure actually helps.

The use of episiotomy during the birthing process is fairly widespread in the United States. Estimates of episiotomy use in hospitals range from 65–95% of deliveries, depending on how many times the mother has given birth previously. This routine use of episiotomy is being reexamined in many hospitals and health care settings. However, an episiotomy is always necessary during a forceps delivery because of the size of the forceps.

Preparation

It may be possible to avoid the need for an episiotomy. Pregnant women may want to talk with their

KEY TERMS

Kegel exercises—A series of contractions and relaxations of the muscles in the perineal area. These exercises are thought to strengthen the pelvic floor and may help prevent urinary incontinence in women.

Perineum—The area between the opening of the vagina and the anus in a woman, or the area between the scrotum and the anus in a man.

Sitz bath—A shallow tub or bowl, sometimes mounted above a toilet, that allows the perineum and buttocks to be immersed in circulating water.

Urinary incontinence—The inability to prevent the leakage or discharge of urine. This situation becomes more common as people age, and is more common in women who have given birth to more than one child.

care providers about the use of episiotomy during the delivery. Kegel exercises are often recommended during the **pregnancy** to help strengthen the pelvic floor muscles. Prenatal perineal massage may help to stretch and relax the tissue around the vaginal opening. During the delivery process, warm compresses can be applied to the area along with the use of perineal massage. Coaching and support are also important during the delivery process. A slowed, controlled pushing during the second stage of labor (when the mother gets the urge to push) may allow the tissues to stretch rather than tear. Also, an upright birthing position (rather than one where the mother is lying down) may decrease the need for an episiotomy.

Aftercare

The area of the episiotomy may be uncomfortable or even painful for several days. Several practices can relieve some of the **pain**. Cold packs can be applied to the perineal area to reduce swelling and discomfort. Use of the **Sitz bath** available at the hospital or birth center can ease the discomfort, too. This unit circulates warm water over the area. A squirt bottle with water can be used to clean the area after urination or defecation rather than wiping with tissue. Also, the area should be patted dry rather than wiped. Cleansing pads soaked in witch hazel (such as Tucks) are very effective for cleaning the area and also feel soothing.

Risks

Several side effects of episiotomy have been reported, including infection, increased pain, prolonged healing time, and increased discomfort once sexual intercourse is resumed. There is also the risk that the episiotomy incision will be deeper or longer than is necessary to permit the birth of the infant. There is a risk of increased bleeding.

Normal results

In a normal and well managed delivery, an episiotomy may be avoided altogether. If an episiotomy is deemed to be necessary, a simple midline incision will be made to extend the vaginal opening without additional tearing or extensive trauma to the perineal area. Although there may be some pain associated with the healing of the episiotomy incision, relief can usually be provided with mild pain relievers and supportive measures, such as the application of cold packs.

Abnormal results

An episiotomy incision that is too long or deep may extend into the rectum, causing more bleeding and an increased risk of infection. Additional tearing or tissue damage may occur beyond the episiotomy incision, leaving a cut and a tear to be repaired.

Resources

OTHER

Childbirth.org. http://www.childbirth.org.

Altha Roberts Edgren

Epispadias *see* **Hypospadias and epispadias**
Epistaxis *see* **Nosebleed**
EPS *see* **Electrophysiology study of the heart**

Epstein-Barr virus

Definition

Epstein-Barr virus, or EBV, is the name given to a member of the herpesvirus family that is associated with a variety of illnesses—from **infectious mononucleosis** (IM) and **multiple sclerosis** to nasopharyngeal cancer and Burkitt's lymphoma. EBV is also known as human herpesvirus 4 or HHV-4. It is named for Anthony Epstein and Yvonne Barr, who identified the virus in 1964 in tissue samples sent to them from Uganda by Denis Burkitt (1911–1993), for whom Burkitt's lymphoma was named.

Demographics

EBV occurs in nearly all regions of the world, and is considered among the most common infectious viruses known to humankind. It is likely as of 2009 that its genetic diversity is greater than was thought when it was first identified. In the United States, the Center for Disease Control (CDC) estimates that 95% of adult Americans between the ages of 35 and 40 years have been infected with EBV, but it is less prevalent in children and teenagers. This pattern of infecting adults more than children persists throughout other prosperous Western countries, but does not hold true in underdeveloped regions such as Africa and Asia. In Africa, most children have been infected by EBV by the age of three years.

About 10% of cancers of the stomach are associated with EBV. The reason for this association is not known as of 2009.

Nasopharyngeal cancer is uncommon in the West but more prevalent in the Far East. It affects three times as many men as women, and usually occurs in adults between the ages of 40 and 50 years. This type of cancer is diagnosed in fewer than 1 in every 100,000 Caucasians but in 10–53 persons per 100,000 in mainland China, Taiwan, Hong Kong, and Malaysia. It also occurs more frequently in Eskimos in Greenland and Alaska, and in Tunisians, with about 20 cases per 100,000 people per year. The prevalence rate for adults of Asian descent in the United States is 3–4.2 cases per 100,000 persons per year. Nasopharyngeal cancer accounts for less than 1% of malignancies in children. It affects 1 in every 100,000 children in North America and Europe each year, but between 8 and 25 of every 100,000 children in Asia.

Description

Herpesviruses have long been known. The name actually comes from the Greek adjective *herpestes*, which means creeping. Many herpesvirus species appear to establish a lifelong presence in the human body, remaining dormant for long periods and becoming active for some, often inexplicable, reason. EBV is only one of several members of the Herpesvirus family that have similar traits. Others include varicella zoster virus—the cause of both **chickenpox** and shingles—,

and the herpes simplex virus responsible for both **cold sores** and **genital herpes**. EBV is usually transmitted through saliva but not blood, and is not normally an airborne infection.

Individuals with EBV infections typically show some elevation in the **white blood cell count** and a noticeable increase in lymphocytes—white blood cells associated with the immune response of the body. IM is a time-limited infection that usually lasts from one to two months. Symptoms include **fever**, malaise, **sore throat, swollen glands** and (sometimes) swollen spleen and/or liver.

EBV infections that lead to Burkitt's lymphoma in Africa typically affect the jaw and mouth area, while the (very rare) incidences of Burkitt's lymphoma found in developed countries are more apt to manifest tumors in the abdominal region, most commonly in the intestines, kidneys, or ovaries.

Causes and symptoms

EBV and mononucleosis

EBV is normally transmitted by contact with the saliva of an infected person; it is not ordinarily transmitted through the air. The virus takes about 4 to 6 weeks to incubate, and thus infected persons can spread the disease to others over a period of several weeks. After entering the patient's mouth and upper throat, the virus infects B cells, which are a certain type of white blood cell produced in the bone marrow. The infected B cells are then carried into the lymphatic system, where they affect the liver and spleen and cause the lymph nodes to swell and enlarge. The infected B cells are also responsible for the fever, swelling of the tonsils, and sore throat that characterize mononucleosis.

Most people who become infected with EBV do not have any symptoms, however. In children, EBV infection is usually asymptomatic; when it does cause symptoms, they are difficult to distinguish from routine mild childhood infections. Teenagers who were not exposed to EBV in childhood have a 35% to 50% chance of developing infectious mononucleosis (IM) from EBV. The most common symptoms of IM in teenagers are fever, sore throat, and swollen lymph glands. The patient may also have an enlarged spleen and liver.

After the symptoms of mononucleosis go away, the EBV virus remains in a few cells in the patient's throat tissues or blood for the rest of the person's life. The virus occasionally reactivates and may appear in samples of the person's saliva, but it does not cause

KEY TERMS

B cell—A type of white blood cell produced in the bone marrow that makes antibodies against viruses.

Lymphocyte—Any of a group of white blood cells of crucial importance to the immune system's production of a tailor-made defense against specific invading organisms.

Lymphoma—A group of cancers in which the cells of tissue usually found in the lymph nodes or spleen multiply abnormally.

Malaria—A serious disease prevalent in the tropics. It is caused by parasites and produces severe fever and sometimes complications affecting the kidneys, liver, brain, and blood. It is spread by the Anopheles mosquito and can be fatal.

Nasopharyngeal—Referring to the passage connecting the nasal cavity behind the nose to the top of the throat behind the soft palate.

new symptoms of illness. EBV infection does not cause any problems during **pregnancy**, such as miscarriages or **birth defects**.

EBV and cancer

EBV has been linked to IM in the Western world for decades. It has also become associated consistently with nasopharyngeal cancers in Asia (especially China) and Burkitt's lymphoma in Africa and Papua New Guinea. According to the CDC, EBV is not the sole cause of these two malignancies, but does play an important role in the development of both cancers. The mechanism that allows Epstein-Barr virus to at least help in producing such diverse illnesses in diverse regions of the world has been the subject of increasing research and scrutiny. One theory regarding the higher rate of nasopharyngeal cancer in Asia is that EBV interacts with chemicals called nitrosamines, used in the preparation of salted fish and other preserved foods popular in the region, to trigger changes in cells that lead to cancer.

It is known that EBV is one of the herpesviruses that remain in the human body for life. Under certain, still not-understood conditions, it alters white blood cells normally associated with the immune system, changing the B cells (white blood cells normally associated with making antibodies), and causing them to reproduce uncontrollably. EBV can bind to these white blood cells to produce a solid mass made up of B cells—called Burkitt's lymphoma—or to the mucous membranes of the mouth and nose and cause nasopharyngeal cancer. Since Burkitt's lymphoma typically occurs in people living in moist, tropical climates, the same regions where people usually contract **malaria**, some doctors speculate that the immune system is altered by its response to malaria. When EBV infection occurs, the altered immune system reacts by producing a tumor.

Special concerns

Though studies about the hereditary tendency of abnormal cell development after EBV infection are incomplete, researchers have found it to be associated with abnormalities on multiple human chromosomes, including chromosomes 1, 2, 3, 4, 5, 6, 8, 9, 11, 13, 14, 15, 16, 17, 22, and the X chromosome.

Diagnosis

The diagnosis of mononucleosis caused by EBV is usually based on the results of blood tests combined with the doctor's examination of the patient's throat and neck. The doctor will also tap on or feel the patient's abdomen to see whether the liver and spleen have become enlarged.

A patient infected by EBV will have an increased number of white blood cells in the blood sample, an increased number of abnormal white blood cells, and antibodies to the Epstein-Barr virus. These antibodies can be detected by a test called the monospot test, which gives results within a day but may not be accurate during the first week of the patient's illness. Another type of blood test for EBV antibodies takes longer to perform but gives more accurate results within the first week of symptoms.

Treatment

Traditional

Drugs

Because EBV infections are viral in origin, **antibiotics** are ineffective against them. Much research is geared toward the development of a vaccines effective against both the virus and cancer.

Treatment for mononucleosis caused by EBV consists of self-care at home until the symptoms go away. Patients should rest in bed if possible and drink plenty of fluids. Nonaspirin **pain** relievers like Advil or Tylenol can be taken to bring down the fever and relieve muscle aches and pains. Throat lozenges or gargling with warm salt water may help ease the discomfort of a sore throat.

Because mononucleosis can affect the spleen, patients should avoid vigorous **exercise** or contact sports for at least one month after the onset of symptoms or until the spleen returns to its normal size. This precaution will lower the risk of rupture of the spleen.

With regard to cancers associated with EBV, such **anticancer drugs** as cyclophosphamide or **radiation therapy** have been shown to be effective against Burkitt's lymphoma in four out of five cases.

Alternative

The goal of alternative treatment is to lower the white blood cell count to normal levels. Treatment often includes such **nutritional supplements** as flaxseed oil or shark cartilage, vitamins—including **vitamins** C and K, and mineral supplements containing magnesium and potassium. Well-conducted randomized clinical trials have not yet been conducted to prove the efficacy of these therapies.

Prognosis

Mononucleosis caused by EBV rarely leads to serious complications. In most patients, the fever goes down in about 10 days but **fatigue** may last for several weeks or months. Some people do not feel normal again for about three months. A patient who feels sick longer than 4 months, however, should go back to the doctor to see whether they have another disease or disorder in addition to mononucleosis. In some cases the patient is diagnosed with **chronic fatigue syndrome** or CFS. The Epstein-Barr virus does not cause CFS; however, it appears to make some patients with mononucleosis more susceptible to developing chronic fatigue syndrome.

The prognosis for nasopharyngeal cancer associated with EBV in adults is poor, because about 60% of these cancers have already metastasized to other regions of the head and neck by the time diagnosis is made. The prognosis for this type of cancer in children is also relatively poor. The survival rates for children treated only with radiation therapy are about 45%. When **chemotherapy** and radiation therapy are used together, long-term survival rates range from 55% to 80%.

Prevention

As of 2009 there is no vaccine that can prevent mononucleosis caused by EBV. In addition, the fact that many people can be infected with the virus and transmit it to others without having symptoms of the disease means that mononucleosis is almost impossible to prevent. The best precautionary measure is for patients who have been diagnosed with mono to avoid kissing or other close personal contact with others, and to wash their drinking glasses, food dishes, and eating utensils separately from those of other family members or friends for several days after the fever goes down. It is not necessary for people with mono to be completely isolated from other people, however.

Because the Epstein-Barr virus remains in the body after the symptoms of mononucleosis go away, people who have had IM should not donate blood for at least 6 months after their symptoms started.

Resources

BOOKS

Gluckman, Toma R. *Herpesviridae Viral Structure, Life Cycle, and Infections*. New York: Nova Science Publishers, 2009.

Krueger, Hans, et al. *HPV and Other Infectious Agents in Cancer: Opportunities for Prevention and Public Health*. New York: Oxford University Press, 2010.

Tao, H. E., ed. *DNA Tumor Viruses*. New York: Nova Science Publishers, 2009.

PERIODICALS

Bagert, B.A. "Epstein-Barr Virus in Multiple Sclerosis." *Current Neurology and Neuroscience Reports* 9 (September 2009): 405–410.

Boysen, T., et al. " EBV-associated Gastric Carcinoma in High- and Low-incidence Areas for Nasopharyngeal Carcinoma." *British Journal of Cancer* 101 (August 4, 2009): 530–33.

Chang, C.M., et al. "The Extent of Genetic Diversity of Epstein-Barr Virus and its Geographic and Disease Patterns: A Need for Reappraisal." *Virus Research* 143 (August 2009): 209–21.

Morris, M. A., et al. "Role of the Epstein-Barr Virus-encoded Latent Membrane Protein-1, LMP1, in the Pathogenesis of Nasopharyngeal Carcinoma." *Future Oncology* 5 (August 2009): 811–25.

Oluwadara, O., and F. Chiappelli. "Biomarkers for Early Detection of High Risk Cancers: From Gliomas to Nasopharyngeal Carcinoma." *Bioinformation* 3 (April 21, 2009): 332–39.

Shinozaki, A., et al. "Epstein-Barr Virus-associated Gastric Carcinoma: A Distinct Carcinoma of Gastric Phenotype by Claudin Expression Profiling." *Journal of Histochemistry and Cytochemistry* 57 (August 2009): 775–85.

OTHER

Centers for Disease Control and Prevention (CDC). *Epstein-Barr Virus and Infectious Mononucleosis*. http://www.cdc.gov/ncidod/diseases/ebv.htm

Lin, Ho-Sheng, and Willard E. Fee, Jr. "Malignant Nasopharyngeal Tumors." *eMedicine*, December 21, 2007.

http://emedicine.medscape.com/article/848163-overview

Paulino, Arnold C., and Stephan A. Grupp. "Nasopharyngeal Cancer." *eMedicine*, October 17, 2008. http://emedicine.medscape.com/article/988165-overview

National Library of Medicine Tutorial. . http://www.nlm.nih.gov/medlineplus/tutorials/epsteinbarrvirusmono/htm/index.htm

Virology Down Under. *Epstein-Barr Virus*. http://www.uq.edu.au/vdu/VDUEBV.htm

ORGANIZATIONS

American Society for Virology (ASV), asv@asv.org, http://www.asv.org/.

Centers for Disease Control and Prevention (CDC), 1600 Clifton Road, Atlanta, GA, 30333, 800-232-4636, cdcinfo@cdc.gov, http://www.cdc.gov.

International Association for Research on Epstein-Barr Virus and Related Diseases, [site hosted at Baylor College of Medicine, Houston, TX], ebv-webmaster@bcm.edu, http://www.bcm.edu/ebvassociation/index.htm.

Joan Schonbeck, RN
Rebecca J. Frey, PhD

Epstein-Barr virus test

Definition

The Epstein-Barr virus test is a blood test, or group of tests, to determine the presence or absence of antibodies in the blood stream directed against proteins of the Epstein-Barr virus, the cause of **infectious mononucleosis**.

Purpose

The test is primarily used to detect whether first time infection (called primary infection) with the Epstein-Barr virus is currently occurring, or has occurred within a short period of time. The pattern of the antibodies detected can, however, tell if the person has never been infected with the Epstein-Barr virus, or if the infection occurred in the more distant past. These tests are mostly utilized in the diagnosis of Epstein-Barr virus-associated infectious mononucleosis when the more common diagnostic test, the heterophile antibody, is negative, or in situations where the infection is manifesting unusual symptoms. Therefore, the tests are often not needed in a situation where a doctor believes that a person has mononucleosis and the heterophile test (also called the monospot test) is positive.

In addition, Epstein-Barr virus testing is usually not needed in the evaluation of a patient who has long-lasting **fatigue**, and may have the **chronic fatigue syndrome**. Initially, it was thought that discovering a particular pattern of antibodies to this virus was helpful in the diagnosis of chronic fatigue syndrome, but this no longer appears to be the case.

Precautions

As in any blood test, standard precautions should be performed to prevent infection at the site where the blood is obtained, and to prevent excess bleeding. Normally, the site is cleaned with an antiseptic liquid prior to the blood being obtained; a sterile non-reusable needle and syringe are used; and, once the needle is removed, pressure is placed at the site until bleeding has stopped.

Description

These tests are more often performed in a consulting laboratory than at a physician's office or in a hospital laboratory. Like most antibody tests, they are performed on serum, the liquid part of the blood obtained after the whole blood is allowed to clot in a tube. Antibodies can be detected against several components of the Epstein-Barr virus (EBV). These components are the EBV early antigen (EA), the viral capsid antigen (VCA), and the nuclear antigen (EBNA). These several antigens are different proteins that are produced in the process (stages) of the virus' growth.

At the time of infection with Epstein-Barr virus, antibodies to EA are found and usually last for four to six months only. This antibody, however, persists substantially longer in about 10% of persons who have had EBV infection in the more remote past. The absence of antibody to EA when other EBV antibodies are present strongly suggests that first time infection with EBV occurred in the past.

Antibody to VCA is found both early and late in EBV infection. At the time of infection, antibody of both the IgM and IgG types are detectable. After four to six months, usually, only the IgG antibody against VCA can be found.

Unlike antibodies to EA and VCA, antibody to EBNA does not usually develop until recovery from first time infection of this virus. Therefore, finding detectable amounts of antibody to EBNA during an illness which might be caused by EBV makes the causal relationship very unlikely.

Preparation

The skin area from which the blood sample will be obtained is wiped with an antiseptic such as alcohol or iodine.

Aftercare

The aftercare is similar to that for any blood test. Usually, pressure is applied to the area for several moments until bleeding stops. If the results are difficult to interpret, it may be necessary to re-test later, after waiting one to three weeks. The change in the amounts of antibody detected between the two tests can be particularly useful, at times, in helping to make a diagnosis.

Risks

There are no risks over and above those of having blood drawn for any other purpose. These tests are more expensive than many other blood tests but are usually covered by medical insurance.

Normal results

The pattern of the three antibodies can be used to determine whether the person has not had infection with EBV to this point (is susceptible to infection); is currently, or recently, infected with EBV for the first time; or has had first time infection with EBV sometime in the past (more than six months ago).

If one defines "normal" results as either not having EBV in the past, and call that category one; or having had it in the past, and call that category two. Most young children below the age of five will fall into category one, while most adults over the age of 20 years will fall into category two.

The results for susceptibility are:

- antibody to EA = negative
- antibody to VCA (either IgM or IgG) = negative
- antibody to EBNA = negative

The results for past infection are:

- antibody to EA = negative (90% of time)
- antibody to VCA IgM = negative
- Antibody to VCA IgG = positive
- Antibody to EBNA = Positive.

It is important to realize that the Epstein-Barr virus, like all the human herpes viruses, does not totally leave the body after the patient recovers from illness. With EBV, the virus will intermittently recur in the saliva of people without any symptoms. Such people will have a test pattern of previous infection. It is

this group of people who can transmit EBV to others without themselves being ill.

Abnormal results

The results for current or recent infection are:

- antibody to EA = positive
- antibody to VCA IgM = positive
- antibody to VCA IgG = positive
- antibody to EBNA = negative.

Without the pattern of the three antibodies, it can be difficult to be accurate in interpretation. The presence of antibody to VCA IgM is the best single test for current or recent first time infection.

Resources

PERIODICALS

Raggam, Reinhard, et al. "Detection and quantitation of Epstein-Barr virus (EBV) DNA in EDTA whole blood samples using automated sample preparation and real time PCR." *Clinical Chemistry and Laboratory Medicine* 48, no. 3 (March 1, 2010): 413–18.

Larry I. Lutwick, MD, FACP

ERCP *see* **Endoscopic retrograde cholangiopancreatography**

Erectile disorder *see* **Impotence**

Erectile dysfunction

Definition

Erectile dysfunction (ED) is the consistent inability to achieve or maintain a penile erection that is sufficient for satisfactory sexual intercourse.

Demographics

It is estimated that 15–30 million American men suffer from some degree of ED. Of these, 10–20 million have severe ED resulting in the complete inability to attain or maintain a penile erection. As the population ages, the number of American men with ED is projected to increase by nearly 10 million by 2025. The worldwide incidence of ED is projected to be more than 320 million by 2025.

The incidence of ED increases with advancing age, along with the incidence of chronic disorders and conditions that are commonly associated with ED, including diabetes, **hypertension**, and cardiovascular disease.

It is estimated that 26% of men in their 50s, 40% of men in their 60s, and 77% of men 75 and older have some degree of ED. However ED is notorious for being underreported, undiagnosed, and under–treated due to its perceived stigma. It is estimated that 70% of ED cases remain undiagnosed. In a survey of general medical practice, less than 12% of men with ED reported having received treatment. Thus, the true incidence of ED may be much higher than most estimates.

Description

ED is defined as the consistent inability to achieve or maintain an erection, usually associated with **fatigue**, anger, depression, or other stressful emotions. However the term "impotence" is now rarely used because of its association with weakness and lack of power.

Penile erection occurs when the penis becomes engorged with blood. The anatomical compartments—the two corpora cavernosa and the corpus spongiosum—can be distended with up to seven times the normal amount of blood. This change results in an erection in association with the relaxation of the penile muscles.

The sequence of events resulting in penile erection is complex. Erection is usually initiated by sexual arousal stimuli in the brain as a result of visual, auditory, or olfactory sensations or erotic thoughts. Tactile (touch) sensations of the penis, acting through the spinal cord, play a similar role. Sexual arousal results in the release of nitric oxide from specialized cells. Nitric oxide causes the formation of cyclic glutamine monophosphate (cGMP), which is responsible for dilating the blood vessels of the penis and relaxing the penile muscles, enabling increased blood flow and erection. Compression of the dilated blood vessels against the firm outer lining of the penis prevents the blood from escaping and perpetuates the erection. An enzyme called phosphodiesterase 5 (PDE5) causes the breakdown of cGMP and, along with nerves from the sympathetic nervous system, enables the penis to return to its flaccid relaxed state. Any defect in this complex cascade of events can result in ED.

Sex is an important quality–of–life issue for adults of all ages and ED usually results in a reduced quality of life. Many affected men experience depression, distress, and relationship difficulties as a result of ED. Despite this, ED sufferers often fail to seek help. Reasons for this failure include:

- ignorance of the availability of safe and effective ED therapies
- inadequate information from physicians about the timing of medications, the need for preliminary sexual arousal, and other factors
- concerns about marital discord and a lack of partner support
- concerns about invasiveness, adverse effects, discomfort, inconvenience, and cost of therapies
- high rates of discontinuation of therapy due to inadequate responses and adverse effects

Risk factors

ED is frequently associated with vascular conditions such as hypertension and coronary artery heart disease and may even serve as marker for detection of cardiovascular disorders. Additionally ED is associated with depression that is distinct from depression resulting from ED. Lifestyle factors—such as **obesity**, physical inactivity, cigarette **smoking**, and excessive intake of alcohol—are also risk factors for ED.

Causes and symptoms

Because of the complicated nature of the human sexual response and the complex physiology of penile erection and relaxation, it is often difficult or even impossible to determine the cause of an individual case of ED precisely. Often ED is the result of multiple factors. Normal erectile function requires the coordination of vascular, neurologic, hormonal, and psychological components and any condition that interferes with one or more of these processes can result in ED.

Although the incidence of ED increases with advancing age it is no longer regarded as an inevitable consequence of **aging**. Likewise, whereas most cases of ED were once considered primarily psychological and/or psychiatric in origin, it is now recognized that organic, non–psychological factors play a much more significant role, with physical causes being responsible for at least 80% of cases. However significant psychological and social factors—such as guilt, depression, **anxiety**, tension, or marital discord—are often present in addition to one or more underlying physical components:

- Diabetes mellitus is the single most common cause of ED, as a result of combined nerve and blood vessel damage. As many as 50% of male diabetics have ED.
- Hardening of the arteries (arteriosclerosis) is the most common vascular (circulation–related) cause of ED. Diseases of the aorta or the arteries supplying the pelvis and penis or damage to arteries from trauma, surgery, or irradiation can cause ED. Surgery involving the prostate gland may affect both arteries and nerves.
- A variety of diseases and factors can influence penile circulation. For example Peyronie's disease, characterized by fibrous tissue and bending of the penis,

KEY TERMS

Dopamine—A chemical in brain tissue that transmits nerve impulses (a neurotransmitter) and helps to regulate movement and emotions.

Hypertension—Abnormally high arterial blood pressure, which if left untreated can lead to heart disease and stroke.

Hypogonadism—Functional incompetence of the male gonads, with impaired production of hormones and germ cells.

Prolactin—A hormone produced by the pituitary gland.

Prostate—The walnut–shaped gland that surrounds the urethra at the neck of the bladder in males and supplies fluid for semen.

Testosterone—The primary male sex hormone.

Urethra—The tube in the penis that discharges urine from the bladder to the outside of the body.

---

limits the expandability of penile tissues and prevents venous compression, enabling blood to exit the penis. Arteriosclerotic plaque, injury to the inner lining blood vessels from trauma, surgery, or irradiation, or aortic occlusion (blockage in a main artery leading out of the heart) can compromise penile blood flow and prevent erection.

- Neurological causes of ED include diseases of the brain and spinal cord, such as Alzheimer's disease or multiple sclerosis, respectively.

- Hormonal or endocrine causes of ED are uncommon, although deficient testicular function and low circulating levels of the male sex hormone testosterone can result in erectile dysfunction. These are referred to as hypogonadism and can be due to congenital abnormalities or testicular disease.

- Various classes of medications can cause ED, although not all drugs within a class have the same effects. For example some antidepressants are associated with ED, whereas the antidepressant trazodone (Desyrel) tends to prolong penile erection. Some high blood pressure medications, central nervous system medications such as methyldopa for **Parkinson's disease**, sedatives or tranquilizers such as barbiturates, and anti–anxiety medications such as diazepam (Valium) also can cause ED.

- Tobacco, alcohol, and illicit drugs, including heroin, can cause ED.

- Psychological factors—including stress, fatigue, depression, guilt, low self–esteem, or negative feelings for or by a sexual partner—can precipitate ED. Depressive symptoms or difficulty coping with anger can be particularly detrimental.

- ED is the main symptom of a mental disorder known as male erectile disorder.

Although the primary ED symptom is the inability to attain or maintain an adequate erection for completed sexual activity, patterns of ED vary. Some men are unable to attain any erection. Others cannot maintain an erection adequate for penetration. Some men lose their erection during sexual intercourse. Others experience an erection only upon awakening or during masturbation.

Diagnosis

Examination

Thorough medical, psychosocial (both psychological and social), and sexual histories are an essential first step in the diagnosis of ED. A general medical history can indicate the existence of ED–associated conditions such as high blood pressure, diabetes, or arteriosclerosis, as well as medications that may contribute to ED and any history of **substance abuse**. A psychosocial history includes current sexual practices, the existence of stresses or performance anxiety, and any special circumstances under which ED occurs. The sexual partner's participation in the taking of a psychosocial history can be beneficial. The sexual history assists in distinguishing ED from other abnormalities in sexual function, such as ejaculatory and orgasmic disturbances or loss of sexual desire. The patient's sexual history includes:

- the frequency and duration of sexual intercourse
- the degree and quality of penile erections
- nocturnal erections
- the success or failure of penetration
- any sexual dysfunction of the partner, such as painful intercourse (dyspareunia) or vaginal dryness

Self–administered questionnaires can assist in the evaluation of sexual function. The International Index of Erectile Function (IIEF) is the most widely used. It addresses:

- sexual desire
- erectile function
- orgasmic function
- intercourse satisfaction
- overall satisfaction

A routine **physical examination** is conducted with special emphasis on the genitourinary, circulatory, and neurologic systems. The physician may look for evidence of **hypogonadism** or congenital conditions causing defective testicular function. The genitalia are examined for testicular size and consistency and penile deformities. A **rectal examination** can evaluate the size and consistency of the prostate gland and certain muscular reflexes. Vital signs such as blood pressure and pulse are measured.

Tests

Blood tests and/or other assessments for high blood cholesterol, hypertension, coronary artery heart disease, and depression may be performed, since ED can be a marker or symptom of such disorders. Blood levels of the hormones testosterone and prolactin may be measured.

Procedures

There are several diagnostic procedures for ED:

- Duplex Doppler ultrasonography provides information about both arterial and venous blood flow.
- Pharmacological testing involves the injection of a small amount of an agent—such as 10 micrograms of alprostadil (prostaglandin E1)—that produces an erection in a patient with normal erectile function.
- Nocturnal studies are used to identify erectile dysfunction due to organic causes. Patients are monitored in a sleep laboratory for nocturnal erections during sleep, since men with physiologically normal erectile function have erections during sleep. A self-test can also be performed.

Treatment

Traditional

There are a variety of treatment options for ED, including a combination of therapies:

- Psychosexual therapy, individual psychotherapy, or couples therapy may be recommended.
- Vacuum constriction device therapy involves a mechanical device for increasing penile blood flow and erection.
- Various types of penile prostheses can be surgically inserted into the penis to produce erections.
- In rare cases surgery may be used to correct a defect that interferes with penile erection.

Drugs

There are various drug treatments for ED:

- Adjustment of prescription or over–the–counter medications may be required.
- PDE5 inhibitors relax the muscles in the penis to increase penile blood flow and produce an erection. This class of drugs includes sildenafil (Viagra), vardenafil (Levitra), and tadalafil (Cialis). These should not be used by men who take nitroglycerin for heart problems because they can cause a sudden drop in blood pressure. PDE5 inhibitors also have been associated with an increased risk for a rare condition called nonarteritic ischemic optic neuropathy, which can lead to sudden vision loss.
- Apomorphine is a morphine derivative that targets dopamine receptors to facilitate erections.
- Alpha–adrenergic blockers target adrenergic receptors in smooth muscles, causing the blood vessels to dilate more easily.
- Intracavernous injection therapy (ICIT) is the injection of penile structures with the drugs alprostadil (Caverject), papaverine (Pavabid), or phentolamine, which promote blood flow.
- Intraurethral therapy is the insertion of alprostadil into the urethra to increase blood flow and muscle relaxation.

Alternative

Herbal remedies for ED include:

- dehydroepiandrosterone (DHEA)
- ginkgo
- ginseng
- L–arginine
- yohimbe
- epimedium (horny goat weed)
- zinc
- folic acid and vitamin E in combination with Viagra

Alternative treatments should be used with care, as the benefits of many such treatments have not been confirmed by scientific research.

Home remedies

A first step in ED treatment is the alteration or elimination of modifiable risk factors or causes, including smoking, obesity, and substance or alcohol abuse.

Prognosis

A better understanding of ED, combined with new, more effective therapies, has markedly improved the prognosis. It is estimated that at least 65% of all ED cases can be treated successfully. The modification of risk factors—such as physical inactivity, smoking, excessive alcohol intake, certain medications, and obesity—improve the prognosis. However other risk factors—including aging and conditions such as diabetes or pelvic surgery affecting nerves—negatively impact the prognosis.

Prevention

Physicians can help prevent ED by prescribing high blood pressure and other medications that are not associated with ED for their at–risk patients. Various lifestyle changes can help prevent ED. These include:

- not smoking
- losing weight
- not abusing alcohol or other substances

Resources

BOOKS

Drake, Elizabeth. *50 plus One Questions to Ask Your Doctor.* Detroit: Thorndike Press, 2008.

Ellsworth, Pamela, and Bob Stanley. *100 Questions & Answers About Erectile Dysfunction,* 2nd ed. Sudbury, MA: Jones and Bartlett, 2008.

Judd, Sandra J. *Men's Health Concerns Sourcebook,* 3rd ed. Detroit: Omnigraphics, 2009.

Morgentaler, Abraham. *Testosterone for Life: Revitalize Your Vitality, Sex Drive, Muscle Mass & Overall Health.* New York: McGraw–Hill, 2009.

Steidle, Christopher P., and Janet Casperson. *Sex and the Heart: How a Healthier Heart Helps Overcome Erectile Dysfunction.* Omaha, NE: Addicus Books, 2008.

PERIODICALS

Heidelbaugh, J. J. "Management of Erectile Dysfunction." *American Family Physician* 81(3) (February 1, 2010): 305–12.

"Information From Your Family Doctor. Erectile Dysfunction." *American Family Physician* 81(3) (February 1, 2010): 313.

Katz, Alan, and Anne Katz. "Erectile Dysfunction." *Canadian Medical Association Journal* 182(4) (March 9, 2010): 381–82.

OTHER

American Diabetes Association. "Erectile Dysfunction." *Living With Diabetes.* http://www.diabetes.org/living-with-diabetes/complications/mens-health/sexual-health/erectile-dysfunction.html (accessed September 25, 2010).

"Erectile Dysfunction." MedlinePlus. http://www.nlm.nih.gov/medlineplus/erectiledysfunction.html (accessed September 25, 2010).

NIDDK. "Erectile Dysfunction." NIH Publication No. 09–3923. http://kidney.niddk.nih.gov/kudiseases/pubs/ED (accessed September 25, 2010).

"Erection Self–Test." MedlinePlus. http://www.nlm.nih.gov/medlineplus/ency/article/003339.htm (accessed September 25, 2010).

ORGANIZATIONS

American Diabetes Association (ADA), 1710 North Beauregard St., Alexandria, VA, 22311, (800) DIABETES, http://www.diabetes.org.

American Urological Association (AUA), 1000 Corporate Blvd., Linthicum, MD, 21090, (410) 689–3700, (866) RING–AUA (746–4282), (410) 689–3800, aua@AUAnet.org, http://www.auanet.org.

National Kidney and Urologic Diseases Information Clearinghouse, 3 Information Way, Bethesda, MD, 20892–3580, (703) 738–4929, (800) 891–5390, (703) 738–4929, nkudic@info.niddk.nih.gov, http://kidney.niddk.nih.gov.

Ralph Myerson, MD
Stephanie Watson
Margaret Alic, PhD

▌Erectile dysfunction treatment

Definition

Erectile dysfunction (ED)—the consistent inability to achieve or maintain an erection long enough to engage in satisfactory sexual intercourse—is most often treated with drugs. However, in some cases, more invasive techniques or devises must be used to treat ED.

Purpose

The purpose of ED treatment is to enable men to achieve and maintain erections of sufficient strength and duration to engage in sexual intercourse. This usually requires maintaining an erection for 30–60 minutes.

Demographics

It is estimated that 15–30 million American men suffer from some degree of ED and 10–20 million of these men are completely unable to attain or maintain a penile erection. About 75% of men in the general population who have tried ED drugs have found them to be helpful. Although these drugs have revolutionized ED treatment, some men—for example **prostate cancer** patients and those with ED stemming from psychological issues—often require alternative treatments.

Description

Sexual arousal normally causes the release of nitric oxide from specialized cells. Nitric oxide causes the formation of cyclic glutamine monophosphate (cGMP), which is responsible for dilating the blood vessels of the penis and relaxing the penile muscles, enabling increased blood flow and erection. Compression of the dilated blood vessels against the firm outer lining of the penis prevents blood from escaping and perpetuates the erection. An enzyme called phosphodiesterase–5 (PDE5) breaks down cGMP, resulting in decreased blood flow to the penis, which then returns to its flaccid relaxed state. The most common drugs for treating ED are PDE5 inhibitors.

A first step in ED treatment is the alteration or elimination of modifiable factors that can cause the disorder. These include **smoking**, **obesity**, and alcohol or other **substance abuse**. An adjustment in prescription or over–the–counter medications that can cause ED also may be required. ED that is caused, at least in part, by psychosocial factors may be treated with psychosexual therapy, individual **psychotherapy**, or couples therapy.

There are three prescription oral PDE5 inhibitors available in the United States for treating physical causes of ED: **sildenafil citrate** (Viagra), vardenafil hydrochloride (Levitra), and tadalafil (Cialis). These drugs increase the supply of nitric oxide to open blood vessels and relax muscles in the penis, thereby increasing penile blood flow and producing an erection. Once sexual activity is completed, blood flow to the penis decreases and the erection is lost.

Available dosages of PDE5 inhibitors are as follows:

- Viagra: 25, 50, and 100 milligrams (mg), with an average recommended dose of 50 mg
- Levitra: 2.5, 5, 10, and 20 mg tablets
- Cialis: 5, 10, and 20 mg tablets, with 10 mg as the recommended starting dose. Some evidence indicates that higher doses of sildenafil and vardenafil, but not tadalafil, provoke better responses than lower doses. ED drugs are covered by most insurance plans.

The three PDE5 inhibitors are very similar and appear to be equally effective. Viagra and Levitra must be taken without food and are effective for up to four hours. Cialis can be taken with or without food and is effective for up to 36 hours.

Other drugs that are sometimes used to treat ED include:

- testosterone, for hypogonadism in which levels of the male sex hormone are low

- apomorphine, a morphine derivative that targets dopamine receptors to facilitate erections
- alpha–adrenergic blockers, which target adrenergic receptors in smooth muscles causing blood vessels to dilate more readily

Herbal remedies that may improve ED in some cases include:

- dehydroepiandrosterone (DHEA)
- ginkgo
- ginseng
- L–arginine
- yohimbe
- epimedium (horny goat weed)
- zinc
- folic acid and vitamin E in combination with Viagra

Alternative treatments should be used with care, as the benefits of many such treatments have not been confirmed by scientific research.

Intracavernous injection therapy (ICIT) is the injection of penile structures with drugs that promote blood flow. The drugs are injected into the corpora cavernosa—the erectile tissues that form the bulk of the penis and that become engorged with blood during an erection. Alprostadil (prostaglandin E1; Caverject) and papaverine hydrochloride (Pavabid) relax the smooth muscle tissue to enhance blood flow into the penis. Injection therapy often involves a three–drug combination commonly referred to as the "Knoxville formula," apparently after the city of its original introduction. Although there are a number of slightly different formulations in use, they all involve alprostadil, papaverine, and phentolamine mesylate.

Intraurethral therapy or MUSE (medical urethral system for erection) involves administering alprostadil into the urethral opening of the penis. A thin tube—about the width of a spaghetti noodle—is inserted into the urethral opening and a plunger is pressed to deliver a tiny pellet containing alprostadil. The drug must be injected shortly before intercourse. It takes about 10 minutes to achieve an erection that lasts about one hour.

Vacuum pump therapy involves inserting the penis into a clear plastic cylinder and pumping air out of the cylinder to form a partial vacuum, which helps draw blood into the corpora cavernosa. A special ring is placed over the base of the penis to trap the blood.

Implanted **penile prostheses** are usually a last resort for treating ED. These are implanted in the corpora cavernosa to make the penis rigid without the need for blood flow. The semi–rigid type of prosthesis consists of a pair of flexible silicone rods that can be bent up or down. An inflatable device consists of cylinders implanted in the corpora cavernosa, a fluid reservoir implanted in the abdomen, and a pump placed in the scrotum. Squeezing the pump moves fluid into the cylinders to inflate them and make them rigid. Squeezing the pump again reverses the process. Men can resume sexual activity six ro eight weeks after implantation surgery.

In rare cases when narrowed or diseased veins are responsible for ED, surgery may be required to reroute the blood flow into the corpora cavernosa or to remove leaking blood vessels that interfere with penile erection.

Origins

Drugs for treating ED are relatively new:

- Alprostadil was first approved for ED by the U.S. Food and Drug Administration (FDA) in 1995.
- Sildenafil was originally developed in 1991 as a treatment for angina (chest pain). Viagra received FDA approval as a treatment for ED in 1998.
- Levitra and Cialis received FDA approval in 2003.

Benefits

It is estimated that at least 65% of all ED cases can be treated successfully. Addressing risk factors, such as physical inactivity, smoking, excessive alcohol intake, certain medications, and obesity, improves the prognosis. Levitra can often improve erectile function even in men with other medical problems, such as diabetes or prostate surgery. Cialis has also been shown to improve erectile function in most men, including those with severe ED. Cialis does not need to be taken on an empty stomach and is not affected by high–fat foods.

Precautions

- PDE5 inhibitors alone do not result in an erection; nor do they increase sexual desire. They require sexual stimulation and arousal to be effective.
- PDE5 inhibitors cannot be taken more than once a day.
- Viagra and Levitra should be taken on an empty stomach to be effective.
- High–fat foods can interfere with the absorption of Viagra.
- Men who experience cardiovascular symptoms—such as dizziness, chest or arm pain, or nausea—after taking a PDE5 inhibitor should cease all sexual activity and consult their physician before taking the drug again.
- PDE5 inhibitors should not be used by women or children or by men without ED.

- Many ED treatments, often labeled as "dietary supplements," are available online. The FDA has warned consumers that these products may contain unlabeled PDE5 inhibitors that should not be used except under a physician's supervision, as well as various other substances that may be harmful.
- Implantable penile prostheses cause the penis to always be erect.
- Although inflatable implants allow for planned erections, they have a slightly higher malfunction rate than silicone rods.
- Implants permanently destroy the ability to achieve a natural erection.

PDE5 inhibitors do not cause side effects in most people; however higher doses increase the risk of side effects. The most common side effects of PDE5 inhibitors are mild to moderate **headache** or **nausea**, which usually disappear within a few hours. Less common side effects include:

- flushing
- indigestion
- stuffy or runny nose
- back pain and muscle aches with Levitra and Cialis
- temporary vision changes, including "blue vision," with Viagra

Geriatric

ED treatments may be less effective in geriatric patients. Men over age 65 should start with the lowest possible dose of a PDE5 inhibitor.

Other conditions and allergies

- Since sexual activity can put stress on the heart, men with heart conditions should talk to their physicians about the advisability of sexual activity prior to using any ED treatment.
- ED treatments may be less effective in men who have had pelvic surgery affecting nerves.
- PDE5 inhibitors are only about 60–65% effective in diabetics.
- Men with kidney or liver impairment should begin with the lowest possible dose of a PDE5 inhibitor.
- PDE5 inhibitors should not be used by men who take nitroglycerin or other nitrate drugs for heart problems.
- Men who use alpha–blockers—sometimes prescribed for high blood pressure or prostate problems—also should not take PDE5 inhibitors, since such combinations can cause an unsafe drop in blood pressure.
- Numerous other drugs can interact with PDE5 inhibitors.

KEY TERMS

Angina—A condition in which lack of blood to the heart causes severe chest pain.

Arrhythmia—An irregularity in the normal rhythm or force of the heartbeat.

Atherosclerosis—Hardening of the arteries; an arterial disease in which raised areas of degeneration and cholesterol deposits (plaques) form on the inner surfaces of the arteries.

Dopamine—A chemical in brain tissue that transmits nerve impulses (a neurotransmitter) and helps to regulate movement and emotions.

Corpora cavernosa—The pair of columns of erectile tissue on either side of the penis that, together with the corpus spongiosum, produce an erection when filled with blood.

Phosphodiesterase-5 (PDE5) inhibitors—The drugs Viagra, Levitra, and Cialis, which are used to treat ED.

Priapism—A prolonged erection lasting more than four hours.

Testosterone—The primary male sex hormone.

Urethra—The tube in the penis that discharges urine from the bladder to the outside of the body.

PDE5 inhibitors are known to increase cardiovascular nerve activity and can trigger temporary **hypotension** (low blood pressure). They may not be safe for patients with:

- atherosclerosis
- heart problems including angina (chest pains), abnormal heart rhythms (arrhythmias), heart failure, or recent heart attack
- uncontrolled high or low blood pressure
- stroke within the past six months
- eye problems, such as retinitis pigmentosa, or relatives with certain eye problems
- sickle cell anemia, leukemia, or other health problems that can cause priapism

Preparation

Viagra is taken 60 minutes or more prior to sexual activity. Levitra and Cialis are taken 30 minutes or more before sex.

Aftercare

Blood pressure should be monitored after taking PDE5 inhibitors.

Risks

Priapism, a prolonged erection, is a very rare side effect of all prescription ED medications. Alprostadil and papaverine sometimes cause painful erections or priapism that must be treated with a shot of epinephrine. Any erection lasting more than four hours requires immediate medical attention because priapism can permanently damage the penis.

There are other risks associated with ED treatments:

- PDE5 inhibitors increase the risk of heart attack in patients with unstable heart disease or who take nitrate medications.
- PDE5 inhibitors may be associated with an increased risk for a rare condition called nonarteritic ischemic optic neuropathy, which can lead to sudden vision loss.
- The injection of ED medications is often painful. Alprostadil injection can cause pain and burning in the urethra for about five to 15 minutes.
- Vacuum pump therapy can cause bruising if the vacuum is left on for too long.

Resources

BOOKS

Carson, Culley C., and Chris G. McMahon. *Erectile Dysfunction,* 4th ed. Abington, UK: Health Press, 2008.

Ellsworth, Pamela, and Bob Stanley. *100 Questions & Answers About Erectile Dysfunction,* 2nd ed. Sudbury, MA: Jones and Bartlett, 2008.

Hanash, Kamal Antwan. *New Frontiers in Men's Sexual Health: Understanding Erectile Dysfunction and the Revolutionary New Treatments.* Westport, CT: Praeger, 2008.

PERIODICALS

Heidelbaugh, J. J. "Management of Erectile Dysfunction." *American Family Physician* 81(3) (February 1, 2010): 305–12.

Katz, Alan, and Anne Katz. "Erectile Dysfunction." *Canadian Medical Association Journal* 182(4) (March 9, 2010): 381–2.

Tonks, Alison. "Evidence Favors Phosphodiesterase-5 Inhibitors for Erectile Dysfunction." *British Medical Journal* 339(7728) (October 31, 2009): 996.

OTHER

American College of Physicians. "Hormonal Testing and Pharmacological Treatment of Erectile Dysfunction." Annals of Internal Medicine: Summaries for Patients. http://www.annals.org/content/151/9/I–44.full.pdf (accessed September 25, 2010).

"Erectile Dysfunction." MedlinePlus. http://www.nlm.nih.gov/medlineplus/erectiledysfunction.html (accessed September 25, 2010).

Mayo Clinic Staff. "Erectile Dysfunction Herbs: A Natural Treatment for ED?" MayoClinic.com. http://www.mayoclinic.com/health/erectile–dysfunction–herbs/MC00064/METHO D = print (accessed September 25, 2010).

Mayo Clinic Staff. "Erectile Dysfunction: Viagra and Other Oral Medications." MayoClinic.com http://www.mayoclinic.com/print/erectile–dysfunction/MC00029/METHOD = print (accessed September 25, 2010).

"Treating Erectile Dysfunction: Lifestyle Changes." Cleveland Clinic. http://my.clevelandclinic.org/disorders/erectile_disorder_impotence/hic_t reating_erectile_dysfunction_lifestyle_changes.aspx (accessed September 25, 2010).

U.S. Food and Drug Administration. "Hidden Risks of Erectile Dysfunction 'Treatments' Sold Online." Consumer Updates. http://www.fda.gov/ForConsumers/ConsumerUpdates/ucm048386.htm (accessed September 25, 2010).

ORGANIZATIONS

American Urological Association (AUA), 1000 Corporate Blvd., Linthicum, MD, 21090, (410) 689–3700, (866) RING–AUA (746–4282), (410) 689–3800, aua@AUAnet.org, http://www.auanet.org.

National Kidney and Urologic Diseases Information Clearinghouse (NKUDIC), 3 Information Way, Bethesda, MD, 20892–3580, (703) 738–4929, (800) 891–5390, (703) 738–4929, nkudic@info.niddk.nih.gov, http://kidney.niddk.nih.gov.

U.S. Food and Drug Administration (FDA), 10903 New Hampshire Ave., Silver Spring, MD, 20993–0002, (888) INFO–FDA, http://www.fda.gov.

Ken R. Wells
Margaret Alic, PhD

Ergotamine *see* **Antimigraine drugs**

Erosive gastritis *see* **Gastritis**

Erysipelas

Definition

Erysipelas is a skin infection that often follows **strep throat**.

Description

Erysipelas, also called St. Anthony's fire, is caused by infection by Group A *Streptococci*. This same type of bacteria is responsible for such infections as strep throat, and infections of both surgical and other kinds of **wounds** in the skin. The infection occurs most often in young infants and the elderly.

Causes and symptoms

Erysipelas usually occurs rather abruptly. When the preceding infection was strep throat, the rash begins on the face. Occasionally, when the preceding infection was of a wound from an injury or operation, the rash will appear on an arm or leg.

Classically, the usual presentation is a bright-red, butterfly-shaped rash appearing across the bridge of the nose and the cheeks. It is hot to the touch, painful, shiny, and swollen, with clearly defined margins. The edges of the rash are a raised ridge, hard to the touch. There may be fluid-filled bumps scattered along the area. The rash spreads rapidly. Some patients have swelling of the eyelids, sometimes so severe that their eyes swell shut. The patient may have **fever**, chills, loss of energy, **nausea and vomiting**, and swollen, tender lymph nodes. In severe cases, walled-off areas of pus (abscesses) may develop beneath the skin. If left untreated, the streptococcal bacteria may begin circulating in the bloodstream (a condition called **bacteremia**). A patient may then develop an overwhelming, systemic infection called **sepsis**, with a high risk of **death**.

Diagnosis

The rash of erysipelas is very characteristic, raising the practitioner's suspicion towards that diagnosis, especially when coupled with a history of recent strep infection. Attempts to culture (grow) the bacteria from a sample of the rash usually fail. When the bacteria are present in the blood, they may be grown in a laboratory, and identified under a microscope. Other laboratory tests involve reacting fluorescently-tagged antibodies with a sample of the patient's infected tissue. This type of test may be successful in positively identifying the streptococcal bacteria.

Treatment

Penicillin is the drug of choice for treating erysipelas. It can usually be given by mouth, although in severe cases (or in cases of diagnosed bacteremia) it may be given through a needle placed in a vein (intravenously).

Even with antibiotic treatment, swelling may continue to spread. Other symptoms, such as fever, **pain**, and redness, usually decrease rapidly after penicillin is started. Cold packs and pain relievers may help decrease discomfort. Within about five to 10 days, the affected skin may begin drying up and flaking off.

Prognosis

With prompt treatment, the prognosis from erysipelas is excellent. Delay of treatment, however, increases the chance for bacteremia and the potential for death from overwhelming sepsis. This is particularly true of people with weakened immune systems (babies, the elderly, and people ill with other diseases, especially Acquired **Immunodeficiency** Syndrome, or **AIDS**). Frequently, an individual who has had erysipelas will have it occur again in the same location.

Prevention

Prevention involves appropriate and complete treatment of **streptococcal infections**, including strep throat and wound infections.

Resources

PERIODICALS

De Godoy, Jose Maria Pereira, et al. "Epidemiological data and comorbidities of 428 patients hospitalized with erysipelas." *Angiology* (July 2010): 492–494.

Rosalyn Carson-DeWitt, MD

Erythema infectiosum *see* **Fifth disease**

Erythema multiforme

Definition

Erythema multiforme is a skin disease that causes lesions and redness around the lesions.

KEY TERMS

Herpes virus—Viruses that can infect the skin, mucous membranes, and brain, and they are responsible for such diseases as herpes simplex, chicken pox, and shingles.

Mycoplasma pneumonia—An incomplete bacterium that infects the lung.

Description

Erythema multiforme appears on the skin and the mucous membranes (the lining of the mouth, digestive tract, vagina, and other organs). Large, symmetrical red blotches appear all over the skin in a circular pattern. On mucous membranes, it begins as blisters and progresses to ulcers. A more advanced form, called Stevens-Johnson syndrome, can be severe and even fatal.

Causes and symptoms

Erythema multiforme has many causes, most commonly are drugs. Penicillin, **sulfonamides**, certain **epilepsy** drugs, **aspirin**, and **acetaminophen** are the most likely medication-induced causes. Erythema multiforme can also be caused by certain diseases. Herpes virus and mycoplasma **pneumonia** are likely infectious causes.

Diagnosis

The appearance of the rash is sufficiently unique to identify it on sight. Having identified it, the physician will determine the underlying cause.

Treatment

Erythema multiforme is inadvertently treated when the causative agent, whether it be a drug or a disease, is treated. In severe cases, cortisone-like medication is often used along with general supportive measures and prevention of infection.

Prognosis

As a rule, the rash abates by itself without damaging the skin. Only in the case of infection, severe blistering, or continued use of an offending drug does complications occur.

Resources

BOOKS

Fauci, Anthony S., et al., eds. *Harrison's Principles of Internal Medicine*. 17th ed. New York: McGraw-Hill Professional, 2008.

J. Ricker Polsdorfer, MD

Erythema nodosum

Definition

Erythema nodosum is a skin disorder characterized by painful red nodules appearing mostly on the shins.

Description

Erythema nodosum is an eruption of tender red lumps on both shins and occasionally the arms and face. Bruising often accompanies the nodule formation. Erythema nodosum is most prevalent in young adults.

Causes and symptoms

Erythema nodosum can be caused by many important and treatable diseases. Among them are **tuberculosis**, several fungal lung infections, **leprosy**, inflammatory bowel disease, and some potentially dangerous bacterial infections. Drugs can also induce erythema nodosum. The most common are penicillin, **sulfonamides**, and birth control pills.

Diagnosis

There are a few other skin eruptions that mimic erythema nodosum, so the physician may have to perform a biopsy to sort them out. There are a few types of *panniculitis,* fat inflammation, that may signal a **cancer** somewhere in the body, and there are other kinds of inflammation that may confuse the diagnosis.

Once the skin problem has been diagnosed, its underlying cause must then be identified. A lengthy evaluation may ensue, and often times the cause remains unknown.

Treatment

Painful nodules can be treated with mild **pain** killers and local application of ice packs. Medical attention will be directed toward the underlying disease.

The nodules will eventually disappear, leaving no trace behind.

Resources

BOOKS

Cecil, Russell L., Lee Goldman, and D. A. Audiello.*Cecil Medicine*. 23rd ed, Philadelphia: Saunders Elsevier, 2008.

J. Ricker Polsdorfer, MD

Erythremia *see* **Polycythemia vera**

Erythroblastosis fetalis

Definition

Erythroblastosis fetalis refers to two potentially disabling or fatal blood disorders in infants: Rh incompatibility disease and ABO incompatibility disease. Either disease may be apparent before birth and can cause fetal **death** in some cases. The disorder is caused by incompatibility between a mother's blood and her unborn baby's blood. Because of the incompatibility, the mother's immune system may launch an immune response against the baby's red blood cells. As a result, the baby's blood cells are destroyed, and the baby may suffer severe anemia (deficiency in red blood cells), brain damage, or death.

Description

Red blood cells carry several types of proteins, called antigens, on their surfaces. The A, B, and O antigens are used to classify a person's blood as type A, B, AB, or O. Each parent passes one A, B, or O antigen gene to their child. How the genes are paired determines the person's blood type.

A person who inherits an A antigen gene from each parent has type A blood; receiving two B antigen genes corresponds with type B blood; and inheriting A and B antigen genes means a person has type AB blood. If the O antigen gene is inherited from both parents, the child has type O blood; however, the pairing of A and O antigen genes corresponds with type A blood; and if the B antigen gene is matched with the O antigen gene, the person has type B blood.

Another red blood cell antigen, called the Rh factor, also plays a role in describing a person's blood type. A person with at least one copy of the gene for the Rh factor has Rh-positive blood; if no copies are inherited, the person's blood type is Rh-negative. In **blood typing**, the presence of A, B, and O antigens, plus the presence or absence of the Rh-factor, determine a person's specific blood type, such as A-positive, B-negative, and so on.

A person's blood type has no effect on health. However, an individual's immune system considers only that person's specific blood type, or a close match, acceptable. If a radically different blood type is introduced into the bloodstream, the immune system produces antibodies, proteins that specifically attack and destroy any cell carrying the foreign antigen.

Determining a person's blood type is very important if she becomes pregnant. Blood cells from the unborn baby (fetal red blood cells) can cross over into the mother's bloodstream, especially at delivery. If the mother and her baby have compatible blood types, the crossover does not present any danger. However, if the blood types are incompatible, the mother's immune system manufactures antibodies against the baby's blood.

Usually, this incompatibility is not a factor in a first **pregnancy**, because few fetal blood cells reach the mother's bloodstream until delivery. The antibodies that form after delivery cannot affect the first child. In later pregnancies, fetuses and babies may be in grave danger. The danger arises from the possibility that the mother's antibodies will attack the fetal red blood cells. If this happens, the fetus or baby can suffer severe health effects and may die.

There are two types of incompatibility diseases: Rh incompatibility disease and ABO incompatibility disease. Both diseases have similar symptoms, but Rh disease is much more severe, because anti-Rh antibodies cross over the placenta more readily than anti-A or anti-B antibodies. (The immune system does not form antibodies against the O antigen.) Therefore, a greater percentage of the baby's blood cells are destroyed by Rh disease.

Both incompatibility diseases are uncommon in the United States due to medical advances over the last 50 years. For example, prior to 1946 (when newborn blood transfusions were introduced) 20,000 babies were affected by Rh disease yearly. Further advances, such as suppressing the mother's antibody response, have reduced the incidence of Rh disease to approximately 4,000 cases per year.

Rh disease only occurs if a mother is Rh-negative and her baby is Rh-positive. For this situation to occur, the baby must inherit the Rh factor gene from the father. Most people are Rh-positive. Only 15% of the Caucasian population is Rh-negative, compared to 5–7% of the African-American population and virtually none of Asian populations.

ABO incompatibility disease is almost always limited to babies with A or B antigens whose mothers have type O blood. Approximately one third of these babies show evidence of the mother's antibodies in their bloodstream, but only a small percentage develop symptoms of ABO incompatibility disease.

Cause and symptoms

Rh disease and ABO incompatibility disease are caused when a mother's immune system produces antibodies against the red blood cells of her unborn child. The antibodies cause the baby's red blood cells to be destroyed and the baby develops anemia. The baby's body tries to compensate for the anemia by releasing immature red blood cells, called erythroblasts, from the bone marrow.

The overproduction of erythroblasts can cause the liver and spleen to become enlarged, potentially causing liver damage or a ruptured spleen. The emphasis on erythroblast production is at the cost of producing other types of blood cells, such as platelets and other factors important for blood clotting. Since the blood lacks clotting factors, excessive bleeding can be a complication.

The destroyed red blood cells release the blood's red pigment (hemoglobin) which degrades into a yellow substance called bilirubin. Bilirubin is normally produced as red blood cells die, but the body is only equipped to handle a certain low level of bilirubin in the bloodstream at one time. Erythroblastosis fetalis overwhelms the removal system, and high levels of bilirubin accumulate, causing hyperbilirubinemia, a condition in which the baby becomes jaundiced. The **jaundice** is apparent from the yellowish tone of the baby's eyes and skin. If hyperbilirubinemia cannot be controlled, the baby develops kernicterus. The term kernicterus means that bilirubin is being deposited in the brain, possibly causing permanent damage.

Other symptoms that may be present include high levels of insulin and low blood sugar, as well as a condition called hydrops fetalis. Hydrops fetalis is characterized by an accumulation of fluids within the

KEY TERMS

Amniocentesis—A procedure in which a needle is inserted through a pregnant woman's abdomen and into her uterus to withdraw a small sample of amniotic fluid. The amniotic fluid can be examined for sign of disease or other problems afflicting the fetus.

Amniotic fluid—The fluid that surrounds a fetus in the uterus.

Anemia—A condition in which there is an abnormally low number of red blood cells in the bloodstream. Major symptoms are paleness, shortness of breath, unusually fast or strong heart beats, and tiredness.

Antibody—A protein molecule produced by the immune system in response to a protein that is not recognized as belonging in the body.

Antigen—A protein that can elicit an immune response in the form of antibody formation. With regard to red blood cells, the major antigens are A, B, O, and the Rh factor.

Bilirubin—A yellow-colored end-product of hemoglobin degradation. It is normally present at very low levels in the bloodstream; at high levels, it produces jaundice.

Cordocentesis—A procedure for delivering a blood transfusion to a fetus. It involves a fine needle being threaded through a pregnant woman's abdomen and into the umbilical cord with the aid of ultrasound imaging.

Hemoglobin—A molecule in red blood cells that transports oxygen and gives the cells their characteristic color.

Hydrops fetalis—A condition in which a fetus or newborn baby accumulates fluids, causing swollen arms and legs and impaired breathing.

Hyperbilirubinemia—A condition in which bilirubin accumulates to abnormally high levels in the bloodstream

Placenta—A protective membrane that surrounds and protects the fetus during pregnancy.

Platelet—A blood factor that is important in forming blood clots.

Rh factor—An antigen that is found on the red blood cells of most people. If it is present, the blood type is referred to as Rh-positive; if absent, the blood type is Rh-negative.

---

baby's body, giving it a swollen appearance. This fluid accumulation inhibits normal breathing, because the lungs cannot expand fully and may contain fluid. If this condition continues for an extended period, it can interfere with lung growth. Hydrops fetalis and anemia can also contribute to heart problems.

Diagnosis

Erythroblastosis fetalis can be predicted before birth by determining the mother's blood type. If she is Rh-negative, the father's blood is tested to determine whether he is Rh-positive. If the father is Rh-positive, the mother's blood will be checked for antibodies against the Rh factor. A test that demonstrates no antibodies is repeated at week 26 or 27 of the pregnancy. If antibodies are present, treatment is begun.

In cases in which incompatibility is not identified before birth, the baby suffers recognizable characteristic symptoms such as anemia, hyperbilirubinemia, and hydrops fetalis. The blood incompatibility is uncovered through blood tests such as the Coombs test, which measures the level of maternal antibodies attached to the baby's red blood cells. Other blood tests reveal anemia, abnormal blood counts, and high levels of bilirubin.

Treatment

When a mother has antibodies against her unborn infant's blood, the pregnancy is watched very carefully. The antibodies are monitored and if levels increase, **amniocentesis**, fetal umbilical cord blood sampling, and ultrasound are used to assess any effects on the baby. Trouble is indicated by high levels of bilirubin in the amniotic fluid or baby's blood, or if the ultrasound reveals hydrops fetalis. If the baby is in danger, and the pregnancy is at least 32–34 weeks along, labor is induced. Under 32 weeks, the baby is given blood transfusions while still in the mother's uterus.

There are two techniques that are used to deliver a blood **transfusion** to a baby before birth. In the first, a needle is inserted through the mother's abdomen and uterus, and into the baby's abdomen. Red blood cells injected into the baby's abdominal cavity are absorbed into its bloodstream. In early pregnancy or if the baby's bilirubin levels are gravely high, cordocentesis is performed. This procedure involves sliding a very fine needle through the mother's abdomen and, guided by ultrasound, into a vein in the umbilical cord to inject red blood cells directly into the baby's bloodstream.

After birth, the severity of the baby's symptoms are assessed. One or more transfusions may be necessary to treat anemia, hyperbilirubinemia, and bleeding. Hyperbilirubinemia is also treated with **phototherapy**, a treatment in which the baby is placed under a special light. This light causes changes in how the bilirubin molecule is shaped, which makes it easier to excrete. The baby may also receive oxygen and intravenous fluids containing electrolytes or drugs to treat other symptoms.

Prognosis

In many cases of blood type incompatibility, the symptoms of erythroblastosis fetalis are prevented with careful monitoring and blood type screening. Treatment of minor symptoms is typically successful and the baby will not suffer long-term problems.

Nevertheless, erythroblastosis is a very serious condition for approximately 4,000 babies annually. In about 15% of cases, the baby is severely affected and dies before birth. Babies who survive pregnancy may develop kernicterus, which can lead to deafness, speech problems, **cerebral palsy**, or **mental retardation**. Extended hydrops fetalis can inhibit lung growth and contribute to **heart failure**. These serious complications are life threatening, but with good medical treatment, the fatality rate is very low. According to the U.S. Centers for Disease Control and Prevention, there were 21 infant deaths in the United States during 1996 that were attributable to hemolytic disease (erythroblastosis fetalis) and jaundice.

Prevention

With any pregnancy, whether it results in a live birth, **miscarriage**, **stillbirth**, or abortion, blood typing is a universal precaution against blood compatibility disease. Blood types cannot be changed, but adequate forewarning allows precautions and treatments that limit the danger to unborn babies.

If an Rh-negative woman gives birth to an Rh-positive baby, she is given an injection of immunoglobulin G, a type of antibody protein, within 72 hours of the birth. The immunoglobulin destroys any fetal blood cells in her bloodstream before her immune system can react to them. In cases where this precaution is not taken, antibodies are created and future pregnancies may be complicated.

Resources

PERIODICALS

Illanes, Sebastian, Peter Soothill. "Noninvasive approach for the management of hemolytic disease of the fetus." *Expert Review of Hematology* (Oct 2009): 577–582.

Julia Barrett

Erythrocyte sedimentation rate

Definition

The erythrocyte sedimentation rate (ESR), or sedimentation rate (sed rate), is a measure of the settling of red blood cells in a tube of blood during a specified period of time. The rate is an indication of inflammation and increases in many diseases.

Purpose

ESR is increased in rheumatoid diseases, most infections, and in **cancer**. An advanced rate does not diagnose a specific disease, but it does indicate that an underlying disease may be present.

A physician can use ESR to monitor a person with an associated disease. When the disease worsens, the ESR may increase; when the disease improves, the ESR may decrease. The ESR does not always follow the course of cancer.

ESR is called an acute-phase reactant test, meaning that it reacts to acute conditions in the body, such as infection or trauma. The rate increase follows a rise in temperature and increase in **white blood cell count**, peaks after several days, and usually lasts longer than the elevated temperature or increased white blood cell count.

Description

The ESR test is a simple test dating back to the ancient Greeks. A specific amount of diluted, unclotted blood is placed in a special narrow tube and left undisturbed for a specified amount of time. The red cells settle towards the bottom of the tube, and the pale yellow liquid (plasma) rises to the top. After the specified time has elapsed, measurements are taken of the distance the red cells traveled to settle at the bottom of the tube. Methods used include the Westergren, the modified Westergren and the Wintrobe methods. Each method produces slightly different results.

KEY TERMS

Acute phase reactant—A substance in the blood that increases as a response to an acute conditions such as infection, injury, tissue destruction, some cancers, burns, surgery, or trauma.

Rouleaux—The stacking up of red blood cells, caused by extra or abnormal proteins in the blood that decrease the normal distance red cells maintain between each other.

Most laboratories use the Westergren or modified Westergren method.

Normally red cells do not settle far toward the bottom of the tube. Many diseases make extra or abnormal proteins that cause the red cells to move close together, stack up, and form a column (rouleaux). In a group, red cells are heavier and fall faster. The faster they fall, the further they settle, and the higher the ESR.

The ESR test is covered by insurance when medically necessary. Results are usually available the same or following day.

Preparation

This test requires about 5mL of blood. A healthcare worker ties a tourniquet on the patient's upper arm, locates a vein in the inner elbow region, and inserts a needle into that vein. Vacuum action draws the blood through the needle into an attached tube. Collection of the sample takes only a few minutes.

Aftercare

Discomfort or bruising may occur at the puncture site. Pressure applied to the puncture site until the bleeding stops reduces bruising. Warm packs to the puncture site relieve discomfort. The patient may feel dizzy or faint.

Risks

There are no major risks associated with this blood test.

Results

A normal value does not rule out disease. Normal values for the Westergren method are:

- Newborns (male or female): 0–2 mm/hr
- Females less than 50 years old: 0–25 mm/hr
- Males less than 50 years old: 0–15 mm/hr
- Females 50 years and older: 0–30 mm/hr
- Males 50 years and older: 0–20 mm/hr

Abnormal results

The highest ESR levels are usually seen in a cancer of a certain type of white blood cell (**multiple myeloma**) and rheumatoid disease, such as **rheumatoid arthritis**. Many other diseases also increase the ESR: infection, **kidney disease**, anemia, diseases involving white blood cells, cancer, and autoimmune and inflammatory diseases.

Any disease that changes the shape and size of red blood cells decreases the ESR. Distorted cells, such as with **sickle cell disease**, do not stack, and consequently do not settle far, even in the presence of an ESR-associated disease. Diseases that cause the body to make less protein or extra red blood cells also decrease the ESR.

Some medications, including anticonvulsants, **oral contraceptives**, and others may cause an increase in the ESR. Drugs such as cortisone and quinine may cause a decrease in ESR values.

Resources

OTHER

"ESR." American Association for Clinical Chemistry. *Lab Tests Online*. May 17, 2010. http://www.labtestsonline.org/understanding/analytes/esr/test.html (accessed October 4, 2010).

Nancy J. Nordenson
Melinda Granger Oberleitner, RN, DNS, APRN, CNS

Erythromycins and macrolide antibiotics

Definition

Macrolides are **antibiotics** that kill bacteria or prevent their growth.

Purpose

Macrolides are used to treat bacterial infections in various sites:

- middle and inner ear
- eyes
- sinuses

- tonsils
- throat and larynx (voice box)
- lungs (pneumonia and bronchitis)
- skin (infected eczema, acne, psoriasis)
- genitalia, sexually transmitted diseases (Chlamydia, gonorrhea)

These antibiotics are used to prevent infections prior to dental and other procedures for patients at risk for developing infections of the heart valves (**endocarditis**).

Macrolide antibiotics can be used as alternatives to penicillin for people with penicillin **allergies**.

These antibiotics will *not* cure colds, flu, and other viral infections.

Description

Members of the macrolide antibiotic family include erythromycin (Erythrocin, Ery-C, E-Mycin, azithromycin (Zithromax) and clarithromycin (Biaxin). They are available by prescription as capsules, tablets (including chewable), liquids, and for injection.

Recommended dosage

Dosage depends on the drug used and the reason for its use.

Antibiotics should always be taken exactly as directed, for as long as they are prescribed. Do not stop antibiotics if symptoms begin improving.

Precautions

These drugs should be used with caution by patients with liver or **kidney disease**.

People who have inherited blood disorders, like porphyria, should not take these antibiotics.

Macrolides increase the risk of heart arrhythmia in patients who have prolonged Q-T interval on EKG.

These antibiotics may aggravate muscle weakness in patients with **Myasthenia Gravis**.

ALLERGIES. Anyone who has had unusual reactions to a macrolide antibiotic previously should avoid taking it again.

PREGNANCY. There are no well controlled studies on these antibiotics and **pregnancy**.

BREASTFEEDING. Macrolide antibiotics pass into breast milk, though no specific dangers have been identified.

KEY TERMS

Bronchitis—Infection of the air passages in the lungs.

Gonorrhea—A sexually transmitted infection with fever and a pussy penile discharge in males and abdominal pain and vaginal discharge in females.

Bacteria—Organisms that can only be seen under a microscope.

Pneumonia—Infection of the lungs caused by bacteria, viruses, or chemical irritants.

Sinus—Air-filled cavities in the bones of the skull.

Side effects

Macrolide antibiotics may widen the Q-T interval on EKG. People who are at risk for developing severe heart **arrhythmias**, or who take drugs that widen the Q-T interval, should avoid taking these antibiotics.

The more common side effects from macrolides include mild **diarrhea**, **nausea**, **vomiting**, and stomach or abdominal cramps that go away as the body adjusts to the drug.

Less commonly, sore mouth or tongue and vaginal **itching** may occur. These rarely require medical attention.

If these, more serious, side effects occur, seek medical help:

- severe abdominal pain, and continued nausea, vomiting, or diarrhea
- fever
- skin rash, redness, or itching
- unusual tiredness or weakness
- swelling of the lips, face or neck

Interactions

Prescribers need to know the medications their patients take; this class of antibiotics may interact with many drugs.

Food may change the effects of erythromycin and clarithromycin (Biaxin), increasing the risks of side or adverse effects.

Grapefruit juice may increase the absorption of macrolide antibiotics, possibly increasing the possibility of adverse or side effects.

St Johns Wort may decrease blood levels of erythromycin.

The effectiveness of combined **oral contraceptives** may be reduced when macrolide antibiotics are taken. It would be wise to use an additional method of preventing pregnancy for up to seven days after discontinuing these antibiotics.

Taking quinolone antibiotics (Tequin, Levaquin, Avelox) with erythromycin increases the potential for fatal heart arrhythmias.

Macrolide antibiotics increase the risk of fatal heart arrhythmias when taken with medications to treat heart arrhythmias, (Cordarone, Norpace, Tikosyn, Sotalol, Bretylium, and Quinidine).

Macrolide antibiotics increase the blood-thinning effects of warfarin (Coumadin).

Macrolide antibiotics increase the adverse, muscle wasting effects of cholesterol-reducing medications (Lipitor, Zocor, Mevacor).

People who take **digoxin** (Lanoxin) and macrolide antibiotics together risk developing digoxin toxicity.

People who take carbamazepine (Tegretol) for seizures, **schizophrenia**, ethanol withdrawal, restless-leg syndrome, or **post-traumatic stress disorder** (PTSD) risk developing carbamazepine toxicity when they take macrolide antibiotics.

Macrolide antibiotics increase the effects of Colchicine used to treat **Gout**, increasing the risk of toxicity.

Macrolide antibiotics increase the effects, and toxicity, of ergot drugs used to treat migraine headaches.

Macrolide antibiotics increase the effects, and toxicity, of pimozide (Orap) and clozapine (Clozaril) used to treat **psychosis**.

Macrolide antibiotics increase the effects, and toxicity, of verapamil (Calan) used to treat **angina** (heart **pain**) and rapid heartbeats.

Macrolide antibiotics increase the sedative effects of anti-anxiety medications Buspar and **benzodiazepines** Xanax, Valium, and Halcion.

Taken together, macrolide antibiotics and theophyllines (Choledyl, Theo-Dur and Uniphyl), used to treat chronic **asthma** and asthma-like conditions, adversely effect each other. Theophyllin levels increase in the blood, increasing the chance of toxicity, and macrolide effectiveness is reduced.

Resources

OTHER

"Antibiotics, macrolide." *NHS Choices*. Nation Health Service (NHS). http://www.nhs.uk.

James Waun, MD, RPh

Erythropoietin *see* **Cancer therapy, supportive; Immunologic therapies**

Erythropoietin test

Definition

Erythropoietin, also called EPO, is a type of protein called a glycoprotein that is formed mainly in the kidneys to stimulate the production of red blood cells.

Purpose

The erythropoietin (EPO) test is used to determine if hormonal secretion is causing changes in the red blood cells. The test has great value in evaluating low hemoglobin (anemia), and another disorder called polycythemia, in which unusually large numbers of red blood cells are found in the blood. The EPO test is also used to identify kidney tumors and identify or assess **kidney disease** It also may be used to evaluate **abuse** by athletes who believe commercially prepared erythropoietin enhances performance.

Precautions

Not every laboratory is equipped to evaluate EPO, so the reference laboratory (a large commercial lab that does tests for hospitals not equipped to do them) performing the test may require as many as four days to complete the analysis. It should also be noted that EPO values increase in **pregnancy**, in which significantly higher levels are found before the twenty-fourth week.

Description

Erythropoietin is produced primarily in the kidneys but interacts with other factors in the bone marrow to increase red cell production. EPO is unique among the blood cell growth factors, because it is the only one that behaves like a hormone.

Erythropoietin acts as the principal regulator in the production of red blood cells (erythrocytes) by controlling the number, the kinds, and the survival of the cells.

KEY TERMS

Anemia—A condition in which the hemoglobin concentration in the blood is below normal.

Polycythemia vera—A condition characterized by an unusually large number of red blood cells in the blood due to increased production by the bone marrow. Symptoms include headaches, blurred vision, high blood pressure, dizziness, and night sweats.

Secondary polycythemia—Secondary polycythemia occurs when the excess of red blood cells is caused by a condition other than polycythemia vera. For example, when low levels of oxygen in the blood stimulate the bone marrow to produce more red blood cells, as in chronic lung disease.

Because of this ability, it is being investigated for use in **cancer** patients to prevent anemia (hemoglobin concentration in the blood is lower than normal), or to treat anemia that has been induced by **chemotherapy** and **bone marrow transplantation** (BMT).

The correction of anemia can result in reduced **transfusion** requirements, so the erythropoietin test is used to diagnose anemia, including the anemia of end-stage renal disease. Erythropoietin determination is also valuable in diagnosing a condition known as polycythemia, when increased numbers of red blood cells occur. Levels of erythropoietin are extremely low in **polycythemia vera** but are normal or high in **secondary polycythemia**. It happens rarely, but cysts in the liver or kidneys, as well as tumors in the kidneys or brain, can also produce erythropoietin. Patients with these conditions can have high levels of erythropoietin and may develop secondary polycythemia.

Kidney disease can cause anemia and many patients on **kidney dialysis** will require monthly EPO tests to check their hemoglobin levels.

Some athletes use EPO to enhance performance, as the increased red cell volume adds more oxygen-carrying capacity to the blood. Adverse reactions to this practice can include clotting abnormalities, **headache**, seizures, high blood pressure, **nausea**, **vomiting**, **diarrhea**, and rash.

Preparation

The EPO test requires a blood sample. The patient is to fast with nothing to eat or drink for at least eight hours before the test. It is also suggested that the patient lie down for 30 minutes before the test.

Risks

Risks for this test are minimal, but may include slight bleeding from the blood-drawing site, **fainting** or feeling lightheaded after venipuncture, and hematoma (blood accumulating under the puncture site).

Normal results

Reference values vary from laboratory to laboratory, but a general normal range is 11–48 mU/mL (milliunits per milliliter).

Abnormal results

Low levels of EPO are found in anemic patients with inadequate or absent production of erythropoietin. Severe kidney disease may decrease production of EPO, and congenital absence of EPO can occur.

Elevated levels of EPO can be found in some **anemias** when the body tries to overcompensate for reduced blood volume. Elevated levels are also seen in polycythemia, and erythropoietin-secreting tumors.

Resources

PERIODICALS

"GP Clinical: Anemia in Kidney Disease." *GP* November 5, 2004: 66.

Janis O. Flores
Teresa G. Odle

ESB *see* **Electrical stimulation of the brain**

Escherichia coli

Definition

Escherichia coli (*E. coli*) is one of several types of bacteria that normally inhabit the intestine of humans and animals (commensal organism). Some strains of *E. coli* are capable of causing disease under certain conditions when the immune system is compromised or disease may result from an environmental exposure to the organism.

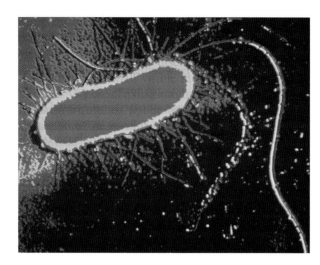

A magnified image of the E. coli bacterium. *(© Howard Sochurek/Corbis.)*

Demographics

Neonatal **meningitis** caused by *E. coli* is associated with a mortality rate of 8%. The organism is the leading cause of urinary tract infections in men and in women. The bacterium also causes approximately 30 to 45% of traveler's **diarrhea** in people traveling to Mexico.

Description

E. coli bacteria may give rise to infections in **wounds**, the urinary tract, biliary tract, and abdominal cavity (**peritonitis**). This organism may cause septicemia, neonatal meningitis, infantile **gastroenteritis**, tourist diarrhea, and hemorrhagic diarrhea. An *E. coli* infection may also arise due to environmental exposure. Infections with this type of bacteria pose a serious threat to public health with outbreaks arising from food and water that has been contaminated with human or animal feces or sewage. This type of bacteria has been used as a biological indicator for safety of drinking water since the 1890s. Exposure may occur during hospitalization, resulting in **pneumonia** in immunocompromised patients or those on a ventilator.

Causes and symptoms

The symptoms of infection and resulting complications are dependent upon the strain of *E. coli* and the site of infection. These bacteria produce toxins that have a wide range of effects. Symptoms caused by some *E. coli* infections range from mild to severe, bloody diarrhea, acute abdominal **pain, vomiting**, and **fever**. Gastrointestinal complications that can cause *E. coli* infections include **irritable bowel syndrome** (IBS), ischemic **colitis**,

appendicitis, perforation of the large bowel, and in some instances **gangrene** in the colon. Other known *E. coli*-causing infections include chronic renal failure, **pancreatitis**, and **diabetes mellitus**. Neurological symptoms such as drowsiness, seizure, and **coma** may occur. In infants, *E. coli* infections are present in cases of infantile gastroenteritis and neonatal meningitis.

Strains of *E. coli* that produce diarrhea were initially distinguished by their O (somatic) antigens found on the bacterial surface. Although there is an overlap in characteristics between strains, they may be classified into four main groups; enterohemorrahagic (0157), enteropathogenic (055,0111), enterotoxigenic (06,078), and enteroinvasive (0124,0164).

E.coli O157 (VTEC)

The O157:H7 strain is the member of the group most often associated with a particularly severe form of diarrhea. (The O indicates the somatic antigen, while the H denotes the flagellar antigen, both of which are found on the cell surface of the bacteria.) The bacterium was discovered in 1977, and first reports of infections followed in 1982. *E. coli* O157:H7, as it is frequently referred to by researchers, causes bloody diarrhea in many infected patients. It accounts for about 2% of all cases of diarrhea in the western world, and at least one-third of cases of hemorrhagic colitis, or about 20,000 cases per year.

E. coli O157:H7 is also the most common cause of unique syndromes, known as **hemolytic-uremic syndrome** (HUS) and thrombocytopenic purpura (TTP), which cause kidney failure, **hemolytic anemia**, and **thrombocytopenia**. Infection with this strain of bacteria often subsides without further complications. However, about 5% of people who are infected develop HUS/TTP. This infection also accounts for the majority of episodes of HUS, especially in children.

This strain of bacteria produces a potent toxin called verotoxin, named for the toxin's ability to kill green monkey kidney or "vero" cells. Bacteria that produce verotoxin are referred to as verotoxin-producing *E. coli* (VTEC). The numbers of bacteria that are necessary to reproduce infectious levels of bacteria are quite small, estimated at 10-100 viable bacteria. These toxins are lethal for intestinal cells and those that line vessels (endothelial cells), inhibiting protein synthesis and causing cell **death**. It is believed that the damage to blood vessels results in the formation of clots, which eventually leads to HUS. HUS/TTP is a serious, often fatal, syndrome that has other causes in addition to *E. coli* O157:H7; it is characterized by the breaking up of red blood cells (hemolysis) and kidney failure (uremia). The syndrome occurs most often in the very young and very old.

KEY TERMS

Antigen—A substance, usually a protein, that causes the formation of an antibody and reacts specifically with that antibody.

Anti-motility medications—Medications such as loperamide (Imodium), dephenoxylate (Lomotil), or medications containing Codeine or narcotics that decrease the ability of the intestine to contract. This can worsen the condition of a patient with dysentery or colitis.

Colitis—Inflammation of the colon or large intestine, usually causing diarrhea that may be bloody.

Food irradiation methods—A process using radiant energy to kill microorganisms in food, to extend the amount of time in which food can be sold and eaten safely.

Oral Rehydration Solution (ORS)—A liquid preparation developed by the World Health Organization that can decrease fluid loss in persons with diarrhea. Originally developed to be prepared with materials available in the home, commercial preparations have recently come into use.

Urea—Chemical formed during the body's metabolism of nitrogen and normally excreted by the kidney. Urea levels rise in the blood when kidney failure occurs.

E. coli O157:H7 is commonly found in cattle and poultry, and outbreaks of disease have been associated with cattle and bovine products. There are reports of contamination from unpasteurized apple juice, hamburger meat, radish sprouts, lettuce, and potatoes, as well as other food sources. Environmental contamination may occur in water drained from cattle pastures or water containing human sewage used for drinking or swimming. Human to human transmission, through contact with fecal matter, has also been identified in daycare centers.

After an incubation period of three to four days on average, watery diarrhea begins, which rapidly progresses to bloody diarrhea in many cases. **Nausea, vomiting**, and low-grade fever are frequently present. Gastrointestinal symptoms last about one week, and recovery is often spontaneous. Symptomatic infection may occur in about 10% of infected individuals. About 5-10% of individuals, usually at the extremes of age develop HUS/TTP, and ultimately, kidney failure. Patients taking **antibiotics** or medications for gastric acidity may also be at risk. Neurological symptoms can occur as part of HUS/TTP and consist of seizures, **paralysis**, and coma. **Rectal prolapse** may be a complication, and in some cases colitis, appendicitis, perforation of the large bowel, and gangrene in the bowel. Systemically, the most prevalent complications of *E. coli* 157 infections are HUS and TTP.

E. coli non-O157 (VTEC)

These strains of *E. coli* produce verotoxin, but are strains other than O157. There have been as many as 100 different types implicated in the development of disease. Strain OH111 was found to be involved in outbreaks in Australia, Japan, and Italy. The O128, O103, and O55 groups have also been implicated in diarrhea outbreaks. In Britain, cases of infantile gastroenteritis in maternity hospitals and neonatal units have been attributed to the *E. coli*) non-0157 group. Many of these organisms have been identified in cattle.

Enterotoxigenic E. coli

Two toxins may be produced by this group, the heat-labile enterotoxin (LT) that can produce enteritis in infants, and a heat stable enterotoxin (ST), the action of which has yet to be determined.

Enteroinvasive E. coli

Some strains of the enteroinvasive *E. coli* have been involved in the development of gastroenteritis in infants. These organisms do not produce an enterotoxin. The cells of the intestine are affected, with the development of symptoms that are typical of a shigellae infection.

Diagnosis

Diagnosis of a specific type of infection is dependent upon the characteristics of the particular strain of the organism.

E. coli O157:H7 (HUS)

This particular strain of *E. coli* is suspected when bloody diarrhea, bloody stools, lack of fever, elevated leukocyte count, and abdominal tenderness are present. Stool cultures are used to tentatively identify the bacteria. Unfortunately, cultures are often negative or inconclusive if done after 48 hours of symptoms. Further tests are usually needed for confirmation of infection. This may include a full blood count, blood film, and tests to determine urea, electrolyte, and LDH (lactate dehydrogenase) levels. Damaged red blood cells and elevated levels of creatinine, urea, and LDH with a drop in **platelet count** may indicate that HUS will develop. Immunomagnetic separation is used for diagnosis as well.

E. coli non-O157 (VTEC)

Diagnosis is often difficult for these types of bacteria, but production of enterohemolysin (Ehly) is used as an indicator. Other diagnostic tests are used to detect verotoxins, including ELISA (enzyme-linked immunosorbent assays), colony immunoblotting, and DNA-based tests.

E. coli 0157 STEC

Methods for detection of this type of bacteria are under development, including culture growth media selective for this organism. Immunomagnetic separation and specific ELISA, latex agglutination tests, colony immunoblot assays, and other immunological-based detection methods are being explored.

Treatment

Traditional

Uncomplicated cases of the *E. coli* O157:H7 infection clear up within ten days. It is not certain that antibiotics are helpful in treating *E. coli* O157:H7. Antimicrobials that may be administered include doxycycline (Vibramycin), trimethoprim/sulfamethoxazole (Bactrim DS, Septra), **fluoroquinolones** (Cipro), and rifaximin (Xifaxan, RedActiv, Flonorm). **Dehydration** resulting from diarrhea must be treated with either Oral Rehydration Solution (ORS) or intravenous fluids. Anti-motility agents that decrease the intestines' ability to contract, should not be used in any patient with bloody diarrhea. Treatment of HUS, if it develops, involves correction of clotting factors, plasma exchange, and **kidney dialysis**. Blood transfusions may be required. Treatment methods for other *E. coli* infections are similar.

Drugs

Antibiotics are often used in the treatment of *E. coli* infections, but their role is controversial. Some antibiotics may enhance the development of HUS/TTP depending upon their action, as well as the use of anti-diarrhea medications that should be avoided. Treatment with third-generation cephalosporin antibiotics such as ceftriaxone (Rocephin) is indicated for neonatal meningitis.

Antibiotic therapy may be complicated by the presence of antibiotic resistant organisms. These organisms appear to be increasing since the late 1990s and are resistant to the **penicillins** and **cephalosporins** as well as to the fluoroquinolones and gentamicin, which in the past, were reserved to treat only the most serious of infections.

Prognosis

In most cases of O157:H7, symptoms last for about a week and recovery is often spontaneous. Ten percent of individuals with *E. coli* O157:H7 infection develop HUS; 5% of those die of the disease. Some who recover from HUS are left with some degree of kidney damage and possibly irritable bowel syndrome. Additionally, there is a possibility of chronic *E. coli* infection.

Infants that develop *E. coli* infections may be permanently affected. Gastroenteritis may leave the child with **lactose intolerance**. Neonates developing meningitis from *E. coli* strains have a high morbidity and mortality rate. Some of these neonates may develop neurological and developmental dysfunction.

Prevention

Thorough cooking of all meat and poultry products and adhering to proper food preparation is the most effective way to avoid infection. More studies are needed to determine the appropriate safety margins for killing these bacteria. Food irradiation methods are also being developed to sanitize food. The enforcement of regulations for meat production and water are critical. Steam pasteurization is used in the United States and is being explored in other countries. Vaccinations to *E. coli* 0157 are under development, as are medications aimed at limiting the effects of the verotoxin.

Prevention of *E. coli* gastroenteritis in infants is best achieved by **breastfeeding**. Breast milk contains antibodies that combat the infection. For bottle-fed infants, care should be taken in the preparation of the milk and bottles. Good hygiene of the umbilical cord area is important. Keeping this area clean and dry may reduce infection.

Resources

PERIODICALS

Harrington, S.M., E.G. Dudley, and J.P Nataro. "Pathogenesis of Enteroaggregative Escherichia Coli Infection." *FEMS Microbiology Letters* 254, no. 1 (January 2006): 12–8.

OTHER

Centers for Disease Control and Prevention. "*E. coli.*" March 16, 2010. http://www.cdc.gov/ecoli (accessed October 4, 2010).

Madappa, Tarun, and Chi Hiong U Go. "Escherichia Coli Infections." *eMedicine*. September 10, 2010. http://emedicine.medscape.com/article/217485-overview (accessed October 4, 2010).

Jill Granger, MS
David Kaminstein, MD
Melinda Granger Oberleitner,
RN, DNS, APRN, CNS

Esophageal acidity test *see* **Esophageal function tests**

Esophageal aperistalsis *see* **Achalasia**

Esophageal atresia

Definition

Esophageal atresia is a serious birth defect in which the esophagus, the long tube that connects the mouth to the stomach, is segmented and closed off at any point. This condition usually occurs with **tracheoesophageal fistula**, a condition in which the esophagus is improperly attached to the trachea, the nearby tube that connects the nasal area to the lungs. Esophageal atresia occurs in approximately 1 in 4,000 live births.

Description

Failure of an unborn child (fetus) to develop properly results in **birth defects**. Many of these defects involve organs that do not function, or function only incidentally, before birth, and, as a result, go undetected until the baby is born. In this case, the digestive tract is unnecessary for fetal growth, since all **nutrition** comes from the mother through the placenta and umbilical cord.

During fetal development, the esophagus and the trachea arise from the same original tissue. Normally, the two tubes would form separately (differentiate); however, in cases of esophageal atresia and tracheoesophageal fistulas, they do not, resulting in various malformed configurations. The most common configuration is the "C" type, in which the upper part of the esophagus abruptly ends in a blind pouch, while the lower part attaches itself to the trachea. This configuration occurs in 85–90% of cases. Esophageal atresia without involvement of the trachea occurs in only 8% of cases.

Causes and symptoms

The cause of esophageal atresia, like that of most birth defects, is unknown.

An infant born with this defect will at first appear all right, swallowing normally. However, the blind pouch will begin to fill with mucus and saliva that would normally pass through the esophagus to the stomach. These secretions back up into the mouth and nasal area, causing the baby to drool excessively. When fed, the baby will also immediately regurgitate what he or she has eaten. **Choking** and coughing may also occur as the baby breaths in the fluid backing up from the esophagus. Aspiration **pneumonia**, an infection of the respiratory system caused by inhalation of the contents of the digestive tract, may also develop.

Diagnosis

Physicians who suspect esophageal atresia after being presented with the above symptoms diagnose the condition using x-ray imaging or by passing a catheter through the nose and into the esophagus. Esophageal atresia is indicated if the catheter hits an obstruction 4–5 in (10–13 cm) from the nostrils.

Treatment

Infants with esophageal atresia are unlikely to survive without surgery to reconnect the esophagus. The procedure is done as soon as possible; however, **prematurity**, the presence of other birth defects, or complications of apiration pneumonia may delay surgery. Once diagnosed, the baby will be fed intravenously until he or she has recovered sufficiently from the operation. Mucus and saliva will also be continuously removed via a catheter until recovery has occured. When surgery is performed, the esophagus is reconnected and, if neccessary, separated from the trachea. If the two ends of the esophagus are too far apart to be reattached, tissue from the large intestine is used to join them.

Prognosis

Surgery to correct esophageal atresia is usually successful. Post-operative complications may include difficulty swallowing, since the esophagus may not contract efficiently, and gastrointestinal reflux, in which the acidic contents of stomach back up into the lower part of the esophagus, possibly causing ulcers.

Resources

BOOKS

Sleisenger, Marvin H., et al.*Sleisenger & Fordtran's Gastrointestinal and Liver Disease: Pathophysiology, Diagnosis, Management.* St. Louis, Mo.: MD Consult, 2009.

J. Ricker Polsdorfer, MD

Esophageal cancer

Definition

Esophageal **cancer** is a malignancy that develops in tissues of the hollow, muscular canal (esophagus) along which food and liquid travel from the throat to the stomach.

Description

Esophageal cancer usually originates in the inner layers of the lining of the esophagus and grows outward. In time, the tumor can obstruct the passage of food and liquid, making swallowing painful and difficult. Since most patients are not diagnosed until the late stages of the disease, esophageal cancer is associated with poor quality of life and low survival rates.

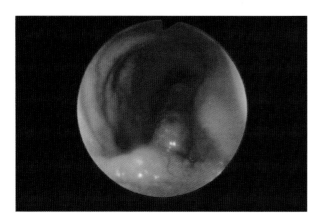

A close-up view of a cancerous esophageal tumor. *(Custom Medical Stock Photo, Inc. Reproduced by permission.)*

Squamous cell carcinoma is the most common type of esophageal cancer, accounting for 95% of all esophageal cancers worldwide. The esophagus is normally lined with thin, flat squamous cells that resemble tiny roof **shingles**. Squamous cell carcinoma can develop at any point along the esophagus but is most common in the middle portion.

Adenocarcinoma has surpassed squamous cell carcinoma as the most common type of esophageal cancer in the United States. Adenocarcinoma originates in glandular tissue not normally present in the lining of the esophagus. Before adenocarcinoma can develop, glandular cells must replace a section of squamous cells. This occurs in Barrett's esophagus, a precancerous condition in which chronic acid reflux from the stomach stimulates a transformation in cell type in the lower portion of the esophagus.

A very small fraction of esophageal cancers are melanomas, **sarcomas**, or lymphomas.

There is great variability in the incidence of esophageal cancer with regard to geography, ethnicity, and gender. The overall incidence is increasing. About 13,000 new cases of esophageal cancer are diagnosed in the United States each year. During the same 12-month period, 12,000 people die of this disease. It strikes between five and ten North Americans per 100,000. In some areas of China the cancer is endemic.

Squamous cell carcinoma usually occurs in the sixth or seventh decade of life, with a greater incidence in African-Americans than in others. Adenocarcinoma develops earlier and is much more common in white patients. In general, esophageal cancer occurs more frequently in men than in women.

Causes and symptoms

The exact cause of esophageal cancer is unknown, although many investigators believe that chronic irritation of the esophagus is a major culprit. Most of the identified risk factors represent a form of chronic irritation. However, the wide variance in the distribution of esophageal cancer among different demographic groups raises the possibility that genetic factors also play a role.

Several risk factors are associated with esophageal cancer.

- Tobacco and alcohol consumption are the major risk factors, especially for squamous cell carcinoma. Smoking and alcohol abuse each increase the risk of squamous cell carcinoma by five-fold. The effects of the two are synergistic, in that the combination of smoking and alchohol increases the risk by 25- to

100- fold. It is estimated that drinking about 13 ounces of alcohol every day for an extended period of time raises the risk of developing esophageal cancer by 18%. That likelihood increases to 44% in individuals who also smoke one or two packs of cigarettes a day. Smokeless tobacco also increases the risk for esophageal cancer.

- Gastroesophageal reflux is a condition in which acid from the stomach refluxes backwards into the lower portion of the esophagus, sometimes causing symptoms of heartburn. In some cases of gastroesophageal reflux, the chronic exposure to acid causes the inner lining of the lower esophagus to change from squamous cells to glandular cells. This is called Barrett's esophagus. Patients with Barrett's esophagus are roughly 30 to 40 times more likely than the general population to develop adenocarcinoma of the esophagus.
- A diet low in fruits, vegetables, zinc, riboflavin, and other vitamins can increase risk of developing to esophageal cancer.
- Caustic injury to the esophagus inflicted by swallowing lye or other substances that damage esophageal cells can lead to the development of squamous cell esophageal cancer in later life.
- Achalasia is a condition in which the lower esophageal sphincter (muscle) cannot relax enough to let food pass into the stomach. Squamous cell esophageal cancer develops in about 6% of patients with achalasia.
- Tylosis is a rare inherited disease characterized by excess skin on the palms and soles. Affected patients have a much higher probability of developing esophageal cancer than the general population. They should have regular screenings to detect the disease in its early, most curable stages.
- Esophageal webs, which are protrusions of tissue into the esophagus, and diverticula, which are outpouchings of the wall of the esophagus, are associated with a higher incidence of esophageal cancer.

Symptoms

Unfortunately, symptoms generally don't appear until the tumor has grown so large that the patient cannot be cured. Dysphagia (trouble swallowing or a sensation of having food stuck in the throat or chest) is the most common symptom. Swallowing problems may occur occasionally at first, and patients often react by eating more slowly and chewing their food more carefully and, as the tumor grows, switching to soft foods or a liquid diet. Without treatment, the tumor will eventually prevent even liquid from passing into the stomach. A sensation of burning or slight mid-chest pressure is a rare, often-disregarded symptom of esophageal cancer. Painful swallowing is usually a symptom of a large tumor obstructing the opening of the esophagus. It can lead to regurgitation of food, weight loss, physical wasting, and **malnutrition**. Anyone who has trouble swallowing, loses a significant amount of weight without dieting, or cannot eat solid food because it is too painful to swallow should see a doctor.

Diagnosis

A barium swallow is usually the first test performed on a patient whose symptoms suggest esophageal cancer. After the patient swallows a small amount of barium, a series of x rays can highlight any bumps or flat raised areas on the normally smooth surface of the esophageal wall. It can also detect large, irregular areas that narrow the esophagus in patients with advanced cancer, but it cannot provide information about disease that has spread beyond the esophagus. A double contrast study is a barium swallow with air blown into the esophagus to improve the way the barium coats the esophageal lining. **Endoscopy** is a diagnostic procedure in which a thin lighted tube (endoscope) is passed through the mouth, down the throat, and into the esophagus. Cells that appear abnormal are removed for biopsy. Once a diagnosis of esophageal cancer has been confirmed through biopsy, staging tests are performed to determine whether the disease has spread (metastasized) to tissues or organs near the original tumor or in other parts of the body. These tests may include computed tomography, endoscopic ultrasound, **thoracoscopy**, **laparoscopy**, and **positron emission tomography**.

Treatment

Treatment for esophageal cancer is determined by the stage of the disease and the patient's general health. The most important distinction to make is whether the cancer is curable. If the cancer is in the early stages, cure may be possible. If the cancer is advanced or if the patient will not tolerate major surgery, treatment is usually directed at palliation (relief of symptoms only) instead of cure.

Staging

Stage 0 is the earliest stage of the disease. Cancer cells are confined to the innermost lining of the esophagus. Stage I esophageal cancer has spread slightly deeper, but still has not extended to nearby tissues, lymph nodes, or other organs. In Stage IIA, cancer has invaded the thick, muscular layer of the esophagus

KEY TERMS

Computed tomography—A radiology test by which images of cross-sectional planes of the body are obtained.

Endoscopic ultrasound—A radiology test utilizing high frequency sound waves, conducted via an endoscope.

Laparoscopy—Examination of the contents of the abdomen through a thin, lighted tube passed through a small incision.

Positron emission tomography—A radiology test by which images of cross-sectional planes of the body are obtained, utilizing the properties of the positron. The positron is a subatomic particle of equal mass to the electron, but of opposite charge.

Synergistic—The combined action of two or more processes is greater than the sum of each acting separately.

Thoracoscopy—Examination of the contents of the chest through a thin, lighted tube passed through a small incision.

that propels food into the stomach and may involve connective tissue covering the outside of the esophagus. In Stage IIB, cancer has spread to lymph nodes near the esophagus and may have invaded deeper layers of esophageal tissue. Stage III esophageal cancer has spread to tissues or lymph nodes near the esophagus or to the trachea (windpipe) or other organs near the esophagus. Stage IV cancer has spread to distant organs like the liver, bones, and brain. Recurrent esophageal cancer is disease that develops in the esophagus or another part of the body after initial treatment.

Surgery

The most common operations for the treatment of esophageal cancer are esophagectomy and esophagogastrectomy. Esophagectomy is the removal of the cancerous part of the esophagus and nearby lymph nodes. This procedure is performed only on patients with very early cancer that has not spread to the stomach. Esophagogastrectomy is the removal of the cancerous part of the esophagus, nearby lymph nodes, and the upper part of the stomach. The resected esophagus is replaced with the stomach or parts of intestine so the patient can swallow. These procedures can significantly relieve symptoms and improve the nutritional status of more than 80% of patients with dysphagia. Although surgery can cure some patients whose disease has not spread beyond the esophagus, but more than 75% of esophageal cancers have spread to other organs before being diagnosed. Less extensive surgical procedures can be used for palliation.

Chemotherapy

Oral or intravenous **chemotherapy** alone will not cure esophageal cancer, but pre-operative treatments can shrink tumors and increase the probability that cancer can be surgically eradicated. Palliative chemotherapy can relieve symptoms of advanced cancer but will not alter the outcome of the disease.

Radiation

External beam or internal radiation, delivered by machine or implanted near cancer cells inside the body, is only rarely used as the primary form of treatment. Post-operative radiation is sometimes used to kill cancer cells that couldn't be surgically removed. Palliative radiation is effective in relieving dysphagia in patients who cannot be cured. However, radiation is most useful when combined with chemotherapy as either the definitive treatment or preoperative treatment.

Palliation

In addition to surgery, chemotherapy, and radiation, other palliative measures can provide symptomatic relief. Dilatation of the narrowed portion of the esophagus with soft tubes can provide short-term relief of dysphagia. Placement of a flexible, self-expanding stent within the narrowed portion is also useful in allowing more food intake.

Follow-up treatments

Regular barium swallows and other imaging studies are necessary to detect recurrence or spread of disease or new tumor development.

Alternative treatment

Photodynamic therapy (PDT) involves intravenously injecting a drug that is absorbed by cancer cells and kills them after they are exposed to specific laser beams. PDT can be used for palliation, but it also cured some early esophageal cancers during preliminary studies. Researchers are comparing its benefits with those of more established therapies.

Endoscopic laser therapy involves delivering short, powerful laser treatments to the tumor through an endoscope. It can improve dysphagia, but multiple treatments are required, and the benefit is seldom long-lasting.

Prognosis

Since most patients are diagnosed when the cancer has spread to lymph nodes or other structures, the prognosis for esophageal cancer is poor. Generally, no more than half of all patients are candidates for curative treatment. Even if cure is attempted, the cancer can recur.

Prevention

There is no known way to prevent esophageal cancer.

Resources

BOOKS

Abeloff, Martin D., et al. *Abeloff's Clinical Oncology*. 4th ed. Philadelphia: Churchill Livingstone/Elsevier, 2008.

Sabiston, David C., et al. *Sabiston Textbook of Surgery: The Biological Basis of Modern Surgical Practice*. Philadelphia: Saunders/Elsevier, 2008.

ORGANIZATIONS

American Cancer Society, 1599 Clifton Rd. NE, Atlanta, GA, 30329, (800) 227-2345, http://www.cancer.org.

National Coalition for Cancer Survivorship, 1010 Wayne Ave., Suite 770, Silver Spring, MD, 20910, (301) 650-9127, (301) 565-9670, (888) 650-9127, info@canceradvocacy.org, http://www.canceradvocacy.org.

Maureen Haggerty
Kevin O. Hwang, M.D.

Esophageal disorders

Definition

The esophagus is a tube that connects the back of the mouth to the stomach. Abnormalities of the esophagus generally fall into one of four categories: structural abnormalities, motility disorders, inflammatory disorders, and malignancies.

Description

The main function of the esophagus is to move food from the back of the mouth to the stomach. The adult esophagus is about 10 in (25 cm) long. It is consists of a layer of cells that secretes mucus and two layers of muscle, one circular and one longitudinal. This combination of muscles allows the esophagus to contract and propel food from the mouth the stomach. This rhythmic contraction is called peristalsis. At the end of the esophagus nearest the mouth is a ring of muscle called the upper esophageal sphincter (UES). A similar muscular ring called the lower esophageal sphincter (LES) is found 1–1.5 in (2–4 cm) above the point where the esophagus enters the stomach. The LES contracts to prevent the contents of the stomach from backflowing into the lower end of the esophagus.

Structural abnormalities

Structural abnormalities of the esophagus can be either congenital or acquired. Congenital abnormalities occur in about 1 of every 3,000–5,000 births. The two most common congenital esophageal abnormalities are **esophageal atresia** (EA) and **tracheoesophageal fistula** (TEF).

EA is a condition in which the esophagus is interrupted and the portion of the tube near the mouth is not connected to the portion that goes into the stomach. Usually the upper part of the tube ends in a blind pouch. This creates a life-threatening condition for the newborn who is unable to eat.

TEF is a condition in which the esophagus is connected to the trachea (windpipe). The trachea and the esophagus lie parallel to each other in the neck. Sometimes during fetal development, a connection called a **fistula** develops between these two tubes. This allows food to enter the trachea and be inhaled into the lungs causing a life-threatening condition called aspiration **pneumonia**. Often TEF and EA are present in the same infant. Both these conditions must be surgically corrected for the infant to survive.

Other, less common congenital structural abnormalities include webs, stenosis, cysts, and diverticula. Webs are thin membranes that lie across the esophagus and cause a partial obstruction. Stenosis is the abnormal reduction in the diameter of the esophagus due to thickening of the esophageal wall Diverticula are pouches of tissue that extend off the esophagus. Both diverticula and stenosis can be either congenital or acquired later in life.

Acquired structural abnormalities of the esophagus include Schatzki ring and **hiatal hernia**. Schatzki ring, sometimes called a **lower esophageal ring**, is a circular band of tissue located where the esophagus empties into the stomach. This ring is found in 6–14% of individuals, and for most people the presence of this ring does not create symptoms. Schatzki ring is found equally in all races and in both men and women. Schatzki rings that cause symptoms usually occur in middle age individuals. The ring can cause intermittent problems swallowing food or food impaction where the esophagus enters the stomach.

The esophagus passes a gap in the diaphragm called the diaphragmatic hiatus in order to reach the stomach. Hiatal hernia (also called hiatus hernia) is a condition that occurs when a portion of the stomach pushes up through this gap next to the esophagus. Although a hiatus hernia is not a direct structural abnormality of the esophagus, it is associated with **gastroesophageal reflux disease** (GERD) or **heartburn** in which the acidic stomach contents backflow into the lower part of the esophagus and erode the cell lining. Hiatal hernia is very common and often causes no symptoms. It is treated as a separate entry.

Lacerations, tears, and ruptures of the esophagus, known as **Mallory-Weiss syndrome** and Boerhaave syndrome, are life-threatening disorders. Mallory-Weiss syndrome usually occurs in alcoholics. In both conditions, tears result from **vomiting** and retching. The resulting bleeding creates a medical emergency that can be fatal.

Motility abnormalities

Motility abnormalities create difficulty in swallowing, called dysphagia. Dysphagia is a symptom of several esophageal motility disorders as well as several obstructive disorders such as esophageal webs or Schatzki ring.

Achalasia is an esophageal motility disorder caused by uncoordinated contractions of the two muscular layers that make up the esophagus. Because muscular contractions are disorganized, peristalsis and the orderly movement of food down the esophagus does not occur. In addition, with achalasia the lower esophageal sphincter remains contracted when food is present in the esophagus which prevents the food from entering the stomach. This causes the esophagus to bulge above the LES, a condition called megaesophagus.

Achalasia is caused by destruction of some of the nerve cells that control muscular contraction of the esophagus. This disorder generally begins in young adults and becomes progressively worse as the individual ages. Individuals with achalasia also have a higher risk of developing **esophageal cancer** at an earlier than usual age.

Individuals can also develop esophageal motility disorders secondary to other muscle diseases. **Scleroderma** is a disorder in which smooth muscle begins to atrophy. The smooth muscle in the esophagus can be affected just like other smooth muscle in the body, making swallowing difficult. Scleroderma esophagus is also associated with GERD and increased risk of **cancer** of the esophagus. Other conditions such as **diabetes mellitus**, **alcoholism**, and some psychiatric disorders can also produce secondary esophageal motility disorders.

Inflammatory disorders

Inflammatory esophageal disorders fall under the general name of esophagitis. Esophagitis causes the esophagus to become swollen and the lining of the esophagus becomes eroded and sore. It is present in about 5% of the population in the United States. There are four main types of esophagitis: reflux, infection, corrosive, and radiation. Reflux esophagitis is caused by GERD when the lower esophageal sphincter does not close tightly and the acidic contents of the stomach enter esophagus. GERD is common and is treated in depth in a separate entry. Infectious esophagitis can be caused fungal, viral, or bacterial infections. Infectious esophagitis occurs frequently in individuals with compromised immune systems, such as those with **AIDS** or leukemia. Corrosive esophagitis occurs when an individual either intentionally or accidentally swallows harsh chemicals such as lye. Radiation esophagitis is a complication of radiation treatments for cancer of the esophagus or lung.

Malignancies

Barrett's esophagus is a pre-cancerous condition which has a high risk of developing into esophageal cancer. It is found most commonly in white males in their 50s and 60s and is usually associated with years of chronic GERD.

Cancers of the esophagus tend to be aggressive and have poor outcomes. Adenocarcinoma is the primary cancer of the esophagus. Esophageal cancers are treated in detail in a separate entry.

Causes and symptoms

The causes of esophageal disorders depend on the type of disorder. Congenital defects are caused by errors in development. It is not clear why some structural disorders, such as Schatzki ring and hiatal hernia, occur. Many more people have these defects than develop symptoms or seek medical care, so that the presence of these asymptomatic structural defects is found only during autopsies. Other individuals develop symptoms that require medical attention.

Obesity and advancing age are thought to be contributing factors in developing symptoms.

Achalasia is caused by **death** of nerve cells that control the muscles that make peristalsis possible. These nerve cells are destroyed by T cells that are part of the body's immune system. It is not clear what triggers these T cells to attack inappropriately. Difficulty swallowing develops slowly, usually beginning in young adults, although the disorder can occur in children. As nerve control is lost, the LES fails to relax, preventing food from entering the stomach. As a result, the lower part of the esophagus becomes stretched creating a condition called megaesophagus. At night, food is often regurgitated and can be inhaled into the lungs, creating the risk of aspiration pneumonia. Achalasia can also be caused by **Chagas' disease**, a disease rare in North America, but common in Central and South America. Individuals with achalasia are also at higher risk to develop esophageal cancer, esophageal infections, and esophageal rupture.

Inflammatory esophagitis is most often caused by GERD. Infectious esophagitis can be caused by fungi, usually *Candida albicans*, bacteria, or viruses. Fungal infections usually occur in individuals who have diabetes, a weakened immune system, or who are taking **antibiotics**. Antibiotics change the balance of naturally occurring bacteria in the esophagus and allow fungi, which are normally present in the digestive tract, to grow unchecked. The most common causes of viral esophagitis are cytomegalovirus (CMV) and *Herpes simplex*. These are usually opportunistic infections in individuals with HIV/AIDS.

Corrosive esophagitis is usually caused by swallowing harsh chemicals, but it can also be caused by certain medications. Radiation esophagus is a side effect of **radiation therapy** for cancer.

Diagnosis

EA and TEF can sometimes be diagnosed in fetal ultrasounds before birth. If not, these defects become obvious soon after birth, because the infant is unable to eat. The inability to pass a tube from the mouth to the stomach is a definite diagnosis for EA. TEF can be detected through x-rays.

A barium swallow x ray with video is the basic method of diagnosing most esophageal disorders. For a barium swallow x ray, the individual drinks a barium, a material that coats the esophagus and shows up on x-ray film. A video camera records the passage of the barium down the esophagus in order to detect **swallowing disorders** or pockets and pouches

(diverticula) bulging from the esophagus. A barium swallow is also used to detect Schatzki rings.

Upper gastrointestinal **endoscopy** is often used in conjunction with a barium swallow to diagnose esophageal disorders. In an endoscopy, a thin, fiberoptic tube with a tiny camera is inserted into the esophagus. This allows the physician to see the lining of the esophagus. Endoscopes are equipped to take samples (biopsies) of any areas that may appear pre-cancerous or cancerous or to collect samples to test for the organism causing infectious esophagitis.

GERD can often be diagnosed from symptoms such as heartburn and regurgitation. Mallory-Weiss tears and Boerhaave syndrome are difficult to diagnose. Individuals with these disorders are often severely ill and have intense chest **pain** and **vomiting**, however chest x rays are normal 10–15% of the time. CT scans may be used in conjunction with chest x rays.

Treatment

Surgery is the only treatment for EA and TEF. It is done as soon as possible, based on the condition of the infant and any other **birth defects** that may be present that could affect the surgery.

Schatzki rings and hiatal hernias often cause no or mild symptoms and need no treatment. In severe cases, Schatzki rings are treated with bougienage. In this treatment, a series of tubes of ever-increasing diameter are inserted through the esophagus to stretch the ring. Stretching can also be done with balloon dilation. Surgery is done when no other treatment succeeds in relieving symptoms. Large hiatal hernias can be repaired surgically, but often there is not need for treatment. GERD accompanies many hiatal hernias. GERD can be treated with drugs to block acid production in the stomach (H2 blockers or **proton pump inhibitors**) and changes in diet. In severe cases of GERD stomach surgery may be necessary.

Mallory-Weiss syndrome and Boerhaave syndrome are medical emergencies. The individual is stabilized and the tear or rupture is repaired surgically. The chance of infection (**sepsis**) is high, so individuals are admitted to intensive care and do not take any food or liquid by mouth for 7–10 days. Hospital stays can last months, and repeated tears are possible.

Achalasia is treated with drugs that relax the smooth muscle and allow the LES to relax and open. When this fails, surgery to may be needed. Individuals that are not good candidates for surgery (the elderly or frail) may be treated by injecting botulinum toxin (botox) into the LES to prevent it from closing. The

KEY TERMS

Atrophy—To wither and become unresponsive.

Congenital—Present at birth.

Diaphragm—A muscle that separates the cavity containing the lungs from the abdomen.

Diverticula—Abnormal pouches of tissue that bulge off the main part of the digestive system.

Peristalsis—A wave of contractions passing through a hollow muscular tube such as the esophagus or intestine.

disadvantage of this treatment is its expense and the fact that more than one injection is needed.

Infectious esophagitis is treated by treating the underlying cause of the disease with antifungal, antiviral or antibiotic medications. These can be given either by mouth or intravenously (IV) depending on the severity of the disease.

Malignancies are treated with **chemotherapy** and radiation. See the entry on esophageal cancer for specific details.

Prognosis

The outcome of treatment depends on the type of disorder, severity, age, and general health of the individual. EA and TEF surgeries are often successful, but infants born with these conditions frequently have other congenital abnormalities that compromise their health.

When needed, treatment for Schatzki rings produces relief of symptoms, but almost always has to be repeated periodically.

Mallory-Weiss and Boerhaave syndromes are often fatal. Thirty to fifty percent of individuals die from these disorders even if they are diagnosed promptly. If diagnosis is delayed, the death rate can be as high as 90%.

Achalasia and scleroderma esophagus are progressive diseases that need continued therapy. They frequently lead to serious weight loss and **malnutrition**.

The outcome for treatment of inflammatory esophagitis depends almost entirely on the success of treating the underlying cause. Where individuals have a weakened immune system, infectious esophagitis can be an ongoing problem. When inflammatory esophagitis is caused by GERD, treatment

along with lifestyle modification is usually successful in providing relief.

Esophageal cancers are aggressive and have generally poor outcomes.

Prevention

Many symptoms of esophageal disorders can be prevented or alleviated by lifestyle changes that include:

- weight loss to control obesity
- eating slowly and chewing food well
- eating smaller and more frequent meals
- not eating several hours before going to bed
- limiting the use of alcohol and caffeine

Resources

OTHER

Ansari, Sajid and Sandeep Mukherjee. *Esophagitis,*22 November 2004 [cited 1 March 2005]. http://www.emedicine.com/med/topic735.htm.

Carey, Martin J. *Esophageal Perforation, Rupture and Tears,*26 July 2002 [cited 1 March 2005]. http://www.emedicine.com/emerg/topic176.htm.

"Esophageal and Swallowing Disorders." *The Merck Manual.* October 2007. http://www.merck.com/mmpe/sec02/ch012/ch012a.html?qt = esophageal disorders&alt = sh.

Fayyad, Abdullah and Eric Gaumnitz. *Esophageal Motility Disorders,*3 September 2004 [cited 1 March 2005]. http://www.emedicine.com/med/topic740.htm.

Minkes, Robert K. and Alison Snyder. *Congenital Anomalies of the Esophagus,*14 June 2004 [cited 1 March 2005]. http://www.emedicine.com/ped/topic2934.htm.

Paik, Nam-Jong. *Dysphagia,*19 August 2004 [cited 1 March 2005]. http://www.emedicine.com/pmr/topic194.htm.

Patti, Marco. *Gastroesophageal Reflux Disease,*29 December 2004 [cited 1 March 2005]. http://www.emedicine.com/med/topic857.htm.

Qureshi, Wagar A. *Hiatal Hernia,*August 24, 2009 [cited October 16, 2010]. http://emedicine.medscape.com/article/178393-overview.

Vossough, Arastoo and Stephen E. Rubesin. *Schatzki Ring,*14 April 2003 [cited 1 March 2005]. http://www.emedicine.com/radio/topic620.htm.

Tish Davidson, A.M.

Esophageal diverticula *see* **Esophageal pouches**

Esophageal function tests

Definition

The esophagus is the swallowing tube through which food passes on its way from the mouth to the stomach. The main function of this organ is to propel food down into the stomach. There is also a mechanism to prevent food from coming back up or "refluxing" from the stomach into the esophagus. Esophageal function tests are used to determine if these processes are normal or abnormal.

Purpose

The esophagus is a long, muscular tube that also has two muscles (or sphincters) at the top and bottom. All of these muscular areas must contract in an exact sequence for swallowing to proceed normally. There are three main symptoms that occur when esophageal function is abnormal: difficulty with swallowing (dysphagia), **heartburn**, and chest **pain**.

Doctors perform a variety of tests to evaluate these symptoms. **Endoscopy**, which is not a test of esophageal function, is often used to determine if the lining of the esophagus has any ulcers, tumors, or areas of narrowing (strictures). Many times, however, endoscopy only shows the doctor if there is injury to the esophageal lining, and the procedure gives no information about the cause of the problem.

Therefore, in addition to endoscopy, several studies are available that measure esophageal function. There are three basic types of tests used to assess esophageal function:

- Manometry is used to study the way the muscles of the esophagus contract, and is most useful for the investigation of difficulty with swallowing.
- Esophageal pH monitoring measures changes in esophageal acidity, and is valuable for evaluating patients with heartburn or gastroesophageal reflux disease (GERD).
- X-ray studies investigate swallowing difficulties. They either follow the progress of barium during swallowing using a fluoroscope, or they use radioactive scanning techniques.

Precautions

Pregnant patients undergoing x-ray exams should carefully review the risks and benefits with their doctors. Most x-ray exams of the gastrointestinal tract do not involve radiation levels that are harmful to the unborn baby.

Description

Manometry

This study is designed to measure the pressure changes produced by contraction of the muscular portions of the esophagus. An abnormality in the function of any one of the segments of the swallowing tube causes difficulty in swallowing. Doctors call this symptom dysphagia. This exam is most useful in evaluating those patients whose endoscopy is negative.

During manometry, the patient swallows a thin tube carrying a device that senses changes in pressures in the esophagus. Readings are taken at rest and during swallowing. Medications are sometimes given during the study to help in the diagnosis. The results are then transmitted to recording equipment. Manometry can best identify diseases that produce disturbances of motility or contractions of the esophagus.

ESOPHAGEAL PH MONITORING. This procedure involves measuring the esophagus' exposure to acid that has "refluxed" from the stomach. The test is ideal for evaluating recurring heartburn or GERD. Too much acid produces not only heartburn, but also ulcers that can bleed or produce areas of narrowing (strictures) when they heal.

Normally, acid refluxes into the esophagus in only small amounts for short periods of time. A muscle called the lower esophageal sphincter prevents excessive reflux. Spontaneous contractions that increase esophageal emptying and production of saliva are other important protective mechanisms.

"pH" is the scientific term that tells just how acidic or alkaline a substance is. Researchers have shown that in the esophagus, the presence of acid is damaging only if it persists for prolonged periods. Therefore, the test has been designed to monitor the level of acidity over 24 hours, usually in the home. In this way, patients maintain their daily routine, documenting their symptoms, and at what point in their activities they occurred. During this period, a thin tube with a pH monitor remains in the esophagus to record changes. After the study, a computer is used to compare changes in acidity with symptoms reported by the patient.

Surgery is an effective and long-lasting treatment for symptoms of recurrent reflux and is the choice of many patients and doctors. pH monitoring is usually performed before surgery to confirm the diagnosis and to judge the effects of drug therapy.

X-RAY TESTS. These fall into two categories: (1) those done with the use of barium and a fluoroscope; and (2) those performed with radioactive materials.

Studies performed with fluoroscopy are of greatest value in identifying a structural abnormality of the esophagus. Although this is not truly an esophageal function test, it does allow doctors to consider other diagnostic possibilities. Often a sandwich or marshmallow coated with barium is used to identify the site of an obstruction.

During fluoroscopy, the radiologist can observe the passage of material through the esophagus in real time, and video recordings can also be done. This is particularly useful when the swallowing symptoms appear to involve mainly the upper region of the esophagus. The most common cause of swallowing difficulties is a previous **stroke**, although other diseases of the neuromuscular system (like **myasthenia gravis**) can produce the same symptoms.

Scans using low-dose radioactive materials are useful because they are able not only to demonstrate that food passes through the esophagus more slowly than normal, but also how slow. These studies involve swallowing food coated with material that is followed by a nuclear medicine scanner. Scans are best used when other methods have failed to make a diagnosis, or if it is necessary to determine the degree of the abnormality. Scans mainly serve as research tools.

Preparation

Patients should not eat or drink for several hours before the exam. Many medications affect the esophagus; doses sometimes need to be adjusted or even stopped for a while. Patients must inform doctors of all medications taken, including over-the-counter medications (purchased without a doctor's prescription), and any known **allergies**.

Aftercare

For most of these studies, no special care is needed after the procedure. Patients can often go about normal daily activities following any of these tests. One exception is for those who undergo an x-ray exam with the use of barium. This can have a constipating effect and patients should ask about using a mild laxative later on.

Risks

Exposure of a fetus to x rays, especially in the first three months, is a potential risk.

Other studies of esophageal function are essentially free of any significant risk. The tubes passed during these procedures are small, and most patients adjust to them quite well. However, since medications cannot be used to relax patients, some may not tolerate the exam.

Abnormal results

Manometry is used to diagnose abnormalities related to contraction or relaxation of the various muscular regions of the esophagus. These studies cannot distinguish whether injury to either the muscle or nerves of the esophagus is producing the abnormal results. Only the final effect on esophageal muscle is identified. Results should be interpreted in light of the patient's entire medical history.

For example, there are many diseases that cause poor relaxation of the lower esophageal sphincter. When no cause is found, the disease is called **achalasia**.

Abnormal results of pH tests can confirm symptoms of heartburn or indicate a cause of chest pain (or rarely, swallowing difficulties). Doctors may want to start or change medications based on these results, or even repeat the test using different doses of medication. As noted above, these studies are indicated before surgical treatment of GERD.

X-ray tests can only serve to document an abnormality, and they are far from perfect. If they are negative, then other studies are often needed.

Resources

PERIODICALS

Lazarescu, A., et al. "Perception of dysphagia: lack of correlation with objective measurements of esophageal function." *Neurogastroenterology and Motility* (Dec 2010): 1292.

David Kaminstein, MD

Esophageal laceration *see* **Mallory-Weiss syndrome**
Esophageal manometry *see* **Esophageal function tests**

Esophageal pouches

Definition

Esophageal pouches, also known as esophageal diverticula, are pocket-like structures formed when the interior space of the esophagus, the tube that connects the mouth to the stomach, protrudes into the walls that surround it.

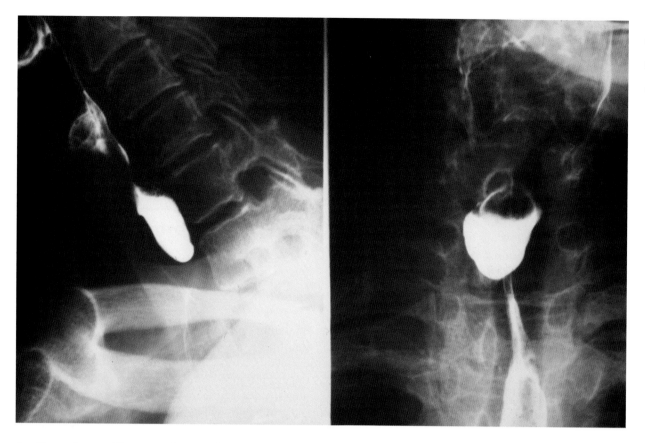

A split x-ray image of the upper chest, neck, and esophagus (left), and chest and esophagus (right). *(Custom Medical Stock Photo, Inc. Reproduced by permission.)*

Description

The esophagus is a muscular tube that propels food into the stomach. A defect in the wall of the esophagus may allow the lining to herniate, creating a space where food can be caught. Pouches can appear anywhere between the throat and the stomach. They occur primarily in men and usually later in life.

Different names for the condition apply to different locations along the esophagus:

• Zenker's diverticula are pharyngeal pouches, or ones that occur in the upper neck area at the top of the esophagus.

• Traction diverticula are a type of mid-esophageal pouch.

• Epiphrenic diverticula occur at the bottom of the esophagus near where it enters the stomach.

Causes and symptoms

To propel food into the stomach (or out of it during **vomiting**) the esophagus generates internal pressure just like the bowel. Under certain circumstances, that pressure can herniate the esophageal lining through a weakness in the wall, creating a pouch (a balloon squeezed in the hand will herniate through the fingers in the same way). Pouches are more common in people who have motility disorders of the esophagus, swallowing that is not well coordinated and may be spastic. A **traction** diverticulum can develop from a scar that pulls the esophagus out of shape. Food and saliva can collect in all of these pouches.

Pouches in the neck usually cause **bad breath** (halitosis) and the regurgitation of swallowed food and saliva. Some patients with Zenker's diverticula can push on their neck and make old food appear in their mouths. Pouches near the stomach may cause swallowing problems, conditions known as *achalasia* or *dysphagia*. Mid-esophageal pouches usually cause no symptoms.

In the most serious cases, a person may be unable to swallow because the esophagus is obstructed, or the esphagus may rupture, spilling its contents into the chest or neck.

KEY TERMS

Achalasia—Failure of the lower end of the esophagus (or another tubular valve) to open, resulting in obstruction, either partial or complete.

Contrast agent—A substance that produces shadows on an x ray so that hollow structures can be more easily seen.

Dysphagia—Difficult swallowing.

Esophagoscopy—Looking down the esophagus with a flexible viewing instrument.

Herniate—To protrude beyond usual limits.

Manometry—Pressure measurement.

Diagnosis

Difficulty swallowing, bad breath, or food reappearing in the back of the mouth are among the signs physicians look for when diagnosing this condition. Sometimes the patient may also experience **pain** in the chest resembling a **heart attack**. A series of x rays taken while swallowing a contrast agent usually demonstrates the diverticulum clearly. An esophagoscopy may also be needed to gather more detail. Manometry, measuring pressures inside the esophagus using a balloon that is passed down it, may help determine the cause of the diverticula.

Treatment

Treatment for this condition is primarily aimed at alleviating symptoms. Physicians direct the patient to eat a bland diet, to chew his or her food thoroughly, and to drink water after eating to clean out the pouches. If the condition is severe, several types of surgery are available to remove the pouches and repair the defects. If a pouch is due to a stenosis (narrowing) in the esophagus it may be possible to relieve it by passing a dilator through it, a process called bougeinage.

Prognosis

The two complications that can render these nuisances dangerous, obstruction and rupture, are emergencies. Both require immediate medical attention. Other than that, diverticula will usually grow slowly over the years, gradually increasing the symptoms they cause.

Resources

BOOKS

Fauci, Anthony S., et al., eds.*Harrison's Principles of Internal Medicine*. 17th ed. New York: McGraw–Hill Professional, 2008.

J. Ricker Polsdorfer, MD

Esophageal ulcers *see* **Ulcers (digestive)**

Esophagogastroduodenoscopy

Definition

An endoscope as used in the field of gastroenterology (the medical study of the stomach and intestines) is a thin, flexible tube that uses a lens or miniature camera to view various areas of the gastrointestinal tract. When the procedure is limited to the examination of the inside of the gastrointestinal tract's upper portion, it is called upper **endoscopy** or esphagogastroduodenoscopy (EGD). With the endoscope, the esophagus (swallowing tube), stomach, and duodenum (first portion of the small intestine) can be easily examined, and abnormalities frequently treated. Patients are usually sedated during the exam.

Purpose

EGD is performed to evaluate or treat symptoms relating to the upper gastrointestinal tract, such as:

- upper abdominal or chest pain
- nausea or vomiting
- difficulty swallowing (dysphagia)
- bleeding from the upper intestinal tract
- anemia (low blood count). EGD can be used to treat certain conditions, such as an area of narrowing or bleeding in the upper gastrointestinal tract

Upper endoscopy is more accurate than x rays for detecting inflammation, ulcers, or tumors. It is used to diagnose early **cancer** and can frequently determine whether a growth is benign (not cancerous) or malignant (cancerous).

Biopsies (small tissue samples) of inflamed or "suspicious" areas can be obtained and examined by a pathologist. Cell scrapings can also be taken by the introduction of a small brush; this helps in the diagnosis of cancer or infections.

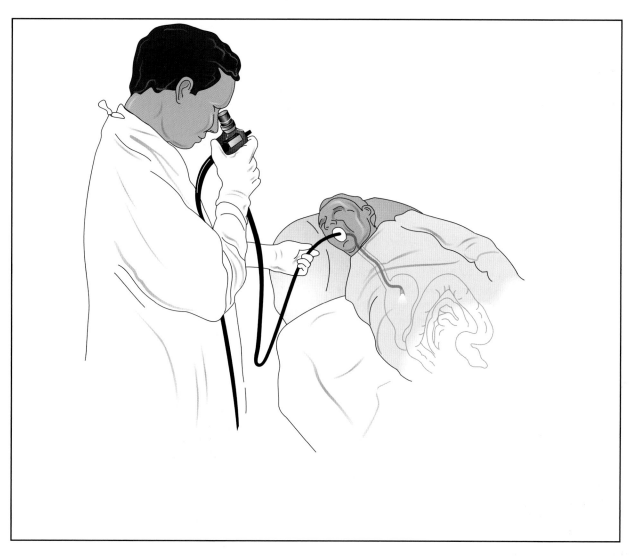

Esophagogastroduodenoscopy (EGD) is performed to evaluate or treat symptoms relating to the upper gastrointestinal tract. By inserting an endoscope into the mouth and guiding it through the gastrointestinal tract, the esophagus, stomach, and duodenum can be examined and abnormalities treated. *(Illustration by Electronic Illustrators Group. Reproduced by permission of Gale, a part of Cengage Learning.)*

When treating conditions in the upper gastrointestinal tract, small instruments are passed through the endoscope that can stretch narrowed areas (strictures), or remove swallowed objects (such as coins or pins). In addition, bleeding from ulcers or vessels can be treated by a number of endoscopic techniques.

Recent studies have shown the usefulness of endoscopic removal of early tumors of the esophagus or stomach. This is done either with injection of certain materials (like alcohol), or with the use of instruments (like lasers) that burn the tumor. Other techniques combining medications and lasers also show promise.

Precautions

Patients should inquire as to the doctor's expertise with these procedures, especially when therapy is the main goal. The doctor should be informed of any **allergies**, medication use, and medical problems.

Description

First, a "topical" (local) medication to numb the gag reflex is given either by spray or is gargled. Patients are usually sedated for the procedure (though not always) by injection of medications into a vein. The endoscopist then has the patient swallow the scope, which is passed

KEY TERMS

Pathologist—A doctor who specializes in the anatomic (structural) and chemical changes that occur with diseases. These doctors function in the laboratory, examining biopsy specimens, and regulating studies performed by the hospital laboratories (blood tests, urine tests, etc). Pathologists also perform autopsies.

through the upper gastrointestinal tract. The lens or camera at the end of the instrument allows the endoscopist to examine each portion of the upper gastrointestinal tract; photos can be taken for reference. Air is pumped in through the instrument to allow proper observation. Biopsies and other procedures can be performed without any significant discomfort.

Preparation

The upper intestinal tract must be empty for the procedure, so it is necessary NOT to eat or drink for at least 6–12 hours before the exam. Patients need to inquire about taking their medications before the procedure.

Aftercare

Someone should be available to take the person home after the procedure and stay with them for a while; patients will not be able to drive themselves due to **sedation**. **Pain** or any other unusual symptoms should be reported immediately.

It is important to recognize early signs of any possible complication. The doctor should be notified if the patient has **fever**, trouble swallowing, or increasing throat, chest, or abdominal pain.

Risks

EGD is safe and well tolerated; however, complications can occur as with any procedure. These are most often due to medications used during the procedure, or are related to endoscopic therapy. The overall complication rate of EGD is less than 2%, and many of these complications are minor (such as inflammation of the vein through which medication is given). However, serious ones can and do occur, and almost half of them are related to the heart or lungs. Bleeding or perforations (holes in the gastrointestinal tract) are also reported, especially when tumors or narrowed areas are treated or biopsied. Infections have also

been rarely transmitted; improved cleaning techniques should be able to prevent them.

Resources

OTHER

"Understanding Upper Endoscopy." *American Society for Gastrointestinal Endoscopy.* http://www.asge.org.

David Kaminstein, MD

Essential tremor *see* **Tremors**

Estradiol *see* **Hormone replacement therapy**

Estrogen *see* **Hormone replacement therapy**

Estrogen fractions test *see* **Sex hormones tests**

Estrogen replacement therapy *see* **Hormone replacement therapy**

Ethambutol *see* **Antituberculosis drugs**

Etodolac *see* **Nonsteroidal anti-inflammatory drugs**

Evoked potential studies

Definition

Evoked potential studies are a group of tests of the nervous system that measure electrical signals along the nerve pathways.

Purpose

Nerves convey information to the body by sending electrical signals down the length of the nerve. These signals can be recorded by wires placed over the nerves on the surface of the skin, in a procedure called an evoked potential (EP) study. The person conducting the test evokes the patient's neural activity by visual or auditory stimulation or using a mild electrical shock. This causes changes in the electrical potential in the nerves. Analysis of the signals can provide information about the condition of nerve pathways, especially those in the brain and spinal cord. They can indicate the presence of disease or degeneration, and can help determine the location of nerve lesions.

There are three major types of EP studies used regularly:

- Visual evoked potentials are used to diagnose visual losses due to optic nerve damage, especially from multiple sclerosis. They are also useful to diagnose "hysterical blindness," in which loss of vision is not due to any nerve damage.

- Auditory evoked potentials are used to diagnose hearing losses. They can distinguish damage to the acoustic nerve (which carries signals from the ear to the brain stem) from damage to the auditory pathways within the brainstem. Most auditory EPs record activity from the brainstem, and are therefore called "brainstem auditory evoked potentials." Disorders diagnosed with auditory EPs include acoustic neuroma (tumors of the inner ear) and multiple sclerosis (chronic disease in which nerves lose patches of their outer covering). They may also be used to assess high frequency hearing ability, to determine brain death, and to monitor brainstem function during surgery

- Somatosensory evoked potentials record transmission of nerve impulses from the limbs to the brain, and can be used to diagnose nerve damage or degeneration within the spinal cord or nerve roots from multiple sclerosis, trauma, or other degenerative disease. Somatosensory EPs can be used to distinguish central versus peripheral nerve disease, when combined with results from a nerve conduction velocity test, which measures nerve function in the extremities.

Precautions

Evoked potential studies are painless, noninvasive, and without any significant risk. Somatosensory EP tests involve very mild electric shocks, usually felt as a **tingling**.

Description

The person performing the test locates and marks specific spots on the patient's head for placement of electrodes. These spots are cleaned, and an adhesive conducting paste is applied. Cup electrodes are attached. For somatosensory EP, spots on the arm or leg are also marked and cleaned; electrodes may be taped in place. The patient sits or reclines in a chair throughout the tests.

For a visual EP, the patient focuses on a TV screen which displays a checkerboard pattern. The eye not being tested is covered with a patch. For children or others whose attention may wander, goggles are used which show the pattern to one eye at a time. Each eye is usually tested twice, and the entire procedure takes approximately 30–45 minutes.

For auditory EP, headphones are used to deliver a series of clicks to one ear at a time. A masking or static sound is played into the other ear. Each ear is usually

tested twice, and the entire procedure takes approximately 30–45 minutes.

For somatosensory EP, mild electrical shocks are delivered to the arm or leg. This may cause some twitching and tingling. The stimulus lasts for about two minutes at a time, and the entire procedure takes approximately 30 minutes.

After the tests, the electrodes are removed with acetone and the scalp is cleaned.

Preparation

Hair must be clean, dry, and free of any braids, pins, or jewelry. The patient should shampoo before the test, and must not use any hair spray, gel, or other hair care products after shampooing. Clothing should be loose and comfortable. The patient may eat and take some medications as usual before the test, although sedative medications should be avoided on the day of the test, if possible. It is best to check with the physician supervising the test for specific instructions.

Aftercare

This test is painless and has no residual effects. The patient may return to work or other activities immediately afterward.

Normal results

EP test results are displayed as jagged electrical tracings (wave forms), which have characteristic shapes, heights, and lengths, indicating the speed and intensity of signal transmission. Results are read by someone trained in evoked potential studies.

Abnormal results

Changes in the electrical tracings may indicate damage to or degeneration of nerve pathways to the brain from the eyes, ears, or limbs. Absence of any activity may mean complete loss of nerve function in that pathway. Other changes may provide evidence of the type and location of nerve damage.

Resources

BOOKS

Husain, Aatif M. *Illustrated Manual of Clinical Evoked Potentials*. New York: Demos Medical Publishing, 2011.

Richard Robinson

Evoked responses *see* **Evoked potential studies**

Exanthema subitum *see* **Roseola**

Exercise

Definition

Exercise can be defined as physical activity that involves planned, structured, and repetitive bodily movements for the purpose of maintaining or improving physical fitness and overall health. Exercise includes cardiovascular training, muscle-strength training, and stretching activities for flexibility and to prevent injury. Typical exercise activities include walking, running, cycling, swimming, weight training, aerobics, and individual and team sports.

Purpose

Regular exercise is important for the physical, mental, and emotional health of people of all ages— from young children to the elderly. Exercise promotes:

- weight maintenance or weight loss
- cardiovascular efficiency
- musculoskeletal strength and flexibility
- improved functioning of the metabolic, endocrine, and immune systems
- bone density
- lower cholesterol levels
- recovery from illness, injury, or surgery
- mental and emotional wellbeing

The beneficial effects of exercise diminish within two weeks of substantially reducing physical activity. Physical fitness is lost completely if exercise is not resumed within two to eight months.

Demographics

The National Institutes of Health (NIH) has identified inactivity as a major public health problem in the United States, and most North American adults would benefit from increasing their level of physical activity. More than 60% of American adults do not get enough physical activity to provide health benefits and more than 25% are inactive during their leisure

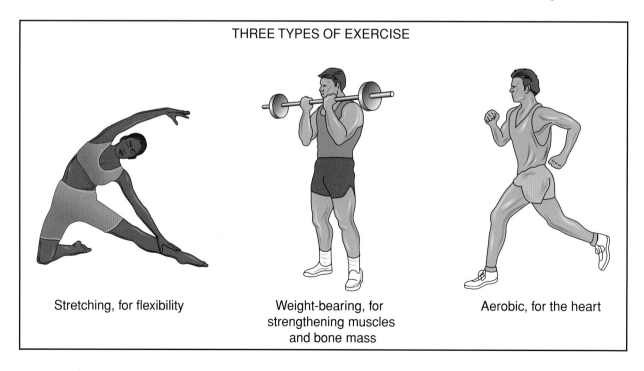

THREE TYPES OF EXERCISE

Stretching, for flexibility

Weight-bearing, for strengthening muscles and bone mass

Aerobic, for the heart

Exercise is utilized to improve health, maintain fitness, and is important as a means of physical rehabilitation. *(Illustration by Electronic Illustrators Group. Reproduced by permission of Gale, a part of Cengage Learning.)*

time. Lack of exercise is a major contributor to the current epidemic of **obesity**, since people burn fewer calories than they take in, resulting in weight gain. Sedentary lifestyles and unhealthy eating patterns are responsible for at least 300,000 deaths from chronic disease each year in the United States. Likewise a recent survey in the United Kingdom found that only one-third of adults meet recommended goals for physical activity.

Insufficient exercise is more prevalent among women than men and among those with lower levels of economic stability and educational achievement. However the number of adult Americans who are exercising regularly is on the increase. According the Centers for Disease Control and Prevention (CDC), between 2001 and 2005 the number of women exercising at least 30 minutes per day increased by 8.6% and the number of men increased by 3.5%.

Geriatric

Exercise generally decreases with age. It is estimated that two-thirds of Americans over age 65 have at least one chronic condition, with 36 million suffering from some form of arthritis. Lack of exercise is a significant contributor to conditions such as **osteoarthritis**, lower back **pain**, and **osteoporosis**. More than 300,000 total joint replacements are performed each year due to osteoarthritis.

Description

Exercise programs should include three types of exercise: strengthening, including weight or resistance training, stretching and flexibility exercises, and cardiovascular exercise. Recent studies have indicated that muscle strength and aerobic fitness make independent contributions to health and that more muscle strength correlates with lower **death** rates, regardless of aerobic fitness. The American College of Sports Medicine recommends two strength-training workouts per week, each consisting of about ten repetitions of ten exercises for strengthening all of the major muscle groups. **Yoga** is often recommended for stretching, bending, and improving overall flexibility.

Chosen exercises should be interesting and appealing: studies have found that people are more likely to stick with an exercise program when they enjoy the activity, whether as an individual, with a partner, or with a group or team. Convenience is also an important consideration. Exercise can take place at home, outdoors, at a health club or fitness center, school, church, or community center. Taking a class, working out with a friend, competing, or setting personal goals can help maintain motivation. Walking for exercise can be combined with various enjoyable activities, such as bird watching, museum visits, window shopping, or exercising the dog. Group exercises and team sports are good ways to socialize. Varying exercise routines every few weeks can benefit different muscle groups and help prevent boredom. In addition, since the human body adjusts rapidly to most exercises, continuing the same routine for too long can result in decreased benefits.

The most efficient cardiovascular exercises for improving physical fitness include:

- brisk walking (3–4 mph), whether outside, in a mall, or on a treadmill
- jogging
- running
- bicycling, either outside or on a stationary bike
- stair climbing
- elliptical cross-training on exercise machines
- aerobics
- swimming
- water exercise or aerobics
- rowing
- cross-country (Nordic) skiing
- jumping rope—a particularly good exercise for children

Other exercises that provide cardiovascular conditioning—but are less endurance-promoting because they usually require frequent starting and stopping—include:

- dancing
- basketball
- soccer
- softball
- badminton
- racquetball
- squash
- tennis
- table tennis
- volleyball
- skating
- golfing, if walking and carrying clubs

Teenagers can get cardiovascular exercise through school sports including:

- baseball
- cross country
- track and field
- cheerleading

- drill team
- field hockey
- football
- lacrosse
- wrestling

People who are generally sedentary can still get exercise through their occupation, housework, home repair, gardening, using stairs instead of an elevator, and various recreational pursuits. People with health problems can find exercises that accommodate their injuries or disorders. The American Council on Exercise suggests specific exercises for the elderly and for adults with problems such as **asthma**, chronic pain, bad knees, shoulder injuries, arthritis, and flat feet.

Regularity and intensity are key elements of exercise. It has generally been recommended that all adults get at least 30 minutes of moderate-intensity exercise on most days of the week. However the most recent consensus is to aim for 150 minutes per week, regardless of how it is divided up. The latest evidence suggests that three ten-minute bouts of exercise are as beneficial as one 30-minute workout. Improving cardiovascular endurance requires at least 20–60 minutes of cardiovascular exercise three to five days per week. The U.S. Department of Health and Human Services recommends at least 60 minutes of physical activity for children and teens on most or all days of the week.

Defining "moderate intensity" can be tricky. Until recently exercise intensity was generally gauged by increased heart rate. However intensity is more accurately measured by metabolic rate, as represented by units of metabolic equivalents or METS. METS is an individual's metabolic rate during exercise divided by the metabolic rate when sitting still. The latter is defined as 1 kilocalorie per kilogram (kg) of body weight per hour or an oxygen uptake of 3.5 milliliters per kg per minute. Moderate activity is defined as 3–6 METS. Although a precise measurement requires determining oxygen intake in a laboratory, charts of average METS for various activities are available. Examples of METS include:

- walking, 2–8
- running, 8–18
- bicycling, 4–16
- stationary bicycling, 3–12.5
- general health-club exercise, 5.5
- calisthenics, 3–8
- weight lifting, 3–6
- swimming, 6–11

- cross-country skiing, 7–16.5
- downhill skiing, 5–8
- volleyball, 3–8
- dancing, 3–10
- basketball, 4.5–8
- tennis, 5–8
- tai chi, 4
- stretching, hatha yoga, 2.5
- household tasks, 2–9
- mowing with a hand mower, 6

Exercise geared to a target heart rate is typically about 70% of the maximum heart rate for one's age. Heart rate is calculated by counting the pulse, usually about halfway through a 20–30-minute workout. Fingers are placed firmly but lightly over the inside of the wrist or on the neck just below the angle of the jaw; however too much pressure on the neck can slow down the heart rate. The palm also can be placed over the heart to count the number of beats. A zero is added to a six-second count or a ten-second count is multiplied by six to obtain the beats per minute (bpm). Maximum bpm is calculated by subtracting one's age from 220. For example:

- Target heart rate during cardiovascular exercise for a healthy 50-year-old might be 170 multiplied by 70% or 119 bpm.
- A particularly fit 50-year-old might have a target heart rate of 80% of maximum or 136 bpm.
- A 50-year-old with a medical condition may have a target exercising heart rate of only 50% or 85 bpm. A bpm above the target rate indicates a need to slow down, whereas a bpm below the target indicates a need to speed up the pace of exercise.

There are other methods for measuring the intensity of cardiovascular exercise:

- Classes and DVDs usually include a timed heart-rate check and a chart of target rates by age.
- Electronic exercise pulse monitors are available.
- A simple "talk test" is based on speaking a complete sentence: the pace of exercise is too high if the sentence cannot be completed and too low if it is overly easy to speak the sentence.
- Cardiovascular exercise usually involves sweating; therefore people who no longer sweat during their exercise routine may need to increase the intensity, duration, or frequency of their workouts.

Improved fitness in response to exercise appears to be genetically determined and to run in families. Some previously sedentary people show less improvement in fitness than would be expected following weeks of a vigorous exercise program and about 10% show no improvement at all. However even those who show no improvement in fitness measures still respond to exercise with lowered blood pressure and cholesterol, improved insulin levels, and less abdominal fat.

Origins

Throughout most of human history, most people had plenty of exercise. Then, early in the twentieth century, the rate of heart attacks in Western countries began to increase dramatically. The first indication that this might be due to lack of exercise came in a landmark 1953 study of London bus conductors: conductors, who spent their days collecting fares from seated passengers and walking up and down the stairs of double-decker buses, had half the number of heart attacks as seated bus drivers. Since then countless studies have confirmed the positive effects of exercise, not just on the heart and circulatory system, but on virtually every system of the body.

Benefits

Exercise promotes:

- cardiovascular fitness, including improved heart function and increased heart, lung, and muscle endurance
- muscle strength and mass
- flexibility
- weight loss
- lowered blood pressure
- bone density and strength, which reduces the risk of fractures and osteoporosis
- mental health and psychological and emotional well-being from the release of brain hormones called endorphins

Additional benefits of cardiovascular exercise include:

- improved immune system function
- improved utilization and control of blood sugar
- decreased cholesterol and triglycerides
- decreased abdominal fat
- increased energy levels
- less fatigue
- improved appetite
- improved sleep
- reduced stress
- pain reduction

Regular exercise lowers the risk of a **heart attack** by 50–80%. Exercise also has been shown to reduce the risk of:

- stroke
- cancer
- diabetes
- liver and kidney disease
- osteoporosis
- depression
- dementia

Even those who are overweight or obese can become aerobically fit with exercise. Studies have found that the risk of dying is more closely related to fitness than to weight. In fact people who are fit but obese have a lower risk of dying than people who are unfit but of normal weight.

More than 30 million Americans undergo surgery each year. Each patient's surgical risk, complications, and outcome depend, at least in part, on their physical fitness: how well their cardiovascular and pulmonary systems withstand the **stress** of anesthesia; how quickly their bones and muscles recover after surgical procedures; and how well their metabolic and immune systems respond to surgery and the risk of infection.

Precautions

- Everyone should have a physical examination before embarking on an exercise program for the first time or after a long period of inactivity.
- Exercise intensity and duration should be increased gradually.
- People who are very weak may need to build strength before they can participate in cardiovascular exercise.
- Warming up before and stretching after exercise are very important.
- People should pace themselves and check their heart rate or otherwise judge their level of exertion.
- If exercising becomes "very hard" or worse, it is important to slow the pace.
- Although some discomfort, such as aches or stiffness, are to be expected during the first few days of a new exercise, if pain is intrusive it is important to stop the activity or get instruction on technique.
- Strenuous cardiovascular exercise should never be halted abruptly without a cool-down, since blood that has concentrated in the working muscles can pool and cause dizziness or lightheadedness.
- Cardiovascular exercise requires a healthy diet with plenty of vegetables.

KEY TERMS

Aerobic exercise—Any exercise that increases the body's oxygen consumption and improves the functioning of the cardiovascular and respiratory systems.

Cholesterol—A fat-soluble steroid alcohol (sterol) found in animal fats and oils and produced in the body from saturated fats. High cholesterol levels contribute to the development of cardiovascular disease.

Endorphins—A class of peptides in the brain that are produced during exercise and bind to opiate receptors, resulting in pleasant feelings and pain relief.

Metabolic equivalent of task; MET—The energy cost of a physical activity, measured as a multiple of the resting metabolic rate, which is defined as 3.5 milliliters of oxygen consumed per kilogram (kg) of body weight per minute, equivalent to 1 kilocalorie per kg per hour.

Obesity—Excessive weight due to accumulation of fat, usually defined as a body mass index (BMI) of 30 or above or body weight greater than 30% above normal on standard height-weight tables.

Physical activity—Any activity that involves moving the body and burning calories.

Physical fitness—A combination of muscle strength, cardiovascular health, and flexibility that is usually attributed to regular exercise and good nutrition.

Sedentary—Inactivity and lack of exercise; a lifestyle that is a major risk factor for becoming overweight or obese and developing chronic diseases.

Stress test—An electrocardiogram recorded before, during, and after a period of increasingly strenuous cardiovascular exercise, usually on a treadmill or stationary bicycle.

Target heart rate—The heart rate, in beats per minute (bpm), that should be maintained during cardiovascular exercise by an individual of a given age.

Triglycerides—Neutral fats; lipids formed from glycerol and fatty acids that circulate in the blood as lipoprotein. Elevated triglyceride levels contribute to the development of cardiovascular disease.

- It is best to wait up to two hours after a full meal before exercising and about an hour after exercising before having a meal, although a small healthy snack before exercising can boost energy levels.
- It is important to drink enough fluid to replace water that is lost as sweat; however coffee, tea, colas, chocolate, or alcohol can cause the body to lose fluid.
- Simple home exercises, such as a balance board, can reduce the risk of recurrent sprained ankles.
- Taking a few days off from cardiovascular exercise every month can help rejuvenate the body.

Geriatric

Both maximum heart rate and cardiac output are lower in older adults, in part due to a decrease in the beta-adrenergic response. Older adults should have a **stress test** before embarking on a cardiovascular exercise program. A good result on a stress test is a bpm that is 80% of the age-adjusted maximum, with 90% considered excellent.

Other conditions

Various medical conditions can affect exercise. For example people with back problems should avoid exercises that require twisting or vigorous forward movements, such as aerobic dancing or rowing. People with spinal disk disease should avoid high-impact activities.

Preparation

Exercise should begin with a light or very light warm-up of five to ten minutes that may include gentle stretching to loosen muscles and joints and help prevent injury. The warm-up may involve slowly beginning the conditioning activity—warming up for a brisk walk or jog by walking slowly or strolling, or warming up to ride a stationary bike by pedaling slowly with no resistance. Warming up increases blood flow to the muscles, increases muscle temperature, and prepares them to work harder.

Aftercare

Cardiovascular exercise should be followed by a light or very light five-or ten-minute cool-down to allow the heart and circulation to gradually return to a resting state. The cool-down can include the same activity as the conditioning phase at a slower pace—slower walking or pedaling with reduced resistance on a stationary bike.

Most doctors encourage patients to become active as soon as possible following surgery. Aftercare is individualized and there may be limitations on physical activity; however the goal is to return the patient to normal daily activities and exercise routines.

Patients should ask for explicit guidelines concerning exercise.

Risks

Exercise poses a risk of injury, particularly if exercises are inappropriate or improperly performed. Too much exercise can be as harmful as too little; overuse of certain muscles and joints can lead to problems such as **tennis elbow** or **shin splints**. High-intensity exercises, such as high-impact aerobics and jogging, are not recommended as frequently as in the past. Running, in particular, is hard on the knees and ankle joints, and there is a risk of sprained ankles and injuries from falls. About one half of all regular runners and players of team sports suffer some type of musculoskeletal injury each year.

Inadequate rest increases the risk of **stroke** and circulatory problems. Injury or illness from overtraining is sometimes indicated by a high resting heart rate, sleeping difficulties, or exhaustion. The risk of a heart attack can rise as much as 100-fold for a completely unfit individual who undertakes vigorous exercise such as jogging or shoveling snow. In contrast, a person who runs five times per week merely doubles their risk of heart attack during vigorous exercise. The risk of heart attack subsides about one-half hour after exercising and pales in comparison to the lifetime benefits of regular exercise.

Pregnant or breastfeeding

Some types of exercise are inappropriate for pregnant women. Pregnant women are generally advised not to exercise for two consecutive days.

Resources

BOOKS

Harper, Bob. *Are You Ready! Take Charge, Lose Weight, Get in Shape, and Change Your Life Forever.* New York: Broadway Books, 2008.

Manocchia, Pat. *Anatomy of Exercise: A Trainer's Inside Guide to Your Workout.* Richmond Hill, ONT: Firefly Books, 2008.

Silver, J. K., and Christopher Morin. *Understanding Fitness: How Exercise Fuels Health and Fights Disease.* Westport, CT: Praeger, 2008.

Ratey, John J., and Eric Hagerman. *Spark: The Revolutionary New Science of Exercise and the Brain.* New York: Little, Brown, 2008.

PERIODICALS

Centers for Disease Control and Prevention. "Prevalence of Regular Physical Activity Among Adults—United States, 2001 and 2005." *MMWR: Morbidity and Mortality Weekly Report* 56 (November 23, 2007): 1209–1212.

Ignelzi, R. J. "Survival of the Fitness: Staying in Shape Without the Gym Easily Doable if You're Disciplined." *San Diego Union-Tribune* (March 24, 2009): D1.

Vanderburg, Helen. "Put Your Heart Health to the Test; Undergo a Stress Test Before Starting Cardiovascular Exercises." *Vancouver Sun* (September 14, 2009): C1.

"What's Your Function?" *Current Health 2* 36, no. 2 (October 2009): 6–7.

OTHER

Hatfield, Heather. "Kick It Up With Cardio Exercise." *WebMD.*http://www.webmd.com/fitness-exercise/guide/kick-up-with-cardio-exercise

"Health and Wellness: Battling Boredom in Your Workout." *American Osteopathic Association.*http://www.osteopathic.org/index.cfm?PageID=you_workoutboredom

"Let's Get Physical: Nine Facts About Fitness." *NewScientist.*http://www.newscientist.com/special/get-physical-nine-facts-about-fitness

"Physical Activity." *Centers for Disease Control and Prevention.* http://www.cdc.gov/physicalactivity/

"Target Heart Rate Calculator." *WebMD.*http://www.webmd.com/fitness-exercise/healthtool-target-heart-rate-calculator

Wilkerson, Rick, ed. "Sports & Exercise." *Your Orthopaedic Connection.*http://orthoinfo.aaos.org/menus/sports.cfm

ORGANIZATIONS

American College of Sports Medicine, PO Box 1440, Indianapolis, IN, 46202-1440, (317) 637-9200, (317) 634-7817, http://www.acsm.org.

American Council on Exercise, 4851 Paramount Drive, San Diego, CA, 92123, (858) 279-8227, (888) 825-3636, (858) 576-6564, support@acefitness.org, http://www.acefitness.org.

American Heart Association, 7272 Greenville Avenue, Dallas, TX, 75231, (800) 242-8721, http://www.americanheart.org.

National Institute of Arthritis and Musculoskeletal and Skin Diseases, Information Clearinghouse, 1 AMS Circle, Bethesda, MD, 20892-3675, (301) 495-4484, (877) 22-NIAMS (226-4267), (301) 718-6366, NIAMSinfo@mail.nih.gov, http://www.niams.nih.gov.

U.S. Centers for Disease Control and Prevention, 1600 Clifton Road, Atlanta, GA, 30333, (800) CDC-INFO (232-4636), cdcinfo@cdc.gov, http://www.cdc.gov.

Margaret Alic, PhD

Exercise electrocardiogram *see* **Stress test**

Exercise stress test *see* **Stress test**

Exhibitionism *see* **Sexual perversions**

Exocrine pancreatic cancer *see* **Pancreatic cancer, exocrine**

Exophthalmos

Definition

When there is an increase in the volume of the tissue behind the eyes, the eyes will appear to bulge out of the face. The terms exophthalmos and proptosis apply. Proptosis can refer to any organ that is displaced forward, while exophthalmos refers just to the eyes.

Description

The eye socket (orbit) is made of bone and therefore will not yield to increased pressure within it. Only forward displacement of the eyeball (globe) will allow more room if tissue behind the eye is increasing.

Causes and symptoms

The most common cause of exophthalmos is Graves' disease, overactivity of the thyroid gland. The contents of the orbits swell due to inflammation, forcing the eyes forward. The inflammation affects primarily the muscles. This combination of muscle impairment and forward displacement reduces eye movement, causing double vision and crossed eyes (**strabismus**). The optic nerves can also be affected, reducing vision, and the clear membrane (conjunctiva) covering the white part of the eyes and lining the inside of the eyelids can swell. Finally, the eyes may protrude so far that the eyelids cannot close over them, leading to corneal damage.

Exophthalmos from Graves' disease is bilateral (occurring on both sides), but not necessarily symmetrical. In contrast, exophthalmos from orbital tumors or a blood clot in the brain happens on only one side.

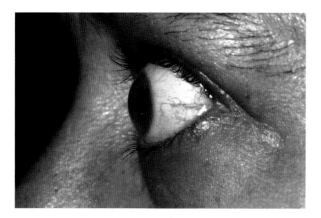

A side view of the bulging eye (exophthalmos) of a person suffering from thytoxicosis. Exophthalmos is caused by swelling of the soft tissue in the eye socket, which forces the eyeball to be pushed forward and the eyelids stretched apart. *(Dr. P. Marazzi/Photo Researchers, Inc.)*

Diagnosis

Exophthalmos is obvious when it is advanced enough to cause complications. When there is doubt in the early stages, a mechanical device called an exophthalmometer can measure the protrusion. **Computed tomography scans** (CT scans) are of great value in examining the bony components of the orbit. **Magnetic resonance imaging** (MRI) scanning is equally valuable for displaying the contents of the orbit, because it "sees through" the bone.

Treatment

If a tumor is growing behind the eye, it needs to be removed. If Graves' disease is the cause, it may subside with treatment of the overactive thyroid, but this is not guaranteed. Local care to the front of the eye to keep it moist is necessary if the eyelid cannot close.

Prognosis

Exophthalmos can be progressive. Its progress must be carefully followed, treating complications as they occur.

Prevention

Vision can usually be preserved with attentive treatment. There is currently no way to prevent any of the underlying conditions that lead to exophthalmos.

KEY TERMS

Asthma—A disease in which the air passages of the lungs become inflamed and narrowed.

Bronchitis—Inflammation of the air passages of the lungs.

Chronic—A word used to describe a long-lasting condition. Chronic conditions often develop gradually and involve slow changes.

Cough suppressant—Medicine that stops or prevents coughing.

Emphysema—An irreversible lung disease in which breathing becomes increasingly difficult.

Mucus—Thick fluid produced by the moist membranes that line many body cavities and structures.

Phlegm—Thick mucus produced in the air passages.

Respiratory tract—The air passages from the nose into the lungs.

Secretion—A substance, such as saliva or mucus, that is produced and given off by a cell or a gland.

Resources

BOOKS

Fauci, Anthony S., et al., eds. *Harrison's Principles of Internal Medicine*. 17th ed. New York: McGraw-Hill Professional, 2008.

J. Ricker Polsdorfer, MD

Expectorants

Definition

Expectorants are drugs that loosen and clear mucus and phlegm from the respiratory tract.

Purpose

The drug described here, guaifenesin, is a common ingredient in **cough** medicines. It is classified as an expectorant, a medicine that helps clear mucus and other secretions from the respiratory tract. However, some debate exists about how effectively guaifenesin does this. In addition, some cough medicines contain other ingredients that may cancel out guaifenesin's effects. **Cough suppressants** such as codeine, for example, work against guaifenesin because they discourage coughing up the secretions that the expectorant loosens.

There are other ways to loosen and clear the respiratory secretions associated with colds. These include using a humidifier and drinking six to eight glasses of water a day.

Description

Guaifenesin is an ingredient in many cough medicines, such as the brand names Anti-Tuss, Dristan Cold & Cough, Guaifed, GuaiCough, and some Robitussin products. Some products that contain guaifenesin are available only with a physician's prescription; others can be bought without a prescription. They come in several forms, including capsules, tablets, and liquids.

Recommended dosage

Adults and children 12 and over

200–400 mg every four hours. No more than 2,400 mg in 24 hours.

Children 6–11

100–200 mg every four hours. No more than 1,200 mg in 24 hours.

Children 2–5

50–100 mg every four hours. No more than 600 mg in 24 hours.

Children under two

Not recommended.

Precautions

Do not take more than the recommended daily dosage of guaifenesin.

Guaifenesin is not meant to be used for coughs associated with **asthma**, **emphysema**, chronic **bronchitis**, or **smoking**. It also should not be used for coughs that are producing a large amount of mucus.

A lingering cough could be a sign of a serious medical condition. Coughs that last more than seven days or are associated with **fever**, rash, **sore throat**, or lasting **headache** should have medical attention. Call a physician as soon as possible.

Some studies suggest that guaifenesin causes **birth defects**. Women who are pregnant or plan to become pregnant should check with their physicians before using any products that contain guaifenesin. Whether guaifenesin passes into breast milk is not known, but no ill effects have been reported in nursing babies whose mothers used guaifenesin.

Side effects

Side effects are rare, but may include **vomiting**, **diarrhea**, stomach upset, headache, skin rash, and **hives**.

Interactions

Guaifenesin is not known to interact with any foods or other drugs. However, cough medicines that contain guaifenesin may contain other ingredients that do interact with foods or drugs. Check with a physician or pharmacist for details about specific products.

Nancy Ross-Flanigan

Exstrophy of the urinary bladder *see* **Congenital bladder anomalies**

External fetal monitoring *see* **Electronic fetal monitoring**

External otitis *see* **Otitis externa**

External sphincter electromyography

Definition

External sphincter **electromyography** helps physicians determine how well the external urinary sphincter muscle is working by measuring the electrical activity in it during contraction and relaxation.

Purpose

The external sphincter muscle is the ring-like muscle that controls urine release from the bladder. When a patient cannot voluntarily control urination (incontinence), a physician may order this test to determine if the problem is caused by the failure of this muscle. The voluntary contraction or release of a muscle such as the external sphincter involves a complex process in which the nerves controlling the muscle signal it to move through the release and uptake of chemicals called neurotransmitters and the generation of electrical impulses. This test records the electrical impulses given off when the muscle contracts or relaxes and allows the physician to determine if the muscle is working properly, if it has been damaged by disease, or some other condition.

Precautions

Patients who are taking **muscle relaxants** or drugs that act like or have an effect on the neurotransmitter acetylcholine (cholinergic or anti-cholinergic drugs) should tell the doctor since they will change the test results. The results will also be altered if the patient moves during the test or if the electrodes are improperly placed.

Description

The patient puts on a surgical gown and lies down on the examining table. The procedure, which takes between 30–60 minutes, may be conducted one of three ways:

- Skin electrodes. This is the most commonly used method of recording information. The skin where the electrodes will be placed is cleaned and shaved and an electrically conductive paste is applied. The electrodes are then taped in place. For female patients, the electrodes are taped around the urethra, while for male patients they are placed between the scrotum and the anus.
- Needle electrodes. This is considered the most accurate method, since the electrodes are inserted directly into the muscle, using needles to guide placement. For male patients, a gloved finger is inserted in the rectum, then needles with wires attached are inserted through the skin between the anus and the scrotum. For female patients, the needles are inserted around the urethra. The discomfort of placing the needles is about the same as that of an injection. The needles are withdrawn, and the wires are taped to the thigh.
- Anal plug electrodes. The tip of an anal plug is lubricated and inserted into the rectum as the patient relaxes the anal sphincter. Electrodes are attached to the anal plug.

Once the electrodes are in place and attached to the recording device, the patient is asked to alternately contract and relax the external sphincter muscle. The electrical activity generated during these contractions and relaxations is recorded on a graph called an electromyogram.

Anti-cholinergic drug—A medication that blocks or subdues the action of the neurotransmitter acetylcholine.

Cholinergic drug—A medication that mimics or enhances the action of the neurotransmitter acetylcholine.

Sphincter—A circular muscle that aids in the opening or closing of an opening in the body.

Preparation

Before the test, the patient should discuss with the doctor whether it is necessary to temporarily discontinue any medications, and follow the doctor's orders. No changes in diet or activity are necessary.

Aftercare

Women may see some blood in their urine the first time they urinate after the test. Blood in the urine of men or blood in the urine of women after the first urination should be reported the doctor. The patient should take a warm bath and drink plenty of fluids to ease any discomfort after the test.

Risks

Complications of external sphincter electromyography are rare. Occasionally patients report blood in their urine after being tested with needle electrodes. Also, the urethra may become mildly irritated causing a change in the normal frequency of urination.

Normal results

In a normally functioning external sphincter muscle, the electromyogram will show increased electrical activity when the patient tightens the muscle and a little or no electrical activity when it is relaxed.

Abnormal results

A diseased external sphincter muscle will produce an abnormal pattern of electrical activity. Conditions that affect the external sphincter may include **multiple sclerosis**, **neurogenic bladder**, **Parkinson's disease**, **spinal cord injury**, and stress incontinence. However, additional tests must be done in order to confirm any of these diagnoses.

Resources

BOOKS

Sultan, Abdul H., Ranee Thakar, and Dee E. Fenner. *Perineal and Anal Sphincter Trauma: Diagnosis and Clinical Management*. London: Springer, 2009.

Tish Davidson, A.M.

Extracorporeal membrane oxygenation

Definition

Extracorporeal membrane oxygenation (ECMO) is a special procedure that uses an artificial heart-lung machine to take over the work of the lungs and sometimes also the heart.

Purpose

In newborns, ECMO is used to support or replace an infant's undeveloped or failing lungs by providing oxygen and removing carbon dioxide waste products so the lungs can rest. Infants who need ECMO may include those with:

- meconium aspiration syndrome, (breathing in of a newborn's first stool by a fetus or newborn, which can block air passages and interfere with lung expansion)
- persistent pulmonary hypertension, (a disorder in which the blood pressure in the arteries supplying the lungs is abnormally high)
- respiratory distress syndrome (a lung disorder usually of premature infants that causes increasing difficulty in breathing, leading to a life-threatening deficiency of oxygen in the blood)
- congenital diaphragmatic hernia, (the profusion of part of the stomach through an opening in the diaphragm)
- pneumonia
- blood poisoning

ECMO also is used to support a child or adult patient's damaged, infected, or failing lungs for a few hours to allow treatment or healing. It is effective for those patients with severe, but reversible, heart or lung problems who have not responded to treatment with a ventilator, drugs, or extra oxygen. Adults and children who need ECMO usually have one of these problems:

- heart failure
- pneumonia
- respiratory failure caused by trauma or severe infection

KEY TERMS

Carotid artery—Two main arteries (passageway carrying blood from the heart to other parts of the body) that carry blood to the brain.

Congenital diaphragmatic hernia—The profusion of part of the stomach through an opening in the diaphragm.

Meconium aspiration syndrome—Breathing in of meconium (a newborn's first stool) by a fetus or newborn, which can block air passages and interfere with lung expansion.

Membrane oxygenator—The artificial lung that adds oxygen and removes carbon dioxide.

Pulmonary hypertension—A disorder in which the blood pressure in the arteries supplying the lungs is abnormally high.

Respiratory distress syndrome—A lung disorder usually of premature infants that causes increasing difficulty in breathing, leading to a life-threatening deficiency of oxygen in the blood.

Venoarterial (V-A) bypass—The type of ECMO that provides both heart and lung support, using two tubes (one in the jugular vein and one in the carotid artery).

Venovenous (V-V) bypass—The type of ECMO that provides lung support only, using a tube inserted into the jugular vein.

The ECMO procedure can help a patient's lungs and heart rest and recover, but it will not cure the underlying disease. Any patient who requires ECMO is seriously ill and will likely die without the treatment. Because there is some risk involved, this method is used only when other means of support have failed.

Demographics

ECMO is used most often in newborns and young children, but it also can be used as a last resort for adults whose heart or lungs are failing.

Description

There are two types of ECMO. Venoarterial (V-A) ECMO supports the heart and lungs, and is used for patients with blood pressure or heart functioning problems in addition to respiratory problems. Venovenous (V-V) ECMO supports the lungs only.

V-A ECMO requires the insertion of two tubes, one in the jugular and one in the carotid artery. In the V-V ECMO procedure, the surgeon places a plastic tube into the jugular vein through a small incision in the neck.

Once in place, the tubes are connected to the ECMO circuit, and then the machine is turned on. The patient's blood flows out through the tube and may look very dark because it contains very little oxygen. A pump pushes the blood through an artificial membrane lung, where oxygen is added and carbon dioxide is removed. The size of the artificial lung depends on the size of the patient; sometimes adults need two lungs. The blood is then warmed and returned to the patient. A steady amount of blood (called the flow rate) is pushed through the ECMO machine every minute. As the patient improves, the flow rate is lowered. Many patients require heavy **sedation** while they are on ECMO to lessen the amount of oxygen needed by the muscles.

if the patient improves, the amount of ECMO support is decreased gradually until the machine is turned off for a brief trial period. If the patient does well without ECMO, the treatment is stopped.

Typically, newborns remain on ECMO for three to seven days, although some babies need more time (especially if they have a diaphragmatic **hernia**). Once the baby is off ECMO, he or she will still need a ventilator (breathing machine) for a few days or weeks. Adults may remain on ECMO for days to weeks, depending on the condition of the patient, but treatment may be continued for a longer time depending on the type of heart or lung disease, the amount of damage to the lungs before ECMO was begun, and the presence of any other illnesses or health problems.

Benefits

ECMO can be a life-saving procedure when time is needed for the lungs to recover.

Precautions

Typically, ECMO patients have daily chest x rays and blood work, and constant vital sign monitoring. They are usually placed on a special rotating bed that is designed to decrease pressure on the skin and help move secretions from the lungs.

After the patient is stable on ECMO, the breathing machine settings will be lowered to "rest" settings, which allow the lungs to rest without the risk of too much oxygen or pressure from the ventilator.

Preparation

Before ECMO is begun, the patient receives medication to ease **pain** and restrict movement.

Aftercare

Because infants on ECMO may have been struggling with low oxygen levels before treatment, they may be at higher risk for developmental problems. They will need to be monitored as they grow.

Risks

Bleeding is the biggest risk for ECMO patients, since blood thinners are given to guard against **blood clots**. Bleeding can occur anywhere in the body, but is most serious when it occurs in the brain. This is why doctors periodically perform ultrasound brain scans of anyone on ECMO. **Stroke**, which may be caused by bleeding or blood clots in the brain, has occurred in some patients undergoing ECMO.

If bleeding becomes a problem, the patient may require frequent blood transfusions or operations to control the bleeding. If the bleeding cannot be stopped, ECMO will be withdrawn.

Other risks include infection or vocal cord injury. Some patients develop severe blood infections that cause irreversible damage to vital organs.

There is a small chance that some part of the complex equipment may fail, which could introduce air into the system or affect the patient's blood levels, causing damage or **death** of vital organs (including the brain). For this reason, the ECMO circuit is constantly monitored by a trained technologist.

Resources

OTHER

Introduction to ECMO for Parents. Stanford Medical Center. undated [accessed June 25, 2010]. http://lane.stanford.edu/portals/cvicu/HCP_CV_Tab_1/ecmo_for_parents.pdf

Rodriguez-Cruz, Edwin and Henry Waters, III. Extracorporeal membrane Oxygenation. eMedicine.com February 19, 2010. http://emedicine.medscape.com/article/1818617-overview

ORGANIZATIONS

American Society of Extra-Corporeal Technology, 2209 Dickens Road, Richmond, VA, 23230-2005, (804) 565-636, (804) 282-0090, amsect@amsect.org, http://www.amsect.org.

Extracorporeal Life Support Organization (ELSO), 2600 Plymouth Road, Building 300, Room 303, Ann Arbor, MI, 48109-2800, (734) 998-6601, (734) 998-6602, http://www.elso.med.umich.edu.

Carol A. Turkington
Tish Davidson, AM

Extracorporeal shock-wave *see* **Lithotripsy**

Extrinsic allergic alveolitis *see* **Hypersensitivity pneumonitis**

Eye and orbit sonograms *see* **Eye and orbit ultrasounds**

Eye and orbit ultrasounds

Definition

Ultrasound imaging equipment allows eye specialists (ophthalmologists) to "see" the eye in great detail without the **pain** and risk of exploratory surgery, or the limitations and uncertainty inherent to traditional visual examination. Ultrasound is used to detect and diagnose many eye diseases and injuries, to measure the eye prior to corrective surgery, and directly as a treatment tool.

Purpose

An ophthalmologist uses ultrasonic imaging to help diagnose the underlying cause(s) of a patient's symptoms, to assess the general condition of an injured eye, and to measure the eye prior to corrective surgery. Situations that may call for ultrasonic imaging include:

- Excessive tearing or visible infection. These external symptoms could indicate a serious underlying problem such as a tumor, an internal infection, the presence of a deeply lodged irritant (foreign body), or the effects of a previously unrecognized injury. When presented with general symptoms, ultrasound can speed diagnosis if a serious condition is suspected.

- Impaired vision. Fuzzy vision, poor night vision, restricted (tunnel) vision, blind spots, extreme light sensitivity, and even blindness can all stem from inner eye conditions ranging from glaucoma and cataracts, to retinitis, detached retina, tumors, or impaired blood circulation. Again, high resolution ultrasound can quickly identify causes and pinpoint their location. A special type of ultrasound, known

KEY TERMS

Cataracts—A clouding of the lens of the eye or the material immediately surrounding it, causing blurred vision. For many people it occurs naturally with aging, but may also result from injury.

Glaucoma—A common eye disease characterized by increased fluid pressure in the eye that damages the optic nerve, which carries sensations to the brain. Glaucoma can be caused by another eye disorder, such as a tumor or congenital malformation, or appear without obvious cause, but if untreated it generally leads to blindness.

Intraocular—Literally, within the eye.

Ophthalmologist—A medical doctor specializing in eye care who is generally, but not necessarily, an eye surgeon.

Retina—The third and innermost membrane of the eye, which contains the light-sensitive nerve tissue that leads into the optic nerve and is the primary instument of vision. Inflammation of the retina (retinitis) has many causes, including over-exposure to intense light, diabetes, and syphilis.

---

as Doppler, can even perceive and measure circulation in the tiny blood vessels of the eye.

- Eye trauma. The eye can be damaged by a direct impact or a puncture wound, as a result of a general head trauma, or by intense light exposure. Even when the cause of injury is obvious, ultrasound can reveal the exact type, extent, and location of damage, from deformations and ruptures to internal bleeding, and help to guide emergency care efforts.

- Lens replacement surgery. Exact measurement of the eye's optical dimensions with ultrasound greatly improves the visual outcome for cataract patients receiving permanent synthetic lenses; and for severely myopic patients receiving implanted corrective lenses.

Ophthalmic ultrasound imaging is also used routinely to guide the precise placement of instruments during surgery, and can be used directly for the treatment of glaucoma and tumors of the eye.

Precautions

Ultrasound of the eye, properly performed by qualified personnel using appropriate equipment, has no risks. There is no evidence to suggest that the procedure itself poses any threat to a healthy eye, or worsens the condition of a diseased or injured eye.

Description

Ophthalmic ultrasound equipment sends high frequency pulses of sound into the eye, where they bounce off the boundaries between different structures in the eye and produce a distinctive pattern of echoes. This echo pattern is received and interpreted by a computer to produce an image on a television screen. The time it takes an echo to return to the receiver corresponds to the depth it traveled into the eye.

Single transducer (the sound transmitter/receiver) ultrasound is used to measure distances within the eye. This is A-mode ultrasound. A linear array of transducers in a single small probe, B-mode, provides a picture of a cross section through the eye. Doppler mode ultrasound combines B-mode with the ability to detect and measure the flow of blood in the tiny vessels of the eye.

As a direct treatment tool, the vibrations of high intensity A-mode ultrasound can be used to heat and erode tumors. The same technique can be used to control glaucoma by selectively destroying the cells which produce the fluid that causes the internal pressure of the eye to rise.

The procedure followed in a regular ultrasonic **eye examination** is relatively simple. The patient relaxes in a comfortable chair in a darkened room. Mild anesthetic eye drops are administered and the head is held secure. The ultrasonic probe, coated with a sterile gel to ensure good contact, is lightly pressed against the eye as the images are made. The probe may be applied to the eyelid or directly to the eye, as necessary. The patient feels nothing else, and the whole office procedure takes about 15 minutes.

Preparation

Preparation by the patient is generally unnecessary, although under special circumstances an ophthalmologist may perform pretest procedures. The ophthalmologist and/or ultrasound technician will conduct all preparations at the time of the test.

Aftercare

Patients may experience partial and temporary blurred vision, as well as "eye strain" headaches. These symptoms usually fade within an hour of the procedure, during which time patients should rest their eyes and avoid all activities that require good eyesight, like driving.

Risks

Improperly focused, high-intensity ultrasound could burn and physically disrupt delicate eye tissue and cause injury. This risk is, however, slight and would arise only from improper use, or as a potential side effect of tumor or glaucoma treatment.

Normal results

A normal ultrasound scan would indicate a fully healthy eye. For therapeutic ultrasound, a normal result would be an improvement in the targeted condition, such as shrinking of a tumor or lessening of pressure inside the eye of a glaucoma patient.

Abnormal results

Because diagnostic ultrasound is generally used to investigate symptoms, the results of a scan will often be abnormal and they will detect evidence of an underlying condition.

ORGANIZATIONS

American Academy of Ophthalmology (AAO), P. O. Box 7424, San Francisco, CA, 94120-7424, (415) 561-8500, (415) 561-8500, http://www.aao.org.

American Institute of Ultrasound in Medicine, 14750 Sweitzer Lane, Suite 100, Laurel, MD, 20707-5906, (301) 498-4100, (301) 498-4450, http://www.aium.org.

National Eye Institue, 2020 Vision Place, Bethesda, MD, (301) 496-5248, http://www.nei.nih.gov/.

Kurt Richard Sternlof

Eye cancer

Definition

Eye **cancer** refers to a cancerous growth in any part of the eye. Some eye cancers are considered to be primary tumors, indicating the tumor originated in the eye or the orbit of the eye. Other eye cancers represent metastases from primary cancers elsewhere in the body. The most common type of primary intraocular cancer in adults is intraocular melanoma or melanoma of the eye. The most common type of eye cancer affecting children is **retinoblastoma**.

Demographics

All types of eye cancer are rare in comparison to other cancerous tumors. According to the American Cancer Society, 2,480 people in the United States will be diagnosed with cancer of the eye or orbit in 2010, and 230 persons will die from the disease. Most of these cases of eye cancer will be caused by melanoma. Lymphomas are the second most common tumors of the eye in adults. Most cases of melanoma and lymphomas of the eye begin elsewhere in the body.

Retinoblastoma in children is an extremely rare type of cancer in the United States with about 300 new cases diagnosed each year. The average age at diagnosis is two years of age. This type of cancer is rarely diagnosed in children older than age six. Most of the time the cancer is confined to one eye. However in about one–third of cases, tumors affect both eyes.

Description

Eye cancers can be grouped into three basic categories according to their location in the eye: tumors of the eyelid and conjunctiva; intraocular tumors; and orbital tumors. This article will focus on retinoblastoma, the most common eye cancer in children, and intraocular melanoma, the most common eye cancer in adults.

Retinoblastoma typically begins as a small tumor in the retina, the tissue that lies at the very back of the eye. In growing children, the retina originates from cells called retinoblasts that grow and divide very quickly. These cells eventually become the mature cells of the retina when they stop growing. In the case of retinoblastoma the retinoblasts do not stop growing but, instead, form a tumor that can continue to grow and cause further complications if not treated quickly.

Retinoblastoma typically has three classifications: intraocular, extraocular, and recurrent retinoblastoma. In the intraocular form the cancer can be found in one or both eyes but not in tissue external to the eye. In the extraocular form the cancer has spread outside the eye. It can spread to the tissue surrounding the eye or it can invade other areas of the body. In the recurrent form the cancer returns after previously being treated. It may recur in the eye, its surrounding tissues, or elsewhere in the body.

Intraocular melanoma is a rare cancer overall, yet it is the most common eye cancer seen in adults. Intraocular melanoma occurs when cancer cells are found in the uvea of the eye. The uvea includes the iris (the colored portion of eye), the ciliary body (an eye muscle

Brachytherapy—A type of radiation treatment for cancer in which the source of the radiation is applied directly to the surface of the body.

Carcinogen—A substance that is known to cause cancer.

Conjunctiva—The thin membrane that lines the eyelids.

Cornea—The transparent front portion of the exterior cover of the eye.

Enucleation—Surgical removal of the eyeball.

Iris (plural, irides)—The circular pigmented membrane behind the cornea of the eye that gives the eye its color. The iris surrounds a central opening called the pupil.

Ocular melanoma—A malignant tumor that arises within the structures of the eye. It is the most common eye tumor in adults.

Ophthalmology—The branch of medicine that deals with the diagnosis and treatment of eye disorders.

Orbit—The bony cavity that contains the eyeball.

Pupil—The opening in the center of the iris of the eye that allows light to enter the eye.

Uvea—The middle of the three coats of tissue surrounding the eye, comprising the choroid, iris, and ciliary body. The uvea is pigmented and well supplied with blood vessels.

---

that focuses the lens) and the choroid (found in the back of the eye next to the retina).

Intraocular cancer of the iris usually grows slowly and usually does not spread. The tumor is seen on the iris as a spot that is darker than the surrounding area. Intraocular cancer of the choroid or ciliary body occurs in the back of the eye. This type of cancer is classified by size with a small tumor being two to three mm or smaller and a medium or large tumor being larger than three mm.

Intraocular cancer can spread and become extraocular as well. If not found and treated early enough it can spread to surrounding tissues, the optic nerve or into the orbit (eye socket).

Causes and symptoms

The causes of intraocular melanoma are not yet fully understood. Individuals who appear to be at high risk for the development of intraocular melanoma include:

- individuals with light skin and eye color
- people diagnosed with dysplastic nevus syndrome
- people with abnormal brown spots in the uvea of the eye
- individuals who have been exposed to the sun and/or sunlamps

The symptoms of this type of cancer usually begin with blurred vision and tenderness of the eye. Other symptoms include appearance of floaters in the eye and changes in the position of the eyeball in the eye socket. Advanced symptoms may include loss of vision. Most of the time, these symptoms are painless.

If symptoms persist a person should make an appointment with an eye specialist.

About 75% of cases of retinoblastoma are of the non–hereditary or sporadic type. This type of retinoblastoma affects only one eye.

A form of hereditary or congenital retinoblastoma has been identified. This form of retinoblastoma is also referred to as bilateral retinoblastoma because most of the cases involve cancer in both eyes. However, about 15% of cases of hereditary or congenital retinoblastoma occur in one eye only.

Signs and symptoms associated with retinoblastoma include:

- leukocoria or white papillary reflex, also referred to as cat's eye reflex, the most common sign observed at time of diagnosis
- strabismus, or improper alignment of the eyes, the second most common finding
- poor vision
- red, painful eyes
- white spots on the iris
- orbital inflammation
- glaucoma
- retinal detachment

Diagnosis

The diagnosis of eye cancer is usually made by an ophthalmologist, a doctor who specializes in treating eye disorders. In the case of cancerous growths, the doctor is usually able to see the tumor through the pupil or directly on the iris if the cancer is intraocular melanoma of the iris. Because the doctor can usually readily see the tumor a biopsy is rarely needed.

An ultrasound or a fluorescein **angiography** are two tests doctors use to further diagnose eye cancers. In an ultrasound, sound waves are pointed at the tumor and, depending on how they reflect off the tumor, the doctor can better diagnose the disorder. In a fluorescein angiography a fluorescent dye is injected into the patient's arm. When this dye circulates through the body and reaches the eye a series of rapid pictures are taken through the pupil. The tumor will show up in these photos.

Most retinoblastomas can be diagnosed as part of a detailed **eye examination** by an experienced ophthalmologist. Once a diagnosis is confirmed, imaging tests such as ultrasound, CT or MRI scans, and bone scans may be ordered to help to determine the size of the tumor and to ascertain to what extent the cancer has spread.

Treatment

The modalities used to treat intraocular melanoma depend on the size of the tumor and on how far the tumor has spread. If the tumor is in the advanced stages and there is little hope of regaining vision, the most effective treatment is an enucleation, the removal of the eye. Enucleation is a drastic treatment option and is avoided if possible. Other eye surgeries include the following:

- choroidectomy: removal of part of the choroid
- iridectomy: removal of part of the iris
- iridocyclectomy: removal of parts of the ciliary body and parts of iris
- iridotrabeculectomy: removal of parts of the supporting tissues around the cornea and iris

In cases in which the tumor is small and there is a good chance that vision will be restored, less drastic measures than the above surgeries are taken. Radiation and **chemotherapy** are two courses of treatment that may help to destroy an existing tumor and prevent its spread to other areas of the body. **Radiation therapy** can utilize external beam radiation therapy or brachytherapy approaches. Most cases of intraocular melanoma respond poorly to chemotherapy, however.

The most common type of laser treatment used for intraocular melanoma is transpupillary thermotherapy. This procedure uses infrared light to heat and destroy the tumor in one to three treatment sessions in most people.

Treatment for retinoblastoma is best performed by health care providers who are experienced in the care of young children with this very rare type of cancer. Most of the time the most experienced practitioners can be found at major children's cancer centers and hospitals.

The treatment options for retinoblastoma depend on the stage of the cancer and can include one or more of the following modalities:

- surgery, which may include enucleation of one or both eyes if the tumor is large and/or if vision has been permanently destroyed
- radiation therapy utilizing brachytherapy or external beam radiation therapy
- photocoagulation, a procedure which employs the use of lasers to treat patients with small tumors
- cryotherapy, a treatment that utilizes probes that have been frozen to very low temperatures. The probes freeze and destroy small tumors
- thermotherapy, which utilizes heat to kill small tumors
- chemotherapy, which may be used to reduce the size of large tumors before other treatment modalities are used. A common chemotherapy regimen used in the treatment of retinoblastoma is a combination of the drugs carboplatin and vincristine. Other chemotherapy drugs which may be utilized include cisplatin, etoposide, teniposide, cyclophosphamide, and doxorubicin.

Prognosis

Most forms of retinoblastoma and intraocular melanoma are treatable. Enucleation can usually be avoided if the tumor is found early enough. In addition, primary cancers of the eye have a relatively low mortality rate if treated promptly.

Up to 90% of children diagnosed with retinoblastoma can be cured if the cancer is diagnosed and treated in early stages.

Prevention

Retinoblastoma is not considered a preventable disease. Individuals with hereditary or congenital retinoblastoma diagnosed in family members should notify their health care providers and may be monitored more frequently to detect any early signs of disease.

As intraocular melanoma is diagnosed more frequently in individuals with light skin and eyes, these individuals should have frequent eye exams conducted by experienced ophthalmologists. Minimizing exposure to the sun and to artificial sources of sunlight such as **tanning** beds and sunlamps is also recommended to decrease the possibility for development of intraocular melanoma. Individuals with abnormal brown spots on the uvea of the eye should also be closely monitored by experienced ophthalmologists for any changes that would indicate a progression to a cancerous tumor in the eye.

Resources

BOOKS

American Joint Committee on Cancer. "Malignant Melanoma of the Uvea." In *AJCC Cancer Staging Manual*, 7th ed. New York, NY: Springer, 2010.

Karcioglu, Z.A., and B.G. Haik. "Eye, Orbit, and Adnexal Structures." In: Abeloff, M.D., et al., editors. *Abeloff's Clinical Oncology*, 4th ed. Philadelphia, PA: Elsevier, 2008.

PERIODICALS

Gear, H., H. Williams, E. G. Kemp, and F. Roberts. "BRAF Mutations in Conjunctival Melanoma." *Investigative Ophthalmology and Visual Science* 45 (August 2004): 2484–88.

Grimm, S.A., et al. "Primary Ocular Lymphoma: An International Primiary Nervous System Lymphoma Collaborative Group Report." *Annals of Oncology*. 18 (2007)1851–55.

Honavar, S.G., and A.D. Singh, A.D. "Management of Advanced Retinoblastoma." *Ophthalmology Clinics of North America*. 18(1) (March 2005): 65–73.

Shields, C. L., H. Demirci, E. Karatza, and J. A. Shields. "Clinical Survey of 1643 Melanocytic and Nonmelanocytic Conjunctival Tumors." *Ophthalmology* 111 (September 2004): 1747–54.

ORGANIZATIONS

American Academy of Ophthalmology, PO Box 7424, San Francisco, CA, 94120–7424, http://www.aao.org.

American Cancer Society, (800) 227–2345, http://www.cancer.org.

Canadian Ophthalmological Society, 610–1525 Carling Ave., Ottawa, ON, K1Z 8R9, http://www.eyesite.ca.

National Eye Institute, Information Office, 31 Center Dr., MSC 2510, Bethesda, MD, 20892–2510, http://www.nei.nih.gov.

Ocular Oncology Service, Wills Eye Hospital, 840 Walnut St., Suite 1440, Philadelphia, PA, 19107, http://www.eyecancerinfo.com.

Thomas Scott Eagan
Ronald Watson, PhD
Rebecca J. Frey, PhD
Melinda Granger Oberleitner,
RN, DNS, APRN, CNS

Eye examination

Definition

An eye examination is a series of tests that measure a person's ocular health and visual status, to detect abnormalities in the components of the visual system, and to determine how well the person can see.

Purpose

An eye examination is performed by an ophthalmologist, (M.D. or D.O. -doctor of **osteopathy**), or an optometrist (O.D.) to determine if there are any pre-existing or potential vision problems. Eye exams may also reveal the presence of many non-eye diseases. Many systemic diseases can affect the eyes, and since the blood vessels on the retina are observed during the exam, certain problems may be uncovered (e.g., high blood pressure or diabetes).

Infants should be examined by a physician to detect any physical abnormalities. Frequency of eye exams then generally differs with age and the health of the person. Eye exams can be performed in infants, and if a problem is noted the infant can be seen, generally by a pediatric ophthalmologist. A child with no symptoms should have an eye exam at age three. Early exams are important because permanent decreases in vision (e.g., **amblyopia**, also called lazy eye) can occur if not treated early (usually by ages 6–9). Again, with no other symptoms, the second exam should take place before first grade. After first grade, the American Optometric Association recommends an eye exam every two years; ages 19–40, every two to three years;

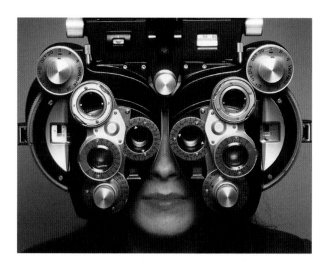

A woman looking through a refractor. *(John Greim/Photo Researchers, Inc.)*

ages 41–60, every two years; and annually after that. However, these are recommendations for healthy people with no risk factors. Patients should ask their doctors how often they should come for exams. Some patients have risk factors for eye disease (e.g., people with diabetes or a family history of eye disease; African Americans, who are at higher risk for glaucoma) and may need more frequent checkups. Also, if children seem to be having trouble in school, problems with reading, rubbing their eyes when reading, etc., an eye exam may be necessary sooner.

Precautions

The examiner needs to know if the patient is taking any medications or has any existing health conditions. Some medications, even over-the-counter (OTC) medications can affect vision or even interfere with the eyedrops the doctor may use during the exam. Certain eyedrops would not be used if the patient has **asthma**, heart problems, or other conditions.

The patient may need someone to drive them home in case the eyes were dilated. Bringing sunglasses to the exam may also help decrease the glare from light until the dilating drops wear off.

Description

An eye examination, given by an ophthalmologist or optometrist, costs about $100. It may or may not be covered by insurance. It begins with information from the patient (case history) and continues with a set of primary tests, plus additional specialized tests given as needed, dictated by the outcomes of initial testing and the patient's age. The primary tests can be divided into two groups, those that evaluate the physical state of the eyes and surrounding areas, and those that measure the ability to see.

The order of the tests for the exam may differ from doctor to doctor, however, most exams will include the following procedures:

Information gathering and initial observations

The examiner will take eye and medical histories that include the patient's chief complaint, any past eye disorders, all medications being taken (e.g., OTC medications, **antibiotics**, and birth control pills), any blood relatives with eye disorders, and any systemic disorders the patient may have. The patient should also tell the doctor about hobbies and work conditions. This information helps in modifying prescriptions and lets the doctor know how the patient uses his or her eyes. For example, using a computer screen vs. construction work, the working distance of a computer screen may affect the prescription; the construction worker needs protective eyewear.

The patient should bring their current pair of glasses to the exam. The doctor can get the prescription from the glasses by using an instrument called a lensometer.

Visual acuity examination

Visual acuity measures how clearly the patient can see. It is measured for each eye separately, with and without the current prescription. It is usually measured with a Snellen eye chart, a poster with lines of different-sized letters, each line with a number at the side denoting the distance from which a person with normal vision can read that line. Other kinds of eye charts with identifiable figures are available for children or anyone unfamiliar with the Roman alphabet. These charts are made to be placed at a certain distance (usually 20 ft) from the person being tested. At this distance, people with normal vision can read a certain line (usually the lowest), marked the 20/20 line; these people are said to have 20/20 vision. For people who can't read the smallest line, the examiner assigns a ratio based on the smallest line they can read. The first number (numerator) of the ratio is the distance between the chart and the patient, and the second number (denominator) is the distance where a person with normal vision would be able to read that line. The ratio 20/40 means the patient can see at 20 ft. what people with normal vision can see at 40 ft. away.

When a patient is unable to read any lines on the chart, they are moved closer until they can read the line with the largest letters. The acuity is still measured the same way. A ratio of 5/200 means the person being tested can see at 5 ft what a normal person can see 200 ft.

When a patient cannot read the chart at all, the examiner may hold up some fingers and ask the patient to count them at various distances, and records the result as "counting fingers" at the distance of recognition. If the patient cannot count the examiner's fingers at any distance, the examiner determines if the patient can see hand movements. If so, the result is recorded as "hand movements." If not, the examiner determines if the patient can detect light from a penlight. If the patient can detect the light but not its direction, the result is recorded at "light perception." If the patient can recognize its direction, the result is recorded as "light projection." If the patient cannot detect the light at all, the result is recorded as "no light perception."

Eye movement examination and cover tests

The examiner asks the patient to look up and down, and to the right and left to see if the patient can move the eyes to their full extent. The examiner asks the patient to stare at an object, then quickly covers one eye and notes any movement in the eye that remains uncovered. This procedure is repeated with the other eye. This, and another similar cover test, helps to determine if there is an undetected eye turn or problem with fixation. The doctor may also have the patient look at a pen and follow it as it is moved close to the eyes. This checks convergence.

Iris and pupil examination

The doctor checks the pupil's response to light (if it dilates and constricts appropriately). The iris is viewed for symmetry and physical appearance. The iris is checked more thoroughly later using a slit lamp.

Refractive error determination-Refraction

The examiner will determine the refractive error and obtain a prescription for corrective lenses for people whose visual acuity is less than 20/20. An instrument called a phoropter, which the patient sits behind, is generally used (sometimes the refraction can be done with a trial frame that the patient wears). The phoropter is equipped with many lenses that allow the examiner to test many combinations of corrections to learn which correction allows the patient to see the eye chart most clearly. This is the part of the exam when the doctor usually says, "Which is better, one or two?" The phoropter also contains prisms, and sometimes the doctor will intentionally make the patient see double. This may help in determining a slight eye turn. The exam will check vision at distance and near (reading).

A prescription for corrective lenses can also be supplied by automated refracting devices, which measure the necessary refraction by shining a light into the eye and observing the reflected light. Another objective way to obtain a prescription is using a hand-held retinoscope. As in the automated method just mentioned, the doctor shines a light in the patient's eyes and can determine an objective prescription. This is helpful in young children or infants.

Sometimes drops will be instilled in the patient's eyes before this part of the exam. The drops may relax accommodation so that the refraction will be more accurate. This is helpful in children and people who are farsighted.

After the refraction and other visual status tests, for example color tests or binocularity tests (can the patient see 3-D, or have depth perception), the doctor will check the health of the eyes and surrounding areas. The main instruments used are the ophthalmoscope and the slit lamp.

Ophthalmoscopic examination

These observations are best accomplished after dilating the pupils and require an ophthalmoscope. The ophthalmoscope most frequently used is a called a *direct ophthalmoscope*. It is a hand-held illuminated 15X multi-lens magnifier that lets the examiner view the inside back area of the eye (fundus). The retina, blood vessels, optic nerve, and other structures are examined.

Slit lamp examination

The slit lamp is a microscope with a light source that can be adjusted. This magnifies the external and some internal structures of the eyes. The lid and lid margin, cornea, iris, pupil, conjunctiva, sclera, and lens are examined. The slit lamp is also used in contact lens evaluations. A little probe called a tonometer may be used at this time to check the pressure of the eyes. A colored eyedrop may be instilled immediately prior to this test. The drop has a local anesthetic so the patient won't feel the probe touch the eye. It is a quick procedure.

Visual field measurement

A perimeter, the instrument for measuring visual fields, is a hollow hemisphere, equipped with a light source that projects dots of light over the inside surface. The patient's head is positioned so that the eye being tested is at the center of the sphere and (about 13 in. 33 cm) from all points on the inside surface of the hemisphere. The patient stares straight ahead at an image on the center of the surface and signals whenever he or she detects a flash of light. The perimeter records which flashes are seen and which are missed and maps the patient's field of vision and blindspots.

Intraocular pressure (IOP) measurement

Tonometers are used to measure IOP. Some tonometers measure pressure by expelling a puff of air (noncontact tonometer) towards the eyeball from a very short distance. Other tonometers are placed directly on the cornea. The noncontact tonometers are not as accurate as the contact tonometers and are sometimes used for screenings.

Amblyopia—Decreased visual acuity, usually in one eye, in the absence of any structural abnormality in the eye.

Conjunctiva—The mucous membrane that covers the white part of the eyes (sclera) and lines the eyelids.

Cornea—Clear outer covering of the front of the eye.

Floaters—Translucent specks that float across the visual field, due to small objects floating in the vitreous humor.

Fundus—The inside of an organ. In the eye, refers to the back area that can be seen with the ophthalmoscope.

Glaucoma—There are many types of glaucoma. Glaucoma results in optic nerve damage and a decreased visual field and blindness if not treated. It is usually associated with increased IOP, but that is not always the case. The three factors associated with glaucoma are increased IOP, a change in the optic nerve head, and changes in the visual field.

Gonioscope—An instrument used to inspect the eye (e.g., the anterior chamber). It consists of a magnifier and a lens equipped with mirrors; it's placed on the patient's cornea.

Iris—The colored ring just behind the cornea and in front of the lens that controls the amount of light sent to the retina.

Macula—The central part of the retina where the rods and cones are densest.

Ophthalmoscope—An instrument designed to view structures in the back of the eye.

Optic nerve—The nerve that carries visual messages from the retina to the brain.

Pupil—The circular opening that looks like a black hole in the middle of the iris.

Retina—The inner, light-sensitive layer of the eye containing rods and cones; transforms the image it receives into electrical messages which are then sent to the brain via the optic nerve.

Sclera—The tough, fibrous, white outer protective covering that surrounds the eye.

Slit lamp—A microscope that projects a linear slit beam of light onto the eye; allows viewing of the conjunctiva, cornea, iris, aqueous humor, lens, and eyelid.

Tonometer—An instrument that measures intraocular pressure (IOP).

Ultrasonography—A method of obtaining structural information about internal tissues and organs where an image is produced because different tissues bounce back ultrasonic waves differently.

Completing the evaluation with additional tests

Depending upon the results other tests may be necessary. These can include, but are not limited to binocular indirect ophthalmoscopy, gonioscopy, color tests, contrast sensitivity testing, ultasonography, and others. The patient may have to return for additional visits.

Results

External observations

INITIAL OBSERVATIONS AND SLIT LAMP EXAM. Some general observations the doctor may be looking for include: head tilt; drooping eyelids (**ptosis**); eye turns; red eyes (injection); eye movement; size, shape, and color of the iris; clarity of the cornea, anterior chamber, and lens. The anterior chamber lies behind the cornea and in front of the iris. If it appears cloudy or if cells can be seen in it during the slit lamp exam an inflammation may be present. A narrow anterior chamber may put the patient at risk for glaucoma. A clouding of the normally clear lens is called a cataract.

Internal observations

OPHTHALMOSCOPIC EXAM. The observations include, but are not limited to the retina, blood vessels, and optic nerve. The optic nerve enters the back of the eye and can be checked for swelling or other problems. The blood vessels can be viewed as can the retina. The macula is a 3–5 mm area in the back of the eye and is responsible for central vision. The fovea is a small area located within the macula and is responsible for sharp vision. When a person looks at something, they are pointing the fovea at the object. Changes in the macular area can be observed with the ophthalmoscope. Retinal tears or detachments can also be seen.

Visual ability

VISUAL ACUITY. The refraction will determine the refractive status for each eye for distance and for near. A prescription for glasses is made after taking many things into consideration. The eye doctor may alter a prescription based upon many factors. Different materials for glasses may be suggested. For example, polycarbonate may be suggested for children or people active in sports because it is very impact resistant. Bifocals, trifocals, single-vision spectacles, and **contact lenses** are also options.

VISUAL FIELDS. A normal visual field extends about 60° upward, about 75° downward, about 65° toward the nose, and about 100° toward the ear and has one blind spot close to the center. Defects in the visual field signify damage to the retina, optic nerve, or the neurological visual pathway.

Seeing clearly does not necessarily mean the eyes are healthy or that the eyes are working together as a team. Regular checkups can detect abnormalities, hopefully before a problem arises. The eye doctor can suggest ways to help protect the eyes and vision (e.g., safety goggles, ultraviolet (UV) coatings on lenses). A person should also have an eye exam if they notice a change in vision, eyestrain, blur, flashes of light, a sudden onset of floaters (little dots), distortion of objects, double vision, redness, **pain** or discharge.

ORGANIZATIONS

American Academy of Ophthalmology (AAO), P. O. Box 7424, San Francisco, CA, 94120-7424, (415) 561-8500, (415) 561-8500, http://www.aao.org.

American Optometric Association, 243 North Lindbergh Blvd., St. Louis, MO, 63141, (314) 991-4100, (314) 991-4101, (800) 365-2219, http://www.aoa.org/.

Lorraine Lica, PhD

Eye exercises *see* **Vision training**

Eye glasses and contact lenses

Definition

Eyeglasses and contact lenses are devices that correct refractive errors in vision. Eyeglass lenses are mounted in frames worn on the face, sitting mostly on the ears and nose, so that the lenses are positioned in front of the eyes. Contact lenses appear to be worn in direct contact with the cornea, but they actually float on a layer of tears that separates them from the cornea.

Purpose

The purpose of eyeglasses and contact lenses is to correct or improve the vision of people with nearsightedness (**myopia**), farsightedness (**hyperopia**), **presbyopia**, and **astigmatism**.

Precautions

People allergic to certain plastics should not wear contact lenses or eyeglass frames or lenses manufactured from that type of plastic. People allergic to nickel should not wear Flexon frames. People at risk of being in accidents that might shatter glass lenses should wear plastic lenses, preferably polycarbonate. (Lenses made from polycarbonate, the same type of plastic used for the space shuttle windshield, are about 50 times stronger than other lens materials.) Also, people at risk of receiving electric shock should avoid metal frames.

People employed in certain occupations may be prohibited from wearing contact lenses, or may be required to wear safety eyewear over the contact lenses. Some occupations, such as construction or auto repair, may require safety lenses and safety frames. Physicians and employers should be consulted for recommendations.

Description

Eyes are examined by optometrists (O.D.) or by ophthalmologists (M.D. or D.O.—doctor of **osteopathy**). Prescriptions, if necessary, are then given to patients for glasses. The glasses are generally made by an optician. A separate contact lens-fitting exam is necessary if the patient wants contact lenses, because an eyeglass prescription is not the same as a contact lens prescription.

Eyeglasses

More than 140 million people in the United States wear eyeglasses. People whose eyes have refractive errors do not see clearly without glasses, because the light emitted from the objects they are observing does not come into focus on their retinas. For people who are farsighted, images come into focus behind the retina; for people who are nearsighted, images come into focus in front of the retina.

LENSES. Lenses work by changing the direction of light so that images come into focus on the retina. The greater the index of refraction of the lens material and the greater the difference in the curvature between the two surfaces of the lens, the greater the change in direction of light that passes through it, and the greater the correction.

Lenses can be unifocal, with one correction for all distances, or they can be correct for more than one distance (multifocal). One type of multifocal, the bifocal, has an area of the lens (usually at the bottom) that corrects for nearby objects (about 14 in from the eyes); the remainder of the lens corrects for distant objects (about 20 ft from the eyes). Another type of multi-focal, a trifocal, has an area in-between that corrects for intermediate distances (usually about 28 in). Conventional bifocals and trifocals have visible lines between the areas of different correction; however, lenses where the correction gradually changes from one area to the other, without visible lines, have been available since the 1970s. Such lenses are sometimes called progressives or no-line bifocals.

To be suitable for eyeglass lenses, a material must be transparent, without bubbles, and have a high index of refraction. The greater the index of refraction, the thinner the lens can be. Lenses are made from either glass or plastic (hard resin). The advantage of plastic is that it is lightweight and more impact resistant than glass. The advantage of glass is that it is scratch resistant and provides the clearest possible vision.

Glass was the first material to be used for eyeglass lenses, and was used for several hundred years before plastic was introduced.

Optical-quality acrylic was introduced for eyeglass use in the early 1940s, but because it was easily scratched, brittle, and discolored rapidly, it did not supplant glass as the material of choice. Furthermore, it wasn't suitable for people with large refractive errors. A plastic called CR-39, introduced in the 1960s, was more suitable. Today, eyeglass wearers can also choose between polycarbonate, which is the most impact-resistant material available for eyewear, and polyurethane, which has exceptional optical qualities and higher refraction than the conventional plastics even glass. Patients with high prescriptions should ask about high index material options for their lenses. Aspheric lenses are also useful for high prescriptions. They are flatter and lighter than conventional lenses.

There are many lenses and lens-coating options for individual needs, including coatings that block the ultraviolet (UV) light or UV and blue light, which have been found to be harmful to the eyes. Such coatings are not needed on polycarbonate lenses, which already have UV protection. UV coatings are particularly important on sunglasses and ski goggles. Sunglasses, when nonprescription, should be labeled with an indication that they block out 99–100% of both UV-A and UV-B rays.

There are anti-scratch coatings that increase the surface hardness of lenses (an important feature when using plastic lenses) and anti-reflective (AR) coatings that eliminate almost all glare and allow other people to see the eyes of the wearer. AR coatings may be particularly helpful to people who use computers or who drive at night. Mirror coatings that prevent other people from seeing the wearer's eyes are also available. There is a whole spectrum of tints, from light tints to darker tints, used in sunglasses. Tint, however, does not block out UV rays, so a UV coating is needed. Polaroid lenses that block out much of the reflected light also allow better vision in sunny weather and are helpful for people who enjoy boating. Photosensitive (photochromatic) lenses that darken in the presence of bright light are handy for people who don't want to carry an extra set of glasses. Photochromatic lenses are available in glass and plastic.

FRAMES. Frames can be made from metal or plastic, and they can be rimless. There is an almost unlimited variety of shapes, colors, and sizes. The type and degree of refractive correction in the lens determine to some extent the type of frame most suitable. Some lenses are too thick to fit in metal rims, and some large-correction prescriptions are best suited to frames with small-area lenses.

Rimless frames are the least noticeable type, and they are lightweight because the nosepiece and temples are attached directly to the lenses, eliminating the weight of the rims. They tend to not be as sturdy as frames with rims, so they are not a good choice for people who frequently remove their glasses and put them on again. They are also not very suitable for lenses that correct a high degree of farsightedness, because such lenses are thin at the edges.

Metal frames are less noticeable than plastic, and they are lightweight. They are available in solid gold, gold-filled, anodized aluminum, nickel, silver, stainless steel, and now titanium and titanium alloy. Until the late 1980s, when titanium-nickel alloy and titanium frames were introduced, metal frames were, in general, more fragile than plastic frames. The titanium frames, however, are very strong and lightweight. An alloy of titanium and nickel, called Flexon, is not only strong and lightweight, but returns to its original shape after being twisted or dented. It is not perfect for everyone, though, because some people are sensitive to its nickel. Flexon frames are also relatively expensive.

Plastic frames are durable, can accommodate just about any lens prescription, and are available in a wide range of prices. They are also offered in a variety of plastics (including acrylic, epoxy, cellulose acetate, cellulose propionate, polyamide, and nylon) and in different colors, shapes, and levels of resistance to breakage. Epoxy frames are resilient and return to their original shape after being deformed, so they do not need to be adjusted as frequently as other types.

Nylon frames are almost unbreakable. They revert to their original shape after extreme trauma and distortion; because of this property, though, they cannot be readjusted after they are manufactured.

FIT. The patient should have the distance between the eyes (PD) measured, so that the optical centers of the lenses will be in front of the patient's pupils. Bifocal heights also have to be measured with the chosen frame in place and adjusted on the patient. Again, this is so the lenses will be positioned correctly. If not positioned correctly, the patient may experience eyestrain or other problems. This can occur with over-the-counter reading glasses. The distance between the lenses is for a "standard" person. Generally, this will not be a problem, but if a patient is sensitive or has more closely set eyes, for example, it may pose a problem. Persons buying ready-made sunglasses or reading glasses should hold them up to see if they appear clear. They should also hold the lenses to see an object with straight lines reflected off of the lenses. If the lines don't appear straight, the lenses may be warped or inferior.

Patients may sometimes need a few days to adjust to a new prescription; however, problems should be reported, because the glasses may need to be rechecked.

Contact lenses

More than 32 million people in the United States wear these small lenses that fit on top of the cornea. They provide a field of view unobstructed by eyeglass frames; they do not fog up or get splattered, so it is possible to see well while walking in the rain; and they are less noticeable than any eyeglass style. On the other hand, they take time to get accustomed to; require more measurements for fitting; require many follow-up visits to the eye doctor; can lead to complications such as infections and corneal damage; and may not correct astigmatism as well as eyeglasses, especially if the astigmatism is severe.

Originally, hard contact lenses were made of a material called PMMA. Although still available, the more common types of contact lenses are listed below:

- Rigid gas-permeable (RGP) daily-wear lenses are made of plastic that does not absorb water but allows oxygen to get from the atmosphere to the cornea. (This is important because the cornea has no blood supply and needs to get its oxygen from the atmosphere through the film of tears that moves beneath the lens.) They must be removed and cleaned each night.

- Rigid gas-permeable (RGP) extended-wear lenses are made from plastic that also does not absorb water but is more permeable to oxygen than the plastic used for daily-wear lenses. They can be worn up to a week.

- Daily wear soft lenses are made of plastic that is permeable to oxygen and absorbs water; therefore, they are soft and flexible. These lenses must be removed and cleaned each night, and they do not correct all vision problems. Soft lenses are easier to get used to than rigid lenses, but are more prone to tears and do not last as long.

- Extended-wear soft lenses are highly permeable to oxygen, are flexible by virtue of their ability to absorb water, and can usually be worn for up to one week. They do not correct all vision problems. There is more of a risk of infection with extended-wear lenses than with daily-wear lenses.

- Extended-wear disposable lenses are soft lenses worn continually for up to six days and then discarded, with no need for cleaning.

- Planned-replacement soft lenses are daily wear lenses that are replaced on a regular schedule, which is usually every two weeks, monthly, or quarterly. They must also be cleaned.

Soft contact lenses come in a variety of materials. There are also different kinds of RGP and soft multifocal contact lenses available. Monovision, where one contact lens corrects for distance vision while the other corrects for near vision, may be an option for presbyopic patients. Monovision, however, may affect depth perception and may not be appropriate for everyone. Contact lenses also come in a variety of tints. Soft contacts are available that can make eyes appear a different color. Even though such lenses have no prescription, they must still be fitted and checked to make sure that an eye infection does not occur. People should never wear someone else's contact lenses. This can lead to infection or damage to the eye.

Tiny, surgically implanted contact lenses may one day replace eyeglasses, contact lenses and **laser surgery** for some patients with extreme nearsightedness. Called intraocular lenses, they were still investigational in the spring of 2004, and although they are surgically installed, they can be removed. Researchers expected FDA approval in 2004.

Aftercare

Contact lens wearers must be examined periodically by their eye doctors to make sure that the lenses fit properly and that there is no infection. Infection and lenses that do not fit properly can damage the cornea. Patients can be allergic to certain solutions that are used to clean or lubricate the lenses. For that reason, patients should not randomly switch products without speaking

KEY TERMS

Astigmatism—Assymetric vision defects due to irregularities in the cornea.

Cornea—The clear outer covering of the front of the eye.

Index of refraction—A constant number for any material for any given color of light that is an indicator of the degree of the bending of the light caused by that material.

Lens—A device that bends light waves.

Permeable—Capable of allowing substances to pass through.

Polycarbonate—A very strong type of plastic often used in safety glasses, sport glasses, and children's eyeglasses. Polycarbonate lenses have approximately 50 times the impact resistance of glass lenses.

Polymer—A substance formed by joining smaller molecules. For example, plastic, acrylic, cellulose acetate, cellulose propionate, nylon, etc.

Presbyopia—A condition affecting people over the age of 40 where the system of accommodation that allows focusing of near objects fails to work because of age-related hardening of the lens of the eye.

Retina—The inner, light-sensitive layer of the eye containing rods and cones; transforms the image it receives into electrical messages sent to the brain via the optic nerve.

Ultraviolet (UV) light—Part of the electromagnetic spectrum with a wavelength just below that of visible light. It is damaging to living material, especially eyes and DNA.

with their doctor. Contact lens wearers should seek immediate attention if they experience eye **pain**, a burning sensation, red eyes, intolerable sensitivity to light, cloudy vision, or an inability to keep the eyes open.

To avoid infection, it is important for contact lens wearers to exactly follow their instructions for lens insertion and removal, as well as cleaning. Soft contact lens wearers should never use tap water to rinse their lenses or to make up solutions. All contact lens wearers should also always have a pair of glasses and a carrying case for their contacts with them, in case the contacts have to be removed due to eye irritation.

Risks

Wearing contact lenses increases the risk of corneal damage and eye infections.

Normal results

The normal expectation is that people will achieve 20/20 vision while wearing corrective lenses. A new technology for customized eyeglasses patented in 2004 claims to achieve exceptional vision assessment and 20/10 acuity by using wavefront measurements and precise parameters to produce measurements such as pupil size and distance, along with other customized lens and frame features.

Resources

PERIODICALS

Asp, Karen. "Implanted Contact Lenses." *Prevention* (June 2004): 68.

"Patent Issued for Z-lens Wavefront Guided, Customized Eyeglasses." *Medical Devices & Surgical Technology Week* (April 18, 2004): 150.

OTHER

Contact Lens Council. http://www.contactlenscouncil.org.

ORGANIZATIONS

American Academy of Ophthalmology (AAO), P. O. Box 7424, San Francisco, CA, 94120-7424, (415) 561-8500, (415) 561-8500, http://www.aao.org.

American Optometric Association, 243 North Lindbergh Blvd., St. Louis, MO, 63141, (314) 991-4100, (314) 991-4101, (800) 365-2219, http://www.aoa.org/.

Optician Association of America, 678 Parkside Drive, Palatine, IL, 60067, (847) 202-1411, http://www.eyewebmasters.com.

Lorraine Lica, PhD
Teresa G. Odle

Eye muscle surgery

Definition

Eye muscle surgery is surgery to weaken, strengthen, or reposition any of the muscles that move the eyeball (the extraocular muscles).

Purpose

The purpose of eye muscle surgery is generally to align the pair of eyes so that they gaze in the same

KEY TERMS

Botulinum toxin (botulin)—A neurotoxin made by *Clostridium botulinum*; causes paralysis in high doses, but is used medically in small, localized doses to treat disorders associated with involuntary muscle contraction and spasms, in addition to strabismus.

Conjunctiva—The mucous membrane that covers the eyes and lines the eyelids.

Extraocular muscles—The muscles (lateral rectus, medial rectus, inferior rectus, superior rectus, superior oblique, and inferior oblique) that move the eyeball.

Orbit—The cavity in the skull containing the eyeball; formed from seven bones: frontal, maxillary, sphenoid, lacrimal, zygomatic, ethmoid, and palatine.

Retina—The inner, light-sensitive layer of the eye containing rods and cones; transforms the image it receives into electrical messages sent to the brain via the optic nerve.

Sclera—The tough, fibrous, white outer protective covering of the eyeball.

Strabismus—A disorder where the two eyes do not point in the same direction.

direction and move together as a team, either to improve appearance or to aid in the development of binocular vision in a young child. To achieve binocular vision, the goal is to align the eyes so that the location of the image on the retina of one eye corresponds to the location of the image on the retina of the other eye.

In addition, sometimes eye muscle surgery can help people with other eye disorders (**nystagmus** and Duane syndrome, for example).

Precautions

Depth perception (stereopsis) develops around the age of three months old. For successful development of binocular vision and the ability to perceive three-dimensionally, the surgery should not be postponed past the age of four. The earlier the surgery the better the outcome, so an early diagnosis is important. Surgery may even be performed before two years old. After surgery, if binocular vision is to develop, corrective lenses and eye exercises (vision therapy) will probably be necessary.

Description

The extraocular muscles attach via tendons to the sclera (the white, opaque, outer protective covering of the eyeball) at different places just behind an imaginary equator circling the top, bottom, left, and right of the eye. The other end of each of these muscles attaches to a part of the orbit (the eye socket in the skull). These muscles enable the eyes to move up, down, to one side or the other, or any angle in between.

Normally both eyes move together, receive the same image on corresponding locations on both retinas, and the brain fuses these images into one three-dimensional image. The exception is in **strabismus** which is a disorder where one or both eyes deviate out of alignment, most often outwardly (exotropia) or toward the nose (esotropia). The brain now receives two different images, and either suppresses one or the person sees double (diplopia). This deviation can be adjusted by weakening or strengthening the appropriate muscles to move the eyes toward the center. For example, if an eye turns upward, the muscle at the bottom of the eye could be strengthened.

Rarely, eye muscle surgery is performed on people with nystagmus or Duane syndrome. Nystagmus is a condition where one or both eyes move rapidly or oscillate; it can sometimes be helped by moving the eyes to the position of least oscillation. Duane syndrome is a disorder where there is limited horizontal eye movement; it can sometimes be relieved by surgery to weaken an eye muscle.

There are two methods to alter extraocular muscles. Traditional surgery can be used to strengthen, weaken, or reposition an extraocular muscle. The surgeon first makes an incision in the conjunctiva (the clear membrane covering the sclera), then puts a suture into the muscle to prevent it from getting lost and loosens the muscle from the eyeball with a surgical hook. During a resection, the muscle is detached from the sclera, a piece of muscle is removed so the muscle is now shorter, and the muscle is reattached to the same place. This strengths the muscle. In a recession, the muscle is made weaker by repositioning it. More than one extraocular eye muscle might be operated on at the same time.

Another way of weakening eye muscles, using botulinum toxin injected into the muscle, was introduced in the early 1980s. Although the botulinum toxin wears off, the realignment may be permanent, depending upon whether neurological connections for binocular vision were established during the time the toxin was active. This technique can also be used to adjust a muscle after traditional surgery.

The cost of eye muscle surgery is about $2,000–$4,000, and about 700,000 surgeries are performed annually in the United States.

Preparation

Patients should make sure their doctors are aware of any medications that they are taking, even over-the-counter medications. Patients should not take **aspirin**, or any other blood-thinning medications for ten days prior to surgery, and should not eat or drink after midnight the night before.

Aftercare

Patients will need someone to drive them home after their surgery. They should continue to avoid aspirin and other non-steroidal anti-inflammatory agents for an additional three days, but they can take **acetaminophen** (e.g., Tylenol). Patients should discuss this with the surgeon to be clear what medications they can or cannot take. **Pain** will subside after two to three days, and patients can resume most normal activities within a few days. Again, this may vary with the patient and the patient should discuss returning to normal activity with the surgeon. They should not get their eyes wet for three to four days and should refrain from swimming for 10 days. Operated eyes will be red for about two weeks.

Risks

As with any surgery, there are risks involved. Eye muscle surgery is relatively safe, but very rarely a cut muscle gets lost and can not be retrieved. This, and other serious reactions, including those caused by anesthetics, can result in vision loss in the affected eye. Occasionally, retinal or nerve damage occurs. Double vision is not uncommon after eye muscle surgery. As mentioned earlier, glasses or vision therapy may be necessary.

Normal results

Cosmetic improvement is likely with success rate estimates varying from about 65–85%. According to the best statistics, binocular vision is improved in young children about 35% of the time. There is no improvement, or the condition worsens 15–35% of the time. A second operation may rectify less-than-perfect outcomes.

Resources

OTHER

Groves, Nancy. "One-step process is beneficial: however, surgical techniques need to be modified and patients chosen carefully." *Ophthalmology Times* (June 15, 2010): 56.

ORGANIZATIONS

American Academy of Ophthalmology (AAO), P. O. Box 7424, San Francisco, CA, 94120-7424, (415) 561-8500, (415) 561-8500, http://www.aao.org.
American Academy of Pediatric Ophthalmology and Strabismus (AAPOS), PO Box 193832, San Francisco, CA, 94119-3832, (415) 561-8505, (415) 561-8531, aapos@aao.org, http://www.aapos.org.

Lorraine Lica, PhD

Eye training *see* **Vision training**

Eyelid disorders

Definition

An eyelid disorder is any abnormal condition that affects the eyelids.

Description

Eyelids consist of thin folds of skin, muscle, and connective tissue. The eyelids protect the eyes and spread tears over the front of the eyes. The inside of the eyelids are lined with the conjunctiva of the eyelid (the palpebral conjunctiva), and the outside of the lids are covered with the body's thinnest skin. Some common lid problems

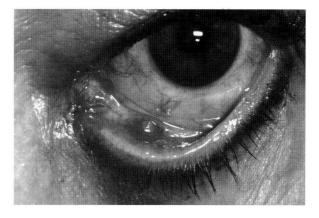

A chalazion on the eyelid. This condition is caused by an obstruction of one of the meibomian glands which lubricate the edge of the eyelid. *(Photo Researchers, Inc.)*

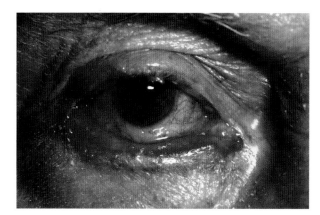

A close-up of the eye of an elderly patient showing ectropion of the lower eyelid. Ectropion is a condition in which the eyelid turns away from the eye. The most common type is senile ectropion (seen here), in which the droop of the eyelid is due to loss of tissue elasticity in old age and weakness in the muscles surrounding the eye. *(Dr. P. Marazzi/Photo Researchers, Inc.)*

include the following: stye, blepharitis, chalazion, entropion, ectropion, eyelid **edema**, and eyelid tumors.

Stye

A stye is an infection of one of the three types of eyelid glands near the lid margins, at the base of the lashes.

Chalazion

A chalazion is an enlargement of a meibomian gland (an oil-producing gland in the eyelid), usually not associated with an infectious agent. More likely, the gland opening is clogged. Initially, a chalazion may resemble a stye, but it usually grows larger. A chalazion may also be located in the middle of the lid and be internal.

Blepharitis

Blepharitis is the inflammation of the eyelid margins, often with scales and crust. It can lead to eyelash loss, chalazia, styes, ectropion, corneal damage, excessive tearing, and chronic **conjunctivitis**.

Entropion

Entropion is a condition where the eyelid margin (usually the lower one) is turned inward; the eyelashes touch the eye and irritate the cornea.

Ectropion

Ectropion is a condition where one or both eyelid margins turn outward, exposing both the conjunctiva that covers the eye and the conjunctiva that lines the eyelid.

Eyelid edema

Eyelid edema is a condition where the eyelids contain excessive fluid.

Eyelid tumors

Eyelids are susceptible to the same skin tumors as the skin over the rest of the body, including noncancerous tumors and cancerous tumors (**basal cell carcinoma**, squamous cell carcinoma, **malignant melanoma**, and sebaceous gland carcinoma). Eyelid muscles are susceptible to sarcoma.

Causes and symptoms

Stye

Styes are usually caused by bacterial **staphylococcal infections**. The symptoms are **pain** and inflammation in one or more localized regions near the eyelid margin.

Chalazion

A chalazion is caused by a blockage in the outflow duct of a meibomian gland. Symptoms are inflammation and swelling in the form of a round lump in the lid that may be painful.

Blepharitis

Some cases of blepharitis are caused by bacterial infection and some by head lice, but in some cases, the cause is unclear. It may also be caused by an overproduction of oil by the meibomian glands. Blepharitis can be a chronic condition that begins in early childhood and can last throughout life. Symptoms can include **itching**, burning, a feeling that something is in the eye, inflammation, and scales or matted, hard crusts surrounding the eyelashes.

Entropion

Entropion usually results from **aging**, but sometimes can be due to a congenital defect, a spastic eyelid muscle, or a scar on the inside of the lid from surgery, injury, or disease. It is accompanied by excessive tearing, redness, and discomfort.

Ectropion

Similar to entropion, the usual cause of ectropion is aging. It also can be due to a spastic eyelid muscle or a scar, as in entropion. It also can be the result of **allergies**. Symptoms are excessive tearing and hardening of the eyelid conjunctiva.

Eyelid edema

Eyelid edema is most often caused by allergic reactions, for example, allergies to eye makeup, eyedrops or other drugs, or plant allergens such as pollen. **Trichinosis**, a disease caused by eating undercooked meat, also causes eyelid edema. However, swelling can also be caused by more serious causes, such as infection, and can lead to **orbital cellulitis** which can threaten vision. Symptoms can include swelling, itching, redness, or pain.

Eyelid tumors

Tumors found on the eyelids are caused by the same conditions that cause these tumors elsewhere on the body. They are usually painless and may or may not be pigmented. Some possible causes include **AIDS** (**Kaposi's sarcoma**) or increased exposure to ultraviolet (UV) rays which may lead to skin **cancer**.

Diagnosis

An instrument called a slit lamp is generally used to magnify the structures of the eyes. The doctor may press on the lid margin to see if oil can be expressed from the meibomian glands. The doctor may invert the lid to see the inside of the lid. Biopsy is used to diagnose cancerous tumors.

Treatment

Stye

Styes are treated with warm compresses for 10–15 minutes, three to four times a day. Chloramphenicol ointment may be used as well. Sometimes **topical antibiotics** may be prescribed if the infection is spreading.

Chalazion

About 25% of chalazia will disappear spontaneously, but warm compresses may speed the process. Chloramphenicol ointment may be used as well. Because chalazia are inside the lid, topical medications are generally of no benefit. Medication may need to be injected by the doctor into the chalazion or if that doesn't help the chalazion may need to be excised. If what appears to be a chalazion recurs on the same site as any previous one, the possibility of sebaceous gland carcinoma should be investigated by biopsy.

Blepharitis

Blepharitis is treated with hot compresses, with antibiotic ointment, and by cleaning the eyelids with a moist washcloth and then with baby shampoo. Good hygiene is essential. Patients can try to keep rooms dry, such as by placing a bowl of water on top of a radiator. Tear film supplements such as hypromellose can help moisten the eyes when dry. If itching, soreness, or redness occurs from the tear film drops, they should be stopped. Topical or systemic **antibiotics** also may be prescribed. If the blepharitis doesn't clear up with treatment or if it seems to be a chronic problem, the patient may have **acne rosacea**. These patients may need to see a dermatologist as well.

Entropion and ectropion

Both entropion and ectropion can be surgically corrected. Prior to surgery, the lower lid of entropion can be taped down to keep the lashes off the eye, and both can be treated with lubricating drops to keep the cornea moist.

Eyelid edema

Patients with swollen eyelids should contact their eye doctor. A severely swollen lid can press on the eye and possibly increase the intraocular pressure. An infection needs to be ruled out. Or, something as simple as an allergy to nail polish and then touching the eyes can cause swelling. The best treatment for allergic eyelid edema is to find and remove the substance causing the allergy. When that is not possible, as in the case of plant allergens, cold compresses and immunosuppresesive drugs such as corticosteroid creams are helpful. However, **steroids** can cause **cataracts** and increase intraocular pressure and patients must be very careful not to get the cream in their eyes. This should not be done unless under a doctor's care. For edema caused by trichinosis, the trichinosis must be treated.

Eyelid tumors

Cancerous tumors should be removed upon discovery, and noncancerous tumors should be removed before they become big enough to interfere with vision or eyelid function. Eyelid tumors require special consideration because of their sensitive location. It is important that treatment not compromise vision, eye movement, or eyelid movement. Accordingly, eyelid reconstruction will sometimes accompany tumor excision.

Prognosis

The prognosis for styes and chalazia is good to excellent. With treatment, blepharitis, ectropion, and entropion usually have good outcomes. The prognosis for nonmalignant tumors, basal cell carcinoma, and squamous cell carcinoma is good once they are properly removed. Survival rate for malignant melanoma depends upon how early it was discovered and if it was completely removed. Sebaceous carcinomas are difficult to detect, so poor outcomes are more frequent.

All of these eyelid disorders, if not treated, can lead to other, possibly serious vision problems—dry eye, **astigmatism**, or even vision loss, for example. An ophthalmologist or optometrist should be consulted.

Prevention

Good lid hygiene is very important. Regular eyelid washing with baby shampoo helps prevent styes, chalazia, blepharitis, and eyelid edema. To avoid these problems, it's also important to refrain from touching and rubbing the eyes and eyelids, especially with hands that have not just been washed.

Blepharitis is associated with dandruff, which is caused by a kind of bacteria that is one of the causes of blepharitis. Controlling dandruff by washing the hair, scalp, and eyebrows with shampoo containing selenium sulfide to kill the bacteria helps control the blepharitis. When using anything near the eyes, it is important to read the label or consult with a doctor first.

Avoiding allergens helps prevent allergic eyelid edema. Staying inside as much as possible when pollen counts are high and eliminating the use of, or at least removing eye makeup thoroughly, or using hypoallergenic makeup may help if the person is sensitive to those substances.

Sunscreen, UV-blocking sunglasses, and wide brimmed hats can help prevent eyelid tumors.

Entropian and ectropian seem to be unpreventable.

Resources

PERIODICALS

"At a Glance: Chalazion Versus Stye." *GP* May 3, 2004: 52.

"Practical Ophthalmology for GPs: The Treatment of Blepharitis." *Pulse* (May 10, 2004): 60.

OTHER

RxMed. http://www.rxmed.com.

ORGANIZATIONS

American Academy of Ophthalmology (AAO), P. O. Box 7424, San Francisco, CA, 94120-7424, (415) 561-8500, (415) 561-8500, http://www.aao.org.

American Optometric Association, 243 North Lindbergh Blvd., St. Louis, MO, 63141, (314) 991-4100, (314) 991-4101, (800) 365-2219, http://www.aoa.org/.

American Society of Ophthalmic Plastic and Reconstructive Surgery, 5841 Cedar Lake Road, Suite 204, Minneapolis, MN, 55416, (952) 646-2038, (952) 545-6073, http://www.asoprs.org.

Lorraine Lica, PhD
Teresa G. Odle

Eyelid edema *see* **Eyelid disorders**
Eyelid plastic surgery *see* **Blepharoplasty**